Cancer Pain

Pharmacologic, Interventional, and Palliative Approaches

Oscar A. de Leon-Casasola, MD

Professor of Anesthesiology and Vice Chair for Clinical Affairs
Department of Anesthesiology, Pain, and Critical Care Medicine
State University of New York at Buffalo
Chief, Pain Medicine
Roswell Park Cancer Institute
Buffalo, New York

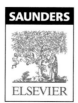

SAUNDERS

ELSEVIER

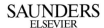

SAUNDERS
ELSEVIER

1600 John F. Kennedy Blvd.
Ste 1800
Philadelphia, PA 19103-2899

CANCER PAIN: PHARMACOLOGIC, INTERVENTIONAL, AND
PALLIATIVE APPROACHES

ISBN-13: 978-0-7216-0261-5
ISBN-10: 0-7216-0261-4

Copyright © 2006 by Elsevier Inc.

Notice

Library of Congress Cataloging-in-Publication Data
Cancer pain : pharmacologic, interventional, and palliative approaches / editor,
 Oscar A. deLeon-Casasola.—1st ed.
   p. ; cm.
  ISBN 0-7216-0261-4
  1. Cancer pain—Treatment.   I. De Leon-Casasola, Oscar A.
  [DNLM: 1. Neoplasms—complications. 2. Pain—therapy. 3. Palliative Care. QZ 200
C21536363 2006]
RC262.C2911922 2006
616.99'406--dc22   2005051657

Executive Publisher: Natasha Andjelkovic
Project Manager: Mary Stermel
Marketing Manager: Dana Butler

Printed in the United States of America

Last digit is the print number: 9 8 7 6 5 4 3 2 1

To God, for the infinite protection and all the blessings I have received.

To my parents, Oscar Humberto and Aura Alicia, who made countless efforts and innumerable sacrifices to give me the appropriate tools to succeed in life.

To my uncle, Ruben Casasola-Roldan, who set a path of unwavering honesty and honor that I have followed throughout my life.

To my wife, Diana, who has given me so much love, support, and happiness.

To my children: Daniel, who made me realize what is truly important in life, adding a new dimension to the meaning of love from the time he was born; and Camilo and Paula, who came to give us so much joy.

To my sister, Priscilla, and my brother, Leonel, for their unconditional love.

Contributors

Ahmed Abdel-Halim, MD
Assistant Professor, Department of Radiology,
State University of New York at Buffalo School
of Medicine and Biomedical Sciences, Buffalo,
New York; Staff Neuroradiologist, Roswell Park
Cancer Institute, Buffalo, New York

Ronald A. Alberico, MD
Director of Neuroradiology/Head and Neck Imaging,
Roswell Park Cancer Institute, Buffalo, New York;
Acting Director of Pediatric Neuroradiology, Women
and Children's Hospital of Buffalo, Buffalo,
New York; Associate Professor of Radiology and
Assistant Clinical Professor of Neurosurgery,
State University of New York at Buffalo School
of Medicine and Biomedical Sciences, Buffalo,
New York

Luis Aliaga, MD, PhD
Pain Unit, Teknon Medical Center, Barcelona, Spain

Nancy A. Alvarez, PharmD
Product Information Manager, Medical Affairs
Department, Endo Pharmaceuticals, Inc.,
Chadds Ford, Pennsylvania

Doralina Anghelescu, MD
Assistant Member, Department of Anesthesiology,
Director of Pain Management Service,
St. Jude Children's Research Hospital,
Memphis, Tennessee

Osvaldo Auad, MD
Pain and Palliative Medicine Department, Sanatorio
Mater Dei, Buenos Aires, Argentina

Annalise Biondolillo, PT
Physical Therapy Department, Roswell Park Cancer
Institute, Buffalo, New York

Stephen C. Brown, MD
Medical Director, Pain Management Center,
The Hospital for Sick Children, Toronto, Ontario;
Assistant Professor, Department of Anesthesia,
University of Toronto, Toronto, Ontario

Eduardo Bruera, MD
Professor and Chair, Department of Palliative Care and
Rehabilitation Medicine, University of Texas MD
Anderson Cancer Center, Houston, Texas

Allen W. Burton, MD
Associate Professor, Section Chief of Pain Management,
Department of Anesthesiology, University of Texas
MD Anderson Cancer Center, Houston, Texas

Paul E. Carns, MD
Assistant Professor of Anesthesiology, Mayo Clinic
College of Medicine, Consultant, Department
of Anesthesiology, Division of Pain Medicine,
Rochester, Minnesota

Daniel B. Carr, MD
Saltonstall Professor of Pain Research, Tufts-New England
Medical Center, Boston, Massachusetts; Professor
of Anesthesiology and Medicine, Tufts University
School of Medicine, Boston, Massachusetts; Chief
Executive Officer and Chief Medical Officer, Javelin
Pharmaceuticals, Inc., Cambridge, Massachusetts

Juan P. Cata, MD
Department of Anesthesiology and Pain Medicine,
University of Texas MD Anderson Cancer Center,
Houston, Texas

Elena Català, MD, PhD
Director, Pain Clinic, Anesthesiology Department,
University Hospital de la Santa Creu i Sant Pau,
Barcelona, Spain

Joseph S. Chiang, MD
Department of Anesthesiology, University of Texas MD
Anderson Cancer Center, Houston, Texas

Nessa Coyle, PhD, FAAN
Supportive Care Program, Pain and Palliative Care
Service, Memorial Sloan-Kettering Cancer Center,
New York, New York

Mellar P. Davis, MD
Director of Research, The Harry R. Horvitz Center for
Palliative Medicine, Cleveland Clinic Foundation,
Cleveland, Ohio

Oscar A. de Leon-Casasola, MD
Professor of Anesthesiology and Vice Chair for Clinical
Affairs, Department of Anesthesiology, Pain, and
Critical Care Medicine, State University of New York
at Buffalo, Buffalo, New York; Chief, Pain Medicine,
Roswell Park Cancer Institute, Buffalo, New York

P. De Negri
Department of Anesthesia, Intensive Care and Pain
Management, Ospedale Oncologico Regionale,
CROB Cancer Center, Rionero in Vulture, Italy

Larry C. Driver, MD
Department of Anesthesiology and Pain Management,
University of Texas MD Anderson Cancer Center,
Houston, Texas

Geoffrey P. Dunn, MD, FACS
Department of Surgery and Palliative Care Consultation
Service, Hamot Medical Center, Erie, Pennsylvania

Anthony Eidelman, MD
Caritas-St. Elizabeth's Medical Center; Clinical
Associate Professor, Tufts University School of
Medicine, Boston, Massachusetts

Naznin Esphani, MD
Adjunct Assistant Professor, Department of Palliative
Care and Rehabilitation Medicine, University of
Texas MD Anderson Cancer Center, Houston, Texas

Robert A. Fenstermaker, MD
Associate Professor, Department of Neurosurgery,
State University of New York at Buffalo School of
Medicine and Biomedical Sciences, Buffalo, New York;
Roswell Park Cancer Institute, Buffalo, New York

Bradley S. Galer, MD
Group Vice President, Scientific Affairs, Endo
Pharmaceuticals, Inc., Chadds Ford, Pennsylvania;
Adjunct Assistant Professor of Neurology, University
of Pennsylvania School of Medicine, Philadelphia,
Pennsylvania

Arnold R. Gammaitoni, PharmD
Director, Medical Affairs Department, Endo
Pharmaceuticals, Inc., Chadds Ford, Pennsylvania

M. Kay Garcia, DrPH, MSN, RN, LAc
Clinical Nurse Specialist, Department of
Anesthesiology, University of Texas MD
Anderson Cancer Center, Houston, Texas

Rodolfo Gebhardt, MD
Assistant Professor of Anesthesiology, Department
of Anesthesiology, State University of New York at
Buffalo, Buffalo, New York; Chief, Pain Management
Services, Veterans Affairs Medical Center, Buffalo,
New York

Jorge Guajardo-Rosas, MD
Department of Anesthesiology and Pain Medicine,
National Institute of Cancer, Mexico City,
Mexico

Maria Del Rocio Guillén-Nuñez, MD
Department of Anesthesiology and Pain Medicine,
National Institute of Cancer, Mexico City,
Mexico

Juan-Diego Harris, MD, CCFP
Assistant Professor of Anesthesiology, Department of
Anesthesiology and Pain Medicine, State University
of New York at Buffalo, Buffalo, New York

Samuel J. Hassenbusch, III, MD, PhD
Professor, Department of Neurosurgery, University
of Texas MD Anderson Cancer Center, Houston,
Texas

Daniel Hinshaw, MD
Medical Director, Palliative Care Consultation Team,
Veterans Affairs Ann Arbor Healthcare System,
Ann Arbor, Michigan

Syed Hamed S. Husain, DO
Resident, Department of Radiology, State University
of New York at Buffalo School of Medicine and
Biomedical Sciences, Buffalo, New York; Veterans
Affairs Medical Center, Buffalo, New York

G. Ivani
Department of Anesthesia and Intensive Care, Regina
Margherita Children's Hospital and S. Anna
Women's Hospital, Turin, Italy

Milind Javle, MD
Department of Medicine, Roswell Park Cancer Institute,
Buffalo, New York

Fayez Kotob, MD
Clinical Fellow in Pediatric Anesthesiology, Department of Anesthesia, Women and Children's Hospital of Buffalo, Buffalo, New York; Research Fellow in Cancer Pain and Neuromodulation, Department of Anesthesiology and Pain Medicine, Roswell Park Cancer Institute, Buffalo, New York

Michael Kuettel, MD, MBA, PhD
Roswell Park Cancer Institute, Buffalo, New York

Allen Lebovits, PhD
Associate Professor, Departments of Anesthesiology and Psychiatry, Co-Director, New York University Pain Management Center, New York University School of Medicine, New York, New York

Mark J. Lema, MD, PhD
Chairman, Department of Anesthesiology and Pain Medicine, Roswell Park Cancer Institute, Buffalo, New York

Mirjana Lovrincevic, MD
Assistant Professor of Clinical Anesthesiology, Department of Anesthesiology and Pain Medicine, Roswell Park Cancer Institute, Buffalo, New York; State University of New York at Buffalo, Buffalo, New York

Patrick W. Mantyh, PhD
Neurosystems Center and Departments of Preventive Sciences, Psychiatry, Neuroscience, and Cancer Center, University of Minnesota, Minneapolis, Minnesota; Veterans Affairs Medical Center, Minneapolis, Minnesota

Mª José Martinez, MD
Clinical Pharmacologist, Service of Clinical Epidemiology—Iberoamerican Cochrane Center; University Hospital de la Santa Creu i Sant Pau, Barcelona, Spain

Rubén Martinez-Castejon, MD
Pain Therapy Unit, Department of Anesthesiology, Teknon Medical Center, Barcelona, Spain

Theresa A. Mays, PharmD, BCOP
Director, Investigational Drug Section, San Antonio, Texas

Brian E. McGeeney, MD, MPH
Assistant Professor of Neurology, Department of Neurology, Boston University School of Medicine, Boston Medical Center, Boston, Massachusetts

Patricia A. McGrath, PhD
Director, Pain Research Center, Senior Associate Scientist, Research Institute, The Hospital for Sick Children, Toronto, Ontario; Professor, Department of Anesthesia, University of Toronto, Toronto, Ontario

Robert J. McQuillan, MD
Associate Professor and Chair, Department of Anesthesiology, Director, Acute and Chronic Pain Therapies, Creighton University Medical Center, Omaha, Nebraska

Laszlo Mechtler, MD
Roswell Park Cancer Institute, Buffalo, New York

Sandra Meyers, MS, OTR/L
Roswell Park Cancer Institute, Buffalo, New York

Rafael V. Miguel, MD
Professor, Chair, and Director of Pain Medicine Program, Department of Anesthesiology, University of South Florida, Tampa, Florida; Attending Pain Physician, Interventional Pain Service, H. Lee Moffitt Cancer Center and Research Institute, Tampa, Florida

Robert A. Milch, MD, FACS
Clinical Professor of Surgery, State University of New York at Buffalo, Buffalo, New York; Medical Director, The Center for Hospice and Palliative Care, Buffalo, New York

P. Modano
Department of Anesthesia, Intensive Care and Pain Management, Ospedale Oncologico Regionale, CROB Cancer Center, Rionero in Vulture, Italy

Joseph Molea, MD
Assistant Professor, Addiction Medicine, Department of Anesthesia, University of South Florida College of Medicine, Tampa General Hospital, Tampa, Florida; Executive Medical Director, Health Care Connection of Tampa, Inc., Tampa, Florida

Timothy J. Ness, MD, PhD
Simon Gelman Endowed Professor of Anesthesiology, Department of Anesthesiology, University of Alabama at Birmingham, Birmingham, Alabama

Linda Oakes, RN, MSN, CCNS
Pain Clinical Nurse Specialist, St. Jude Children's Research Hospital, Memphis, Tennessee

Phillip C. Phan, MD
Department of Anesthesiology and Pain Medicine, University of Texas MD Anderson Cancer Center, Houston, Texas

Ricardo Plancarte-Sanchez, MD
Department of Anesthesiology and Pain Medicine,
National Institute of Cancer, Mexico City, Mexico

Mark Popenhagen, PsyD
Clinical Psychologist—Pain, Specialist for the Pain
Service, St. Jude Children's Research Hospital,
Memphis, Tennessee

Arun Rajagopal, MD
Assistant Professor, Section of Cancer Pain
Management, Department of Anesthesiology,
University of Texas MD Anderson Cancer Center,
Houston, Texas

C. Reato
Department of Anesthesia, Intensive Care and Pain
Management, Ospedale Oncologico Regionale,
CROB Cancer Center, Rionero in Vulture, Italy

Suresh Reddy, MD, FFARCS
University of Texas MD Anderson Cancer Center,
Houston, Texas

Lucia L. Scarpino, MS, RN, CWOCN
Certified Wound Ostomy Continence Nurse, Roswell
Park Cancer Institute, Buffalo, New York

Stephen D. Schwabish, PhD
Research Fellow, Division of Psychology, Roswell Park
Cancer Institute, Buffalo, New York

T. Tirri
Department of Anesthesia, Intensive Care and Pain
Management, Ospedale Oncologico Regionale,
CROB Cancer Center, Rionero in Vulture, Italy

F. Tonetti
Department of Anesthesia and Intensive Care, Regina
Margherita Children's Hospital and S. Anna
Women's Hospital, Turin, Italy

Patrick Tripp, MD
Roswell Park Cancer Institute, Buffalo, New York

Ricardo Vallejo, MD
Bloomington, Illinois

G Varma, MD
Department of Medicine, Roswell Park Cancer Institute,
Buffalo, New York

Luis Vascello, MD
Associate Professor, Department of Anesthesiology,
Director, Acute Pain Service, Medical Director,
Palliative Care Service, Consultant, Shriner's Hospital
Pain Care Center, Samaritan Hospital Pain Care
Center, University of Kentucky, Lexington, Kentucky

Mark S. Wallace, MD
Associate Professor of Clinical Anesthesiology, University
of California, San Diego, San Diego, California

Michael A. Weitzner, MD
Medical Director, Helios Pain and Psychiatry
Center, Tampa, Florida; Professor of Oncology
and Psychiatry, Department of Interdisciplinary
Oncology, University of South Florida College of
Medicine, Tampa, Florida

Cheryl White, MD
Cancer Pain Management Fellow, Section of Cancer
Pain Management, Department of Anesthesiology,
University of Texas MD Anderson Cancer Center,
Houston, Texas

Gilbert Y. Wong, MD
Assistant Professor of Anesthesiology, Mayo Clinic
College of Medicine, Consultant, Department
of Anesthesiology, Division of Pain Medicine,
Rochester, Minnesota

Michael A. Zevon, PhD
Chairman, Department of Psychosocial Oncology,
Director, Division of Psychology, Roswell Park
Cancer Institute, Buffalo, New York; Associate
Research Professor, Department of Natural Sciences,
State University of New York at Buffalo, Buffalo,
New York

Preface

The objective of this book is to provide a comprehensive discussion of the mechanisms involved in generating pain in cancer, the steps that should be taken to diagnose the source of the pain adequately, and the therapeutic modalities that can be implemented to treat it adequately. Unlike other books on cancer pain, this book intends to provide those interested with a mechanistic approach to the different problems that may be encountered when dealing with cancer-related pain. This is particularly important when one considers the potential side effects associated with specific therapies. The hope is that this approach will contribute to changing trends such as the use of opioids as first-line agents for the treatment of neuropathic pain. Additionally, the readership is given updated and complete information on the use of opioids and adjuvants for the pharmacologic treatment of cancer-related pain, the management and prophylactic treatment of their side effects, and guidelines for the judicious implementation of invasive techniques in patients who are either not responding to the pharmacologic approach or whose side effects are limiting their ability to titrate their doses to a therapeutic level.

The book consists of eight sections: I. General Considerations (Chapters 1-4); II. Cancer Pain Resulting from Tumor Extension (Chapters 5-8); III. Cancer Pain Resulting from Therapy (Chapters 9-12); IV. Multidisciplinary Approach to the Patient with Cancer Pain (Chapters 13-15); V. Pharmacologic Management of Cancer Pain (Chapters 16-26); VI. Nonpharmacologic Management of Cancer Pain (Chapters 27-30); VII. Interventional Techniques for Cancer Pain Management (Chapters 31-43); and VIII. Palliative Care (Chapters 44-47).

Section I deals with the mechanisms of cancer-related pain and the physical evaluation of both the adult and pediatric cancer patient. I believe that the readership will find Chapter 1, Taxonomy of Cancer Pain, very stimulating, as it sets the tone for the rest of the book. Dr. Anthony Eidelman and Dr. Daniel B. Carr formulate a description of cancer pain that should help guide clinicians into thinking mechanistically when obtaining the history and performing the physical evaluation of a patient and ordering laboratory workup. This approach has been used at Roswell Park Cancer Institute for several years and has helped us create specific treatments for specific problems as opposed to the "pharmacologic shotgun approach." Although clinical studies documenting the efficacy of this method are lacking, I truly believe this approach can not only directly influence the success in therapy but also limit the incidence of side effects and failures seen with both pharmacologic therapy and interventional techniques.

Section II covers cancer pain syndromes due to tumor extension. A chapter on neurologic pain syndromes due to tumor extension and metastasis to the base of the skull is included in this section and serves as a reminder of the different clinical manifestations that these problems may have.

Section III details the pain syndromes produced or developed due to the implementation of anticancer therapy, detailing the surgical procedures, chemotherapeutic agents, and other therapies associated with these problems.

Section IV discusses the neuroradiologic evaluation of the patient with cancer pain, behavioral assessment, and the diagnosis and treatment of psychiatric complications. These sections should prove very useful for residents and medical students, as they give perspective on the multidisciplinary assessment of these patients.

Section V explores the basic and advanced principles of drug therapy that have proved to be useful in the treatment of cancer-related pain. This section is complemented by Section VI, which includes chapters on the pitfalls of implementing behavioral, physical, occupational, and acupuncture therapies and the alternative ways of managing them, thus reinforcing the modern concept of total support for patients with severe pain. Although a detailed discussion of the nutritional aspects of the cancer patient is beyond the integral management of pain and thus beyond the scope of this book, I encourage those interested to think about nutritional services when dealing with patients with cancer pain.

Section VII explains all the techniques used by pain specialists, including neurosurgical ones, in the treatment of cancer-related pain unresponsive to pharmacologic therapy. It also covers the role of radiation and chemotherapy and the alternative approaches for the management of a patient with intestinal obstruction and pain when surgery is not an option. This section has two chapters on the use of invasive techniques, such as hypophysectomy and epidural and intrathecal neurolysis, that have historical value in the United States and may be useful in other parts of the world with more limited resources for pain management in the face of advanced cancer. It also has a chapter that deals with both "forgotten" invasive techniques and "forgotten" drugs that may prove useful in areas where medical resources are limited. In the section's final chapter, Dr. Osvaldo Auad gives us a historical account of sociological events that may have changed the future of his country, Argentina, as a preamble and a justification for the current use of what he discusses in his chapter. Although this chapter may generate controversy, after seeing the conditions under which

medicine is practiced in some underdeveloped parts of the world, I found enough justification for including it in this book as a historical account, a source, a reference, and a reminder to all of us who practice in environments offering plentiful resources.

The book could not have been complete without Section VIII. The terminal phase in a patient with cancer-related pain is probably the most challenging, as every aspect of care focuses on patient comfort at that point. Thus, the judicious use of drug combinations, comfort measures, and family support are paramount at this stage. The four chapters in this section will be very useful for practitioners dealing with these patients and will also give a significant amount of philosophical insight.

It is my hope that practitioners who treat patients with cancer in their daily practice will find this book a useful reference, as it was created with them in mind. Thus, medical and surgical oncologists, nurse practitioners, physician assistants, family physicians, internists, neurologists, neurosurgeons, radiation therapists, anesthesiologists, psychologists and psychiatrists, rehabilitation physicians and therapists, medical students, and others may consult it for current information.

OSCAR A. DE LEON-CASASOLA, MD

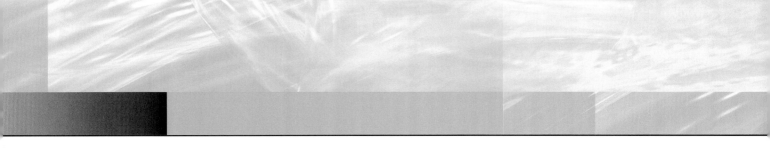

Acknowledgments

To all the contributors who made this book possible.

To the University of San Carlos, the Roosevelt Hospital, and the Military Hospital of Guatemala, where I was taught very early on that it is an honor to be a physician, and where I was branded with a strict code of medical conduct.

To Dr. Mark J. Lema, who created the academic environment for me to forge my career as an anesthesiologist and pain specialist by providing me with support, counsel, and philosophical direction through all these years.

To Roswell Park Cancer Institute, where I have been privileged to practice medicine and fulfill my American dream.

To my patients, who have been the constant source of inspiration to improve myself as a physician not only in the academic sense but also as a human being.

To the Plotkin and Wank families, who helped me during the transition from Guatemala to the United States of America.

Contents

General Considerations

CHAPTER 1

Taxonomy of Cancer Pain

ANTHONY EIDELMAN, MD, AND DANIEL B. CARR, MD

Taxonomy, a compound word formed from the Greek *taxis,* meaning arrangement, and *nomos,* meaning law, is the science of systematic classification. The 18th century scientist Carolus Linnaeus is often cited as the father of taxonomy for his deductive system of naming, ranking, and classifying all living organisms. His work had a profound impact, as he developed a common nomenclature to enable scientists around the world to precisely and consistently, across space and time, communicate about existing flora and fauna and add newly discovered ones into the existing framework. Similarly, the establishment of a taxonomy, or hierarchical classification of cancer pain, is of great preclinical and clinical importance. A widely accepted organizational framework provides a standard system for clinicians and scientists to share insights as to the etiology, biology, and response to therapies for various neoplasias. In other words, it facilitates collection, synthesis, and discussion of scientific information. Clearly, the exchange of information concerning the etiology and pathophysiology of cancer pain will influence the selection of optimal, mechanism-based analgesic therapy as well as primary antitumor therapy. Yet, unlike the challenges facing Linnaeus, the construction of a taxonomic approach faces bigger hurdles because pain is a sensory and emotional experience; has no shape, size, or organs; and lacks an ontogeny.

In the past five years, new light has been directed on the biologic mechanisms of nociceptive activation by many forms of neoplasia. At present, this field is advancing quite rapidly because of the strength of current cellular and molecular research techniques. Soon, the concept of a clinician-based, sign- and symptom-derived taxonomy may become less clinically relevant than objective tests that reveal the neurochemical and genetic signatures of tumor and host, thereby guiding individualized therapy. We will discuss progress toward such a day at the end of this chapter, but until that day arrives, clinicians will continue to rely on careful appraisal of signs and symptoms. And for much of the world, limitations on health care resources will preclude the translation of preclinical approaches into individualized pain therapy indefinitely. Among the many parallels that may be drawn with the diagnosis of nonmalignant conditions, one might contrast the precision of magnetic resonance imaging (MRI) to visualize an emerging cerebrovascular accident with the classic neurologic examination, whose diagnostic specificity is often impressive but always intrinsically inferior to that of MRI.

This chapter describes several current approaches to the categorization of cancer pain, each of which is valuable didactically, in a particular clinical or organizational context, or in the face of certain resource limitations. It closes with an eye toward the future, when the neurochemical signature of an individual's cancer pain may permit analgesic therapy that is biologically if not spatially targeted.

All current taxonomies of pain owe a debt to the International Association for the Study of Pain (IASP), which organized a task force on taxonomy to develop a classification for chronic pain.[1] This scheme, most recently revised in 1994, categorized pain according to five axes: (1) location of the pain; (2) involved organ or tissue system; (3) temporal pattern of pain; (4) pain intensity and time since onset of pain; and (5) etiology of pain. However, the IASP classification does not formally distinguish cancer pain from nonmalignant causes of chronic pain, nor do other diagnostic schema advanced by the U.S. Department of Health and Human Services or the World Health Organization (WHO), discussed later. Grond and colleagues applied the IASP taxonomy of chronic pain to evaluate more than 2200 cancer patients with pain.[2] Substantial information regarding the etiology and pathophysiology of these patients' cancer pain could not be captured using the IASP system. A distinct taxonomy of cancer pain is therefore warranted, because a unique group of syndromes, therapies, and other etiologies of pain occur in this setting.[2–4] In this chapter we review a variety of current approaches for the classification of cancer pain. Several schemes for categorizing cancer pain are summarized in Table 1-1, including etiology, pathophysiology, location, temporal pattern, and severity. The classification of cancer pain may have important diagnostic and therapeutic implications. For example, a mechanism-based treatment approach that determines the sequence of analgesic agents based on the underlying etio-pathology of cancer pain is a promising concept.

ETIOLOGIC CLASSIFICATION OF CANCER PAIN

The four predominant etiologies of cancer pain are: (1) that directly produced by the tumor; (2) that due to the various modalities of cancer therapy; (3) that related to chronic debility; and (4) that due to an unrelated, concurrent disease process.[2,5,6] It is important to clinically distinguish the different etiologies because of their distinct therapeutic and prognostic implications.

Tumor-Related Pain

Most cancer-related pain is directly produced by the malignancy itself.[2,5] The neoplasm may extend into surrounding tissue and exert pressure on nociceptors in diverse organs, as well as nerves. Tumors involving luminal organs may cause pain by obstructing hollow viscera, while locally invasive and erosive cancers directly produce tissue destruction. Furthermore, recent studies have found evidence that pain-generating mediators are directly released from certain tumors or from surrounding

tissue in response to tumor invasion or metastasis such as to bone.[7-12] Notable analgesic substances include prostaglandins, cytokines, interleukins, substance P, histamine, tumor necrosis factor, and endothelins and are discussed later.[7-12]

Treatment-Related Pain

The various modalities of cancer therapy may paradoxically cause pain. Cancer patients may experience acute discomfort following surgery or other invasive procedures. Also, there are numerous postsurgical chronic pain syndromes, including postmastectomy pain, postthoracotomy pain, phantom limb pain, and unintentional severing of peripheral nerves.[13-15] The administration of chemotherapy itself may cause immediate acute pain (e.g., intravenous infusion pain, abdominal discomfort during intraperitoneal infusion) or painful sequelae such as mucositis, arthralgias, and headaches. Moreover, chemotherapeutic agents, including vinca alkaloids, cisplatin, and paclitaxel, are associated with peripheral neuropathies.[16,17] Radiation therapy may injure soft tissue or neuronal structures, resulting in mucositis, proctitis, enteritis, osteonecrosis, peripheral neuropathies, or plexopathies.[18-22] Furthermore, novel anticancer agents such as hormonal or immunotherapy may produce pain.

Debility-Related Pain

Many cancer patients may be inactive or suffer debilities that are associated with painful conditions. For instance, patients who have received immunosuppressive therapy

TABLE 1–1 Various Schemes for Classifying Cancer Pain	
Etiologic classification	Primarily caused by cancer Treatment of malignancy Debility Concurrent pathology
Pathophysiologic classification	Nociceptive (somatic, visceral) Neuropathic Mixed pathophysiology Psychogenic
Location of cancer pain syndromes	Head and neck pain Chest wall syndromes Vertebral and radicular pain Abdominal or pelvic pain Extremity pain (e.g., brachial plexopathy or bony spread)
Temporal classification	Acute Breakthrough Chronic
Severity-based classification	Mild Moderate Severe

or have hematologic malignancies are at increased risk for developing postherpetic neuralgia.[23-25] Also, many malignancies are associated with an increased incidence of thrombosis, which may present as pain and swelling in the affected site.[26]

Non-Malignant Concurrent Disease

Patients with cancer may experience discomfort as a direct consequence of a concurrent, benign disease process (e.g., degenerative joint disease or diabetic neuropathy). Therefore, it is important to review patients' past medical histories and to consider any coexisting nonmalignant condition as a potential source of symptoms.

PATHOPHYSIOLOGIC CLASSIFICATION OF CANCER PAIN

The three classic pathophysiologic types of cancer pain are summarized in Table 1–2, including nociceptive, neuropathic, and psychogenic pain.[27-29] Nociceptive pain results from the stimulation of afferent nociceptive pathways in visceral or somatic tissue, including as a result of inflammation. Neuropathic pain is caused by dysfunction of, or lesions involving, the central or peripheral nervous systems.[1] Psychogenic pain is primarily due to psychological factors and is infrequently seen in cancer patients. Accurate assessment and identification of the pathophysiological types of cancer pain are essential because they may influence the selection of specific therapy.

Nociceptive Somatic Cancer Pain

Somatic pain arises from soft tissue structures that are non-neurological and nonvisceral in origin, including bone, muscle, skin, and joints. The pain is usually well localized and the character of the discomfort is often described as a sharp, aching, or throbbing. Somatic pain usually correlates well with the extent of tissue damage. It may be further classified into deep and superficial somatic pain.

Nociceptive Visceral Cancer Pain

Visceral pain arises from the deep organs of the thorax, abdomen, or pelvis. The underlying mechanisms are less understood than somatic pain. Visceral pain is typically a vague, dull discomfort.[30] The pain is difficult to localize and is often referred to somatic structures. Malignancy may induce visceral pain by causing obstruction of hollow viscera, distension of the organ walls, or stretching of the capsule of solid organs such as the pancreas or liver, or by extension into mesentery (the latter sometimes with an inflammatory reaction). Peritoneal metastasis, usually arising from primary abdominal or pelvic tumors, is one of the more common causes of visceral pain. Other frequent visceral pain syndromes include hepatic distension, midline retroperitoneal syndrome, intestinal obstruction, urethral obstruction, and perineal pain.

Neuropathic Cancer Pain

Neuropathic pain is caused by pathology affecting the nervous system, rather than activation of nociceptors by

---

TABLE 1–2 Clinical Characteristics of the Pathophysiologic Classes of Cancer Pain

Nociceptive Pain	
Somatic Pain	Character of somatic pain is aching, stabbing, throbbing
	Pain is usually well localized
Visceral Pain	Character of pain usually gnawing or cramping when due to obstruction of hollow viscus
	Pain typically described as aching, sharp, throbbing when due to tumor involvement of organ capsule
	Usually diffuse and difficult to localize
	Visceral pain may be referred to somatic structures
Neuropathic Pain	
Nerve Compression	Character of pain often described as burning, pricking, electric-like
	Pain usually located in the area innervated by the compressed peripheral nerve, plexus or nerve root
	Radiographic imaging may show the malignancy compressing the neuronal structure
Deafferentation Nerve Injury	Character of pain similar to that of nerve compression may also be shooting or stabbing in nature
	Dysesthesia or allodynia may be present
	Often associated with loss of afferent sensory function in the painful region
	Superficial burning pain with allodynia, may also have deep aching component
Sympathetically Mediated	Associated symptoms include cutaneous vasodilation, increased skin temperature, abnormal pattern of sweating, trophic changes and allodynia
	Hallmark is nondermatomal pattern of pain
	Confirmed with diagnostic sympathetic block

a noxious stimulus. The dysfunction may be centrally located (brain, spinal cord) or may involve peripheral components of the nervous system (spinal nerve roots, plexuses, peripheral nerves). Neuropathic pain is a heterogeneous entity that can be produced by multiple etiologies.[31] In the setting of malignancy, neuropathic pain can be generated by nerve compression, deafferentation nerve injury, and sympathetically induced pain.[27,32] Stute and colleagues found nerve compression to be the most common cause of neuropathic pain in cancer patients (79%), followed by nerve injury (16%) and sympathetically mediated pain (5%).[32]

Neuropathic pain is clinically distinct from nociceptive pain.[33] The character of neuropathic pain is often described as burning, electric, pricking, or shooting. It may be associated with motor, sensory, and autonomic deficits. Specific sensory abnormalities, including dysesthesia, hyperalgesia, or allodynia may be present. Neuropathic pain is classically located in a dermatomal pattern or in the area innervated by the pathologic spinal root or nerve plexus. The characteristics of the three types of cancer-related neuropathic pain are described in Table 1–2. These different conceptual categories of neuropathic pain are often clinically similar and thus may be a challenge to differentiate. Neuropathic pain is believed to be relatively less responsive to opioids.[34–36] Nonopioid adjuvant drugs, including antiepileptics, antidepressants, and antiarrhythmic agents, are important therapeutic options.[31,37]

Nerve Compression

Tumors may infiltrate or compress sections of the peripheral nervous system, resulting in significant pain and neurologic deficits. Neoplasms may invade or distort spinal nerve roots, producing radicular symptoms.[38,39] Furthermore, cancer may extend into more distal parts of the nervous system, including the various plexuses (e.g., cervical, brachial, or lumbosacral), peripheral nerves, or cranial nerves.[40–44] Some authors believe that tumor compression or invasion of nerves, often accompanied by a perineural inflammatory reaction, initially produces nociceptive pain.[33,45,46] However, neuropathic pain almost certainly develops once the malignancy injures the nerve and disrupts neuronal transmission.[47] The terms *nociceptive nerve pain* and *neuropathic nerve pain* have been proposed to differentiate the two types of neuropathic cancer pain.[45]

Deafferentation Nerve Injury

Nerve injury in cancer patients is a complex process that is caused by multiple mechanisms. Prolonged tumor infiltration or compression of the neuronal structures eventually damages the nerve fibers, causing degenerative changes and deafferentation.[47] In cancer patients, many noncompressive causes of nerve damage are iatrogenic in nature, including inadvertent nerve trauma during surgical procedures, phantom limb pain, or treatment-induced peripheral neuropathy. Furthermore, malignancy can involve the central nervous system, including spinal cord compression or direct cancerous involvement of the brain or spinal cord.

Deafferentation nerve injury typically results in loss of sensation in the area innervated by the damaged peripheral nerve, plexus, or spinal root. Nerve injury also results in a cascade of complex changes within the peripheral and central nervous system. Peripheral sensitization after nerve injury is associated with an increased density of sodium channels in the damaged axons and the associated dorsal root ganglion.[48]

There are ectopic foci of activity in the injured axons, and the stimulus threshold to produce membrane depolarization is decreased. Central sensitization is mediated by release of excitatory amino acids (e.g., glutamate) and neuropeptides (e.g., substance P, neurokinin A) from activated peripheral nociceptors.[49] These excitatory neurotransmitters cause an increase in intracellular calcium and subsequent up-regulation of *N*-methyl-D-aspartate (NMDA) receptors. Moreover, increases in intracellular calcium activate enzymatic reactions and cause the expression of genes that ultimately lower the excitatory threshold of dorsal horn neurons, exaggerate their response to noxious stimuli, and enlarge the size of their receptor fields.

Sympathetically Mediated Cancer Pain

Cancer may induce sympathetic pain by direct or indirect involvement of the sympathetic chain. Sympathetically dependent pain may be associated with vasodilation, increased skin temperature, an abnormal pattern of sweating, trophic changes, and allodynia.[50] In contrast to the other forms of neuropathic pain, the location of the discomfort may not coincide with the distribution of a specific peripheral nerve or dermatome.[5] Rather, sympathetically mediated pain is perceived according to the pattern of sympathetic-vascular innervation. Confirmation of the diagnosis can be made with a selective sympathetic block, which also can be used for therapeutic purposes.

Mixed Pathophysiologic Classes of Pain

A significant percentage of cancer patients have more than one identifiable pathophysiologic class of cancer pain.[51] One study reported that 31% of subjects had mixed nociceptive-neuropathic cancer pain.[2] Moreover, Ashby and colleagues identified two or more pathophysiologic classes of pain in 70% of patients presenting with advanced cancer.[52]

Psychogenic Pain

Psychogenic pain can only be diagnosed after pathology in pain-generating tissues is excluded. Although psychological factors certainly can contribute to pain and suffering, a pure psychogenic etiology of pain is rare in cancer patients. A comprehensive clinical evaluation and workup of the cancer patient almost always results in identification of tumor-related pathology.[53,54]

ANATOMIC CLASSIFICATION OF CANCER PAIN

Cancer pain may involve virtually any anatomic region of the body.[55] Several authors have organized malignancy-related discomfort according to the location of the involved structures or tissues.[6] Cancer pain may originate from the head and neck region, chest wall, abdomen or pelvis, vertebral structures, or the extremities. There is a lack of consensus regarding the utility of an anatomic-based classification because it lacks specificity as to the mechanism of pain. Nonetheless, the site of origin of cancer pain clearly influences whether, and how, certain invasive therapies such as external radiation, neurolytic blocks, electrical stimulation, or targeted drug delivery may be best applied.

TEMPORAL CLASSIFICATION OF CANCER PAIN

As mentioned earlier, a variety of circumstances can potentially cause acute pain in cancer patients, including diagnostic or therapeutic procedures and other modalities of cancer therapy (e.g., chemotherapy, radiation therapy). Often, the presence of acute pain may signal a new metastasis or a serious cancer-related complication such as a pathologic fracture. Therefore, comprehensive evaluation to determine the source of acute pain is necessary in cancer patients.[53] An important type of acute cancer pain is breakthrough pain, the flare-up of discomfort in patients whose baseline pain is well controlled on a by-the-clock analgesic regimen.[56-58] There is a high prevalence of breakthrough pain in cancer patients. Furthermore, poorly controlled breakthrough pain is associated with more severe discomfort and functional impairment.[59] Pain is often termed "chronic" if it has persisted for longer than three months. Typically, chronic cancer pain is directly due to the tumor. However, chronic post-therapy syndromes include phantom limb pain (including postmastectomy pain), chronic chemotherapy-associated neuropathies, and radiation-induced proctitis or enteritis. Chronic pain often has profound psychologic and physical impact on the cancer patient.[55,60]

SEVERITY-BASED CLASSIFICATION OF CANCER PAIN

The severity of cancer pain may reflect the size of the tumor, its location, and the extent of tissue destruction. The mechanism of pain is also an important determinant, as metastatic bone lesions and injury to nerves are notoriously more severe than pain arising from tumor growth within soft tissue. Absent compression of nerves or obstruction of lumens, for example, retroperitoneal masses may grow quite large before they become symptomatic.

Pain intensity is frequently used to guide analgesic therapy. The WHO three-step cancer pain ladder, discussed in detail later in the chapter, recommends a progressive sequence of analgesic drugs based primarily on pain intensity. Valid tools to quantify pain intensity include the visual analog pain scale (VAS), numerical rating scale, verbal descriptors of pain severity (e.g., none, mild, moderate, severe), and the Faces Pain Scale.[60] Pain intensity should be assessed using the subject's own pain rating because nonconcordance has long been recognized between patients' and health care practitioners' assessments of pain. The severity of cancer pain is dynamic, often fluctuates as the disease progresses and as different therapies are administered. Therefore, it is necessary to reevaluate and determine the severity of the pain on a serial basis.

EVALUATION OF CANCER PAIN

It is essential to perform a comprehensive evaluation of pain in the cancer patient.[53,54] Assessment of the cancer pain may alert physicians about malignancy-related complications (e.g., spinal cord compression, fractures), disease progression, or new metastatic lesions.[55] A study performed at the Memorial Sloan-Kettering Cancer Center reported that consultations by the pain service identified a previously undiagnosed metastasis or etiology in 64% of cases.[53] Furthermore, an understanding of the pathophysiology of cancer pain may have therapeutic implications and may influence the selection of pharmaceutical or nonpharmaceutical treatments such as bisphosphonates or external radiotherapy, respectively. In the same Memorial Sloan-Kettering study, 18% of patients received surgery, chemotherapy, or radiotherapy based on the assessment by the pain service.[53]

In addition to a detailed medical history, a specific pain history is paramount to accurate evaluation of the cancer pain patient. Information regarding the pain, including location, character, severity, onset, duration, temporal pattern, relieving and exacerbating factors, associated symptoms, previous analgesic therapy, and specific cancer treatments, should be obtained. The patient's psychological state, including the presence of depression or anxiety, should also be assessed. The most important parts of the physical examination are assessment of the neurologic and musculoskeletal systems. Laboratory studies may be of value in certain cases. Serum tumor markers, including carcinoembryonic antigen (CEA), prostate specific antigen (PSA), and CA-125, may confirm the diagnosis of a specific type of malignancy, particularly in the setting of an unknown primary tumor, or may confirm the suspicion of recurrent cancer.

Imaging studies play a significant role in the evaluation of malignancy-related pain. Computed tomography (CT) is especially useful for evaluating oncologic processes involving the mediastinum or abdominal organs.[61-63] Moreover, CT may be used to guide diagnostic or therapeutic interventional procedures such as percutaneous stent placement or neurolytic blocks. MRI is the technique of choice for imaging the brain or spinal cord.[64] Also, MRI is a sensitive modality for evaluating head and neck tumors, breast masses, or malignancy involving the musculoskeletal tissue.[65-67] The positron emission tomography (PET) scan is a functional imaging technique that has been playing an increasingly significant role in the workup of cancer.[68] The PET scan can be used to detect diverse malignancies, including lung cancer, metastasis to lymph nodes, and head and neck tumors.[69-71] There are several radionuclide studies that can detect primary or metastatic cancers. The nuclear bone scan identifies abnormal foci of bone formation that may be malignant in origin. Other relevant nuclear medicine studies include lymphoscintigraphy, nuclear thyroid scans, and radiolabeled antibody imaging. Invasive diagnostic testing may be indicated if clinical examination and imaging are unable to yield definitive results. Common diagnostic interventions include percutaneous needle biopsy, bronchoscopy, mediastinoscopy, colonoscopy, upper gastrointestinal endoscopy, laparoscopic intervention, or even surgical laparotomy.

THE WHO CANCER PAIN LADDER: APPLICATION OF A SEVERITY-BASED PAIN CLASSIFICATION

The WHO developed a simple, three-step, analgesic ladder for treatment of cancer pain that relies on widely available, inexpensive analgesic agents.[72-74] The method was originally introduced in 1986 and advocates an approach based on pain intensity to manage cancer-related discomfort. The first step of the algorithm manages mild pain with nonopioid analgesics, including nonsteroidal anti-inflammatory drugs (NSAIDs) or acetaminophen. The second step for persistent discomfort or mild to moderate levels of pain advises adding a "weak" opioid such as codeine to the nonopioid analgesic regimen. The third tier recommends combination of a "strong" opioid (e.g., morphine, hydromorphone) and nonopioid agents for moderate to severe pain. Moreover, adjuvant drugs, including antidepressants, corticosteroids, or anticonvulsants, are recommended when appropriate at any step of the ladder.

The WHO drug therapy ladder has been globally distributed and is currently considered the standard for the management of cancer pain. Furthermore, this guideline has facilitated efforts by the WHO and other groups to promote the acceptance and availability of opioids for patients with cancer pain or pain from HIV/AIDS. The effectiveness of the analgesic ladder has been confirmed by multiple studies.[75-78] However, the quality of the supportive evidence has been challenged.[79,80] The WHO three-step method has primarily been evaluated by uncontrolled trials, which may be distorted by bias[80] and which lack comparisons with other sequences of analgesic pharmacotherapy.

The analgesic efficacy of NSAIDs, which are recommended in the initial tier of the WHO regimen, has been well established.[81,82] However, there is controversy regarding the sequence of analgesics recommended by the later steps of the algorithm. It has been recommended that perhaps "strong" opioids should be used in the second step of the WHO ladder.[81,82] Furthermore, Marinangeli and colleagues conducted a randomized controlled trial of cancer patients that found initial therapy with "strong" opioids to be more effective than the analgesia provided by the regimen recommended by the current WHO guidelines.[83]

There are additional analgesic agents that may expand the current WHO analgesic ladder. For instance, selective NSAIDs that inhibit the COX-2 (cyclooxygenase) enzyme are associated with a lower incidence of gastrointestinal adverse effects than traditional NSAIDs.[84] Unfortunately, the increased incidence of cardiovascular and cerebrovascular complications during prolonged use of COX-2 inhibitors has recently led to more and more widespread removal of such agents from the marketplace or other restrictions on their use. As a result, they are less and less accessible for patients with cancer, in whom long-term cardiovascular risks are of less concern than immediate pain relief with minimal gastrointestinal side effects. Also, ketamine, a phencyclidine derivative that acts on numerous classes of receptors and in particular is an NMDA receptor antagonist, may be an effective agent for relief of cancer pain, especially in patients who are opioid-resistant or tolerant.[85,86]

Modified versions of the WHO method for cancer pain control, also based on pain intensity, have been applied for relief of acute postoperative pain, burns, and trauma.[87] Similarly, an analgesic pyramid that consists of a separate treatment arm for nociceptive and neuropathic pain has been devised for management of AIDS discomfort.[88] Comparable to the WHO cancer ladder, each arm recommends selections among analgesic drug options according to the severity of the pain.

A MECHANISM-BASED TREATMENT STRATEGY FOR MANAGEMENT OF CANCER PAIN

The benefits and challenges of a potential mechanism-based taxonomy of pain have been described.[89,90] Likewise, a mechanistic guideline recommends analgesic therapy according to the underlying pathogenesis of the pain. Ashby and colleagues described a mechanism-based treatment algorithm for cancer pain.[52] The pathophysiology of each patient's cancer pain was classified as superficial somatic, deep somatic, visceral, pure neuropathic, or mixed neuropathic/nociceptive. The dominant mechanism of pain, rather than its intensity, was used to determine the sequence of analgesic therapy. For instance, pure neuropathic pain was treated with antidepressants and anticonvulsants. Opioids were selected as a third option only if the previous two drug classes were ineffective. Visceral pain was initially managed with opioids, followed by antispasmodics (only if the pain was colicky) and then anti-inflammatory agents. In the treatment algorithm, none of the analgesics were referred to as adjuvant drugs. Intriguingly, all 20 patients who were studied required an opioid to achieve satisfactory pain relief; concurrent therapy with a mean of 3 drug classes was also necessary to achieve satisfactory pain control. One may conclude that while the concept of matching agent to mechanism is an attractive one, the heterogeneity of mechanisms in actual practice, and the only partial effectiveness of currently available agents, dictates that multiple agents be applied simultaneously.

A mechanism-based algorithm is based on the premise that the various pathophysiologic types of pain may have different sensitivities to distinct classes of analgesics. Nociceptive pain typically responds to opioids; however, there is lack of consensus regarding the effectiveness of opioids for treatment of neuropathic pain.[34] Some authors believe that neuropathic pain is intrinsically unresponsive to opioids.[91] However, other trials suggest opioid responsiveness is a continuum and that neuropathic pain is only somewhat less sensitive to opioids than nociceptive pain.[34-36] An analysis of patients treated at the Memorial Sloan-Kettering Cancer Center assessed

the effectiveness of a single dose of opioid, according to the underlying pathophysiology of cancer pain.[92] Although neuropathic cancer pain responded to the opioids, the pain relief was relatively less compared to the patients with strictly nociceptive discomfort. Therefore, practical evidence trumps taxonomy in that a trial of opioid therapy is warranted and should not be withheld because neuropathic pain is suspected.

Also with regard to the interactions among taxonomy, mechanisms, and optimal therapy, a prospective trial compared the analgesic efficacy of NSAIDs for cancer pain produced by strictly visceral mechanisms with pure somatic pain caused by bone metastases.[93] After 14 days of therapy, no difference in pain intensity was demonstrated between the two groups, although patients with visceral pain consumed greater doses of opioids.

In summary, although it is logical that a taxonomy-driven, mechanism-based analgesic approach may one day be the most effective, current evidence does not unequivocally support a mechanism-based treatment.[55] In fact, no difference in pain relief has been found in cancer patients with neuropathic, nociceptive, or mixed neuropathic–nociceptive cancer pain treated according to the WHO guidelines.[94] Furthermore, the results of a trial by Rasmussen and colleagues did not support a mechanism-based analgesic treatment strategy for patients with benign etiologies of neuropathic pain.[95] A recent systematic review of the opioid responsiveness of chronic noncancer neuropathic pain supports opioids' efficacy, with sustained declines in pain intensity during long-term opioid therapy comparable to those seen for tricyclic antidepressants or anticonvulsants.[96] Nevertheless, a mechanistic approach of cancer pain taxonomy and analgesic therapy remains a promising concept, even though it is at present confounded by several factors.[46] As described above, the pathogenesis of malignancy-associated pain is often heterogeneous and a significant percentage of cancer patients have pain that is produced by multiple mechanisms.[2,51,52] Also, many analgesic agents are nonselective and act on a variety of targets to alleviate different types of pain. Moreover, there is lack of consensus regarding the classification of neuropathic cancer pain. Tumor compression of nerves, for example, may be considered a form of nociceptive pain.[33,45] As mentioned earlier, the terms *nociceptive nerve pain* and *neuropathic nerve pain* have been coined to distinguish subtypes of neuropathic cancer pain.[45]

THE FUTURE OF TAXONOMY: FROM PROFILE TO FINGERPRINT?

In the past several years, tremendous progress has been made in understanding the underlying mechanisms of malignancy-associated pain.[12,97] Animal models have been developed that may provide important insights into the tumor biology and cellular etiologies of cancer pain.[98] One of the first preclinical models by Schwei and colleagues simulated metastatic bone cancer by injecting murine osteolytic sarcoma cells into the marrow space of the mouse femur.[99] Recently, several of the specific mediators of cancer pain have been identified. It has been discovered that certain tumors release factors that sensitize or stimulate primary afferent neurons. Many tumors express high levels of COX-2 and secrete prostaglandins.[99-101] Therefore, drugs, including NSAIDs, that inhibit the COX enzymes provide particularly effective analgesia for certain types of cancer pain. Selective inhibitors of COX-2 may have benefit not only for analgesia but also for inhibition of angiogenesis. Unfortunately, the results of one recent trial of the long-term administration of a COX-2 inhibitor prophylactically in patients with familial polyposis extended prior suspicions of increased cardio- and cerebrovascular risk in patients treated with this class of agents, leading to the withdrawal of rofecoxib from the marketplace. At present, the future therapeutic availability of the entire class of COX-2 inhibitors is in question. Certain metastatic tumors, including prostate cancer, secrete the peptide endothelin-1.[11,102-104] There is increasing evidence that endothelin-1 is a significant mediator of pain in both animals and humans.[12,102-104] Moroever, a selective endothelin receptor antagonist has been found to relieve pain in a mouse model.[11] Malignant cells have been shown to secrete several other pain-producing mediators, including nerve growth factors, interleukins, and cytokines.[10,12] Furthermore, malignancy-induced acidosis may exacerbate cancer pain.[12,97] Two classes of pH-sensitive ion channels are expressed on subsets of afferent nerve terminals, the vanilloid receptor TRPV1[105,106] and the acid-sensing ion channel 3 (ASIC-3).[107] It has been postulated that tumor-induced acidosis and release of protons may activate the TRPV1 and ASIC-3 channels, exacerbating pain.[12] Therefore, antagonists of the TRPV1 and ASIC-3 channels may potentially provide analgesia in certain types of cancer pain.[105]

As our understanding of the specific cellular mechanisms of cancer pain increases, more effective therapy can be developed that targets the precise mediators of pain, both according to the nature of the specific tumor and the individual suffering from pain. An important step is to replace the broad, clinically based profiles that now form the basis for current taxonomic classifications—akin to profiling of criminal suspects—with precise molecular characterization of the mediators involved in a specific individual's tumor, along with the neurochemical signatures produced in the peripheral and central nervous systems in response to distinct forms of nociceptive input.[108-111] To extend the forensic metaphor, the newer approach replaces broad, imprecise profiling with more specific fingerprints or genetic information.

CONCLUSION

Thirty years ago, Loeser and Black observed in the first volume of the journal *Pain* that "semantic problems [which] occur when physiologists talk to clinicians, anatomists or psychologists… often preclude meaningful interchange…. It is imperative that we develop a new taxonomy of the phenomena related to pain."[112] This call was taken up by Merskey and others of the International Association for the Study of Pain, which instituted a Task Force on Taxonomy whose classification of terms related to chronic pain[1] has been immensely valuable to researchers and clinicians alike. A well-defined, valid, and widely accepted taxonomy of cancer pain would likewise be of great importance in preclinical and clinical research and clinical practice. Current classification systems of cancer pain are predominantly based on the etiology, pathophysiology, and location of the symptoms. As the mechanisms of nociception and pain become more evident, especially at the cellular level, perhaps a true mechanistic taxonomy can be developed. The latter will have significant clinical implications and may potentially guide analgesic drug therapy that targets the precise pain mechanisms. When that day arrives, pain clinicians may look back on current therapies as reminiscent of therapies for pneumonia based on physical signs and symptoms, as opposed to the rapid DNA typing that increasingly guides clinical antibiotic therapy. Currently, the WHO three-step analgesic ladder is the gold standard for therapy of cancer pain. However, a treatment approach that determines the sequence of analgesic therapy based primarily on an individualized taxonomy of the cancer pain, rather than an epidemiologically based approach dictated solely by the intensity of pain, is inevitable. We have elsewhere written[55] of replacing the three-step ladder with a more complex approach keeping with the 21st century. "Optimally matching the options for cancer pain control with individual needs, preferences, and likely responses may require evolution of the three-step analgesic ladder into an 'elevator' that delivers patients promptly and with ease to their chosen destinations within a multistoried edifice, and 'escalators' to reposition them subsequently between nearby levels."[55] If we who practice pain medicine and palliative care follow the same path as our oncology colleagues—as is likely—then taxonomy will likely maintain its didactic importance but may play less of a role in informing the practical therapeutic choices confronting individual clinicians caring for one patient at a time. Already in an era of combination analgesic chemotherapy,[113] we will look toward individual responses to refine our therapeutic choices just as our colleagues in oncology now do.

REFERENCES

1. Merskey H, Bogduk N (eds): Classification of Chronic Pain, 2nd ed. Seattle, IASP Press, 1994.
2. Grond S, Zech D, Diefenbach C, et al: Assessment of cancer pain: A prospective evaluation in 2266 cancer patients referred to a pain service. Pain 64:107–114, 1996.
3. Ventafridda V, Caraceni A: Cancer pain classification: A controversial issue. Pain 46:1–2, 1991.
4. Bruera E, MacMillan K, Hanson J, et al: The Edmonton staging system for cancer pain: Preliminary report. Pain 37:203–209, 1989.
5. Twycross R: Cancer pain classification. Acta Anaesthesiol Scand 41:141–145, 1997.
6. Caraceni A, Weinstein S: Classification of cancer pain syndromes. Oncology 15:1627–1640, 2001.
7. Cain D, Wacnik P, Eikmeier L, et al: Functional interactions between tumor and peripheral nerve in a model of cancer pain in the mouse. Pain Med 2:15–23, 2001.
8. Sabino M, Ghilardi J, Jongen J, et al: Simultaneous reduction in cancer pain, bone destruction, and tumor growth by selective inhibition of cyclooxygenase-2. Cancer Res 62:7343–7349, 2002.
9. Tobinick E: Targeted etanercept for treatment-refractory pain due to bone metastasis: Two case reports. Clin Ther 25:2279–2288, 2003.
10. Lee B, Dantzer R, Langley K, et al: A cytokine-based neuroimmunologic mechanism of cancer-related symptoms. Neuroimmunomodulation 11:279–292, 2004.
11. Yuyama H, Koakutsu A, Fujiyasu N, et al: Effects of selective endothelin ETa receptor antagonists on endothelin-1 induced potentiation of cancer pain. Eur J Pharmacol 492:177–182, 2004.
12. Mantyh P, Hunt S: Mechanisms that generate and maintain bone cancer pain. Novartis Found Symp 260:221–238, 2004.
13. Macrae WA: Chronic pain after surgery. Br J Anesth 87:88–98, 2001.
14. Smith W, Bourne D, Squair J, et al: A retrospective cohort study of post mastectomy pain syndrome. Pain 83:91–95, 1999.
15. Marchettini P, Formaglio F, Lacerenza M: Iatrogenic painful neuropathic complications of surgery in cancer. Acta Anaesthesiol Scand 45:1090–1094, 2001.
16. Verstappen C, Heimans J, Hoekman K, et al: Neurotoxic complications of chemotherapy in patients with cancer: Clinical signs and optimal management. Drugs 63:1549–1563, 2003.
17. Cavaletti G, Boqliun G, Marzorati L, et al: Early predictors of peripheral neurotoxicity in cisplatin and paclitaxel combination chemotherapy. Ann Oncol 15:1439–1442, 2004.
18. Monceaux G, Perie S, Montravers F, et al: Osteoradionecrosis of the hyoid bone: A report of 3 cases. Am J Otolaryngol 20:400–404, 1999.
19. McFarlane V, Clein G, Cole J, et al: Cervical neuropathy following mantle radiotherapy. Clin Oncol 14:468–471, 2002.
20. Krabbenhoff D, Hoang C, Morris A, et al: Complications of chronic pelvic radiation injury. J Am Coll Surg 198:1022–1023, 2004.

21. Schierle C, Winograd J: Radiation-induced brachial plexopathy. Complication without a cure. J Reconstr Microsurg 20:149–152, 2004. Review.
22. Scully C, Epstein J, Sonis S: Oral mucositis: A challenging complication of radiotherapy, chemotherapy and radiochemotherapy. Part 2: Diagnosis and management of mucositis. Head Neck 26:77–84, 2004.
23. Rusthoven J, Ahlgren P, Elhakim T, et al: Risk factors for varicella zoster disseminated infection among adult cancer patients with localized zoster. Cancer 15:1641–1646, 1988.
24. Pruitt A: Central nervous system infection in cancer patients. Neurol Clin 9:867–888, 1991.
25. Modi S, Pereira J, Mackey J: The cancer patient with chronic pain due to herpes zoster. Curr Rev Pain 4:429–436, 2000.
26. Kirkova J, Fainsinger R: Thrombosis and anticoagulation in palliative care: An evolving clinical challenge. Palliat Care 20:101–104, 2004.
27. Portenoy R: Cancer pain: Pathophysiology and syndromes. Lancet 339:1026–1031, 1992.
28. Caraceni A: Clinicipathological correlates of common cancer pain syndromes. Hematol Oncol Clin North Am 10:57–78, 1996.
29. Caraceni A, Portenoy R: An international survey of cancer pain characteristics and syndromes. Pain 82:263–274, 1999.
30. Gebhart G (ed): Visceral pain: Progress in pain research and management, vol 5. Seattle, IASP Press, 1995.
31. Chong M, Bajwa Z: Diagnosis and treatment of neuropathic pain. J Pain Symptom Manage 25:S4–S11, 2003.
32. Stute P, Soukup, Menzel M: Analysis and treatment of different types of neuropathic cancer pain. J Pain Symptom Manage 26:1123–1130, 2003.
33. Martin L, Hagen N: Neuropathic pain in cancer patients: Mechanism, syndromes and clinical controversies. J Pain Symptom Manage 14:99–117, 1997.
34. Portenoy R, Foley K, Inturrisi C: The nature of opioid responsiveness and its implications for neuropathic pain: New hypotheses derived from studies of opioid infusions. Pain 43:273–286, 1990.
35. Jadad A, Carroll D, Glynn C, et al: Morphine responsiveness of chronic pain: Double-blind randomized crossover study with patient-controlled analgesia. Lancet 339:1367–1371, 1992.
36. McQuay H, Jadad A, Carroll D, et al: Opioid sensitivity of chronic pain: A patient- controlled analgesic method. Anaesthesia 47:757–767, 1992.
37. Caraceni A, Zecca E, Martini C, et al: Gabapentin as an adjuvant to opioid analgesia for neuropathic cancer pain. J Pain Symptom Manage 17:441–445, 1999.
38. Coles M: S1 radiculopathy due to adenocarcinoma: A case study. J Neurosci Nurs 36:40–41, 2004.
39. Yamamoto T, Fujita I, Kurosaka M, et al: Sacral radiculopathy secondary to multicentric osteosarcoma. Spine 26:1729–1732, 2001.
40. Kori S: Diagnosis and management of brachial plexus lesions in cancer patients. Oncology 9:756–760, 1995.
41. Hawley R, Patel A, Lastinger L: Cranial nerve compression from breast cancer metastasis. Surg Neurol 52:431–432, 1999.

42. Grisold W, Piza-Katzer H, Jahn R, et al: Intraneural nerve metastasis with multiple mononeuropathies. J Peripher Nerv Syst 5:163–167, 2000.
43. Zingale A, Ponzo G, Ciavola G, et al: Metastatic breast cancer delayed brachial plexopathy: A brief case report. J Neurosurg Sci 46:147–149, 2002.
44. Abraham P, Capobianco D, Cheshire W: Facial pain as the presenting symptom of lung carcinoma with normal chest radiograph. Headache 43:499–504, 2003.
45. Vecht C: Cancer pain: A neurological perspective. Curr Opin Neurol 13:649–653, 2000.
46. Ventafridda V, Caraceni A: Cancer pain classification: A controversial issue. Pain 46:1–2, 1991.
47. Tasker R: The problem of deafferentation pain in the management of the patient with cancer. J Palliat Care 2:8–12, 1987.
48. England J, Happel L, Kline D, et al: Sodium channel accumulation in humans with painful neuromas. Neurology 47:272–276, 1996.
49. Beydoun A, Backonja M: Mechanistic stratification of antineuralgic agents. J Pain Symptom Manage 25:S18–S30, 2003.
50. Churcher M, Ingall J: Sympathetic dependent pain. Pain Clinic 1:217–218, 1987.
51. Twycross R, Harcourt J, Bergl S: A survey of pain in patients with advanced cancer. J Pain Symptom Manage 2:273–282, 1996.
52. Ashby M, Fleming B, Brooksbank M, et al: Description of a mechanistic approach to pain management in advanced cancer. Preliminary report. Pain 51:153–161, 1992.
53. Gonzales G, Elliot K, Portenoy R, et al: The impact of a comprehensive evaluation in the management of cancer pain. Pain 47:141–144, 1991.
54. Jacox AK, Carr DB, Payne R, et al: Management of Cancer Pain. Clinical Practice Guideline No. 9. Rockville, MD: Agency for Health Care Policy and Research, Public Health Service, U.S. Department of Health & Human Services, 1994. AHCPR Pub. No. 94-0592.
55. Goudas LC, Carr DB, Bloch R, et al: Management of Cancer Pain. Vol 1 & Vol 2 Evidence Tables. Evidence Report/ Technology Assessment No. 35. (Prepared by the New England Medical Center Evidence-based Practice Center under Contract No. 290-97-0019). AHRQ Publication No. 02-E002. Rockville, MD: Agency for Healthcare Research and Quality. October 2001.
56. Portenoy R: Breakthrough pain: Definition, prevalence and characteristics. Pain 41:273–281, 1990.
57. Patt R, Ellison N: Breakthrough pain in cancer patients: Characteristics, prevalence, and treatment. Oncology 12:1035–1046, 1998.
58. Simmonds, M: Management of breakthrough pain due to cancer. Oncology 13:1103–1108, 1999.
59. Caraceni A, Martini C, Zecca E, et al: Breakthrough pain characteristics and syndromes in patients with cancer pain. An international survey. Palliat Med 18:177–183, 2004.
60. Carr DB, Goudas LC, Lawrence D, et al: Management of Cancer Symptoms: Pain, Depression, and Fatigue. Evidence

Report/Technology Assessment No. 61. (Prepared by the New England Medical Center Evidence-based Practice Center under Contract No. 290-97-0019). AHRQ Publication No. 02-E032. Rockville, MD: Agency for Healthcare Research and Quality. July 2002.

61. Glazer G, Orringer M, Gross B, et al: The mediastinum in non-small cell lung cancer: CT-surgical correlation. AJR Am J Roentgenol 142:1101–1105, 1984.

62. Heiken J, Weyman P, Lee J, et al: Detection of focal hepatic masses: Prospective evaluation with CT, delayed CT, CT during arterial portography, and MR imaging. Radiology 171:47–51, 1989.

63. Tabuchi T, Itoh K, Ohshio G, et al: Tumor staging of pancreatic adenocarcinoma using early- and late-phase helical CT. AJR Am J Roentgenol 173:375–380, 1999.

64. Higer H, Pedrosa P, Schuth M: MR imaging of cerebral tumors: State of the art and work in progress. Neurosurg Rev 12:91–106, 1989.

65. Tien R, Robbins K: Correlation of clinical, surgical, pathologic, and MR fat suppression results for head and neck cancer. Head Neck 14:278–284, 1992.

66. Warner E, Plewes D, Hill K, et al: Surveillance of BRCA1 and BRCA2 mutation carriers with magnetic resonance imaging, ultrasound, mammography, and clinical breast examination. JAMA 292:368–370, 2004.

67. Parsons T, Filzen T: Evaluation and staging of musculoskeletal neoplasia. Hand Clin 20:137–145, 2004.

68. Hillner B, Tunuguntla R, Fratkin M: Clinical decisions associated with positron emission tomography in a prospective cohort of patients with suspected or known cancer at one United States center. J Clin Oncol 22:4147–4156, 2004.

69. Goldsmith S, Kostakoglu L, Somrov S, et al: Radionuclide imaging of thoracic malignancies. Thorac Surg Clin. 14:95–112, 2004.

70. McGuirt W, Greven K, Williams D: PET scanning in head and neck oncology: A review. Head Neck 20:208215, 1998.

71. Teknos T, Rosenthal E, Lee D, et al: Positron emission tomography in the evaluation of stage III and IV head and neck cancer. Head Neck 23:1056–1060, 2001.

72. World Health Organization. Cancer Pain Relief, Geneva, World Health Organization, 1986.

73. World Health Organization. Cancer Pain Relief and Palliative care, Geneva, World Health Organization, 1990.

74. World Health Organization. Cancer Pain Relief, 2nd ed. With a guide to opioid availability. Geneva, World Health Organization, 1996.

75. Ventafridda V, Tamburini M, Caraceni A, et al: A validation study of the WHO method for cancer pain relief. Cancer 59:850–856, 1987.

76. Walker V, Hoskin P, Hanks G: Evaluation of WHO analgesic guidelines for cancer pain in a hospital-based palliative care unit. J Pain Symptom Manage 3:145–149, 1988.

77. Schug S, Zech D, Dorr U: Cancer pain management according to WHO analgesic guidelines. J Pain Symptom Manage 5:27–32, 1990.

78. Zech D, Grond S, Lynch J, et al: Validation of World Health Organization Guidelines for cancer relief: A 10-year prospective study. Pain 63:65–76, 1995.

79. Lawrence D, Lipman A, Goudas LC, et al: Management of cancer pain. In Chang AE, Ganz PA, Hayes DF, Kinsella T, Pass HI, Schiller JH, Stone R, Stecher V (eds). Oncology: An Evidence-Based Approach. New York, Springer-Verlag (in press).

80. Jadad A, Browman G: The WHO analgesic ladder for cancer pain management. JAMA 274:1870–1873, 1995.

81. Eisenberg E, Berkley C, Carr D, et al: Efficacy and safety of nonsteroidal anti-inflammatory drugs for cancer pain: A meta-analysis. J Clin Oncol 12:2756–2765, 1994.

82. McNicol E, Strassels S, Goudas L, et al: Nonsteroidal anti-inflammatory drugs, alone or combined with opioids, for cancer pain: A systematic review. J Clin Oncol 22:1975–1992, 2004.

83. Marinangeli F, Ciccozzi A, Leonardis M, et al: Use of strong opioids in advanced cancer pain: A randomized trial. J Pain Symptom Manage 27:509–516, 2004.

84. Mamdani M, Rochon P, Juurlink D, et al: Observational study of upper gastrointestinal haemorrhage in elderly patients given selective cyclo-oxygenase-2 inhibitors or conventional non-steroidal anti-inflammatory drugs. BMJ 325:607–608, 2002.

85. McDonnell F, Sloan J, Hamann S: Advances in cancer pain management. Curr Pain Headache Rep 5:265–271, 2001.

86. Carr DB, Goudas LC, Denman WT, et al: Safety and efficacy of intranasal ketamine for the treatment of breakthrough pain in patients with chronic pain: A randomized, double blind, placebo-controlled, crossover study. Pain 108:17–27, 2004.

87. De Smet J, Charlton JE, Meynadier J: Pain and rehabilitation from landmine injury. Pain: Clinical Updates Volume VI, Issue 2, July 1998.

88. Breitbart W, Patt R, Passik S: Pain in AIDS: A call for action. Pain: Clinical Updates Volume IV, Issue 1, March 1996.

89. Woolf C, Bennett G, Doherty M, et al: Towards a mechanism-based classification of pain? Pain 77:227–229, 1998.

90. Max M: Is mechanism-based treatment attainable? Clinical trial issues. J Pain 1:2–9, 2000.

91. Arner S, Meyerson B: Lack of analgesic effect of opioids on neuropathic and idiopathic forms of pain. Pain 33:11–23, 1988.

92. Cherny N, Thaler H, Friedlander-Klar M, et al: Opioid responsiveness of cancer pain syndromes caused by neuropathic or nociceptive mechanisms: A combined analysis of controlled, single-dose studies. Neurology 44:857–861, 1994.

93. Mercadante S, Casuccio A, Agnello A, et al: Analgesic effects of nonsteroidal anti- inflammatory drugs in cancer pain due to somatic or visceral mechanisms. J Pain Symptom Manage 17:351–356, 1999.

94. Grond S, Radbruch L, Meuser T, et al: Assessment and treatment of neuropathic cancer pain following WHO guidelines. Pain 79:15–20, 1997.

95. Rasmussen P, Sindrup S, Jensen T, et al: Therapeutic outcome in neuropathic pain: Relationship to evidence of nervous system lesion. Eur J Neurol 11:545–553, 2004.

96. Eisenberg E, McNicol ED, Carr DB. Efficacy and safety of opioid agonists in the treatment of neuropathic pain of non-malignant origin: Systematic review and meta-analysis of randomized controlled trials. JAMA, 2005; 293:3043-3052.

97. Mantyh PW, Clohisy DR, Koltzenburg M, et al: Molecular mechanisms of cancer pain. Nat Rev (Cancer) 2:201–209, 2002.

98. Medhurst SJ, Walker K, Bowes M, et al: A rat model of bone cancer pain. Pain 96:129–140, 2002.

99. Schwei M, Honore P, Rogers S, et al: Neurochemical and cellular reorganization of the spinal cord in a murine model of bone cancer pain. J Neurosci 19: 10886–10897, 1999.

100. Molina M, Sitja-Arnau M, Lemoine M, et al: Increased cyclooxygenase-2 expression in human pancreatic carcinomas and cell lines: Growth inhibition by nonsteroidal anti-inflammatory drugs. Cancer Res 59:4356–4362, 1999.

101. Shappell S, Manning S, Boeflin W, et al: Alterations in lipoxygenase and cyclooxygenase-2 catalytic activity and mRNA expression in prostate carcinoma. Neoplasia 3:287–303, 2001.

102. Davar G: Endothelin-1 and metastatic cancer pain. Pain Med 2:24–27, 2001.

103. Peters C, Lindsay T, Pomonis J, et al: Endothelin and the tumorigenic component of bone cancer. Neuroscience 126: 1043–1052, 2004.

104. Pomonis J, Rogers S, Peters C, et al: Expression and localization of endothelin receptors: implications for the involvement of peripheral glia in nociception. J Neurosci 21:999–1006, 2001.

105. Bleh K: Recent developments in transient receptor potential vanilloid receptor 1 agonist-based therapies. Expert Opin Investig Drugs 13:1445–1456, 2004.

106. Nagy I, Santha P, Jancso G, et al: The role of the vanilloid (capsaicin) receptor (TRPV1) in physiology and pathology. Eur J Pharmacol 500:351–369, 2004.

107. Bassler E, Ngo-Anh T, Geisler H: Molecular and functional characterization of acid-sensing ion channel (ASIC) 1b. J Biol Chem 276:33782–33787, 2001.

108. Villar MJ, Wiesenfeld-Hallin Z, Xu X-J, et al: Further studies on galanin-, substance P-, and CGRP-like immunoreactivities in primary sensory neurons and spinal cord: Effects of dorsal rhizotomies and sciatic nerve lesions. Exp Neurol 112:29–39, 1991.

109. Wiesenfeld-Hallin Z, Xu X-J, Hokfelt T. The role of spinal cholecystokinin in chronic pain states. Pharmacol Toxicol 91: 398–403, 2002.

110. Honore P, Rogers SD, Schwei MJ, et al: Murine models of inflammatory, neuropathic and cancer pain each generates a unique set of neurochemical changes in the spinal cord and sensory neurons. Neuroscience 98:585–598, 2000.

111. Sabino MA, Luger NM, Mach DB, et al: Different tumors in bone each give rise to a distinct pattern of skeletal destruction, bone cancer-related pain behaviors and neurochemical changes in the central nervous system. Int J Cancer 104:550–558, 2003.

112. Loeser JD, Black RG: A taxonomy of pain. Pain 1:81–84, 1975.

113. Walker SM, Goudas LC, Cousins MJ, Carr DB. Combination spinal analgesic chemotherapy: A systematic review. Anesth Analg 95:674–715, 2002.

CHAPTER 2

Current Trends in Cancer Pain Management

NAZNIN ESPHANI, MD, AND EDUARDO BRUERA, MD

Quality of life is influenced by pain. Unrelieved pain can impair a patient's functional status and quality of life deteriorates. A major fear of cancer patients is the fear of unmitigated pain. Cancer-related pain has been estimated to afflict 30% to 60% of patients at the time of diagnosis and 55% to 95% of patients at advanced disease stages.[1-4] Some authors have indicated that approximately 28% of cancer patients die without adequate pain relief.[5,6] According to the World Health Organization (WHO),[7] "palliative care provides relief from pain and other distressing symptoms; affirms life and regards dying as a normal process; integrates the psychological and spiritual aspects of patient care; offers a support system to help patients live as actively as possible until death; and offers a support system to help the family cope during the patient's illness and in their own bereavement."

Palliative care requires a team approach to meet the needs not only of the patient but also of his or her family, including counseling. This not only enhances quality of life, but also influences the course of illness in a very positive way. The current trend is increasingly moving toward instituting palliative care much earlier in the course of disease, resulting in the application of palliative care lasting for months or even years.

Vigorous attention to pain is the cornerstone of good palliative care. This translates into constant monitoring of the adequacy of treatment. Although this is a time-consuming and difficult task, it is essential in managing cancer pain. Emphasis is placed on maintaining an ambulatory state with the patient being as physically active as possible, while continuing to maintain an excellent cognition and clarity of mind. Side effects related to pain medications should be reduced to the minimum.

In palliative care patients, it remains extremely important to carefully determine the cause of pain, because management options may vary markedly according to the mechanisms of pain. Even at the end of life, invasive procedures may be appropriate if they allow increased mobility, more comfortable nursing, or improved cognitive function. The etiology and classification of cancer pain is discussed extensively in Chapter 1. This chapter discusses the current trends in delivering successful palliative care both at the institutional level and in the health care community in general.

ASSESSMENT OF SYMPTOMS

One of the areas that has revolutionized palliative care is the careful assessment of symptoms. Cancer patients present with complex and troubling symptoms. Palliative care has incorporated pain as one of the main and very important symptoms of cancer to be managed. The health care provider faces a dual challenge in managing pain manifestations of cancer. The first and often understated goal is diagnostic—appropriately identifying the source and cause of pain. The importance of history taking cannot be overemphasized. A careful review of medical history and the chronology of cancer pain is important to place the pain complaint in the appropriate context. The pain-related history must include the characteristics of pain and the responses of the patient to various analgesic therapies in the past. Individual assessment must be carefully done in the presence of multiple pain complaints, which are quite common. Validated pain assessment instruments are invaluable tools that are helpful not only in monitoring the adequacy of therapy, but also in serving as a means of communication between the patient and the health care provider. The clinician must evaluate the many different aspects of pain, including impairment in activities of daily living,[8-10] interacting with others,[11] appetite,[11-13] and vitality giving rise to fatigue in cancer patients,[14] sleep disturbance,[15,16] financial concerns, and psychological, familial, and professional dysfunction. It is equally important to evaluate the patient's mental status, including depression, anxiety, and the discernible level of pain. The meaning of pain in relation to a particular illness has a great bearing on the pain severity and may actually exacerbate the perceived pain intensity.[17,18]

MULTIDIMENSIONAL PAIN ASSESSMENT

In palliative care, one often encounters the finding that the expression of pain is not directly proportional to the pathophysiology of pain. Behavior and psychology play an important role in the expression of pain. Most clinicians tend to ignore this and treat only the pathophysiologic aspects. The spinoreticular pathway is the current focus in the literature on the motivational components of pain. The biologic substrates for the sensory discriminative qualities of pain and cortical mechanisms play a role in the cognitive and sensory aspects of pain mechanisms. Mood swings, psychological well-being, or contrary feelings can suppress or exacerbate perception of pain.[19,20]

Assessment is the cornerstone of adequate pain management. It is an oversimplification to say pain is "whatever the patient says it is." Pain, especially in cancer patients, is a complex symptom influenced by the patient's coping skills, financial burden, caregiver burden, social or family adjustments, and spiritual issues. No single health care provider, regardless of his or her professional expertise, can manage complex pain symptomatology in a cancer patient. A multidimensional approach for patient screening and assessment is essential for managing pain.[21,22] This is also referred to as "whole person" care. A multidimensional assessment delves thoroughly into physical, psychological, social, cultural, and spiritual components of pain.[21] The components of multidimensional pain assessment include the following:

- Detailed history and physical examination, including pain and medication history, social and family history.
- Cognitive assessment. Patients should be questioned about the actual implication of "pain" and also their attitudes and beliefs (including cultural influences) about pain, including misconceptions of pain and its treatment. Patients need to be assessed for the presence of cognitive impairment. Cognitive failure poses difficulties in accurate assessment of symptoms and must be taken into account while managing cancer patients with pain.[23-27]
- Thorough psychological evaluation.
- Spiritual assessment.

ASSESSMENT TOOLS

Clear communication of findings between clinicians and patients and between clinicians themselves can smooth the delivery of broad-based care. Various assessment tools

are used for appropriate cancer pain management.[28-33] Assessment includes the following:

- Causes (cancer, treatment related or not related to cancer).
- Intensity (visual-analog scale, numerical, verbal, etc.). These may be recorded and can be placed in front of the chart for ongoing assessment. The rating is proportional to symptoms that the patient experiences.
- Use of alcohol or drugs (CAGE questionnaire, etc.).
- Psychosocial distress (somatization).
- Cognitive function (MMSE, etc.).
- Mechanisms of pain (neuropathic, non-neuropathic).
- Nature (continuous, incidental).
- Other related symptoms (ESAS, etc.).

The Edmonton Symptom Assessment System (ESAS) is based on nine visual-analog scales measuring pain, activity, nausea, appetite, depression, anxiety, shortness of breath, drowsiness, and well-being, which are completed every day for assessment of the patient's symptoms. Its validity and reliability are yet to be thoroughly studied (Figure 2–1).[28]

Mini Mental Status Examination (MMSE) is a validated, widely used screening tool for evaluation of cognitive function.[29] The MMSE assesses five general cognitive areas in a patient: orientation to time and place, attention and calculation, registration, language, and recall. It includes test for short-term memory, language, and ability to understand and perform simple construction tasks. The unadjusted maximum score is 30. An adjusted score, which considers age and education level and is calculated using a chart included in the MMSE, should be used as a maximum for an individual patient. A score of 24 or higher is considered normal, and a score of 23 or lower generally indicates cognitive impairment.[29] In the presence of cognitive impairment, the numerical assessment of symptoms may not be valid, and clinicians may refer to prior assessment or other cues to manage symptoms.

Delirium and Cancer Pain

Delirium is a common and often serious medical complication in patients with advanced cancer and AIDS.[23-27,33-35] Delirium has been defined as a transient global disorder of cognition and attention. It represents a neuropsychiatric manifestation[23-27,36] of an underlying generalized disorder of cerebral metabolism and neurotransmission. Delirium is highly prevalent in cancer patients with advanced disease, particularly in the last weeks of life.[37] Depending on the populations and assessment methods, prevalence rates range from 25% to 85%.[23,27,33,38,39] Levine and others found that between 15% and 20% of 100 hospitalized cancer patients had organic mental disorders.[40] Massie and others found delirium in 25% of 334 hospitalized cancer patients requiring

Edmonton Symptom Assessment System Graph
(ESAS)

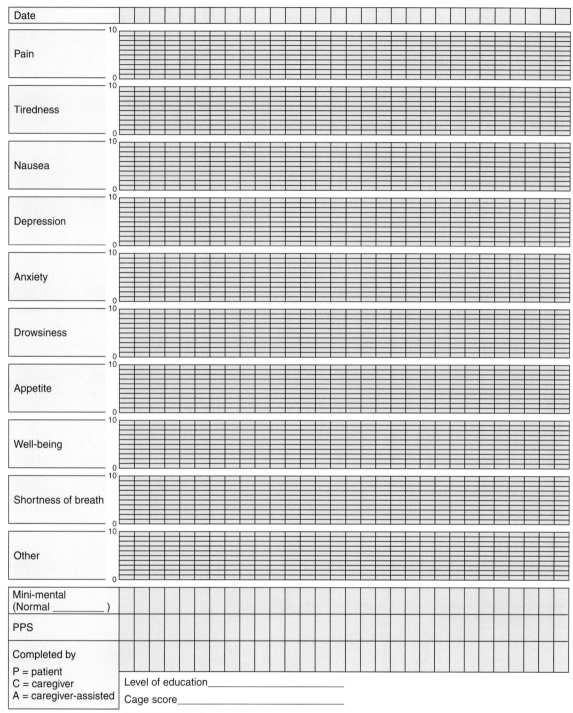

FIGURE 2–1   Edmonton Symptom Assessment System (ESAS).

psychiatric referrals and in 85% (11 of 13) of terminal cancer patients.[23] Approximately 90% of patients with advanced cancer experience delirium in the hours to days before death.[23,24,27,34] The incidence of delirium is on the rise.[25,26] Delirium is very distressful to patients, family members, and staff because it is associated with increased morbidity in the terminally ill.[27,41]

The MMSE[29] and confusion assessment method (CAM)[42] are simple assessment tools that can be performed even by nonphysicians. The MMSE and CAM impose relatively little burden on patients, while facilitating the diagnosis of delirium.[29,30,42] These tools can be used by the nursing staff in the care of patients with delirium. The Memorial Delirium Assessment Scale is a great tool for assessing cognition, but requires a trained physician.[30]

In palliative care it is essential to monitor delirium in patients with cancer pain. Delirium portends significant pathophysiologic disturbances, usually related to multiple medical etiologies (Figure 2–2).[23-25,27,43-45] Occasionally a cause may not be identified. However, this should not deter health care providers from looking for potentially reversible causes of delirium, because the majority of causes are reversible, once identified and treated. Delirium may be an early sign of opioid toxicity.[36,43,44] Opioids are a major cause of delirium, used for the treatment of cancer-related pain.[35,36,38,43-46] Other etiologies include infection, organ failure, rare paraneoplastic syndromes, nonopioid medications.[23,24,27,46-49]

Delirium is underdiagnosed or misdiagnosed and inadequately treated or untreated in terminally ill patients. Delirium shortens the survival of cancer patients and makes pain and other symptom assessment difficult. Delirium may influence not only assessment, but treatment of pain as well.[37,39,50] Opioid-induced delirium can be exacerbated by tricyclic antidepressants, other opioids, other drugs[41,47,48,50] or by coexisting factors as shown in Figure 2–2. Cognitive disorders, and delirium in particular, have enormous relevance to symptom control and palliative care. Delirium not only modifies the expression of pain, but also the use of analgesic medication. In a study, it was reported that patients without delirium used more analgesic doses for breakthrough pain in the morning, whereas patients with delirium tended to use breakthrough analgesic doses in the evening and at night.[51] The clinical features of delirium include various neuropsychiatric manifestations. Prodromal symptoms of restlessness, irritability, sleep disturbances, and anxiety precede reduced attention, altered arousal, altered psychomotor activity, emotional lability, altered perceptions, hallucinations, delusions, disorganized thinking, and memory impairment.[52,53]

Differential diagnosis of delirium would include other psychiatric disorders, keeping in mind that the clinical manifestations overlap in delirium, and other psychiatric disorders may coexist with delirium. The early manifestations of delirium, such as anxiety, mood changes, and insomnia, may be misdiagnosed and treated wrongly with anxiolytics and antidepressants, which may actually worsen the delirium.

Prevention of delirium involves the recognition of risk factors. These include severe illness, level of comorbidity, prior dementia, advanced age, medications (including opioids and other psychoactive medications), hypoalbuminemia, infection, dehydration, and azotemia. In addition, the poor prognostic factors for pain management, including incidental pain, somatization of psychological distress, prior history of alcohol or drug abuse, tolerance, and neuropathic pain, also pose as risk factors for induction of opioid-related delirium in advanced cancer patients.[54] In the presence of cachexia and impaired functional status[55-57] in patients with advanced cancer, the precipitating factors such as medications are often superimposed on a relatively high level of baseline vulnerability to the development of delirium.[36,44,57,58]

Management of delirium requires a stepwise approach. First and foremost is to search for and correct the

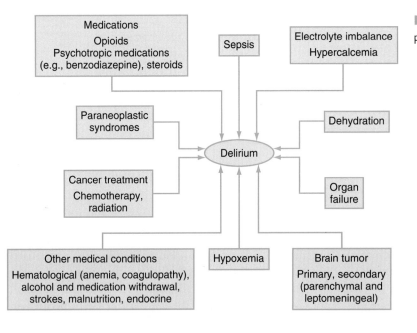

FIGURE 2–2 Causes of delirium in cancer patients.

underlying reversible cause of delirium and manage the symptoms and signs of delirium.[59-61] A disciplined, multi-dimensional assessment is crucial to identify the baseline predisposing and precipitating factors and to identify the potentially reversible underlying causes such as opioid toxicity, infection, dehydration, metabolic disturbances, and medications. For opioid toxicity, either dose reduction or switching to another opioid may help.[62,63]

In the palliative care setting, baseline irreversible vulnerable factors for delirium such as cachexia, impaired functional status, and hepatic impairment are generally related to progressive disease. Correction of precipitating factors such as medications and dehydration may cause the delirium to resolve or improve. Although reversibility rates of 50% to 60% have been reported in patients in some studies, the study population may actually represent select patient populations and settings likely to be reversible.[34,64]

Although environmental control for symptomatic treatment of delirium such as reorientation and reducing noise stimulation has been advocated, it has not been evaluated.[30] Psychotropic agents may be used, but not necessarily in all cases of delirium. They are commonly indicated for hyperactive or mixed type delirium. The drug of choice in such cases is haloperidol, a potent neuroleptic with dopamine-blocking properties and fewer anticholinergic properties.[25,35] In a double-blind trial of haloperidol, chlorpromazine, and lorazepam, the efficacy of haloperidol and chlorpromazine was similar, with minimal extrapyramidal side effects.[33] Lorazepam in this study[33] proved to be ineffective and has treatment-limiting side effects.[33,65] Newer agents such as risperidone and olanzapine have not been extensively studied in the treatment of delirium.[66,67]

CAGE Questionnaire

The CAGE questionnaire is a screening tool for alcoholism.[26] CAGE positivity suggests the possibility of a patient using chemical means to cope with stress. The clinicians face a challenge when attempting to manage a CAGE-positive patient's symptoms, especially as complex as pain. The CAGE questionnaire should be completed during the initial assessment of a patient, even prior to asking routinely about the amounts of alcohol or illicit drugs ingested. This improves the validity of the CAGE results. In a retrospective study[68] it was shown that alcoholism is frequently underdiagnosed, and with a multidimensional approach using the CAGE questionnaire, the prevalence of alcoholism was much more.

Alcoholism is a poor prognostic factor for pain control, as well for patient and family coping skills.[69,70] CAGE positivity implies that patients may chemically cope to deal with symptoms such as pain. There is a cross-addiction

between ethanol, opioids, and other drugs. The reward mechanisms of ethanol involve endorphin release. Therefore, we are interested in CAGE positivity not as a marker of ethanol use, but as a marker of aberrant use of opioids and other psychoactive drugs.[71,72] Patients with cancer pain should never be denied opioids if they have a positive CAGE, but frank discussions with the patients and the family with regard to the difference between the nociceptive and overall suffering will help prevent inappropriate opioid dose escalation. The CAGE questionnaire queries patients on four topics: **c**utting down on alcohol consumption, **a**nnoyance from possible criticism about drinking, **g**uilty feelings about drinking, and **e**ye-openers to avoid hangovers.

STAGING OF CANCER PAIN

The simple definition of "pain due to cancer" is not enough to define the pain adequately based on our current knowledge of the mechanisms and response of cancer pain to treatments. The Edmonton Staging System[28] provides a clinical staging system for cancer pain (Table 2-1). The system allows accurate prediction of the outcome of patients with cancer pain. It has an excellent sensitivity (>90%), but poor specificity (<50%).[54]

The pain in all patients with cancer is staged on admission. There are two stages of prognosis for cancer pain control. Stage 1 indicates a good prognosis. Patients with stage 1 cancer pain achieve more than 90% of relief with simple analgesics. Stage 2 indicates poor prognosis for pain control. Patients with this staging of cancer pain achieve moderate relief with analgesics.

There are some poor prognostic factors for pain management. In patients with one or more of these factors, it may be difficult to achieve adequate pain control.[28, 54,73] Mnemonic RAPIDN (**r**apid **a**cceleration of **p**ain **i**ndicates **d**amaged **n**erves) helps remember these poor prognostic factors, which are the following:

Rapid tolerance
Alcoholism
Psychological (history of affective disorders such as anxiety and depression)
Incidental pain (pain related to activity or movement)
Delirium or cognitive failure
Neuropathic pain

The cancer pain prognostic scale (CPPS) proposed by Hwang and others[74] is an excellent tool for the accurate prediction of the likelihood of achieving adequate pain relief for patients with moderate to severe cancer within 2 weeks. Both of these tools, the EDSS[28,54] and the CPPS,[74] are important as well for prognostication of pain management outcomes.

TABLE 2-1 Edmonton Staging System for Cancer Pain

A. Mechanism of Pain
A1. Visceral
A2. Bone or soft tissue
A3. Neuropathic
A4. Mixed
A5. Unknown

B. Pain Characteristics
B1. Nonincidental
B2. Incidental

C. Psychological Distress
C1. No major psychological distress
C2. Major psychological distress

D. Opiate Tolerance
D1. Increase of <5% of initial dose/day
D2. Increase of >5% of initial dose/day

E. Past history
E1. Negative history for alcoholism or drug addiction
E2. Positive history for alcoholism or drug addiction

Stage 1: Good prognosis
A1, A2, B1, C1, D1, E1

Stage 2: poor prognosis
A3 (any B- C- D- E)
A4 (any B- C- D- E)
A5 (any B- C- D- E)

Scoring: (Results would indicate Stage 1 or 2)

MULTIDIMENSIONAL MANAGEMENT OF CANCER PAIN

There is a definite association between pain and its treatment and other symptoms in cancer patients. It is important to know in palliative care that heavy emphasis is laid on excellent symptom control. The patient's somnolent status is not acceptable. In the process of treating cancer pain, we may aggravate other symptoms, such as opioid-related side effects. Any therapeutic intervention should aim to control the whole plethora of symptoms, when feasible. In the following paragraphs we will discuss special challenges presented in advanced cancer pain.

Nausea,[55,75] cachexia,[55-58] and cognitive failure[23-27,59] have an important bearing on pain assessment, and may make it more difficult. An important aspect is appropriate assessment of all these symptoms in the patient who is depressed[76-78] or fatigued.[79-81] Multiple symptom assessment is different from simple assessment.[16] Cognitive failure prevents accurate assessment of symptoms and should be corrected if possible.[9,23-25,27] Psychological distress often affects symptom expression.[8,11,13,75] In cancer patients, whenever severe symptoms emerge, new pain symptoms develop, or the existing pain intensity changes, clinicians who practice palliative care continually monitor and manage complex symptomatology and functional disturbances. Symptom control and psychological adaptation[11,13] are the usual concerns during the period of active disease therapies. As end of life approaches, however, needs intensify and broaden.

It is imperative for clinicians to be skilled in pain management.[82-85] In several studies of pain relief among cancer patients in the United States[86] and in France,[1] the discrepancy between patient and physician evaluation of the severity of the pain problem was a major predictor of inadequate relief. The inadequacy was due to the physician's suboptimal evaluations. In another study by Grossman, while evaluating the correlation between patient's and clinician's assessment of pain severity it was found that when patients rated their pain as moderate to severe, oncology fellows failed to appreciate the severity of the problem in 73% of cases.[87] Oncology clinicians recognize that suboptimal assessment is one of the most important causes of inadequate pain relief in cancer patient.[88-90]

During the course of illness, a subset of cancer patients becomes demanding, angry, and manipulative.[91]Although anger has compounding effects on pain, depression, and psychosocial functioning, clinicians tend to ignore the clinical relevance of anger in appropriate pain management.[92] Clinicians should specifically assess for anger and, when warranted, target it for intervention. Treatment of anger leads to improved reports of pain intensity, pain behavior, and activity level.[92-94]

The McGill pain questionnaire[32] and self-report methods[94] are available, prompting attention to them. However, these methods have their own limitations, as they require candid self-report, have the potential for situational biases, and need to be validated on the reliability of their measurement tools and strategies.

Delirium and Opioid Use

Delirium is reversible in a large percentage of patients, and opioids have a role in newly recognized delirium. Recognition of opioid-induced toxicity is essential to manage patients with pain.[34,36,38,61] Delirium precipitated by opioids and other psychoactive drugs and dehydration are frequently reversible with opioid rotation, dose reduction, discontinuation of the offending unnecessary psychoactive medication, or hydration.[34,61-63]

With the increased availability and use of opioids for cancer pain, we see a surge in the detection of opioid-related adverse effects, primarily neuropsychiatric manifestations.[36] Most of the commonly used opioids, such as morphine, oxycodone, hydromorphone, and fentanyl have been implicated in the development of neurotoxicities. These include myoclonus, visual, auditory, or tactile (most frequent) hallucinations, grand-mal seizures, delirium, late-onset sedation hyperalgesia, and allodynia.[34,36,38,43,44] Patients at high risk who are susceptible to developing those toxicities include those with renal impairment and dehydration; patients with neuropathic pain; those with baseline impaired cognition; patients on high doses of opioids, especially for prolonged periods; and patients on concurrent psychoactive medications.[36,38,43,44,61,95,96] The onset and recognition of these side effects should not deter a clinician from using opioids for treating cancer pain. With different strategies, these toxicities could be prevented, improved, or reversed. These strategies include reduction of the opioids if possible, opioid rotation, hydration, and removal of other offending drugs as and where appropriate.[61,63,97,98]

Anorexia, Cachexia, and Hydration

Anorexia, cachexia, or both occur in up to 80% to 90% of patients with advanced cancer (Figure 2–3).[56-58] Patients with these syndromes have poor quality of life and are susceptible to side effects of opioids or respond poorly to

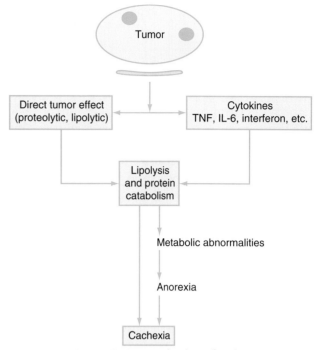

FIGURE 2–3   Mechanism of cachexia.

therapy.[55,58] Hydration influences assessment and treatment of cancer pain. Health care professionals have to be aware that due to cachexia, the determined doses of opioids for cancer pain have to be lowered. Some level of hydration is required to eliminate the active metabolites of opioids completely.[95,96] In those patients with mild to severe dehydration, opioid-related toxicity in the form of nausea, vomiting, drowsiness, somnolence, and delirium would be either precipitated or worsened.[95,96] Also look for coexisting metabolic conditions such as hypercalcemia that could be corrected.[60-62]

Dehydration can affect the outcomes of pain assessment and control for different reasons, as it exacerbates (or precipitates) existing confusion and renal failure. Accumulation of opioid metabolites may cause nausea, restlessness, myoclonus, seizures, and even hyperalgesia.[95,96] Dehydration may also pose a risk for development of pressure sores. The clinical manifestations include fatigue, confusion, lethargy, constipation, and dry mouth. Dry mouth or thirst usually reflects side effects related to opioids or other drugs and oral complications related to disease progression. Since the clinical presentation of dehydration overlaps with that of opioid-induced toxicity, it may at times be difficult to clinically delineate the etiology. In such circumstances, a short trial of hydration may help to distinguish dehydration from other etiology. Hydration can be given orally to those patients who are able to take large amounts of fluids by oral dose. If not, it can be given intravenously or subcutaneously.[99]

Fatigue

Patients with cancer pain definitely have fatigue, which incapacitates them completely or partially (Figure 2–4). Fatigue results in not only declined physical functioning, but also diminished mental functioning, which has a profound bearing on impairment of quality of life. Fatigue can aggravate cancer (and its complications) or its treatment-related symptoms. Opioids, other treatments, and metastases contribute greatly to fatigue. Attempts to minimize fatigue should be made if possible.[79-81]

It is important to remember that uncontrolled pain and fatigue are interrelated. Pain giving rise to fatigue and treatment of pain may contribute to fatigue. Also anorexia-cachexia syndrome contributes to fatigue and may worsen opioid-related side effects when patients are treated.

Fatigue can be treated like most other cancer-related symptoms, by mainly treating the correctable underlying factors. With aggressive treatment of concurrent symptoms, fatigue can be greatly mitigated, and hence cancer pain, in cases in which they are interrelated.[79-81]

Opioid Rotation

When the side effect profile and effective analgesic dose relationship is compromised, switching from one opioid to another is a useful strategy. This allows for elimination of possibly accumulated toxic opioid metabolites, since opioids have different effects on selective subsets of opioid receptors in the central nervous system.[97,98,100,101] Usually hydromorphone is used as an alternative agent if it has not already been used.[95-98] The disadvantage for

this is that it may not be effective in the presence of renal impairment. The opioid of choice would be the one with inert metabolites, such as methadone.[98,101-105] Alternative opioids with high intrinsic potency such as methadone and fentanyl may be a more effective choice when there is a neuropathic component of pain or evidence of rapid development of tolerance.[63,97,101]

The current advantage for opioid switch is the availability of methadone for cancer pain management.[97,100,101] When patients require rapid dose escalation of opioids, there is a possibility of activation of the N-methyl-D-aspartate (NMDA) receptors. Methadone not only has a high potency compared to morphine, but it also has the added advantages of being an NMDA receptor antagonist and having unique pharmacokinetic properties.[97,98,101-103] From different studies it is evident that a highly individualized approach and conversion ratios have to be followed when switching to methadone in patients on high morphine doses.[105,106] Different methods have been proposed by different authors to overcome this problem of methadone toxicity, which may evolve if the current conversion ratios are strictly followed without tailoring to the individual patient's dose requirements.[106-108]

CURRENT CONCEPTS IN MANAGING OPIOID SIDE EFFECTS

Traditional opioid side effects include sedation, nausea, constipation, respiratory depression, pruritus, urinary retention, and anaphylaxis.[100] Patients with opioid-induced nausea and vomiting should receive prokinetic agents such as metoclopramide. Patients who receive opioids for the first time should receive scheduled antiemetics at least for the first few days.[109]

Constipation occurs in approximately 90% of patients treated with opioids. Patients require laxative therapy as long as they are receiving opioids. These include contact cathartics and bulk agents such as senna, docusate, and bisacodyl; saline laxative preparations such as magnesium hydroxide or sulfate and sodium sulfate; and osmotic laxatives, including lactulose, mannitol, and sorbitol.[110,111]

In cancer pain, sedation is a major issue related to either opioids or the disease.[36,44,100] Assessment should be ongoing for other potential reversible causes of sedation and corrected when possible. If patients still have persisting sedation while on opioids, other psychostimulants can be tried.[112,113]

Methylphenidate

Methylphenidate is a mild central nervous system stimulant. Although its exact mode of action is not known, it presumably activates the cortex and reticular activating system to produce its stimulant effect. Few pilot studies

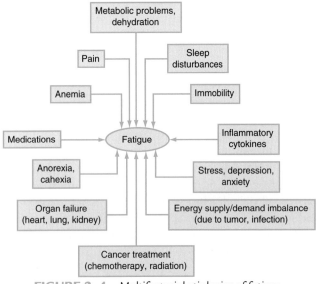

FIGURE 2–4   Multifactorial etiologies of fatigue.

have shown the beneficial effects of methylphenidate for combating fatigue.[112,113] Methylphenidate is attractive because it not only antagonizes sedation, but also helps to fight fatigue and depression simultaneously. More prospective randomized studies are being done to elucidate the effectiveness of methylphenidate, but the effects appear to be short term.

Donepezil

Donepezil is a central-acting, reversible inhibitor of the enzyme acetylcholinesterase, which acts by enhancing cholinergic function. A preliminary study[114] has shown it to be effective in mitigating opioid-related sedation. This study assessed the effectiveness of donepezil in opioid-induced sedation and related symptoms in patients with cancer pain. In 20 patients, sedation, fatigue, anxiety, well-being, depression, and anorexia significantly improved. Gastrointestinal side effects included nausea, vomiting, diarrhea, muscle and abdominal cramps, and anorexia. Overall, however, the treatment was well tolerated.[114] Randomized controlled trials of this agent are needed.

Role of Corticosteroids

Many of the uncontrolled studies have shown the beneficial effects of corticosteroids in the cancer population, which include improved analgesia especially for refractory neuropathic pain, pain associated with ductal obstruction or capsular distension, osseous pain, bowel obstruction, ascites, lymphedema, or headache caused by elevated intracranial tension. It also improves appetite and reduces nausea and malaise, thereby improving the overall quality of life. In spite of the favorable outcomes, the effects are short-lived.[115,116]

CONCLUSION

Pain occurs in a vast majority of patients who ultimately die of cancer. The control of cancer pain has the highest priority in palliative care. However, instituting palliative care earlier in the course of illness has made health care professionals aware of the needs while maintaining function and providing comfort to the patient and family as well as possible. It is important for health care professionals to deliver effective palliative care service with awareness of complexity of cancer pain and assessment of major symptoms that occur in cancer pain. The two critical issues related to cancer pain, awareness and assessment, must be addressed by every health care professional who evaluates patients with cancer-related pain and other symptoms for effective cancer pain management.

REFERENCES

1. Larue F, Colleau SM, Breasseur L, et al: Multicenter study of cancer pain and its treatment in France. Br Med J 310: 1034–1037, 1995.
2. Bonica JJ, Ventafridda V, Twycross RG: Cancer Pain. In Bonica JJ (ed) The Management of Pain, vol 1, 2nd ed. Philadelphia, Lea & Febiger, 1990, pp 400–460.
3. Jacox A, Carr DB, Payne R, et al: Management of cancer pain. Clinical Practice Guideline No 9. AHCPR Publication N.94-0592. Rockville, Md. Agency for Health Care Policy and Research, U.S. Department of Health and Human Services, Public Health Service; March 1994, 8.
4. Sela RA, Bruera E, Conner-Spady B, et al: Sensory and affective dimensions of advanced cancer pain. Psycho-Oncology 11:23–34, 2002.
5. Westwell P, Johnson NF: A comparison of pain vocabulary and affective symptoms in patients with malignant and non malignant disorders. Med Sci Res 16:583–584, 1988.
6. Wagner G: Frequency of pain in patients with cancer. Recent Results in Cancer Res 89:64–71, 1984.
7. World Health Organization: National Cancer Control Programmes: Policies and Managerial Guideline, 2nd ed. Geneva, World Health Organization, 2002.

8. Folkman S, Lazarus RS, Dunkel-Schetter C, et al: Dynamics of a stressful encounter: Cognitive appraisal, coping, and encounter outcomes. J Pers Soc Psychol 50:992–1003, 1986.
9. Fishman B: The cognitive behavioral perspective on pain management in terminal illness. Hosp J 8:73–88, 1992.
10. Syrjala KL, Chapko ME: Evidence for a biopsychosocial model of cancer treatment-related pain. Pain 61:69–79, 1995.
11. Massie MJ, Holland JC: The cancer patient with pain: Psychiatric complications and their management. J Pain Symptom Manage 7:99–109, 1992.
12. Feuz A, Rapin CH: An observational study of the role of pain control and food adaptation of elderly patients with terminal cancer. J Am Diet Assoc 94:767–770, 1994.
13. Ferrell BR: The impact of pain on quality of life: A decade of research. Nurs Clin North Am 30:609–624, 1995.
14. Burrows M, Dibble SL, Miaskowski C: Differences in outcomes among patients experiencing different types of cancer-related pain. Oncol Nurs Forum 25: 735–741, 1998.
15. Thorpe DM. The incidence of sleep disturbance in cancer patients with pain. In 7th World Congress on Pain: Abstracts. IASP Publications, Seattle, Abstract 451, 1993.

16. Cleeland CS, Nakamura Y, Mendoza TR, et al: Dimensions of the impact of cancer pain in a four country sample: new information from multidimensional scaling. Pain 67:267–273, 1996.
17. Barkwell DP: Ascribed meaning: A critical factor in coping and pain attenuation in patients with cancer-related pain. J Palliat Care 7:5–14, 1991.
18. Bond MR, Pearson IB: Psychological aspects of pain in women with advanced cancer of the cervix. J Psychosom Res 13:13–19, 1969.
19. Ventafridda V: Continuing care: A major issue in cancer pain management. Pain 36:137–143, 1989.
20. Shegda LM, McCorkle R: Continuing care in the community. J Pain Symptom Manage 5:279–286, 1990.
21. Muir CJ, McDonagh A, Gooding N: Multidimensional patient assessment. In Berger A, Portenoy RK, Weissman DE (eds): Principles and Practice of Palliative Care & Supportive Oncology, 2nd ed. Philadelphia, Lippincott Williams & Wilkins, 2002, pp 651–660.
22. McHugh M, West P, Assatly C, et al: Establishing an interdisciplinary patient care team: Collaboration at the bedside and beyond. J Nurs Adm; 26:21–27, 1996.

23. Massie MJ, Holland J, Glass E. Delirium in terminally ill cancer patients. Am J Psychiatry 140:1048–1050, 1983.

24. Lawlor PG, Bruera E: Delirium in patients with advanced cancer. Hematol Oncol Clin North Am 16:701–714, 2002.

25. Lipowski ZJ, Delirium (acute confusional states). JAMA 285:1789–1792, 1987.

26. Gillick MR, Serrel NA, Gillick LS: Adverse consequences of hospitalization in the elderly. Soc Sci Med 16:1033–1038, 1982.

27. Bruera E, Miller MJ, McCallion J, et al: Cognitive failure in patients with terminal cancer: A prospective study. J Pain Symptom Manage 7:192–195, 1992.

28. Bruera E, Kuehn N, Miller MJ, et al: The Edmonton Symptom Assessment System (ESAS): A simple method for the assessment of palliative care patients. J Palliat Care 7:6–9, 1991.

29. Williams MA. Delirium/acute confusional states: Evaluation devices in nursing. Int Psychogeriatr 3:301–308, 1991.

30. Breitbart W, Rosenfeld B, Roth A, et al: The Memorial Delirium Assessment Scale J Pain Symptom Manage 13:128–137, 1997.

31. Daut RL, Cleeland CS, Flannery RC: Development of the Wisconsin Brief Pain Questionnaire to assess pain in cancer and other diseases. Pain 17:197–210, 1983.

32. Melzack R: The McGill pain questionnaire. In Melzack R (ed): Pain Measurement and Assessment. New York, Raven, 1983, pp 41–48.

33. Breitbart W, Marotta R, Platt M, et al: A double-blind trial of haloperidol, chlorpromazine, and lorazepam in the treatment of delirium in hospitalized AIDS patients. Am J Psychiatr 153:231–237, 1996.

34. Lawlor PG, Gagnon B, Mancini IL, et al: Occurrence, causes, and outcome of delirium in advanced cancer patients: A prospective study. Arch Intern Med 160: 786–794, 2000.

35. Breitbart W, Passik S: Psychiatric aspects of palliative care. In Doyle D, Hanks GWC, MacDonald N (eds): Oxford Textbook of Palliative Medicine, 2nd ed. Oxford, Oxford University Press, 1998, pp 933–954.

36. Bruera E, Pereira J: Neuropsychiatric toxicity of opioids. In Jensen TS, Turner JA, Wiesenfeld-Hallin Z (eds): Proceedings of the 8th World Congress on Pain. Seattle, IASP Press, 1996, pp 717–738.

37. Fainsinger R, MacEachern T, Hanson J, et al: Symptom control during the last week of life in a palliative care unit. J Palliat Care 7:5–11, 1991.

38. Leipzig R, Goodman H, Gray G, et al: Reversible narcotic associated mental status impairment in patients with metastatic cancer. Pharmacology 35:47–54, 1987.

39. Bruera E, Fainsinger R, Miller MJ, Kuehn N: The assessment of pain intensity in patients with cognitive failure: A preliminary report. J Pain Symptom Manage 7:267–270, 1992.

40. Levine PM, Silverfarb PM, Lipowski ZJ: Mental disorders in cancer patients: A study of 100 psychiatric referrals. Cancer 42:1385–1391, 1978.

41. Trzepacz PT, Teague GB, Lipowski ZJ: Delirium and other organic mental disorders in a general hospital. Gen Hosp Psychiatry 7:101–106, 1985.

42. Inouye SK, Van Dyck CH, Alessi CA: Clarifying confusion: The Confusion Assessment method. Ann Intern Med 113:941–948, 1990.

43. Daeninck PJ, Bruera E: Opioid use in cancer pain: Is a more liberal approach enhancing toxicity? Acta Anesthesiol Scand 43(9): 924–938, 1999.

44. Bruera E, Macmillan K, Hanson J, et al: The cognitive effects of the administration of narcotic analgesics in patients with cancer pain. Pain 39:13–16, 1989.

45. Posner JB. Delirium and exogenous metabolic brain disease. In Beeson PB, McDermott W, Wyngarden JB (eds): Cecil Textbook of Medicine. Philadelphia, Saunders, 1979, pp 644–651.

46. Cherny N, Ripamonti C, Pereira J, et al: Strategies to manage the adverse effects of oral morphine: An evidence-based report. J Clin Oncol 19:2542–2554, 2001.

47. Silberfarb PM: Chemotherapy and cognitive defects in cancer patients. Annu Rev Med 34:35–46, 1983.

48. Stiefel F, Breitbart WS, Holland JC: Corticosteroids in cancer: Neuropsychiatric complications. Cancer Invest 7:479–491, 1989.

49. Stiefel F, Fainsinger R, Bruera E: Acute confusional states in patients with advanced cancer. J Pain Symptom Manage 7:94–98, 1992.

50. Stiefel F, Holland J: Delirium in cancer patients. Int Psychogeriatr 3:333–336, 1991.

51. Gagnon B, Lawlor PG, Mancini IL, et al: The impact of delirium on the circadian distribution of breakthrough analgesia in advanced cancer patients. J Pain Symptom Manage 22:826–833, 2001.

52. Wise MG, Brandt GT: Delirium. In Yudofsky SC, Hales RE (eds): Textbook of Neuropsychiatry, 2nd ed. Washington, DC, American Psychiatric Press, 1992, pp 363–423.

53. Ross CA: CNS arousal systems: Possible role in delirium. Int Psychogeriatr 3:353–371, 1991.

54. Bruera E, Schoeller T, Wenk R, et al: A prospective multi-center assessment of the Edmonton Staging System for cancer pain. J Pain Symptom Manage 10:348–355, 1995.

55. Pereira J, Bruera E: Chronic nausea. In Bruera E, Higginson I (eds): Cachexia-Anorexia in Cancer Patients. New York, Oxford University Press, 1996, pp 23–37.

56. Vigano A, Watanabe S, Bruera E: Anorexia and cachexia in advanced cancer patients. Cancer Surv 21:99–115, 1994.

57. MacDonald N, Alexander R, Bruera E: Cachexia-anorexia-asthenia. J Pain Symptom Manage 10:151–155, 1995.

58. Bruera E, Fainsinger R: Clinical management of cachexia and anorexia. In Doyle D, Hanks G, MacDonald N (eds): Oxford Textbook of Palliative Medicine, 2nd ed. Oxford, Oxford University Press, 1998.

59. Breitbart W: Diagnosis and management of delirium in the terminally ill. In Bruera E, Portenoy RK (eds): Topics in Palliative Care, vol 5. Oxford, Oxford University Press, 2001, pp 303–321.

60. Fainsinger RL, Tapper M, Bruera E: A perspective on the management of delirium in terminally ill patients on a palliative care unit. J Palliat Care 9:4–8, 1993.

61. Lawlor PG: Delirium. In Fisch MJ, Bruera E (eds): Handbook of Advanced Cancer Care, 1st ed. Cambridge, Cambridge University Press, 2003, pp 390–396.

62. Lawlor PG, Bruera E. Side effects of opioids in chronic pain treatment. Curr Opin Anaesthesiol 11:539–545, 1998.

63. d' Stoutz ND, Bruera E, Suarez-Almazor M. Opioid rotation for toxicity in terminal cancer patients. J Pain Symptom Manage 10(5):378–384, 1995.

64. Tuma R, DeAnngelis LM: Altered mental status in patients with cancer. Arch Neurol 57:1727–1731, 2000.

65. Breitbart W: Psychiatric complications of cancer. In Brain MC, Carbone PP (eds): Current Therapy in Hematology Oncology, 3rd ed. Toronto and Philadelphia, B.C. Decker Inc, 1988, pp 268–274.

66. Sipahimalani A, Massand PS. Olanzapine in the treatment of delirium. Psychosomatics 39:422–430, 1998.

67. Sipahimalani A, Sime RM, Massand PS: Treatment of delirium with risperidone. Int J Geriatr Psychopharmacol 1:24–26, 1997.

68. Bruera E, Moyano J, Seifert L, Fainsinger RL, Hanson J, Suarez-Almazor M: The frequency of alcoholism among patients with pain due to terminal cancer. J Pain Symptom Manage 10: 599–603, 1995.

69. Ewing J: Detecting alcoholism: The CAGE questionnaire. JAMA 252:1905–1907, 1984.

70. Mansky P: Reminiscence of an addictionalogist: Thoughts of a researcher and clinician. Psychiatr Q 64:81–106, 1993.

71. Franklin JE, Frances RJ: Alcohol and other psychoactive substance disorders. In Hales RE, Yudofsky SC, Talbott JA (eds): Text book of Psychiatry, 3rd ed. Washington, DC, The American Psychiatry Press Inc., 1999, pp 363–423.

72. Kessler RC, Crumb, Warner LA, et al: Lifetime ccO-occurrence of DSM -111 R alcohol abuse and dependence with other psychiatric disorders in the national comorbidity survey. Arch Gen Psychiatry 54:313–321, 1997.

73. Skykes J, Johnson R, Hanks GW: Difficult pain problems. Br Med J 315:867–869, 1997.

74. Hwang SS, Chang VT, Fairclough DL, et al: Development of cancer pain prognostic scale. J Pain Symptom Manage 24(4): 366–378, 2002.

75. Lichter I: Nausea and vomiting in patients with cancer. Hematol Oncol Clin North Am 10:207–220, 1996.

76. Gamsa A: Is emotional disturbance a precipitator or a consequence of chronic pain. Pain 42:183–195, 1990.

77. Massie MJ, Holland JC: The cancer patient with pain: Psychiatric complications and their management. J Pain Symptom Manage 7:99–109, 1992.

78. Ferrell BR: The impact of pain on quality of life: A decade of research. Nurs Clin North Am 30:609–624, 1995.

79. Stone P, Richards M, Hardy J: Fatigue in patients with cancer. Eur J Cancer 34(11):1670–1676, 1998.

80. Cella D, Peterman A, Passik S, et al: Progress toward guidelines for the management of fatigue. Oncology 12(11A):369–377, 1998.

81. Portenoy RK, Itri LM: Cancer-related fatigue: Guidelines for evaluation and management. Oncologist 4(1):1-10, 1999.

82. Cherny NI, Catane R: Professional negligence in the management of cancer pain: A case for urgent reforms [editorial; comment]. Cancer 76:2181-2185, 1995.

83. Edwards RB: Pain management and the values of health care providers. In Hill C S, Fields W S (eds): Drug Treatment of Cancer Pain in a Drug Oriented Society: Advances in Pain Research and Therapy, vol 11. New York, Raven, 1989, pp 101-112.

84. Emanuel EJ: Pain and symptom control: Patient rights and physician responsibilities. Hematol Oncol Clin North Am 10(1): 41-56, 1996.

85. Haugen PS: Pain relief. Legal aspects of pain relief for the dying. Minn Med 80:15-18, 1997.

86. Cleeland CS, Gonin R, Hatfield AK, et al: Pain and its treatment in outpatients with metastatic cancer. N Engl J Med 330: 592-596, 1994.

87. Grossman SA, Sheidler VR, Swedeen K, et al: Correlation of patient and caregiver ratings of cancer pain. J Pain Symptom Manage 6:53-57, 1991.

88. Von Roenn JH, Cleeland CS, Gonin R, et al: Physician attitudes and practice in cancer pain management. A survey from the Eastern Cooperative Oncology Group. Ann Intern Med 119(2):121-126, 1993.

89. Cherny NI, Ho MN, Bookbinder M, et al: Cancer pain: Knowledge and attitudes of physicians at a cancer center (meeting abstract). Proceedings of the Annual Meeting of the American Society of Clinical Oncologists 13, 1994.

90. Sapir R, Catane R, Cherny NI: Cancer pain: Knowledge and attitudes of physicians in Israel (meeting abstract). Proceedings of the Annual Meeting of the American Society of Clinical Oncologists 16, 1997.

91. Wade JB, Price DD, Hamer RM, et al: An emotional component analysis of chronic pain. Pain 40:303-310, 1990.

92. Fernandez E, Turk DC: The scope and significance of anger in the experience of chronic pain. Pain 61:165-175, 1995.

93. Kerns RD, Rosenberg R, Jacob MC: Anger expression and chronic pain. J Behavioral Med 17:57-70, 1994.

94. Jensen MP: Validity of self-report and observation measures. In: Jensen RS, Turner JA, Weisenfeld-Halleb Z (eds): Proceedings of the 8th World Congress on Pain. IASP Press, Seattle, 1997, 637-661.

95. Osborne RJ, Joel SP, Grebinik K, et al: The pharmacokinetics of morphine and morphine glucoronides in kidney failure. Clin Pharmacol Ther 54:158-167, 1993.

96. D'Honneur G, Gilton A, Sandouk P, et al: Plasma and cerebrospinal fluid concentrations of morphine and morphine glucuronides after oral morphine: The influence of renal failure. Anaesthesiology 81:87-93, 1994.

97. Mercadante S: Opioid rotation in cancer pain: Curr Rev Pain 3:131-142, 1998.

98. Bruera E, Pereira J, Watanabe S, et al: Opioid rotation in patients with cancer pain: A retrospective comparison of dose ratios between methadone, hydromorphone, and morphine. Cancer 78:852-857, 1996.

99. Fainsinger R, Mac Eachern T, Miller M, et al: The use of hypodermoclysis for rehydration in terminally ill cancer patients. J Pain Symptom Manage 9(5):298-302, 1994.

100. Cherney NJ, Chang V, Frager G, et al: Opioid pharmacotherapy in the management of cancer pain. Cancer 76: 1288-1293, 1995.

101. Mercadante S. Methadone in cancer pain. Eur J Pain 1:77-85, 1997.

102. Crews JC, Sweeney N, Denson DD: Clinical efficacy of methadone in patients refractory to other Mu-opioid receptor agonist analgesics for the management of terminal cancer pain. Cancer 72: 2266-2272, 1993.

103. Lawlor P, Turner K, Hanson J, et al: Dose ratio between morphine and methadone in patients with cancer pain: A retrospective study. Cancer 82:1167-1173, 1998.

104. Ripamonti C, Groff L, Brunelli C, et al: Switching from morphine to oral methadone in treating cancer pain: What is the equianalgesic dose ratio? J Clin Oncol 16:3216-3221, 1998.

105. Galer BS, Coyle N, Pasternak GW, et al: Individual variability in the response to different opioids: Report of five cases. Pain 49:87-91, 1992.

106. Vigano A, Fan D, Bruera E: Individualized use of methadone and opioid rotation in the comprehensive management of cancer pain associated with poor prognostic indicators. Pain 67:115-119, 1996.

107. Morley JS, Makin MK: Comments on Ripamonti, et al Pain 73:14, 1997.

108. Bruera E, MacEachern T, Sachynski K, et al: Comparison of the efficacy, safety and pharmacokinetics of controlled release and immediate release metoclopramide for the management of chronic nausea in advanced cancer patients. Cancer 74(12):3204-3211, 1994.

109. Mancini I, Bruera E: Constipation in advanced cancer patients. Support Care Cancer 6(4):356-364, 1998.

110. Sykes NP: Constipation and diarrhea. In Doyle D, Hanks GWC, MacDonald N (eds): Oxford Textbook of Palliative Medicine, 2nd ed. Oxford, Oxford University Press, 1998, pp 513-526.

111. Bruera E, Miller MJ, Macmillan K, et al: Neuropsychological effects of methylphenidate in patients receiving a continuous infusion of narcotics for cancer pain. Pain 48:163-166, 1992.

112. Bruera E, Driver L, Barnes E, et al: Patient controlled methylphenidate (PCM) for the management of fatigue in patients with advanced cancer. J Clin Oncol 21: 4439-4443, 2003.

113. Bruera E, Strasser F, Shen L, et al: The effect of donepezil on sedation and other symptoms in patients receiving opioids for cancer pain: A pilot study. J Pain Symptom Manage 26(5): 1049-1054, 2003.

114. Bruera E, Roca E, Cedaro L, et al: Action of oral prednisolone sodium succinate on quality of life in preterminal cancer patients: A placebo-controlled Multicenter Study. The Methylpredinisolone Preterminal Cancer Study Group. Eur J Cancer 25:1817-1821, 1989.

115. Tannock I, Gospodarowicz M, Makin W, et al: Treatment of metastatic prostate cancer with low dose prednisone: Evaluation of pain and quality of life as prognostic indices of response. J Clin Oncol 7:590-597, 1989.

CHAPTER 3

Initial Approach to the Patient with Cancer Pain

RAFAEL V. MIGUEL, MD

Patients with cancer commonly have complaints of pain. Historically, these patients had been routinely undertreated. Physicians caring for cancer pain patients would not uncommonly adopt a "you have to learn to live with it" posture with resultant unnecessary patient suffering. This inadequate pain relief was surveyed by Von Roenn and others in 1993.[1] In a survey of 1800 Eastern Cooperative Oncology Group (ECOG) physicians, 86% reported that they felt their patients' pain was undertreated. Seventy-six percent of the physicians surveyed felt that the most common reason was that there was an inadequate assessment of the cancer patient in pain. Cleeland surveyed cancer patients and their physicians from 54 cancer centers.[2] He found that 42% of patients surveyed reported inadequate analgesia with a higher incidence reported by females, the elderly, and members of minority groups. Effective communication of pain status was felt to be a significant factor contributing to effective analgesia.

There are a variety of misconceptions that impede patients' desire to report pain. These include the belief that pain is inevitable and the old adage "suffer in silence" is the required appropriate behavior. Patients may be fearful that pain indicates advanced disease and do not want to admit that their cancer may be recurring. Patients may feel that by reporting pain symptoms, they may be distracting their physicians from active treatment of their cancer.

Some patients manifest a reluctance to take medications, especially opioids. This reluctance may be due to a fear of addiction, cultural barriers or religious concerns, discomfort with route of administration, or fear of unmanageable side effects. This was underscored in a recent study by Anderson and others assessing pain and related perceptions in 31 African American and Hispanic cancer patients.[3] While the patients reported their physicians as the most trusted and reliable source of information, they felt that communication difficulties and a reluctance to complain of pain were barriers to improved pain relief.

It is imperative that the pain physician have a frank and open discussion with the cancer patient that includes family members and caregivers whenever possible. This will provide the best situation to elicit valuable information necessary to formulate a treatment strategy and modify it in an expeditious manner if necessary.

Enormous strides have been made in the past decade to decrease the pain complaints of cancer patients. A thorough understanding of the cancer status, type of cancer, and type of pain is essential to implementing an effective pain management strategy.

COMPREHENSIVE EVALUATION AND ESTABLISHMENT OF TREATMENT PLAN

The success of any implemented cancer pain prescription is improved with an in-depth understanding of the patients' complete medical condition, extent of disease, and characteristics of the pain complaints. Furthermore, it is important that all complaints of pain be elicited and addressed. In a review of 2266 cancer patients with pain, Grond and others found that 70% of the patients they assayed had pain in at least two sites.[4]

Initial Consultation

While attention to cancer and its status is essential, a thorough history and physical examination is mandatory. It may appear unnecessary to the pain practitioner to perform a complete history and physical examination, especially when the cause for pain is obvious (e.g., upper abdominal pain in patient with unresectable pancreatic cancer); however, it provides valuable insight. A review of organ function may reveal dysfunction and alert the physician to conditions that may affect certain approaches to pain relief. Many commonly used chemotherapeutic agents produce toxicities that affect pain management, either by producing painful syndromes or by affecting analgesic interventions (Table 3–1).

On initial evaluation it may be discovered that the chemotherapy regimen has induced renal dysfunction (e.g., cisplatin,[5] high-dose methotrexate[6]) which, for example, may preclude nonsteroidal anti-inflammatory drug (NSAID) use in a patient with bony metastases. Chemotherapy-induced renal dysfunction may decrease renal reserve and preclude the use of contrast media in diagnostic studies. Furthermore, NSAIDs possess the potential to worsen high blood pressure or interfere with the action of some antihypertensives (Table 3–2),[7,8] so a detailed cardiovascular history is essential. Reversible airway disease may be present in heavy cigarette smokers with lung cancer, and concern about triggering a bronchospastic event or worsening an already compromised lung function needs to be considered prior to prescribing NSAIDs. A list of common clinical conditions that may be present in cancer patients and their potential impact on analgesic therapy is presented in Table 3–3.

Medication History

Specific attention should be paid to all medications taken by the patient. The cancer pain patient is frequently on multiple medications, including antitumor therapy, which influences the selection of analgesic medications

and techniques. Knowledge of the type of chemotherapeutic regimens the patient has received and their associated side effects profile will often lead to the pain diagnosis and facilitate establishment of an effective treatment plan. Side effects such as thrombocytopenia or neutropenia are not uncommon, and the timing of a round of chemotherapy and the planning of an interventional pain procedure or implantation of an analgesic device need to be considered.

Patients with malignancy often have a prothrombic state due to the ability of almost all types of cancer cells to activate the coagulation system. Hypercoagulability syndrome is frequently associated with some cancers (e.g., breast and prostate). Unfortunately, none of the hemostatic markers of coagulation have any predictive value for the occurrence of thrombotic events in a particular patient. While not all mechanisms are clearly understood, the prothrombic state of a cancer patient is characterized by some general tumor-host responses (i.e., acute phase, inflammation, and angiogenesis), decreased levels of inhibitors of coagulation, and impaired fibrinolysis.[9] In addition, this prothrombic tendency is enhanced by anticancer therapy such as surgery, chemotherapy, hormone therapy, and radiotherapy by indwelling central venous catheters and by hemodynamic compromise (i.e., venous stasis). Due to this state of hypercoagulability, some patients may require antiplatelet therapy.

TABLE 3–1 Chemotherapy-Induced Dysfunction and Pain Syndromes

Chemotherapeutic agent	Toxicity	Impact on pain
Vinca alkaloids (vincristin, vinblastin)	Neurologic	Peripheral neuropathy (glove and stocking distribution), autonomic neuropathy (abdominal pain, constipation, paralytic ileus, urinary retention, and orthostatic hypotension)
Paclitaxel/Docetaxel	Bone marrow depression, neurologic	Neutropenia, mucositis (painful mouth ulcerations), peripheral neuropathy
Platinum complexes (cisplatin, carboplatin)	Renal, bone marrow depression, neurologic	Decrease creatinine clearance, peripheral neuropathy (cisplatin)
Etoposide	Bone marrow depression	Leukopenia, thrombocytopenia, mucositis (high dose)
Nitrogen mustards (mechlorethamine, chlorambucil, cyclophosphamide, ifosphamide)	Bone marrow depression	Leukopenia, thrombocytopenia, hemorrhagic cystitis (cyclophosphamide)
Anthracycline antibiotics	Bone marrow suppression, cardiac	Leukopenia, thrombocytopenia/anemia (less severe), stomatitis, cardiac arrhythmias, congestive heart failure
Mitoxantrone	Bone marrow suppression	Mucositis
Cytarabine	Bone marrow suppression, neurologic	Granulocytopenia/thrombocytopenia, peripheral neuropathy (high doses)
Methotrexate	Bone marrow suppression, renal	Pancytopenia, mucositis (early indicator of toxicity), chronic renal failure
Bleomycin	Pulmonary	Mucositis (dose-related), lung fibrosis

TABLE 3–2 Nonsteroidal Anti-inflammatory Agents in Hypertension

No effect	aspirin, sulindac
Mild elevation	celecoxib, rofecoxib
Intermediate elevation	Ibuprofen
Significant elevation	Indomethacin, piroxicam, naproxen

Adapted from Brook RD, Kramer MB, Blaxall BC, Bisognano JD: Nonsteroidal anti-inflammatory drugs and hypertension. J Clin Hypertens 2:319–323, 2000.

This will often require modifying the anticoagulation regimen (e.g., discontinuing coumadin and starting enoxaparin, whose shorter half-life allows more flexibility to schedule procedures around the anticoagulant effect) when planning an interventional analgesic technique.

Extent of Disease and Cancer Status

An in-depth knowledge of the type of cancer and its status is imperative. Pain is more frequently associated with tumors arising in noncompliant tissue (e.g., bone) than in hematologic malignancies. A patient may have a very small mass in bone causing severe pain compared to one in a compliant organ such as the lung or pancreas with few signs or symptoms until progression involves other structures (e.g., pleura or biliary tract, respectively). It is important to know whether one is evaluating a patient with primary, potentially curable disease or a patient with an incurable, metastatic process. While one may select a medical regimen with a patient in the early stages of disease with no evidence of metastases, a patient with metastatic or recurrent disease warrant more aggressive measures, such as neurolysis, as early as the initial consultation.

Patients may present to the pain clinic years after their cancer diagnosis and treatment have occurred. A new pain complaint has arisen and the unsuspecting physician may be misled and opt to treat a more likely and common condition, such as osteoarthritis. *Any new pain in a patient with a history of cancer is a recurrence until ruled out!* A frank discussion of the cancer type, treatment received, and last evaluation by the oncologist must be held at initial evaluation. If it has been more than 3 months since the last oncologic evaluation, serious consideration should be given to referral for reevaluation or ordering the necessary workup (e.g., bone scan, carcinoembryonic antigen, computed tomography scans) to rule out recurrent or metastatic disease. Delays in diagnosing a recurrence may have grave consequences on treatment and

TABLE 3–3 Clinical Conditions in the Cancer Patient

Dysfunctional Organ System	Etiology	Impact on Pain Therapy
Constitutional	Tumor-induced wasting, anorexia, nausea/vomiting chronic fatigue syndrome, anemia of cancer/chemotherapy	Hypoalbuminemia (decreases protein binding, increases plasma free fraction), tolerate oral medications
Hematologic	Anemia, thrombocytopenia, neutropenia	Excessive fatigue, coagulopathy and interventions, infections with analgesic implants
Head, eyes, ear, nose, and throat	Irradiation, postsurgical (laryngectomy)	Difficulty/inability swallowing oral medications, xerostomia (oral transmucosal medications)
Lung	Smoking history, asthma, chemotherapy (bleomycin [pulmonary fibrosis])	NSAIDs, central alveolar hypoventilation (opioids)
Cardiac	Hypertension, coronary artery disease/prior myocardial infarction, prior mediastinal irradiation, chemotherapy (daunorubicin, doxorubicin)	NSAIDs hypertension, edema, congestive heart failure, adrenergic antidepressants, electrocardiogram changes
Renal	Idiopathic, chronic (e.g., long-standing hypertensive), chemotherapy/NSAID-induced	Drug elimination/toxicity, diagnostic studies with contrast
Neurologic	Postsurgical, chemotherapy (cisplatin, vinca alkaloids, peripheral neuropathy), central nervous system irradiation, sleep disturbances	
Gastrointestinal	Postsurgical (e.g., "short gut," ostomies)	Drug absorption (e.g., slow release opioids)

NSAID, nonsteroidal anti-inflammatory drug.

survival and be the cause of needless pain and suffering due to suboptimal pain treatment.

Pain Characteristics

Cancer pain may be described in many ways, and it is imperative that the type of pain be categorized into the appropriate group. Somatic, visceral, and neuropathic pains are generally identified by their clinical presentation, and that will direct their treatment. While questioning the patient regarding the *quantity* of pain (i.e., numerical scales, visual analog scale, Faces Pain Scale) is important to get an initial impression of severity and obtain a baseline from which to compare the efficacy of subsequent treatment, specific questioning regarding the *quality* of the pain is essential toward implementing a directed and effective treatment plan.

Nociceptive pain arises from activation of nociceptors in somatic or visceral structures. Somatic pain can be due to mechanical, thermal, or electrical stimuli. It is usually well localized (i.e., the patient can point to painful spot) and is commonly described by the patient as sharp, achy, throbbing, constant, pressure-like. It generally responds well to endogenous and exogenous opioids.

Visceral pain occurs due to injury to sympathetically innervated organs, such as that seen with pain that emanates from soft organs of the thorax, abdomen, and pelvis. It is generally poorly defined (i.e., generalized area of pain rather than fingertip localization). It not uncommonly has a referred component due to dual innervation, central convergence of afferent impulses, or chemical irritation by tumor-mediated algesics. It is classically described as deep, dull, gnawing, or vague. A cramping nature is often reported when involvement of hollow viscus is present. Aching and sharp descriptors are generally present with solid organ capsule stretching. It also responds well to opioids in the majority of cases.

Neuropathic pain is more complicated and has been reported to exist in 34% of cancer patients with pain.[4] It may present as the initial complaint but is commonly seen as the tumor progresses. Some estimate that neuropathic pain syndromes make up more than 50% of new pain diagnoses in a cancer pain patient.[10] The clinical picture may change and a different symptom complex may appear. This is usually due to damage to the sympathetic nerve fibers, peripheral nerves, or direct central nervous system involvement. Pathologic neurofunctional changes (e.g., "wind-up," abnormal *N*-methyl-D-aspartate (NMDA) receptor activation, abnormal sympathetic-somatic activation) are also frequently implicated in the development of neuropathic pain. Clinically, patients describe it as localized, with radiations following a dermatomal distribution. It possesses particular characteristics that distinguish it from other types of pain. Patients will commonly report burning, tingling, and shooting sensations. Neuropathic pain has been generally considered to be opioid-unresponsive. While it is commonly treated with adrenergic antidepressants and antiepileptic drugs (AEDs), more recent research indicates that opioids may indeed play a role in its management.[11-13] While neuropathic pain certainly has a rightward shift in its opioid-responsiveness compared with pain arising from nociceptor stimulation, the diagnosis of neuropathic pain should not preclude an opioid trial for analgesia. A variety of neuropathic pain syndromes are well described related to particular oncologic processes and should be sought out in patients with these cancers presenting with pain. These are presented in Table 3–4.

The patient must be interrogated with regard to other characteristics of pain. The patient must report if there are any factors that improve or worsen the pain complaint or if there are any positions that affect the intensity of the pain. It would be important to note whether there is a mechanical component to the pain, which may speak of bony or articular involvement. The natural course of most cancer-related pain is a waxing and waning nature, and one must know whether the pain is constant with intermittent peaks or is only associated with episodic bouts. This would affect the selected medical pain regimen (e.g., selection of sustained-release opioids and immediate release for breakthrough versus a treatment plan based on breakthrough pain only). It is also important to know how long the painful episodes last, as that would influence the type of breakthrough agent used. There may be secondary features that the cancer pain patient may report on questioning. These include localized weakness or numbness, which usually indicate nerve compression. Another important query to present to the patient is whether there are any temperature or vasomotor changes. This may indicate sympathetic involvement and is an important consideration when formulating a treatment strategy.

Idiopathic pain is pain for which there is no known origin. This may occur, for example, in psychogenic pain, which occurs very rarely in cancer patients. It is not uncommon that pain arises before biologic markers and imaging studies are able to identify a cause. A thorough psychiatric evaluation is mandatory, and even in the presence of a psychiatric diagnosis, extreme caution should be taken prior to making this diagnosis.

Measurement of Pain

Pain is always a subjective finding and is influenced by the specific patient's degree of stoicism. For this reason, while useful as supplemental information, dependence on observations such as grimacing, postural accommodations, or even sympathetic outflow signs (i.e., heart rate increases, hypertension) may be unreliable. Nowhere in the pain physician's practice should a complaint of pain be accepted more than when caring for a cancer patient.

TABLE 3–4 Cancer-Related Neuropathic Pain

Tumor invasion/compression of peripheral nerves
Radiculopathy
Obliteration of epidural space by direct tumor growth
Bony metastases
Plexopathies by compression
Brachial (lung cancer in superior sulcus syndrome "Pancoast tumor")
Lumbosacral (cervical cancer, pelvic/retroperitoneal sarcomas)
Peripheral neuropathy
Chemotherapy (e.g., cisplatin, vinca alkaloids), "glove/stocking" distribution
Surgically induced (e.g., postthoracotomy, postmastectomy [rare in sentinel node lymphadenectomies], postnephrectomy, post-neck dissection, stump pain, postabdomino-perineal resection)
Postradiotherapy syndromes
Viscera (enteritis, cystitis)
Plexitis (brachial, lumbosacral)
Myelopathy
Postherpetic neuralgia in immunocompromised patients

Because of this dependence on the patient reporting pain, it is essential that clear lines of communication be established. This is particularly important in those patients in which communication is affected, such as children, older adults, patients from different cultural or language backgrounds, and those developmentally or cognitively impaired or with emotional disturbances.

There are a multitude of pain intensity scales to assist the patient in reporting, and the pain physician in assessing, pain intensity. These will help in initiating an analgesic regimen and indicate its ongoing effectiveness. Whichever scale is used, it should be appropriate for the patient's age and level of understanding. No one scale will accommodate everyone, but there are scales for everybody. Most adults and children over the age of 7 will be able to score their pain on a numerical 0 to 10 scale (no pain to worst pain imaginable), but some will require a specialized method of pain scoring. A few of the available simple pain scales are presented in Figure 3-1.

More elaborate pain assessment tools exist that have proven efficacy in cancer pain patients. The Brief Pain Inventory (BPI) is one such questionnaire.[14] The BPI

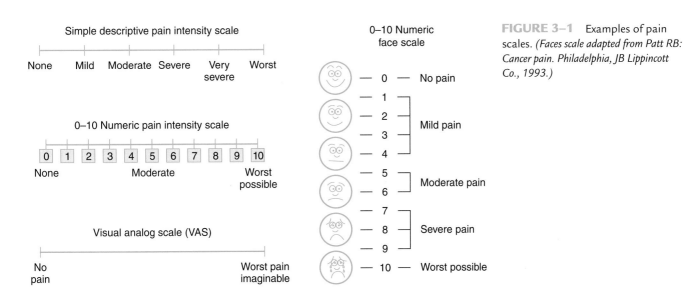

FIGURE 3–1   Examples of pain scales. *(Faces scale adapted from Patt RB: Cancer pain. Philadelphia, JB Lippincott Co., 1993.)*

measures both the intensity of pain (sensory dimension) and interference of pain in the patient's life (reactive dimension). It also queries the patient about pain relief, pain quality, and patient perception of the cause of pain. The BPI has demonstrated reliability and validity across cultures and languages and is being adopted in many countries for clinical pain assessment, epidemiologic studies, and studies of the effectiveness of pain treatment.[15-20]

The relationship of pain and its interference with function and the activities of daily life (ADLs) is a valuable assessment query. While the improved ability to perform ADLs is important, it is equally important that both of these factors be evaluated independently, as there is evidence that interference of function does not follow linearly with pain.[21]

Sleep and Cancer

Sleep disturbances are commonly seen in patients with cancer.[22] Adults who survive cranial irradiation as adolescents for medulloblastoma have demonstrated persistent sleep alterations compared to unradiated cohorts.[23] Mercadante and others surveyed 123 consecutive patients admitted to a pain and palliative care unit.[22] They found that 30% of the patients surveyed slept less than 5 hours at night and these patients more commonly had anxiety, difficulty falling asleep, awakening, and getting back to sleep, and nightmares.[24] However, patients may not be aware of the presence of many of these sleep problems or may consider them secondary to their cancer diagnosis and pain and fail to mention them during the pain consultation. Specific questioning regarding hours of sleep, night awakenings (and the reasons why) as well as the sensation of daytime fatigue and tiredness as an index of sleep quality needs to be done. Daytime functioning, daytime sleepiness, and altered circadian rhythms should be considered salient outcomes in addition to severity of cancer-related fatigue. Clinicians should consider whether a patient's sleep problem has been chronic and unrelated to cancer or precipitated by diagnosis and treatment. The specific type of sleep problem should be ascertained so that appropriate interventions (i.e., analgesia versus sleep aids versus psychiatric consultation) can be prescribed.

Psychosocial Evaluation

Cancer-related pain is not only characterized by location, quality, and intensity but also by affective, cognitive, and behavioral responses.[25] In a study comparing 40 patients with cancer-related pain to 37 pain-free cancer patients matched on diagnosis, stage of disease, age, sex, and inpatient versus outpatient status, Ahles et al. found that cancer pain patients had significantly more psychological disorders warranting a greater multidimensional conceptualization of their pain. In another study, 215 new admissions to three collaborating cancer centers were assessed for psychiatric disorders.[26] Forty-seven percent of the patients received a DSM-III diagnosis. Of these, approximately 68% of the psychiatric diagnoses consisted of adjustment disorders, with 13% representing major affective disorders (depression). Approximately 85% of those patients with a positive psychiatric condition were experiencing a disorder with depression or anxiety as the central symptom. The large majority of conditions were judged to represent highly treatable disorders. Modifying these responses is part of treating the cancer patient's pain, and adequate pain control will be difficult to achieve without addressing these issues.[27]

When faced with a life-threatening illness such as cancer, patients frequently demonstrate unnatural responses in their behavior, such as depression and adjustment disorder with depressed mood.[28] Cancer patients evaluated with the Minnesota Multiphasic Personality Inventory have demonstrated symptoms consistent with depressive personality with marked introversion and dependence.[29] The aggressivity test on these patients showed that self-aggressiveness coincides with inhibition and lethargy tone. While the cancer pain physician should certainly address these issues with the patient and their family, when appropriate, the cancer pain physician should recognize the limits of his or her neuropsychiatric training and knowledge, practice in a multi- or interdisciplinary manner, and secure psychological or psychiatric consultation as needed.

The American Society of Anesthesiologists Task Force on Pain Management has recommended that each cancer pain patient's psychosocial evaluation include a variety of symptoms and situational queries.[30] These are summarized in Table 3–5. The patient may have had a preexisting neuropsychiatric condition that is now exacerbated by the cancer diagnosis. This makes appropriate responses to therapy difficult. A patient may report a dramatic increase in opioid use, and one should not be surprised to discover that patients (and some physicians unknowingly) will self-treat depression with opioids. A targeted multidisciplinary approach toward the underlying psychiatric illness will enhance the treatment regimen.

The support system at home is critical for the cancer pain patient and frequently this will directly affect the selection of analgesic therapies. For example, if one is contemplating implanting an intrathecal pump, one has to be certain that reliable transportation for continuing evaluations and refills is present. Similarly, if a procedure is contemplated that may make a limb useless and the patient lives alone; it may be an absolute contraindication to its performance. Specific questioning about home life should be included in the initial consultation to guide the pain physician in the task of selecting the most appropriate analgesic prescription.

TABLE 3–5   Components of Initial Psychosocial Evaluation

Presence of psychological symptoms (e.g., depression, anxiety)
Indicators of psychiatric disorder (e.g., delirium, major depression)
Investigation of the "meaning" of the pain
Changes in mood
Current coping mechanisms
Family interaction
Availability of psychosocial support systems
Assessment of patient expectations and preconceptions regarding pain care (e.g., fear of addiction, loss of faculties)

Modified from Ferrante MF, Capla RA, Chang H, et al: Practice guidelines for cancer pain management: A report by the American Society of Anesthesiologists Task Force on Pain Management, Cancer Pain Section. Anesthesiology 84(5);1243–1257, 1996.

CONCLUSION

The cancer pain patient presents multiple challenges to controlling pain and improving quality of life. A systematic and comprehensive approach to the cancer patient, taking into consideration not only the cancer and its impact on various organs, but also the patient's preexisting and present physical and psychiatric condition will maximize success. Comorbid psychiatric conditions complicate pain management frequently but should be able to be controlled satisfactorily by obtaining psychosocial consultation when appropriate. Interestingly, cancer patients facing end-of-life scenarios usually have come to terms with their mortality and are more concerned with not dying a painful death. It is a reasonable request that deserves our complete attention and will be optimized by a multidisciplinary approach in evaluating and managing cancer pain and its associated disturbances.

REFERENCES

1. Von Roenn JH, Cleeland CS, Gonin R, Hatfield AK, Pandya KJ: Physician attitudes and practice in cancer pain management: A survey from the Eastern Cooperative Oncology Group. Ann Intern Med 119: 121–126, 1993.
2. Cleeland CS, Gonin R, Hatfield AK, et al: Pain and its treatment in outpatients with cancer. N Engl J Med 330:592, 1994.
3. Anderson KO, Richman SP, Hurley J, et al: Cancer pain management among underserved minority outpatients: Perceived needs and barriers to optimal control. Cancer 15;94(8):2295–2304, 2002.
4. Grond S, Zech D, Diefenbach C, et al: Assessment of cancer pain: A prospective evaluation in 2266 cancer patients referred to a pain service. Pain 64:107–114, 1996.
5. Pinzani V, Bressolle F, Haug IJ, et al: Cisplatin-induced renal toxicity and toxicity-modulating strategies: A review. Cancer Chemother Pharmacol 35(1):1–9, 1994.
6. Widemann BC, Balis FM, Kempf-Bielack B, et al: High-dose methotrexate-induced nephrotoxicity in patients with osteosarcoma. Cancer 15;100(10):2222–2232, 2004.
7. Wolfe F, Zhao S, Pettitt D: Blood pressure destabilization and edema among 8538 users of celecoxib, rofecoxib, and nonselective nonsteroidal antiinflammatory drugs (NSAID) and nonusers of NSAID receiving ordinary clinical care. J Rheumatol 31(6):1143–1151, 2004.

8. Brook RD, Kramer MB, Blaxall BC, Bisognano JD: Nonsteroidal anti-inflammatory drugs and hypertension. J Clin Hypertens 2: 319–323, 2000.
9. De Cicco M: The prothrombotic state in cancer: Pathogenic mechanisms. Crit Rev Oncol Hematol 50(3):187–196, 2004.
10. Gonzales GR, Elliot KJ, Portenoy RK, Foley KM: The impact of a comprehensive evaluation in the management of cancer pain. Pain 41:141–144, 1990.
11. Eisenach et al: Alfentanil, but not amitriptyline, reduces pain, hyperalgesia, and allodynia from intradermal injection of capsaicin in humans. Anesthesiology 86:1279–1287, 1997.
12. Gilron I, Bailey JM, Tu D, Holden RR, Weaver DF, Houlden RL: Morphine, gabapentin, or their combination for neuropathic pain. N Eng J Med 352:1324–1334, 2005.
13. Eisenberg E, McNicol ED, Carr DB: Efficacy and safety of opioid agonists in the treatment of neuropathic pain of nonmalignant origin: Systematic review and metaanalysis of randomized controlled trials. JAMA, 293:3043–3052, 2005.
14. Cleeland CS, Ryan KM: Pain assessment: Global use of the Brief Pain Inventory. Ann Acad Med Singapore 23(2):129–138, 1994.
15. Badia X, Muriel C, Gracia A, et al: Validation of the Spanish version of the Brief Pain Inventory in patients with oncological pain. Med Clin (Barc) 25;120(2):52–59, 2003.

16. Klepstad P, Loge JH, Borchgrevink PC, et al: The Norwegian brief pain inventory questionnaire: Translation and validation in cancer pain patients. J Pain Symptom Manage 24(5):517–525, 2002.
17. Mystakidou K, Mendoza T, Tsilika E, et al: Greek brief pain inventory: Validation and utility in cancer pain. Oncology 60(1): 35–42, 2001.
18. Ger LP, Ho ST, Sun WZ, et al: Validation of the Brief Pain Inventory in a Taiwanese population. J Pain Symptom Manage 18(5):316–322, 1999.
19. Caraceni A, Mendoza TR, Mencaglia E, et al: A validation study of an Italian version of the Brief Pain Inventory (Breve Questionario per la Valutazione del Dolore). Pain 65(1):87–92, 1996.
20. Wang XS, Mendoza TR, Gao SZ, Cleeland CS: The Chinese version of the Brief Pain Inventory (BPI-C): Its development and use in a study of cancer pain. Pain 67(2–3): 407–416, 1996.
21. Serlin RC, Mendoza TR, Nakamura Y, et al: When is cancer pain mild, moderate or severe? Grading pain severity by its interference with function. Pain 61(2):277–284, 1995.
22. Mercadante S, Girelli D, Casuccio A: Sleep disorders in advanced cancer patients: Prevalence and factors associated. Support Care Cancer 12(5):355–359, 2004.

23. Van Someren EJ, Swart-Heikens J, Endert E, et al: Long-term effects of cranial irradiation for childhood malignancy on sleep in adulthood. Eur J Endocrinol 150(4): 503–510, 2004.
24. Lee K, Cho M, Miaskowski C, Dodd M. Impaired sleep and rhythms in persons with cancer. Sleep Med Rev 8(3):199–212, 2004.
25. Ahles TA, Blanchard EB, Ruckdeschel JC: The multidimensional nature of cancer-related pain. Pain 17(3):277–288, 1983.

26. Derogatis LR, Morrow GR, Fetting J, et al: The prevalence of psychiatric disorders among cancer patients. JAMA 249(6):751–757, 1983.
27. Spiegel D: Cancer and depression. Br J Psychiatry 168(30):109–116, 1996.
28. Cleeland CS: The impact of pain on the patient with cancer. Cancer 54(11): 2635–2641, 1984.
29. Delgado Martin ME, Llorca Ramon G, Blanco Gonzalez AL, et al: Psychosomatics

and cancer. Actas Luso Esp Neurol Psiquiatr Cienc Afines 17(3):169–175, 1989.
30. Ferrante MF, Capla RA, Chang H, et al: Practice guidelines for cancer pain management: A report by the American Society of Anesthesiologists Task Force on Pain Management, Cancer Pain Section. Anesthesiology 84(5);1243–1257, 1996.

CHAPTER 4

Evaluation and Control of Cancer Pain in the Pediatric Patient

STEPHEN C. BROWN, MD, AND PATRICIA A. MCGRATH, PHD

Pain control is an integral component of caring for all children with cancer. In 1993 the World Health Organization (WHO) and the International Association for the Study of Pain (IASP) invited experts in the fields of oncology, palliative care, anesthesiology, neurology, pediatrics, nursing, palliative care, psychiatry, psychology, and pastoral care to attend a conference on the management of pediatric cancer pain and palliative care. This landmark conference resulted in the 1998 publication Cancer Pain Relief and Palliative Care in Children that was instrumental in not only addressing the issue but also in guiding future research and study in this area.[1] Children may experience many different types of pain from invasive procedures, the cumulative effects of toxic therapies, progressive disease, or from psychological factors. The pain is often complex with multiple sources, composed of nociceptive and neuropathic components. In addition, several situational factors usually contribute to children's pain, distress, and disability. Thus, to adequately treat pain in children with cancer, we must evaluate the primary pain sources and also ascertain which situational factors are relevant for which children and families. Treatment emphasis should shift accordingly from an exclusive disease-centered framework to a more child-centered focus.

In this chapter, we describe a child-centered framework for understanding and controlling pain for children with cancer. Although the goal in cancer care is to minimize morbidity (such as pain) on the road to a cure, at times, even with the best of care, we fail at this goal and thus we also address the issue of palliative pain management. Pain control should include regular pain assessments, appropriate analgesics administered at regular dosing intervals, adjunctive drug therapy for symptom and side effects control, and nondrug interventions to modify the situational factors that can exacerbate pain and suffering.[2] Parents concerned about medication centered on their children's comfort are calling for improved communication, standardization of nursing procedures and techniques, and a guide for a clear understanding of what to expect and from whom.[3] Basic information on pathophysiology, pharmacology, and physical interventions is beyond the scope of this chapter. Instead, this chapter provides a complementary focus to the other contributions in this textbook by describing the unique nature of children's pain including the primary factors that affect their pain and quality of life, presenting guidelines for selecting and administering drug therapy in accordance with the nociceptive and neuropathic components, and recommending practical nondrug therapies for integration within a hospital, home, or hospice setting.

THE NATURE OF A CHILD'S PAIN

Throughout the past decade, we have gained an increasing appreciation for the plasticity and complexity of a child's pain. As with adults, a child's pain is often initiated by tissue damage caused by noxious stimulation, but the consequent pain is neither simply nor directly related to the amount of tissue damage. Perhaps even more than in adults, differing pain responses to the same tissue damage are noted. The eventual pain evoked by a relatively constant noxious stimulus can be different depending on children's expectations, perceived control, or the significance that they attach to the pain.[4] Children do not sustain tissue damage in an isolated manner, devoid of a particular context, but actively interpret the strength and quality of any pain sensations, determine the relevance of any hurting, and learn how to interpret the pain by observing the general environment, especially the behavior of other people. Children's perceptions of pain are defined by age and cognitive level; previous pain experiences, against which they evaluate each new pain; the relevance of the pain or disease causing pain; expectations for obtaining eventual recovery and pain relief; and ability to control the pain themselves. While plasticity and complexity are critical features for all pain perception, plasticity seems an even more important feature for controlling children's pain.[3]

Much research has been conducted to identify the critical factors responsible for the plasticity of pain perception.[4,5] Animal behavior studies, in which the physiologic responses activated by a noxious stimulus are directly recorded, have demonstrated that certain factors, such as the primate's attention, the predictability of a painful stimulus, and the relevance of the stimulus, can directly modify the intensity of the physiologic responses evoked by a constant noxious stimulus. Parallel psychophysical studies, in which adults rate the painfulness of constant noxious stimuli in different contexts, have demonstrated that these same factors can modify the perceived intensity and unpleasantness of the consequent pain sensations. Psychologically mediated modulation of pain can occur not only at the earliest levels of pain processing, but also at the highest levels. Recent positron emission tomography (PET) and functional magnetic resonance imaging (MRI) studies have demonstrated that painful stimulation activates different cortical regions—depending on an individual's expectations and attention.[6] Human studies evaluating the impact of environmental and psychological factors on the perception of experimentally induced pain have been conducted primarily in adults. However, results from the few laboratory studies conducted with children are consistent with those from adult studies.[3,7,8] In addition, much compelling evidence about the powerful mediating role of psychological factors in children's pain derives from clinical studies of acute, recurrent, and chronic pain. These studies highlight the need to recognize and evaluate the mediating impact of these factors in order to optimally control children's pain.

The model illustrated in Figure 4-1 provides a framework for assessing the common factors that affect pain in a child with cancer. Some factors are relatively stable for a child, such as sex, temperament, and cultural background, whereas other factors change progressively, such as age, cognitive level, previous pain experience, and family learning.[2] These characteristics shape how children generally interpret and experience the various sensations caused by tissue damage. In contrast, the cognitive, behavioral, and emotional factors are not stable. They represent a unique interaction between the child and the situation in which the pain is experienced.[9,10] These situational factors can vary dynamically throughout the course of a child's illness, depending on the specific circumstances in which children experience pain. For example, a child receiving treatment for cancer will have repeated injections, central port access, and lumbar

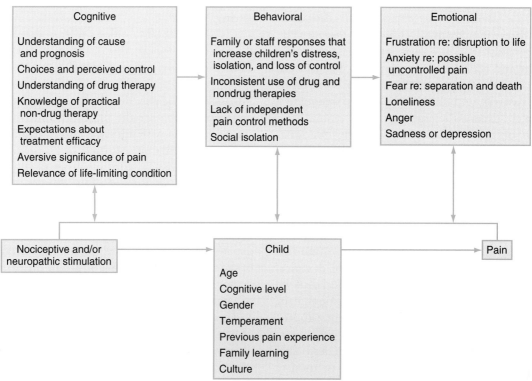

FIGURE 4–1   The situational factors that affect pain in children with cancer. *(Adapted from McGrath PA, Brown SC: Paediatric palliative medicine: Pain control. In Doyle D, Hanks GWC, Cherny NI, Calman K (eds): Oxford Textbook of Palliative Medicine, 3rd ed. Oxford, Oxford University Press, 2004, p.776, with permission.)*

punctures—all of which may cause some pain depending on the analgesics, anesthetics, or sedatives used. Even though the tissue damage from these procedures is the same each time, the particular set of situational factors for each treatment is unique for a child—depending on a child's (and parent's) expectations, a child's (and parent's and staff's) behaviors, and on a child's (and family's) emotional state. Although the causal relationship between an injury and a consequent pain seems direct and obvious, what children understand, what they do, and how they feel all affect their pain. Certain factors can intensify pain, exacerbate suffering, or affect adversely a child's quality of life.[3] Although parents and health care providers may be unable to change the more stable child characteristics, they can modify situational factors and dramatically improve children's pain and lives.

THE IMPACT OF SITUATIONAL FACTORS ON A CHILD'S PAIN

Cognitive factors include children's understanding about the pain source, their ability to control what will happen, their expectations regarding the quality and strength of pain sensations that they will experience, their primary focus of attention (that is distracted away from or focused primarily on the pain), and their knowledge of pain control strategies. In general, children's pain can be lessened by providing accurate age-appropriate information about pain, for example, emphasizing the specific sensations that children will experience (such as the stinging quality of an injection, rather than the general hurting aspects), by increasing their control and choices, by explaining the rationale for what can be done to reduce pain, and by teaching them some independent pain-reducing strategies.[9,11] For children with any life-threatening illness, key cognitive factors also include the relevance or meaning of their illness—particularly its life-threatening potential, their beliefs about death, and their understanding of the significance of their lives.

Behavioral factors refer to the specific behaviors of children, parents, and staff when children experience pain and also encompass parents' and children's wider behaviors in response to a course of repeated painful treatments, chronic pain, or progressive illness. Common behavioral factors include children's distress or coping reactions (e.g., crying, using a pain control strategy, withdrawing from life) and parents' and health staff's subsequent reactions to them (e.g., displaying frustration, calmly providing encouragement for children to use pain control strategies, engaging them in conversation and activities).[3,8] They also include the extent to which children are physically restrained during invasive or aversive treatments and the broader physical and social restrictions on children's and family's lives if children become sicker.

Distress behaviors and some altered behavioral patterns may initiate, exacerbate, or maintain children's pain. In general, as children's mental or physical activity increases, as children use coping and pain control methods, as their distress and disability behaviors decrease, and as staff and parental responses become more consistent in encouraging them to use pain control methods, their pain should lessen. Children receiving treatment for cancer seem to report less pain, feel less distressed by pain, and have a higher quality of life when families and staff encourage them to remain engaged in life and to live as fully as possible.[9]

Emotional factors include parents' and children's feelings in response to pain and to the daily effects of the underlying illness or condition. Children's emotions affect their ability to understand what is happening, their ability to cope positively, their behaviors, and ultimately their pain.[12] Children's immediate emotional reactions to pain may vary from a relatively neutral acceptance to annoyance, anxiety, fear, frustration, anger, or sadness. The specific emotions depend on the nature of the pain—type, cause, intensity, and duration—and the pain's impact on their lives. In general, the more emotionally distressed children are, the stronger or more unpleasant their pain. When children do not understand what is happening, when they lack control and do not know independent pain control strategies, their emotional distress increases and their pain intensifies. Similarly, when children's behaviors are restricted, when they are physically restrained during medical procedures, or when their usual daily activities and social interactions are disrupted, their emotional distress and pain can intensify. Children with life-threatening conditions may not understand what they are feeling or may be unable to verbalize their fears and anxieties. Yet, almost all children will become aware of differences in how their parents and families respond to them if they progress from receiving active curative treatments to receiving only palliative therapies. Even very subtle behavioral cues can still evoke fear, uncertainty, apprehension, or depression depending on children's ages and what they understand about their cancer. Thus, an essential component of pain control should be evaluating whether these emotions are exacerbating children's pain and distress and impairing the quality of their lives.

If the disease progresses, cognitive and emotional factors become the most salient situational factors that affect pain for children. Children probably often endure a prolonged period of intermittent pain, physical disability, and multiple aversive treatments. Children receiving curative therapies are more focused on the future consequences of their disease. Their thoughts, behaviors, and feelings change if their care becomes palliative. If this should happen, the type of support, information, and guidance children require changes. While the impact of palliation is profound for all children and families, each child and family is unique with respect to psychological, medical, social, and spiritual needs. All families experience anguish and grief, but they may also experience denial, anxiety, anger, guilt, frustration, and depression. It is essential that health professionals listen attentively and observe carefully not only to ensure that all the needs of both the child and family are met but also to resolve the myriad factors that can exacerbate children's pain and suffering.

A shift in care from curative to palliative therapies may signify to some children and families that health professionals are giving up on the child. Children and families must understand that stopping ineffective therapies is not giving up but represents a rational decision based on children's best interests. Pain control is an essential component of cancer care and of palliative care.[1,13-18] Children and parents should not fear that health professionals have given up on controlling pain and aversive symptoms. Pain and all symptoms must be treated aggressively from the dual perspective of targeting the primary source of tissue damage and modifying the secondary contributing factors. Although most families receive accurate information about their disease and required treatments, few children or their parents receive concrete information about their pain, the factors that can attenuate or exacerbate it, a rationale for the interventions they receive, and training in effective nondrug pain control methods. The latter may be particularly important for children in palliative care, who have diminishing control in their lives. Children and their parents often do not understand that pain control therapies may vary in efficacy due to changing disease, the effects of other drugs, and situational factors. Thus, their confidence in certain pain control therapies can decrease, even though these therapies would effectively alleviate pain at another time. The fear of inadequate pain control places an enormous emotional burden on an already distressed child and family and can create a situation in which children's pain and disability intensifies.

Generally, children's physical activity has been progressively restricted due to the disability caused by their condition. Parents who encourage children to adopt passive patient roles, to behave differently than other children, and to depend primarily on others for pain control will undoubtedly create a situation wherein children's pain is maximized. Even when children are somnolent, it is possible to create some normal environment in which children can participate and actively involve themselves during their alert periods. Children should live as fully as possible, even if they are in a palliative phase of their care.

Children who experienced adverse physical effects from medication, such as hair loss and weight gain, may have become acutely self-conscious about their appearance. As a result, these children may have progressively withdrawn from social interactions with their peers because they anticipated negative reactions. Children become more distant from the people and activities that they had enjoyed. Moreover, many children may lose the opportunity to be regarded as unique individuals by the friends and classmates they value; instead, they are regarded increasingly as sick, different, or even dying. Their peers and their daily accomplishments (whether social, academic, or athletic) had provided special meaning about children's unique value in the world. While families emphasize children's value to them and to the world, children often lose the objective feedback they routinely received. The increased withdrawal and social isolation can exacerbate their pain and emotional distress. Their withdrawal may increase when treatment emphasis shifts from cure to palliation alone. Parents may close in, spending even more exclusive time with the dying child as a closed family unit. While important for children and families, the exclusive focus on the family increases a child's social isolation and may cause more anxiety for some children—particularly when the family does not openly address the child's concerns about death and dying. Inadvertently, the family may prevent the child from interacting both with peers who can lessen anxiety through play and conversation and also with health professionals who can help resolve anxiety and fears about dying.

Children seem to know intuitively, even when dying has not been discussed directly with them. They fear separation and abandonment; some children may fear that their illness is a punishment. Dying children may feel frightened, isolated, and guilty unless they are able to openly express and resolve their concerns. Many observers have noted that children who are dying have a level of maturity far beyond their years. It is essential to acknowledge and resolve their fears. Children should receive accurate information that is consistent with their spiritual beliefs and presented in a calm, reassuring manner. They may need concrete reassurance that they will not suffer when they die, that they will not be alone, and that their families will remember them. Unresolved emotions add anguish and may intensify their pain. (For the comprehensive care of the dying child, please see references 16 and 19 to 23.)

EVALUATING THE FACTORS THAT INTENSIFY A CHILD'S PAIN

Pain assessment is an integral component of diagnosis and treatment. The differential diagnosis of a child's pain is a dynamic process that guides our clinical management. We should select specific therapies to target the responsible central and peripheral mechanisms and to mitigate the pain-exacerbating impact of situational factors, recognizing that the multiple causes and contributing factors will vary over time. Drug therapies—analgesics, analgesic-adjuvants, and anesthetics—are essential for pain control; in addition, nondrug therapies—cognitive, physical, and behavioral—are also essential. As we monitor the child's improvement in response to the therapies initiated, we refine our pain diagnosis and treatment plan accordingly. Pain control is achieved practically by adjusting both drug and nondrug therapies in a rational child-centered manner based on the assessment process, as outlined by the treatment algorithm in Figure 4–2.[24] Controlling children's pain requires an integrated approach because many factors are responsible, no matter how seemingly clear-cut the etiology. Adequate analgesic prescriptions, administered at regular dosing intervals, must be complemented by a practical cognitive–behavioral approach to ensure optimal pain relief.

Because children may experience complex pains due to myriad physical and psychological factors, pain control must be child-centered rather than disease-centered. Health care providers must carefully evaluate the varied causes and contributing factors to select the most effective therapies for each child's pain. Onset, location, intensity, quality, duration (or frequency, if recurring), spatial extent, temporal pattern, and accompanying physical symptoms are the key pain characteristics for assessment, as listed in Table 4–1. All these characteristics should be evaluated as part of the initial clinical examination, with pain intensity and any other characteristics that are clinically relevant for children monitored regularly.

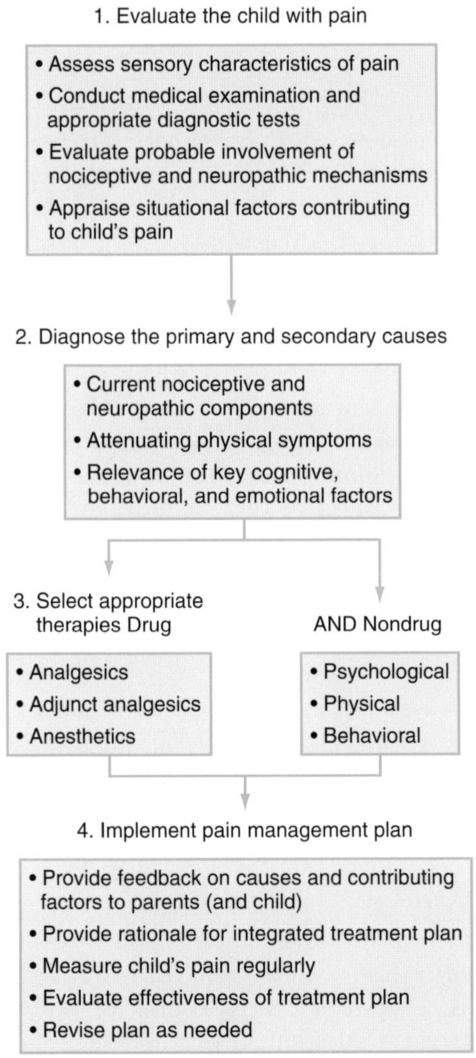

Children's descriptions about the nature of their pain (when self-report is available) complete the information obtained through radiologic and laboratory investigations. Because several situational factors usually contribute to children's pain, distress, and disability, health care providers should evaluate the extent to which these may be relevant for a child—building on their knowledge of the child and family's previous experiences throughout the child's illness and their observations of the current situation.

A thorough medical history, physical examination, and assessment of pain characteristics and contributing factors are necessary to establish a correct clinical diagnosis. Subsequent assessments of pain intensity enable us to determine when treatments are effective and to identify those children for whom they are most effective. Health care providers need pain measures that are convenient to administer and whose resulting pain scores provide meaningful information about children's pain experiences. An extensive array of pain measures have been developed and validated for use with infants, children, and adolescents.[25-27]

Like adult pain measures, children's pain measures are classified as physiologic, behavioral, or psychological, depending on what is monitored—physical parameters (e.g., heart rate, sweat index, blood pressure, cortisol level), distress behaviors (e.g., grimaces, cries, protective guarding gestures), or children's own descriptions of what they are experiencing (e.g., words, drawings, numerical ratings). Physiologic and behavioral measures provide indirect estimates of pain because health care providers must infer the location and strength of a child's pain solely from his or her responses. In contrast, psychologic measures can provide direct information about the location, strength, quality, affect, and duration.

The criteria for an accurate pain measure are similar to those required for any measuring instrument. A pain measure must be valid, in that it measures a specific aspect of pain so that changes in pain ratings reflect meaningful differences in a child's pain experience. The measure must be reliable, in that it provides consistent and trustworthy pain ratings regardless of the time of testing, the clinical setting, or who is administering the measure. The measure must be relatively free from bias, in that children should be able to use it similarly, regardless of differences in how they may wish to please adults. The pain measure should be practical and versatile for

1. Evaluate the child with pain

- Assess sensory characteristics of pain
- Conduct medical examination and appropriate diagnostic tests
- Evaluate probable involvement of nociceptive and neuropathic mechanisms
- Appraise situational factors contributing to child's pain

2. Diagnose the primary and secondary causes

- Current nociceptive and neuropathic components
- Attenuating physical symptoms
- Relevance of key cognitive, behavioral, and emotional factors

3. Select appropriate therapies Drug   AND Nondrug

- Analgesics
- Adjunct analgesics
- Anesthetics

- Psychological
- Physical
- Behavioral

4. Implement pain management plan

- Provide feedback on causes and contributing factors to parents (and child)
- Provide rationale for integrated treatment plan
- Measure child's pain regularly
- Evaluate effectiveness of treatment plan
- Revise plan as needed

FIGURE 4–2   Treatment algorithm for controlling children's pain.

TABLE 4–1 Key Components of Evaluating a Child's Pain

Sensory features	Pain onset
	Location
	Intensity
	Quality
	Duration
	Spread to other sites (consistent with neurologic pattern)
	Radiation
	Temporal pattern
	Accompanying symptoms
Medical/surgical appraisal	Investigations conducted
	Radiologic and laboratory results
	Consult results
	Analgesic and adjuvant medications (type, dose, frequency, route, length of medication trial)
Clinical and situational factors	Roles of medical and associated health professionals
	Documentation of pain
	Criteria for determining analgesic efficacy
	Cognitive factors (understanding, expectations, control)
	Behavioral factors (child, parents, staff)
	Emotional factors (child, parents)

assessing different types of pain (e.g., disease-related, procedural pain) in many different children (according to age, cognitive level, cultural background) and for use in diverse clinical and home settings.

PHYSIOLOGIC AND BEHAVIORAL PAIN SCALES

Although physiologic parameters can provide valuable information about a child's distress state, more research is required to develop a sensitive system for interpreting how these parameters reflect pain strength. At present, there are no valid physiologic pain scales for children. Health care providers must use behavioral or self-report scales.

Behavioral pain scales include lists of the different distress behaviors that children generally exhibit when they experience a certain type of pain.[25,26,28,29] To develop these scales, trained health care providers carefully observe children when they are in pain (e.g., after surgery) and document any behaviors that seem caused by the pain. They then list these presumed pain behaviors (e.g., crying, facial expression, limb rigidity) on an itemized checklist. Parents or health care providers complete the pain scale by checking which of the listed behaviors they see when children are ill. On many scales, parents also rate the intensity of the behaviors. The intensity scores for each of the observed behaviors are summed to produce a composite pain score. Recent attention has

focused on the need to develop sensitive measures for children who are cognitively or physically impaired.[30]

The current behavioral scales should be adequate for many children under treatment for cancer but may not be adequate for children who are very ill or receiving palliative care. The complexity of a child's disease or health condition, concomitant drug therapy, and the other distress sources in the health care environment may limit children's ability to behave so that the pain score is not meaningful. Their pain behaviors may be very different from those of the children studied to develop the original scales. Moreover, the most salient pain behavior might be very child-dependent and vary widely among different children or change throughout the course of their illness. At present, health care providers must use their content expertise and consult with parents to carefully consider which behavior or behaviors are the most relevant indices of pain for a particular child. They can chart the presence and intensity of these behaviors (it is likely that these will be more subtle indices than on current standardized scales) and interpret them as an indirect measure of pain.

SELF-REPORT PAIN MEASURE

Self-report measures, often referred to as psychological measures, capture a child's subjective experience of pain. Interviews, questionnaires, adjective checklists, and numerous pain intensity scales are available for children, each with some evidence of validity and reliability.[25,31] Clinical interviews are ideally suited for learning about the sensory characteristics of pain, the aversive component, and contributing cognitive, behavioral, and emotional factors. Interviews should also include a simple rating scale to document pain strength. Children choose a level on the scale that best matches the strength of their own pain (i.e., a level on a number or thermometer scale, a number of objects, a mark on a visual analog scale, face from a series of faces varying in emotional expression, or a particular word from adjective lists). Pain intensity scales are easy to administer, requiring only a few seconds once children understand how to use them. Many of these scales yield pain scores on a 0 to 10 scale. Visual and colored analog scales are versatile for use with acute, recurrent, and chronic pain and provide a convenient and flexible pain measure for use in hospital and at home.

Health care providers must consider the age and cognitive ability of a child when selecting a pain scale. Most toddlers (approximately 2 years old) can communicate the presence of pain, using words learned from their parents to describe the sensations they feel when they hurt themselves. They use concrete analogies to describe their perceptions. Gradually, children learn to differentiate and describe three levels of pain intensity—a little, some or medium, and a lot. By age 5, most children can differentiate a wider range of pain intensities and many can use simple pain intensity scales.

Children's understanding and descriptions of pain naturally depend on their age, cognitive level, and previous pain experience. Children begin to understand pain through their own hurting experiences; they learn to describe the different characteristics of their pains (intensity, quality, duration, and location) in the same way that they learn specific words to describe different sounds, tastes, smells, and colors. Most children can communicate meaningful information about their pain. Gradually, they develop an increasing ability to describe specific pain features—the quality (aching, burning, pounding, sharp), intensity (mild to severe), duration and frequency (a few seconds to years), location (from a diffuse location on their skin to more precise internal localization), and unpleasantness (mild annoyance to an intolerable discomfort). Children's understanding of pain and the language that they use to describe pain comes from the words and expressions used by their families and peers and from characters depicted in books, videos, and movies. (For a more extensive review of developmental factors in children's pain, see references 9, 10, and 32 to 36).

Physicians should always ask children directly about their pain. Pain onset, location, frequency (if recurring), quality, intensity, accompanying physical symptoms, and pain-related disability should be assessed as part of children's clinical examination. Health care providers

should also assess relevant situational factors in order to modify their pain-exacerbating impact, especially the factors listed in Figure 4–1.

ANALGESIC SELECTION AND ADMINISTRATION

Pain control should include regular pain assessments, appropriate analgesics, and adjuvant analgesics administered at regular dosing intervals, adjunctive drug therapy for symptom and side effects control, and nondrug therapies to modify the situational factors that can exacerbate pain and suffering. Analgesics include acetaminophen, nonsteroidal anti-inflammatory drugs, and opioids. Adjuvant analgesics include a variety of drugs with analgesic properties, such as anticonvulsants and antidepressants that were initially developed to treat other health problems. Adjuvant analgesics are especially crucial when pain has a neuropathic component.

The guiding principles of analgesic administration are "by the ladder," "by the clock," "by the child," and "by the mouth." "By the ladder" refers to a three-step approach for selecting drugs according to their analgesic potency based on the child's pain level—acetaminophen to control mild pain, codeine to control moderate pain, and morphine for strong pain.[37] The ladder approach was based on our scientific understanding of how analgesics affect pain of nociceptive origins. If pain persists despite starting with the appropriate drug, recommended doses, and dosing schedule, move up the ladder and administer the next more potent analgesic. Even when children require opioid analgesics, they should continue to receive acetaminophen (and nonsteroidal anti-inflammatory drugs, if appropriate) as supplemental analgesics. The analgesic ladder approach is based on the premise that acetaminophen, codeine, and morphine should be available in all countries and that doctors and health care providers can relieve pain in the majority of children with a few drugs.

However, increasing attention is focusing on thinking beyond the ladder in accordance with our improved understanding of pain of neuropathic origins.[38,39] Children should receive adjuvant analgesics to more specifically target neuropathic mechanisms. Regrettably, two of the main classes of adjuvant analgesics, antidepressants and anticonvulsants, have unfortunate names. Proper education of health care providers, parents, and children should lead to a wider acceptance and use of these medications for pain management. For example, amitriptyline may require 4 to 6 weeks to affect depression, but often requires only 1 to 2 weeks to affect pain. The newer classes of antidepressants, the selective serotonin reuptake inhibitors (SSRIs), may be beneficial to treat depression for a child with pain but have not been shown to be beneficial for pain management. The other main class of adjuvant analgesics is the anticonvulsants. The two principal medications used for this purpose in pediatrics are carbamazepine and gabapentin. With gabapentin, the main dose-limiting side effect is sedation so that a slow titration to maximal dose is required. Because of its greater number of significant side effects, the use of carbamazepine has decreased recently and the use of gabapentin has increased. We still await published studies to support the wide use of gabapentin.

Nonsteroidal anti-inflammatory drugs (NSAIDs) are similar in potency to aspirin. NSAIDs are used primarily to treat inflammatory disorders and to lessen mild to moderate acute pain. They should be used with caution in patients with hepatic or renal impairment, compromised cardiac function, hypertension (since they may cause fluid retention, edema), and a history of gastrointestinal bleeding or ulcers. NSAIDs may also inhibit platelet aggregation and thus must be monitored closely in patients with prolonged bleeding times. Indications for NSAIDs are much narrower for children with cancer (due to the concern for bleeding problems) than for children with other painful conditions. Although acetaminophen should be considered the routine nonopioid analgesic for children with cancer, NSAIDs are effective for patients with bony metastases, who have adequate platelets.

Although the specific drugs and doses are determined by the needs of each child, general guidelines for drug therapies to control pain for children in palliative care have been developed through a Consensus Conference on the Management of Pain in Childhood Cancer, published as a supplement to Pediatrics,[40] in a monograph,

Cancer Pain Relief and Palliative Care for Children,[1] and in clinical practice guidelines.[41-43] The drugs listed in this chapter are based on these sources and guidelines from our institution.[44] Recommended starting doses for analgesic medications to control children's disease-related pain are listed in Tables 4-2 and 4-3; starting doses for adjuvant analgesic medications to control pain, drug-related side effects, and other symptoms are listed in Table 4-4. (For further review of analgesics and adjuvant analgesics in children, see references 39 and 45-50.)

Analgesic doses should be adjusted "by the child." There is no one dose that will be appropriate for all children with pain. The goal is to select a dose that prevents children from experiencing pain before they receive the next dose. It is essential to monitor the child's pain regularly and adjust analgesic doses as necessary to control the pain. The effective opioid dose to relieve pain varies widely among different children or in the same child at different times. Some children require massive opioid doses at frequent intervals to control their pain. If such large doses are necessary for effective pain control and the side effects can be managed by adjunctive medication so that children are comfortable, then the doses are appropriate. Children receiving opioids may develop altered sleep patterns so that they are awake at night, fearful and complaining about pain, and they sleep intermittently throughout the day. They should receive adequate analgesics at night with antidepressants or hypnotics as necessary to enable them to sleep throughout the night. To relieve severe ongoing pain, opioid doses should be increased steadily until comfort is achieved, unless the

TABLE 4–2 Nonopioid Drugs of Cancer Pain Relief in Children

Drug	Dosage	Comments
Acetaminophen	10–15 mg/kg PO, every 4–6 h Dose limit of 65 mg/kg/day or 4 g/day, whichever is less	Lacks gastrointestinal and hematologic side effects; lacks anti-inflammatory effects (may mask infection-associated fever)
Ibuprofen	5–10 mg/kg PO, every 6–8 h Dose limit of 40 mg/kg/day; max dose of 2400 mg/day	Anti-inflammatory activity. Use with caution in patients with hepatic or renal impairment, compromised cardiac function or hypertension (may cause fluid retention, edema), history of GI bleeding or ulcers, may inhibit platelet aggregation
Naproxen	10–20 mg/kg/day PO, divided every 12 h Dose limit of 1 g/day	Anti-inflammatory activity. Use with caution and monitor closely in patients with impaired renal function. Avoid in patients with severe renal impairment
Diclofenac	1 mg/kg PO, every 8–12 h Dose limit of 50 mg/dose	Anti-inflammatory activity. Similar GI renal and hepatic precautions as noted above for ibuprofen and naproxen

Note: Increasing the dose of nonopioids beyond the recommended therapeutic level produces a ceiling effect (i.e., there is no additional analgesia but there are major increases in toxicity and side effects).

PO, per os; *GI*, gastrointestinal.

From McGrath PA, Brown SC: Paediatric palliative medicine: Pain control. In Doyle D, Hanks GWC, Cherny NI, Calman K (eds): Oxford Textbook of Palliative Medicine, 3rd ed. Oxford, Oxford University Press, 2004, p 781, with permission.

TABLE 4–3   Starting Doses for Opioid Analgesics

Drug	Equianalgesic dosage (parenteral)	Starting dosage IV	IV:PO ratio	Starting dosage PO/Transdermal	Duration of action
Morphine	10 mg	Bolus dose = 0.05 mg/kg 0.1 mg/kg every 2–4 h Continuous infusion = 0.01–0.04 mg/kg/h	1:3	0.15–0.3 mg/kg/dose every 4 h	3–4 h
Hydromorphone	1.5 mg	0.015–0.02 mg/kg every 4 h	1:5	0.06 mg/kg every 3–4 h	2–4 h
Codeine	120 mg	Not recommended		1 mg/kg every 4 h (dose limit 1.5 mg/kg/dose)	3–4 h
Oxycodone	5–10 mg	Not recommended		0.1–0.2 mg/kg every 3–4 h	3–4 h
Meperidine[a]	75 mg	0.5–1 mg/kg every 3–4 h	1:4	1–2 mg/kg every 3–4 h (dose limit 150 mg)	1–3 h
Fentanyl[b]	100 µg	1–2 µg/kg/h as continuous infusion		25 µg patch	72 h (patch)
Controlled-release morphine[c,d]				0.6 mg/kg every 8 h or 0.9 mg/kg every 12 h	
Controlled-release hydromorphone[d]				0.18 mg/kg every 12 h	
Controlled-release codeine[d]				3 mg/kg every 12 h	
Controlled-release oxycodone[d]				0.3–0.6 mg/kg every 12 h	
Methadone	10 mg	0.1 mg/kg every 4–8 h	1:2	0.2 mg/kg every 4–8 h	12–50 h

Doses are for opioid naive patients. For infants under 6 months, start at one-quarter to one-third the suggested dose and titrate to effect.

Principles of opioid administration:
1. If inadequate pain relief and no toxicity at peak onset of opioid action, increase dose in 50% increments.
2. Avoid IM administration
3. Whenever using continuous infusion, plan for hourly rescue doses with short onset opioids if needed. Rescue dose is usually 50% to 200% of continuous hourly dose. If greater than 6 rescues are necessary in 24-h period, increase daily infusion total by the total amount of rescues for previous 24 h divided by 24. An alternative is to increase infusion by 50%.
4. To change opioids — because of incomplete cross-tolerance: if changing between opioids with short duration of action, start new opioid at 50% of equianalgesic dose. Titrate to effect. If changing between opioids from short to long duration of action (i.e., morphine to methadone), start at 25% of equianalgesic dose and titrate to effect.
5. To taper opioids — anyone on opioids over 1 week must be tapered to avoid withdrawal: taper by 50% for 2 days, and then decrease by 25% every 2 days. When dose is equianalgesic to an oral morphine dose of 0.6 mg/kg/day, it may be stopped. Some patients on opioids for prolonged periods, may require much slower weaning.
   (a) Avoid use in renal impairment. Metabolite may cause seizures.
   (b) Potentially highly toxic. Not for use in acute pain control.
   (c) Use may be hampered by child's difficulty in swallowing large tablets.
   (d) The widely equianalgesic doses in adults are used as guidelines in pediatric practice but have not been substantiated in children.

PO, per os; *IV*, intravenous.

From McGrath PA, Brown SC: Paediatric palliative medicine: Pain control. In Doyle D, Hanks GWC, Cherny NI, Calman K (eds): Oxford Textbook of Palliative Medicine, 3rd ed. Oxford, Oxford University Press, 2004, p 781, with permission.

child experiences unacceptable side effects such as somnolence or respiratory depression.

"By the mouth" refers to the oral route of drug administration. Medication should be administered to children by the simplest and most effective route, usually by mouth. If children are afraid of painful injections they may deny that they have pain or they may not request medication. When possible, children should receive medications through routes that do not cause additional pain. Although optimal analgesic administration for children requires flexibility in selecting routes according to children's needs, parenteral administration is often the most efficient route

for providing direct and rapid pain relief. Since intravenous, intramuscular, and subcutaneous routes cause additional pain for children, serious efforts have been expended on developing more pain-free modes of administration that still provide relatively direct and rapid analgesia. Attention has focused on improving the effectiveness of oral routes. As an example, oral transmucosal fentanyl citrate (OTFC) provides rapid-onset analgesia via a pleasant route for children with cancer receiving painful medical procedures. OTFC produces significant serum concentrations after 15 to 20 minutes.[51] Children aged 2 to 14 years have shown good cooperation and sedation when given OTFC

TABLE 4–4 Adjuvant Analgesic Drugs

Drug Category	Drug, Dosage	Indications	Comments
Antidepressants	Amitriptyline Initial dose 0.2–0.5 mg/kg PO Titrate upward by 0.25 mg/kg every 2–3 days Maintenance: 0.2–3 mg/kg Alternatives: nortriptyline, doxepin, imipramine	Neuropathic pain (i.e., vincristine-induced, radiation plexopathy, tumor invasion, CRPS-1), insomnia	Usually improved sleep and pain relief within 3–5 days. Anticholinergic side effects are dose-limiting. Use with caution for children with increased risk for cardiac dysfunction
Anticonvulsants	Gabapentin Initial dose 5 mg/kg/day PO Titrate upward over 3–7 days Maintenance: 15–50 mg/kg/day PO divided TID Carbamazepine Initial dose 10 mg/kg/day PO divided OD or BID Maintenance: up to 20–30 mg/kg/day PO divided every 8 h. Increase dose gradually over 2–4 weeks Alternatives: clonazepam	Neuropathic pain, especially shooting, stabbing pain.	Monitor for hematologic, hepatic, and allergic reactions. Side effects include gastrointestinal upset, ataxia, dizziness, disorientation, and somnolence
Sedatives, hypnotics, anxiolytics	Diazepam, 0.025–0.2 mg/kg PO every 6 h Lorazepam, 0.05 mg/kg/ dose SL Midazolam, 0.5 mg/kg/ dose PO administered 15–30 min prior to procedure; 0.05 mg/kg/ dose IV for sedation	Acute anxiety, muscle spasm; premedication for painful procedures	Sedative effect may limit opioid use. Other side effects include depression and dependence with prolonged use
Antihistamines	Hydroxyzine, 0.5 mg/kg PO every 6 h Diphenhydramine, 0.5–1 mg/kg PO/IV every 6 h	Opioid-induced pruritus, anxiety, nausea	Sedative side effects may be helpful
Psychostimulants	Dextroamphetamine, Methylphenidate, 0.1–0.2 mg/kg BID Escalate to 0.3–0.5 mg/kg as needed	Opioid-induced somnolence Potentiation of opioid analgesia	Side effects include agitation, sleep disturbance, and anorexia. Administer second dose in the afternoon to avoid sleep disturbances
Corticosteroids	Prednisone, prednisolone, and dexamethasone dosage depends on clinical situation Dexamethasone initial dose: 0.2 mg/kg IV. Dose limit 10 mg. Subsequent dose 0.3 mg/kg/day IV divided every 6 h	Headache from increased intracranial pressure, spinal, or nerve compression; widespread metastases	Side effects include edema, dyspeptic symptoms, and occasional gastrointestinal bleeding

CRPS-1, complex regional pain syndrome type 1; *PO*, per os; *IV*, intravenous; *SL*, sublingual.
From McGrath PA, Brown SC: Paediatric palliative medicine: Pain control. In Doyle D, Hanks GWC, Cherny NI, Calman K (eds): Oxford Textbook of Palliative Medicine, 3rd ed. Oxford, Oxford University Press, 2004, p 782, with permission.

as a premedication.[52,53] OTFC produced safe and effective analgesia for outpatient wound care in children and the taste was preferred to oral oxycodone.[54]

Many hospitals have restricted the use of intramuscular injections because they are painful and drug absorption is not reliable; they advocate the use of intravenous lines into which drugs can be administered directly without causing further pain. Topical anesthetic creams should also be applied prior to the insertion of intravenous lines in children. The use of central venous ports has become the gold standard in pediatrics, particularly for children with cancer who require administration of multiple drugs at weekly intervals.

Continuous infusion has several advantages over intermittent subcutaneous, intramuscular, or intravenous routes. This method circumvents repetitive injections, prevents delays in analgesic drug administration, and provides continuous levels of pain control without children experiencing increased side effects at peak level and pain breakthroughs at trough level. Continuous infusion should be considered when children have pain for which oral and intermittent parenteral opioids do not provide satisfactory pain control, when intractable vomiting prevents oral medications, and when children would like to remain at home despite severe pain. Children receiving a continuous infusion should continue to receive "rescue doses" to control breakthrough pain as necessary. As outlined in Table 4–3, the rescue doses should be 50% to 200% of the continuous infusion hourly dose. If children experience repeated breakthrough pain, the basal rate can be increased by 50% or by the total amount of morphine administered through the rescue doses over a 24-hour period (divided by 24 hours).

Patient-controlled analgesia (PCA) enables children to administer analgesic doses according to their pain level. PCA provides children with a continuum of analgesia that is prompt, economical, not nurse dependent and a lower overall narcotic use.[55-60] It has a high degree of safety, allows for wide variability between patients, and there is no delay in analgesic administration (for review, see reference 55). It can now be regarded as a standard for the delivery of analgesia in children older than 5 years.[61] However, there are opposing views about the use of background infusions with PCA. Although they may improve efficacy, they may increase the occurrence of adverse effects such as nausea and respiratory depression. In a comparison of PCA with and without a background infusion for children having lower extremity surgery, the total morphine requirements were reduced in the PCA only group and the background infusion offered no advantage.[62] In another study comparing background infusion and PCA, children between 9 and 15 achieved better pain relief with PCA while children between 5 and 8 showed no difference.[63] Although data on the use of background infusions in combination with PCA for the pediatric palliative care patient is limited, our current standard is to add a background infusion to the PCA if the pain is not controlled adequately with PCA alone. The selection of opioid used in PCA is perhaps less critical than the appropriate selection of parameters such as bolus dose, lockout and background infusion rate. The opioid choice may be based on adverse effect profile rather than efficacy. Clearly, PCA offers special advantages to children who have little control and who are extremely frightened about uncontrolled pain. PCA is as it states, patient-controlled analgesia. When special circumstances require that alternate people administer the medication, we do allow both nurse- and parent-controlled analgesia. Under these circumstances, parents require our nurse educators to fully educate them on the use of PCA.

Fentanyl is a potent synthetic opioid, which, like morphine, binds to mu receptors. However, fentanyl is 75 to 100 times more potent than morphine. The intravenous preparation of fentanyl has been used extensively in children. A transdermal preparation of fentanyl was introduced in 1991 for use with chronic pain. This route provides a noninvasive but continuously controlled delivery system. Although limited data is available on transdermal fentanyl (TF) in children, its use is increasing for children with stable and chronic cancer pain. In a 2001 study, TF was well tolerated with effective pain relief in 11 of 13 children and provided an ideal approach for children where compliance with oral analgesics was problematic.[64] When children in palliative care were converted from oral morphine doses to TF; the investigators noted diminished side effects and improved convenience with TF.[65] The majority of parents and investigators considered TF to be better than the previous treatment. No serious adverse events were attributed to fentanyl, suggesting that TF was both effective and acceptable for children and their families. Similarly, no adverse effects were noted in a study of TF for children with pain due to sickle cell crisis.[66] This study showed a significant relationship between TF dose and fentanyl concentration; pain control with the use of TF was improved in 7 of 10 patients in comparison to PCA alone. In a multicenter crossover study in adults, TF caused significantly less constipation and less daytime drowsiness in comparison to morphine, but greater sleep disturbance and shorter sleep duration.[67] Of those patients able to express a preference, significantly more preferred fentanyl patches. Of special note, fatal adult complications have been noted with the use of multiple transdermal patches.[68]

ADDICTION AND TOLERANCE

The fear of opioid addiction in children has been greatly exaggerated. While physical dependence is common, gradual tapering protocols can control the withdrawal syndromes caused by an abrupt cessation of the medication. Physical dependence may develop in as short a period as 7 to 10 days. Tolerance is also an expected change to be seen and anticipated in children. There is no empirical evidence that children receiving opioid analgesics for pain control are at risk for addiction. In contrast, children who do not receive appropriate analgesic medications are probably more at risk for pseudo-addiction by becoming excessively concerned about receiving their next medication dose in the hope that they might eventually have relief from their suffering.

Parents, and occasionally staff, may have misconceptions about the use of potent opioids. Although the sensory characteristics of children's pain should be consistent with the known pattern from the presumed source of tissue injury, the source is not easily identified for all children. This is particularly true for children who have cancer because there may be multiple sources of noxious stimulation due to disease and the effects of curative therapies. Yet, children's pain must be controlled, even when the specific etiology is not yet determined. Otherwise, children become increasingly anxious, fearful, and distressed—beginning a cycle of increasing pain that will be more difficult to alleviate.

Parents are often anxious about opioids for their children, particularly when children require increased dose increments. Staff must educate parents that physical dependence and tolerance are very different from addiction. Parents will then understand that physical dependence and tolerance are normal drug effects; they do not mean that their children with pain have become addicted. Physical drug dependence is well recognized. When opioids are suddenly withdrawn, children may suffer from irritability, anxiety, insomnia, diaphoresis, rhinorrhea, nausea, vomiting, abdominal cramps, and diarrhea. These withdrawal symptoms can be prevented by the gradual tapering of an opioid. Even though children with severe pain require progressively higher and more frequent opioid doses due to drug tolerance, they should receive the doses they need to relieve their pain. However, children who require increased opioids to relieve previously controlled pain should be assessed carefully to determine whether the disease has progressed, since pain may be the first sign of advancing disease.

Therapists can use familiar analogies to explain dependence, tolerance, and addiction. For example, parents are often accustomed to drinking coffee in the morning. They know that they will experience some noticeable effects without their usual caffeine intake, but they also know that they can withdraw from coffee by gradually lowering their daily consumption. The fact that their body is used to a certain amount of caffeine at certain times of the day means that they are dependent. Similarly, many people become accustomed to a certain level of salt for a food to taste salty. After a while they may need to increase their salt intake if they want foods to taste the same because their bodies have adjusted to or now tolerate the previous amount of salt so that it no longer has the same effect. In the same way, their children can become tolerant to a morphine dose so that they require a slightly higher dose to achieve the same pain reduction. These benign examples of a body's normal responses to substances often help parents understand that when opioids are prescribed for their children the effects of those drugs are well known, well understood, and will not lead to adverse effects, including addiction.

OPIOID-RELATED SIDE EFFECTS

The safe, rational use of opioid analgesics requires an understanding of their clinical pharmacology. The potent opioids that we use to treat children for cancer and palliative pain control have no fixed upper dosage limit. The dose can be increased as necessary to maximize pain control as long as children do not experience dose-limiting side effects (i.e., vomiting, respiratory depression). The goal should be titrating medication either up or down for maximum clinical effect. Side effects must be anticipated and treated aggressively. Since opioids produce physical dependence and tolerance, doses must be increased over time to control pain. Doses must be adjusted according to the child's need depending on pain severity, prior analgesic medication use, and the bioavailability and drug distribution of the medication.

All opioids have a similar spectrum of side effects. These well-known problems should be anticipated and treated whenever opioids are administered, so that children can receive pain control without suffering untoward effects. Children may not report all side effects (e.g., constipation, dysphoria) voluntarily, so they should be asked specifically about these problems. Some side effects may resolve within the first one or two weeks of initiating therapy as the child develops tolerance to them (e.g., nausea, vomiting, and drowsiness). The clinician must educate the patient about these problems and encourage them to give the medication an adequate trial. Slow titration may minimize this problem. Other side effects may require aggressive treatment. If they persist despite appropriate interventions, conversion to an alternative opioid may be indicated. There is generally incomplete cross-tolerance between opioids, so that the guidelines for converting from one opioid to another are to begin at the lower dosing range, considering the presence or absence of central nervous system side effects, and titrate upward. When used in therapeutic doses, opioids have not been demonstrated to cause long-term permanent organ toxicity. This makes them a safe choice for use in children. There is evidence that untreated severe chronic pain may cause cognitive impairment, which is improved with opioid therapy. The treatment of opioid side effects is summarized in Table 4–5.

COMPLEMENTARY AND ALTERNATIVE THERAPIES

An extensive array of nondrug therapies are available to treat children's pain, including counseling, guided imagery, hypnosis, biofeedback, behavioral management, acupuncture, massage, homeopathic remedies, naturopathic approaches, and herbal medicines. In a 2002 self-report questionnaire of 1013 pediatric patients seeking primary care, the most common types of complementary and alternative therapies (CAM) were herbs (41%), prayer healing (37%), folk and home remedies (28%), massage therapy (19%), and chiropractic therapy (18%).[69]

TABLE 4–5 Opioid Side Effects

Side Effect	Management
Respiratory depression	Reduction in opioid dose by 50%, titrate to maintain pain relief without respiratory depression
Respiratory arrest	Naloxone, titrate to effect with 0.01 mg/kg/dose IV/ETT increments or 0.1 mg/kg/ dose IV/ETT, repeat PRN. Small, frequent doses of diluted naloxone or naloxone drip preferable for patients on chronic opioid therapy to avoid severe, painful withdrawal syndrome. Repeated doses often required until opioid side effect subsides.
Drowsiness/sedation	Frequently subsides after a few days without dosage reduction; methylphenidate or dextroamphetamine (0.1 mg/kg administered twice daily, in the morning and mid-day so as not to interfere with nighttime sleep). The dose can be escalated in increments of 0.05-0.1 mg/kg to a maximum of 10 mg/dose for dextroamphetamine and 20 mg/dose for methylphenidate
Constipation	Increased fluids and bulk, prophylactic laxatives as indicated
Nausea/vomiting	Administer an antiemetic (e.g., ondansetron, 0.1 mg/kg IV/PO every 8 h). Antihistamines (e.g., dimenhydrinate 0.5 mg/kg/dose every 4-6 h IV/PO) may be used. Prechemotherapy, Nabilone 0.5-1 mg PO and then every 12 h may also be used
Confusion, nightmares, hallucinations	Reassurance only, if symptoms mild. A reduced dosage of opioid or a change to a different opioid or add neuroleptic (e.g., haloperidol 0.1 mg/kg PO/IV every 8 h to a maximum of 30 mg/day)
Multifocal myoclonus, seizures	Generally occur only during extremely high-dose therapy; reduction in opioid dose indicated if possible. Add a benzodiazepine (e.g., clonazepam 0.05 mg/kg/day divided BID or TID increasing by 0.05 mg/kg/day every 3 days PRN up to 0.2 mg/kg/day. Dose limit of 20 mg/day)
Urinary retention	Rule out bladder outlet obstruction, neurogenic bladder, and other precipitating drugs (e.g., tricyclic antidepressant). Particularly common with epidural opioids. Change of opioid, route of administration, and dose may relieve symptom. Bethanechol or catheter may be required.

IV, intravenous; *PO*, per os; *ETT*, endotracheal tube; *PRN*, as needed.

From McGrath PA, Brown SC: Paediatric palliative medicine: Pain control. In Doyle D, Hanks GWC, Cherny NI, Calman K (eds): Oxford Textbook of Palliative Medicine, 3rd ed. Oxford, Oxford University Press, 2004, p 783, with permission.

Nondrug therapies are generally regarded as safe, with few contraindications for their use in otherwise healthy children. However, little is known about the safety and effectiveness of certain therapies for children undergoing treatment for cancer or for palliative care. The problem of major adverse events and the high degree of uncertainty regarding a causal relationship of these events and the therapy is frequently noted. The size of the problem and its importance relative to the well-documented risks of conventional treatments is currently unknown.[70] Although Sampson[71] reports 908 randomized controlled trials (RCTs) in the field of CAM and Moher[72] has assessed the quality of 47 CAM systematic reviews in which they found the overall quality of reporting similar to conventional therapy, researchers continue to call for more studies in this area.[73] Thus, the efficacy of complementary therapies for treating children's pain is unclear, even though children are increasingly using complementary therapies.[74] Madsen[75] reported in 2003 that 53% of pediatric patients had tried CAM as a supplement to conventional medicine, compared with an Australian study in which 33% of parents used CAM for their inpatient child.[76] The percentages were even higher for children with cancer using CAM (65%) as compared with a control group (51%).[77] In contrast, the evidence supporting the efficacy of cognitive and behavioral approaches is strong.[1,3,7,78-89] These methods can mitigate some of the factors that intensify pain, distress, and disability for children.

COGNITIVE AND BEHAVIORAL THERAPIES

The primary cognitive and behavioral therapies are listed in Table 4-6. Cognitive therapies are directed at a child's beliefs, expectations, and coping abilities. They encompass a wide range of approaches from basic patient education to formal psychotherapy. Most children and families benefit from supportive counseling. Accurate information about what will happen and what children may feel should improve children's understanding, increase their control, lessen their distress, and reduce their pain. In addition, health care providers can teach children how to use a few pain control methods to lessen pain and guide families to recognize the particular circumstances that exacerbate pain and distress. These methods provide children with some independent strategies—either to

TABLE 4–6 Cognitive and Behavioral Therapies

Cognitive
Information
Choices and control
Supportive counseling
Counseling
Stress management
Attention and distraction
Guided imagery
Hypnosis
Behavioral
Simple exercise
Participation in activities
Desensitization training
Relaxation training
Biofeedback
Behavioral modification

relieve mild pain or to complement the medication needed to relieve strong pain. Children seem more adept than adults at using nondrug therapies, presumably because they are usually less biased than adults about their potential efficacy.

Distraction is a simple and effective pain control method. When children intently attend to something other than their pain, they can lessen its intensity and unpleasantness. Distraction is often incorrectly perceived as a simple diversionary tactic; the implication is that the pain is still there but the child is momentarily focused elsewhere. However, when children's attention is fully absorbed in some engaging topic or activity, distraction is a very active process that can reduce the neuronal responses to a noxious stimulus. Children do not simply ignore their pain, but are actually reducing it. The essential feature for achieving pain relief is a child's ability to attend fully to and concentrate on something else besides the pain. Therefore, the choice of a distraction is crucial and varies according to children's ages and interests. Young children usually need to be actively involved with their parents or peers, whereas older children and adolescents can distract themselves more independently. Children should work with their parents or a therapist to choose distracting activities that children can practically incorporate into their lives.

There is considerable overlap among the interventions of attention and distraction, guided imagery, and hypnosis.

Hypnosis usually begins with an induction procedure in which a child's full attention is focused gradually on the therapist and his or her suggestions. The therapist guides the child into a very relaxed physical and mental state, an altered level of consciousness distinct from an alert or sleep state. The induction procedure typically includes guided imagery for children and progressive muscle relaxation for adolescents. The induction can be very simple for young children. They can be guided into a hypnotic state as they vividly imagine their favorite television shows, movies, books, or cartoon characters.[90-92] As they imagine an activity, scene, or character, they gradually receive suggestions for relaxation, reduced anxiety, increased control, and pain reduction. The therapist provides consistent positive suggestions, rather than authoritative commands. The emphasis is on the child's own natural abilities, as in "notice that your back, legs (painful body areas) feel lighter; the heaviness and pain are starting to lessen. It seems as if your back doesn't hurt as much as before. You are doing well at turning down the pain switch."

During a hypnotic state, individuals become extremely susceptible to suggestions, including suggestions for pain relief. Children become so involved in thoughts or ideas that they dissociate from a reality orientation.[91] Hypnosis enables children to redirect attention from the painful sensation or to reinterpret the sensation as something more pleasant and less aversive or less bothersome.[92] Like adults, children differ in their ability to be hypnotized. Children's ability to use their imagination is the key component in determining their hypnotic susceptibility.

Behavior therapy is often used in combination with cognitive therapy. The goals are to lessen the specific behaviors (i.e., child, family, and staff) that may increase pain, distress, or disability, while concomitantly increasing healthy behaviors that engage children in living as fully as possible. Relaxation training is a common method used for children who require painful procedures or who experience chronic pain. Therapists train children how to achieve a state of mental and physical relaxation so that children can eventually relax independently when they experience pain or feel stressed and fearful about their condition. Therapists may use guided imagery, hypnosis, deep breathing, or progressive relaxation exercises to train children.

PRACTICAL PAIN CONTROL METHODS

Specific pain control methods that require the child to concentrate and focus attention should always be used for children with cancer pain. Beales noted critical differences between adults and children in their perceptions of pain, especially cancer pain.[93] Children's cancer pain seemed even less positively correlated with pathology than adults' cancer pain. Beales suggested that some of the psychological mechanisms involved in pain perception may be manipulated more easily in children than in adults, consistent with our clinical observations that children's cancer pain is more plastic than that of adults.[9,86] Children seem to possess an enhanced ability to absorb themselves completely in a task, game, or imagined event and thus, might be more able than adults to trigger endogenous pain-inhibitory mechanisms. Even very young children can easily learn to use a variety of practical pain control methods. The goals of therapy are to enable children to understand what is happening and to have something that they can actively do to lessen their anxiety, distress, and pain.

The specific methods selected depend on the age of the child, the type of pain experienced, and the resources available. Simple methods such as deep breathing, blowing bubbles, alternately tightening and relaxing their fists, squeezing their mother's hand, listening to stories or music, and imagining that they are in a pleasant setting can be very effective for reducing procedural-related pain, when used with appropriate analgesics. When possible, children should learn a few basic methods to reduce their pain and distress. They should not be encouraged to develop a false reliance on the magical benefits of any one method. Instead, they should understand that these practical methods relieve pain because they change the factors that usually increase pain and they help to restore normal sensory input.

All children should learn that pain from some procedures is generally less when they are able to choose the site and rub the area before and after the injection or finger prick. They should learn that pain is less when they are very relaxed. Progressive muscle relaxation with simple exercises in which they tense and relax their body limbs and biofeedback can help to show them that any type of pain can be intensified if the muscles are always tightened. Children should learn that fear and anxiety can make them tense and increase pain. Then they need practical tools to alleviate their fear about the cancer or their anxiety toward necessary treatments. Families must learn that what they think, how they behave, and how they feel affects their children's pain. Then they can begin to work independently and with staff to create additional nondrug pain control methods based on the child's interest, the cultural setting, and the availability of resources. Specific interventions should be selected and administered to children as part of a comprehensive pain program, in the same manner as the most appropriate analgesics are selected and administered in adequate doses, at regular dosing intervals, through the most efficient routes.

INTERVENTIONAL TECHNIQUES

Anesthesia, ranging from topical to full general anesthetics, is more frequently used to sedate children with cancer during invasive procedures. Moderate sedation is a medically controlled state of depressed consciousness,[94] wherein protective reflexes are maintained, the child maintains a patent airway independently and continuously, and the child is able to respond appropriately to physical stimulation or verbal commands (e.g., "Open your eyes.").[95] In contrast, deep sedation is a medically controlled state of depressed consciousness from which a child may not be aroused, has partial or complete loss of protective reflexes, is unable to maintain a patent airway independently, and is unable to respond purposefully to physical stimulation or verbal command.[95] General anesthesia refers to a medically controlled state of unconsciousness accompanied by a loss of protective reflexes including the inability to maintain a patent airway independently and respond purposefully to physical stimulation or verbal command.[95] For all levels of sedation, proper facilities must be available to administer the sedation. Staff fully qualified in the administration of the various medications and with a thorough knowledge and training in airway management is mandatory. Full monitoring and resuscitative equipment must be immediately available at all sites in which sedation is administered. (For a full description see reference 96.)

Myriad techniques are available for the pediatric patient from the most simple and noncomplex to the invasive that may be associated with pain. To begin with, the child with cancer often has to undergo multiple procedures in the course of investigation and treatment of their cancer. Simple techniques lessen and often eliminate the pain that a child experiences.

The use of topical anesthetics such as topical tetracaine HCl (Ametop) or topical Lidocaine-Prilocaine (EMLA) often eliminate the pain associated with the frequent procedures these children experience such as blood taking, intravenous insertions and lumbar punctures if after application, sufficient time is allowed for their full benefit. Some oncology groups have made the use of local anesthetics their primary source of analgesia to control procedural pain.[97]

Midazolam is frequently used for various hematology and oncology procedures. Sandler and others[98] compared the use of fentanyl with midazolam and found that 72% preferred the midazolam to fentanyl. Preprocedural anxiety, adverse behavioral symptoms, and visual analog scales all improved and side effects were minimal with midazolam. Ketamine has also been studied and compared to midazolam with children showing significantly less distress during the procedure when given ketamine.[99] Finally, intravenous midazolam and ketamine in combination also provided effective levels of sedation in children for invasive procedures.[100]

Full general anesthesia is used more frequently for procedures such as intrathecal chemotherapy and bone marrow aspirates and for activities such as radiation oncology, stereotactic radiosurgery, computed tomography, and magnetic resonance imaging. (For a full discussion of this area see reference 96.) While the techniques and medications employed may change over time, patients and families and oncologists prefer general anesthesia for these procedures, as evidenced from a study at Memorial Sloan-Kettering in 1990.[101] It was especially helpful for newly diagnosed patients, small children, infants and uncooperative patients. McDowall and others in 1995 reported a series of 971 patients receiving total intravenous anesthesia for procedural pain.[102] Over the course of the study the main anesthetic agent administered changed to propofol. Propofol was associated with hypoxemia (15.7%), which was easily managed with supplemental oxygen but occasionally required manually assisted ventilation via facemask. Hypoxemia was defined as an oxygen saturation less than 94%. Other complications with propofol were minimal. Propofol's low incidence of nausea and vomiting was noteworthy, especially in the children receiving intrathecal chemotherapy. Rapid recovery and the low incidence of agitation are beneficial characteristics of propofol, particularly for these often ambulatory patients. At the Hospital for Sick Children, propofol is the drug of choice for general anesthesia in these patients. They are fully monitored, often receive supplemental oxygen, and are always attended to by a pediatric anesthesiologist.

There is another option for these patients—the use of inhalational anesthesia. Patients who do not have central line access because they may be on a different protocol or therapy often request an inhalational induction to avoid peripheral venous cannulation. Fisher and others[103] examined the use of enflurane, halothane, and isoflurane in pediatric patients undergoing invasive procedures. They found that halothane especially allowed a rapid induction time with minimal airway-related complications, making it an excellent choice for these procedures. At the Hospital for Sick Children, Sevoflurane has essentially replaced other agents because of its speed and ease of use in inhalational inductions. All the necessary anesthetic equipment, monitors, scavengers, and so on, are required, and this makes the technique of inhalational anesthesia potentially more difficult for some institutions. At the Hospital for Sick Children, clinicians have overcome this obstacle through the development of off-site procedure rooms dedicated to anesthesia. These sites are constructed to meet OR standards and are equipped with appropriate anesthetic machines and drugs. A cornerstone of care must be the presence of a skilled individual who has the responsibility of monitoring these patients,

especially with regard to hypoventilation and hypoxemia.[104] In those patients who will be undergoing numerous procedures, adequate preparation of these patients and parents ahead of time and maximal pharmacologic management during the initial procedure will optimize them for the course of therapy.[105] An anesthesiologist is optimal for this purpose, especially in off-site areas.[106]

The use of regional techniques (epidural and spinal) for the administration of local anesthetics and analgesics for children continues to be an integral part of pain control in children.[107] Experience from many centers suggests that these techniques can be extremely useful for children with advanced cancer with resulting pain that may be difficult to control by more conventional means. It is also feasible for children to receive epidural and spinal infusions at home on an extended basis. A variety of medications may be employed for use in these blocks including local anesthetics, narcotics, and clonidine. For a full description of this topic, see references 108 and 109.

Appropriate monitoring is paramount for the safety of patients during administration of potent analgesics and anesthetics. This involves the education and training of staff; immediate availability of resuscitative drugs and equipment; and an accurate and timely pain record consisting of vital signs and pain and sedation scores. A complete set of intravenous and epidural monitoring guidelines has been included in Table 4–7.

CONCLUSION

Optimal pain control for children with cancer and for palliative care requires an integrated treatment plan with both drug and nondrug therapies. Publications from various specialties and countries continue with an emphasis on addressing pharmacologic and nonpharmacologic interventions to make alleviation of pain a primary goal.[110] Although some areas of the world appear to be succeeding in attaining the goals of the WHO,[111] a 2003 paper from a survey of pediatric cancer pain management in China clearly reveals that optimal pain control for these patients still requires dissemination of present pain knowledge to bring down barriers and thus create improvement in that part of the world.[112]

However, the specific interventions must be selected after determination of the primary and secondary sources of noxious stimulation and after a thorough assessment of the unique situational, behavioral, emotional, and familial factors that affect a child's pain. It is impossible to adequately relieve children's pain from a unidimensional perspective, in which pain is considered as synonymous with the nature and extent of tissue damage. Childhood pain must be viewed from a multidimensional perspective because multiple sensory, environmental, and emotional factors are responsible for the pain—no matter how

TABLE 4–7 Analgesia Monitoring Guidelines
Baseline assessment
Obtain RR, HR, BP, O₂ saturation, sedation score, and pain score before administering a single or intermittent dose or initiating continuous infusion
Intermittent intravenous administration
RR, HR, BP, and sedation score every 5 min X 4, then every 30 min X 2, and then as per child's condition/preexisting orders
Pain score every 20–30 min
Continuously monitor O₂ saturation only for children whose underlying condition predisposes them to respiratory depression.
Intravenous additive (to run over 15–20 min)
RR, HR, BP, and sedation score every 10 min X 2, then every 30 min X 2, and then as per child's condition
Pain score at completion of the flush, then every 30 min X 2, and then as per child's condition/preexisting orders
Continuously monitor O₂ saturation only for children whose underlying condition predisposes them to respiratory depression
Continuous IV infusion/PCA
RR, HR, BP, pain score, and sedation score every 1 h X 4, then RR and sedation score every 1 h, and then HR, BP, and pain score every 4 h
Continuously monitor O₂ saturation and document reading every 1 h
Intermittent epidural administration
RR, HR, and BP every 5 min for the first 20 min following a bolus dose, and then RR and sedation score every 1 h
HR, BP, pain score, and motor block score every 4 h
Continuously monitor only for children whose underlying condition predisposes them to respiratory depression
Continuous epidural infusion[a,b]
RR, HR, BP, sedation score, pain score, and motor block score every 1 h X 4 h, then RR and sedation score every 1 h, and HR, BP, pain score, and motor block score every 4 h.
Continuously monitor O₂ saturation and document reading every 1 h

[a]Opioids used with bupivicaine.

[b]Note: After any change in drug dose, infusion rate or if transferred between patient care areas, return to assessments every 1 h for 4 h.

Continuous respiratory rate/apnea monitoring may provide additional benefits for certain children who are receiving continuous opioid infusions by alerting the nurse to a decreasing respiratory rate. Respiratory rate monitoring is not, however, a substitute for frequent patient observation and vital sign monitoring.

ECG monitoring is not routinely required, but may be ordered if the child's underlying condition predisposes them to ECG abnormalities.

Adapted from 2001–2002 Drug Formulary, the Hospital for Sick Children, Toronto, Ontario.

seemingly clear cut an etiology. Treatment begins with a thorough assessment of these multiple factors, using structured interviews and standardized measures. Pharmacologic, physical, and psychological strategies must be incorporated into a flexible intervention program for children, in which parents and siblings form an essential component of treatment.

All analgesics should be selected "by the ladder" and administered "by the clock," "by the child," and in an effective and painless route. Dosing intervals should be frequent enough to adequately control pain, so that children do not experience an alternating cycle of pain, drowsy analgesia, pain, and so on. Children should also learn some simple pain control strategies so that they can reduce acute pain caused by invasive treatments and disease or therapy-related pain. Adjuvant medications should be administered to control aversive symptoms and side effects. Nondrug therapies should also be used to control pain.

Special problems in palliative pain control may arise when children die at home, unless parents and medical and nursing teams communicate openly about the availability of potent analgesics and the flexibility of dosing routes and regimens. Parents may be unduly anxious because even small children, like adults with cancer, may require larger opioid doses at more frequent intervals. Parents' fears can lead them to deny the extent to which their children are in pain or children may fail to report pain because they do not want to further distress parents or because they fear injections.

Multiple sources of noxious stimulation are usually responsible for pain in dying children, as the disease progressively affects many systems. Increased disability, toxic side effects of medication, physical impairment, and the emotional adjustment of children and their families can intensify pain and suffering. Like adults, children's pain affects the entire family and must be viewed within a broader context. Effective pain control is possible when the goals are to reduce or block nociceptive activity by attenuating responses in peripheral afferents and central pathways, activate endogenous pain inhibitory systems, and modify situational factors that exacerbate pain. Thus, the choice for pain control is not merely drug versus nondrug therapy, but rather a therapy that mitigates both the causative and contributing factors for pain. Pain management is a continuous dynamic process, since the disease state and factors that influence pain are not static. Different combinations of drug and nondrug therapies will be required at different times over the course of the cancer. Thus, health professionals must continually assume as much responsibility for monitoring and relieving children's pain as for medically managing their diseases. We have the knowledge to ensure that children receive adequate pain control, from the time they are diagnosed with cancer throughout their treatment protocol.

REFERENCES

1. World Health Organization: Cancer Pain Relief and Palliative Care in Children. Geneva, World Health Organization, 1998.
2. McGrath PA, Brown SC: Paediatric palliative medicine: Pain control. In Doyle D, Hanks GWC, Cherny NI, Calman K (eds): Oxford Textbook of Palliative Medicine, 3rd ed. Oxford, Oxford University Press, 2004, pp. 775–789.
3. McGrath PA, Hillier LM: Modifying the psychological factors that intensify children's pain and prolong disability. In Schechter NL, Berde CB, Yaster M (eds): Pain in Infants, Children, and Adolescents, 2nd ed. Philadelphia, Lippincott Williams & Wilkins, 2003, pp 85–104.
4. Price DD: Psychological Mechanisms of Pain and Analgesia. Seattle, IASP Press, 1999.
5. Price DD, Bushnell CM, eds: Psychological Modulation of Pain: Integrating Basic Science and Clinical Perspectives. Seattle, IASP Press (in press).
6. Casey K, Bushnell M, (eds): Pain Imaging. Seattle, IASP Press, 2000.
7. Schechter NL, Berde CB, Yaster M, (eds): Pain in Infants, Children, and Adolescents. Philadelphia, Lippincott Williams & Wilkins, 2003.
8. McGrath PA, Dade LA: Effective strategies to decrease pain and minimize disability. In Price DD, Bushnell CM (eds): Psychological Modulation of Pain: Integrating Basic Science and Clinical Perspectives. Seattle, IASP Press, pp 73–96.
9. McGrath PA: Pain in Children: Nature, Assessment and Treatment. New York, Guilford Press, 1990.
10. Ross DM, Ross SA: Childhood Pain: Current Issues, Research, and Management. Baltimore, Urban & Schwarzenberg, 1988.
11. McGrath PA, de Veber LL: The management of acute pain evoked by medical procedures in children with cancer. J Pain Symptom Manage 1:145–150, 1986.
12. Brown SC, McGrath PA, Krmpotic KR: Pain in children. In Pappagallo, M. (ed): The Neurologic Basis of Pain. New York, McGraw-Hill, pp 225–242.
13. Chafee S: Pediatric palliative care. Primary Care 28:365–390, 2001.
14. American Academy of Pediatrics: Committee on Bioethics and Committee on Hospital Care. Palliative care for children. Pediatrics 106:351–357, 2000.
15. Goldman A: ABC of palliative care: Special problems of children. BMJ 316:49–52, 1998.
16. Goldman A, (eds): Care of the Dying Child. New York, Oxford University Press, 1994.

17. Goldman A, Frager G, Pomietto M: Pain and palliative care. In Schechter NL, Berde CB, Yaster M (eds): Pain in Infants, Children, and Adolescents, 2nd ed. Philadelphia, Lippincott Williams & Wilkins, 2003, pp 539–562.
18. Frager G: Palliative care and terminal care of children. Child Adoles Psychiatr Clin North Am 6:889–900, 1997.
19. Howell D, Martinson I: Management of the dying child. In Pizzo P, Poplack D (eds): Principles and Practice of Pediatric Oncology, 2nd ed. Philadelphia, J.B. Lippincott, 1993, pp 1115–1124.
20. Davies B, Howell D: Special services for children. In Doyle D, Hanks G, MacDonald N (eds): Oxford Textbook of Palliative Medicine, 2nd ed. Oxford, Oxford University Press, 1998, pp 1078–1084.
21. Sourkes BM: The broken heart: Anticipatory grief in the child facing death. J Palliat Care 12:56–59, 1996.
22. Stevens M: Care of the dying child and adolescent: Family adjustment and support. In Doyle D, Hanks G, MacDonald N (eds): Oxford Textbook of Palliative Medicine, 2nd ed. Oxford, Oxford University Press, 1998, pp 1045–1056.
23. Stevens M: Psychological adaptation of the dying child. In Doyle D, Hanks G, MacDonald N (eds): Oxford Textbook of Palliative Medicine, 2nd ed. Oxford, Oxford University Press, 1998, pp 1045–1056.
24. McGrath PA, Brown SC: Special Considerations in Pediatric Pain Management. In Lipman AG (ed): Pain Management for Primary Care Clinicians. Bethesda, Maryland, American Society of Health-System Pharmacists, pp 199–217.
25. McGrath PA, Gillespie JM: Pain assessment in children and adolescents. In Turk DC, Melzack R (eds): Handbook of Pain Assessment, 2nd ed. New York, Guilford Press, 2001, pp 97–118.
26. Finley GA, McGrath PJ, (eds): Measurement of Pain in Infants and Children. Seattle, IASP Press, 1998.
27. Royal College of Nursing Institute: Clinical Guideline for the Recognition and Assessment of Acute Pain in Children: Recommendations. Royal College of Nursing Institute, 1999.
28. Sweet SD, McGrath PJ: Physiological measures of pain. In Finley GA, McGrath PJ (eds): Measurement of Pain in Infants and Children. Seattle, IASP Press, 1998, pp. 59–81.
29. Collins JJ, Devine TD, Dick GS, et al: The measurement of symptoms in young

children with cancer: The validation of the Memorial Symptom Assessment Scale in children aged 7–12. J Pain Symptom Manage 23: 10–16, 2002.
30. Hunt AM, Goldman A, Mastroyannopoulou K, Seers K: Identification of pain cues of children with severe neurological impairment. In Devor M, Rowbotham MC, Wiesenfeld-Hallin Z (eds): Proceedings of the 9th World Congress on Pain. Seattle, IASP Press, Abstract 84, 1999.
31. Champion GD, Goodenough B, von Baeyer CL, Thomas W: Measurement of Pain by Self-Report. In Finley GA, McGrath PJ: Measurement of Pain in Infants and Children. Seattle, IASP Press, 1998, pp 123–160.
32. Bush JP, Harkins SW (eds.): Children in Pain Clinical and Research Issues from a Developmental Perspectives. New York, Springer-Verlag, 1991.
33. Gaffney A, McGrath PJ, Dick B: Measuring pain in children: Developmental and instrument issues. In Schechter NL, Berde CB, Yaster M (eds): Pain in Infants, Children, and Adolescents, 2nd ed. Philadelphia, Lippincott Williams & Wilkins, 2003, pp. 128–141.
34. McGrath PJ, Unruh AM: Pain in Children and Adolescents. Amsterdam, Elsevier, 1987.
35. Peterson I, Harbeck C, Farme RJ, Zink M: Developmental contributions to the assessment of children's pain: Conceptual and methodological implications. In Bush JP, Harkins SW (eds): Children in Pain: Clinical and Research Issues from a Developmental Perspective. New York, Springer-Verlag, 1991, pp 33–58.
36. Pichard-Leandri E, Gauvain-Piquard A, eds.: La Douleur Chez l'Enfant. Paris, Medsi/McGraw-Hill, 1989.
37. World Health Organization: Cancer Pain Relief and Palliative Care. Geneva, World Health Organization, 1990.
38. Staats P: Cancer pain: Beyond the ladder. J Back Musculoskeletal Rehabil 10:67–80, 1998.
39. Galloway KS, Yaster M: Pain and symptom control in terminally ill children. Pediatr Clin North Am 47: 711–746, 2000.
40. Schechter NL, Altman A, Weisman S: Report of the Consensus Conference on the Management of Pain in Childhood Cancer. Pediatrics 86, 1990.
41. Acute Pain Management Guideline: Clinical Practice Guideline: Acute pain management in infants, children, and adolescents: Operative and medical procedures. Agency for Health Care Policy and Research, 1992.

42. Consensus Panel: Pediatric Pain and Symptom Algorithms for Palliative Care. Seattle, Children's Hospital, 1999.

43. Jacox A, Carr DB, Payne R, et al: Management of Cancer Pain. Rockville, Md: U.S. Department of Health and Human Services, Public Health Service, Agency for Health Care Policy and Research, 1994.

44. Hulland SA, Freilich MM, Sandor GK: Nitrous oxide-oxygen or oral midazolam for pediatric outpatient sedation. Oral Surg Oral Med Oral Pathol Oral Radiol Endod 93:643–646, 2002.

45. Collins JJ, Weisman SJ: Management of pain in childhood cancer. In Schechter NL, Berde CB, Yaster M (eds): Pain in Infants, Children, and Adolescents, 2nd ed. Philadelphia, Lippincott Williams & Wilkins, 2003, pp 517–538.

46. Krane EJ, Leong MS, Golianu B, Leong YY: Treatment of pediatric pain with non-conventional analgesics. In Schechter NL, Berde CB, Yaster M (eds): Pain in Infants, Children, and Adolescents, 2nd ed. Philadelphia, Lippincott Williams & Wilkins, 2003, pp 225–240.

47. Maunuksela E-L, Olkkola KT: Nonsteroidal anti-inflammatory drugs in pediatric pain management. In Schechter NL, Berde CB, Yaster M (eds): Pain in Infants, Children, and Adolescents, 2nd ed. Philadelphia, Lippincott Williams & Wilkins, 2003, pp 171–180.

48. Yaster M, Kost-Byerly S, Maxwell LG: Opioid agonists and antagonists. In Schechter NL, Berde CB, Yaster M (eds): Pain in Infants, Children, and Adolescents, 2nd ed. Philadelphia, Lippincott Williams & Wilkins, 2003, pp 181–224.

49. Yaster M, Tobin J, Kost-Byerly S: Local anesthetics. In Schechter NL, Berde CB, Yaster M (eds): Pain in Infants, Children, and Adolescents, 2nd ed. Philadelphia, Lippincott Williams & Wilkins, 2003.

50. Anghelescu D, Oakes L: Working toward better cancer pain management for children. Cancer Pract 10(Suppl 1):S52–S57, 2002.

51. Schutzman SA, Liebelt E, Wisk M, Burg J: Comparison of oral transmucosal fentanyl citrate and intramuscular meperidine, pro-methazine, and chlorpromazine for conscious sedation of children undergoing laceration repair. Ann Emerg Med 28:385–390, 1996.

52. Dsida RM, Wheeler M, Birmingham PK, et al: Premedication of pediatric tonsillectomy patients with oral transmucosal fentanyl citrate. Anesth Analg 86:66–70, 1998.

53. Malviya S, Voepel-Lewis T, Huntington J, et al: Effects of anesthetic technique on side effects associated with fentanyl Oralet pre-medication. J Clin Anesth 9:374–378, 1997.

54. Sharar SR, Carrougher GJ, Selzer K, et al: A comparison of oral transmucosal fentanyl citrate and oral oxycodone for pediatric outpatient wound care. J Burn Care Rehabil 23:27–31, 2002.

55. Gaukroger P: Patient-controlled analgesia in children. In Schechter NL, Berde CB, Yaster M (eds): Pain in Infants, Children, and Adolescents. Baltimore, Lippincott Williams & Wilkins, 1993, pp 203–212.

56. Hill HF, Chapman CR, Kornell JA, et al: Self-administration of morphine in bone marrow transplant patients reduces drug require-ment. Pain 40:121–129, 1990.

57. Rodgers BM, Webb CJ, Stergios D, Newman BM: Patient-controlled analgesia in pediatric surgery. J Pediatr Surg 23: 259–262, 1988.

58. Shapiro B, Cohen D, Howe C: Use of patient-controlled analgesia for patients with sickle cell disease. J Pain Symptom Manage 6:176, 1991.

59. Tahmooressi J, Schmalzle S, Tobin J: Patient-controlled analgesia in the adolescent undergoing Cotrel-Dubosset Rod. J Pain Symptom Manage 6:160, 1991.

60. Webb C, Paarlberg J, Sussman M: The use of a PCA device by parents or nurses for postoperative pain in children with cerebral palsy. J Pain Symptom Manage 6:160, 1991.

61. McDonald AJ, Cooper MG: Patient-con-trolled analgesia: An appropriate method of pain control in children. Paediatr Drugs 3:273–284, 2001.

62. McNeely JK, Trentadue NC: Comparison of patient-controlled analgesia with and with-out nighttime morphine infusion following lower extremity surgery in children. J Pain Symptom Manage 13:268–273, 1997.

63. Bray RJ, Woodhams AM, Vallis CJ, Kelly PJ, Ward-Platt MP: A double-blind comparison of morphine infusion and patient controlled analgesia in children. Paediatr Anaesth 6:121–127, 1996.

64. Noyes M, Irving H: The use of transdermal fentanyl in pediatric palliative care. Am J Hosp Palliat Care 18:411–416, 2001.

65. Hunt A, Goldman A, Devine T, Phillips M: Transdermal fentanyl for pain relief in a paediatric palliative care population. Palliat Med 15:405–412, 2001.

66. Christensen ML, Wang WC, Harris S, Eades SK, Wilimas JA: Transdermal fentanyl administration in children and adolescents with sickle cell pain crisis. J Pediatr Hematol Oncol 18:372–376, 1996.

67. Ahmedzai S, Brooks D: Transdermal fentanyl versus sustained-release oral morphine in cancer pain: Preference, efficacy, and quality of life. The TTS-Fentanyl Comparative Trial Group. J Pain Symptom Manage 13: 254–261, 1997.

68. Edinboro LE, Poklis A, Trautman D, Lowry S, Backer R, Harvey CM: Fatal fentanyl intoxication following excessive transdermal application. J Forensic Sci. 42:741–743, 1997.

69. Sawni-Sikand A, Schubiner H, Thomas RL: Use of complementary/alternative therapies among children in primary care pediatrics. Ambul Pediatr 2:99–103, 2002.

70. Ernst E: Serious adverse effects of uncon-ventional therapies for children and adolescents: A systematic review of recent evidence. Eur J Pediatr 162:72–80, 2003.

71. Sampson M, Campbell K, Ajiferuke I, Moher D: Randomized controlled trials in pediatric complementary and alternative medicine: Where can they be found? BMC Pediatr 3:1, 2003.

72. Moher D, Soeken K, Sampson M, Ben-Porat L, Berman B: Assessing the quality of reports of randomized trials in pediatric complementary and alternative medicine. BMC Pediatr 2:2, 2002.

73. Scrace J: Complementary therapies in palliative care of children with cancer: A literature review. Paediatr Nurs 15:36–39, 2003.

74. Spigelblatt L, Laine-Ammara G, Pless IB, Guyver A: The use of alternative medicine by children. Pediatrics 94:811–814, 1994.

75. Madsen H, Andersen S, Nielsen RG, Dolmer BS, Host A, Damkier A: Use of complementary/alternative medicine among paediatric patients. Eur J Pediatr 162: 334–341, 2003.

76. Fong DP, Fong LK: Usage of complemen-tary medicine among children. Aust Fam Physician 31:388–391, 2002.

77. Friedman T, Slayton WB, Allen LS, et al: Use of alternative therapies for children with cancer. Pediatrics 100:E1, 1997.

78. Dahlquist LM, Gil KM, Armstrong FD, et al: Behavioral management of children's distress during chemotherapy. J Behav Ther Exp Psychiatr 16:325–329, 1985.

79. Dash J: Hypnosis for symptom ameliora-tion. In Kellerman J (ed): Psychological Aspects of Childhood Cancer. Springfield, Ill, Thomas, 1980, pp 215–230.

80. Hartman GA: Hypnosis as an adjuvant in the treatment of childhood cancer. In Spinetta JJ, Deasy-Spinetta P (eds): Living with Childhood Cancer. St. Louis, Mosby, 1981, pp 143–152.

81. Hilgard JR, LeBaron S: Relief of anxiety and pain in children and adolescents with cancer: Quantitative measures and clinical observations. Int J Clin Exp Hypn 30: 417–442, 1982.

82. Hilgard JR, LeBaron S: Hypnotherapy of Pain in Children with Cancer. Los Altos, Calif, Kaufmann, 1984.

83. Jay SM, Elliott CH, Ozolins M, et al: Behavioral management of children's distress during painful medical procedures. Behav Res Ther 23:513–520, 1985.

84. Katz ER, Kellerman J, Ellenberg L: Hypnosis in the reduction of acute pain and distress in children with cancer. J Pediatr Psychol 12:379–394, 1987.

85. LaBaw W, Holton C, Tewell K, Eccles D: The use of self-hypnosis by children with cancer. Am J Clin Hypn 17:233–238, 1975.

86. McGrath PA, Hillier LM: A practical cognitive-behavioral approach for treating children's pain. In Turk DC, Gatchel RJ (eds): Psychological Approaches to Pain Management: A Practitioner's Handbook, 2nd ed. New York, The Guilford Press, 2002, pp 534–552.

87. Olness K: Imagery (self-hypnosis) as adjunct therapy in childhood cancer: Clinical experience with 25 patients. Am J Pediatr Hematol Oncol 3:313–321, 1981.

88. Olness K: Hypnosis in pediatric practice. Curr Probl Pediatr 12:1–47, 1981.

89. Zeltzer L, LeBaron S: Hypnosis and non-hypnotic techniques for reduction of pain and anxiety during painful procedures in children and adolescents with cancer. J Pediatr 101:1032–1035, 1982.

90. Hall H: Hypnosis and pediatrics. In Temes R (eds): Medical Hypnosis: An Introduction and Clinical Guide. New York, Churchill Livingstone, 1999, pp 79–93.

91. LeBaron S, Zeltzer LK: Children in pain. In Barber J (ed): Hypnosis and Suggestion in the Treatment of Pain: A Clinical Guide, 1st ed. New York, W.W. Norton, 1996, pp 305–340.

92. Olness K, Kohen DP: Hypnosis and Hypnotherapy with Children. New York, Guilford Press, 1996.

93. Beales J: Pain in children with cancer. In Bonica J, Ventafridda V (eds): Advances in Pain Research and Therapy. New York, Raven Press, 1979, pp 89–98.

94. Maxwell LG, Yaster M: The myth of conscious sedation. Arch Pediatr Adolesc Med 150:665–657, 1996.

95. American Academy of Pediatrics Committee on Drugs: Guidelines for monitoring and management of pediatric patients during and after sedation for diagnostic and therapeutic procedures: Addendum. Pediatrics 110:836–838, 2002.

96. Brown SC, Roy WL: Anesthesia and sedation for satellite and remote locations. In Bissonnette B, Dalens B (eds): Pediatric Anesthesia: Principles and Practice. New York, McGraw Hill, 2002, pp 627–642.

97. Bouffet E, Douard MC, Annequin D, et al: Pain in lumbar puncture: Results of a 2-year discussion at the French Society of Pediatric Oncology. Arch Pediatr 3:22–27, 1996.

98. Sandler ES, Weyman C, Conner K, et al: Midazolam versus fentanyl as premedication for painful procedures in children with cancer. Pediatrics 89:631–634, 1992.

99. Tobias JD, Phipps S, Smith B, Mulhern RK: Oral ketamine premedication to alleviate the distress of invasive procedures in pediatric oncology patients. Pediatrics 90:537–541, 1992.

100. McMillan CO, Spahr-Schopfer IA, Sikich N, et al: Premedication of children with oral midazolam. Can J Anaesth 39:545–550, 1992.

101. Ferrari L, Barst S, Pratila M, Bedford RF: Anesthesia for diagnostic and therapeutic procedures in pediatric outpatients. Am J Pediatr Hematol Oncol: 12:310–313, 1990.

102. McDowall RH, Scher CS, Barst SM: Total intravenous anesthesia for children undergoing brief diagnostic or therapeutic procedures. J Clin Anesth 7:273–280, 1995.

103. Fisher DM, Robinson S, Brett CM, et al: Comparison of enflurane, halothane, and isoflurane for diagnostic and therapeutic procedures in children with malignancies. Anesthesiology 63:647–650, 1985.

104. Broennle AM, Cohen DE: Pediatric anesthesia and sedation. Curr Opin Pediatr 5:310–314, 1993.

105. Zeltzer LK, Altman A, Cohen D, et al: American Academy of Pediatrics Report of the Subcommittee on the Management of Pain Associated with Procedures in Children with Cancer. Pediatrics 86:826–831, 1990.

106. Roy WL: Anaesthetizing children in remote locations: Necessary expeditions or anaesthetic misadventures? Can J Anaesth 43:764–768, 1996.

107. Wilder R: Regional anesthetic techniques for chronic pain management in children. In Schechter NL, Berde CB, Yaster M (eds): Pain in Infants, Children, and Adolescents, 2nd ed. Philadelphia, Lippincott Williams & Wilkins, 2003.

108. Swarm R, Karanikolas M, Cousins M: Anaesthetic techniques for pain control. In Doyle D, Hanks G, Cherny N, Calman K (eds): Oxford Textbook of Palliative Medicine. Oxford, Oxford University Press, 2004, 378–396.

109. Liossi C: Procedure-Related Cancer Pain in Children. Abingdon, Radcliffe Medical, 2002.

110. Hooke C, Hellsten MB, Stutzer C, Forte K: Pain management for the child with cancer in end-of-life care: APON position paper. J Pediatr Oncol Nurs 19:43–47, 2002.

111. Ellis JA, McCarthy P, Hershon L, et al: Pain practices: A cross-Canada survey of pediatric oncology centers. J Pediatr Oncol Nurs 20:26–35, 2003.

112. Wang XS, Tang JY, Zhao M, et al: Pediatric cancer pain management practices and attitudes in China. J Pain Symptom Manage 26:748–759, 2003.

Cancer Pain Resulting from Tumor Extension

CHAPTER 5

Pain Due to Tumors of the Skull Base

LASZLO MECHTLER, MD

As new imaging techniques are coupled with advances in medical, interventional, and surgical techniques, pain specialists have an increasingly important role in the evaluation of skull base tumor–related pain syndromes. An accurate assessment of both the type and the cause of pain is important in the differential diagnosis of skull base tumors as these lesions may initially present with pain. Additionally, the nature of the pain may assist the clinician in determining appropriate treatment for the underlying disease.

The complex anatomy of the skull base has long been a challenge to clinicians. In the past, conservative modes of treatment such as external beam radiation have been the standard of care for skull base tumors. This is largely due to the deep location and surrounding critical neurovascular structures in this anatomic site, with the result that, until recently, most surgical attempts have been associated with significant morbidity. The exquisite bone detail provided by computerized tomography (CT) and the soft tissue definition obtained with magnetic resonance imaging (MRI) have dramatically improved preoperative planning and postoperative assistance, resulting in significantly improved results with skull base surgery.[1] Moreover, noninvasive stereotactically focused radiation treatment has improved control of tumor growth and pain-related symptoms.

SKULL BASE ANATOMY

Anatomically, the skull base can be divided into three territories (Figure 5–1): (a) anterior cranial fossa, (b) middle cranial fossa, and (c) posterior cranial fossa. Each cranial fossa can be further divided into subterritories according to laterality. Pain-sensitive structures of the head and face include the skin and blood vessels of the scalp, the dura, the venous sinuses, the arteries, and the sensory fibers of the fifth, ninth, and tenth nerves. The trigeminal nerve is a mixed nerve conveying sensory, motor, and autonomic impulses. Sensory neurons of the trigeminal nerves V_1 to V_3 lie in the gasserian ganglion, which is

embedded within the temporal bone within the middle cranial fossa, also known as Meckel's cave. From the gasserian ganglion, three trigeminal divisions proceed forward and exit from the skull-base foramina: V_1 (ophthalmic nerve) exits the superior orbital fissure, V_2 (maxillary nerve) exits via the foramen rotundum, and V_3 (mandibular nerve) exits via the foramen ovale. In addition, branches of the trigeminal nerve, vagus (X) nerve, and the sympathetic nerves supply the dura mater. Ethmoidal nerves of the ophthalmic division of V supply part of the falx cerebri and the anterior cranial fossa. Recurrent tentorial branches of the ophthalmic division of V innervate the tentorium cerebelli and the posterior falx cerebri. Branches of the maxillary and mandibular divisions of V innervate the middle cranial fossa. Recurrent meningeal branches of the vagus nerve innervate the posterior cranial fossa. Sympathetic autonomic fibers follow the middle meningeal arteries to innervate the dura mater but not the cerebral blood vessels.

MECHANISMS OF PAIN GENERATION

Tumors affect cranial nerves by compression, without directly breaching the epineurium, or by invasion along perineural and endoneural planes. Typically, squamous cell carcinoma of the face, certain melanomas, and adenoid cystic carcinomas can be neurotropic, tracking microscopically along the course of the nerve. A blood–nerve barrier that is similar to the blood–brain barrier may exclude water-soluble chemotherapeutic agents from the nerve and provide a "sanctuary" for tumor cells. With compressive lesions of cranial nerves, pain is usually the first symptom. The pain may be felt locally at the site of compression or more distally in the sensory distribution of the nerve involved. Pain usually precedes other neurologic deficits by weeks to months. In invasive lesions of nerves, pain and neurologic deficits often occur simultaneously. In general, when mixed nerves are involved, motor function is affected out of proportion to sensory loss, regardless of the mechanism of nerve involvement.

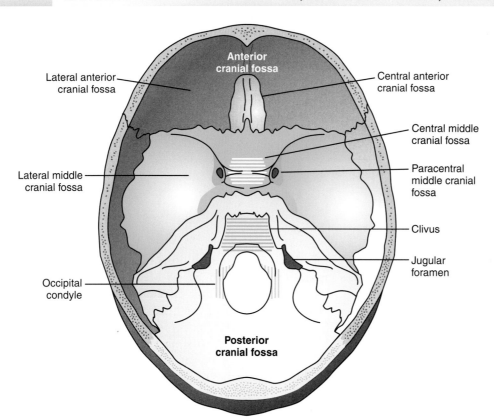

FIGURE 5–1 Diagrammatic sketch of the major anatomic regions of the base of the skull.

The mechanisms by which the tumors found at the base of the skull can cause pain include direct stimulation of nerve endings in the mucosa and submucosa, ulceration and infection, compression and invasion of the sensory nerves, and bone invasion.[2] Pain reported by cancer patients can be categorized as nociceptive somatic, nociceptive visceral, neuropathic (non-nociceptive) and psychogenic.[3,4] Pain secondary to infiltration of bone is classified as nociceptive somatic. Nerve root compression from tumors manifests itself as neuropathic pain.[3,4]

ANATOMIC CLASSIFICATION OF SKULL BASE PAIN CAUSED BY TUMORS

Skull base tumors may originate from the neurovascular structure at the base of the brain, the meninges, the cranial base proper, or the subcranial structures of the head and neck. Although the diversity of tumor types affecting this site have thus far defied development of a unified classification system, tumors located in a specific region of the skull base often are associated with a specific constellation of signs and symptoms. Furthermore, certain tumor pathologies tend to have regional specificity. Therefore, classifications based on location within the skull base are useful for clinical pathologic correlation.

Tumors of the skull base are classified histopathologically as primary or metastatic, and as benign or malignant.[5] A number of systemic tumors—especially breast, prostate, and lung tumors—frequently metastasize to bone, including the base of the skull.[6] Metastatic tumors arising at this anatomic site usually compromise the cranial nerves that exit through the basal foramina. The resulting clinical presentation depends on the location, involved neurovascular structure, and the extent and aggressiveness of the tumor. Constant localized aching pain resulting from bone destruction and neurologic deficits due to progressive cranial nerve palsies are cardinal manifestations of skull base tumors. Slow-growing primary benign tumors (i.e., meningioma, schwannoma) may also cause dramatic neurologic signs and symptoms as well as pain.

Although the tissue diagnosis of a lesion requires biopsy, the neuroradiologist is usually called on to predict the identity of the pathologic lesion preoperatively. Based on the site of origin, MRI, and CT appearance, the neuroradiologist can reduce quite accurately the types of lesions to a small number of possibilities. For example, some tumor types have a strong tendency to arise or even exclusively arise in a particular location. Pain syndromes that have been associated with the appearance of tumors in a particular locus of the skull base are listed in Tables 5–1 and 5–2.

TABLE 5–1   Common Skull Base Pain Syndromes

Syndrome	Cranial Nerves Involved	Pain Characteristics	Symptoms and Signs (in Addition to Pain) and Clinical Commentary
Occipital condyle syndrome	XII	Severe, localized, continuous unilateral occipital pain aggravated by neck flexion and rotation of the head to the side contralateral to the pain. Tenderness to palpation over affected occipital or suboccipital area. In some patients the pain can radiate anteriorly toward the ipsilateral ear, temple, vertex, or forehead.	Unilateral cranial nerve XII paralysis—paralysis of tongue, weakness of sternocleidomastoid, stiff neck, dysarthria, and dysphagia. Patients should stay in bed, head rotated ipsilateral to the pain, keeping the position with the help of their hand.
Jugular foramen syndrome	IX, X, XI, (XII)	Occipital pain radiating often to the vertex and ipsilateral shoulder or neck. Head movement often exacerbates the pain. Chronic, unilateral pain occurs behind the ear on the involved side. It can be accompanied by local tenderness and exacerbation with movement of the head. Lancinating throat pain (glossopharyngeal neuralgia) has been associated with this syndrome.	Most common are dysarthria, dysphagia, weakness of the palate/pharynx/larynx, hoarseness, and voice changes. Less common are either weakness and atrophy ("wasting") of the ipsilateral sternocleidomastoid and upper portion of the trapezius muscle, or tongue wasting. Glossopharyngeal neuralgia is sometimes accompanied with syncope. Expansion of tumor through the roof of the jugular fossa followed by invasion of the middle ear can cause conductive deafness. Expansion into the posterior cranial fossa may raise the intracranial pressure, causing headache. The headaches are worse in the morning and pain is increased by coughing or stooping.
Orbital syndrome	III, IV, VI, first division of V	Progressively severe, dull, aching pain in the retro-orbital and supraorbital area of the affected eye, including headache. Lancinating pain in distribution of the ophthalmic nerve is occasionally seen.	Diplopia or ophthalmoplegia, proptosis, chemosis of the involved eye, red eye, periorbital swelling, external ophthalmoparesis, ipsilateral papilledema, and a decreased sensation in the ophthalmic division of the trigeminal nerve V_1. Occasionally, binocular vision is blurred. Decreased vision is unusual and occurs late. The tumor sometimes is palpable.
Cavernous sinus (para-sellar) syndrome	III, IV, V, VI	Unilateral, dull, aching headache in the supraorbital and frontal area. There may also be maxillary regional pain, and occasionally sharp, shooting, episodic lancinating pain.	Patients may present with paresis in any of the III–VI cranial nerves, and may have diplopia, ophthalmoparesis, exophthalmos, or papilledema. Formal visual testing may show hemianopsia or quadrantanopsia. Unilateral or bilateral sudden total visual loss can occur. There can be sensory disturbance, sometimes in V_1 cranial nerve, less often in V_2 or the entire trigeminal region. Signs may also include diabetes insipidus or anterior hypopituitarism.
Clivus syndrome	VI–XII	Vertex headache which is often exacerbated by neck flexion	Symptom may include lower cranial nerve (VI–XII) dysfunction that usually begins unilaterally and often can become bilateral.

Continued

TABLE 5–1 Common Skull Base Pain Syndromes—cont'd

Syndrome	Cranial Nerves Involved	Pain Characteristics	Symptoms and Signs (in Addition to Pain) and Clinical Commentary
Sphenoid sinus syndrome	VI	Severe bifrontal headache radiating to both temples and/or retroorbital pain, which may radiate to the temporal regions.	Nasal stuffiness or sense of fullness of the head; diplopia caused by unilateral or bilateral sixth nerve palsy can be present.
Gasserian syndrome (middle fossa syndrome)	V_2, V_3 (V_1)	Facial pain with paresthesias and/or numbness referred to the distribution of V_2 or V_3, referred to the cheek or jaw. Pain is usually dull, and aching continual, but it can be paroxysmal or lancinating. Pain is similar to trigeminal neuralgia but without trigger points. 25% of the patients have headaches.	Hypoesthesia, numbness in a trigeminal nerve distribution and weakness in the ipsilateral muscles of mastication. Occasionally with anterior lesions; abducens nerve palsy, diplopia, posterior lesion, facial nerve palsy, combination of extraocular palsies or dysarthria, or dysphagia can occur. Symptoms may begin close to the midline on the upper lip or chin subsequently progressing laterally to the anterior part of the ear (numb chin syndrome).

TABLE 5–2 Rare Skull Base Pain Syndromes

Syndrome	Nerves Involved	Pain Characteristics	Symptoms and Signs (in Addition to Pain) and Clinical Commentary
Superior orbital fissure syndrome (Rochon-DuVigneaud syndrome)	III–V_1	Severe ache in the distribution of the ophthalmic nerve (eye; supraorbital, and root and lateral part of the nose)	Sensory loss in V_1, ophthalmoplegia, exophthalmos without vision loss
Retropharyngeal syndrome (Villaret's syndrome) Cerebellopontine angle syndrome	Lower cranial and sympathetic nerves V, VII–XII	Severe ache in the retroparotid region, glossopharyngeal neuralgia Trigeminal and glossopharyngeal neuralgias	Dysfunction of the lower cranial nerves, Bernard–Horner syndrome with ptosis, miosis, and enophthalmos secondary to tumors in the retroparotid Dysfunction of VIII cranial nerve, cerebellar disturbances, sensory disturbances of V, IX cranial nerves, signs of elevated intracerebral pressure, brainstem symptoms
Garcin–Hartmann syndrome	I–XII (unilateral)	Neuralgia or similar type of pains in V nerve, nervus intermedius, or IX cranial nerve	Loss of function of all cranial nerves on one side secondary to nasopharyngeal carcinomas and metastases
Sinus of Morganini syndrome	V_3 and VIII	Aching sharp pain in distribution of V_3 (lower jaw, lateral tongue, ear, temporal region), headache	Unilateral deafness; anesthesia of the lower jaw; deviation of the palate; defective mobility of the palatal and internal pterygoid muscles, trismus, fullness in the lateral wall of nasopharynx, cervical and retropharyngeal adenopathy secondary to tumors deep in the lateral wall of the nasopharynx
Gradenigo-Lannois syndrome	V, VI, (II, IV, VII)	Neuralgia in the division of V_1, V_2, and V_3, frontal headache	Symptoms, signs beside pain are persistent diplopia, internal strabismus, sometimes sensory disturbances in V_2 and V_3 due to tumors that involve the apex of the petrous pyramid

TABLE 5–2 Rare Skull Base Pain Syndromes—cont'd

Pterygopalatine fossa syndromew	II, V	Typical of secondary neuralgia with continuous severe aching, burning pain in the upper jaw, upper back molar teeth, the face and later extension to the lower jaw	Unilateral deafness, paralysis and anesthesia of the palate, the pterygoid muscles, with deviation of jaw opening and homolateral blindness; fullness of temporal fossa and unilateral/bilateral cervical adenopathy due to tumors of the pterygopalatine fossa
Retrosphenoidal syndrome (Jacob's syndrome)	III–V	Trigeminal neuralgia, headache	Symptoms, signs beside pain are total unilateral ophthalmoplegia; amaurosis, deafness, palatal muscle paralysis, unilateral and bilateral adenopathy due to tumors of the medial cranial fossa expanding to under the foramen of rotundum, foramen ovale, and superior orbital fossa

BIOLOGIC POTENTIAL

Skull base tumors can also be graded by their biologic progressiveness. The three pathologic entities are benign, low-grade, and high-grade malignancies (Table 5–3). Benign tumors grow in an expansive fashion and thus they induce clinical symptoms by exerting pressure on specific neurovascular structures. Slow-growing malignancies, such as chondrosarcomas, chordomas, and adenoid cystic carcinomas, are best treated with a combined mode of surgical debulking and radiotherapy. Highly malignant tumors can be removed en bloc if critical structures can be avoided. However, in most situations, piecemeal resection or sacrifice of a significant structure may be involved. Hence, radiotherapy, specifically radiosurgery, with or without chemotherapy, is the main treatment modality when surgery may cause a loss of sensitive cranial structures.

Metastases to the base of the skull often cause characteristic syndromes combining headache and cranial nerve deficits. Early diagnosis is important because antitumor therapy may be effective and may reverse symptoms completely. Neuroimaging is relied on for the accurate diagnosis and mapping of the extent of tumor. Axial and coronal contrast-enhanced CT scanning performed with bone and soft tissue windows provides optimal information on tumor-induced bone erosion or destruction.[1] MRI demonstrates superior soft tissue resolution, and in addition it can visualize anatomy in multiple planes.[7] To attain the greatest amount of useful information, it is important to view CT and MRI as complementary, rather than mutually exclusive, techniques. Thus, when used together, MRI and CT clearly identify base of skull metastases in 81% of patients.[8] Presently, single photon emission computer tomography (SPECT) is recommended

TABLE 5–3 Biologic Behavior of Skull Base Tumors

Benign Tumors	Low-grade Malignancy	High-grade Malignancy
Meningiomas	Chordomas	Adenocarcinomas
Schwannomas/Neurofibromas	Chondrosarcomas	Sarcomas
Pituitary adenomas	Adenoid cystic carcinomas	Rhabdomyosarcoma
Paragangliomas	Fibrosarcomas	Ewing's sarcoma
Epidermoid cysts	Esthesioneuroblastomas	Fibrosarcomas
Juvenile angiofibromas	Hemangiopericytomas	Esthesioneuroblastomas
Cholesterol granulomas	Atypical meningioma	Lymphomas
Osteomas		Multiple myelomas
		Metastases

when MRI and CT are nondiagnostic. Bone SPECT was able to identify a hot spot in the appropriate region of the skull base in 78% of patients. In symptomatic patients who had normal CT and MRIs, a SPECT scan commonly reveals abnormal lesions.[8]

PAIN SYNDROMES ASSOCIATED WITH TUMORS IN SPECIFIC SKULL BASE LOCATIONS

Anterior Cranial Fossa Pain Syndromes

This section presents pain syndromes that have been associated with the appearance of tumors in a specific anatomic location within the base of the skull. Table 5–4 outlines pain syndromes according to anatomic location in the base of the skull. The anterior cranial fossa boundaries include the anterior inner surface of the frontal bone and extend posteriorly to the edge of the lesser wing of the sphenoid bone. Located within it are the frontal lobes of the brain and cranial nerve I, which exits the cranial cavity here through the cribriform plate. Subterritories include the central anterior skull and the lateral anterior skull base.[9]

Tumors involving the central anterior cranial fossa may cause olfactory groove syndrome, which typically consists of anosmia, frontal headaches, visual disturbance, and when large enough, cognitive changes. An uncommon form of anterior cranial fossa syndrome, the Foster–Kennedy syndrome, and is a triad of anosmia, ipsilateral optic atrophy, and contralateral papilledema, is most likely related to olfactory groove meningiomas.[10]

Olfactory groove meningiomas are almost always benign tumors, originate from the meninges, and cause displacement of the adjacent structures such as the brain. Figure 5–2 shows MRIs of a 56-year-old female who presented with bifrontal headaches and cognitive changes; the headaches, dementia, and loss of smell completely resolved following surgery and radiation.

Other tumors in this location include esthesioneuroblastoma and paranasal sinus carcinomas. Esthesioneuroblastoma is thought to arise from olfactory neuroepithelial cells high in the nasal cavity and has also been called olfactory neuroblastoma. The most common presenting symptoms in esthesioneuroblastoma are nasal obstruction in 55%, epistaxis in 44%, anosmia in 8% and headache in 8% of patients.[11] Primary tumors of the nasal cavity include squamous cell carcinoma, adenocarcinoma, adenoid cystic carcinoma, and rarely, a variety of other lesions such as melanoma, lymphoma, and plasmacytoma.[12] Loss of olfactory nerve function occurs uncommonly in nasopharyngeal carcinoma and even more rarely with metastatic tumors. Rhabdomyosarcoma, usually seen in children, can extend from the sinonasal region to the exterior skull base.[9]

Lateral anterior skull base tumors infiltrate the orbit causing visual changes and the so-called orbital syndrome.[13] Exophthalmos, superorbital pain, and diplopia are characteristic of this syndrome.[13,14] The third nerve passes through the superior orbital fissure in its passage from the cavernous sinus into the orbit. This fissure may be infiltrated by several different primary or secondary tumors such as meningiomas, nasopharyngeal carcinomas, multiple myelomas, and lymphomas. In the superior orbital fissure syndrome, a localized variant of orbital syndrome, tumors may cause deep orbital and unilateral frontal headache with progressive VI, III, and IV cranial nerve palsies with sensory disturbances in the area of V_1. Adenoid cystic carcinomas arise from the minor salivary glands and have a tendency to invade perineural spaces which may occur long after the primary lesion has been removed. An example is shown in Figure 5–3, which depicts a 40-year-old patient with infiltration of the superior orbital fissure and ethmoid sinus causing orbital pain, ophthalmoparesis, and proptosis.

An unusual symptom complex, the Tolosa-Hunt syndrome, mimics some of the symptoms of skull base tumors, although histologically it is more consistent with an inflammatory pseudotumor.[15] This is an uncommon cause of painful ophthalmoplegia, usually appearing in the fourth through the sixth decades of life. The syndrome slowly evolves over several weeks as a steady, boring, unilateral, orbital pain caused by nonspecific granulomatous tissue in the superior orbital fissure or orbital apex. Palsies of the third, fourth, and sixth nerves, in any combination, are possible. The first division of the trigeminal sensory nerve (V_1) may be involved. This entity is diagnosed by exclusion of other space-occupying lesions in an area of the superior orbital fissure. Corticosteroid responsiveness is the rule.

Middle Fossa Cranial Pain Syndromes

The middle cranial fossa consists of the sphenoid bone and its contiguous tissues. Its subterritories include: (a) the central middle fossa, which includes the sphenoid sinus and the sella turcica, (b) the paracentral middle fossa, which is the cavernous sinus, and (c) the lateral middle fossa, which includes the sphenoid wing and infratemporal fossa.

Central middle cranial fossa syndromes are caused by masses involving the pituitary fossa (sella turcica) and the sphenoid sinus. Pain syndromes within the sella turcica are usually due to pituitary tumors. Headache may be an early finding and is attributed to the stretching of the enveloping dura and diaphragma sellae. Pituitary tumors may directly provoke headaches by eroding laterally into the cavernous sinus, which contains the first and second divisions of the trigeminal nerve, by involvement of the dural lining of the sella or diaphragma sellae

TABLE 5–4	Anatomic Locations and Histologic Types of Tumors Associated with Pain Syndromes in the Base of the Skull	
Location	**Syndrome**	**Tumor (Primary and Secondary)**
Anterior Cranial Fossa	Olfactory Groove Syndrome (central)	Meningioma Esthesioneuroblastoma Nasopharyngeal carcinoma
	Orbital Syndrome (lateral)	Meningioma, multiple myeloma Nasopharyngeal carcinoma Lymphoma Metastases from breast cancer Orbital tumors *In children*: Neuroblastoma Ewing's sarcoma Wilms tumor Leukemia
Middle Cranial Fossa	Central Middle Fossa Syndrome Sella Turcica Syndrome	Pituitary adenoma Craniopharyngioma Meningioma
	Sphenoid Sinus Syndrome	Adenoid cystic carcinoma Juvenile nasal angiofibroma Meningioma Pituitary adenoma
	Cavernous Sinus (parasellar) Syndrome	Meningioma Schwannoma Chordoma Adenoid cystic carcinoma Nasopharyngeal carcinoma Metastases (breast, prostate, lung cancers)
	Gasserian Ganglion Syndrome (middle fossa syndrome)	Nasopharyngeal carcinoma Adenocystic carcinoma Metastases (breast, lung, prostate) Meningioma Trigeminal schwannoma
Posterior Cranial Fossa	Clivus Syndrome	Chordoma Meningioma Nasopharyngeal carcinoma Chondrosarcoma Schwannoma Metastases
	Occipital Condyle Syndrome	Metastases Meningioma Schwannoma Chordoma
	Cerebellopontine Angle Syndrome (upper lateral)	Schwannoma Meningioma Lipoma Epidermoid Metastases Schwannoma
	Jugular Foramen Syndrome (lower lateral)	Paraganglioma Metastases Nasopharyngeal carcinoma

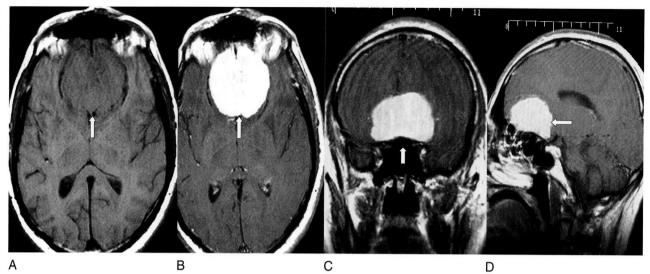

FIGURE 5–2 Typical olfactory groove meningioma in a 56-year-old female presenting with bifrontal headaches and cognitive changes. *A*, Non-contrast T1-weighted axial MRI shows an isointense large extra-axial mass distorting the frontal lobe. *B*, With gadolinium (Gd) contrast there is homogenous enhancement. Postoperatively, headaches and dementia completely resolved. *C*, T1-weighted coronal Gd contrast MRI confirming the location of the meningioma within the floor of the anterior cranial fossa. *D*, Sagittal contrast T1-weighted MRI.

or via sinusitis, particularly after transsphenoidal surgery. Headache is typically characterized by steady bifrontal or unilateral frontal aching (ipsilateral to tumor). In some instances, the pain is localized in the mid-face, either because of involvement of the second division

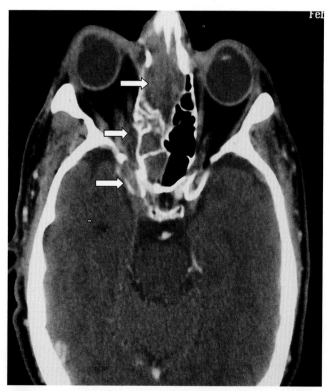

FIGURE 5–3 Adenoid cystic carcinoma eroding the orbital apex and the ethmoid sinus on the right. This contrast axial CT scan was seen in a patient with superior orbital fissure syndrome associated with orbital and frontal pain and ophthalmoparesis.

of the trigeminal nerve (V_2) or secondary to sinusitis. In contrast to the insidious subacute development of headache in most patients with pituitary tumors, patients with pituitary apoplexia may experience acute severe headache perhaps associated with symptoms and signs of meningeal irritation, cerebrospinal fluid (CSF) pleocytosis or oculomotor paresis. One to two percent of pituitary adenomas undergo symptomatic hemorrhagic infarction, producing the often dramatic clinical syndrome of pituitary apoplexy. The headache is sudden and postural due to the stretching and irritation of the dura mater within the walls of the sella supplied by the meningeal branches of cranial nerve V. Frequently it is retroorbital in location and may be unilateral at onset, eventually becoming generalized. Vomiting occurs in 69% of patients, while visual acuity or field defects occur in 64% of patients.[16]

Inferior to the sella turcica is the sphenoid sinus. Sphenoid sinus syndrome symptoms are caused by tumors residing in that sinus, including metastases as well as nasopharyngeal tumors. Tumors in this location commonly cause severe bifrontal headaches radiating to both temples with intermittent retroorbital pain.[17] At times, bilateral cranial nerve VI palsy occurs, causing diplopia. This is associated with some nasal stuffiness and sense of fullness in the head. The most common cause of isolated sphenoid sinus disease is infection followed by neoplasias.

Paracentral middle fossa syndromes refer to cranial nerve deficits and pain due to tumors infiltrating the cavernous sinus. In addition to tumors, carotid artery aneurysm, carotid cavernous fistulas, and inflammatory processes are the principle causes of cavernous sinus syndrome. The cavernous sinuses are paired venous structures located on either side of the sella turcica. The cavernous sinus contains the carotid artery, its sympathetic plexus, and the ocular motor nerves (cranial nerves III, IV, and VI). In addition, the ophthalmic branch of the fifth nerve traverses the cavernous sinus. The most characteristic manifestations of lesions in the cavernous sinus are ophthalmoplegia, orbital congestion, and proptosis. Cavernous sinus syndrome, also called parasellar syndrome, causes pain that is characterized by a unilateral frontal headache with ocular paresis, initially without proptosis.[18,19] Headache is usually the initial complaint in these patients and is localized to the supraorbital and frontal areas. Most patients describe the pain as dull and aching, although some patients experience an episodic sharp shooting pain.[13] Diplopia results from involvement of the ocular motor nerves as they traverse the cavernous sinus. The most common nerve involvement is the oculomotor nerve (III). Figure 5–4 shows a meningioma in a 60-year-old female who complained of supraorbital pain and partial third nerve palsy.

Metastatic cavernous sinus syndrome is relatively common and is caused predominantly by breast, prostate, and lung cancers.[20] Carcinomas arising in the face, usually squamous but occasionally basal cell carcinoma, may extend microscopically along the first or second division of the trigeminal nerve to the cavernous sinus. In such instances, facial pain or sensory loss is the first symptom and diplopia occurs later. Adenoid cystic

carcinoma is also a common cause of cavernous sinus syndrome but is due to perineural extension.

The gasserian ganglion syndrome (middle fossa syndrome) is usually due to metastatic lesions involving Meckel's cave where the ganglion for the trigeminal nerve is located.[13] Facial pain with or without numbness is a common symptom of tumors involving the trigeminal nerve. When cancer causes facial pain, the tumor site can be at the most peripheral branches of the trigeminal nerve in the subcutaneous tissues of the face, the entry of the trigeminal nerve in the brainstem, or anywhere along those tracts, as well as lesions involving the brainstem. Typical presenting complaints in gasserian ganglion syndrome patients are numbness, paresthesias, and usually, pain referred to the trigeminal distribution. The numbness at times occurs without pain, usually begins close to the midline on the upper lip or chin, and progresses laterally to the anterior part of the ear. The pain consists of either a dull ache in the cheek, jaw, or forehead or lightning-like pain very similar to trigeminal neuralgia but unaccompanied by trigger points. Definitive differentiation from idiopathic trigeminal neuralgia can be made by the subsequent appearance of numbness and sensory loss. Headache is present in about 28% of patients, in marked contrast to the cavernous sinus syndrome in which 83% of patients suffer headache as an early and severe symptom. Three-fourths of cancers in this site typically originate from nasopharyngeal carcinomas as well as breast, lung, and prostate metastases. Figure 5–5 shows

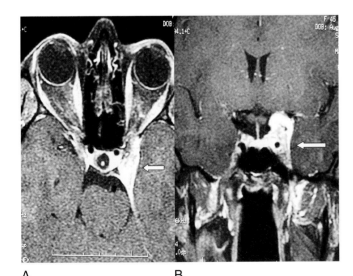

A   B

FIGURE 5–4 Meningioma infiltrating the left cavernous sinus causing a left cavernous sinus syndrome with supraorbital pain and partial third nerve palsy. *A*, T1-weighted fat suppression (STIR) MRI in the axial plane with gadolinium (Gd) contrast. *B*, Coronal T1-weighted Gd contrast MRI with extension of the tumor into the suprasellar cistern.

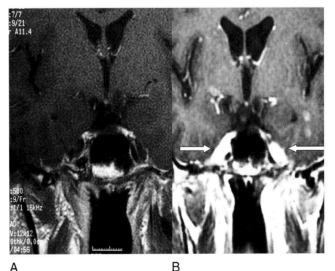

A   B

FIGURE 5–5 T1-weighted Gd contrast coronal MRIs in a 25-year-old with bifrontal headaches, facial numbness, and sixth nerve paresis bilaterally. Patient has metastatic adenocarcinoma to Meckel's cave causing a gasserian ganglion syndrome, which completely resolved after base of the skull radiation. *A*, Coronal contrast MRI shows normal Meckel's cave. *B*, One year later, patient developed significant frontal headaches and multiple cranial nerve deficits (V, VI).

MRIs in a 25-year-old patient with bifrontal headaches, facial numbness, and sixth nerve paresis bilaterally. This patient had CSF-positive metastatic colon adenocarcinoma extending to both Meckel's caves causing a gasserian ganglion syndrome, which completely resolved after base of the skull radiation. Primary benign tumors such as meningiomas and trigeminal schwannomas are also commonly seen. Tumors of the trigeminal nerve, predominantly schwannomas, most often present with facial pain described as burning. Sensory paresthesias and diminished cornea reflex also may be encountered. Motor dysfunction of the muscles of mastication occurs late as the tumor enlarges.[21]

Numb chin syndrome results from dysfunction of the inferior alveolar nerve, which is a distal branch of the V_3 (mandibular) nerve compressed by metastases of the mandible.[22] This pain syndrome has also has been described in patients with leptomeningeal disease as well as those with metastases to the skull base. Patients complain of numbness, although almost always there is pain involving the chin and lower lip. Lymphoma, leukemia, and breast cancer are relatively common causes. The importance of numb chin syndrome is that it may be the first sign of systemic cancer or metastasis.[23]

Posterior Cranial Fossa Pain Syndromes

The posterior cranial fossa can be subclassified into four different regions: (a) clivus, (b) foramen magnum (occipital condyle), (c) cerebellopontine angle, and (d) jugular foramen. Each of these anatomic regions is associated with characteristic syndromes involving cranial nerves and their related pain.

In the upper central posterior cranial fossa lies the clivus. Clivus syndrome is typically caused by chordomas or metastases.[24] Clivus chordomas have been reported in all age-groups including children and adolescents, with a median age at diagnosis of 46 years. Diplopia is the most common reported symptom at presentation and headache is the second most common. Cranial nerve VI is the most likely to be involved at presentation. Other common tumors in this location are metastases and nasopharyngeal carcinoma. The clivus syndrome is characterized by pain at the vertex that is increased by neck flexion. As the tumor advances, lower cranial palsies, especially hypoglossal paresis, may become evident. Lower cranial nerve dysfunction (VI-XII) usually begins on one side but often progresses to bilateral. Figures 5-6 to 5-8 show a clivus chordoma in a patient who presented with lower cranial nerve dysfunction and headaches. A noteworthy comment concerning management of these patients is that it is prudent to stabilize the neck of any patient before they undergo neuroimaging.[25,26]

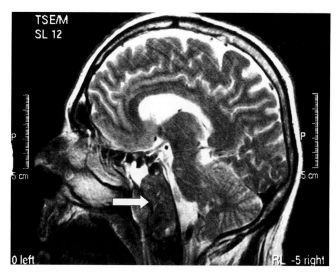

FIGURE 5-6 T2-weighted sagittal MRI showing an isointense mass replacing the normal bone marrow of the clivus. This patient has a clivus syndrome with headache worsened by neck flexion. The diagnosis is chordoma.

Tumors growing in the lower central posterior fossa, which is in the region of the foramen magnum, can cause a rare but stereotypical pain syndrome, the occipital condyle syndrome.[27,28] This syndrome is associated with unilateral occipital pain and ipsilateral hypoglossal paralysis and most often is caused by metastases. The pain is usually severe and aggravated by neck flexion. Tenderness to palpation over the affected occipital condyle area is noted. Unilateral cranial nerve XII paralysis leads to loss of tongue mobility. There is also stiffness in the neck with occasional dysarthria, dysphagia, and weakness in the sternocleidomastoid. Often the pain becomes unbearable with head rotation to the nonpainful side and with unilateral suboccipital palpation. The onset of this pain occurs at times up to 2½ months prior to the hypoglossal paralysis.[13]

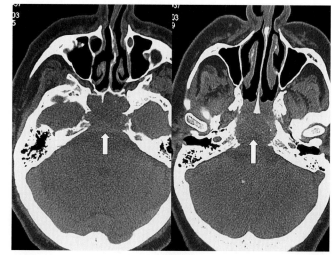

FIGURE 5-7 Axial CT scan showing a mass eroding the clivus. Histology was consistent with a chordoma.

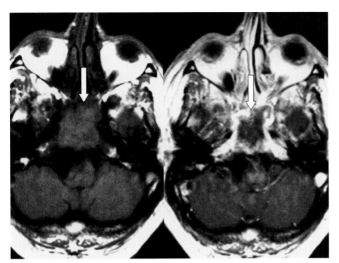

FIGURE 5–8   T1-weighted axial MRIs showing a mass involving the clivus without and with gadolinium contrast.

In the upper lateral posterior cranial fossa is the cerebellopontine angle. Often masses in this area will cause seventh and eighth nerve involvement as well as at times spread to involve the fifth and lower cranial nerves, eventually compressing the adjacent brainstem.[29] Three quarters of the tumors in this location are schwannomas with cerebellopontine angle meningiomas a distant second. Trigeminal and glossopharyngeal neuralgia are common with compression of these nerves. Dysfunction of cranial nerve VIII will cause hearing loss, vertigo, and nystagmus. The adjacent cerebellar peduncle may cause ataxia and cerebellar syndromes. Other masses that may be found in these locations include metastases, epidermoids and arachnoid cysts.

Within the lower lateral posterior cranial fossa is the jugular foramen. Jugular foramen syndrome is associated with occipital pain that is usually referred to the vertex of the head.[13] Ipsilateral shoulder and arm pain is often exacerbated by head movement. There may be tenderness of the occipital condyle and occasionally, glossopharyngeal neuralgia either by itself or together with syncope. Hoarseness and dysphagia are the most common symptoms after pain. Objective signs of abnormalities of cranial nerves IX–XI have been seen. When the tumor is not confined to the jugular foramen, other findings such as weakness and atrophy of the tongue or Horner's syndrome may be present indicating involvement of the hypoglossal canal and extracranial sympathetics. Jugular foramen syndrome is characterized by loss of taste of the posterior third of the tongue and posterior pharyngeal wall anesthesia, paralysis of the vocal cord and weakness of the trapezius/sternocleidomastoid. When the hypoglossal nerve is involved, paralysis of all four nerves IX–XII is known as the Collet–Sicard syndrome, whereas involvement of the cranial nerves IX–XI is called Vernet's syndrome.[30,31] Pain in or behind the ear

is attributable to irritation of the auricular branches of the ninth and tenth nerves. Whenever an adult complains of constant pain in one ear without evidence of middle ear disease, cancer of the pharynx must be suspected. Metastases, neuromas, chondromas, meningiomas, and nasopharyngeal carcinoma are tumors that commonly are seen in patients with jugular foramen syndrome.

Pain Secondary to Atlantoaxial Tumors

Although not strictly belonging to the skull base, the diagnosis and management of tumors involving the atlantoaxial spine is extremely important. The most common symptom of atlantoaxial metastases is neck pain. In one study, rotational neck pain was a major component in 91% of patients with tumors in this site.[32] One-third of patients had occipital neuralgia and 10% had lower cranial neuropathies resulting from extensive tumor at the base of the skull. Most patients who receive external beam radiation have significant resolution of this pain. Interestingly, the radiosensitivity of the tumor did not affect treatment choices or outcome. Patients with metastatic infiltration of the atlantoaxial spine and who have normal spine alignment or minimal fracture subluxation can be managed successfully with external beam radiation therapy and hard collar immobilization, regardless of the tumor histology. Surgical stabilization should be considered for odontoid fracture with atlantoaxial displacement larger than 5 mm.

Neuralgic Pain Syndromes

Tumors of the skull base occasionally will cause neuralgia. Neuralgia is defined as an intense, burning, or stabbing pain caused by irritation of or damage to a nerve. The pain is usually brief, but may be quite severe and disabling. Two forms of neuralgia are known, one of which is idiopathic, and other is secondary. The most common cranial and facial neuralgias from tumors include trigeminal neuralgia, glossopharyngeal neuralgia, geniculate neuralgia, and occipital neuralgia.

Trigeminal neuralgia (tic douloureux) is a brief lancinating pain that occurs in the distribution of the trigeminal nerve. The pain is described as paroxysmal, electric shock-like, shooting pain that only lasts a few seconds, but the pain may be repetitive at short intervals so that the individual attacks blur into one another. Most cases tend to occur in patients over 50 years of age, and they are idiopathic, although there are secondary causes including multiple sclerosis, cerebellopontine angle tumors, schwannomas, and vascular compression. The pain typically occurs in the second and third trigeminal divisions. Trigeminal neuralgia has also been reported as a presentation of lymphomatous meningitis and with tumor infiltration of the trigeminal nerve.

This pain can accompany head and neck cancers including adenoid cystic carcinoma and facial skin tumors. Retrograde perineural spread of tumor into the cavernous sinus, gasserian ganglion, the trigeminal nerve and the pons may be seen. In patients with nasopharyngeal cancer, facial pain and paresthesias were observed in 24% of 110 patients.[33] The clinical presentation differs between the two origins of trigeminal neuralgias. Patients who have tumor-related trigeminal neuralgia usually experience continuous pain, although there may be bouts of intensification, whereas patients having idiopathic trigeminal neuralgia are afflicted by short attacks of severe pain, with painless periods in between. Skull base malignancy should be suspected in patients presenting with facial pain and cranial nerve involvement. In a patient with neurofibromatosis-2, who presented with trigeminal paresthesias and neuralgic pain, as well as hearing loss, multiple schwannomas were observed (Figure 5–9).

An unusual referred facial pain syndrome has been seen in patients with lung carcinoma. Many of these patients describe a constant, aching, sometimes sharp pain, which may have a paroxysmal component. This pain is usually located in the ear and temporal region and occasionally the jaw. The etiology of the pain referral pattern is felt to be vagal in origin, which may also explain the right-sided predominance, because of the close anatomic relationship of the right vagus to the trachea and mediastinal lymph nodes.[34]

Glossopharyngeal neuralgia is pain within the IX cranial nerve distribution. The pain is lancinating and episodic and may be quite severe. Pain in the throat,

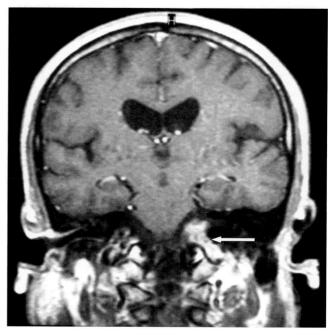

FIGURE 5–10   T1-weighted coronal Gd contrast study in a 52-year-old male presenting with glossopharyngeal neuralgia and dysphagia. A left dumbbell enhancing mass consistent with a glossopharyngeal schwannoma is seen.

the tonsil region, and in the posterior third of the tongue, the larynx, the nasopharynx, and the pinna of the ear is often described by patients. The pain is usually triggered by swallowing, chewing, speaking, laughing, or coughing. Glossopharyngeal neuralgia may also be associated with syncope and hypotension in patients with leptomeningeal metastases, jugular foramen syndrome, and head and neck malignancies. Figure 5–10 illustrates a 52-year-old musician who presented with dysphagia and dysphonia as well as neuralgia. He was found to have a left dumbbell mass enhancing the jugular foramen, consistent with a glossopharyngeal schwannoma.[35]

Geniculate neuralgia (nervous intermedius neuralgia) is an uncommon syndrome characterized by sharp pain deep within in the ear. The sharp pain is sometimes associated with a contrasting dull, burning pain extending to the ipsilateral face.

Occipital neuralgia is characterized by paroxysmal pain in the suboccipital region in the back of the head, in the distribution of the greater or lesser occipital nerves. Known causes of neuralgic pains in this area include trauma to the greater or lesser occipital nerves, or compression of these nerves or the upper cervical roots by arthritic changes in the spine and by tumors involving C2 and C3 cervical dorsal roots. Occipital neuralgia characteristically presents with continuous aching and throbbing pain on which shock-like jabs can be superimposed. Pressure over the occipital nerves can lead

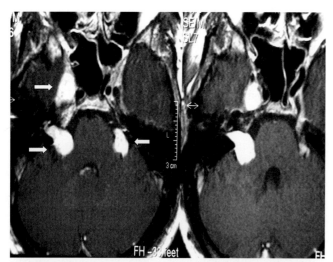

FIGURE 5–9   Multiple schwannomas in a patient with neurofibromatosis type 2. Bilateral vestibular and right-sided Meckel's cave schwannomas are evident on these T1-weighted axial contrast MRIs. Patient presented with trigeminal paresthesias and neuralgic pain, as well as hearing loss.

to exacerbation. Percussion over the occipital nerves (Tinel's sign) should reproduce the symptoms, and discrete tenderness should be evident in the area of the nerve low in the occipital region. Local anesthetic can be infiltrated around the nerve as a diagnostic procedure.

Pain Related to Leptomeningeal Metastases

Leptomeningeal metastases (LM) occur when tumor cells infiltrate the arachnoid and the pia mater (leptomeninges), causing focal or multifocal infiltration. LM develop in approximately 5–8% of patients with non-Hodgkin lymphoma and up to 70% of patients with leukemia. Adenocarcinomas are the most common solid tumors causing LM, including, in decreasing order of frequency, breast, lung, melanoma, and gastrointestinal cancers. Untreated primary central nervous system tumors, such as medulloblastoma, ependymoma, and glioblastoma multiforme also have a high frequency of leptomeningeal seeding. The clinical features of LM are referable to the cerebrum, cranial nerves, and spinal nerve roots. Features of cranial nerve involvement, in order of frequency, are oculomotor palsies, facial weakness, hearing loss, vision loss, facial numbness, and tongue deviation. Headache and encephalopathy are common. Pain is the initial symptom in 25% of patients, and may occur in 40% of patients with LM infiltration.[36,37] In most cases the pain is a dull, constant headache and may be one of two types: either with or without neck stiffness and back pain, the latter usually localizing to the lower back and buttocks. The pain results from traction on tumor-infiltrated nerves in the meninges. A clue that cranial nerve involvement is secondary to LM rather than to epidural tumor at the base of the brain is that multiple cranial nerves are usually affected. If the involvement is bilateral, it is even more likely that the pathology lies in the subarachnoid space rather than at the base of the brain.

CT continues to be used as a screening tool in the metastatic work-up for many cancer patients, but it is relatively insensitive compared to MRI, particularly in the detection of LM. MRI depicts LM well, particularly when magnetization transfer or post-contrast T1-weighted or FLAIR techniques are used.[38] Examination of the CSF is the most important test for LM. Only 3% of initial lumbar punctures yield normal CSF, but positive cytology is seen on initial CSF examination in 54% of LM patients, and the yield increases to above 90% when three separate spinal taps are performed.[39] The best yield is obtained when the CSF is taken from the symptomatic area. LM should be suspected when headaches are posturally induced or occur upon awakening, especially in cancer patients with normal CT or MR scans.

Pain Syndromes Caused by Tumors of the Skull Base in Children

Skull base tumors in the pediatric population differ from adult tumors in a number of aspects, including surgical considerations and epidemiologic differences.[40] The surgeon must consider carefully the different anatomy and the involvement of growth centers in children. In addition, a better prognosis is often reported for children compared to adults with skull base tumors. In part, this may be a result of a higher rate of complete resection, as tissue planes are reportedly better defined in children. Also contributing to the better prognosis is the high proportion of childhood tumors which are benign. In the pediatric population, there are proportionately fewer skull base lesions than adults, and more males (69%) than females are affected. In the anterior cranial fossa, esthesioneuroblastoma are often seen. Tumors common in the middle cranial fossa include craniopharyngioma and in contrast to adults, juvenile nasopharyngeal angiofibroma. Most posterior cranial fossa tumors such as meningioma, schwannoma, epidermoid, cholesteatoma, chordoma, and chondrosarcoma are more common in adults, whereas other rare tumors, such as Ewing's sarcoma, are more common in children. Ewing's sarcoma is a primitive neuroectodermal tumor that involves the pediatric skull base. Cholesteatomas are tumors with stratified squamous epithelium and keratinous debris derived from the sloughing epithelium, and are categorized as congenital or acquired. Chordomas and chondrosarcomas are typically slow-growing, locally invasive tumors.

Medical and Surgical Patient Management and Risks

Skull-base tumors are usually managed by surgery, radiation therapy (fractionated external beam or stereotactically focused), or careful observation in follow-up. Chemotherapy has been proven to be effective only for certain malignant tumors such as nasopharyngeal carcinomas, Ewing's sarcoma, lymphomas, and some benign tumors such as prolactinomas.[41] Risk of cranial-base surgery includes injury to the cranial nerve, neurovascular structures (stroke), infections, CSF leakage, and brain or brainstem injury. The highest surgical risks are associated with skull base meningiomas because of the nature of the invasion in the perineurium of the cranial nerves and adventitia of the arteries. In regard to location, cavernous sinus tumors are associated with a 30% risk of cranial nerve deficits. The incidence of CSF leak in skull-base surgery is reported to be 5–28%. Fractionated external beam radiation therapy shows considerable success in managing paragangliomas, meningiomas, and radio-sensitive tumors such as lymphomas. Better success is obtained with radiosurgery or stereotactic radiotherapy, which consists of delivering a high dose of radiation in single or multiple fractions to an accurately localized small target volume. In managing high-grade malignant tumors, radiotherapy is a central part of treatment modalities. Tumor size, involvement of multiple foci, invasion of the pia mater (edema of the brain), encasement of arteries, and prior radiotherapy are known to be important factors in predicting surgical outcome and complication rates.

REFERENCES

1. Curtin HD, Chavali R: Imaging of the skull base. Radiol Clin North Am 36: 801–817, 1998.
2. Boerman RH, Maassen EM, Joosten J, et al: Trigeminal neuropathy secondary to perineural invasion of head and neck carcinomas. Neurology 53:213–216, 1998.
3. Vecht CJ, Hoff AM, Kansen PJ, et al: Types and causes of pain in cancer of the head and neck. Cancer 70:178–184, 1992.
4. Regan JM, Peng P: Neurophysiology of cancer pain. Cancer Control 7:111–119, 2000.
5. Bernstein M, Berger M: Neuro-Oncology: The Essentials. New York, Thieme, 2000, pp. 419–433.
6. Stark AM, Eichmann T, Mehdorn HM: Skull metastases: Clinical features, differential diagnoses and review of the literature. Surg Neurol 60:219–226, 2003.
7. West MS, Russell EJ, Breit R, et al: Calvarial and skull base metastases: Comparison of non-enhanced and Gd-DTPA-enhanced MR images. Radiology 174:85–91, 1990.
8. Jansen BP, Pillay M, de Bruin HG, et al: 99mTc SPECT in the diagnosis of skull base metastasis. Neurology 48:1326–1330, 1997.
9. Bulsara KR, Fukushima T, Friedman AH: Management of malignant tumors of the anterior skull base: Experience with 76 patients. Neurosurg Focus 13, Article 5, 2002.
10. Obeid F, Al-Mefty O: Recurrence of olfactory groove meningiomas. Neurosurgery 53: 534–542, 2003.
11. Dulguerov P, Calcaterra T: Esthesioneuroblastoma: The UCLA Experience 1970-1990. Laryngoscope 102:843–849, 1992.
12. Bradley PJ, Jones NS, Robertson I: Diagnosis and management of esthesioneuroblastoma. Curr Opin Otolaryngol Head Neck Surg 11:112–118, 2003.
13. Greenberg HS, Deck MD, Vikram B, et al: Metastases to the base of the skull: Clinical findings in 43 patients. Neurology 31: 530–537, 1981.
14. Holland D, Maune S, Kovacs G, et al: Metastatic tumors of the orbit: A retrospective study. Orbit 22:15–24, 2003.

15. Kline LB, Hoyt WF: The Tolosa-Hunt syndrome. J Neurol Neurosurg Psychiatry 71:577–582, 2001.
16. Majos C, Coll S, Aguilera C, et al: Imaging of giant pituitary adenomas. Neuroradiology 40:651–655, 1998.
17. Kelly JB, Payne R: Pain syndromes in a cancer patient. Neurol Clin 9:937–953, 1991.
18. Johnston J: Parasellar syndromes. Curr Neurol Neurosci Rep 2:423–431, 2002.
19. Spell DW, Gervais DS, Ellis JK, et al: Cavernous sinus syndrome due to metastatic renal cell carcinoma. South Med J 91:576–579, 1998.
20. Yi HJ, Kim CH, Bak KH, et al: Metastatic tumors in the sellar and parasellar regions: Clinical review of four cases. J Korean Med Sci 15:363–367, 2000.
21. Eldevik OP, Gabrielson TO, Jacobson EA: Am J Neuroradiol 21:1139–1144, 2000.
22. Lossos A, Siegal T: Numb chin syndrome in cancer patients: Etiology, response to treatment, and prognostic significance. Neurology 42:1181–1184, 1992.
23. Brown J: Mechanism of cancer invasion of the mandible. Curr Opin Otolaryngol Head Neck Surg 11:96–102, 2003.
24. Keane JR: Combined VIth and XIIth cranial nerve palsies: A clival syndrome. Neurology 54:1540–1541, 2000.
25. St. Martin M, Levine SC: Chordomas of the skull base: Manifestations and management. Curr Opin Otolaryngol Head Neck Surg 11:324–327, 2003.
26. Lanzino G, Dumont AS, Lopes BM, et al: Skull-based chordomas: Overview of disease, management options, and outcome. Neurosurg Focus 10 Article 12, 2001.
27. Capobianco JD, Brazis WP, Rubino AF, et al: Occipital condyle syndrome. Headache 42:142–146, 2002.
28. Moris G, Roig C, Misiego M, et al: The distinctive headache of the occipital condyle syndrome: A report of four cases. Headache 38:308–311, 1998.
29. Marzo SJ, Leonetti JP, Petruzzelli G: Facial paralysis caused by malignant skull base neoplasms. Ear Nose Throat J 81:845–849, 2002.

30. Paparounas K, Gotsi A, Apostolou F, et al: Collet-Sicard syndrome disclosing glomus tumor of the skull base. Eur Neurol 49: 103–105, 2003.
31. Prashant R, Franks A: Collet-Sicard syndrome: A report and review. Lancet Oncol 4:376–377, 2003.
32. Bilsky MH, Shannon F, Sheppard S, et al: Diagnosis and management of a metastatic tumor in the atlantoaxial spine. Spine 27: 1062–1069, 2002.
33. Cheng TM, Cascino TL, Onofrio BM: Comprehensive study of diagnosis and treatment of trigeminal neuralgia secondary to tumors. Neurology 43:2298–2302, 1993.
34. Bongers KM, Willigers MM, Koehler PJ: Referred facial pain from lung carcinoma. Neurology 42:1841–1842, 1992.
35. MacDonald DR, Strong E, Nielsen S, et al: Syncope from head and neck cancer. J Neurooncol 1:257–267, 1983.
36. Balm M, Hammack J: Leptomeningeal carcinomatosis: Presenting features and prognostic factors. Arch Neurol 53: 626–632, 1996.
37. Kaplan JG, DeSouza TG, Farkash A, et al: Leptomeningeal metastases: comparison of clinical features and laboratory data of solid tumors, lymphomas, and leukemias. J Neurooncol 9:225–229, 1990.
38. Nemzek WR, Hecht S, Gandour-Edwards R, et al: Perineural spread of head and neck tumors: How accurate is MR imaging? Am J Neuroradiol 19:701–706, 1998.
39. Wasserstrom WR, Glass JP, Posner JB: Diagnosis and treatment of leptomeningeal metastases from solid tumors: Experience with 90 patients. Cancer 49:759–772, 1982.
40. Tsai EC, Santoreneos S, Rutka J: Tumors of the skull base in children: Review of tumors and types and management of strategies. Neurosurg Focus 12: Article 1, 2002.
41. Jacob HE: Chemotherapy for cranial base tumors. J Neurooncol 20:327–335, 1994.

CHAPTER 6

Pain Due to Epidural Metastases and Spinal Cord Compression

MIRJANA LOVRINCEVIC, MD

There are two proposed mechanisms by which epidural metastases and spinal cord compression occur: Hematogenic spread to bone marrow that leads to vertebral body collapse and epidural mass formation; and direct tumor invasion through the intervertebral foramina, from a paravertebral source (Figures 6–1 and 6–2).[1] Most epidural spinal cord compressions come from a solid tumor metastasis (lung, breast, prostate, kidney) to the vertebral body, which spreads posteriorly to the epidural space. Other tumors (lymphomas, neuroblastomas) invade the epidural space per continuitatem. Untreated, epidural metastases with spinal cord compression lead inevitably to neurologic damage, including paraplegia. The most important prognostic factor is the degree of neurologic injury at the time of presentation: 75% of patients who begin treatment while ambulatory remain ambulatory; the success of treatment declines to 30% to 50% in patients who are paretic on presentation and to 10% to 20% in patients who present plegic.[2] Virtually all patients with confirmed epidural metastases experience pain at some time during the course of the disease, and in a striking 10% of cases back pain is the only symptom at the time of diagnosis. The treatment of epidural metastases with spinal cord compression involves the administration of corticosteroids, radiation therapy, or surgical decompression.[3]

CLINICAL PRESENTATION

Pain is the predominant symptom in most patients with epidural metastatic disease. When back pain and radiculopathy or myelopathy occur in the setting of known malignancy, the diagnosis is generally straightforward. However, in about 20% of cases, spinal cord compression is the initial manifestation of the disease.[4] Radicular pain is usually unilateral in the cervical and lumbosacral regions and bilateral in the thorax, where it is often experienced as a tight band around the chest or abdomen.[5] Lhermitte's

sign is very suggestive of epidural extension of the disease, although these electric shock-like sensations that spread down the spine usually occur in patients with multiple sclerosis, cervical spondylotic myelopathy, cisplatin neurotoxicity, cervical radiation injury, and neck trauma.[6] A sudden onset of pain with minimal trauma or applied force to the vertebrae may indicate a pathologic fracture: Weakened bony fragments invade the epidural space or nerve roots giving rise to dysesthesias that follow dermatomal pattern. Local pain over the involved vertebral body is exacerbated with the recumbency, while the radicular pain gets worse with increases in intraspinal pressure (straining, coughing, sneezing).

After a period of progressive pain, weakness, sensory loss, autonomic dysfunction, and reflex abnormalities develop. Certain spinal tracts appear to be more vulnerable to compression than the others. Because the corticospinal tracts and posterior columns are particularly vulnerable, weakness, spasticity, and hyperreflexia tend to be the earliest signs. Spinothalamic tracts and descending autonomic fibers are less vulnerable, so loss of pain and temperature sensation and bowel and bladder function occur later in course of the disease.[7] The rate of the progression of the disease is variable, and the prognosis for the neurologic recovery depends on the time interval from the initial presentation of symptoms to the institution of treatment. Studies have shown that the likelihood of regaining ambulation increased if treatment began less than 12 h after loss of ambulation, and if patients had bladder and bowel function and sacral sensory sparing.[8]

DIAGNOSTIC INVESTIGATIONS

The initial evaluation of patients with symptoms suggestive of metastatic epidural disease includes plain radiographic examination. Although useful for demonstrating a destructive lesion, they do not reliably rule out

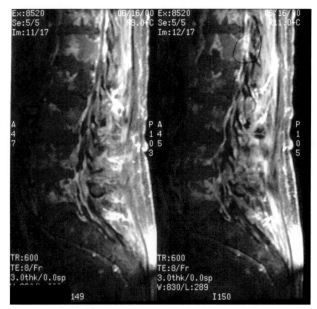

FIGURE 6–1   Hematogenic spread to bone marrow that leads to vertebral body collapse and epidural mass formation.

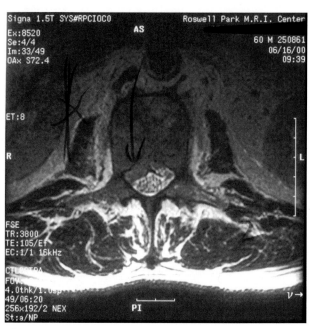

FIGURE 6–2   Direct tumor invasion from a paravertebral source.

the presence of the epidural engagement. When destructive changes are present, they may include loss of visualization of the pedicle, osteolysis of vertebral body with or without collapse, spinous process erosion, and elevation of soft tissue shadows. Plain radiographs are especially important in patients with a history of a cancer, in whom the possibility of metastatic disease must be strongly considered. However, the bone may not be sufficiently damaged to change the radiograph, or the tumor may involve the epidural space with little or no involvement of the adjacent bone, such as occurs in patients with lymphoma in strikingly more than 60% of the time.[9]

For patients with known primary cancer, bone scintigraphy is an excellent screening test for identifying metastatic disease. Although lacking specificity and ability to provide detailed anatomic description of the area that is being investigated, bone scanning is useful in detection of a high bone turnover state. Computed tomography alone or in combination with myelography allows direct visualization of the bone anatomy and spinal canal. Magnetic resonance imaging (MRI) is, however, a preferred method because it is noninvasive and offers accurate soft tissue imaging and multiplanar views. In addition to its convenience, ability to visualize the entire spine regardless of complete subarachnoid block, and superiority to myelography in demonstrating bone and intramedullary lesions, make it a study of choice for patients without contraindications.[10] MRI can provide direct evidence of cord compression and the degree of spinal stenosis present based on the intrinsic contrast effect of the high signal intensity cerebrospinal fluid on T2 weighted imaging. Metastatic lesions to the vertebral bodies

replace normal marrow fat with tumor tissue, which can be detected on MR scanning. The use of gadolinium on T1 weighted images may further enhance differentiation between normal and pathologic processes.

MANAGEMENT

The treatment of patients with epidural metastases and spinal cord compression requires an aggressive multidisciplinary approach (Table 6-1). When recommendations for the type of treatment are being made, several factors need to be taken into consideration: spinal stability, neurologic compromise, sensitivity of the tumor to radiation and chemotherapy, amount of pain, and overall prognosis.

Radiation therapy is the preferred form of treatment when the patient presents with severe pain or neurologic

TABLE 6–1 Treatment Options for Epidural Metastases and Spinal Cord Compression
Radiation therapy
• External beam radiation
• Brachytherapy
Surgery
• Decompression (anterior, posterior, combined)
• Stabilization
Chemotherapy
• Alone
• Adjuvant

deficit and without the evidence of bony instability. Primary tumor needs to be radiosensitive, and adequate manipulation of the dosage and fractionation of the delivered radiation needs to be done. There are numerous radiation dosage protocols, but no consensus about the ideal regimen. Current controversy surrounds the issue of using radiotherapy prior to surgery. The studies have shown that spinal radiation before surgical decompression for metastatic spinal cord compression is associated with a significantly higher major wound complication rate, in addition to adversely affecting surgical outcome,[11] while postoperative radiation does not have major effects on the healing, if it is delayed for 3 to 6 weeks after surgery.

Intraoperative paraspinal brachytherapy using 125I has also shown good results in a large population of patients with malignant tumors resulting in spinal cord compression.[12] Permanent 125I seeds in absorbable suture are placed with open exposure after resection in this, generally well-tolerated procedure, resulting in durable local control and ambulatory function. Brachytherapy might be used with or without external beam radiotherapy.

Surgery is indicated in case of progressive neurologic deficit during or after radiation therapy, intractable pain unresponsive to conservative treatment, need for histologic diagnosis, radioresistant tumors, and spinal instability or vertebral collapse, with or without neurologic deficit. Survival time is one factor that must be considered. Although no absolute value has been established, a minimum life expectancy of 3 to 6 months has been accepted as a prerequisite for surgery.[13] Surgical treatment usually involves anterior, posterior, or combined decompression and stabilization procedures. Palliative laminectomy with total or subtotal tumor reduction results in amelioration of motor function, pain, and continence and significantly improves the patients' quality of life in all but severe cases.[14]

Chemotherapy alone is an alternative to surgery or radiation therapy in the management of epidural metastases with spinal cord compression from chemosensitive tumors such as lymphoma, myeloma, breast, prostate, or germ cell tumors. It can also be used as an adjuvant. Response has been shown in both adults and children.[15-17] Patients, however, should be monitored closely so that early signs of neurologic injury can be recognized and emergency treatment instituted.

PAIN TREATMENT OPTIONS

Pain treatment options are summarized in Table 6-2. Opioid analgesics are the mainstay of therapy for any cancer pain. When the epidural metastatic disease is diagnosed, it is very likely that patients have been exposed to some of them before. However, in case of an occasional

TABLE 6–2 Pain Treatment Options
Oral and Parenteral Analgesia
• Steroids
• Opioids
• Adjuvants (tricyclic antidepressants, antiepileptics)
Transcutaneous Delivery Systems
Patient-Controlled Analgesia
Neuraxial Analgesia

opioid-naive patient, the following principles should be followed:

- Know the pharmacology of a few drugs and use them first
- Administer drugs at regular intervals; give the next dose before the effect of the previous dose has diminished
- "As needed" administration should be avoided except to treat breakthrough pain
- The therapeutic goal should be titration of the dose until a pain-free state is achieved
- If one drug is ineffective, a stronger or different one should be prescribed
- Use adjuvant drugs early and when necessary, especially in presence of radiculopathy
- Do not confuse tolerance or physiologic dependence with addiction

Medications and dosages that can be administered intrathecally are listed in Table 6-3. High-dose steroid protocol is often used in the acute stages of cord compression. Steroids have been shown to reduce edema, relieve the pain, and help preserve neurologic function.[18,19] The use of dexamethasone as the steroid of choice for treatment of spinal epidural metastases is based in part on the low mineralocorticoid activity of dexamethasone and in part on tradition. One of the common regimens is dexamethasone 100 mg intravenous bolus followed by 24 mg orally four times daily for 3 days, then tapered

TABLE 6–3 Medications and Their Doses Used Intrathecally	
Morphine	1–23.5 mg/day
Hydromorphone	0.5–25 mg/day
Fentanyl	60–775 µcg/day
Sufentanil	10–100 µcg/day
Clonidine	55–800 µcg/day
Bupivacaine	5–30 mg/day

over 10 days. It has been reported that administration of intravenous dexamethasone reduced pain levels within 3 h for patients with spinal epidural metastases who had complete blockade on myelography.[20] Lower-dose regimens are indicated in patients without neurologic deficits, and they usually consist of dexamethasone 10 mg intravenous bolus followed by 4 mg intravenously four times daily, then tapered over 14 days.

Adjuvant therapy includes different medications that are combined with analgesics to potentiate their effect, to provide inherent analgesic action, and to improve mood, sleep, nausea, anxiety, or somnolence.[21] Considering the epidural metastatic disease and spinal cord compression typical presentation, we will mention tricyclic antidepressants and antiepileptics. Tricyclic antidepressants have been indicated to treat neuropathic pain syndromes, especially dysesthesias. Tertiary amines (amitriptyline, doxepine) are often used as a first line of therapy because of their greater analgesic effect. If excessive sedation is an issue, a secondary amine (desipramine, nortriptyline) would be more appropriate. Antiepileptics are particularly useful in treatment of lancinating, shooting, electrical shock-like pain and paroxysmal dysesthesias. Gabapentin and oxcarbazepine have been shown to be effective in neuropathic pain unresponsive to carbamazepine, clonazepam, or phenytoin.[22]

The development of long-acting controlled-release transcutaneous opioid analgesic, fentanyl, has revolutionized pain management in cancer patients. The continuous mode of administration made possible by this formulation permits blood and cerebrospinal fluid (CSF) opioid concentrations to be sustained, so that peak and trough effects are minimized. Patients do not experience recurrent pain at the end of a dosing interval, which is the case in administration of drug on an as needed basis.

Patient-controlled analgesia allows the patient, by means of programmable pump, to self-administer predetermined boluses of opioids at a minimum time interval, until satisfactory analgesia is reached. The intravenous route is the most commonly prescribed, but intramuscular, subcutaneous, and epidural routes have also been used. All pumps permit the use of a baseline infusion, which eliminates frequent patient usage. Patient-controlled analgesia has found its place in managing acute pain, such as in epidural metastatic disease with spinal cord compression, where rapid relief and titration of dosage is needed.[23]

When the pain control cannot be adequately controlled anymore with oral or parenteral medications, or when severe side effects develop that preclude their further use, the epidural/intrathecal route is considered.[24,25] When opioids alone are used, profound analgesia is achieved at a much lower dose, without the motor, sensory, or sympathetic block associated with intrathecal local anesthetic administration. However, in cancer patients the presence of neuropathic pain is the most frequent reason to use an intrathecal technique, and the addition of a local anesthetic, clonidine, or both is necessary to achieve adequate pain control. Combinations of low-dose opioid with local anesthetic or clonidine act synergistically to produce effective analgesia while decreasing the side effects of compounds.[26]

Neuropathic pain associated with compression of spinal cord and exiting nerve roots can be extraordinarily difficult to manage in spite of all measures mentioned previously. Some studies have shown that epidural metastases were associated with refractory pain in approximately 70% of this patient population[27] where "refractory" means that the pain dominates the patient's life totally, other methods fail to provide acceptable pain relief, and the patients are intolerant to or have unacceptable side effects from opioids.

As epidural and intrathecal analgesia using opioids in combination with local anesthetics or clonidine can often control neuropathic pain associated with cancer that does not respond to systemic opioids or adjuvant analgesics, this approach was presumed to be effective in painful epidural metastatic disease as well. Imaging studies in those patients, especially MRI, can help in planning catheter placement.[28] Tumor involvement of the posterior bony elements of the spinal canal or the posterior aspect of the epidural space can be clearly seen and avoided, since spinal or epidural catheter placement directly through areas of tumor may lead to sudden neurologic deterioration due to bleeding into the tumor, spinal cord, and subarachnoid spaces. The occurrence and severity of complications during insertion of epidural or intrathecal catheters are related to the location of the tumor, its relation to the puncture site, and the degree of spinal canal stenosis. Commonly encountered complications include the need for multiple attempts to achieve dural puncture, likely due to reduction of the posterior subarachnoid space or tumorous infiltration of the dura; aspiration of bloody CSF, probably due to accidental puncture of the tumor located in the path of the needle; aspiration of air bubbles from the catheter, usually encountered in the presence of only a thin layer of CSF in the subarachnoid space so that air bubbles are drawn out into the catheter through the holes of the catheter tip; catheter occlusion, which occurs more commonly in cancer patients treated with epidural then intrathecal catheter, secondary to extravasation of blood proteins and formation of fibrin in the epidural space after accidental tumor puncture. The major complication of epidural or intrathecal pain management in this patient population is neurologic deterioration after catheterization and it occurred only in patients with spinal canal stenosis.

REFERENCES

1. Loeser JD, Butler SH, Chapman CR, Turk DC: Bonica's Management of Pain, 3rd ed. Philadelphia, Lippincott, Williams & Wilkins, 2001.
2. Wall PD, Melzack R: Textbook of Pain, 4th ed. Edinburgh, Churchill-Livingstone, 1999.
3. Greenberg HS, Kim J, Posner JB: Epidural spinal cord compression from metastatic tumor: Results with a new treatment protocol. Ann Neurol 8:361–366, 1980.
4. Schiff D, O'Neill BP, Suman VJ: Spinal epidural metastasis as the initial manifestation of malignancy: Clinical features and diagnostic approach. Neurology 49(2): 452–456, 1997.
5. Jenis LG, Dunn EJ, Howard SA: Metastatic disease of the cervical spine: A review. Clin Orthoped Relat Res 359:89–103, 1999.
6. Newton HB, Rea GL: Lhermitte's sign as a presenting symptom of primary spinal cord tumor. J Neuro-Oncol 29:183–188, 1996.
7. Tarlov IM: Acute spinal cord compression paralysis. J Neurosurg 36:10–20, 1972.
8. Zaidat OO, Ruff RL: Treatment of spinal epidural metastasis improves patient survival and functional state. Neurology 58:1360–1366, 2002.
9. Haddad P, Thaell JF, Kiely JM, Harrison EG, et al: Lymphoma of the spinal extradural space. Cancer 38:1862–1866, 1976.
10. Schiff D, O'Neill BP, Wang CH, O'Fallon JR: Neuroimaging and treatment implications of patients with multiple epidural spinal metastases. Cancer 83:1593–1601, 1998.
11. Ghogawala Z, Mansfield FL, Borges, Lawrence F: Spinal radiation before surgical decompression adversely affects outcomes of surgery for symptomatic metastatic spinal cord compression. Spine 26: 818–824, 2001.
12. Rogers CL, Theodore N, Dickman CA, et al: Surgery and permanent 125I seed paraspinal brachytherapy for malignant tumors with spinal cord compression. Int J Radiat Oncol Biol Phys 54:505–513, 2002.
13. Wise JJ, Fischgrund JS, Herkowitz HN, et al: Complications, survival rates, and risk factors of surgery for metastatic disease of the spine. Spine 24:1943, 1999.
14. Schoeggl A, Reddy M, Matula C: Neurological outcome following laminectomy in spinal metastases. Spinal Cord 40:363–366, 2002.
15. Mora J, Wollner N: Primary epidural non-Hodgkin lymphoma: Spinal cord compression syndrome as the initial form of presentation in childhood non-Hodgkin lymphoma. Med Pediatr Oncol 32: 102–105, 1999.
16. Pashankar FD, Steinbok P, Blair G, Pritchard S: Successful chemotherapeutic decompression of primary endodermal sinus tumor presenting with severe spinal cord compression. J Pediatr Hematol Oncol 23: 170–173, 2001.
17. De Bernardi B, Pianca C, Pistamiglio P, et al: Neuroblastoma with symptomatic spinal cord compression at diagnosis: Treatment and results with 76 cases. J Clin Oncol 19:183–190, 2001.
18. Abrahm JL: Management of pain and spinal cord compression on patients with advanced cancer. Ann Intern Med 131: 37–46, 1999.
19. Sorensen S, Helweg-Larsen S, Mouridsen H, Hansen HH: Effect of high-dose dexamethasone in carcinomatous metastatic spinal cord compression treated with radiotherapy: A randomized trial. Eur J Cancer 30A:22–27, 1994.
20. Vecht CJ, Haaxma-Reiche H, Van Putten WLJ, et al: Initial bolus of conventional versus high-dose dexamethasone in metastatic spinal cord compression. Neurology 39:1255–1257, 1989.
21. Hewitt DJ, Portenoy RK: Adjuvant drugs for neuropathic cancer pain. In: Topics in Palliative Care. vol 2. Bruera E, Portenoy RK, eds. New York, Oxford University Press, 1998, pp 41–61.
22. Caraceni A, Zecca E, Martini C, De Conno F: Gabapentin as an adjuvant to opioid analgesia for neuropathic cancer pain. J Pain Symptom Manage 17:441–445, 1999.
23. Ferrel BR, Nash CC, Warfield CC: The role of patient-controlled analgesia in the management of cancer pain. J Pain Symptom Manage 7:149–154, 1992.
24. Miguel R: Interventional treatment of cancer pain: The fourth step in the World Health Organization Analgesic Ladder? Cancer Control 7:149–156, 2000.
25. Lema MJ: Invasive analgesia techniques for advanced cancer pain. Surg Oncol Clin North Am 1:127–136, 2001.
26. Hassenbuch SJ, Portenoy RK: Current practices in intraspinal therapy: A survey of clinical trends and decision making. J Pain Symptom Manage 20:S4–S11, 2000.
27. Appelgren I, Nordborg C, Sjoberg M, et al: Spinal epidural metastasis: Implications for spinal analgesia to treat "refractory" cancer pain. J Pain Symp Manage 13: 25–42, 1997.
28. Rathmel JP, Roland T, Du Pen SL: Management of pain associated with metastatic epidural spinal cord compression: Use of imaging studies in planning epidural therapy. Reg Anes Pain Med 25:113–116, 2000.

CHAPTER 7

Pain Due to Bone Metastases: New Research Issues and Their Clinical Implications

PATRICK W. MANTYH, PhD

Recently, the first animal models of bone cancer pain have been developed. In the mouse femur model, bone cancer pain is induced by injecting murine osteolytic sarcoma cells into the intramedullary space of the femur (Figure 7–1).[1] Critical to this model is ensuring that the tumor cells are confined within the marrow space of the injected femur and that they do not invade adjacent soft tissues, which would directly affect the joints of the muscle, making behavioral analysis problematic.[2,3] Following injection the tumor cells proliferate, and ongoing, movement-evoked, and mechanically evoked pain-related behaviors develop that increase in severity with time (Table 7–1). These pain behaviors correlate with the progressive tumor-induced bone destruction that ensues, which appears to mimic the condition in patients with primary or metastatic bone cancer. These models have allowed us to gain mechanistic insights into how cancer pain is generated and how the sensory information it initiates is processed as it moves from sense organ to the cerebral cortex under a constantly changing molecular architecture. As detailed later, these insights promise to fundamentally change the way cancer pain is controlled.

PRIMARY AFFERENT SENSORY NEURONS

Primary afferent sensory neurons are the gateway by which sensory information from peripheral tissues is transmitted to the spinal cord and brain (Figure 7–2), and these neurons innervate the skin and every internal organ of the body, including mineralized bone, marrow, and periosteum. The cell bodies of sensory fibers that innervate the head and body are housed in the trigeminal and dorsal root ganglia, respectively, and can be divided into two major categories: myelinated A fibers and smaller-diameter unmyelinated C fibers. Nearly all large-diameter myelinated A beta fibers normally conduct non-noxious stimuli applied to the skin, joints, and muscles, and thus these large sensory neurons usually do not

conduct noxious stimuli.[4] In contrast, most small-diameter sensory fibers—unmyelinated C fibers and finely myelinated A fibers—are specialized sensory neurons known as nociceptors, whose major function is to detect environmental stimuli that are perceived as harmful and convert them into electrochemical signals that are then transmitted to the central nervous system (CNS). Unlike primary sensory neurons involved in vision or olfaction, which are required to detect only one type of sensory stimulus (light or chemical odorants, respectively), individual primary sensory neurons of the pain pathway have the remarkable ability to detect a wide range of stimulus modalities, including those of physical and chemical nature.[5,6] To accomplish this, nociceptors express an extremely diverse repertoire of transduction molecules that can sense forms of noxious stimulation (thermal, mechanical, and chemical), albeit with varying degrees of sensitivity.

The past few years have seen remarkable progress toward understanding the signaling mechanisms and specific molecules that nociceptors use to detect noxious stimuli. For example, the vanilloid receptor TRPV1 (formerly known as VR1), which is expressed by most nociceptors, detects heat[7] and also appears to detect extracellular protons[8-10] and lipid metabolites.[11,12] To detect noxious mechanical stimuli, nociceptors express mechanically gated channels that initiate a signaling cascade on excessive stretch.[13] The cells also express several purinergic receptors capable of sensing adenosine triphosphate (ATP), which may be released from cells on excessive mechanical stimulation.[14,15]

To sense noxious chemical stimuli, nociceptors express a complex array of receptors capable of detecting inflammation-associated factors released from damaged tissue. These factors include protons,[8,9] endothelins,[16] prostaglandins,[17] bradykinin,[17] and nerve growth factor.[18] Aside from providing promising targets for the development of more selective analgesics, identification of receptors expressed on the nociceptor surface has increased our

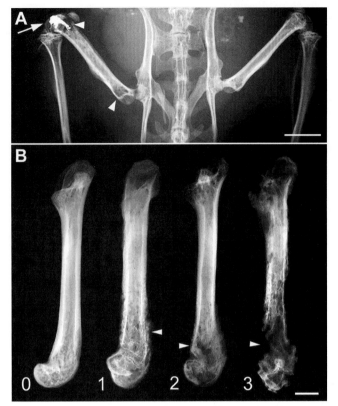

FIGURE 7–1   Progressive destruction of mineralized bone in mice with bone cancer. (*A*) Low-power anterior-posterior radiograph of mouse pelvis and hindlimbs after a unilateral injection of sarcoma cells into the distal part of the femur and closure of the injection site with an amalgam plug (arrow), which prevents the tumor cells from growing outside the bone.[2] Radiographs of murine femora (*B*) show the progressive loss of mineralized bone caused by tumor growth. These images are representative of the stages of bone destruction in the murine femur. At week 1 there is a minor loss of bone near the distal head (arrow); at week 2, substantial loss of mineralized bone at both the proximal and distal (arrow) heads; and at week 3, loss of mineralized bone throughout the entire femur and fracture of distal head (arrow). Scale bar: 2 mm. (*Modified from Schwei MJ, Honore P, Rogers SD, et al: Neurochemical and cellular reorganization of the spinal cord in a murine model of bone cancer pain. J Neurosci 19[24]:10886–10897, 1999.*)

understanding of how different tumors generate cancer pain in the peripheral tissues they invade and destroy.

In addition to expressing channels and receptors that detect tissue injury, sensory neurons are highly "plastic" in that they can change their phenotype in the face of a sustained peripheral injury. Following tissue injury, sensory neuron subpopulations alter patterns of signaling peptide and growth factor expression.[19] This change in phenotype of the sensory neuron in part underlies peripheral sensitization, whereby the activation threshold of nociceptors is lowered so that a stimulus that would normally be mildly noxious is perceived as highly noxious (hyperalgesia). Damage to a peripheral tissue also activates previously "silent" or "sleeping"

nociceptors, which then become highly responsive both to normally non-noxious stimuli (allodynia) and to noxious stimuli (hyperalgesia).

There are several examples of nociceptors that undergo peripheral sensitization in experimental cancer models.[1-3] In normal mice, the neurotransmitter substance P is synthesized by nociceptors and released in the spinal cord in response to a noxious, but not to a non-noxious, palpation of the femur. In mice with bone cancer, normally non-painful palpation of the affected femur induces the release of substance P from primary afferent fibers that terminate in the spinal cord. Substance P in turn binds to and activates the neurokinin-1 receptor that is expressed by a subset of spinal cord neurons.[20,21] Similarly, normally non-noxious palpation of tumor-bearing limbs of mice with bone cancer also induces the expression of c-fos protein in spinal cord neurons. In normal animals that do not have cancer, only noxious stimuli will induce the expression of c-fos in the spinal cord.[22] Thus, peripheral sensitization of nociceptors appears to be involved in the generation and maintenance of bone cancer pain.

PROPERTIES OF TUMORS THAT EXCITE NOCICEPTORS

Tumor cells and tumor-associated cells that include macrophages, neutrophils, and T-lymphocytes secrete a wide variety of factors that sensitize or directly excite primary afferent neurons (see Figure 7–2). These include prostaglandins,[23,24] endothelins,[16,25] interleukins 1 and 6,[26-28] epidermal growth factor,[29] transforming growth factor,[30,31] and platelet-derived growth factor.[32-34] Receptors for many of these factors are expressed by primary afferent neurons. Each of these factors may play an important role in generating pain in particular forms of cancer, and therapies that block two of these factors, prostaglandins and endothelins, are currently approved for use in patients with other (noncancer) indications.

Prostaglandins are proinflammatory lipids that are formed from arachidonic acid by the action of cyclooxygenase (COX) and other downstream synthetases. There are two distinct forms of the COX enzyme, COX-1 and COX-2. Prostaglandins are involved in the sensitization or direct excitation of nociceptors by binding to several prostanoid receptors.[35] Several tumor cells and tumor-associated macrophages express high levels of COX-2 and produce large amounts of prostaglandins.[36-40]

The COX enzymes are a major target of current medications, and COX inhibitors are commonly administered for reducing both inflammation and pain. A major problem with using COX inhibitors such as aspirin or ibuprofen to block cancer pain is that these compounds inhibit both COX-1 and COX-2, and inhibition of the constitutively expressed COX-1 can cause bleeding

TABLE 7–1 Mechanically Evoked Pain-Related Behaviors in the Murine Femur Model of Bone Cancer Pain

Pain Behavior	Naive	Sham	Sarcoma		
			day 6	day 10	day 14
I. Ongoing Plan					
• Guarding (sec) over 2-min observation period	0.4 ± 0.2	1.4 ± 0.5	2.1 ± 0.5	4.3 ± 0.8	15.2 ± 3.3
• Flinches (count) over 2-min observation period	1.7 ± 0.7	3.1 ± 0.7	7.7 ± 1.6	13.0 ± 2.0	24.5 ± 3.8
II. Movement-Evoked Pain					
A. AMBULATORY PAIN					
• Forced ambualtion on rotarod (score) 5 (normal) to 0 (impaired)	4.7 ± 0.3	4.4 ± 0.3	3.8 ± 0.4	2.5 ± 0.3	2.3 ± 0.3
• Limb use during normal ambulation (score) 4 (normal) to 0 (impaired)	4.0 ± 0.0	3.9 ± 0.1	3.7 ± 0.2	3.5 ± 0.3	2.7 ± 0.3
B. PALPATION-EVOKED PAIN (over 2-min. period)					
• Guarding (sec) following nonpainful palpation	0.4 ± 0.4	1.4 ± 0.5	1.9 ± 0.6	7.1 ± 0.6	18.1 ± 4.0
• Flinches (count) following nonpainful palpation	2.0 ± 1.2	3.1 ± 1.7	7.0 ± 2.1	19.0 ± 1.1	30.5 ± 5.1

☐ $P < 0.05$ vs. sham

From Honore P, Rogers SD, Schwei MJ, et al: Murine models of inflammatory, neuropathic and cancer pain each generates a unique set of neurochemical changes in the spinal cord and sensory neurons. Neuroscience 98(3):585–598, 2000.

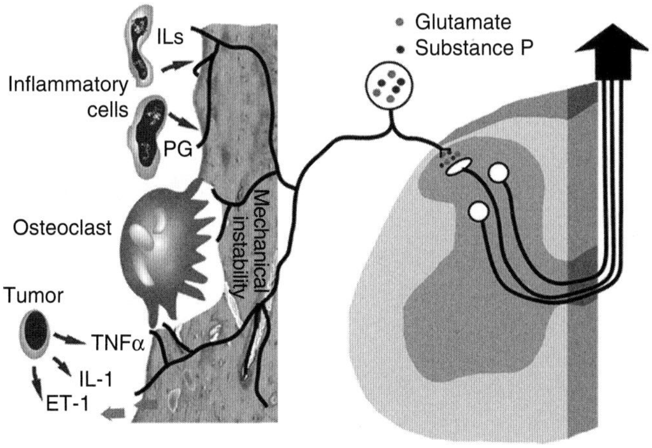

FIGURE 7–2 Sensory neurons and detection of noxious stimuli due to tumor cells. Nociceptors use a diversity of signal-transduction mechanisms to detect noxious physiologic stimuli, and many of these mechanisms may be involved in driving cancer pain. Thus, when nociceptors are exposed to products of tumor cells, tissue injury, or inflammation, their excitability is altered and this nociceptive information is relayed to the spinal cord and then to higher centers of the brain. Some of the mechanisms that appear to be involved in generating and maintaining cancer pain include activation of nociceptors by factors such as extracellular protons (+), endothelin-1 (ET-1), interleukins (ILs), prostaglandins (PG), and tumor necrosis factor (TNF).

and ulcers. In contrast, the new COX-2 inhibitors, or coxibs, preferentially inhibit COX-2 and avoid many of the side effects of COX-1 inhibition, which may allow their use in treating cancer pain. Other experiments have suggested that COX-2 is involved in angiogenesis and tumor growth,[41,42] so in cancer patients, in addition to blocking cancer pain, COX-2 inhibitors may have the added advantage of reducing the growth and metastasis of the tumor. COX-2 antagonists show significant promise for alleviating at least some aspects of cancer pain, although clearly more research is required to fully define the actions of COX-2 in different types of cancer.

A second pharmacologic target for treating cancer pain is the peptide endothelin-1 (Figure 7–3). Several tumors, including prostate cancer, express high levels of endothelins,[16,43,44] and clinical studies have reported a correlation between the severity of the pain in patients with prostate cancer and plasma levels of endothelins.[45] Endothelins could contribute to cancer pain by directly sensitizing or exciting nociceptors, given that a subset of small unmyelinated primary afferent neurons express receptors for endothelin.[46] Direct application of endothelin to peripheral nerves activates primary afferent fibers and induces pain behaviors.[47] Like prostaglandins, endothelins that are released from tumor cells are also

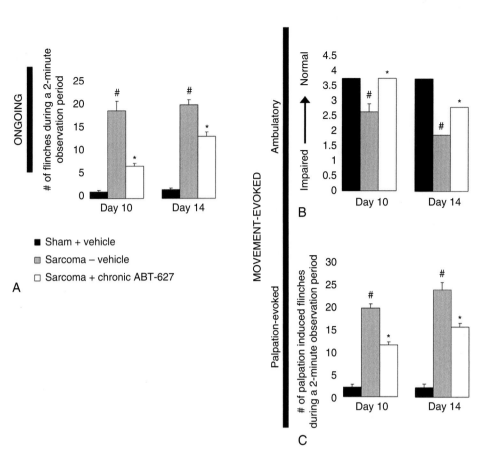

FIGURE 7–3   Selective ET_AR inhibition attenuates ongoing and movement-evoked bone cancer pain behaviors. The number of spontaneous flinches of the cancerous limb over a 2-minute observation period was used as a measure of ongoing pain (*A*). Parameters of movement-evoked pain include assessment of the sarcoma-bearing limb during normal ambulation in an open field (*B*). Quantification of the number of flinches evoked by normally non-noxious palpation of the sarcoma-bearing limb over a 2-minute observation period following palpation was used as a measure of palpation-evoked pain (*C*). All pain behaviors were significantly reduced 10 and 14 days after sarcoma injection with chronic administration of ABT-627 beginning at 6 days after sarcoma injection: bars, ± SEM. # $P <$ 0.05 versus sham; *$P <$ 0.05 versus sarcoma + vehicle group. Note that the ability of chronic ET_AR inhibition to attenuate ongoing pain was significantly reduced from day 10 to day 14 postsarcoma injection.

thought to be involved in regulating angiogenesis[48] and tumor growth,[49] suggesting again that endothelin antagonists may be useful not only in inhibiting cancer pain but in reducing the growth and metastasis of the tumor.

TUMOR-INDUCED RELEASE OF PROTONS AND ACIDOSIS

Tumor cells become ischemic and undergo apoptosis as the tumor burden exceeds its vascular supply.[50] Local acidosis, a state in which an accumulation of acid metabolites is present, is a hallmark of tissue injury.[6,51] In the past few years the concept that sensory neurons can be directly excited by protons or acidosis has generated intense research and clinical interest. Studies have shown that subsets of sensory neurons express different acid-sensing ion channels.[6,52] The two major classes of acid-sensing ion channels expressed by nociceptors are TRPV1[11,53] and the acid-sensing ion channel-3 (ASIC-3).[52,54,55] Both these channels are sensitized and excited by a decrease in pH. More specifically, TRPV1 is activated when the pH falls below 6.0, whereas the pH that activates ASIC-3 appears to be highly dependent on the coexpression of other ASIC channels in the same nociceptor.[56]

There are several mechanisms by which a decrease in pH could be involved in generating and maintaining cancer pain. As tumors grow, tumor-associated inflammatory cells invade the neoplastic tissue and release protons that generate local acidosis.[50] A second mechanism by which acidosis may occur is apoptosis of the tumor cells. Release of intracellular ions may generate an acidic environment that activates signaling by acid-sensing channels expressed by nociceptors.

Tumor-induced release of protons and acidosis may be particularly important in the generation of bone cancer pain. In both osteolytic (bone-destroying) and osteoblastic (bone-forming) cancers there is a significant proliferation and hypertrophy of osteoclasts.[57] Osteoclasts are terminally differentiated, multinucleated cells of the monocyte lineage that are uniquely designed to resorb bone by maintaining an extracellular microenvironment of acidic pH (4.0 to 5.0) at the interface between osteoclast and mineralized bone.[58] Studies have shown significant expression of ASIC[52] and TRPV1[11,59] in peptidergic afferent fibers, and we have localized peptidergic fibers in bone marrow and cortical bone.[60] This evidence suggests that exposure of these sensory fibers to the osteoclast's acidic extracellular microenvironment could activate resident proton-sensitive ion channels, stimulating pain sensation. Recent experiments in a murine

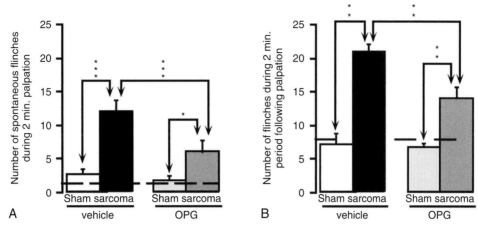

FIGURE 7–4 Attenuation of bone cancer pain by osteoprotegerin (OPG). Histograms show that administration of OPG beginning 6 days after tumor implantation attenuated both (*A*) spontaneous and (*B*) palpation-evoked pain in mice at day 17 following tumor implantation. OPG is a naturally occurring protein that is a secreted decoy receptor that inhibits osteoclast differentiation, proliferation, and hypertrophy, resulting in reduced osteoclast activity and bone resorption. *(Honore P, Luger NM, Sabino MA, et al: Osteoprotegerin blocks bone cancer-induced skeletal destruction, skeletal pain and pain-related neurochemical reorganization of the spinal cord. Nat Med 6:521–528, 2000.)*

model of bone cancer pain reported that osteoclasts play an essential role in cancer-induced bone loss, and that osteoclasts contribute to the etiology of bone cancer pain.[3,61] Recent work has shown that osteoprotegerin[61] and a bisphosphonate,[62,63] both of which are known to induce osteoclast apoptosis, are effective in decreasing osteoclast-induced bone cancer pain (Figure 7-4). Similarly, TRPV1 or ASIC antagonists may be used to reduce pain in patients with soft tumors or bone cancer by blocking excitation of the acid-sensitive channels on sensory neurons.

RELEASE OF GROWTH FACTORS BY TUMOR CELLS

One of the most important discoveries in the past decade has been the demonstration that the biochemical and physiological status of sensory neurons is maintained and modified by factors derived from the innervated tissue. Changes in the periphery associated with inflammation, nerve injury, or tissue injury are mirrored by changes in the phenotype of sensory neurons[64] After peripheral nerve injury, expression of a subset of neurotransmitters and receptors by damaged sensory neurons is altered in a highly predictable fashion. These changes are caused, in part, by a change in the tissue level of several growth factors released from the environment local to the injury site, including nerve growth factors (NGF)[65-67] and glial-derived neurotrophic factor (GDNF).[68,69] These neurochemical changes can be reversed in a receptor-specific fashion by intrathecal or peripheral application of NGF or GDNF.[70-73]

Although the level of NGF expression reportedly correlates with the extent of pain in pancreatic cancer,[74,75] relatively little is known about how other tumors affect the synthesis and release of growth factors. However, one certainty is that the repertoire of growth factors to which the sensory neuron is exposed will change as the developing tumor invades the peripheral tissue that the neuron innervates. Thus, in addition to a disruption of the growth factors normally released by the intact peripheral tissue, one can expect release of a variety of additional growth factors by tumor cells as well as by tumor-infiltrating leukocytes, which can comprise up to 80% of the total tumor mass.[76] Activated leukocytes synthesize and release high levels of several growth factors,[29-34,77,78] and thus one would expect a significant change in the phenotype and response characteristics of the sensory neurons following tumor invasion of a peripheral organ.

Although tumor growth alters the invaded tissue, it is also clear that the affected tissue influences the phenotype of the invading tumor cell.[79] Because the local environment can influence the molecules that tumor cells express and release, it follows that the same tumor in the same individual may be painful at one site of metastasis but not at another. Clinical observations reveal that pain from cancer can be quite perplexing because the size, location, or type of cancer tumor does not necessarily predict symptoms. Different patients with the same cancer may have vastly different symptoms. Kidney cancer may be painful in one person and asymptomatic in another. Metastases to bone in the same individual may cause pain at the site of a rib lesion, but not at that of a humeral lesion. Small cancer deposits in bone may be very painful, whereas large soft-tissue cancers may be painless.[80] Important areas for future research include identification of tissue-specific mechanisms of cancer pain, comparing soft tissue with bone and site-specific mechanisms, comparing flat bones (ribs) with tubular bones (femurs). It will also be of interest to determine patient-specific factors that influence disease progression and its relationship to pain perception.

TUMOR-INDUCED DISTENSION AND DESTRUCTION OF SENSORY FIBERS

In general, previous reports have suggested that tumors are not highly innervated by sensory or sympathetic neurons.[81-83] However, in many cancers, rapid tumor growth frequently entraps and injures nerves, causing mechanical injury, compression, or ischemia or direct proteolysis.[84] Proteolytic enzymes produced by the tumor can also injure sensory and sympathetic fibers, causing neuropathic pain.

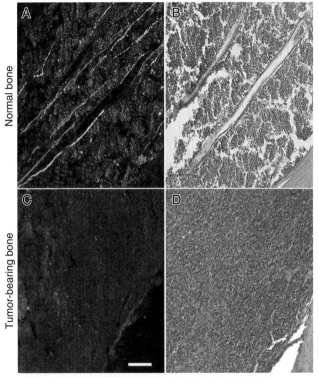

FIGURE 7–5   Sensory nerve fibers in the marrow of the mouse femur are destroyed by invading sarcoma tumor cells. Confocal (*A* and *C*) images show calcitonin gene related peptide (CGRP, green) and neurofilament-200 (RT-97, red) and serially adjacent sections (*B* and *D*) stained with hematoxylin and eosin in the normal (*A* and *B*) and tumor-bearing (*C* and *D*) marrow. In the normal marrow CGRP and RT-97 expressing sensory fibers are generally associated with the vasculature, whereas 14 days following injection and confinement of the tumor cells to the marrow space few if any CGRP or RT-97 expressing sensory fibers can be detected. Scale bar = 150 μm.

The capacity of a tumor to injure and destroy peripheral nerve fibers has been directly observed in an experimental model of bone cancer. Following injection and containment of lytic murine sarcoma cells in the intramedullary of the mouse femur, tumor cells grow in the marrow space and disrupt innervating sensory fibers (Figures 7–5 and 7–6). As the tumor cells grow they first compress and then destroy both the hematopoietic cells of the marrow and the sensory fibers that normally innervate the marrow, mineralized bone, and periosteum.[1]

Although the mechanisms by which any neuropathic pain is generated and maintained are still not well understood, several therapies that have proven useful in the control of other types of neuropathic pain may also be useful in treating tumor-induced neuropathic pain. For example, gabapentin, which was originally developed as an anticonvulsant but whose mechanism of action remains unknown, is effective in treating several forms of neuropathic pain and may also be useful in treating cancer-induced neuropathic pain.[85]

CENTRAL SENSITIZATION IN CANCER PAIN

A critical question is whether the spinal cord and forebrain also undergo significant neurochemical changes as a chronic cancer pain state develops. The murine cancer pain model revealed extensive neurochemical reorganization within spinal cord segments that receive input from primary afferent neurons innervating the cancerous bone.[3,86] These changes included astrocyte hypertrophy (Figure 7–7) and up-regulation of the prohyperalgesic peptide dynorphin. Spinal cord neurons that normally would only be activated by noxious stimuli were activated by non-noxious stimuli. These spinal cord changes were attenuated by blocking the tumor-induced tissue destruction and pain.[3,86] Together, these neurochemical changes suggest that cancer pain induces and is at least partially maintained by a state of central sensitization, in which an increased transmission of nociceptive information allows normally non-noxious input to be amplified and perceived as noxious stimuli.

Once nociceptive information has been transmitted to the spinal cord by primary afferent neurons, it can travel via multiple ascending "pain" pathways that project from the spinal cord to higher centers of the brain. Classically, the main emphasis in examining the ascending conduction of pain has been placed on spinothalamic tract neurons. However, data from recent clinical studies have necessitated a reassessment of this position by showing significant attenuation of some forms of difficult-to-control visceral cancer pain following lesion of the axons of non-spinothalamic tract neurons.[87,88] Together these data suggest that one reason that cancer pain is frequently

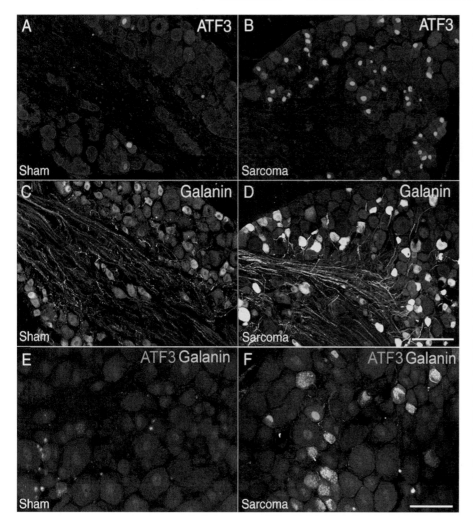

FIGURE 7–6   Tumor-induced destruction of sensory nerve fibers in the tumor-bearing bone results in the up-regulation of activated transcription factor-3 (ATF-3) and galanin in the cell body of sensory neurons that innervate the tumor-bearing femur. Neurons in the normal L2 dorsal root ganglia express low levels of both ATF-3 (*A*) or the neuropeptide galanin (*C*) whereas 14 days following injection and confinement of sarcoma cells to the marrow space there is a marked up-regulation of both ATF-3 and galanin in sensory neurons in the L2 dorsal root ganglia ipsilateral to the tumor-bearing bone. Many sensory neurons which show an up-regulation of galanin in response to tumor-induced destruction of sensory fibers in the bone also show up-regulation of ATF-3 in their nucleus (compare *E* with *F*). These data suggest that as tumor cells invade the bone sensory nerve fibers that normally innervate the bone are destroyed with a resulting generation of the neurochemical signature of neuropathy in sensory neurons that innervate the tumor-bearing bone. Scale bar = 100 μm. *(Modified from Luger NM, Honore P, Sabino MAC, et al: Osteoprotegerin diminishes advanced bone cancer pain. Cancer Res 61:4038–4047, 2001.)*

perceived as such an intense and disturbing pain is that it ascends to higher centers of the brain via multiple parallel neuronal pathways. Importantly for cancer patients, many of whom frequently experience anxiety or depression, it is clear that higher centers of the brain can modulate the ascending conduction of pain. Descending pathways that modulate the ascending conduction of cancer pain may play an important role in either enhancing or inhibiting the patient's perception of pain. The general mood and attention of the patient thus may be significant factors in determining the pain's intensity and degree of unpleasantness.

A CHANGING SET OF FACTORS MAY DRIVE CANCER PAIN WITH DISEASE PROGRESSION

Cancer pain frequently becomes more severe as the disease progresses, and adequate control of cancer pain becomes more difficult to achieve without encountering significant unwanted side effects.[89-91] Although tolerance may contribute to the escalation of the dose of analgesics required to control cancer pain, a compatible possibility is that with the progression of the disease, different factors assume a greater importance in driving cancer pain. For example, in the mouse model of bone cancer, as tumor cells first begin to proliferate, pain-related behaviors start to occur long before any significant bone destruction is evident. This pain may be due to prohyperalgesic factors such as prostaglandins and endothelin that are released by the growing tumor cells and subsequently activate nociceptors in the marrow. Pain at this stage might be attenuated by COX-2 inhibitors and endothelin antagonists. As the tumor continues to grow, sensory neurons innervating the marrow are compressed and destroyed, causing a neuropathic pain to develop that may best respond to treatment with drugs such as gabapentin that are known to attenuate noncancer–induced neuropathic pain. When the tumor begins to induce proliferation and hypertrophy of osteoclasts,[92,93] the pain due to excessive osteoclast activity might be largely blocked by antiosteoclastogenic drugs such as bisphosphonates or osteoprotegerin (see Figure 7–4). As the tumor cells completely fill the intramedullary space, tumor cells begin to die, generating an acidic environment;

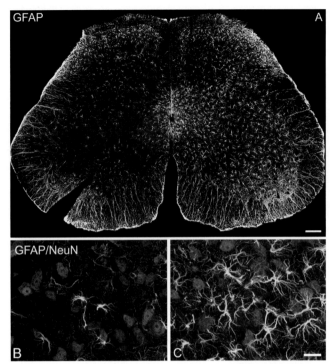

FIGURE 7–7   Cancer-induced reorganization of the central nervous system. Chronic cancer pain not only sensitizes peripheral nociceptors, but also can induce significant neurochemical reorganization of the spinal cord. This reorganization may participate in the phenomenon of central sensitization, that is, an increased responsiveness of spinal cord neurons involved in transmission of pain. (A) Confocal image of a coronal section of the mouse L4 spinal cord showing glial fibrillary acidic protein (GFAP) positive astrocytes (white) which have undergone hypertrophy on the side ipsilateral to the tumor-bearing bone. B and C show higher magnification of the ipsilateral and contralateral dorsal horn seen in A, with colocalization of the neuron-specific antibody NeuN. Note that although the astrocytes (spindle-shaped cells) have undergone a massive hypertrophy, there does not appear to be any significant loss of NeuN positive neurons. Scale bars: A, 200 μm; B and C, 30 μm. *(Modified from Schwei MJ, Honore P, Rogers SD, et al: Neurochemical and cellular reorganization of the spinal cord in a murine model of bone cancer pain. J Neurosci 19:10886–10897, 1999.)*

antagonists to TRPV1 or ASICs may attenuate the pain induced by this acidosis. Finally, as bone destruction compromises the mechanical strength of the bone, antagonists that block the mechanically gated channels and ATP receptors in the richly innervated periosteum may attenuate movement-evoked pain.

Although this pattern of tumor-induced tissue destruction and nociceptor activation may be unique to bone cancer, an evolving set of nociceptive events probably occurs in other cancers. This complex pattern may in part explain why cancer pain is frequently difficult to treat and why it is so heterogeneous in nature and severity.[94,95] Changes in tumor-induced tissue injury, in nociceptor activation, and in the brain areas involved in transmitting these nociceptive signals as the disease progresses suggest that different therapies will be efficacious at particular stages of the disease.[96-100] Understanding how tumor cells differentially excite nociceptors at different stages of the disease, and how the phenotype of nociceptors and CNS neurons involved in nociceptive transmission change as the disease progresses, should allow a mechanistic approach to designing more effective therapies to treat cancer pain.

FUTURE DIRECTIONS

For the first time, animal models of cancer pain are available that mirror the clinical picture of patients with cancer pain. Information generated from these models should elucidate the mechanisms that generate and maintain different types of cancer pain. Many of these cancer models have been developed in mice and rats, but implantation of human tumors in immunocompromised rodent strains should allow examination of the pain that different human tumors generate. These animal models may also offer insight into one of the major conundrums of cancer pain: that the severity of cancer pain is variable from patient to patient, from tumor to tumor, and even from site to site. Newer molecular techniques using microarrays and proteomics should reveal which specific features of different tumors are important in inducing cancer pain. Once we have determined the mechanisms by which the different types of cancer induce pain, we can identify molecular targets and develop mechanism-based therapies. Ultimately, the key will be to integrate information about tumor biology and the host's response to neoplasia with our understanding of how chronic pain is generated and maintained. These studies should improve the quality of life of all those who suffer from cancer pain.

ACKNOWLEDGMENTS

Supported by National Institutes of Health grants from the National Institute of Neurologic Disorders and Stroke (NS23970) and the National Institute for Drug Abuse (DA11986), National Institute of Dental and Craniofacial Research Dentist Scientist Award (DSA) DE00270 and training grant DE07288, and a merit review from the Veterans Administration.

REFERENCES

1. Schwei MJ, Honore P, Rogers SD, et al: Neurochemical and cellular reorganization of the spinal cord in a murine model of bone cancer pain. J Neurosci 19: 10886–10897, 1999.

2. Honore P, Luger NM, Sabino MA, et al: Osteoprotegerin blocks bone cancer-induced skeletal destruction, skeletal pain and pain-related neurochemical reorganization of the spinal cord. Nat Med 6: 521–528, 2000.

3. Luger NM, Honore P, Sabino MAC, et al: Osteoprotegerin diminishes advanced bone cancer pain. Cancer Res 61:4038–4047, 2001.

4. Djouhri L, Bleazard L, Lawson SN: Association of somatic action potential shape with sensory receptive properties in guinea-pig dorsal root ganglion neurones. J Physiol 513(Pt 3):857–872, 1998.

5. Basbaum AI, Jessel TM: The perception of pain. In: Kandel ER, Schwartz JH, Jessell TM (eds): Principles of Neural Science. New York, McGraw-Hill, 2000, pp 472–490.

6. Julius D, Basbaum AI: Molecular mechanisms of nociception. Nature 413:203–210, 2001.

7. Kirschstein T, Greffrath W, Busselberg D, Treede RD: Inhibition of rapid heat responses in nociceptive primary sensory of rats by vanilloid receptor antagonists. J Neurophysiol 82:2853–2860, 1999.

8. Bevan S, Geppetti P: Protons: Small stimulants of capsaicin-sensitive sensory nerves. Trends Neurosci 17:509–512, 1994.

9. Caterina MJ, Leffler A, Malmberg AB, et al: Impaired nociception and pain sensation in mice lacking the capsaicin receptor. Science 288:306–313, 2000.

10. Welch JM, Simon SA, Reinhart PH: The activation mechanism of rat vanilloid receptor 1 by capsaicin involves the pore domain and differs from the activation by either or heat. Proc Natl Acad Sci USA 97:13889–13894, 2000.

11. Tominaga M, Caterina MJ, Malmberg AB, et al: The cloned capsaicin receptor integrates multiple pain-producing stimuli. Neuron 21:531–543, 1998.

12. Nagy I, Rang H: Noxious heat activates all capsaicin-sensitive and also a sub-population of capsaicin-insensitive dorsal root ganglion neurons. Neuroscience 88:995–997, 1999.

13. Price MP, McIlwrath SL, Xie JH, et al: The DRASIC cation channel contributes to the detection of cutaneous touch and acid stimuli in mice. Neuron 32:1071–1083, 2001.

14. Krishtal OA, Marchenko SM, Obukhov AG: Cationic channels activated by extracellular ATP in rat sensory neurons. Neuroscience 27:995–1000, 1988.

15. Xu GY, Huang LYM: Peripheral inflammation sensitizes P2X receptor-mediated responses in dorsal root ganglion neurons. J Neurosci 22:93–102, 2002.

16. Nelson JB, Carducci MA: The role of endothelin-1 and endothelin receptor antagonists in prostate cancer. BJU Int 85 (suppl 2):45–48, 2000.

17. Alvarez FJ, Fyffe RE: Nociceptors for the 21st century. Curr Rev Pain 4:451–458, 2000.

18. McMahon SB: NGF as a mediator of inflammatory pain. Philos Trans R Soc Lond B Biol Sci 351:431–440, 1996.

19. Woolf CJ, Salter MW: Neuronal plasticity: Increasing the gain in pain. Science 288:1765–1769, 2000.

20. Mantyh PW, DeMaster E, Malhotra A, et al: Receptor endocytosis and dendrite reshaping in spinal neurons after somatosensory stimulation. Science 268:1629–1632, 1995.

21. Hunt SP, Mantyh PW: The molecular dynamics of pain control. Nat Rev Neurosci 2:83–91, 2001.

22. Hunt SP, Pini A, Evan G: Induction of c-fos-like protein in spinal cord neurons following sensory stimulation. Nature 328:632–634, 1987.

23. Nielsen OS, Munro AJ, Tannock IF: Bone metastases: Pathophysiology and management policy. J Clin Oncol 9:509–524, 1991.

24. Galasko CS: Diagnosis of skeletal metastases and assessment of response to treatment. Clin Orthop 64–75, 1995.

25. Davar G: Endothelin-1 and metastatic cancer pain. Pain Med 2:24–27, 2001.

26. Watkins LR, Goehler LE, Relton J, et al: Mechanisms of tumor necrosis factor-alpha (TNF-alpha) hyperalgesia. Brain Res 692:244–250, 1995.

27. Leskovar A, Moriarty LJ, Turek JJ, et al: The macrophage in acute neural injury: Changes in cell numbers over time and levels of cytokine production in mammalian central and peripheral nervous systems. J Exp Biol 203:1783–1795, 2000.

28. Opree A, Kress M: Involvement of the proinflammatory cytokines tumor necrosis factor-alpha, IL-1 beta, and IL-6 but not IL-8 in the development of heat hyperalgesia: Effects on heat-evoked calcitonin gene-related peptide release from rat skin. J Neurosci 20:6289–6293, 2000.

29. Stoscheck CM, King Jr LE: Role of epidermal growth factor in carcinogenesis. Cancer Res 46:1030–1037, 1986.

30. Poon RT, Fan ST, Wong J: Clinical implications of circulating angiogenic factors in cancer patients. J Clin Oncol 19:1207–1225, 2001.

31. Roman C, Saha D, Beauchamp R: TGF-beta and colorectal carcinogenesis. Microsc Res Tech 52:450–457, 2001.

32. Daughaday WH, Deuel TF: Tumor secretion of growth factors. Endocrinol Metab Clin North Am 20:539–563, 1991.

33. Radinsky R: Growth factors and their receptors in metastasis. Semin Cancer Biol 2:169–177, 1991.

34. Silver BJ: Platelet-derived growth factor in human malignancy. Biofactors 3:217–227, 1992.

35. Vasko MR: Prostaglandin-induced neuropeptide release from spinal cord. Prog Brain Res 104:367–380, 1995.

36. Dubois RN, Radhika A, Reddy BS, Entingh AJ: Increased cyclooxygenase-2 levels in carcinogen-induced rat colonic tumors. Gastroenterology 110:1259–1262, 1996.

37. Molina MA, Sitja-Arnau M, Lemoine MG, et al: Increased cyclooxygenase-2 expression in human pancreatic carcinomas and cell lines: Growth inhibition by nonsteroidal anti-inflammatory drugs. Cancer Res 59:4356–4362, 1999.

38. Kundu N, Yang QY, Dorsey R, Fulton AM: Increased cyclooxygenase-2 (COX-2) expression and activity in a murine model of metastatic breast cancer. Int J Cancer 93:681–686, 2001.

39. Ohno R, Yoshinaga K, Fujita T, et al: Depth of invasion parallels increased cyclooxygenase-2 levels in patients with gastric carcinoma. Cancer 91:1876–1881, 2001.

40. Shappell SB, Manning S, Boeglin WE, et al: Alterations in lipoxygenase and cyclooxygenase-2 catalytic activity and mRNA expression in prostate carcinoma. Neoplasia 3:287–303, 2001.

41. Masferrer JL, Leahy KM, Koki AT, et al: Antiangiogenic and antitumor activities of cyclooxygenase-2 inhibitors. Cancer Res 60:1306–1311, 2000.

42. Moore BC, Simmons DL: COX-2 inhibition, apoptosis, and chemoprevention by nonsteroidal anti-inflammatory drugs. Curr Med Chem 7:1131–1144, 2000.

43. Shankar A, Loizidou M, Aliev G, et al: Raised endothelin 1 levels in patients with colorectal liver metastases. Br J Surg 85:502–506, 1998.

44. Kurbel S, Kurbel B, Kovacic D, et al: Endothelin-secreting tumors and the idea of the pseudoectopic hormone secretion in tumors. Med Hypotheses 52:329–333, 1999.

45. Nelson JB, Hedican SP, George DJ, et al: Identification of endothelin-1 in the pathophysiology of metastatic adenocarcinoma of the prostate. Nat Med 1:944–999, 1995.

46. Pomonis JD, Rogers SD, Peters CM, et al: Expression and localization of endothelin receptors: Implication for the involvement of peripheral glia in nociception. J Neurosci 21:999–1006, 2001.

47. Davar G, Hans G, Fareed MU, et al: Behavioral signs of acute pain produced by application of endothelin-1 to rat sciatic nerve. Neuroreport 9:2279–2283, 1998.

48. Dawas K, Laizidou M, Shankar A, et al: Angiogenesis in cancer: The role of endothelin-1. Ann R Coll Surg Engl 81:306–310, 1999.

49. Asham EH, Loizidou M, Taylor I: Endothelin-1 and tumour development. Eur J Surg Oncol 24:57–60, 1998.

50. Helmlinger G, Sckell A, Dellian M, et al: Acid production in glycolysis-impaired tumors provides new insights into tumor metabolism. Clin Cancer Res 8:1284–1291, 2002.

51. Reeh PW, Steen KH: Tissue acidosis in nociception and pain. Prog Brain Res 113: 143–151, 1996.

52. Olson TH, Riedl MS, Vulchanova L, et al: An acid sensing ion channel (ASIC) localizes to small primary afferent neurons in rats. Neuroreport 9:1109–1113, 1998.

53. Caterina MJ, Schumacher MA, Tominaga M, et al: The capsaicin receptor: A heat-activated ion channel in the pain pathway. Nature 389:816–824, 1997.

54. Bassilana F, Champigny G, Waldmann R, et al: The acid-sensitive ionic channel subunit ASIC and the mammalian degenerin MDEG form a heteromultimeric H+-gated Na+ channel with novel properties. J Biol Chem 272:28819-28822, 1997.

55. Sutherland S, Cook S, Ew M: Chemical mediators of pain due to tissue damage and ischemia. Prog Brain Res 129:21-38, 2000.

56. Lingueglia E, Weille JR, Bassilana F, et al: A modulatory subunit of acid sensing ion channels in brain and dorsal root ganglion cells. J Biol Chem 272:29778-29783, 1997.

57. Clohisy DR, Perkins SL, Ramnaraine ML: Review of cellular mechanisms of tumor osteolysis. Clin Orthop Res 104-114, 2000.

58. Delaisse J-M, Vaes G: Mechanism of mineral solubilization and matrix degradation in osteoclastic bone resorption. In Rifkin BR, Gay CV (ed): Biology and Physiology of the Osteoclast. Ann Arbor, CRC, 1992, pp 289-314.

59. Guo A, Vulchanova L, Wang J, et al: Immunocytochemical localization of the vanilloid receptor 1 (VR1): Relationship to neuropeptides, the P2X3 purinoceptor and IB4 binding sites. Eur J Neurosci 11: 946-958, 1999.

60. Mach DB, Rogers SD, Sabino MC, et al: Origins of skeletal pain: Sensory and sympathetic innervation of the mouse femur. J Neurosci 113:155-166.

61. Honore P, Menning PM, Rogers SD, et al: Neurochemical plasticity in persistent inflammatory pain. Prog Brain Res 129:357-363, 2000.

62. Fulfaro F, Casuccio A, Ticozzi C, Ripamonti C: The role of bisphosphonates in the treatment of painful metastatic bone disease: A review of phase III trials. Pain 78:157-169, 1998.

63. Mannix K, Ahmedazai SH, Anderson H, et al: Using bisphosphonates to control the pain of bone metastases: Evidence based guidelines for palliative care. Palliat Med 14:455-461, 2000.

64. Honore P, Rogers SD, Schwei MJ, et al: Murine models of inflammatory, neuropathic and cancer pain each generates a unique set of neurochemical changes in the spinal cord and sensory neurons. Neuroscience 98:585-598, 2000.

65. Fu SY, Gordon T: The cellular and molecular basis of peripheral nerve regeneration. Mol Neurobiol 14:67-116, 1997.

66. Koltzenburg M: The changing sensitivity in the life of the nociceptor. Pain (suppl 6): S93-102, 1999.

67. Fukuoka T, Kondo E, Dai Y, et al: Brain-derived neurotrophic factor increases in the uninjured dorsal root ganglion neurons in selective spinal nerve ligation model. J Neurosci 21:4891-4900, 2001.

68. Boucher TJ, McMahon SB: Neurotrophic factors and neuropathic pain. Curr Opin Pharmacol 1:66-72, 2001.

69. Hoke A, Gordon T, Zochodne DW, Sulaiman OA: A decline in glial cell-line-derived neurotrophic factor expression is associated with impaired regeneration after long-term Schwann cell denervation. Exp Neurol 173:77-85, 2002.

70. Bennett DL, French J, Priestley JV, McMahon SB: NGF but not NT-3 or BDNF prevents the A fiber sprouting into lamina II of the spinal cord that occurs following axotomy. Mol Cell Neurosci 8:211-220, 1996.

71. Bennett DL, Michael GJ, Ramachandran N, et al: A distinct subgroup of small DRG cells express GDNF receptor components and GDNF is protective for these neurons after nerve injury. J Neurosci 18:3059-3072, 1998.

72. Boucher TJ, Okuse K, Bennett DL, et al: Potent analgesic effects of GDNF in neuropathic pain states. Science 290: 124-127, 2000.

73. Ramer MS, Priestley JV, McMahon SB: Functional regeneration of sensory axons into the adult spinal cord. Nature 403: 312-316, 2000.

74. Zhu ZW, Friess H, diMola FF, et al: Nerve growth factor expression correlates with perineural invasion and pain in human pancreatic cancer. J Clin Oncol 17: 2419-2428, 1999.

75. Schneider MB, Standop J, Ulrich A, et al: Expression of nerve growth factors in pancreatic neural tissue and pancreatic cancer. J Histochem Cytochem 49:1205-1210, 2001.

76. Zhang F, Lu W, Dong Z: Tumor-infiltrating macrophages are involved in suppressing growth and metastasis of human prostate cancer cells by INF-beta gene therapy in nude mice. Clin Cancer Res 8:2942-2951, 2002.

77. Leon A, Buriani A, Dal Toso R, et al: Mast cells synthesize, store, and release nerve growth factor. Proc Natl Acad Sci USA 91:3739-3743, 1994.

78. Caroleo MC, Costa N, Bracci-Laudiero L, Aloe L: Human monocyte/macrophages activate by exposure to LPS overexpress NGF and NGF receptors. J Neuroimmunol 113:193-201, 2001.

79. Mundy GR: Metastases to bone: Causes, consequences, and therapeutic opportunities. Nat Rev Cancer 2:584-593, 2002.

80. Mantyh PW, Clohisy DR, Koltzenburg M, Hunt SP: Molecular mechanisms of cancer pain. Nat Rev Cancer 2:201-209, 2002.

81. O'Connell JX, Nanthakumar SS, Nielsen GP, Rosenberg AE: Osteoid osteoma: The uniquely innervated bone tumor. Modern Pathol 11:175-180, 1998.

82. Seifert P, Spitznas M: Tumours may be innervated. Virchows Archiv 438: 228-231, 2001.

83. Terada T, Matsunaga Y: S-100-positive nerve fibers in hepatocellular carcinoma and intrahepatic cholangiocarcinoma: an immunohistochemical study. Pathol Int 51: 89-93, 2001.

84. Mercadante S: Malignant bone pain: Pathophysiology and treatment. Pain 1997; 69:1-18, 1997.

85. Ripamonti C, Dickerson ED: Strategies for the treatment of cancer pain in the new millennium. Drugs 61:955-977, 2001.

86. Honore P, Schwei J, Rogers SD, et al: Cellular and neurochemical remodeling of the spinal cord in bone cancer pain. Prog Brain Res 129:389-397, 2000.

87. Willis WD, Al-Chaer ED, Quast MJ, Westlund KN: A visceral pain pathway in the dorsal column of the spinal cord. Proc Natl Acad Sci USA 1999; 96:7675-7679.

88. Nauta HJW, Soukup VM, Fabian RH, et al: Punctate midline myelotomy for the relief of visceral cancer pain. J Neurosurg 92 (suppl 2S):125-130.

89. Payne R. Practice guidelines for cancer pain therapy. Issues pertinent to the revision of national guidelines. Oncology 12:169-175, 1998.

90. Foley KM: Advances in cancer pain. Arch Neurol 56:413-417, 1999.

91. Portenoy RK, Lesage P: Management of cancer pain. Lancet 353:1695-1700, 1999.

92. Clohisy DR, Ramnaraine ML, Scully S, et al: Osteoprotegerin inhibits tumor-induced osteoclastogenesis and bone growth in osteopetrotic mice. J Orthop Res 18: 967-976, 2000b.

93. Clohisy DR, O'Keefe PF, Ramnaraine ML: Pamidronate decreases tumor-induced osteoclastogenesis in mice. J Orthop Res 19:554-558, 2001.

94. Coyle NJ, Adelhardt KM, Foley KM, Portenoy RK: Character of terminal illness in the advanced cancer patient: Pain and other symptoms during the last four weeks of life. J Pain Symptom Manage 5: 83-93, 1990.

95. de Wit R, van Dam F, Loonstra S, et al: The Amsterdam Pain Management Index compared to eight frequently used outcome measures to evaluate the adequacy of pain treatment in cancer patients with chronic pain. Pain 91:339-349, 2001.

96. Mercadante S, Arcuri E: Breakthrough pain in cancer patients: Pathophysiology and treatment. Cancer Treat Rev 24: 425-432, 1998.

97. Meuser T, Pietruck C, Radbruch L, et al: Symptoms during cancer pain treatment following WHO guidelines: A longitudinal follow-up study of symptom prevalence, severity and etiology. Pain 93:247-257, 2001.

98. Payne R: Mechanisms and management of bone pain. Cancer 80(suppl 8): 1608-1613, 1997.

99. Payne R, Mathias SD, Pasta DJ, et al: Quality of life and cancer pain: Satisfaction and side effects with transdermal fentanyl versus oral morphine. J Clin Oncol 16:1588-1593, 1998.

100. Portenoy RK, Payne D, Jacobsen P: Breakthrough pain: Characteristics and impact in patients with cancer pain. Pain 81:129-134, 1999.

CHAPTER 8

Visceral Pain

TIMOTHY J. NESS, MD, PHD

Cancer produces a diffuse disruption of normal physiological processes. Uncontrolled growth leads to the compression and invasion of neighboring structures. Because the site of origin for many cancers is an internal organ, they may often be silent or asymptomatic until a critical event occurs producing ischemia, compression, or obstruction of the organ of origination or neighboring structures. When this happens, the symptom of visceral pain becomes manifest. Poorly localized and vague in multiple dimensions of description, it is a symptom that worries medical specialists who treat or diagnose cancer. It is a symptom that may be a sequelae of antineoplastic treatments or may indicate recurrence of cancer. As a consequence, a report of visceral pain prompts an examination and evaluation to rule out malignancy. Anxiety is evoked by visceral pain and at the same time exacerbates visceral symptoms. Caught in a positive feedback loop of pain-producing anxiety that increases pain, patients with visceral pain may present with symptoms that seem out of proportion to their pathology.

Recently, scientific studies have defined some of the qualities and mechanisms of visceral pain. These studies have demonstrated that visceral pain is uniquely different from pain that arises from superficial structures of the body both in substrate and in response to environmental factors. At the same time, it has determined that there are underlying similarities in multiple visceral sensory systems such that an understanding of one particular system may improve understanding of other systems. This chapter will summarize what is known about the phenomenon of visceral pain, particularly in the context of cancer, and will contrast and compare it with what is known about other pains. A particular effort will be made to incorporate new information related to the accentuation of visceral pain responses that is produced by physiologic and psychologic variables. Much of what is known about visceral pain is clinical lore that is derived from observations of the uncontrolled experiments of life. Multiple general statements are therefore

referenced to several reviews of these observations.[1–3] General statements related to anatomy and neurobiology of visceral pain are referenced to several basic science reviews and primary sources found therein.[4–7]

SOURCES OF VISCERAL PAIN

Based on clinical experience, stimuli that can produce visceral pain in cancer can be lumped into four groups: (1) acute mechanical stretch of visceral structures; (2) ischemia of visceral structures; (3) chemical stimuli from an infiltrating tumor or the body's reaction to the infiltration; and (4) a compressive form of neuropathic pain that occurs due to direct invasion of nervous structures subserving the viscera (Figure 8–1). Visceral pains may also occur secondary to the treatment of cancer because there may be iatrogenic damage of the viscera and their associated nerves produced by surgery, chemotherapy, or radiation.

Stimuli that produce tissue damage or predict potential tissue damage (e.g., cutting, burning, pinching) universally produce reports of pain when applied to most surfaces of the body but unreliably evoke reports of pain when applied to deeper, visceral structures. Stimuli that can produce pain from visceral structures such as distension of the gallbladder are also stimuli that occur naturally and normally evoke no sensations at all. In controlled studies, the most commonly employed mechanical stimulus used to produce visceral pain has been the distension of hollow organs using fluids or distension balloons. This is because such mechanical stimuli are easily quantified, easily controlled, can be isolated to a particular organ, and are related to a natural stimulus. That natural stimulus is bowel, biliary, or urinary tract obstruction that occurs secondary to the expansion of a cancer or other disruptive processes acutely or subacutely. Mechanical stretch of the hepatic, renal, or splenic capsules or other compartments within the abdominal and chest cavities

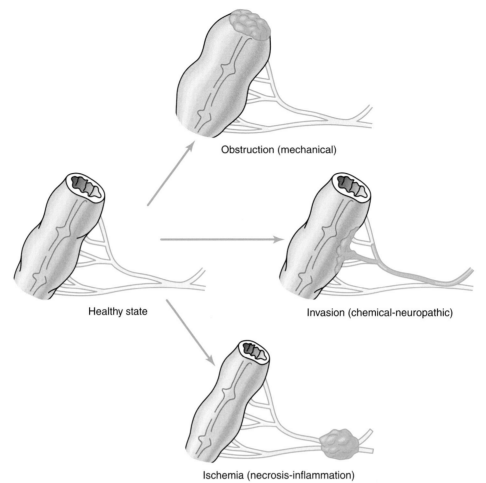

Obstruction (mechanical)

Healthy state

Invasion (chemical-neuropathic)

Ischemia (necrosis-inflammation)

FIGURE 8–1   Sources of visceral pain. Cancer can disrupt normal visceral systems, producing alterations that lead to pain. This occurs with obstruction of a hollow viscus leading to the mechanical stimulus of distension (top right); with invasion of parenchymal structures and release of algogenic substances (chemical stimulation, middle right) or invasion of neural structures producing compression (neuropathic, middle right); or compromise of blood flow to the viscera, producing ischemia with secondary necrosis and inflammation (bottom right).

can also produce profound pain and autonomic alterations. Torsion or stretch on mesenteric structures or omentum has also been noted to evoke severe pain and visceral ischemia with subsequent necrosis and inflammatory changes. Slow obstructive processes may not be pain-producing until a critical obstruction occurs even after profound tissue adaptation and expansion.

Abnormal chemical stimuli are also present in association with neoplastic processes. Certain tumors may secrete algogenic substances such as serotonin and prostaglandin E2 and so produce pain on their invasion of other structures even at a microscopic level. In experimental visceral pain studies chemical stimuli have been applied topically, intravascularly or via physiologic pathways (e.g., systemic cyclophosphamide-induced cystitis) to evoke nociceptive responses. Quantification, control, isolation, and modality-specificity of chemical stimuli are unfortunately very preparation-dependent

leading to significant ambiguity related to precise mechanisms associated with chemically induced visceral pain. Ischemia has been produced in a controlled fashion by occlusion of vasculature or in an uncontrolled fashion by tumor compression. The effects of such occlusion are dependent on collateral blood flow and metabolic activity of the selected organ. As a consequence, the stimulus itself is not readily controlled and is coupled with a mechanical stimulus. This has made its use limited experimentally despite its obvious and profound clinical importance.

Necrosis occurs when rapidly growing tissue exceeds its source of metabolic nutrients. Secondary inflammatory processes may then produce either focal or diffuse changes throughout the abdomen. The "evil humors" produced by inflammation and ischemia (acidosis, kinins, prostanoids, leukotrienes, and other cytokines) are presumed to be chemical initiators and maintainers of visceral pain, although there is some suggestion that they may be just sensitizers that make low-intensity mechanical stimuli sufficient to activate normally silent neurological elements. The disruptions of normal function associated with cancer are multifactorial with pathologic changes leading to the generation of combinations of stimuli, the sum result of which is the phenomenon of pain. The actual qualities of visceral pain and what distinguishes it from other types of pain are discussed in the following section.

CLINICAL DIFFERENCES BETWEEN SUPERFICIAL AND VISCERAL PAIN

When the viscera are healthy they are insensate or, at best, minimally sensate. However, as noted earlier, when diseased, they can create an overwhelmingly disruptive sensation that stops all activity and demands all attention. In contrast, the surface of the body is always sensate, though it can become more sensitive with pathology. Injury of the surface of the body inspires motion with fight or flight the typical reflex behavioral response—visceral pain tends to invoke immobility. Both types of pain produce emotional responses, but it is clinical lore that visceral pains produce emotional responses that may appear greater than that expected for the perceived intensity of the pain. It is common for patients to be highly distressed by a visceral pain rated as only 2 or 3 on a scale of 1 to 10. Nausea and dyspnea appear more commonly with visceral pains than superficial pains. Sweating (diaphoresis) and other autonomic responses can be profound with visceral pains such as angina, but appear of a lesser magnitude when evoked by superficial pains.

Overall, there is a poor correlation between the amount of visceral pathology and the intensity of visceral pain. Cancer can be very extensive throughout the abdomen but may produce little or no pain in some individuals, whereas hard-to-detect, minimally discernable pathology may produce out-of-control pain in others. There is obvious variability in individuals' responses to any stimulus, but this variability appears greater for visceral pains. The observation that pathology and symptomatology may not correlate is not unique to cancer-related pain as it is readily apparent in numerous visceral pain disorders. Some disorders such as chronic pancreatitis have definable pathology, but alterations in pain appear out of proportion to changes in radiographic or laboratory findings.[8] Other disorders such as irritable bowel syndrome, noncardiac chest pain, and postcholecystectomy syndrome appear to lack a definitive histopathologic basis for the discomfort and pain. Instead, visceral discomfort or pain in such conditions is termed *functional* and is often associated with altered motility, production of gas,

and triggers that may include the ingestion of food or beverage. In short, hypersensitivity to natural visceral stimuli in the physiologic range can be associated with discomfort and pain in the absence of obvious visceral pathology. In contrast, hypersensitivity to stimulation of the surface of the body is always associated with tissue damage and inflammation or nerve injury.

The greatest differences between visceral and superficial pain as derived by clinical lore can be summarized in three statements: (1) the viscera are minimally sensate, whereas the surface of the body is always highly sensate; (2) visceral pain has poorer localization than superficial pain; and (3) visceral pain is more strongly linked to emotion than superficial pain. Any valid description of the neurobiology of visceral pain must be able to explain these noted differences or prove that the clinical lore is not correct. Each of these observations will be addressed individually with psychophysical and basic science data that may or may not support the general clinical observations following a brief discussion of the animal pain models used to generate the basic science data.

PAIN MODELS

There are more than 50 different models of visceral pain that have been described, but only a few have been well characterized.[9] These include the common pharmaceutical screening model, the writhing test, which consists of the intraperitoneal injection of a chemical irritant (e.g., acetic acid, phenylquinone, or hypertonic saline) followed by counting the number of writhes produced. Writhes are a characteristic contraction of abdominal muscles accompanied by a hindlimb extensor motion. Variations have been described in primates, cats, dogs, and guinea pigs, but the model has been predominantly used in rodents. Methodologic and ethical concerns have presented significant constraints to use of this model. Distension of hollow organs has also been employed in multiple models of visceral pain. Most commonly, distension of the distal gastrointestinal tract (caecum, colon, rectum) has been used to evoke respiratory, cardiovascular, visceromotor, behavioral, and neurophysiologic responses in multiple species including horses, dogs, cats, rabbits, and rats. Studies have been performed in multiple laboratories in Europe, Asia, and the Americas with consistent findings among sites. Distension of the gallbladder and associated biliary system produces pathologic pain when the gallbladder is inflamed or associated ducts obstructed and has been experimentally used. Distention or chemical stimulation of the urinary bladder and other urinary tract structures has also been commonly employed. Distension, compression, or traction on reproductive organs also produces nocifensive responses, and chemical activation of cardiac afferents using bradykinin or other pain-producing chemicals has been demonstrated to produce robust neurophysiologic alterations in activity.[10]

Due to the often protean nature of many visceral pathologic processes, most models of visceral pain are not models of these processes, but simply models of pain arising from a particular viscera. There are, however, exceptions that are representative of specific pathophysiologic processes. Such is the case in relation to the work of Giamberardino and colleagues,[11,12] who modeled urolithiasis by creating a model of artificial ureteral calculosis. Following surgical exposure, an artificial stone is placed into the ureter and rats are then continuously observed for behaviors similar to those observed in the writhing test. These same researchers have also demonstrated that artificial endometriosis leads to a hormonally sensitive exacerbation of the same behaviors.[13]

There are significant limitations to what models of visceral pain can tell us about the overall phenomenon. Apart from aversion to a stimulus, there is little about the emotional aspects of pain that can be determined and qualitative descriptors or site and degree of pain localization are limited to humans who can feel and describe pain at multiple levels. That said, animal models of visceral pain have proven predictive of analgesic effects of various drugs and surgical manipulations. They have also led to an improved understanding of the wiring of visceral pain and expanded our understanding of neurochemical changes that result from persistent and deep forms of pain. To understand the neurobiology of visceral pain requires use of the dual approach of animal investigation coupled with investigations in humans.

VISCERA ARE MINIMALLY SENSATE

Historical Observations

In 1628, Sir William Harvey examined the exposed heart of a boy who had suffered a chest injury. Harvey was able to pinch and prick the surface of the heart and determined that the boy could not reliably identify such stimuli. He concluded that the viscera were insensate.[14] Two and a half centuries later the great surgeon Lennander pioneered new surgical techniques thanks to the then newly discovered local anesthetic effects of cocaine. He carefully cataloged his patients' reports of intraoperative sensation (or the lack thereof) while scratching, probing, pinching, burning, tugging, distending, and stretching various internal organs of the body. His patients, liberally treated with cocaine and morphine, felt no pain.[15] Subsequent surgeons performing similar studies but with less cocaine and morphine demonstrated some sensitivity of the viscera. One of these, Kinsella,[16] identified that inflammation and spatial and temporal summation were all requirements for visceral sensation.

Based on numerous additional studies in unanesthetized patients in which catheters or balloons were placed into internal organs via natural or man-made orifices,[17] it is the consensus that the viscera are not insensate, but are rather minimally sensate when healthy and can become exquisitely sensitive following an event that moves sensation from a subconscious realm to the conscious.

Controlled Psychophysical Studies

To confirm or refute clinical observations in an experimental fashion, sophisticated, controlled studies have examined sensations evoked by visceral sensation. An example of this is a recent study by Kwan et al.[18] that examined the sensations evoked by rectal distension in normal subjects. In these individuals a balloon assembly was placed into the rectum. Using a commercially available device that can simultaneously measure and control volumes and pressures of distension within the balloon (a barostat), a series of isobaric distensions were administered and reports of sensation evoked using a real-time, computer-driven visual analog scale and verbal perception ratings for three items: intensity of urge to defecate, intensity of pain, and intensity of unpleasantness. The evocation of reports of pain required higher pressures of rectal distension than the evocation of an urge to defecate. Mean ratings of intensity for the very first distensions were in the range of "strong" for urge to defecate, "mild to moderate" for pain intensity, and "distressing" for unpleasantness. After five distensions, the mean ratings for urge to defecate were still "strong," pain ratings had become "intense" and unpleasantness ratings were "excruciating." The compliance of the rectum was also noted to change with repeated distension with increasing volumes of distension produced by identical isobaric stimuli.

Other psychophysical studies have also demonstrated that a sensitization process can occur with sequentially repeated stimuli. Specifically, repeated distension of the gut or of the urinary bladder may lead to increasing intensities of pain and discomfort when the same organ is distended[19-21] and may also sensitize neighboring visceral structures.[22] In normal subjects initial visceral stimuli are generally nonpainful or of low intensity but they become painful with repeated presentation of the visceral stimulus. Stated differently, a nearly insensate organ becomes hypersensitive with the presentation of abnormal afferent input. Psychophysical studies have demonstrated evidence for similar hypersensitivity in virtually all clinically relevant visceral pain disorders. This includes hypersensitivity to gastric distension in patients with functional dyspepsia,[23] intestinal and rectal distension in patients with irritable bowel syndrome,[24,25] biliary and pancreatic duct distension in patients with postcholecystectomy syndrome, or chronic pancreatitis[26] and bladder distension in patients with interstitial cystitis.[27] In all cases, pain and discomfort (e.g., bloating) were experienced at intensities of stimulation lower than required to produce the same quality and intensity of sensation in a healthy population. A more sophisticated testing of visceral sensitivity using random-order, graded distension of the rectum in irritable bowel patients suggests that the population of subjects is heterogeneous.[28] One subgroup appears to be physiologically hypersensitive and another subgroup appears to be psychologically hypervigilant. Dissociating potential psychologic modifiers of sensory reports from other more functional pathologies has proved to be a difficult and sometimes insurmountable methodologic problem.

Basic Science: Sensitization of Visceral Sensory Elements

Correlates to the sensitization process that occurs secondary to the repeated presentation of visceral stimuli noted in the psychophysical studies previously described occur in animals, whereby repeated presentation of the same visceral stimuli produce increasing vigor of neuronal, cardiovascular, and visceromotor reflex responses. Inflammation of visceral structures also produces an increased vigor of responses with decreasing stimulation thresholds for the evocation of nociceptive responses.[29,30] Inflammation of visceral structures has proven to be a potent modifier of behavioral, neuronal, autonomic, and motor responses to visceral stimulation in experimental models.[9] The clinical correlate to this is that the presence of inflammation in visceral structures frequently, but not universally, leads to reports of pain. Cystitis, esophagitis, gastritis, duodenitis, ileitis, colitis, and proctitis all have as a hallmark finding evidence of mucosal inflammatory changes.

Inflammation produces profound changes in certain primary afferents, and the term *silent afferents* has been coined to describe them. These afferents are normally nonreactive to most stimuli, but in the presence of products of inflammation become spontaneously active and highly reactive to mechanical stimuli such as distension. Silent afferents have been frequently noted in visceral structures forming up to 50% of the neuronal sample[31] but are only infrequently noted in cutaneous structures. The lack of sensitivity of the viscera at baseline may also relate to the sparsity of the visceral afferents themselves, which are quantitatively fewer per unit area than similar measures of cutaneous afferents. Because they are few, increased activity may be necessary to cross a threshold for perception. The diffuse nature of the visceral afferent sensory pathway will be discussed more fully in the next section.

Spinal neurons responsive to visceral stimuli also change their responsiveness to visceral stimuli in the presence of inflammation and when other sensitizing manipulations have been performed.[32] Whether this is due to increased afferent activity, altered intrinsic properties of dorsal horn neurons, or altered modulatory influences within the central nervous system is unknown. It is likely that all of these separate mechanisms contribute in some way to the final sensitized state. Recent studies have demonstrated an important role of the dorsal column pathways in visceral nociception, but not in cutaneous nociception. In particular, Palacek and Willis[33] have demonstrated that this pathway is necessary for augmented reflex responses following visceral inflammation. Taken together, these findings suggest that visceral pain requires a sensitization process that involves the neuronal substrates encoding for visceral events and that occurs both peripherally and within the spinal cord.

VISCERAL PAIN IS POORLY LOCALIZED

Clinical Observations

It is standard clinical practice that asserts that visceral pains are deep and diffuse. The source of pain generation may only be localized by physical examination manipulations, which directly stimulate the painful organ. This is in contrast to superficial pains, which are highly localizable. Depending on the site of the body surface tested, painful stimuli can be localized to within millimeters. Perhaps more importantly, evoked superficial sensations from a specific site are always reliably localized to the same site and do not migrate to other body areas in the absence of nerve injury. The same cannot be said for visceral pain. Pain can be felt in several different areas at the same time or can migrate throughout a region even though pathology appears to be localized. Unless highly recurrent, pain is not normally perceived as localized to the organ itself but to somatic structures that receive afferent inputs at the same spinal segments as visceral afferent entry. For this reason, visceral pain is classically described as either wholly unlocalized pain or as referred pain that may have two separate components: (1) the sensation of the diseased viscera is transferred to another site (e.g., an ischemic myocardium can be felt in neck and arms) or (2) other sites become hypersensitive to inputs applied directly to those other sites (e.g., flank muscle becomes sensitive to palpation with urolithiasis). This latter phenomenon is also described as secondary somatic hyperalgesia.

Psychophysical Studies: Visceral Stimuli are Poorly Localized

Direct psychophysical studies of internal organ sensation have been very basic using simple stimuli.[17] As noted before, results of these studies were mainly associated with the determination of stimuli that produce visceral pain. Other psychophysical studies using visceral stimuli examined the localization of referred sensations described by the subjects themselves but did not directly contrast them with cutaneous sensations. It is notable that patient drawings related to sites of referred sensation generally extend over large surface areas (Figure 8–2A), whereas studies using cutaneous stimuli generate pinpoint localization to highly precise sites.

Some of the oldest formal psychophysical studies related to pain were dedicated to the topic of visceral sensation. Head, in his classic 1893 treatise titled "On disturbances of sensation with especial reference to the pain of visceral disease,"[34] examined the phenomenon of secondary somatic hyperalgesia produced by visceral pathology (Figure 8–2B) and compared these sites of sensitivity with lesions produced by herpes zoster. Using this information, Head was able to generate one of the dermatomal charts that we use today. For any particular visceral disease process, multiple dermatomes were involved indicating that the phenomenon of secondary somatic hyperalgesia is widely distributed (i.e., poorly localized).

Only recently have psychophysical studies attempted to determine more complex information that compares visceral with nonvisceral pains. A unique study by Strigo et al.[35] compared sensations evoked by balloon distension of the esophagus with thermal stimulation of the midchest skin. Consistent with clinical lore, visceral sensations were poorly localized as subjects indicated significantly

larger areas of perceived sensation for the esophageal distension-evoked sensation than for intensity-matched, heat-evoked sensation when asked to indicate areas of sensation on body maps. Notably, there was a tight temporal link between the heat stimulus and the evoked sensations but a poor temporal correlation with the esophageal stimulus. A sustained, relatively high intensity of visceral discomfort lingered after termination of the distending esophageal stimulus but not after the cutaneous stimulus. Hence, the visceral sensation was not only diffuse in the spatial realm, but also in the temporal realm. These same researchers[36] also compared the effects of esophageal distension with chest thermal stimulation on cerebral blood flow measures as an indicator of sites of central activation and observed that many similar sites were activated by both stimuli. In addition, the visceral stimulus activated the inferior somatosensory cortex bilaterally, the primary motor cortex bilaterally, and an anterior site within the anterior cingulate cortex that was not activated by the cutaneous stimulus. In summary, the psychophysical studies of visceral sensations have identified these sensations to be diffusely perceived and to lead to large areas of central nervous system activation.

Basic Science: Visceral Neuroanatomy is Diffusely Organized

Sensations begin with primary afferent nerve fibers, and visceral primary afferents differ significantly from cutaneous primary afferents in both number and pattern

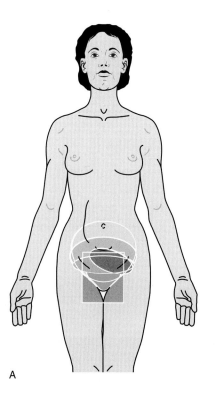
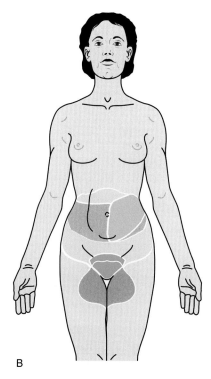

A

B

FIGURE 8–2 Poor localization of visceral pain. *A,* Examples of patient drawings of site of pain localization produced by urinary bladder distension. *B,* Representative drawings of areas of secondary somatic hyperalgesia to pinprick produced by visceral disease. *(A modified from Ness TJ, Richter HE, Varner RE, Fillingim RB: A psychophysical study of discomfort produced by repeated filling of the urinary bladder. Pain 76:61–69, 1998; B modified from Head H: On disturbances of sensation with especial reference to the pain of visceral disease. Brain 16: 1-133, 1893.)*

of distribution. Grossly, visceral sensory pathways are diffusely organized into conglomerations of nerve fascicles and cell body groupings that extend from the prevertebral region to reach the viscera by predominantly perivascular routes. This is in contrast to superficial sensory structures that form distinct peripheral nerve entities with reliable anatomy. The cell bodies of many primary afferent nerve fibers associated with visceral sensation reside in the dorsal root ganglia of the thoracic and upper lumbar spine, but the peripheral axons of these neurons follow a serpentine path to the internal organs that includes passage through the paravertebral sympathetic chain and ganglia and loose gatherings of nerve fascicles that are termed the cardiac and splanchnic nerves (Figure 8–3). The splanchnic nerves are divided into the greater, lesser, least, thoracic, and lumbar divisions. The pelvic nerve also arises from dorsal root ganglia but at sacral levels and in its peripheral path accepts contributions from the sympathetic chain before innervating urogenital visceral structures.

Visceral sensory processing is uniquely different from cutaneous sensory processing in that there are peripheral sites of visceral neuronal synaptic contact that occur with the cell bodies of prevertebral ganglia such as the celiac ganglion, superior mesenteric ganglion, and pelvic ganglion. This synaptic contact can lead to alterations in local visceral function that is outside central control. The gut also carries the enteric nervous system as a self-contained "little brain" regulating the complex functions of digestion and absorption. The weblike combinations

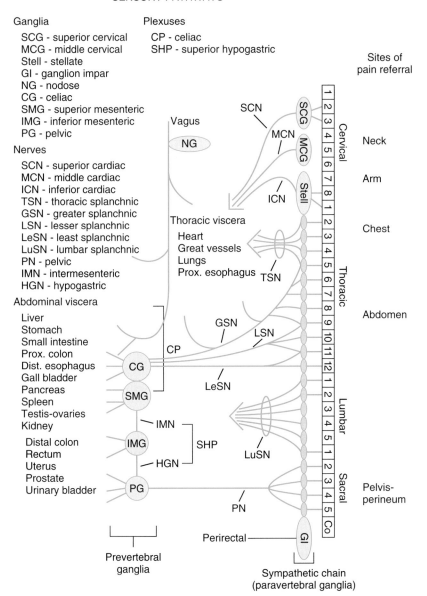

SENSORY PATHWAYS

FIGURE 8–3 Schematic of visceral nerve pathways. Abbreviations are defined at top left, and sites of referred pain are shown at right. (*Modified from Ness TJ, Gebhart GF: Visceral pain: A review of experimental studies. Pain 41:167–234, 1990.*)

of nerves and ganglia that lead to the central nervous system coat the retroperitoneal wall and wrap around the major vascular structures feeding the viscera.

The location of the dorsal root ganglion neurons innervating the viscera appears to follow the original location of the structural precursors of the viscera during embryological development. Thoracic organs arose near somites corresponding to thoracic segments. Most abdominal organs arose from somites corresponding to mid-to-low thoracic and upper lumbar spinal segmental structures. Organization appears more complicated in the realm of urogenital and pelvic structures where a dual innervation is apparent with afferents from lower thoracic–upper lumbar segments and from sacral segments. The testes and ovaries both originate relatively high in the abdomen and so carry with them a thoracic innervation. The urinary bladder arises from structures that traverse the developing umbilicus and is still connected to it by the residual urachus. It has a similar thoracolumbar innervation with sensory inputs extending up to the T10 level. However, like all structures that physically open their orifices to sacral dermatomes (rectum, genital structures), it also has a dual spinal innervation that includes local sacral inputs (the pelvic nerve; S2-4). An apparent gap in the innervation of urogenital structures is simply the absence of those nerves associated with somites, which selectively grew to be the hindlimb bud (L3-S1). Mixed with spinal innervations are the wandering inputs and outputs of the vagus nerve and an elaborate local ganglionic circuitry. The result is that pelvic organs such as the urinary bladder, gynecologic structures, and the lower gastrointestinal tract have a complex and diffuse neuroanatomy.

In addition to the diffuse appearance of visceral sensory systems on a macroscopic level, there is an even greater dispersal of sensory information on a microscopic level. Afferents with endings in a focal visceral site may have cell bodies in the dorsal root ganglia of 10 or more spinal levels in a bilaterally distributed fashion. In contrast, cutaneous afferents from a particular body surface arise from only three to five unilaterally located dorsal root ganglia. Cell body localization into dorsal root ganglia indicates the level of spinal entry; however, Sugiura and colleagues[37] have demonstrated that individual viscero-ceptive afferent fibers branch once they enter the spinal cord and may spread over a dozen or more spinal segments interacting with neurons in at least five different dorsal horn laminae on both sides of the spinal cord. The same researchers demonstrated that individual cutaneous afferents form tight baskets of input to localized spinal cord sites unilaterally limited to one or two laminae. The fact that visceral afferents selectively terminate in a different spinal laminar pattern than cutaneous afferents suggests that they may also interact with different spinal neuronal populations. When quantitatively examined, spinal dorsal horn neurons with visceral inputs have multiple inputs, from the viscera, from joints, from muscle, and from cutaneous structures. Convergent receptive fields for these neurons are therefore large with diffuse inputs. In contrast, neurons with exclusively cutaneous input are commonly identified in the dorsal horn, in particular from glabrous skin with small localized areas that produce excitation. Taken together, from a macro- to microscopic level, there is an imprecise and diffuse organization of visceral primary inputs that would be consistent with an imprecise and diffuse localization by the central nervous system.

VISCERAL PAIN IS STRONGLY LINKED TO EMOTION

Visceral Pain, Unpleasantness, and Anxiety

When nervous, one feels "butterflies" or "a pit" in the stomach. "Gut wrenching" emotions can also evoke profound changes in heart rate, breathing, and all other visceral functions such that a rapid trip to a lavatory may be a necessity. There is little doubt that emotional state can alter sensations from and function of the viscera,[38] but the reverse situation also appears to be true: visceral pain evokes strong emotions, stronger than those evoked by equal intensities of superficial pain. This has been demonstrated in numerous observational studies, but was most definitively demonstrated by the study by Strigo et al.[35] discussed in the previous section, which compared balloon distension of the esophagus with thermal stimulation of the midchest skin. Using graded intensities of both distending and thermal stimuli, these investigators were able to match the intensity of evoked sensations produced at the two different sites. The magnitude of emotional responses was then quantified using several tools designed to dissect the affective components of clinical pain. Equal intensities of reported sensation produced greater emotional responses when the visceral stimulus was employed as evidenced by unpleasantness ratings that were higher than intensity rating when the esophageal stimulus was administered but lower than intensity ratings when the thermal stimulus was utilized. Word selection from the McGill Pain Questionnaire suggested a stronger affective component to the sensation evoked by esophageal distension compared with the thermal stimulus. Greater anxiety was evoked by esophageal distension as measured by the Spielberg State-Trait Anxiety Inventory. Multiple measures led to consistent findings: visceral stimuli evoke more emotion than cutaneous stimuli. As noted previously, stressful life events have been viewed as classic triggers for the evocation of diffuse abdominal complaints of presumed visceral origin. As a consequence, the findings of Strigo and colleagues suggest that a positive feedback phenomenon can occur where visceral pain produces anxiety, which increases visceral pain that increases anxiety in an unending cycle.

Animal Models: Aversiveness and Stress-Induced Changes

There are severe limitations to the interpretation of emotional experiences of animals. As a consequence, there is only limited basic science data that can address issues related to the emotional impact of visceral stimuli. We can demonstrate aversion to a stimulus by demonstrating alterations in behavior performed by an animal so that it might avoid the experience of such a stimulus.[39,40] It is possible to compare relative levels of aversion between visceral and cutaneous stimuli and to show that visceral stimuli produce more motivation than cutaneous stimuli, but the simple reality is that we would be attempting to compare apples with oranges. For this reason, there is a greater literature related to the easier-to-interpret effects of experimental manipulations known to induce changes in pain-related behavioral, reflex, and neuronal responses. This is particularly true to manipulations related to anxiety or stress in nonhuman subjects.

Stress-induced analgesia (or hypoalgesia) has been a long-recognized phenomenon associated with cutaneous pain sensation. Soldiers in war may sustain severe wounds but only feel pain after the battle subsides. However, it would appear that stress-induced hyperalgesia is the correlate phenomenon associated with visceral pain sensation. In animal models, classic behavioral stressors such as a cold-water swim or restraint stress produce an elevation in thresholds for the evocation of responses to thermal stimuli (stress-induced analgesia), but the same animals have an increased vigor of visceromotor responses to visceral stimuli.[41,42] This phenomenon appears to be associated with early-in-life events and can be modified by gonadal hormones, neurokinins, corticotrophin-releasing factor, and mast cell function. Genetic factors also play a part as demonstrated by Gunter et al.,[43] who observed that rats with high measures of anxiety on experimental testing also had increased responsiveness to visceral stimuli. Mechanisms that underlie this phenomenon may include central nervous system changes. This same research group also demonstrated that experimentally induced alterations of the central nervous system by injections of corticosteroids or mineralocorticoids into the amygdala produced increased measures of anxiety and also produced augmented responses to visceral stimuli.[44-46] A hypersensitivity to visceral stimulation was measured as an increased vigor of visceromotor responses and as

increased responses of spinal dorsal horn neurons to colon or urinary bladder distension. Given the multiple interaction effects that have been noted between manipulations known to alter emotional state and visceral sensitivity, there can be little doubt that the two are linked at a basic neurophysiologic level.

TREATMENT OF VISCERAL PAIN

The goal of this chapter was to describe the phenomenon of visceral pain in association with cancer. Other chapters address specific therapeutics that can be used for its treatment ranging from behavioral interventions to opioid pharmacotherapeutics to neurolytic techniques. It is a moral imperative that all appropriate means of treatment be used to ease the suffering of those with cancer-related pain. However, even basic therapies such as nonsteroidal anti-inflammatory drug use[47] or neurolysis[48] may carry their own risks such as gastrointestinal or renal toxicity or unplanned neural damage. The sensory consequence of controlled nerve injuries can be highly beneficial but neuropathic sequelae due to such treatments may serve as another source of pain related to cancer.

There are some general treatment issues related to cancer-related visceral pain that appear obvious given the observations noted in this chapter. Foremost of these issues is that one should not ignore the emotional factors that may accompany or exacerbate other symptoms. Because anxiety is both induced by visceral pain and at the same time produces an increase in visceral pain sensation, it would appear prudent to include an anxiolytic in any regimen of pharmacotherapeutics. The diffuse nature of the neuroanatomy of visceral pain would argue that highly localized treatments such as precise ganglionic injections of neurolytic solutions should be expected to have only morphine-sparing effects rather than producing an absolutely pain-free state. Realistic expectations on the part of both patients and care providers lead to optimized treatment rather than disappointment. Sequelae of treatments are not always benign, so the multimodal therapies put forward by the rest of this text are not only ideal, but necessary.

CONCLUSION

Pain of visceral origin is a common clinical entity with multiple etiologies both known and unknown. One of these known etiologies is cancer, which produces a recurrent, acute pain when mechanical, chemical, ischemic, or neuropathic stimuli awaken a normally silent system. The organization of visceral sensory systems is diffuse on both macroscopic and microscopic levels. Strong emotions such as anxiety are evoked by visceral stimuli and at the same time may exacerbate visceral symptoms. As a consequence, our treatments for visceral pain related to cancer need to address emotional as well as physical factors and need to maintain a realistic assessment of the effect of our interventions.

ACKNOWLEDGMENTS

The generation of this manuscript was supported by funding from the National Institute of Diabetes and Digestive Kidney Diseases (DK51413). The secretarial assistance of Mary Ann Nelson is gratefully acknowledged.

REFERENCES

1. Rigor BM Sr: Pelvic cancer pain. J Surg Oncol 75:280–300, 2000.
2. Regan JM, Peng P: Neurophysiology of cancer pain. Cancer Control 7:111–119, 2003.
3. Payne R: Cancer pain: Anatomy, physiology and pharmacology. Cancer 63(Suppl): 2266–2274, 1989.
4. Joshi SK, Gebhart GF: Visceral pain. Curr Rev Pain 4:499–506, 2000.
5. Cervero F, Laird, JMA: Visceral pain. Lancet 353:2145–2148, 1999.
6. Cervero F: Sensory innervation of the viscera: Peripheral basis of visceral pain. Physiol Revs 74:95–138, 1994.
7. McMahon SB, Dmitrieva N, Koltzenburg M: Visceral pain. Br J Anaesth 75:132–144, 1995.
8. Walsh TN, Rode J, Theis BA, Russell RCG: Minimal change chronic pancreatitis. Gut 33:1566–1571, 1992.
9. Ness, TJ: Models of visceral nociception. ILAR Journal 40:119–128, 1999.
10. Euchner-Wamser I, Meller ST, Gebhart GF: A model of cardiac nociception in chronically instrumented rats: Behavioral and electrophysiological effects of pericardial administration of algogenic substances. Pain 58:117–128, 1994.
11. Giamberardino MA, Valente R, de Bigontina P, Vecchiet L: Artificial ureteral calculosis in rats: Behavioural characterization of visceral pain episodes and their relationship with referred lumbar muscle hyperalgesia. Pain 61:459–469, 1995.
12. Giamberardino MA, Vecchiet L, Albe-Fessart D: Comparison of the effects of ureteral calculosis and occlusion on muscular sensitivity to painful stimulation in rats. Pain 43:227–234, 1990.
13. Giamberardino MA, Berkley KJ, Affaitati G, et al: Influence of endometriosis on pain behaviors and muscle hyperalgesia induced by a ureteral calculosis in female rats. Pain 95:247–257, 2002.
14. Bonica JJ: History of pain concepts and pain theory. Mt Sinai J Med 58:191–202, 1991.
15. Lennander KG: Abdominal pain, especially in connection with ileus. JAMA 1013, 1907.
16. Kinsella VJ: Sensibility in the abdomen. Br J Surg 27:449–463, 1940.
17. Ness TJ, Gebhart GF: Visceral pain: A review of experimental studies. Pain 41:167–234, 1990.
18. Kwan CL, Mikula K, Diamant NE, Davis KD: The relationship between rectal pain, unpleasantness, and urge to defecate in normal subjects. Pain 97:53–63, 2002.
19. Ness TJ, Metcalf AM, Gebhart GF: A psychophysiological study in humans using phasic colonic distension as a noxious visceral stimulus. Pain 43:377–386, 1990.

20. Ness TJ, Richter HE, Varner RE, Fillingim RB: A psychophysical study of discomfort produced by repeated filling of the urinary bladder. Pain 76:61–69, 1998.
21. Mayer EA, Munakata J, Mertz H, et al: Visceral hyperalgesia and irritable bowel syndrome. In Gebhart GF (ed): Visceral Pain. Seattle, IASP Press, 1995, pp 429–468.
22. Munakata J, Naliboff B, Harraf F, et al: Repetitive sigmoid stimulation induces rectal hyperalgesia in patients with irritable bowel syndrome. Gastroenterology 112:55–63, 1997.
23. Salet GA, Samsom M, Roelofs JM, et al: Responses to gastric distension in functional dyspepsia. Gut 42:823–829, 1998.
24. Ritchie J: Pain from distension of the pelvic colon by inflating a balloon in the irritable colon syndrome. Gut 14:125–132, 1973.
25. Mertz H: Review article: Visceral hypersensitivity. Alimentary Pharmacol Ther 17: 623–633, 2003.
26. Corazziari E, Shaffer EA, Hogan WJ, et al: Functional disorders of the biliary tract and pancreas. Gut 45(suppl 2):1148–1154, 1999.
27. Pontari MA, Hanno PM, Wein AJ: Logical and systematic approach to the evaluation and management of patients suspected of having interstitial cystitis. Urology 49(suppl 5A):114–120, 1997.
28. Naliboff BD, Munakata J, Fullerton S, et al: Evidence for two distinct perceptual alterations in irritable bowel syndrome. Gut 41:505–512, 1997.
29. Coutinho SV, Meller ST, Gebhart GF: Intracolonic zymosan produces visceral hyperalgesia in the rat that is mediated by spinal NMDA and non-NMDA receptors. Brain Res 736:7–15, 1996.
30. Morteau O, Hachet T, Causette M, Bueno L: Experimental colitis alters visceromotor response to colorectal distension in awake rats. Dig Dis Sci 39:1239–1248, 1994.
31. Habler HJ, Janig W, Koltzenburg M: Activation of unmyelinated afferent fibres by mechanical stimuli and inflammation of the urinary bladder in the cat. J Physiol (Lond) 425:545–562, 1990.
32. Olivar T, Cervero F, Laird JM: Responses of rat spinal neurons to natural and electrical stimulation of colonic afferents: Effects of inflammation. Brain Res 866:168–177, 2000.
33. Palacek J, Willis WD: The dorsal column pathway facilitates visceromotor responses to colorectal distension after colon inflammation in rats. Pain 104:501–507, 2003.
34. Head H: On disturbances of sensation with especial reference to the pain of visceral disease. Brain 16:1–133, 1893.

35. Strigo IA, Bushnell MC, Boivin M, Duncan GH: Psychophysical analysis of visceral and cutaneous pain in human subjects. Pain 97:235–246, 2002.
36. Strigo IA, Duncan GH, Boivin M, Bushnell MC: Differentiation of visceral and cutaneous pain in the human brain. J Neurophysiol 89:3294–3303, 2003.
37. Sugiura Y, Terui N, Hosoya Y, et al: Quantitative analysis of central terminal projections of visceral and somatic unmyelinated (C) primary afferent fibers in the guinea pig. J Comp Neurol 332:315–325, 1993.
38. Mertz H: Review article: Visceral hypersensitivity. Alimentary Pharmacol Ther 17: 623–633, 2003.
39. Berkley KJ, Wood E, Scofield SL, Little M: Behavioral responses to uterine or vaginal distension in the rat. Pain 61:121–131, 1995.
40. Ness TJ, Randich A, Gebhart GF: Further behavioral evidence that colorectal distension is a noxious visceral stimulus in rats. Neurosci Lett 131:113–116, 1991.
41. Coutinho SV, Plotsky PM, Sablad M, et al: Neonatal maternal separation alters stress-induced responses to viscerosomatic nociceptive stimuli in rats. Am J Physiol 282: G307–G316, 2002.
42. Bradesi S, Eutamene H, Fioramonti J, Bueno L: Acute restraint stress activates functional NK1 receptor in the colon of female rats: Involvement of steroids. Gut 50:349–354, 2002.
43. Gunter WD, Shepard JD, Foreman RD, et al: Evidence for visceral hypersensitivity in high-anxiety rats. Physiol Behav 69:379–382, 2000.
44. Qin C, Greenwood-Meerveld B, Foreman RD: Spinal neuronal responses to urinary bladder stimulation in rats with corticosterone or aldosterone onto the amygdala. J Neurophysiol 90:2180–2189, 2003.
45. Qin C, Greenwood-Meerveld B, Foreman RD: Visceromotor and spinal neuronal responses to colorectal distension in rats with aldosterone onto the amygdala. J Neurophysiol 90:2–11, 2003.
46. Greenwood-Van Meerveld B, Gibson M, Gunter W, et al: Stereotaxic delivery of corticosterone to the amygdale modulates colonic sensitivity in rats. Brain Res 893:135–142, 2001.
47. Mercante SM, Casuccio A, Agnello A, et al: Analgesic effects of nonsteroidal anti-inflammatory drugs in cancer pain due to somatic or visceral mechanisms. J Pain Sympt Manage 17:351–356, 1999.
48. DeLeon-Casasola OA: Critical evaluation of chemical neurolysis of the sympathetic axis for cancer pain. Cancer Control 7:142–148, 2003.

Cancer Pain Resulting from Therapy

CHAPTER 9

Pain Following Mastectomy, Thoracotomy, and Radical Neck Dissection

SURESH REDDY, MD, FFARCS

Postsurgical pain syndromes are well-known entities that may result after simple, as well as complicated surgeries, in various regions of the body. Some are well studied and well defined, such as postmastectomy pain syndromes and postthoracotomy pain syndromes, whereas others are not well studied, such as postradical neck pain syndromes.[1]

POSTMASTECTOMY PAIN SYNDROME

Postmastectomy pain syndrome (PMPS) is a well-known entity, defined as persistent pain in the anterior chest, axilla, and medial and posterior parts of the arm that follows any surgical procedure on the breast. It can result from simple procedure, such as lumpectomy, to radical mastectomy and axillary lymph node dissection. The incidence is variable and quoted as 4% by Granek and colleagues,[2] 20% by Stevens and colleagues,[3] and 30% in a study by Vecht and colleagues.[4] The time of onset varies between 2 weeks and 6 months after the procedure. The general term PMPS is used to describe pain after the mastectomy, but it fails to specify the type and pathophysiology of pain. The type of pain can vary between somatic or neuropathic, but most commonly it is of mixed type.

Pathophysiology

The exact mechanism is uncertain but generally results from damage to the intercostobrachial nerve, which is the lateral cutaneous branch of the second intercostal nerves. During radical mastectomy or extensive dissection of the axilla, this nerve can be injured leading to a neuropathy or neuromata, causing pain in some patients. PMPS may occur more frequently in patients who have postoperative complications, such as wound infection or fluid retention, which may lead to increased fibrosis around the nerve.[5] Sometimes it may be caused by and complicated by axillary hematoma.[6] The pain can start anytime after surgery and persist beyond the normal healing time, with the long-term prognosis being unclear.[7] The pain is neuropathic in character and is described as sensations of burning, electric shock, or stabbing.[8] The pain is usually felt in the region innervated by the damaged nerve, in the axilla, arm or shoulder of the affected side. The variations of PMPS can range from phantom breast sensations[9] to other somatic pain sequelae resulting from surgery in localized breast cancer.[10] In a preliminary study by Queinnec and colleagues, a total of 1023 patients were followed for 1 year and the existence and extent of pain, as well as quality of life score (0 to 10), were evaluated by the patients themselves. Three mail questionnaires (MQ) were evaluated at 6 weeks, 6 months, and 1 year. They noted increasing frequency of somatic pain and decreasing frequency of neuropathic pain over the course. The treatment that generated the most pain was surgery with axillary dissection and reconstructive surgery. This study allowed the investigators to elaborate a classification of 12 pain syndromes related to treatment.

Clinical Presentation

Pain is typically characterized by tight, constricting, or burning sensations in the anterior chest, axilla, and medial and posterior aspect of the arm. It is often associated with bouts of lancinating pain, paresthesias, and hyperpathia in the nerve distribution. Pain is increased with arm movement, leading to restriction of motion of the shoulder, and subsequently leading to frozen shoulder. Occasionally PMPS may lead to complex regional pain syndrome (CRPS) type 1.[11] Many patients experience severe pain on contact with undergarments, and palpation of the skin aggravates the pain. The palpation of neuroma, if formed, may result in excruciating pain.

Diagnosis

The diagnosis is usually established from the history and physical examination of the patient. The pain is usually shooting, sharp, stabbing, pulling, tight, or burning, and it significantly interferes with daily activities. The range of motion of the shoulder is limited secondary to pain, as well as frozen shoulder in long-standing cases. Areas of allodynia, hypesthesia, and hyperalgesia may be noted in intercostobrachial nerve distribution. This pain syndrome is sometimes complicated by lymphedema of the extremity.

Treatment

The treatment of PMPS depends on the pathophysiology of pain. Initial aggressive physical therapy should be undertaken to prevent frozen shoulder, as well as disuse atrophy. Studies have shown relief using pharmacologic approaches.[12] If the pain is mostly nociceptive in nature, then a nociceptive pain algorithm should be employed (Table 9–1). If the neuropathic component of pain is high, then a neuropathic treatment algorithm should be employed (Table 9–2). Mostly, the pain is a combination of neuropathic and nociceptive, in which case a balanced analgesia technique is employed, along with physical therapy measures (Table 9–3). A long-standing pain can result in anxiety and depression, in which case they should be treated aggressively with both counseling and pharmacotherapy. Interventions may range from simple trigger point injections, intercostals nerve blocks, by either local anesthetic agents or radiofrequency lesioning. Intrathecal or epidural therapy in intractable pain may be useful, but lack evidence. Topical treatment with capsaicin has been reported.[13,14] In extreme cases dorsal root entry zone lesions have also been employed.

TABLE 9–1   Treatment for Nociceptive Pain Syndromes
Nonsteroidal anti-inflammatory drugs (NSAIDs)
Mild opioids
Physical measures
Strong opioids

Adjuvant medications
    Tricyclic antidepressants (TCAs)
    Antiepileptic drugs

Behavioral techniques
Muscle relaxants

TABLE 9–2   Treatment for Neuropathic Pain Syndromes
Tricyclic antidepressants (TCAs)
Antiepileptic drugs
Mild opioids
Strong opioids

Topical agents
    Capsaicin
    Lidocaine patch

Physical techniques
Behavioral techniques

POSTTHORACOTOMY PAIN

Postthoracotomy pain syndrome may occur after thoracotomy for malignant or nonmalignant lesions. It is characterized by moderate to severe pain in the distribution of one or more intercostals nerves, which persists beyond the usual course of the postoperative pain.[15,16] The majority of the pain after thoracotomy ceases after 6 to 10 days, but in a small percentage of patients the pain persists for weeks and months secondary to damage to soft tissues but, more specifically, to the damage to intercostals nerves during surgery.[17] In the majority of patients pain is usually mild and only slightly or moderately interferes with normal daily living. In a small subset of patients, pain can be severe and can be described as a true disability to the extent that these patients are incapacitated. The exact mechanism for the pathogenesis of PTPS is still not clear, but cumulative evidence suggests that it is a combination of neuropathic and

TABLE 9–3 Treatment for Combination Pain Syndromes	
If Neuropathic Component Predominates	**If Nociceptive Component Predominates**
Adjuvant medications	NSAIDS
Tricyclic antidepressants (TCAs) Antiepileptic drugs Opioids	Mild opioids Strong opioids Physical therapy
NSAIDs	Behavioral therapy
Physical therapy	Nerve blocks
Behavioral therapy	
Nerve blocks	
NSAIDs, nonsteroidal anti-inflammatory drugs	

nonneuropathic (myofascial) pain.[18] Trauma to the intercostal nerve during thoracotomy is the most likely cause. In patients who have undergone thoracotomy, the recurrence of pain may indicate recurrence of tumor, and this needs to be excluded.[19] Kranner and colleagues prospectively followed 126 cancer patients for 5 months after thoracotomy to define the pattern of the pain. Three groups of patients were identified. In the first group of 79 patients, pain eventually disappeared, but 17% (13/79) of this group had recurrence of pain because of recurrence of tumor locally, or in the pleura, chest wall, bone, or other site. Group 2 consisted of 20 patients; pain persisted and increased in intensity during the follow-up period. The increasing pain was caused by local recurrence in the pleura, chest wall, or spine. There was also infection in two patients, and one patient had superior vena cava syndrome. In group 3, 18 patients had a stable or declining pain and resolved over time. In this study a total of 33 out of 117 patients (28%) had persistent pain secondary to tumor recurrence or infection, and 31 of these patients at the time of surgery had tumor in the pleura or chest wall or residual disease; hence, they represented a high-risk group for tumor recurrence. Hence the authors concluded that persistent pain in the distribution of thoracotomy scar in patients with cancer is most commonly associated with recurrent tumor.

Pathophysiology

The possible explanation is the deafferentation pain caused by the nerve severance or neuroma formation. As the study of the pathophysiology of chronic pain with regard to the plasticity of the central nervous system advances, new insights are being gained into not only the potential origins of chronic postthoracotomy pain, but also its potential treatment options. Pain that is originally nociceptive in nature in the acute postoperative period after thoracotomy may become neuropathic in time. The ongoing research into the development of chronic pain, including that observed after thoracic surgery, portends the development of further advances in options for its control. A myofascial pain component results in some patients.[18] The employment of multidisciplinary strategies of pharmacologic, behavioral, and interventional procedural techniques provide the current foundation for the management of this challenging condition.

Clinical Presentation

The characteristics of pain depend on underlying pathophysiology. Pain is usually restricted to one or more dermatomes and may exhibit features of allodynia or hyperalgesia if a neuropathic component is involved. There may be some local tenderness caused by soft tissue damage or neuroma formation. Sensory loss is usually present as well. Pain is described as mild discomfort in the specific dermatomes to diffuse in nature. Pain is described commonly in terms of numbness, tingling, burning, shooting, and sometimes itching. It commonly results in sensitivity to touch, especially to clothes. Physical examination may reveal hypesthetic areas, as well as allodynia in the involved dermatomes. Occasionally, a painful neuromata in the surgical scar area may result in severe shooting pain.

Treatment

Preemptive analgesia initiated before surgery shows promise and might help reduce the incidence of PTPS.[20] Scientific evidence is steadily growing, but there is still a need for large, prospective, randomized trials evaluating PTPS.[21] Patients must be warned preoperatively about the possibility of developing PTPS and how it might affect their quality of life after surgery. Measures such as selecting the least traumatic and painful surgical approach,[22] avoiding intercostal nerve trauma, and adopting an aggressive preoperative pain management regimen, which should include thoracic epidural analgesia commenced before the surgical incision, may prevent postthoracotomy pain syndrome.

Treatment includes identifying the underlying cause and treating tumor recurrence by anticancer treatment. The pharmacologic management will depend on the type of pain. Mostly a balanced analgesia technique that employs opioids, as well as adjuvant medications, to treat neuropathic pain is satisfactory. Early mobilization and physical therapy to prevent frozen shoulder should be done aggressively. Transcutaneous electrical nerve stimulation may be useful in some patients.[23] Specific nerve blocks that relieve pain include intercostals nerve blocks with local anesthetics, as well as with neurolytic agents on occasion.[24] Radiofrequency lesioning[25] of these intercostals nerves may be carried out after the successful local anesthetic blocks of the same nerves. Intrathecal therapy also can be tried in refractory cases.

Because pain does not cause disability in the majority of patients, management is usually conservative. If pain is causing disability, then multidisciplinary pain management involving the pain specialist, social worker, physical therapist, and a psychologist is required. It is mandatory to exclude recurrence of disease or malignancy as a cause for the pain before initiating treatment.

POSTRADICAL NECK PAIN SYNDROME

The literature on this subject is sparse, but it has been described as a postsurgical, primarily neuropathic condition.[26-28] The incidence is unknown, but one study reported incidences as 50% following surgery.[29] In a study by Sist and colleagues[30] all of the 25 patients in the study experienced neuropathic pain and 72% experienced regional myofascial pain. They concluded that criteria for postradical neck pain syndrome involves persistent, nonprogressive neuropathic pain involving one or more branches of the superficial cervical plexus (SCP), which may be accompanied by regional nonprogressive somatic pain associated with myofascial pain triggers in head and neck muscles. Hence, it appears that a combination of neuropathic and myofascial pain syndrome is more common than one specific type of pain. With this combination, pain is described as spontaneous, continuous burning pain (81%), shooting pain (69%), or allodynia (88%). Neuropathic pain sites were within the distribution of the SCP. The postsurgical variable clinical picture of shoulder disability is related not only to the accessory nerve injury, but also to the secondary glenohumeral stiffness resulting from the scapulohumeral girdle muscles' weakness and postoperative forced immobility.[31,32] A recurrent pain after regional treatment of cancer heralds recurrence of the disease, and hence, should be excluded.[33]

Pathophysiology

The pathophysiology is unclear, but again points to deafferentation pain caused by resection of SCP, combined with myofascial triggers in the head and neck muscles. Radiation-induced fibrosis may complicate the pain syndrome. Shoulder pain secondary to spinal accessory nerve damage may result in neuropathic pain syndrome.

Clinical Presentation

Pain is described in terms of neuropathic to nociceptive caused by trigger points in the head and neck muscles. Range of motion of the neck and shoulder, with abduction difficulty, on the surgical side may be restricted. Areas of hypoesthesia, allodynia, and hyperalgesia in the distribution of SCP may be noted. Skin hardening may be identified as a complication of radiation treatment.

Treatment

The treatment is aimed at preventing trigger points and improving the range of motion of the neck with physical therapy. The pharmacologic treatment should be based on the type of pain syndrome (see Tables 9-1 to 9-3). Sist and colleagues[30] showed that local anesthetic injection of the SCP temporarily eliminated all neuropathic pain in the 17/25 patients who underwent the procedure. The 10 patients who also had myofascial pain reported temporary relief of their somatic pain after myofascial trigger point injections (TPI). They also suggested that early physical therapy aimed at recovering passive motion and avoiding the occurrence of joint fibrosis has been shown to have a real contributory role in decreasing shoulder complaints and improving the patients' quality of life.[31]

REFERENCES

1. Kanner R: Postsurgical pain syndromes. In Foley K (ed): Management of Cancer Pain. New York, Memorial Sloan Kettering Cancer Center, 1985, pp 65-69.
2. Granek I, Ashikari R, Foley KM: Postmastectomy pain syndrome: Clinical and Anatomic correlates. Proc Am Soc Clin Oncol, 3:122, 1983.
3. Stevens PE, Dibble SL, and Miaskowski C: Prevalence, characteristics, and impact of postmastectomy pain syndrome: An investigation of women's experiences. Pain 61, pp 61-68, 1995.
4. Vecht CJ, Van de Brand HJ, Wajer OJM: Post axillary dissection pain in breast cancer due to a lesion of the intercostobrachial nerve. Pain 38:171-176, 1989.
5. Carpenter JS, Sloan P, Andrykowski MA, et al: Risk factors for pain after mastectomy/lumpectomy. Cancer Pract 7:66-70, 1999.
6. Blunt C, Schmiedel A: Some cases of severe post-mastectomy pain syndrome may be caused by an axillary haematoma. Pain 108:294-396, 2004.
7. Kwekkeboom K: Postmastectomy pain syndrome. Cancer Nurs 19:37-43.
8. Wallace SW, Wallace AM, Lee J, Dobke MK: Pain after breast surgery: A survey of 282 women. Pain 66:195-205, 1996.
9. Kroner K, Krebs B, Skov J, Jorgensen HS: Immediate and long-term phantom breast syndrome after mastectomy: Incidence, clinical characteristics and relationship to pre-mastectomy breast pain. Pain: 36:327-334, 1989.
10. Queinnec E, Pichard B, George M, et al: Prospective evaluation of treatment-related pain in patients with localized breast cancer. Preliminary report. American Society of Clinical Oncology, 2005, No 8021.
11. Graham LE, McGuigan C, Kerr S, Taggart AJ: Complex regional pain syndrome post mastectomy. Rheumatol Int 21:165-166, 2002.
12. Eija K, Tiina T, Pertii N: Amitriptyline effectively relieves neuropathic pain following treatment of breast cancer. Pain 64:293-302, 1995.
13. Watson CP, Evans RJ: The postmastectomy pain syndrome and topical capsaicin: A randomised trial. Pain 51:375-379, 1992.
14. Dini D, Bertelli G, Gozza A, Forno GG: Treatment of the post-mastectomy pain syndrome with topical capsaicin. Pain 54:223-226, 1993.
15. Karmakar MK, Ho AM: Postthoracotomy pain syndrome. Thorac Surg Clin 14:345-352, 2004.
16. Erdek MA, Staats PS: Chronic pain and thoracic surgery. Thorac Surg Clin 15:123-130, 2005.
17. Dajczman E, Gordon A, Kreisman H, Wolkove N: Long-term postthoracotomy pain. Chest 99:270-274, 1991.
18. Hamada H, Moriwaki K, Shiroyama K, et al: Myofascial pain in patients with postthoracotomy pain syndrome. Reg Anesth Pain Med 25:302-305, 2000.
19. Kanner R, Martini N, Fole KM: Nature and incidence of postthoracotomy pain. Proc Am Soc Clin Oncol 1:152, 1982.

20. Senturk M, Ozcan PE, Talu GK, et al: The effects of three different analgesia techniques on long-term postthoracotomy pain. Anesth Analg 94:11–15, 2002.

21. Hu JS, Lui PW, Wang H, et al: Thoracic epidural analgesia with morphine does not prevent postthoracotomy pain syndrome: A survey of 159 patients. Acta Anaesthesiol Sin 38:195–200, 2000.

22. Rogers ML, Duffy JP: Surgical aspects of chronic post-thoracotomy pain. Eur J Cardiothorac Surg 18:711–716, 2000.

23. Carrol EN, Badura AS: Focal intense brief transcutaneous electric nerve stimulation for treatment of radicular and postthoracotomy pain. Arch Phys Med Rehabil 82:262–264, 2001.

24. Swerdlow M: Role of nerve blocks and pain involving the chest and brachial plexus. In Bonica JJ, Ventafridda (eds): Advances in Pain Research and Therapy, Vol. 2. New York, Raven Press, 1979, pp 567–576.

25. Forouzanfar T, van Kleef M, Weber WE: Radiofrequency lesions of the stellate ganglion in chronic pain syndromes: Retrospective analysis of clinical efficacy in 86 patients. Clin J Pain 16:164–168, 2000.

26. Portenoy RK: Cancer pain: Pathophysiology and syndromes. Lancet 339:1026–1031, 1992.

27. Foley KM: Pain syndromes in patients with cancer. Med Clin North Am 71:169–184, 1987.

28. Vecht CJ, Hoff AM, Kansen PJ, et al: Types and causes of pain in cancer of the head and neck. Cancer 70:178–184, 1992.

29. Keefe FJ, Manuel G, Brantley A, Crisson J: Pain the head and neck cancer patient: Changes over treatment. Head Neck Surg 8:169–176, 1986.

30. Sist T, Miner M, Lema M: Characteristics of post radical neck pain syndrome: A report of 25 cases. J Pain Symptom Manage 18:95–102, 1999.

31. Salerno G, Cavaliere M, Foglia A, et al: The 11th nerve syndrome in functional neck dissection. Laryngoscope 112(7 Pt 1): 1299–1307, 2002. J Pain Symptom Manage 18:95–102, 1999.

32. Van Wilgen CP, Dijkstra PU, van der Laan BF, Plukker JT, Roodenburg JL: Shoulder complaints after neck dissection: Is the spinal accessory nerve involved? Oral Maxillofac Surg 41:7–11, 2003.

33. Smit M, Balm AJ, Hilgers FJ, Tan IB: Pain as sign of recurrent disease in head and neck squamous cell carcinoma. Head Neck 23:372–375, 2001.

CHAPTER 10

Pain Following Extremity Amputation

RODOLFO GEBHARDT, MD

It is important to distinguish among three distinct but interconnected pathophysiologic entities following extremity amputation:

- Phantom limb: feeling of the amputated limb as still present.
- Stump pain: pain in the stump of an amputated limb, usually originating from a neuroma.
- Phantom limb pain: pain originating from an amputated extremity.

Phantom limb was first mentioned by Silas Weir Mitchell,[1] who provided its first clear clinical description. Patients with this syndrome feel an amputated extremity as still present, and in some cases also experience pain or cramping in the missing limb. This term is also used to designate a dissociation between the felt position of an extremity and its actual position. It is important to note that the patient recognizes that what he or she experiences is an illusion, not a delusion.

Lord Nelson lost his right arm during an unsuccessful attack on Santa Cruz de Tenerife; he subsequently developed phantom limb pain. These sensations lead the sea veteran to proclaim that his phantom pain was a direct proof of the existence of the soul.[2] If an arm can survive physical annihilation, why can't an entire person?

INCIDENCE AND DURATION OF PHANTOM LIMB PAIN

A majority of all patients (90%–98%) experience a vivid phantom immediately following the loss of a limb. The incidence might be even higher in cases of traumatic loss of limb or if there was preexisting pain in the involved limb, compared to a planned surgical amputation of a nonpainful limb.

Phantoms are seen less frequently in early childhood. This might be due to the lack of sufficient time to consolidate an image of the body. Simmel reported that the incidence of phantoms in child amputees was 20% in those younger than 2 years old, 25% in children between 2 and 4 years, 61% in those between 4 and 6 years, 75% between 6 and 8 years, and 100% of children older than 8.[3] Phantoms can also occur in patients born without limbs.[4-6]

In 75% of cases phantoms develop as soon as the anesthetic wears off and the patient is conscious, and the remaining 25% develop it in a few days or weeks.[7] A more recent report by Carlen et al. found that 33% of soldiers after an amputation had immediate phantoms, 32% within a day, and 34% within a few weeks.[8] The onset of phantoms is not affected by the limb amputated or the place where the amputation is made.[9]

Duration of phantom limb is variable; it might last for a few days or weeks and then fade away gradually. It may also persist for years and even decades in up to 30% of patients.[9]

Some patients have phantoms after mastectomy,[10] some have sensations of bowel movement or flatus after a colectomy,[11] some have phantom erections after having had the penis removed,[9] and some have had menstrual cramps after hysterectomy. These findings suggest that very elaborate sensory memories can reemerge in the phantom, probably due to deafferentation. Phantoms are more vivid and persist longer after a traumatic limb loss or after the amputation of a previously painful limb, when compared with the planned surgical amputation of a nonpainful limb. This could be due to a greater attention paid to the mutilated or painful limb before amputation, or it could represent the survival of preamputation pain memories in the phantom.[12]

Sherman et al.[13] found that more than 70% of amputees continued to experience phantom limb pain as long as 25 years after the amputation. Common descriptions of the pain include shooting pains that travel up and down the limb, burning sensations, and intense cramping sensations.

In some amputees the pain is continuous but with variable intensity, and others experience intermittent but high-intensity pain.[14] Few patients experience a reduction in pain intensity over time, and most of them continue to have pain, which after 6 months becomes very difficult to treat.

PATHOPHYSIOLOGY OF PHANTOM LIMB PAIN

The pathophysiology of phantom limb and stump pain is not completely understood. Both peripheral and central mechanisms have been thought to contribute to the pain. Peripheral mechanisms include ectopic neural activity originating from afferent fibers in a neuroma and spontaneous activity in dorsal root ganglion neurons resulting from activation of tetrodotoxin-resistant sodium channel subtypes that are expressed in injured neurons.[15,16] Central mechanisms that may generate and maintain postamputation pain states include cortical reorganization and spinal cord sensitization.[17-19]

According to Katz,[20] a cycle of sympathetic-efferent somatic-afferent activity may be responsible for the maintenance and amplification of phantom limb pain. Spontaneous activity in the sympathetic system or excitatory input from the cortex begins the cycle by increasing the discharge rate of preganglionic sympathetic neurons with cell bodies in the lateral horn of the spinal cord and terminals in a sympathetic ganglion. These neurons then excite postganglionic noradrenergic cutaneous vasoconstrictor and cholinergic sudomotor fibers that impinge on vascular smooth muscle and the sweat glands in the stump. They also excite sprouts from large-diameter primary afferent fibers trapped in neuromas. The release of acetylcholine and noradrenaline in the neuroma then activates primary afferents to the dorsal horn cells in the spinal cord, which had innervated the amputated limb. From there the cycle is completed when activity reaches the sympathetic ganglia, and also excitation reaches the cortex, contributing to paresthesias.[18] This model may also help explain the triggering of phantom limb pain by emotional distress, which may trigger hypothalamic activation of the spinal cord, leading to the release of acetylcholine and noradrenaline by postganglionic sympathetic efferents, which then excite somatic afferent in the neuromas.[21]

Another theory is that of central sensitization or pain memory, in which local anesthetic block of the injured site does not stop the increase in firing from spinal cord motoneurons.

As described by Woolf,[22] N-methyl-D-aspartate antagonists can prevent, and sometimes even reverse, this sensitization process.

Lastly, there is a remapping in the cerebral cortex as shown by Ramachandran.[18]

TREATMENT OPTIONS

Treatment of phantom limb pain is difficult and often frustrating for both physicians and patients. Multiple therapies have been tried, including opioids, anticonvulsants, tricyclic antidepressants, transcutaneous electrical nerve stimulation, N-methyl-D-aspartate antagonists, clonazepam, and spinal cord stimulation.

Blocking the spinal cord before and during surgical amputation may reduce the incidence of phantom pain by preventing this sensitization process from affecting the spinal cord.

Under the preemptive analgesia scheme, analgesic agents are administered before surgical incision to prevent nerve impulses arising from noxious intraoperative events from reaching and sensitizing central neural structures involved in the perception of pain.[23] It is still possible that even if a preemptive analgesic approach to amputation is effective in the short term, neural impulses generated at an abnormal site may induce a state of central sensitization after the short-term effects of the regional anesthesia have worn off.[24]

Placing an epidural before and continuing the infusion during surgery,[25] or for several days after amputation of lower extremities,[26,27] seems to confer protection from long-term pain.

It is interesting to note that a study by Lambert et al.[28] showed no difference in preventing phantom limb pain between an epidural block started 24 hours before surgery and a perineural catheter implanted during surgery.

Gabapentin was better than placebo in relieving postamputation phantom limb pain, although no differences were found in mood, sleep interference, or activities of daily living.[29] There are case reports describing the benefit of methadone for phantom limb pain[30] and some benefits from the treatment with clonazepam.

REFERENCES

1. Mitchell SW: Phantom limbs. Lippincott's Magazine 8:563–569, 1871.
2. Ridodoch G: Phantom limbs and body shape. Brain 64:197–222, 1941.
3. Simmel M: The reality of phantom sensations. Social Res 29:337–356, 1962.
4. Saadah ES, Melzach R: Phantom limb experiences in congenital limb-deficient adults. Cortex 30:479–485, 1994.
5. Ramachandran VS, Stewart M, Rogers-Ramachandran DC: Perceptual correlates of massive cortical reorganization. Neuroreport 3:583–586, 1992.
6. La Croix R, Melzack R, Smith D, Mitchell N. Multiple phantom limbs in a child. Cortex 28: 503–507, 1992.
7. Moser H: Schmerzzustande nach amputation. Arztl Mh 11:977, 1948.
8. Carlen PL, Wall PD, Nadvorna H, Steinbach T: Phantom limbs and related phenomena in

recent traumatic amputations. Neurology 28:211–217, 1978.

9. Sunderland S: Nerves and nerve injuries, 2nd ed. Edinburgh, Churchill Livingstone, 1978.

10. Scholz MJ: Phantom breast pain following mastectomy. RN 56:78, 1993.

11. Ovesen P, Kroner K, Ornsholt J, Bach K: Phantom related phenomena after rectal amputation: Prevalence and clinical characteristics. Pain 44:289–291, 1991.

12. Katz J, Melzack R. Pain memories in phantom limbs: Review and clinical observations. Pain 43:319-36, 1990.

13. Sherman RA, Sherman CJ, and Parker L. Chronic phantom and stump pain among American veterans: Results of a survey. Pain 18:83–95, 1984.

14. Serman RA, Sherman CJ: Prevalence and characteristics of chronic phantom limb pain among American veterans. Am J Phys Med 62:227–238, 1983.

15. Akopian AN, Sivilotti L, Wood JN: A tetrodotoxin-resistant voltage-gated sodium channel expressed by sensory neurons. Nature 379:257–262, 1996.

16. Coward K, Plumpton C, Facer P, et al: Immunolocalization of SNS/PN3 and NaN/SNS2 sodium channels in human pain states. Pain 85: 41–50, 2000.

17. Nikolajsen L, Jensen TS: Phantom limb pain. Curr Rev Pain 4:166–70, 2000.

18. Ramachandran VS, Hirstein W: The perception of phantom limbs. Brain 121:1603–1630, 1998.

19. Woolf CJ, Thompson SW: The induction and maintenance of central sensitization is dependent on N-methyl-D-aspartic acid receptor activation: Implications for the treatment of post injury pain hypersensitivity states. Pain 44:293–299, 1991.

20. Katz J: Psycho physiological contributions to phantom limbs. Can J Psychiatr 37: 282–298, 1992.

21. Jensen TS, Krebs B, Nielsen J, Rasmussen P: Immediate and long-term phantom limb pain in amputees: Incidence, clinical characteristics and relationship to pre-amputation limb pain. Pain 21:267–278, 1985.

22. Woolf CJ: Evidence for a central component of post injury pain hypersensitivity. Nature 306:686–688, 1983.

23. Katz J, Clairoux M, Kavanagh BP, et al: Preemptive lumbar epidural anaesthesia reduces postoperative pain and patient-controlled morphine consumption after lower abdominal surgery. Pain 59:395–403, 1994.

24. Devor M: The pathophysiology of damaged peripheral nerves. In Wall PD, Melzack R (eds): The textbook of pain. Edinburgh, Churchill Livingstone, 1994, pp 79–100.

25. Bach S, Noreng MF, Tjellden NU: Phantom limb pain in amputees during the first 12 months following limb amputation, after preoperative lumbar epidural blockade. Pain 33:297–301, 1988.

26. Jahangiri M, Bradley JWP, Jayatunga AP, Dark CH: Prevention of phantom limb pain after major lower limb amputation by epidural infusion of diamorphine, clonidine and bupivacaine. Ann R Coll Surg Engl 76:324–326, 1994.

27. Schug SA, Burrell R, Payne J, Tester P: Pre-emptive epidural analgesia may prevent phantom limb pain. Reg Anesthes 20:256, 1995.

28. Lambert AW, Dashfiled AK, Cosgrove C, et al: Randomized prospective study comparing preoperative epidural and intraoperative perineural analgesia for the prevention of postoperative stump and phantom limb pain following major amputation. Regional Anesth Pain Med 26:316–321, 2001.

29. Bone M, Critchley P, Buggy DJ: Gabapentin in post amputation phantom limb pain: A randomized, double blind, placebo controlled, crossover study. Regional Anesth Pain Med 27:481–486, 2002.

30. Bergmans L, Snijdelaar DG, Datz J, Crul BJ: Methadone for phantom limb pain. Clinical J Pain 18:202–205, 2002.

CHAPTER 11

Peripheral Neuropathy Due to Chemotherapy and Radiation Therapy

LARRY C. DRIVER, MD, JUAN P. CATA, MD, AND PHILLIP C. PHAN, MD

CHEMOTHERAPY-INDUCED PERIPHERAL NEUROPATHIES

Chemotherapy agents have been used for many years in the treatment of different solid and nonsolid malignant tumors. Cancer patients can complain of a wide range of cancer-related symptoms and chemotherapy-induced side effects, such as pain, fatigue, depression, nausea, vomiting, diarrhea, constipation, cardiac arrhythmias, vascular and pulmonary toxicity, skin changes, mucositis, and sensory-motor disturbances.[1-4] Sometimes chemotherapy-induced symptoms are transient, but in other cases they may persist for long periods of time, affecting the quality of life of the patients. As described by Markman, many patients "have learned to live with the discomfort or dysfunction."[5]

Tuxen and Hansen classified the chemotherapy-induced neurotoxic effects in four groups: peripheral neuropathy, autonomic neuropathy, cranial neuropathy, and encephalopathy.[6] Postma and Heimans defined peripheral neuropathy as "a derangement in structure and function of peripheral motor, sensory, and autonomic neurons, causing peripheral neuropathic symptoms and signs."[7] Painful or nonpainful neuropathies in cancer patients can have different origins. Neural structures can be damaged by multiple mechanisms, such as tumor infiltration or invasion, chemotherapy agents, radiation or nerve compression secondary to vertebral bone collapse.[8] Chemotherapy-induced peripheral neuropathy (CIPN) symptoms can present as pure sensory or motor disturbances or, more commonly, as a mixed sensory-motor neuropathy. Other atypical manifestations like Lhermitte's sign or urinary dysfunction have been reported.[9,10]

Cranial nerve neuropathy can be present in patients treated with antineoplastic drugs such as cisplatin or carboplatin.[11] Ototoxicity seems to be dose dependent, usually bilateral, irreversible, and frequency dependent. The mechanism of ototoxicity is still unclear. Patients at higher risk are those with previous cochlear damage, the elderly, or those simultaneously receiving other potential ototoxic drugs. Possibly, oxaliplatin has the least ototoxic side effect of the platine-related compounds. Patients treated with cisplatin had clinical signs of peripheral neuropathy at a cumulative dose of 417 mg/m^2, but at this dose the patients did not develop auditory impairment.[12] Therefore, it is likely that high cumulative doses of cisplatin are needed to induce ototoxicity when compared with cumulative doses that produce peripheral sensory changes.

Autonomic neuropathy was reported as another neurotoxic side effect seen in vincristine-treated patients.[13] Fifty-one percent of the subjects had clinical and electrocardiographic signs of cardiovascular autonomic dysfunction, and 53% of them had depressed deep-tendon reflexes.[14] Two studies found autonomic dysfunction in patients who received Taxol alone and Taxol plus cisplatin.[15,16] Impotence can be another manifestation of autonomic dysfunction in young adult patients who are receiving or have received chemotherapy treatment in the past.[17]

At present, many different nonpharmacologic-related cytotoxic agents have been recognized as potential inducers of painful or nonpainful peripheral neuropathies. Neuropathic symptoms and signs are often related to the cumulative dose or dose-intensity of the administered anticancer drug. Among the most common antitumor agents, paclitaxel, vinca alkaloids, and cisplatin can be mentioned, but the recent development of new drugs for cancer treatment has increased the list of anticancer agents with neurotoxic effects. Not only the traditional cytotoxic agents but also bioimmunomodulator molecules such as IL-2 and antibodies against specific targets can be responsible for the induction of neuropathic symptoms in cancer patients.

The incidence of chemotherapy-induced painful neuropathy depends not only on the specific anticancer drug used but also on many other factors, such as the previous or simultaneous administration of cytotoxic agents and the presence of coexisting diseases.[18] The dose, regimen of infusion, and cumulative dose of the anticancer agent have been postulated as important points that can influence the onset of the symptoms. It is generally accepted that higher doses and greater cumulative doses are related to higher incidence and earlier onset of the sensory-motor disturbances.[19,20]

Pathophysiology

The exact mechanism of neurotoxicity of the different taxanes is still unclear. The antitumor activity of Taxol is due to a direct binding to the beta-subunit of tubulin in the microtubules. Docetaxel is a Taxol-related drug more potent than Taxol as an inhibitor of microtubule depolymerization. Pharmacologic data taken from animals have shown that taxanes crossed the blood–brain barrier in very small concentrations[4]; therefore, it has been suggested that peripheral nerve damage could be responsible for most taxane-induced sensory symptoms. Different studies have suggested that axonal degeneration secondary to a direct effect of cytotoxic agents on nerves would be the key factor in the pathogenesis of the CIPN.[21] But demyelination has also been demonstrated in electrotrophysiologic and histopathologic observations. Rowinsky et al. speculated that Taxol would induce an axonopathy or neuronopathy. It was hypothesized that Schwann cells would be secondarily affected after axon damage, and the administration of high doses of paclitaxel or the combination with other antitumor agents would later induce lesions of the dorsal root ganglia (DRG).[22] Lipton et al. suggested that Taxol would affect dorsal ganglion neurons or Schwann cells due to its ability to induce microtubule dysfunction.[23] Histopathologic observations of the DRG of Taxol-treated animals did not show pathologic changes, although high levels of paclitaxel were present. Sciatic nerve specimens of these animals demonstrated axonal degeneration with microtubule aggregation and Schwann cell abnormalities. These last cells were "activated" in response to possible axon changes. Signs of demyelination were not found. These and other authors suggested that alteration in the neuropeptide content could play an alternative role in the induction of sensory changes.[24,25] Taxol induces a dose-dependent peripheral neuropathy, not only in humans but also in animals.[26,27] Thermal and mechanical hyperalgesia and allodynia have been found in animals treated with Taxol. Interestingly, animals recovered after Taxol was discontinued.[21] Two different research groups

reported that Taxol produced axon caliber and density changes in the sensory nerves of rats. No alterations were observed in the ventral roots.[24,27] The administration of a smaller cumulative dose of Taxol did not produce any morphologic abnormality in peripheral nerves and DRG when compared with nontreated animals. Only endoneurial edema was found in the sciatic nerves.[28] Therefore, it is possible that the Taxol-induced axonal damage also follows a dose-dependent pattern.

Along with the morphologic abnormalities, electrophysiologic studies showed decreased evoked sensory amplitudes without affecting motor amplitudes. Velocity conduction in motor and sensory nerves was slower than in vehicle-treated groups.[27] In another study, in which the animals received a lower dose of Taxol, increased evoked C-fiber firing was found, but the velocity of conduction of the nerves was preserved.[21] These authors found that protein kinase C (PKC) and protein kinase A (PKA) participate in the induction and maintenance of Taxol-induced hyperalgesia. Quasthoff and Hartung found that Taxol induced acute membrane depolarization in human peripheral nerves.[29] Therefore, it seems possible that Taxol-induced peripheral neuropathy could be related to axonal transport changes secondary to microtubule dysfunction and to other non–well-defined mechanisms that could alter the excitability of sensory nerves.

Taxol has been shown to induce enzymes such as cyclooxygenase-2 in human mammary epithelial cells,[30] and it demonstrated a lipopolysaccharide-mimetic activity in peripheral human macrophages. This was appreciated due to increased levels of cytokines such as tumor necrosis factor-alpha and interleukin-1 beta in the tissue culture of murine monocytes and murine and breast cancer cells.[31,32] Prostaglandins, tumor necrosis factor-alpha, and interleukin-1 beta have been demonstrated to induce pain when administered to animals.

The mechanism of neurotoxicity of vincristine is also not well understood. This drug is a vinca alkaloid and, along with paclitaxel, it belongs to the group of so-called microtubule-interfering agents. Many authors have hypothesized that vincristine induces peripheral neurotoxicity because of its ability to alter the axonal transport of neurons.[33-35] Green et al. demonstrated that the fast axonal transport was perturbed in the vagus nerves of vincristine-treated cats.[36] A model of vincristine-induced peripheral neuropathy in rats and mice was also developed to get a better knowledge of this condition in humans. In rats, Tanner et al. demonstrated that vincristine induced microtubule disorientation in unmyelinated axons without loss of myelinated or unmyelinated fibers.[37] Another finding reported by these authors was an increase in the axonal caliber, and they suggested that this axonal change would be secondary to microtubule alterations or to osmotic changes in the cellular environment. In another study, histopathologic specimens from vincristine-treated animals showed axonal degeneration of myelinated axons with figures of cellular infiltration and myelin ovoid formation in peripheral nerves, dorsal nerve roots, and spinal cord.[38] Vincristine crosses the brain–blood barrier in small amounts. Very low concentrations were found in the cerebrospinal fluid of vincristine-treated patients[39,40]; however, Ogawa et al. found dose-dependent spinal cord toxic damage when rabbits received high doses of vincristine. They suggested that the concentration of vincristine found in the central nervous system would be high enough to induce neuronal toxicity in animals[38] and humans.[35] However, no alterations were seen in the DRG and spinal cord of patients with peripheral neuropathy.[13] The administration of vincristine to cultured DRG and superior cervical ganglia neurons[41] caused axonal degeneration in a dose-dependent manner and reduction in the length of the neurite axons. The authors found that, as is similar with Wallerian degeneration, the axonal changes were calcium dependent and mediated; and they hypothesized that calcium entry into the cell would be part of a common mechanism of neuronal damage seen in other models of neurotoxicity.[42] Schwann cells were damaged after the administration of vincristine in mice. The histopathological abnormalities were dose dependent, and Schwann cells of myelinated fibers presented more important toxic changes.[43] Apfel et al. did not find alterations of neuropeptides, substance P, and CGRP levels in cervical dorsal roots of vincristine-treated mice.[44]

Electrophysiologic extracellular recordings of spinal cord neurons of vincristine-treated rats that had previously exhibited mechanical hyperalgesia, showed alteration in the pain sensory process. Prolonged afterdischarges were present after noxious stimuli were applied on the rat hind limbs. These changes suggest that central sensitization can participate in vincristine-induced hyperalgesia. Tanner et al. found altered responsiveness of a subgroup of C-fiber nociceptors; therefore, the authors suggested that vincristine-induced hyperalgesia would be a consequence of changes in nociceptor excitability, and that this would occur in response to vincristine-induced cytoskeleton abnormalities.[37] Weng et al. hypothesized that A-fiber dysfunction in the presence of well-functioning C-fibers as seen in patients with CIPN would drive central disinhibition and secondarily would be responsible for the central changes in sensory processing.[45]

The antitumor activity of platinum compounds is exerted on the cellular nucleus, where they bind to the cellular DNA. The platinum-induced damage on the DNA causes apoptosis of the tumor cells. The mechanism of neurotoxicity is unknown. In vivo and in vitro studies demonstrated apoptosis in dorsal root ganglia neurons of cisplatin-treated rats[46] and in cultured N18D3 hybrid neurons.[47] However, Tredici et al. could not demonstrate apoptosis in DRG of cisplatin-treated rats.[48]

Cisplatin-induced apoptosis was mediated by oxygen radical–mediated p53 activation.[47] Also, cisplatin decreased the nerve-fiber density and the neurite outgrowth of spinal cervical ganglion and DRG neurons co-cultured with Schwann cells.[25,41,49] In carboplatin-treated rats, Cavaletti et al. found evidence of nuclear neuronal alterations; but they could not show signs of cell death. In the same study, the authors reported axonopathy without signs of demyelination. Unmyelinated fibers were normal. Parallel to previous findings, where it was shown that the highest levels of cisplatin were found in DRG, the carboplatin concentrations were higher in the DRG than in other neural tissues.[50] Carboplatin-treated animals had dose-dependent behavioral sensory changes compared with controls.[26] It was demonstrated that cisplatin altered the distribution of neurofilament in the DRG of rats that had presented nerve-conduction velocity reduction. Therefore, some authors have concluded that platinum compounds alter the metabolism and axonal transport of neurons.[29,51,52] Different authors have found significant loss of calcitonin-related peptide neurons in the DRG of cisplatin-treated rats, postulating that these changes would be secondary to axonal degeneration.[25,53] The sciatic nerve of rats intoxicated with cisplatin showed a decreased mean diameter of large myelinated fiber without affecting small cells; however, there were not morphologic abnormalities in the rat saphenous nerves. Loss of large fiber was behaviorally demonstrated in cisplatin-treated mice, which developed difficulty in maintaining their balance in the rotarod test.[53] Interestingly, in this last study cisplatin caused disturbances in the thermal threshold perception that could be related to the neuropeptide sensory level changes found in previously cited studies. Therefore, the authors suggested that mainly large proprioceptive fiber would be selectively damaged by cisplatin; however, it is difficult to rule out a small-fiber dysfunction.[48,54] Resultant discrepancies among different authors can be explained by methodology or interspecies animal differences in the different studies.

Electrophysiologic studies have found that Taxol plus cisplatin induced alterations of the membrane excitability in patients with CIPN.[16] It was demonstrated in different works that the nerve conduction velocity, sensory amplitudes, and distal latencies were abnormal in cisplatin-treated human subjects and in animals.[48,50,54,55] It was reported that cisplatin increased the production of IL-1 beta and TNF in cultured peripheral blood mononuclear cells.[56] Therefore, it could be hypothesized that the presence of these inflammatory mediators in peripheral nerves could contribute to the induction or maintenance of the hyperalgesic behavior manifested by cisplatin-treated animals.

Oxaliplatin can induce acute or persistent dysesthetic sensations, but most of them recover after the drug is discontinued. A different situation is found with cisplatin, which causes sensory disturbances in a dose-dependent manner, and the symptoms can persist longer after cessation of the treatment. Therefore, it has been postulated that the mechanism of neurotoxicity of cisplatin and oxaliplatin would be different. In vitro, oxaliplatin has been demonstrated to induce changes in membrane excitability after its application on peripheral rat nerves or on dorsal unpaired median neurons of *Periplaneta americana*.[57] It has been suggested that oxaliplatin causes an "acute channelopathy,"[58] because it was shown that this antitumor agent altered the normal physiologic kinetics of Na channels. This effect was reversed after the administration of the antiepileptic drug carbamazepine.[59]

Antitumor Agents

Taxol was extracted from the Pacific yew *Taxus brevifolia* in 1963, and in 1979 its mechanism of action as an anti-cancer agent was discovered. To date, it is used as an antitumor drug in patients with different solid malignant tumors such as ovarian, breast, lung, and head and neck cancer. As previously mentioned, its cytotoxic activity is performed by its ability to interfere with microtubule function by inducing the polymerization of tubulin.[4,60] Taxol induces peripheral neuropathy in a dose-dependent manner.[4] It was reported that 84% of the patients who received an average cumulative dose of Taxol of 371.5 mg/m^2 developed neuropathic symptoms at 1.7 cycles, and 26% of them complained of pain. The initial administration of high doses of Taxol (>250 mg/m^2) induced symptoms in the short-term treatment, but when this dose was reduced (135 to 250 mg/m^2) patients could receive multiple infusion of the drug. Lipton et al. found that 55% of the patients developed peripheral neuropathy after a cumulative dose of 200 mg/m^2 and 31% complained of painful symptoms.[23] Rohl et al. showed that chronic administration of paclitaxel (median number of cycles, 20) at a dose ranging from 135 to 175 mg/m^2 did not cause grade 3 to 4 neuropathy in any treated patients. Ten percent developed grade 2 peripheral neuropathy. The authors did not mention the incidence of grade 1 neurotoxic symptoms.[61] Forsyth et al. reported that six patients with mild-to-moderate Taxol-induced peripheral neuropathy showed partial or complete recovery after Taxol was discontinued.[62] Recovery after combination of Taxol-cisplatin or Taxol-carboplatin was seen in the patients after several months following treatment cessation.[15,63] Two different studies found partial recovery of symptoms in patients treated with Taxol and cisplatin.[64,65] Connelly et al. reported similar findings but they found that some patients had sensory disturbances more than 1 year after combined treatment with cisplatin and Taxol had been withdrawn.[66]

Docetaxel is a semisynthetic analog of Taxol that causes dose-dependent peripheral neuropathy, although the incidence of this side effect is possibly lower than Taxol-induced neurotoxicity.[3,4] About 50% of the patients treated with cumulative doses of docetaxel ranging from 110 to 1375 mg/m^2 (mean 300 mg/m^2) complained of neuropathic symptoms. Those who received cumulative doses higher than 600 mg/m^2 manifested moderate-to-severe sensory neuropathy.[67-69] New et al. found the incidence of docetaxel-induced peripheral neuropathy to be 11%, and the symptoms began with a cumulative dose of 50 mg/m^2. In this last study, and in other published by Hilkens et al., most patients manifested improvement of the symptoms a few weeks after docetaxel had been discontinued.[69,70]

Platine-compound cytotoxic agents also cause peripheral neuropathy in a dose-dependent manner.[71-73] Cisplatin has antibiotic and antitumor activity. It was introduced in clinical trials in 1972 and shown to be effective as an antineoplastic drug against different malignancies.[74] Cisplatin-induced peripheral neuropathy has an incidence between 50% and 100%, and it is a rate-limiting toxicity that prevents dose escalation or long-term schedules of treatment.[75] It has been shown that cisplatin (100 mg/m^2) is more neurotoxic than carboplatin (300 mg/m^2) and iproplatin (240 mg/m^2).[11,76] In a large trial, cisplatin-treated patients reported neuropathic symptoms in 58% of the cases[77]; and in another study, when patients received a cumulative dose of 383 mg/m^2 of cisplatin, 49% of them developed neurosensory changes. A very similar incidence was reported by van der Hoop et al., who found that 47% of 292 patients had peripheral neuropathy, and 4% had severe sensory-motor abnormalities. In this last study, the median number of courses was between five and six, and the cumulative dose received by patients was between 500 and 600 mg/m^2.[78] Gregg et al. found an interesting relationship among the cumulative dose, the duration of the therapy, the levels of cisplatin in the DRG, and the clinical presence of the symptoms. The authors reported that the higher levels of cisplatin in the DRG were found in patients with more severe complaints and that there was a positive correlation between the DRG levels of cisplatin and the cumulative dose received by the patients. In this study, the general incidence of peripheral neuropathy was 45%,[51] but when higher doses were used the incidence was 100%.

Coasting phenomenon is progression of the neuropathy after cessation of cisplatin therapy, and it can be present for a long time.[19,29] Siegal and Haim reported that 31% of patients had worsening of peripheral neuropathy after cisplatin was discontinued.[79] Interestingly, 35% of these patients developed symptoms after withdrawal of cisplatin. Most patients with coasting had received high cumulative doses of cisplatin (552.7 mg/m^2).

Mollman et al. suggested that the paraneoplastic dorsal root ganglionitis should be considered in patients with late-onset symptoms, and the cisplatin-induced coasting phenomenon should begin within 2 months of drug cessation, and it should last no more than 3 to 4 months.[80]

Sixty-five percent of the patients showed gradual recovery from symptoms after high-dose cisplatin treatment was discontinued.[19] In a prospective study, Mollman et al. reported that cisplatin-induced peripheral neuropathy was partially reversible because none of the patients returned to their pretreatment neurologic status.[81] Siegal and Haim reported that 4 of 10 patients who presented with coasting after cisplatin showed symptomatic recovery.[79]

Carboplatin is a platine-compound that has been used in patients with solid malignancies like ovarian cancer, lung cancer, and neck cancer.[82] As mentioned above, different studies in humans have shown that carboplatin is less neurotoxic than cisplatin, being an alternative therapy in noncured patients who still are able to receive chemotherapy.[77,83] Swenerton et al.[77] published an incidence of 17% of peripheral neuropathy in a large population of patients who received six cycles of 300 mg/m² of carboplatin. Mangioni et al. reported an incidence of 1%.[11] However, when a combination of a single dose of paclitaxel plus escalated doses of carboplatin was used in patients with advanced solid tumors, about 30% of the patients developed peripheral neuropathy.[63] A similar regimen of treatment with carboplatin plus paclitaxel was significantly more neurotoxic than the administration of vinorelbine plus cisplatin.[84] These last studies showed the synergistic neurotoxic effect of carboplatin when it is associated with other drugs with nerve-damage potential.

Oxaliplatin is an analog of cisplatin. Oxaliplatin-induced peripheral neuropathy can develop as an acute or persistent (cisplatin-like) or less frequently as an atypical peripheral neuropathy. Oxaliplatin has been used in the treatment of gastric and colorectal cancer and, similarly to cisplatin, the persistent neuropathy is dose dependent.[9,10,85,86] About 90% of the patients treated with this agent presented acute neurosensory disturbances; in other cases, atypical neurologic manifestations such as Lhermitte's sign and urinary retention can be present.[10] The presence of Lhermitte's sign has been usually associated with moderate-to-severe forms of peripheral neuropathy. De Gramont et al. found that 68% of the 34 patients suffered from neurosensory toxicity, 18% of treated patients developed peripheral neuropathy grade 3, and 10.5% complained of painful paresthesia.[9] Lhermitte's sign is an electric-like paresthesia that occurs during spinal cervical flexion. It was associated with other atypical neurologic manifestations in patients treated with oxalipaltin[10] or cisplatin.[73] The acute sensory symptoms induced by oxaliplatin are generally transient and reversible, but

cisplatin-like neuropathy can be present as chronic complication.

Vincristine is a microtubule-interfering agent that is administered to patients with hematologic malignancies. The neurotoxic potential of the vinca-alkaloids vinblastine and vinorelbine is lower than vincristine but when combined with other neurotoxic agents can show a synergistic toxic effect.[6] The incidence of vincristine-induced peripheral neuropathy is between 50% and 100%. It has been suggested that older patients exposed to doses of 2 mg or higher would have a greater risk of developing vincristine-induced neuropathy.[8] However, age-related toxicity is still an unclear point.

Vincristine has been demonstrated to cause dose-dependent neurotoxicity.[13,87] Peripheral neuropathy was found in 27 of 40 patients treated with a cumulative dose of 12 mg of vincristine, and 13 of them manifested long-term complaints. Fifty-four percent of the patients with recurrent low-grade non-Hodgkin lymphoma presented with grade 1 and 2 paresthesias after receiving vincristine treatment.[88] Bradley reported that 100% of patients who received 0.05 mg/kg/week for an average of 15 weeks developed sensory loss,[13] and another study also a found a high incidence (84%) of vincristine-induced paresthesia.[87]

It has been shown that vincristine-induced peripheral neuropathy is reversible in some patients and that in others symptoms are long lasting. About 60% of the patients who reported transient symptoms demonstrated abnormal vibratory or touch detection thresholds. Thirty-two percent of the patients developed persistent symptoms, and all of them had altered vibratory or touch threshold. Seventy-six percent of the patients with chronic symptoms improved.[20] Casey et al. found that patients reported improvement of paresthesias after treatment cessation. However, clinical examination showed that in most of them sensory or reflex loss was still present.[87] This would indicate that subjects with peripheral neuropathy should be evaluated carefully after they stop taking antitumor drugs.

Ifosfamide is a cyclophosphamide-related drug that is used in children and young patients with sarcomas and lymphomas and in adults with lung cancer. The main neurotoxic effect is on the central nervous system, and it is manifested by hallucinations, confusion, mutism, or cranial nerve dysfunction.[6] Patel et al. reported that ifosfamide had caused severe painful peripheral neuropathy in four patients. Three of them had been previously treated with other neurotoxic agents, and all of them had received high doses of ifosfamide.[89] Frisk et al. reported a case of a patient with Ewing's sarcoma who had received cisplatin and vincristine before therapy with ifosfamide. The patient developed a severe painful neuropathy that was refractory to conventional opioid and nonopioid analgesics.[90]

Antiganglioside-G-D2 monoclonal antibody has been used in children with neuroblastoma. This drug is administrated after hemopoietic stem-cell transplantation in order to eradicate minimal residual disease. Sixty-eight percent of the children complained of severe pain during the first course of the treatment, and grade 4 neuropathy occurred in 2 of the 13 patients.[91]

Bortezomib is a proteozome inhibitor that is administered to patients with multiple myelomas and other hematologic or nonhematologic malignancies.[92,93] Bortezomib-induced peripheral neuropathy was found in phase I trials.[92,93] It has been recently reported that 31% of the bortezomib-treated patients had symptoms of peripheral neuropathy, and 12% of the subjects developed grade 3 neuropathy. Bortezomib withdrawal secondary to neurotoxicity occurred in 4% of the subjects.[93] The mechanism of bortezomib-induced neurotoxicity has not been studied yet.

Cytarabine is a pyrimidine nucleoside analog used in the treatment of hematologic malignancies. Its mechanism of action is exerted at nuclear level, where it inhibits DNA polymerase. Cytarabine-induced peripheral neuropathy has been reported in a few studies. In one of these reports, one of the patients had received vincristine as a previous treatment, and the nerve biopsy showed signs of axonal degeneration and demyelination.[94]

The combination of different anticancer drugs has been used as a modality of treatment in patients with advanced malignant tumors. As pointed out above, the administration of two or more cytotoxic agents can aggravate or accelerate the induction of the neuropathic manifestation.[18,95,96] Discrepancy exists among different authors about the incidence of CIPN when combined regimens are used, and this is probably related to the use of different schedules of therapy. Rowinsky et al. suggested that the maximum tolerated dose (MTD) of Taxol was 250 mg/m² over 24 hour with 75 mg/m² of cisplatin. In a phase I trial, they found that Taxol (initial dose of 110 mg/m²) plus cisplatin (50 mg/m²) produced mild-to-moderate peripheral neuropathy in 27% of the patients.[15] Considering the low initial doses of the agents, it could be suggested that these agents had a synergistic neurotoxic effect.[15] Gordon et al.[64] recommended an MTD of 225 mg/m² of Taxol with cisplatin at 75 mg/m²; and Schiling et al.[16] using a similar schedule reported that 2 of the 25 patients with neck and head cancer developed grade III/IV peripheral neuropathy.

In patients with coexisting diseases such as diabetes mellitus and alcoholism, the onset of neuropathic manifestations can appear earlier, and the symptoms can be more devastating.[18] Rowinsky et al. found that patients with previous alcohol-induced peripheral neuropathy showed worsening of symptoms after the administration of cisplatin plus paclitaxel.[15] Peripheral neuropathy can be part of paraneoplastic disorders caused by different malignant tumors. Therefore, the clinical identification of this syndrome before chemotherapy infusion should be taken into consideration as another potentially contributing factor in the severity of chemotherapeutic-induced peripheral neuropathy. Most paraneoplastic neurologic syndromes are immunologically mediated, and the detection of anti-Hu antibodies can help the physician to establish the diagnosis of some of them. An asymmetric and painful sensory neuropathy can be found associated to small cell lung cancer and it was associated with the presence of anti-Hu antibodies. Another sensory-motor polyneuropathy has been diagnosed in patients with monoclonal gammopathies such as multiple myeloma.[97,98] In the pediatric cancer population, a family history of Charcot-Marie-Tooth disease or other hereditary or nonhereditary neuropathies should be considered in patients who develop severe neurotoxicity after vincristine treatment.[18,99-101]

It is also very important to know the pharmacokinetic profile of the administered cytotoxic agent because alteration in the metabolism of the agent can produce higher serum level of the infused drug.

Clinical Manifestations and Diagnosis

The symptoms of CIPN can be manifested as sensory- or motor-related disturbances. Neurosensory changes are usually reported as paresthetic or dysesthetic sensations. They usually start distally on toes and fingertips and then spread proximally, resembling a distal stocking and glove pattern of distribution.[12,62,64,70,72,87,102] Taxol, docetaxel, and platine-compound agents seem to induce in most cases a sensory neuropathy.[11,22,60] The most common dysesthesias are reported as numbness, burning, pins-and-needles pain, tingling, and electric-like shock.[13,15,16,19,55,62,81,102] Fifty-eight percent of patients complained of distal numbness after administration of a cumulative dose of 300 mg/m² of cisplatin,[103] and this sensory abnormality was present in 34% of patients who developed docetaxel-induced peripheral neuropathy.[68] Rowinsky et al. found that patients treated with paclitaxel plus cisplatin complained of dysesthesias and paresthesias in the plantar surface of their feet.[15] Cold dysesthesias are an interesting finding manifested by 67.5% of patients treated with oxaliplatin.[9]

Pain usually accompanies and in most cases follows the mapping of distribution of the previously mentioned neuropathic sensations.[68] de Gramont et al.[9] found that 10.5% of patients complained of painful paresthesias after the administration of oxaliplatin. About 20% of subjects treated with paclitaxel[62] or docetaxel[67] had painful sensations, and these were described as "burning," "aching," "cramping," and "like needles."[62] Electric-shock sensations or Lhermitte's sign was reported by 31% of patients treated with a cumulative dose of 556.9 mg/m² of cisplatin.[79] Siegal and Haim believed that electric-like sensations are manifestations of demyelination of peripheral nerves.

Muscle pain is another symptom that might be present in patients with CIPN. Cramps can be reported by patients as muscle "spasms." Patients around the fourth week of vincristine treatment reported muscle pain. Thirty-one of the patients who were treated with a cumulative dose of 416.2 mg/m^2 complained of muscle cramps. These decreased after cisplatin was discontinued.[79] A lower incidence of cramps (5.7%) has been found in the oxaliplatin-treated patients.[9] It is still unclear whether the cramps are related to a direct toxic effect of the antitumor agents on the muscle fiber or whether they are manifestations of a sensory neuropathy.

In a small study, in which patients were treated with a cumulative dose of Taxol higher than 200 mg/m^2, pain was present in 56%. But in this study were diabetic patients, a patient with renal failure, and a patient who had previously received cisplatin.[23] A severe sensory painful neuropathy has been reported in patients treated with ifosfamide.[89,90] Neurologic examination of patients who are receiving chemotherapy should be performed previous to and/or early in the treatment because physical signs such as deep tendon reflex could be altered before the onset of paresthetic or dysesthetic sensations are felt by patients. The clinical scoring systems give the physician an approach to neurologic function and can help to quantify the severity of the neuropathy. Clear grading systems could be used to follow patients, and different examiners or clinicians could interpret the scores. Also, these are useful tools in clinical research. Forsyth et al. used a grading of symptoms and grading of signs score to assess the severity of paclitaxel-induced neuropathy.[62] Both scoring systems used a scale form from 0 to 4. Probably one of the most common scales of severity used by many authors is the one proposed by the World Health Organization.[104] In this system, five grades of severity ranging from 0 to 4 are assigned according to the sensorimotor symptoms and signs found in the clinical examination. Treatment-related pain can also be rated using the same scale. The Eastern Cooperative Oncology Group defined a 0 to 5 severity scale, in which grade 5 was the death of the patient, so grades 0 to 4 were used to establish the severity of the neuropathic symptoms and signs.[105] It is known that symptoms such as pain or paresthesias can disturb the daily function of patients more than other physical or electrophysiologic signs. Therefore, in addition to the assessment of peripheral neuropathy, physicians should evaluate the impact of the motor-sensory or autonomic dysfunction on the quality of life of the patients.[7]

Quantitative sensory testing (QST) has been used to determine the characteristics of the different types of neuropathies and painful conditions.[106] QST is used to explore "the status of somatosensory afferents all the way between cutaneous receptor and brain/mind, without providing clues as to the precise locus of dysfunction along the channels."[107] Vibratory, touch, and pin detection thresholds are clinically used to test the function of myelinated fibers. A-delta fine myelinated nociceptors are responsible for pricking pain discrimination. Thermal thresholds are tested to test C-fiber function and A-delta fine myelinated fibers.[107,108] Forsyth et al. found that 100% of patients who had altered QST had signs of CIPN, and there was a positive correlation between the cumulative dose of paclitaxel and the alteration in the vibratory and thermal thresholds.[62] These authors conclude that QST was less sensitive than neurologic clinical examination in detecting CIPN. However, as suggested in diabetic patients, QST could be useful as a measure of longitudinal evaluation and follow-up in patients with chemotherapy-induced sensory disturbances. A level C recommendation has been given to QST in the evaluation of patients with small-fiber neuropathy. In other words, the usefulness of QST in the assessment of patients with pain syndromes is not clear (level U recommendation). In chemotherapy-induced painful neuropathy, the recommendation is level C. QST could be used to demonstrate chemotherapy-induced sensory disturbances.[109]

Neurologic examination of patients with CIPN usually shows decreased or absent tendon reflexes as one of the first signs,[12,55,81] and this was found to be present in 50% to 100% of patients.[23,72] Hyporeflexia can be present even before paresthetic or dysesthetic sensations appear, and it begins distally, involving ankles and, less commonly, knees and arms.[23,68,87,103] Cavaletti et al. found that depressed deep tendon reflexes were dose dependent in patients treated with Taxol.[55] A positive Romberg's sign indicates proprioceptive loss; therefore, it is considered a manifestation of large-fiber dysfunction. This sign was present in 3% of patients after the administration of docetaxel,[68] but a higher percentage of the patients (89%) had a positive Romberg's sign after treatment with Taxol and/or cisplatin.[65]

As previously mentioned, vibratory detection is a function related to large myelinated fibers. A decreased vibratory threshold initially appears in the toes and fingertips, and it is present early in the development of CIPN.[22,23,70,81] Using the vibration perception threshold, Hilkens et al. found that a decreased threshold was present in 30% of patients treated with docetaxel; but they could not show that the changes in the vibratory threshold were dose dependent.[68] Vibration sensation was also altered in 77% of patients who received a ranging dose of 9 to 48 mg of vincristine. A similar finding was found by Forsyth et al., who found that 73% of subjects treated with paclitaxel had decreased toe vibratory thresholds.[62] In this last study, vibratory detection abnormalities were not correlated to the cumulative dose of paclitaxel received by the patients. Cisplatin-treated patients also have alterations in the vibratory detection[103] after receiving a cumulative dose of 300 mg/m².

As pointed out previously, detection of light touch and pin-prick sensations can be clinically used as parameters of the somatosensory status. Light touch discrimination is considered a function of large myelinated fibers (alpha beta), and pin-prick detection is related to medium-caliber myelinated fiber (alpha delta) function. Both sensations were affected in patients treated with cisplatin,[103] paclitaxel,[62] and docetaxel.[65,68,70] Pin-prick detection was impaired in a dose-dependent manner in the patients treated with cisplatin plus paclitaxel.[15] Roelofs et al. found that cisplatin-treated patients had a progressive alteration on the pin and touch thresholds from the baseline point of examination to the end of the study.[103]

Thermal thresholds have also been measured on patients with chemotherapy-induced sensory disturbances. It was found that 57% of the patients had elevated thermal thresholds at the index finger and 43% at the great toe.[62] Patients treated with oxaliplatin[9] reported cold-induced dysesthesias.

Motor abnormalities can present as mild weakness or clumsiness of the hand to a severe deficit, sometimes causing difficulty in walking or climbing stairs.[70,87] It is important to consider that difficulty in walking can be a manifestation of proprioceptive fiber alterations. Motor symptoms due to muscular wasting usually appear distally. A high incidence (92%) of weakness was found in patients who were treated with a ranging dose of 10 to 34 mg of vincristine.[87] As pointed out previously, cisplatin and other platine analogs induce motor system alterations in a low percentage of patients, being the platine-induced peripheral neuropathy, a predominantly sensory dysfunction.[11,51,66,72-86] Taxol and docetaxel also seem to induce in most cases a sensory neuropathy.[11,22] After receiving docetaxel and paclitaxel, 5% and 24% of the patients developed, respectively, motor impairment.[68] Forman has suggested that the patients with severe motor deficit should be carefully investigated for other possible or coexistent causes,[8] and serum creatine kinase levels or muscle biopsy should be determined to rule out myopathy.[70]

The clinical diagnosis of peripheral neuropathies such as diabetic neuropathy is performed by physical examination, QST, and nerve-conduction studies. It is considered that abnormal findings on two of these tests are required for the diagnosis of diabetic peripheral neuropathy. Therefore, this criterion could help physicians in the diagnosis of CIPN.

Electrophysiologic tests, such as nerve-conduction studies (NCS) and electromyography (EMG), can be used as diagnostic tools in patients with CIPN. The former test measures the ability of peripheral nerves to conduct electrical signals. The sural nerve is the most frequently studied to detect sensory neuropathy.[29] Nerve conduction can be affected by abnormalities in the axons, myelin, and Ranvier's node. The parameters that are analyzed during nerve-conduction studies are velocity of conduction (meter per second), motor amplitude (millivolts), and sensory amplitude (microvolts). Vincristine decreased the amplitude of sensory and motor action potentials, and it produced a fall in the conduction velocity of motor and sensory nerves.[13,87,96] The reduction in nerve-conduction velocity recorded by the authors did not correlate with the severity of the neuropathy.[87] Fibrillation potentials and positive sharp waves at rest were also found in vincristine-treated patients with peripheral neuropathy. These electrical abnormalities were present before the clinically small muscle wasting was present. Cavaletti et al. reported that Taxol-treated patients who had been previously exposed to cisplatin had abnormal sensory electrophysiologic findings that were less severe than the clinical findings.[55] Similar results were reported by others,[15] Cavaletti et al. hypothesized that the clinical examination could be more sensitive than electrophysiologic parameters in the early stage of the CIPN. According to this, in a study performed on patients with docetaxel-induced peripheral neuropathy, abnormal electrophysiologic findings were found in 77% of subjects who developed clinical CIPN, and altered QST parameters were even less sensitive in detecting neuropathy than clinical and neurophysiologic studies.[70] In this study, the most common abnormalities were low-amplitude motor and sensory potentials.[70] In cisplatin-treated patients, altered velocity of conduction and decreased sensory amplitude were reported in different studies; therefore, in addition to clinical and QST findings, cisplatin-induced neuropathy is considered as predominantly sensory type.[12,71,72] The findings reported in previous studies would suggest that axonal degeneration is the predominant nerve lesion, and the presence of early motor distal abnormalities would be a manifestations of a dying back-type process.[6,87] Bradley et al. speculated that this pattern or process would be related to a decreased diameter of terminal fibers that would be manifested by a proximal preservation of the conduction velocity.[13] It is important to consider that in "pure" demyelinating neuropathies slowing of the nerve conduction velocity is also a key finding. This last abnormality, along with depressed deep tendon reflexes, is commonly found in CIPN. Rowinsky et al. suggested that decreased sensory velocities of conduction would be a manifestation of demyelination, and they found the presence of this electrophysiologic abnormality in some asymptomatic patients.[15] Therefore, demyelination would also be present. Hilkens at al. described a mixed axonal-demyelinating neuropathy in patients treated with a cumulative dose of 150 to 1100 mg/m² docetaxel. Summarizing, it seems possible that a mixed axonal-demyelinating neuropathy would be a common pattern found in patients with CIPN. The different electrophysiologic results reported by authors are probably manifestations of early or long-term changes or severity in the course of the neuropathy.

Nerve biopsy is an invasive diagnostic method that has been used in different ways to evaluate the extension of the nerve damage. This technique is not used routinely in the study of patients with CIPN. In early stages of the neuropathy, axonal degeneration and other pathologic changes may not be present, or the distribution of the pathologic findings may not be symmetric. However, Gregg at al. reported that nerve biopsy was very sensitive for diagnosis of peripheral neuropathy in patients treated with cisplatin.[51] Large myelinated fiber loss was found in all five subjects treated with cisplatin. Axonal and myelin abnormalities were seen in large fibers; on the other hand, unmyelinated fibers appeared unaffected. No alteration of the spinal cord was seen.[12]

Prevention

To date there is no specific drug or method for preventing the development of CIPN. The ideal neuroprotective agent should protect nerves from the neurotoxic effects of the antitumor agents; it should not interfere with the cytotoxic activity of the chemotherapeutic agents on malignant cells, and it should have minimal side effects.[11,52] Amifostine (WR-2721), Org2766, leukemia inhibitor factor, lithium, alpha-lipoic acid, folinic acid, glutathione, pyridoxine, and a calcium plus magnesium infusion have been administered to cancer patients receiving chemotherapy treatment (Table 11–1). But most of these drugs have been tested only in small clinical trials.

Amifostine is a cysteine derivative prodrug that reduced the incidence of cisplatin-induced peripheral neuropathy from 25% to 49%.[81] Glover et al. reported in two studies that amifostine reduced the incidence of cisplatin-induced neurologic dysfunction and nephrotoxicity, allowing the clinicians to administer higher

doses of cisplatin.[110] In other randomized, open-label trials, amifostine showed promising neuroprotective results in patients with germ-cell tumors receiving combined regimens of paclitaxel-ifosfamide and carboplatin-etopised-thiotepa.[111] In a pilot study, where patients with metastatic colorectal disease received oxaliplatin, the subcutaneous administration of amifostine showed neuroprotective properties in 10 of 15 subjects.[112] Contrary to these previous studies, amifostine did not show any beneficial effect in a small population of patients with gynecologic cancers treated with paclitaxel (175 mg/m^2) plus cisplatin (75 mg/m^2).[113] Therefore, to determine the actual beneficial effects of amifostine more well-designed investigations are needed.

In one study, glutathione significantly reduced the oxaliplatin-induced neuropathy in patients with colorectal cancer. In a nonrandomized trial, patients with colorectal cancer received carbamazepine simultaneously with oxaliplatin. No patients developed grade 2 to 4 peripheral neuropathy.[114]

Org2766 is an adrenocorticotrophic analog that has been used in animals with CIPN. In clinical trials, the efficacy of this agent has been shown to be controversial. Petrini et al. conducted a small trial in which they showed that lithium partially reversed vincristine-induced neuropathic symptoms in humans.[34]

Leukemia inhibitor factor (LIF) is a cytokine with pleiotropic actions. The subcutaneous injections of LIF to rats reversed the cisplatin- or Taxol-induced tail-flick threshold changes without affecting the growth of control tumors.[26] In another study, LIF prevented Taxol-induced axonal damage; but it was not effective against Taxol-induced CGRP and substance P changes in the DRG.[24]

Alpha-lipoic acid was effective in 53% of patients with colorectal cancer who were receiving oxaliplatin-treatment. It was hypothesized that the mechanism of action of alpha-lipoic acid would be related to improvement of endoneural blood flow and reduction of the oxidative stress.[115] In a randomized, placebo-controlled trial, the administration of reduced glutathione statistically prevented, after 12 cycles, grade 4 oxaliplatin-induced neuropathy and reduced grade 1 to 3 neuropathic symptoms.[85] In vitro, administration of two different antioxidants, *N*-acetylcysteine and Trolox, reversed cisplatin-induced apoptosis on N18D3 hybrid neurons; and this effect was mediated by preventing the accumulation of p53.[47] Therefore, as pointed out previously, the induction of free oxygen radicals could participate in cisplatin-induced neurotoxicity.

The administration of BGP-15 has been shown to improve sensory nerve velocity conduction of the sciatic nerves of rats treated with cisplatin or paclitaxel. The authors conclude that the neuroprotective effect of BGP-15 was related to its inhibitory activity on

TABLE 11–1	Agents That Have Been Used for Prevention of Chemotherapy-Induced Peripheral Neuropathy	
Amifostine	Glutathione
Org2766	Pyridoxine
Leukemia inhibitor factor	Calcium-magnesium solution
Lithium	IGF-1
Alpha-lipoic acid	Nimodipine
Folinic acid	Glutamate

the poly(ADP-ribose) polymerase enzyme.[116] SR 57746A is a nonpeptide compound that, in vitro, has been shown to have protective properties against the neurotoxic effects of cisplatin, vincristine, and Taxol. The mechanism of action of this drug involves enhancing the release of nerve growth factor (NGF) by Schwann cells.[49] As mentioned previously, the administration of cisplatin or Taxol not only altered the content levels of CGRP and substance P in the DRG of treated rats and caused electrophysiologic alterations but also produced behavioral thermal and mechanical threshold changes. All these were reversed by the systemic coadministration of NGF.

Glutathione is an intracellular nonprotein sulfhydryl that naturally protects cells against the endogenous production of reactive oxygen intermediates. It has been suggested that glutathione could protect nontumoral cells against the toxic effects of some chemotherapeutic agents.[117]

The experimental administration of glutamate to rats significantly prevented gait disturbances and rotarod performance deterioration caused by vincristine. Thermal thresholds also improved in glutamate-treated rats. The possible mechanism of glutamate neuroprotection has not been elucidated. Boyle et al. proposed that a direct or indirect action of glutamate on the microtubule dynamics or modulation of associated microtubule proteins could be responsible for its protective neural effect.[118]

Nimodipine is a calcium channel blocker that failed to prevent the neuropathic symptoms caused by cisplatin in ovarian cancer patients. Cassidy et al. reported that nimodipine exacerbated cisplatin-induced neurotoxicity.[119]

Treatment

To date, there is not a mechanistic-based treatment of CIPN, and the clinical management of the neuropathic symptoms is still difficult. NT-3 is a neurotrophin family member that binds to the Trk C receptor. This is located mainly on myelinated axons, which seem to be the most affected in cisplatin-induced peripheral neuropathy. In rats, the experimental injection of NT-3 was able to reverse NCV disturbances, neurofilament protein alterations and the loss of myelinated fibers caused by cisplatin.[54]

RADIATION-INDUCED PERIPHERAL NEUROPATHIES

Neuropathy is a common finding in cancer patients. In patients with a known cancer diagnosis, efforts should be made to elucidate the etiologies of such neuropathy. The most common cause of new-onset neuropathy is progression of tumor or recurrence of such tumor.[120,121] Cancer can directly cause neuropathies or indirectly result in paraneoplastic neuropathies.[122] Signs and symptoms

from neuropathies attributable to cancer can help with cancer diagnosis and contribute to oncologic prognosis. Neuropathies can be directly caused by oncologic treatments, including chemotherapy and radiation therapy. The remainder of this chapter focuses on neuropathies arising from radiation therapy.

Incidence and Prevalence

The exact incidence or prevalence of radiation-induced neuropathies in cancer patients has not been well established. The current literature on this topic is sparse, consisting mostly of case reports or series. The incidence of radiation-induced neuropathies is variable, dependent on location of radiation focus, radiation dosage, and modalities of radiation delivery.[123,124] For example, a case series of 739 patients in whom intraoperative radiation therapy was used reported peripheral neuropathy as the predominant toxicity in 12% of those patients.[125] Another study of patients with colorectal cancer receiving intraoperative radiation reported a higher incidence of neuropathy of 23% with a higher radiation dosage.[126]

Pathophysiology

To understand how radiation can induce neuropathic changes in the peripheral nerves, it is helpful to examine how ionizing radiation affects normal tissues. Radiation kills cells by causing irreversible DNA damage.[127] There is a direct relationship between the amount of physical energy deposited, the degree of DNA damage, the number of cells killed, and the extent of tissue injury.[128] In addition, other factors, including hypoxia, cytokines, and cell–cell interaction, may play a role in promoting cell death or survival.[129] Cells lethally injured by radiation energy may undergo cell death by either apoptosis or necrosis. With apoptosis, cells commit "suicide" by breaking down into apoptotic bodies and being resorbed by neighboring cells.[130] In necrosis, cells break down into fragments, release lysosomal enzymes, and generate inflammatory response. This inflammatory reaction involves release of cytokines and inflammatory mediators. Initial nonspecific changes at tissue level can include fibrosis, atrophy, and ulceration.[131]

Tissue responses can further be broken down into two categories of early effects and late effects. Early tissue changes occur within days or weeks of radiation treatment, while late tissue changes can appear months or even years after radiation treatment. Early effects are often seen in tissues with cell populations that have high turnover rate, that is, gastrointestinal mucosa, bone marrow, skin, and oropharyngeal, and esophageal mucosa.[132] Late radiation effects are seen typically in tissues that are nonproliferating or slowly proliferating such as oligodendroglia, Schwann cells, kidney tubules, and vascular endothelium.[133] Pathogenesis of late effects involves necrotic cell death, production of proinflammatory and profibrotic cytokines, and alteration of gene expression in local cells.[134]

Radiation-induced peripheral neuropathies result from late effects of radiation treatment. The peripheral nerves consist of axon bundles. Thus, the axons of the nerve cells are less likely affected by radiation to the peripheral nerve. But the axons are supported by myelinated sheaths of Schwann cells as well as local blood vessels. These supporting cells are more vulnerable to the ionizing irradiation. Late effects can include myelin destruction, degenerative changes of Schwann cells, and vascular changes, such as endothelial cell loss, capillary occlusion, degeneration, and hemorrhagic exudates. Surrounding tissue changes in regions of the peripheral nerve lead to development of fibrosis around the nerve trunks.[124] Such fibrosis with subsequent compression of nerve bundles is suspected to be the primary etiology of peripheral neuropathies.[125]

Clinical Presentation

Patients with neuropathies can present with many different signs and symptoms, depending on the nerves affected. With radiation delivered close to the spinal cord where the nerve roots emerge, the patient may experience radiculopathies. At the level of the cervical and lumbar spine, the patient often complains of back pain, headaches, extremity pain, numbness, paresthesia, and weakness. Radiation to the thoracic area may cause noncardiac chest pain and abdominal pain.

With radiation therapy for breast cancer, lung cancer, and Hodgkin's lymphoma, the patient receives ionizing irradiation to the superior thorax covering the brachial plexus anatomic location.[121] With brachial plexopathy, the patient experiences chronic neuropathic pain of the affected extremity and also limb paralysis in severe cases.[135] If radiation is closer to the proximal brachial plexus, the patient exhibits characteristic cervical radiculopathy.[136] Any nerve root in the cervical region can be affected, but most commonly the C5, C6, C7, and C8 nerve roots are involved in cervical neuropathies, with related clinical signs and symptoms. For example, in C5 radiculopathy, pain is usually felt radiating into the shoulder and posterior scapular areas. Weakness of deltoid and possibly the biceps is also seen with C5 radiculopathy. The patient also complains of dysesthesia over the lateral aspect of the forearm. With C7 radiculopathy, the patient complains of pain radiating into the triceps, forearm, and hand. Paresthesia is also present in index and long fingers. Weakness of triceps is also prominent with C7 radiculopathy.

Radiation into the abdominal and pelvic regions for cancer of abdominal and pelvic organs will cause significant lumbosacral neuropathies.[137,138] The ionizing radiation will affect the lumbar and sacral nerve roots as they arise from the vertebral foramens and descend into the lower extremities. In L4 radiculopathy, the patient will experience pain in the hip with radiation into the groin, anterior thigh, and knee. Paresthesia may be experienced over the medial aspect the knee. Knee jerk will be diminished, and weakness of the quadriceps is noticeable. In L5 radiculopathy, the patient often reports pain from the back to the lateral hip and thigh and anterior tibial region. In addition, paresthesia over the dorsum of the foot and weakness of ankle and toe dorsiflexion are characteristic. With L5 radiculopathy, weakness of hip abduction is also possible. In S1 radiculopathy, the patient often reports pain radiation to the hip, posterior thigh, and calf. Paresthesia of the lateral aspect of the foot is also a characteristic sign of S1 neuropathy.

Assessment

As mentioned previously, most common neuropathies in cancer patients can be resulting from direct tumor growth and proliferation. That is why patients with known cancer diagnosis presenting with new onset of pain or significant increase in severity of pain should be vigilantly worked up for tumor progression. A complete history and physical examination is the first essential step. The clinical interview should be focused on questions about onset, duration, progression, and nature of neuropathic symptoms such as pain, numbness, and weakness. The physical examination is focused on the site of complaint and also the whole body to rule out other possible noncancer etiologies for neuropathies. This entails a thorough neurologic examination, including sensory and motor testing at the relevant dermatomes or muscle groups. The most prominent findings with neuropathies are abnormal sensory signs and symptoms. The patient often reports paresthesia (painless abnormal sensation), dysesthesia (pain from noxious stimuli), allodynia (pain from non-noxious stimuli), hyperalgia (exaggerated pain response), and hyperpathia (delayed and extreme pain response). These sensory findings usually follow neuroanatomical patterns of distribution.[139]

A thorough diagnostic workup of the neuropathies is essential in eliciting the etiology and possible mechanism of neuropathic pain. This includes laboratory, imaging, and functional neurophysiologic studies. Laboratory workup may include complete blood count, fasting blood glucose, sedimentation rate, general chemistry profile, thyroid function tests, vitamin B_{12} and folate levels, hepatitis viral titers, antinuclear antibodies and rheumatoid factor. Imaging studies, including plain radiographs, computed tomography scan, and magnetic resonance imaging scan, are valuable to determine any tumor involvement of the neurologic structures or postchemotherapy and radiation changes of surrounding tissues. Magnetic resonance imaging studies are extremely helpful in evaluating degree of fibrosis around the nerve trunk.[140] Radiation-induced fibrosis can have both low and high signal intensities on T2-weighted images, and that fibrosis can enhance even 21 years after radiation injury.[140] Additional studies including electromyographic and nerve-conduction studies may be employed to evaluate the functional integrity of the affected muscle groups and the relevant nerve function.

Differential Diagnosis

The etiologies of peripheral neuropathies are diverse and can be multifold.[21,23] They include metabolic or endocrinologic disorders, infections, inflammation, malignancy, autoimmune disorders, immunoglobulinemias, dietary or absorption disorders, nerve entrapment due to anatomic abnormalities, and exposure to drugs or toxins.[141] We will focus on cancer-related differential diagnosis for neuropathies in cancer patients. There are multiple cancer-related mechanisms responsible for causing neuropathies.[142] The growing cancer can cause compression, inflammation, and infiltration of nerve trunks or plexuses. For example, nasopharyngeal carcinomas may cause painful facial neuropathies by direct nerve compression on the facial or trigeminal nerve branches. Breast or lung cancers can infiltrate the brachial plexus and cause painful brachial plexopathies. Pelvic or retroperitoneal cancer can involve the lumbosacral plexus and cause painful lumbosacral neuropathies. Paraneoplastic autoimmune syndromes can also cause painful neuropathies because of the presence of antineuronal antibodies that directly attack nerves.

As stated earlier, neuropathies in cancer patients can be directly related to oncologic treatments, including surgery, chemotherapy, and radiation therapy. Surgical resection of tumor often causes traumatic injury to nerves in the resected region. We see this in post-thoracotomy pain syndrome in which intercostals nerves have been damaged. Chemotherapy with agents such as cisplatinum, taxoids, and vincristine may cause painful neuropathies. Lastly, radiation therapy, especially at higher dosage, leads to development of postradiation plexopathies.

Prognosis

Most neuropathies present later, weeks after radiation treatment. The severity and location of neuropathic symptoms is variable, dependent on the area of cancer. Most patients are able to tolerate the minor symptoms of paresthesia such as minor tingling or numbness. However, with more significant symptoms, such as severe pain or dysesthesia, patients need pharmacologic or interventional treatments to manage neuropathic pain. Medications such as antiepileptic drugs, opioids, nonsteroidal anti-inflammatory drugs, tricyclic antidepressants, local anesthetics, and topical analgesics have proven to have some benefits with neuropathic pain.[121] Additional modalities such as physical therapy, occupational therapy, and electrical nerve stimulation may help patients to improve their neuropathic symptoms. Most patients will experience improvement of their neuropathic pain with time, in a matter of months. Some, however, will continue to experience such neuropathic pain for years after treatment.

CONCLUSION

Peripheral neuropathies are an unfortunate consequence of cancer treatment. Although not yet fully understood, the pathophysiology of radiation-induced peripheral neuropathies involves the late effects of radiation on the peripheral nerves and surrounding tissues. Subsequent tissue changes result in inflammation and fibrosis affecting the peripheral nerves, leading to peripheral neuropathies. In cancer patients presenting with new-onset neuropathies, a full diagnostic workup is recommended to rule out other etiologies, such as progression or metastasis of cancer. Treatment of such peripheral neuropathies requires a multimodality approach, including medications and supportive therapy.

REFERENCES

1. Hartmann JT, Kollmannsberger C, Kanz L, Bokemeyer C: Platinum organ toxicity and possible prevention in patients with testicular cancer. Int J Cancer 83:866–869, 1999.
2. National Institutes Health State-of-the-Science Panel, National Institute of Health State-of-the-Science Conference Statement: Symptom management in cancer: Pain, depression, and fatigue, July 15–17, 2002. J Natl Cancer Inst 95:1110–1117, 2002.
3. Vaishampayan U, Parchment RE, Jasti BR, et al: An overview of the pharmacokinetics and pharmacodynamics. Urology 54:22–29, 1999.
4. Verwei J, Clavel M, Chevalier B: Paclitaxel (Taxol™) and docetaxel (Taxotere™): Not simply two of a kind. Ann Oncol 5:495–505, 2003.
5. Markman M: Chemotherapy-associated neurotoxicity: An important side effect-impacting on quality, rather than quality, of life. J Cancer Res Clin Oncol 122: 511–512, 1996.
6. Tuxen MK, Hansen SW: Complications of treatment: Neurotoxicity secondary to antineoplastic drugs. Cancer Treat Rev 20:191–214, 1994.
7. Postma TJ, Heimans JJ: Grading of chemotherapy-induced peripheral neuropathy. Ann Oncol 11:509–513, 2003.

8. Forman AD: Peripheral neuropathy in cancer patients: Clinical types, etiology, and presentation. Oncology 4:85–89, 1990.

9. de Gramont A, Figer A, Homerin M, et al: Leucovorin and fluorouracil with or without oxaliplatin as first-line treatment in advanced colorectal cancer. J Clin Oncol 18:2938–2947, 2000.

10. Taieb S, Trillet-Lenoir V, Rambaud L, et al: Lhermitte sign and urinary retention. Cancer 94:2434–2440, 2002.

11. Mangioni C, Bolis G, Pecorelli, et al: Randomized trial in advanced ovarian cancer comparing cisplatin and carboplatin. J Natl Cancer Inst 81:1464–1471, 1989.

12. Thompson SW, Davis LE, Kornfeld M, et al: Cisplatin neuropathy: Clinical, electrophysiology, morphology and toxicologic studies. Cancer 54:1269–1275, 1984.

13. Bradley WG, Lassman L, Pearce GW, Walton JN: The neuropathy of vincristine in man: Clinical, electrophysiological and pathological studies. J Neurol Sci 10:107–131, 1970.

14. Roca E, Bruera E, Politi PM, et al: Vinca alkaloid-induced cardiovascular autonomic neuropathy. Cancer Treat Rep 69:149–151, 1985.

15. Rowinsky EK, Gilbert MR, McGuire WP, et al: Sequences of taxol and cisplatin: A phase I and pharmacological study. J Clin Oncol 9:1692–1703, 1991.

16. Schilling T, Heinrich B, Kau R, et al: Paclitaxel administered over 3 h followed by cisplatin in patients with advanced head and neck squamous cell carcinoma: A clinical phase I study (abstract). Oncol 54:89–95, 1997.

17. Hansen SW: Autonomic neuropathy after treatment with cisplatin, vinblastine, and bleomycin for germ cell cancer. Br Med J 300:511–512, 1990.

18. Chaudry V, Chaudry M, Crawford TO, et al: Toxic neuropathy in patients with pre-existing neuropathy. Neurology 60:337–340, 2003.

19. Panici BP, Greggi S, Scambia G, et al: Efficacy and toxicity of very high-dose cisplatin in advanced ovarian carcinoma: 4-year survival analysis and neurological follow-up. Int J Gynecol Cancer 3:44–53, 1993.

20. Postma TJ, Benard BA, Huijgens PC, et al: Long term effects of vincristine on the peripheral nervous system (abstract). J Neuro-Oncol 15:23–27, 1993.

21. Dina OA, Chen X, Reichling D, Levine JD: Role of protein kinase Cε and protein kinase A in a model of paclitaxel-induced painful peripheral neuropathy in the rat. Neuroscience 108:507–515, 2001.

22. Rowinsky EK, Chaudry V, Cornblath DR, Donehower RS: Neurotoxicity of Taxol. Monogr Natl Cancer Inst 15:107–115, 1993.

23. Lipton RB, Apfel SC, Dutcher JP, et al: Taxol produces a predominantly sensory neuropathy. Neurology 39:368–373, 1989.

24. Kilkpatrick TJ, Phan S, Reardon K, et al: Leukaemia inhibitor factor abrogates paclitaxel-induced axonal atrophy in the Wistar rat. Brain Res 911:163–167, 2001.

25. Schmidt Y, Unger JW, Bartke I, Reiter R: Effect of nerve growth factor on peptide neurons in dorsal root ganglia after Taxol or cisplatin treatment and diabetic (db/db) mice. Exp Neurol, 132:16–23, 1995.

26. Boyle FM, Beatson C, Monk R, et al: The experimental neuroprotectant leukaemia inhibitor factor (LIF) does not compromise antitumour activity of paclitaxel, cisplatin and carboplatin. Cancer Chemother Pharmacol 48:429–434, 2001.

27. Cliffer KD, Siuciak J.A, Carson SR, et al: Physiological characterization of Taxol-induced large-fiber sensory neuropathy in the rat. Ann Neurol 43:46–55, 1998.

28. Polomano RC, Mannes AJ, Clark US, Bennet GJ: A painful peripheral neuropathy in the rat produced by the chemotherapeutic drug, paclitaxel. Pain 94:293–304, 2001.

29. Quasthoff S, Hartung HP: Chemotherapy-induced peripheral neuropathy. J Neurol 249:9–17, 2002.

30. Subbaramaiah K, Hart JC, Norton L, Dannenberg AJ: Microtubule-interfering agents stimulate the transcription of cyclooxygenase-2. J Biol Chem 275:14838–14845, 2000.

31. Byrd-Leifer CA, Block EF, Takeda K, et al: Akira S, Ding A. The role of MyD88 and TLR4 in the LPS-mimetic acitivity of Taxol. Eur J Immunol 31:2448–2457, 2001.

32. Zaks-Zilberman M, Zaks TZ, Vogel SN:. Induction of proinflammatory and chemokine genes by lyipopolysaccharide and paclitaxel (Taxol™) in murine and human breast cancer cells lines. Cytokine 15:156–165, 2001.

33. Aley KO, Reichling D, Levine JD: Vincristine hyperalgesia in the rat: A model of painful vincristine neuropathy in humans. Neuroscience 73:259–265, 1996.

34. Petrini M, Vaglini F, Cervetti G, et al: Is lithium able to reverse neurological damage induced by vinca alkaloids? J Neur Transm 106:569–575, 1999.

35. Shelanski ML, Wisniewski H: Neurofibrillary degeneration. Arch Neurol 20:199–206, 1969.

36. Green LS, Donoso JA, Heller-Bettinger IE, Samson FE: Axonal transport disturbances in the vincristine-induced peripheral neuropathy. Trans Am Neurol Assoc 100:195–196, 1975.

37. Tanner KD, Levine JD, Topp KS: Microtubule disorientation and axonal swelling in unmyelinated sensory axons during vincristine-induced painful neuropathy in rats. J Comp Neurol 395:481–492, 1998.

38. Ogawa T, Mimura Y, Kato H, et al: The usefulness of rabbits as an animal model for the neuropathological assessment of neurotoxicity following the administration of vincristine. Neurotoxicology 21:501–512, 2000.

39. Jackson DV, Sethi VS, Spurr CL, McWhorte, JM: Pharmacokinetics of vincristine in the cerebrospinal fluid of humans. Cancer Res 41:1466–1468, 1981.

40. Kellie SJ, Barbaric D, Koopmans P, et al: Cerebrospinal fluid concentrations of vincristine after bolus intravenous dosing. Cancer 94:1815–1820, 2002.

41. Hayakawa K, Itoh T, Niwa H, et al: Nerve growth factor prevention of aged-rat sympathetic neurons injury by cisplatin, vincristine and Taxol: in vitro explant study. Neurosci Lett 274:103–106, 1999.

42. Wang MS, Wu Y, Culver DG, Glass JD: Pathogenesis of axonal degeneration: Parallels between Wallerian degeneration and vincristine neuropathy. J Neuropathol Exp Neurol 59:599–606, 2000.

43. Djaldetti R, Hart J, Alexandrova S, et al: Vincristine-induced alterations in Schwann cells of mouse peripheral nerve. Am J Hematol 52:254–257, 1996.

44. Apfel SC, Arezzo JC, Lewis ME, Kessler JA: The use of insulin-like growth factor I in the prevention of vincristine neuropathy in mice. Ann NY Acad Sci 692:243–245, 1993.

45. Weng H-R, Cordella JV, Dougherty PM: Changes in sensory processing in the spinal dorsal horn accompany vincristine-induced hyperalgesia and allodynia. Pain 2003.

46. Fischer SJ, McDonald ES, Gross L, Windebank AJ: Alterations in cell cycle regulation underlie cisplatin induced apoptosis of dorsal root ganglion neurons in vivo. Neurobiol Dis 8:1027–1035, 2001.

47. Park SA, Choi KS, Bang JH, et al: Cisplatin-induced apoptotic cell death in mouse hybrid neurons is blocked by antioxidants through suppression of cisplatin-mediated accumulation of p53 but not of Fas/Fas ligand. J Neurochem 75:946–953, 2000.

48. Tredici G, Braga M, Nicolini G, et al: Effect of recombinant human nerve growth factor on cisplatin neurotoxicity in rats. Exp Neurol 551–558, 1999.

49. Ruigt GSF, Makkink WK, Konings PNM: SR 57746 attenuates cytostatic drug-induced reduction of neurite outgrowth in co-cultured rat dorsal root ganglia and Schwann cells. Nuerosci Lett 203:9–12, 1996.

50. Cavaletti G, Fabbrica D, Minoia C, et al: Carboplatin toxic effects on the peripheral nervous system of the rats. Ann Oncol 9:443–447, 1998.

51. Gregg RW, Molepo JM, Monpetit JA, et al: Cisplatin neurotoxicity: The relationship between dosage, time, and platinum concentration in neurologic tissues, and morphologic evidence of toxicity. J Clin Oncol 10:795–803, 1992.

52. Verstappen CCP, Heimans JJ, Hoekman K, Postma TJ: Neurotoxic complication of chemotherapy in patients with cancer. Drugs 63:1549–1563, 2003.

53. Apfel SC, Arezzo JC, Lipson LA, Kessler JA: Nerve growth factor prevents experimental cisplatin neuropathy. Ann Neurol 31:76–80, 1992.

54. Gao W-Q, Dybdal N, Shinsky N, et al: Neurotrophin-3 reverses experimental cisplatin-induced peripheral sensory neuropathy. Ann Neurol 38:30–37, 1995.

55. Cavaletti G, Bogliun G, Marzorati L, et al: Peripheral neurotoxicity of Taxol in patients previously treated with cisplatin. Cancer 75:1141–1150, 1995.

56. Sodhi A, Pai K: Increased production of interleukin-1 and tumor necrosis factor by human monocytes treated in vitro with cisplatin or other biological response modifiers. Immunol Lett 34:183–188, 1992.

57. Grolleau F, Gamelin L, Boisdron-Celle M, et al: A possible explanation for a neurotoxic effect of the anticancer agent oxaliplatin on neuronal voltage-gated sodium channels. J Neurophysiol 85:2293–2297, 2001.

58. Grothey A: Oxaliplatin-safety profile: Neurotoxicity. Semin Oncol 30:5–13, 2003.

59. Adelsberger H, Quasthoff S, Grosskreutz J, et al: The chemotherapeutic oxaliplatin alters voltage-gated Na+ channels kinetics on rat sensory neurons. Eur J Pharmacol 406:25–32, 2003.

60. Rowinsky EK, Donehower RS: Paclitaxel (Taxol), N Engl J Med 332:1004–1013, 1995.

61. Rhol J, Kushner D, Markman: Chronic administration of single-agent paclitaxel in gynecologic malignancies 81:205, 2001.

62. Forsyth PA, Balmaceda C, Peterson K, et al: Prospective study of paclitaxel-induced peripheral neuropathy with quantitative sensory testing. J Neuro-Oncol 35:47–53, 1997.

63. Shea T, Graham M, Bernard S, et al: A clinical and pharmacokinetic study of high-dose carboplatin, paclitaxel, granulocyte colony-stimulating factor, and peripheral blood stem cells in patients with unresectable or metastatic cancer. Semin Oncol 22:80–85, 1995.

64. Gordon AN, Stringer CA, Matthews CM, Nemunaitis J: Phase I dose escalation of paclitaxel in patients with advanced ovarian cancer receiving cisplatin: Rapid development of neurotoxicity is dose-limiting. J Clin Oncol 15:1965–1973, 1997.

65. Verstappen CCP, Postma TJ, Hoekman K, Heimans JJ: Peripheral neuropathy due to therapy with paclitaxel, gemcitabine, and cisplatin in patients with advanced ovarian cancer. J Neuro-Oncol 63:201–205, 2003.

66. Connelly E, Markman M, Kennedy A, et al: Paclitaxel delivered as 3-hr infusion with cisplatin in patients with gynecologic cancers: Unexpected incidence of neurotoxicity. Gynecol Oncol 62:166–168, 1996.

67. Aamadal S, Wolff I, Kaplan S, et al: Docetaxel (Taxotere) in advanced malignant melanoma: A phase II study of the EORTC early clinical trials. Eur J Cancer 30A:1061–1064, 1994.

68. Hilkens PHE, Verweij J, Stoter G, et al: Peripheral neurotoxicity induced by docetaxel. Neurology 46:104–108, 1996.

69. Hikens PHE, Verweij J, Vecht ChJ, et al: Clinical characteristics of severe peripheral neuropathy induced by docetaxel (taxotere). Ann Oncol 8:1–4, 1997.

70. New PZ, Jackson CE, Rinaldi D, et al: Peripheral neuropathy secondary to docetaxel (Taxotere). Neurology 46:108–111, 1996.

71. Cowan JD, Kies MS, Roth JL, Joyce RP: Nerve conduction studies in patients treated with cis-diamminedichloroplatinum(II): A preliminary report. Cancer Treat 64:1119–1122, 1980.

72. Boogerd W, ten Bokkel Huinink WW, Dalesio O, et al: Cisplatin induced neuropathy: Central, peripheral and autonomic nerve involvement, J Neuro-Oncol 9:255–263, 1990.

73. Hamers FPT, Gispen WH, Neijt JP: Neurotoxic side-effects of cisplatin. Eur J Cancer 27:376, 1991.

74. Prestayko AW, D'Aoust JC, Issell BF, Crooke ST: Cisplatin (cis-diamminedichloroplatinum II). Cancer Treat Rev 6:17–39, 1979.

75. Screnci D, McKeage MJ: Platinum neurotoxicity: Clinical profiles, experimental models and neuroprotective approaches. JIB 77:105–110, 1999.

76. Gurney H, Crowther D, Anderson H, et al: Five year follow-up and dose delivery analysis of cisplatin, iroplatin or carbopolatin in combination with cyclophosphamide in advanced ovarian carcinoma. Ann Oncol 1:427–433, 1990.

77. Swenerton K, Jeffrey J, Stuart G, et al: Cisplatin-cyclophosphamide versus carboplatin-cyclophosphamide in advanced ovarian cancer: A randomized phase III study of the national cancer institute of Canada clinical trial group, J Clin Oncol 10:718–726, 1992.

78. van der Hoop RG, van der Burg MEL, ten Bokkel Huinink WW, van Houwelingen J, Neijt JP. Incidence of neuropathy in 395 patients with ovarian cancer treated with or without cisplatin. Cancer 66:1697–1702, 1990.

79. Siegal T, Haim N: Cisplatin-induced peripheral neuropathy. Cancer 66:1117–1123, 1990.

80. Mollman JE, Hogan WM, Glover DJ, McCluske LF: Unusual presentation of cis-platinum neuropathy. Neurology 38:488–490, 1988.

81. Mollman JE, Glover DJ, Hogan WM, Furman RE: Cisplatin neuropathy. Cancer 61:2192–2195, 1988.

82. Ruckdeschel JC: The future role of carboplatin. Semin Oncol 21:114–118, 1994.

83. Alberts DS, Green S, Hannigan EV, et al: Improved therapeutic index of carboplatin plus cyclophosphamide versus cisplatin plus cyclophosphamide: Final report by the Southwest Oncology Group of a phase III randomized trial in stages III and IV ovarian cancer, J Clin Oncol 10:706–717, 1992.

84. Kelly K, Crowley J, Bunn PA, et al: Randomized phase III trial of paclitaxel plus carboplatin versus vinorelbine plus cisplatin in the treatment of patients with advanced non-small-cell lung cancer: A southwest oncology group trial. J Clin Oncol 19:3210–3218, 2001.

85. Cascinu S, Catalano V, Cordella L, et al: Neuroprotective effect of reduced glutathione on oxaliplatin-based chemotherapy in advanced colorectal cancer: A randomized, double-blind, placebo-controlled trial. J Clin Oncol 20:3478–3483, 2002.

86. Kim DY, Kim H, Lee S-H, et al: Phase II study of oxaliplatin, 5-fluorouracil and leucovorin in previously platinum-treated patients with advanced gastric cancer. Ann Oncol 14:383–387, 2003.

87. Casey EB, Jellife AM, Le Quesne PM, Millett YL: Vincristine neuropathy. Clinical and electrophysiological observations. Brain 96:69–86, 1973.

88. Klasa RJ, Meyer RM, Shustik C, et al: Randomized phase III study of fludarabine phosphate versus cyclophosphamide, vincristine, and prednisone in patients with recurrent low-grade non-Hodgkin's lymphoma previously treated with alkylating agent of alkylator-containing regimen. J Clin Oncol 20:4649–4654, 2002.

89. Patel SR, Forman AD, Benjamin RS: High-dose ifosfamide-induced exacerbation of peripheral neuropathy. J Natl Cancer Inst 86:305–306, 1994.

90. Frisk P, Stalberg E, Strömberg B, Jakobson A: Painful peripheral neuropathy after treatment with high-dose ifosfamide. Med Ped Oncol 37:379–382, 2001.

91. Ozkaynak F, Sondel PM, Krailo MD, et al: Phase I study of chimeric human/murine anti-ganglioside Gd2 monoclonal antibody (ch14.18) with granulocyte-macrophage colony-stimulating factor in children with neuroblastoma immediately after hematopoietic stem-cell transplantation: A children's cancer group study. J Clin Oncol 18:4077–4085, 2000.

92. Lenz H-J: Clinical update: Proteosome inhibitors in solid tumors. Cancer Treat Rev 29(suppl 1):41–48, 2003.

93. Richardson PG, Barlogie B, Berenson J, et al: A phase 2 study of bortezomib in relapsed, refractory myeloma. N Engl J Med 348:2609–2617, 2003.

94. Borgeat A, De Muralt B, Stalder M: Peripheral neuropathy associated with high-dose Ara-C therapy. Cancer 58:852–854, 1986.

95. Sakai H, Yoneda S, Tamura T, et al: A phase II of paclitaxel plus cisplatin for advanced non-small-cell lung cancer in Japanese patients. Cancer Chemother Pharmacol 48:499–503, 2001.

96. Thant M, Hawley RJ, Smith MT, et al: Possible enhancement of vincristine neuropathy by VP-16. Cancer 49:849–864, 1982.

97. Darnell RB, Posner JB: Mechanisms of disease: Paraneoplastic syndromes involving the nervous system. N Engl J Med 349:1543–1554, 2003.

98. Voltz R: Paraneoplastic neurological syndromes: An update on diagnosis, pathogenesis, and threapy. Lancet Neurol 1:294–305, 2002.

99. Chauvenet A, Shashi V, Selsky C, et al: Vincristine-induced neuropathy as the initial presentation of Charcot-Marie-Tooth disease in acute lymphoblastic leukemia: A pediatric oncology group study. J Ped Hemat Oncol 25:316–320, 2003.

100. McGuire SA, Gospe SM, Dahl G: Acute vincristine neurotoxicity in the presence of hereditary motor and sensory neuropathy type I. Med Ped Oncol 17:520–523, 1989.

101. Norman N, Elinder G, Finkel Y: Vincristine neuropathy and Guillain-Barre Syndrome: A case with acute lymphatic leukemia and quadriparesis. BUSCAR 75–76, 1986.

102. Sarosy G, Kohn E, Stone DA, et al: Phase I study of Taxol and granulocyte colony-stimulating factor in patients with refractory ovarian cancer. J Clin Oncol 10:1165–1170, 1992.

103. Roelofs RI, Hrushesky W, Rogin J, Rosenberg L: Peripheral sensory neuropathy and cisplatin chemotherapy. Neurology 34:934–938, 1984.

104. Miller AB, Hoogstraten B, Staquet M, Winkler A: Reporting results of cancer treatment. Cancer 47:207–214, 1981.

105. Oken MM, Greech RH, Torney DC, et al: Toxicity and response criteria of the Eastern Cooperative Oncology Group. Am J Clin Oncol 5:649–655, 1982.

106. Boivie J: Central pain the role of quantitative sensory testing (QST) in research and diagnosis. Eur J Pain 7:339–343, 2003.

107. Verdugo R, Ochoa JL: Quantitative somatosensory thermotest: A key method for functional evaluation of small calibre afferent channels. Brain 115:893–913, 1992.

108. Willis WD: Nociceptors. In: Gildenberg Ph.L. (ed): The Pain System: The Neural Basis of Nociceptive Transmission in the Mammalian Nervous System. New York, Karger, 1985, pp 22–77.

109. Shy ME, Frohman EM, So YT, et al: Quantitative sensory test. Neurology 60:898–904, 2003.

110. Glover DJ, Glick JH, Weiler C, et al: Phase I/II trials of WR-2721 and cisplatin. Int J Radiat Oncol Biol Phys 12:1309–1312, 1986.

111. Rick O, Beyer J, Schwella N, et al: Assessment of amifostine as protection from chemotherapy-induced toxicities after conventional-dose and high-dose chemotherapy in patients with germ cell tumor. Ann Oncol 12:1151–1155, 2003.

112. Penz M, Kornek GV, Raderer M, et al: Subcutaneous administration of amifostine: A promising therapeutic option in patients with oxaliplatin-related peripheral sensitive neuropathy. Ann Oncol 12: 421–422, 2001.

113. Moore DH, Donnelly J, McGuire WP, et al: Limited access trial using amifostine for protection against cisplatin- and three-hour paclitaxel-induced neurotoxicity: A phase II study of the gynecologic oncology group. J Clin Oncol 21:4207–4213, 2003.

114. Lersch C, Schmelz R, Eckel R, et al: Prevention of oxaliplatin-induced peripheral sensory neuropathy by carbamazepine in patients with advanced colorectal cancer. Clin Colorect Cancer 2:54–58, 2002.

115. Gedlick C, Scheithauer W, Schüll B, Korneck GV: Effective treatment of oxaliplatin-induced cumulative polyneuropathy with alpha-lipoic acid. J Clin Oncol 20:3356–3361, 2002.

116. Bardos G, Moricz K, Rabloczky G, et al: BPG-15, a hydroxamic acid derivative, protects against cisplatin- or Taxol-peripheral neuropathy in rats. Toxicol Appl Pharmacol 190:9–16, 2003.

117. Arrick BA, Nathan CF: Glutathione metabolism as a determinant of therapeutic efficacy: A review. Cancer Res 44: 4224–4232, 1984.

118. Boyle FM, Wheeler H, Shenfield GM: Glutamate ameliorates experimental vincristine neuropathy. J Pharmacol Exp Ther 279:410–415, 1996.

119. Cassidy J, Paul J, Soukop M, et al: Clinical trials of nimodipine as a potential neuroprotector in ovarian cancer patients treated with cisplatin. Cancer Chemother Pharmacol 41:161–166, 1998.

120. Kammer R: Diagnosis and management of neuropathic pain patients with cancer. Cancer Investigation 19:324–333, 2001.

121. Kori SH: Diagnosis and management of brachial plexus lesions in cancer patients. Oncology 9:756–760, 1995.

122. Maslovsky I, Volchek L, Blumental R: Persistent paraneoplastic neurologic syndrome after successful therapy of Hodgkin's disease. Eur J Haematol 66:63–65, 2001.

123. Johansson S, Svensson H, Larsson LG: Brachial plexopathy after postoperative radiotherapy of breast cancer patients: A long term followup. Acta Oncologia 39:373–382, 2000.

124. Johansson S, Svensson H, Denckamp J: Timescale of late radiation injury after post-operative radiotherapy of breast cancer patients. Int J Radiat Oncol Biol Phys 48:745–750, 2000.

125. Azinovic I, Calvo FA, Puebla F: Long-term normal tissue effects of intraoperative electron radiation therapy (IOERT): Late sequelae, tumor recurrence, and second malignancies. Int J Radiat Oncol Biol Phys 49:597–604, 2001.

126. Gunderson LL, Nelson H, Martenson JA: Locally advanced primary colorectal cancer: Intraoperative electron and external beam irradiation +/− F-U. Int J Radiat Oncol Biol Phys 37:601–614, 1997.

127. McBride WH, Withers HR: Biological basis of radiation therapy. In Perez CA (ed): Principles and Practice of Radiation Oncology. Philadelphia, Lippincott, 2004, pp 96–136.

128. Emami B, Lyman J, Brown A, et al: Tolerance of normal tissue therapeutic irradiation. Int J Radiat Oncol Biol Phys 21:109, 1991.

129. Hallahan DE, Haimovitz FA, Kufe DW, et al: The role of cytokines in radiation oncology. Important Adv Oncol 71, 1993.

130. Kerr JF, Winterford CM, Harmon BV: Apoptosis: Its significance in cancer and cancer therapy. Cancer 13:2013, 1994.

131. Withers HR, Peters LJ, Taylor JMG, et al: Late normal tissue sequelae from radiation therapy for carcinoma of the tonsil. Int J Radiat Oncol Biol Phys 33:549, 1995.

132. Michalowski AS: The pathogenesis and conservative treatment of radiation injuries. Neoplasma 42:289, 1995.

133. Turesson I: The progression of late radiation effects in normal tissue and its impact on dose-dependent relationships. Radiother Oncol 15:217, 1998.

134. Neta R: Modulation with cytokines of radiation injury: Suggested mechanisms of action. Env Health Perspect 105s: 1463–1465, 1997.

135. Pritchard J, Anand P, Broome J, et al: Double-blind randomized phase II study of hyperbaric oxygen in patients with radiation-induced brachial plexopathy. Radiother Oncol 58:279–286, 2001.

136. McFarlane VJ, Clein GP, Cole J: Cervical neuropathy following mantle radiotherapy. Clin Oncol 14:468–471, 2002.

137. Anezaki T, Harada T, Kawachi I, et al: A case of post-irradiation lumbosacral radiculopathy successfully treated with corticosteroid and warfarin. Clin Neurol 39:825–829, 1999.

138. Alektiar KM, Hu K, Anderson L, et al: High-dose-rate intraoperative radiation therapy (HDR-IORT) for retroperitoneal sarcomas. Int J Radiat Oncol Biol Phys 47:157–163, 2000.

139. Backonja MM, Galer BS: Pain assessment and evaluation of patients who have neuropathic pain. Neurol Clin 16:775–790, 1998.

140. Wouter van Es H, Engelen AM, Witkamp TD, et al: Radiation-induced brachial plexopathy: MR imaging. Skeletal Radiol 26:284–288, 1997.

141. Bosch EP, Smith BE: Disorders of the peripheral nerves. In Bradley WG et al (eds). Neurology in Clinical Practice. Boston, Butterworth-Heinemann, 2000, pp 2045–2130.

142. Amato AA, Collins MP: Neuropathies associated with malignancy. Semin Neurol 18:125–144, 1998.

CHAPTER 12

Postherpetic Neuralgia in the Cancer Patient

Nancy A. Alvarez, PharmD, Bradley S. Galer, MD, and Arnold R. Gammaitoni, PharmD

Chronic cancer pain may unmercifully plague patients and challenge the health care professionals who care for them. Patients are often afflicted with several pain conditions concurrently, which all may require specific and distinct therapies.[1] Often these pain conditions involve both nociceptive and neuropathic mechanisms further complicating management. Cancer pain syndromes are most often caused as a direct result of the underlying malignancy (e.g., tumor infiltration, nerve impingement, bone metastases). Some patients may experience additional pain due to the presence or development of concurrent diseases. Postherpetic neuralgia (PHN), a well-characterized, difficult to treat, neuropathic pain syndrome, is an example of a concurrent medical condition that may afflict the cancer patient.

Following the development of acute herpes zoster (AZH or "shingles"), some patients may develop PHN, which can become a chronic neuropathic pain condition in the unlucky minority of patients. The pain of PHN often results in a significant decrement in quality of life of the afflicted individual, not uncommonly manifesting in the inability to wear clothing due to hypersensitive, allodynic skin, and reclusiveness.[2-4] There are multiple aspects that affect patients' overall well-being or suffering and may include a combination of physical, psychologic, social, spiritual, and societal factors. Pain may result in decreased functional abilities and diminished strength, interruption in sleep, eating, and concentration. Pain may heighten the severity of worry, anxiety, and depression already experienced by these patients. Conversely, collective suffering may preoccupy patients' thoughts and further exacerbate the perception of pain as they fluctuate among the different stages (e.g., denial, anger, depression, bargaining, and acceptance) of grief trying to cope with the news of their disease, treatment failures, or reemergence of the cancer.[5] There is an urgency to work to alleviate pain in an effort to diminish the suffering experienced by cancer pain patients. For these patients, their pain is a constant reminder of their underlying condition and exacerbations may heighten fear of worsening disease and their own mortality. The objective of this chapter will focus on risk factors for the development of PHN, its clinical presentation, and treatment approaches. In addition, AHZ will be initially but briefly reviewed as it relates to the cancer pain patient.

ACUTE HERPES ZOSTER

Individuals who have had chickenpox (varicella zoster) during their lifetime are at risk for herpes zoster. In fact, over 90% of adults in the United States have serologic evidence of varicella-zoster virus infection.[6,7] In the United States, the overall incidence of herpes zoster ("shingles") is estimated to occur in 600,000 to 850,000 people per year[8,9] and may affect up to 20% of the general population over time, as extrapolated from herpes zoster epidemiology studies.[9-11] The best identified risk factor for the development of herpes zoster is age; that is, as one ages, the risk increases, with the sharpest increase occurring between ages 50 and 60.[9,12,13] Other investigators have observed similar relationships and noted ever-increasing incidence rates as patients grow older beyond 60 and 70 years of age.[10,11] Authorities believe that the overall percentage affected with herpes zoster will increase as the population continues to age.[2,12,14] It is projected that the proportion of the U.S. population greater than 65 years of age will increase from 12.4% in 2000 to 19.6% by 2030; the number of persons aged greater than 65 years is expected to increase from approximately 35 million in 2000 to an estimated 71 million in 2030.[15] In addition to age, one other well-cited risk factor for the development of herpes zoster is an alteration in cell-mediated immunity.[11,12]

Patients with malignancies (especially lymphoproliferative cancers) who are treated with chemotherapy, radiotherapy, or other immunosuppressive modalities for reduction of tumor load or in preparation for bone marrow transplantation, are at increased risk for herpes zoster.[12] Multiple investigations have illustrated that the incidence of herpes zoster infection is greater in those with hematologic malignancies (e.g., Hodgkin's disease, leukemia, non-Hodgkin's lymphoma) versus those with solid tumors (e.g., breast and lung cancer).[12,16-18]

Hodgkin's disease is believed to be the malignancy with the highest incidence rate for the development of herpes zoster.[18] Several investigators have documented the occurrence of herpes zoster in cancer patients receiving radiation and/or chemotherapy treatments but bias introduced by the underlying disease was difficult to control for in the study design. Therefore, data describing the magnitude (if it exists) of risk and the specific treatment regimens associated with the greatest risk is lacking.[12] Organ transplantation (e.g., bone marrow) has been associated with the development of herpes zoster despite study design limitations.[18] Extensive reviews published recently have evaluated these factors and describe the difficulty in ascertaining the degree of risk associated with herpes zoster development.[3,12] It should be noted, however, that the development of herpes zoster or PHN is not a potential sign of an undiagnosed cancer.[12]

The pain associated with AHZ is due to the presence of the varicella zoster virus (VZV), which is reactivated from its dormant state in the dorsal root ganglion (DRG). On reactivation, VZV travels unilaterally along one or two dermatomes from the dorsal root ganglion toward the skin surface where the typical skin rash of "shingles" erupts. In addition, postmortem studies in some PHN patients have also demonstrated direct damage and inflammation in the ipsilateral dorsal horn of the spinal cord,[19,20] thus suggesting that VZV can also travel from the DRG along the spinal root and also simultaneously into the spinal cord, at least in some patients.

Some patients experience a painful prodrome of varied length while others experience pain only after the appearance of vesicles. Rarely patients have been reported to experience pain accompanied by no characteristic rash (zoster sine herpete).[21,22] The affected dermatomes are most often located in the thoracic region but cranial, cervical, and lumbar dermatomes may also be involved.[3,10,23] Three weeks after herpes zoster onset, the rash typically begins to heal, while pain gradually diminishes for most patients.

While all authorities agree that persistent pain in the area of AHZ is PHN, there is a lack of consensus in the literature as to when exactly this conversion period takes place. Varied time frames are cited in the literature in terms of defining when herpes zoster pain ends and postherpetic neuralgia actually begins, with no widespread

acceptance of any one defined time period.[24-30] It has been suggested recently by international authorities that there are typically 3 phases associated with the pain of herpes zoster. Phase 1 is described as an acute herpetic neuralgia paired with the characteristic rash of about 30 days in duration following its onset. The next phase, a subacute herpetic neuralgia lasts for 30 to 120 days following rash onset and postherpetic neuralgia describes persistent pain of greater than 120 days post rash onset.[13,31]

An in-depth discussion of the treatment of acute herpes zoster is beyond the scope of this chapter. Limiting the amount of neural damage caused by the proliferation of VZV is one approach undertaken to attenuate the development of PHN addressed by the use of antiviral therapy (acyclovir, famcicyclovir, and valacyclovir) during acute herpes zoster infection. Aggressive treatment of AHZ reduces the degree of neural damage sustained during the AZH phase, thereby decreasing the likelihood of the development of PHN, the severity of PHN that does develop and the risk of prolonged pain.[13] Despite the growing body of literature demonstrating the effectiveness of antiviral therapy, proper and timely antiviral treatment is not guaranteed to prevent PHN. Unfortunately, many patients continue to develop PHN.[13] Corticosteroids, administered during the AHZ phase, have been used to potentially reduce the incidence and or severity of PHN; however, they do not appear to be effective in preventing PHN despite results from smaller trials that suggest benefit,[32] and are thus not recommended. Neuropathic pain medications, such as the tricyclic antidepressants, administered during the AHZ phase have been hypothesized to also potentially reduce the incidence and/or severity of PHN[33,34] though data is currently being generated to assess this hypothesis. It seems reasonable to attempt to lessen the severity of herpes zoster pain using analgesics such as opioids and this is supported by the well-accepted relationship between herpes zoster pain severity and the development of PHN.[3,13] In addition, it has been suggested that early treatment with sympathetic nerve blocks may also prevent the development of PHN but this data is uncontrolled and most PHN authorities dispute this contention. Most recently, ongoing trials will determine whether the administration of a varicella-zoster vaccine to older adults at risk (i.e., infected with latent VZV) for herpes zoster will be spared viral reactivation.[35]

POSTHERPETIC NEURALGIA

Definition and Prevalence

As eluded to previously, the determination of when herpes zoster ends and postherpetic neuralgia begins evades researchers and clinicians. The definitions range from persistent pain 1 month after herpes zoster outbreak,[26] to persistent pain lasting 3 months or 6 months after the outbreak[27,28] to a classification system that segments herpetic neuralgia temporally (acute, subacute, and chronic).[31] Others, yet, use rash healing as an interval baseline that pain must exceed in order to be classified as PHN (e.g., pain 1 month after rash healing).[29] The estimate of the proportion of patients who go on to develop PHN has been difficult to determine based on the plethora of definitions cited in the literature.

According to the FDA, the prevalence of PHN is less than 200,000. A high estimate, however, projects that the prevalence of PHN may be up to 1 million cases in the United States; to date, there have been no systematic attempts to quantify a more accurate picture of prevalence of this disorder.[13] Most patients are elderly and as an increase in the number of AZH cases as the aged population increases, it is reasonable to expect the number of PHN cases to increase as well.

Risk Factors

While risk factors are delineated for AZH, there is no evidence of strong predictive risks in terms of which patients will go on to develop PHN. Age is universally cited as a primary risk factor for the development of PHN; the incidence of occurrence increases, as patients grow older.[36,37] deMorgas et al. reported that up to 50% of patients aged 70 or greater have pain that persists for over 1 year after the herpes zoster rash heals, although younger herpes zoster patients (i.e., 40 years old or less) rarely progressed to chronic pain status.[36] Subsequent studies generally support this finding.[37,38]

Other risk factors described in the literature include greater acute pain severity (during the AZH phase), greater rash severity, the presence of prodromal pain, more pronounced immune response, fever greater than 38 degrees and the presence of other neurologic abnormalities.[3,37] Psychosocial risk factors (i.e., recent negative life events) trend toward predisposing patients to developing PHN, as well.[39] Cancer patients are often faced with a myriad of psychologic distress surrounding their disease and their potential morbidity (e.g., mastectomy) or mortality, which, though not confirmed, may put them at risk for development of PHN. Study results do not suggest that differences in gender add to the risk of developing PHN.[37,40] Further studies are required to determine whether the distribution of herpes zoster can be used to determine risk of PHN. Ophthalmic dermatomal involvement giving rise to PHN more often has been suggested, but not consistently substantiated.[3,41] Additional consideration of the added burden of cancer treatment is warranted for the cancer pain patient who develops AHZ. Many chemotherapy agents may cause neuronal damage, thus, at least theoretically, making the threat of PHN development more ominous.

Pathophysiology

Persistent pain following AHZ is thought to be a reflection of neuronal damage caused by VZV and may manifest in a variety of forms. Clinical features have been carefully evaluated in the hopes of determining a pathologic origin.[42] As with other neuropathic pain conditions, the pathophysiology underlying PHN is multifaceted and not uniform among patients. An understanding of the mechanisms that contribute to the development and maintenance of PHN pain will further permit the discovery of effective pain treatments. This section will briefly summarize purported pain mechanisms associated with PHN; an extensive review of the range of pain mechanisms can be found elsewhere.[42,43]

Reactivation of the virus results in inflammation and damage to the dorsal root ganglion and primary afferent neurons as the virus travels to the skin surface, as well as possible dorsal horn damage in some patients. During this time of inflammation and neural injury, peripheral sensitization occurs. Peripheral sensitization is characterized by lowered nociceptor activation threshold, exaggerated response to noxious stimuli (e.g., hyperalgesia), and spontaneous discharge. While this is a normal part of pain processing, its ongoing maintenance secondary to neural injury is abnormal and leads to further deleterious changes within both the peripheral and central nervous system. An example of these further changes includes spontaneous, ectopic pain signal generation in an area proximal to the dorsal root ganglion. The damaged areas on the primary afferent neuron express an increased number of abnormally functioning sodium channels that are also believed to be another origin of spontaneous pain signal generation.

Abnormal peripheral nervous system activity increases the amount of pain signal information transmitted to the central nervous system. Constant bombardment of the dorsal horn may cause secondary afferent neurons to become sensitized in a fashion similar to the periphery (lower activation thresholds, exaggerated responses to primary afferent neuron input, and spontaneous discharge). In the presence of central sensitization, A-beta mechanoreceptors (which normally transmit innocuous sensory information) are capable of activating secondary afferent neurons, in the superficial layers of the dorsal horn, eliciting a sensation of pain from a normally nonpainful producing stimulus (allodynia). Furthermore, the discriminatory role of the secondary afferent neurons (regulating pain signal transmission to the high neural structures) may be compromised allowing greater numbers of pain signals to pass through to the higher levels of the CNS.

Moreover, it is possible that some primary afferent neurons atrophy in the wake of neural damage, thus disconnecting (e.g., deafferentation) the line of neural communication with the dorsal horn. In an effort to reestablish central nervous system contact with the deafferented regions, dorsal root axons may develop sprouts. Alternatively, A-beta axons terminating in the dorsal horn may begin to grow into areas normally populated with primary afferent neuron axons. This type of reorganization permits A-beta mechanoreceptors (which normally communicate continuous, innocuous stimuli) direct access to areas that exclusively process pain signals; hence, sensory information can now be processed as pain information and perceived as such. In some patients with completely severed peripheral connections or damaged dorsal horn neurons, pain may result from central neuronal changes, where the pain signal generator is solely located in the CNS; that is, "central neuropathic pain."

Another proposed mechanism is disinhibition. Normally, A-beta fibers are thought to contribute indirect inhibitory input in the dorsal horn by exciting interneurons that inhibit secondary afferent neuron activity; hence pain signal transmission is interrupted or altered. It is also possible that interneurons may be impaired, resulting in a net increase in pain signal transmission. More research is required to further delineate the contribution disinhibition makes toward initiating and maintaining PHN pain. Peripheral sensitization and hyperactivity of primary afferent neurons, central sensitization, and deafferentation (sprouting, A-beta fiber infiltration into pain receptive areas, and central hyperactivity) may exist in a variety of combinations in PHN patients.

Importantly, the variability in the existence of any combination of these underlying mechanisms most likely explains why some medications alleviate the pain of PHN in some patients, may only partially relieve PHN in others, and why most patients often require multiple pharmacotherapeutic agents in order to attain optimal pain relief. Researchers and clinicians alike continue to seek to better understand the underlying pathophysiology in order to effectively treat patients afflicted with this challenging pain syndrome and to identify potential targets for pharmacotherapy.

Postherpetic Neuralgia Subtypes

Fields and Rowbotham have proposed that PHN patients may be subgrouped into three types based on distinct underlying pain pathophysiology: irritable nociceptors, deafferentation with allodynia, and deafferentation without allodynia.[42] Irritable nociceptors describe intact, abnormally functioning primary afferent neurons that generate and maintain pain. These hyperactive neurons (including the nociceptor) contribute to spontaneous pain and allodynia reported by many patients. Allodynia is thought to be supported by central sensitization in these patients. Patients with deafferentation-type pain with allodynia often describe profound sensory loss in the area of greatest pain. Allodynia in these cases is believed to be supported by the development of A-beta primary afferent sprouts on to the dorsal horn areas that have lost their normal pain fiber input. Finally, deafferentation-type pain without allodynia is believed to be supported by CNS hyperactivity secondary to neuroplastic changes that have occurred in the spinal cord. Allodynia is not present because there is a complete primary afferent neuron disconnection from the central structures.

Clinical Presentation

PHN is multifaceted as evidenced by the different types of pathophysiology involved. In addition, clinical presentations vary among PHN patients. The size of the PHN region can be one or several entire dermatomes or can only be the size of a small coin. Patients often report different pain qualities: consistent or intermittent pains, deep or superficial pains, throbbing or burning pains, and so forth.[44] Allodynia, pain as a result of non-noxious mechanical or thermal stimuli (e.g., weight or rubbing of clothing or changes in temperature), is frequently experienced by PHN patients.[2] Allodynia has been described as one if not the most debilitating aspect of PHN and causes tremendous patient distress. PHN patients may become isolated, depressed, and/or anxious, due to the unrelieved pain and the inability to wear clothing over the involved region.

Besides having allodynia, some PHN patients report regions of sensory deficit often described as "numbness." Other patients may report skin pigmentation changes or scarring left over after rash healing.[45,46] Motor weakness, including loss of muscle tone seen on examination, and autonomic dysfunction (e.g., abnormal skin temperature and color and sweating) in the affected area has also been described.[47]

PHARMACOLOGIC THERAPY FOR POSTHERPETIC NEURALGIA

PHN is often difficult to treat based on the complexity of the underlying pathophysiology and highly variable presentation among patients. Although there are a number of treatments with proven efficacy, there has yet to be one medication that consistently treats every aspect of PHN pain in all patients. Therefore, a rational polypharmacy approach to designing a therapeutic plan should be used for cancer (and noncancer) patients afflicted with PHN.

Treating PHN in cancer patients can be even more challenging for the clinician than caring for PHN patients without concomitant cancer. Cancer patients may already be on complex therapeutic regimens to attack the primary malignancy. Additional medications may be necessary to relieve the symptoms that result from the administration of complex chemotherapy regimens (i.e., pain of oral mucositis, fatigue, nausea, and vomiting). Patients may also be receiving treatment to address depression and anxiety. Clinicians should be sensitive to the potential for introducing additional adverse event or drug–drug interaction risk when agents are considered to address the PHN pain. The potential for drug–drug interactions can be minimized by considering pharmacotherapy choices that best complement the current regimen of systemic chemotherapeutic and adjunct medications. Topical analgesic medications, "targeted peripheral analgesics," target delivery of medication directly to pathophysiologic site(s) in the peripheral nervous system while minimizing the absorption of the active ingredient into the bloodstream. Oral, rectal, and transdermal formulations are preferred over subcutaneous, intravenous, and other injectable medications as a means to limit the therapy invasiveness, however, agents delivered via all of these routes result in substantial absorption into the bloodstream.

Lidocaine Patch 5%

The lidocaine patch 5% (Lidoderm® Patch, Endo Pharmaceuticals Inc., Chadds Ford, PA) was the first medication approved by the United States Food and Drug Administration (FDA) for the treatment of the neuropathic pain associated with PHN. The lidocaine patch 5% is the first true analgesic topical patch approved by the FDA.[47–50] This unique lidocaine formulation has recently been included as one of two first-line

choices for PHN and has been cited as one of five first-line medication choices in international recommendations for the pharmacologic treatment of neuropathic pain.[51]

Local anesthetics, such as lidocaine, are believed to bind to sodium channels, inhibit the influx of sodium into the nerve cell, and interrupt pain signal generation and conduction, and thus to be true analgesics. Abnormal sodium channels that develop following damage to the peripheral nerves, such as in neuropathic pain states, have an unusually high binding affinity for drugs such as lidocaine and therefore minimal levels of lidocaine delivered to these nerve membranes (as produced by the lidocaine patch 5% formulation) will preferentially bind to these abnormal channels and reduce their ectopic discharges. Interruption of peripheral nerve pain signal generation also has an indirect effect on the CNS by reducing the receipt of ongoing peripheral input into the spinal cord, which contributes to development and maintenance of central sensitization.

The lidocaine patch 5% is available as a 10×14, nonwoven polyethylene patch containing 700 mg of lidocaine per patch. This novel patented formulation permits the topical delivery of lidocaine to the area where aberrant activity sustains the generation and transmission of pain signals in PHN. When used as directed, minute amounts of lidocaine are detected in the systemic circulation. Table 12–1 contains various traits to assist clinicians in distinguishing the key differences between topical and transdermal patch delivery systems. The patch itself also protects sensitive skin areas from further mechanical stimulation (e.g., touch or rubbing of clothing), thus offering a second line of defense for those patients with allodynia.

Due to its minimal systemic absorption, lack of drug–drug interactions, lack of the need for titration to effective dose and ease of use, many pain authorities have

TABLE 12–1 Comparison of Topical and Transdermal Route of Administration

	Topical	Transdermal
Titration required	No	Yes
Application area	Skin application where pain is reported	Away from painful area
Site of medication activity	Structures directly beneath application (peripheral soft tissue and nerves)	Systemic
Serum drug concentrations achieved	Minimal, clinically insignificant	Required for drug activity
Systemic side effect	None expected	Likely to occur
Drug–drug interactions	Minimal to none expected	Likely to occur
Elimination from system	Dependent on drug characteristics	Dependent on drug characteristics and depot effect (possibly prolonged)

recommended that the lidocaine patch 5% is a logical first choice for the treatment of pain associated with PHN.[13,52,53] International PHN authority Peter Watson wrote in his 2000 New England Journal of Medicine editorial that the lidocaine patch 5% is recommended as the first-line treatment for PHN.[2] PHN cancer patients may particularly benefit from using the lidocaine patch 5% since many have highly complex medication regimens with a need to minimize potential drug–drug interactions and/or systemic side effects.

Three randomized, vehicle-controlled studies have demonstrated that topical lidocaine patch 5% is efficacious with no systemic activity and thus no systemic side effects.[49,50,54] During these studies, patients were permitted to continue therapy with stable doses of opioid and nonopioid medications. As previously mentioned, most PHN patients require different medications with different mechanisms of action to effectively treat pain; however, Davies reported results for patients who used the lidocaine patch 5% as monotherapy (56%) during the trial, which establishes support for the use of the patch alone as well as add-on therapy.[55]

A recent vehicle-controlled study demonstrated that lidocaine patch 5% is statistically more effective than a vehicle patch in alleviating all pain qualities associated with neuropathic pain, such as "burning," "aching," "shooting," and "deep," in addition to "skin sensitivity" and allodynia.[44] A large open-label 4-week trial of 332 PHN patients demonstrated statistical improvement, as well as clinically meaningful improvements in daily functioning, which only further verifies results that gained this agent its PHN indication in 1999. Furthermore, about 75% of patients experienced pain relief improvement as measured by a 4-point (0 = no change; 3 = complete relief) categorical patient and physician global assessment of pain.[56]

Studies have shown that the serum levels achieved with 3 patches on the skin for 12 hours per day result in minimal lidocaine blood levels that are well below those necessary to produce an antiarrhythmic effect.[49] The amount of lidocaine absorbed is directly proportional to the surface area covered and the length of application. Recent data have shown that increasing the dosage to 4 patches (560 sq cm) on for 18 hours per day[57] or 24 hours per day (dosed either daily or BID)[58] resulted in relatively low systemic lidocaine levels versus those required to produce either cardiac or toxic effects. Thus, the use of 4 patches of q24h for extended periods of time resulted in only marginally greater serum lidocaine blood levels and maintained a wide margin of nonsystemic activity, and was well tolerated.

The 24-hour pharmacokinetic study included skin sensory testing, which revealed that patients did not report loss of sensation (light touch and pinprick stimulation)

underneath the patch area at any time point; in other words the lidocaine patch 5% provides analgesia without causing anesthesia. Hence, the unique formulation of lidocaine patch 5% is not expected to result in altered skin sensitivity; that is, numbness. This expectation has been generally supported in clinical trials of other pain states as well, although there have been a few instances of skin sensitivity alteration.[59] The mechanism behind the "numbness" phenomenon typically observed in other formulations of topical lidocaine is not clear. In general, it is thought that the amount of lidocaine topically delivered via the topical lidocaine patch 5% (Lidoderm®) to the dysfunctional or damaged nerve fibers is not sufficient to affect larger, myelinated A-beta sensory neurons.[58] Therefore, the lidocaine patch 5% is analgesic but not anesthetic, unlike the topical local anesthetic cream preparation, Eutectic Mixture of Local Anesthetics Cream (EMLA® Cream, AstraZeneca Pharmaceuticals, Wilmington, DE).

As directed in the current package insert, patients should use up to 3 patches (420 cm²) to cover the entire or most painful region. The patch is applied directly to the painful area (intact skin) and worn for 12 consecutive hours followed by removal for 12 hours. Mild and transient local skin reactions (erythema or edema) may occur in some patients and have been the most reported adverse events in clinical trials.[49,50,56-58] The mean serum levels seen (average of 0.13 µg/mL) in patients are 1/10 the value required for therapeutic antiarrhythmic use.[48] Katz' open-label trial demonstrated that while a majority (66%) report some relief within 1 week of treatment, an additional 43% of those not reporting relief in week 1 begin to experience relief by week 2.[56] Thus, it is recommended to allow for at least 2 weeks of daily treatment as an adequate drug trial.

Anticonvulsants

The use of anticonvulsants for the treatment of neuropathic pain syndromes, including PHN, has been cited in the literature for decades, beginning with their usefulness for the treatment of trigeminal neuralgia.[60-63] Over the past decade, the quality of study design has improved enabling meaningful clinical interpretation as compared with criticized trials evaluating phenytoin and carbamazepine conducted in the 1960s.[64] Anticonvulsants have been evaluated for usefulness to treat neuropathic pain due to the similarities exhibited between neuropathic pain and epilepsy (e.g., shared pathophysiologic and neurochemical mechanisms).[65] The exact mechanism of action for anticonvulsants has yet to be elucidated; however, for neuropathic pain, it is generally believed for many anticonvulsants (but not gabapentin) that sodium channel blockade primarily contributes to their analgesic activity.[65] Serum levels of drug have not been shown to correlate to response; hence it is not necessary to draw and follow them to guide the use of anticonvulsants as analgesics. Furthermore, the administration of loading doses of these medications for pain treatment in hopes of achieving rapid pain relief response has not been demonstrated. Loading doses may unnecessarily position patients to experience greater incidences of side effects and are not recommended.

Gabapentin

Gabapentin has become a first-line therapeutic choice for the treatment of neuropathic pain[51] based on its established efficacy in a number of neuropathic pain syndromes,[62,63,66,67] its adverse events profile, patient tolerability, and its lack of documented drug–drug interactions. The mechanism of action of gabapentin remains unknown although it has been suggested that this agent is involved in calcium channel blockade.[68] Its effectiveness for the treatment of PHN pain has been established, gaining it recent approval from the Food and Drug Administration in 2002 for this indication.[62,63,69]

In 1998, Rowbotham and colleagues published the results of a multicenter, randomized, double-blind, placebo-controlled, parallel design study evaluating the efficacy and safety of gabapentin to treat PHN pain.[62] A total of 229 patients were randomized in this 8-week trial, which included a 4-week titration phase during which patients were titrated to a maximum dose of 3600 mg/day or the maximum tolerable dose. Treatment was maintained for the remaining 4 weeks at the maximum tolerated dose. Gabapentin demonstrated superior analgesia as compared with placebo; the gabapentin group's pain was reduced from 6.3/10 to 4.2/10, as compared with placebo's 6.5 to 6.0 ($P < 0.001$). In terms of pain relief, 43.2% of those who received gabapentin reported at least "moderate" pain relief, as compared with 12.1% of placebo group. The most common adverse effects in the gabapentin group included somnolence, dizziness, ataxia, peripheral edema, and infection, but withdrawal rates were comparable among groups.

Rice and colleagues published the results of a multicenter, randomized, double-blind, placebo-controlled study to evaluate the efficacy and safety of gabapentin 1800 or 2400 mg/day in treating PHN pain.[63] The investigator sought to demonstrate efficacy at a lower dose and simpler regimen than the one described by Rowbotham. Three hundred and thirty-four patients were randomized in this 7-week study, which included a force titration schedule lasting 2 to 3 weeks depending on the dosage assigned to the patient. The gabapentin treatment was maintained at the stable dose of either 1800 or 2400 mg/day through the end of the study. Gabapentin demonstrated superior analgesia compared

with placebo ($P < 0.01$); placebo = 6.4/10 to 5.3/10 (15.7% reduction), gabapentin 1800 mg = 6.5/10 to 4.3/10 (34.5% reduction), gabapentin 2400 mg = 6.5/10 to 4.2/10 (34.4% reduction). The proportion of patients exhibiting a 50% or greater decrease in mean pain scores (baseline to week 7) was significantly higher for both gabapentin groups compared with placebo ($P = 0.001$; placebo 14%, gabapentin 1800 mg 32%, gabapentin 2400 mg 34%). Based on the results of this trial it appears that doses beyond 1800 mg/day do not offer greater improvements in pain relief. The recommended dosing approved by the FDA is up to 1800 mg/day. The most common adverse events reported in the gabapentin group included dizziness, drowsiness, asthenia, peripheral edema, dry mouth, and diarrhea. There was more than double the number of withdrawals due to adverse events compared with placebo: 7 (6.3%) placebo, 15 (13%) gabapentin 1800 mg, and 19 (17.6%) gabapentin 2400 mg. Placebo withdrawals were evenly distributed; gabapentin withdrawals occurred primarily during the forced titration period.

The results of these two randomized, double-blind, placebo-controlled studies, gained gabapentin approval for the treatment of PHN pain. As seen in the lidocaine patch 5% studies, patients in these two trials were allowed to continue to receive concomitant analgesic medications (e.g., antidepressants, opioids, nonsteroidal anti-inflammatory agents, and acetaminophen [alone or in combination with a mild opioid]). Only 15% of patients in the Rice trial took no medication for their PHN pain other than gabapentin.[63]

While gabapentin is recognized as a first-line treatment, it is not without its share of potential limitations. As with other anticonvulsants, some patients do report intolerable or bothersome side effects with gabapentin, including sedation, dizziness, and peripheral edema. As seen in the two trials described above, side effects were most problematic during the initiation and dose escalation period. A modest titration period may be necessary to help patients tolerate the high doses required for efficacy.

The current manufacturer-recommended dosing guidelines are as follows: initial dose as a single 300 mg dose on day 1; 600 mg/day on day 2 (divided dose BID); and 900 mg/day (divided dose TID) on day 3. If a patient is not experiencing any significant pain relief or side effects, the dose can continue to be titrated up to a daily dose of 1800 mg/day (divided dose TID).[69] Many clinicians manage dose titration less aggressively to try to minimize side effects experienced by patients during the dose stabilization period; they increase the dose by 300 mg every 7 days as titrated to pain relief despite the fact that this approach is not outlined in the package insert. Serum levels do not correlate to response (rate or extent); therefore, it is not necessary to follow serum levels. Furthermore, it is not necessary to use loading dose strategies as they do not appear to be predictive of response and may increase the intensity of the expected side effects experienced during the titration period. This is especially true for elderly patients who may not tolerate dizziness, somnolence, or peripheral edema side effects on the way toward establishing a therapeutic dose. Gabapentin is eliminated entirely by the kidneys; therefore, dosage adjustment based on renal function is warranted. Another potential clinical problem with gabapentin is the needed time for titration to reach a therapeutic dose; thus, it is recommended to maintain close and regular patient follow-up and monitoring while titrating to the optimal dose.

Pregabalin

As no one treatment approach adequately addresses the neuropathic pain of PHN, investigators are vigorously searching for additional options. Dworkin et al. recently published the results of an 8-week, randomized, placebo-controlled trial of pregabalin, which was recently approved by the FDA for the treatment of PHN and painful diabetic neuropathy.[68] This study randomized 173 patients into one of two groups of pregabalin ($n = 89$) based on renal function (600 mg/day [$n = 59$] or 300 mg/day [$n = 30$]) or placebo ($n = 84$) if their pain was rated as moderate to severe in intensity. Patients were permitted to continue concomitant analgesics but were held stable during the trial. The primary endpoint was change in pain intensity following 8 weeks using an 11-point scale and reported to show a statistically significant reduction in mean pain intensity for pregabalin (two groups collapsed into one based on steady-state concentrations achieved) over placebo (2.8 vs. 1.0; $P = 0.0001$).

Most adverse events reported were as mild to moderate in severity. Despite this, one third (31.5%) of patients withdrew from the treatment group based on adverse events compared with less than 5% for the placebo group. The most commonly reported adverse events were dizziness and somnolence.

Similar to gabapentin in its structure and its inactivity at the GABA receptor, pregabalin has been shown to be an alpha-2 subtype ligand of voltage gated calcium channels. It is thought that by blocking calcium channels, pain signal transmission may be interrupted. Furthermore, blocking these channels would also impact the release of neurotransmitters such as glutamate and norepinephrine, which are also involved in pain signal transmission. Hence, it is hypothesized that neuronal hyperexcitation may be reduced as demonstrated in animal models of pain, both nociceptive and neuropathic in nature.

Carbamaepine

Carbamazepine has been used as an anticonvulsant for the treatment of neuropathic pain for several decades and was the first anticonvulsant to receive FDA approval for the treatment of a specific neuropathic pain condition: trigeminal neuralgia, previously referred to as tic doloroux. It has also been studied for the treatment of painful diabetic neuropathy. This agent has recently been relegated to second-line therapy, based on evidence generated under less rigorous study design and reporting criteria as compared with state-of-the-art clinical trials today, in addition to its poor side effect profile.[51] As far as carbamazepine for the treatment of PHN, the evidence is not well established. One study found carbamazepine, in combination with clomipramine, was effective versus transcutaneous nerve stimulation in an unblinded study, but the two medications are structurally similar to tricyclic antidepressants and, hence, to each other, which makes it difficult to interpret carbamazepine's contribution to the results.[70]

It is thought that carbamazepine analgesic activity is via sodium channel blockade at the site of ectopic pain signal generation presented by damaged nerves, thereby interrupting pain signal generation. When appropriate, carbamazepine dosing is typically initiated at 100 mg twice daily and titrated every 3 to 7 days to establish a balance between efficacy and tolerable side effects. The most commonly reported side effects include sedation, dizziness, ataxia, confusion, and nausea. Blood dyscrasias and Stevens Johnson syndrome have been associated with the agent and patients should be monitored closely for the potential development of these more severe problems.[53,65] Carbamazepine is also a potent hepatic enzyme inducer and clinicians need to be mindful of potential drug–drug interactions (i.e., theophylline), which may reduce the effectiveness of concomitant medications.

Opioids

Opioids are cornerstone agents in the armamentarium for most cancer pain treatment. Up until most recently, it was once believed, even by pain authorities, that opioids were generally ineffective for the treatment of neuropathic pain. However, advances in our understanding of pain pathophysiology and a growing number of controlled studies have shown that this old, widely held belief is invalid.[71-74] The ongoing debate concerning the first-line use of opioids for the treatment of neuropathic pain may be laid to rest with the anticipated publication of international treatment recommendations for neuropathic pain.[51]

Opioids exert their analgesic effects by interfering with pain signal transmission when activating specific opioid receptors identified to mediate analgesia. Opioid receptors are located throughout the body with primary residence within the central nervous system, peripheral nervous system, and gastrointestinal tract.[75,76] Opioids also alter patients' perceptions of pain.[77]

Several randomized placebo-controlled trials examining the effectiveness of opioids for the treatment of PHN have clearly demonstrated the potential benefit of opioids. Rowbotham and colleagues initially demonstrated in a controlled trial that an intravenous infusion of morphine to PHN patients was efficacious.[78] In 1998, Watson et al. conducted a double-blind, placebo-controlled trial to examine the efficacy of controlled release oxycodone when compared with placebo. This trial demonstrated that controlled release oxycodone was statistically superior to placebo.[71]

Most recently, in 2002, Raja et al. published the findings of a randomized, placebo-controlled trial evaluating the analgesic and cognitive effects among opioids (morphine, primary or methadone, secondary), tricyclic antidepressants (nortriptyline, primary or desipramine, secondary), or placebo.[72] Alternatives were offered instead of the primary treatments if they were intolerable (reflecting clinical practice). Three treatment periods scheduled to last 8 weeks each (with a 1-week washout period in between) were established for 76 PHN patients. Each period was designed to permit adequate titration, maintenance, and taper administration. All medications were discontinued 1 week prior to study enrollment. Dosages were increased or decreased as dictated by inadequate pain relief or intolerable side effects, respectively. Pain intensity was measured by assessing a patient's overall pain during the previous 24 hours using a 0 to 10 numerical rating scale (0 = no pain; 10 = most intense pain imaginable). Mean pain intensity reductions for opioids and tricyclic antidepressants (TCAs) were statistically significant (1.9 and 1.4, respectively) over placebo (0.2, $P < 0.001$). In general, opioids performed better than TCAs in terms of pain intensity reduction, but this finding did not reach significance ($P = 0.06$). In terms of cognitive impairment, results did not show any appreciable effect for either class; opioid treatment did not negatively influence any measure evaluated, unlike the TCAs. Mean percentage pain relief scores were also superior over placebo for both opioids and TCAs (38% and 32% on a 0–100 scale versus 11% for placebo, $P < 0.001$). Side effects reported were what would be expected from these agents: constipation, nausea, dizziness, drowsiness, loss of appetite, and dry mouth. Opioids produced a greater incidence of side effects, but patients preferred them over TCAs and placebo.

Opioid Selection and Dosing

If one opioid does not provide effective pain relief or results in intolerable side effects, consideration of an alternative opioid can be made due to incomplete cross tolerance (e.g., due to differential opioid receptor affinities).[79] While a full discussion of opioid rotation (i.e., changing from morphine to oxymorphone at an equianalgesic dose) is beyond the scope of this chapter, opioid conversion information can be found elsewhere.[80] Over the past decade, the advent of new extended-release formulations of many opioids affords multiple options for the treating physician or other health care professionals including morphine, oxycodone, hydromorphone, and oxymorphone.

Common opioid-related side effects include constipation, nausea and vomiting, and sedation. The latter three tend to be most problematic during initiation of therapy and dosage increases but decrease in intensity as a patient becomes tolerant to the prescribed opioid dose. Constipation, resulting from the stimulation of opioid receptors in the GI tract, can be alleviated with proactive initiation of bowel regimens consisting of a stimulant laxative and stool softener). Other side effects include pruritus and orthostatic hypotension, both thought to be mediated by the release of histamine and respiratory depression. The risk of respiratory depression is minimal when opioids are introduced under proper titration conditions, despite often being the most feared of opioid side effects. Patients who may be predisposed to develop depressed respiration (e.g., COPD patients or patients who have only one lung) may require a more conservative titration approach and aggressive monitoring, but generally do well as they acclimate to their required dosage.

Neuropsychiatric effects such as myoclonus, hallucinations, or dysphoria may be the result of the accumulation of opioid metabolites due to high dose therapy, dehydration, or renal impairment. These side effects can be particularly frightening for the patient and their caregivers. Dosage decreases or opioid rotation may be effective strategies to combat this problem.[81]

Patients receiving long-term therapy with opioids are expected to develop physical dependence despite appropriate use. Patients receiving opioids for legitimate medical purposes do not develop an opioid addiction.[82] Suboptimal use of opioids, due to a lack of accurate understanding of drug tolerance, physical dependence, addiction, and the resulting fear, may pose a real clinical threat; although this may be less problematic in the cancer pain patient afflicted with PHN. Definitions for these terms can be found in Table 12-2.

Tramadol

While tramadol is considered a first-line treatment for the management of chronic neuropathic pain,[51] the published evidence for its effectiveness for the treatment of PHN pain is limited to open label pilot study.[83] Tramadol is believed to exert its action by binding weakly to mu-opioid receptors. It also exhibits serotonin and norepinephrine activity. When used, the manufacturer titration schedule recommends starting at 25 mg daily

TABLE 12–2 Definitions Related to the Use of Opioids for the Treatment of Pain

	Classification	Description
Tolerance	State of adaptation	Exposure to a drug induces changes that results in a diminution of one or more of the drug's effects over time
Physical dependence	State of adaptation	Manifests by drug class specific withdrawal syndrome that can be produced by abrupt cessation, rapid dose reduction, decreasing blood level of the drug, and/or administration of an antagonist
Addiction	Primary, chronic, neurobiologic disease	Manifestation and development influenced by genetic, psychosocial, and environmental factors. Characterized by behaviors including one or more of the following: impaired control over drug use, compulsive use, continued use despite harm, and craving
Pseudoaddiction	Temporary adaptation: distinguished from addiction as behaviors resolve when pain is effectively treated	Referred to as patient behaviors that may occur when pain is undertreated. Characterized by patient focus on obtaining medication, "clock watching" and otherwise seemingly inappropriate "drug seeking" behavior. Behavior may include illicit drug use and deception as patients seek to obtain pain relief

Adapted from Consensus Document of the American Academy of Pain Medicine, the American Pain Society, and the American Society of Addiction Medicine, 2001.

and titrating in 25-mg separate doses every 3 days until patients achieve 100 mg/day (25 mg qid), followed by titration in 50-mg increments every 3 days up to 200 mg/day (50 mg QID). If a patient requires a further dosage increase, 50- to 100-mg increments may be administered in divided doses (every 4 to 6 hours) until a maximum dosage of 400 mg daily is achieved (300 mg if the patient is older than 75 years).[84] If patients have more immediate pain relief needs, it is possible that a more aggressive titration schedule might be necessary. Dosing adjustments are recommended for patients who have renal impairment.

The most commonly reported adverse events associated with tramadol closely resemble those of opioids: constipation, nausea, dizziness, somnolence, and vomiting. Some patients may experience orthostatic hypotension, which may be difficult for an elderly patient to tolerate. Tramadol has been reported to cause seizures during therapy, but the risk is increased when dosages exceed 400 mg daily. Tramadol may be problematic in a patient with a known seizure history or epilepsy or if administered concomitantly with medications that lower an individual's seizure threshold (e.g., TCAs and antipsychotic agents). Tramadol may be incompatible with medications that increase serotonin levels (e.g., selective serotonin reuptake inhibitors [SSRIs], serotonin/norepinephrine reuptake inhibitors [SNRIs], monoamine oxidase inhibitors [MAOIs]), requiring consideration of drug–drug interaction development risk.

Tricyclic Antidepressants

TCAs have been used for several decades to treat neuropathic pain conditions despite the lack of an FDA approval for this indication. Human and animal studies repeatedly demonstrate that the TCAs are analgesics independent of their ability to alleviate depression.[85-87] Many controlled trials evaluating efficacy in PHN[88-92] have demonstrated the benefits of several different tricyclic antidepressants, including amitriptyline, nortriptyline, and desipramine. Support for the overall efficacy of TCAs has earned this class first-line inclusion in published neuropathic pain guidelines.[51,67,93-96]

The exact mechanism for the analgesic efficacy of the TCAs is unknown. It has been widely assumed that efficacy of these agents is based on norepinephrine and serotonin activity on a descending series of neuronal networks originating in the brainstem and synapsing in the dorsal horn. The existence of this "pain-modulating system," however, remains a widely held hypothesis, unsupported with definitive clinical data.[97] Recent data have revealed the importance of the TCAs' local anesthetic pharmacologic activity. Data from peripheral neuropathic pain animal models have demonstrated that these agents reduce animal pain behavior via their sodium channel blocking activity.[98,99] It has been suggested that agents with a mixture of neurotransmitter reuptake inhibition are superior for the treatment of PHN, followed by selectivity for norepinephrine rather than serotonin.[100] It should be noted that SSRIs are generally not recommended as a treatment for PHN[32,101] as clinical experience has been disappointing. Placebo-controlled trials have not been conducted to date evaluating SSRI for the treatment of PHN. In fact, most controlled trials evaluating the treatment of SSRI in other neuropathic pain syndromes have reported negative results[95,102] or marginal efficacy with paroxetine and citalopram.[103,104]

Amitriptyline is the prototypical TCA and the most widely studied agent for the treatment of pain. However, it also has the greatest potential for causing dose-limiting side effects. Other tricyclic antidepressants also have been shown to be analgesic in controlled trials and tend to have fewer side effects, such as nortriptyline, desipramine, and imipramine.[87,90,94,95] Watson et al. conducted a small randomized, double-blind, crossover trial amitriptyline versus nortriptyline in 33 patients with PHN. While patients reported fewer side effects with nortriptyline, a metabolite of amitriptyline, the two therapies were essentially equal in their ability to effectively treat pain, thereby offering an alternative with less anticholinergic and sedative activity.[90] Using secondary amine tricyclic antidepressants such as nortriptyline and desipramine, which have relatively fewer anticholinergic side effects, may be advantageous when dealing with highly susceptible patients and may improve patient tolerability and acceptance.

Specifically, initiating TCA therapy should begin with a 10 mg/day dose administered at bedtime. Conservative dose escalation should occur weekly until titration to adequate pain relief or intolerable side effects occur. There is no specific analgesic dose; a typical effective dose resides between 25 mg and 75 mg (range between 10 and 150 mg/day). Response to analgesic therapy occurs much sooner than response to the antidepressant effects, often within 1 to 2 weeks of achieving a therapeutic dose. Serum levels of drug do not correlate to response; hence it is not necessary to follow serum levels.[100]

Most patients report side effects with TCAs. Weight gain, sedation, dizziness, constipation, urinary retention, dry mouth, and orthostatic hypotension are common TCA class side effects. Dry mouth may pose a problem for patients already experiencing difficulty due to salivary damage from radiation due to head and neck cancers. Anticipated constipation may be compounded by the use of opioids (for PHN or other cancer pain syndromes), requiring introduction of yet additional medications for bowel care. Patients at risk for seizures (e.g., patients with primary brain tumors, brain metastases, or receiving high-dose busulfan regimens) are not good candidates for amitriptyline as the seizure threshold may be reduced. Furthermore, patients with cardiac dysfunction (e.g., arrhythmias or heart failure) or using

chemotherapy known to cause cardiac damage (e.g., anthracene derivatives such as doxorubicin) may be at risk for the occurrence of cardiotoxicity; baseline cardiac screening EKGs may be prudent to monitor chronic therapy with TCAs for high-risk patients.

Side effects may or may not be intolerable. In fact, TCAs are often used specifically for their sedating effects and thus a treatment for insomnia, a common comorbid condition of chronic pain. If the patient is additionally depressed, using TCAs may simplify a patient's drug treatment regimen. If, however, a patient is using an SSRI for depression, adding a TCA for analgesia could result in an unwanted drug–drug interaction, manifesting in excessive serotonin amounts and leading possibly to serotonin syndrome. Procarbazine, used to treat Hodgkin disease, exhibits weak MAO inhibitor activity and may interact with TCAs to cause hypertensive crisis.[105] Careful use and vigilant monitoring can permit PHN patients to benefit from the efficacy of the TCAs for the treatment of pain associate with their condition.

Capsaicin

Capsaicin, contained in various over-the-counter ointment, gel, and lotion formulations, is a natural substance derived from the chili pepper. The mechanism of action for capsaicin is not yet determined, which is similar to other agents discussed previously, although it is hypothesized that capsaicin renders skin insensitive to pain by depleting substance P from sensory nerve endings. Substance P is known as a pain mediator, not responsible for causing pain directly, but instead facilitating pain signal generation by lowering the pain stimulation threshold. In addition, a recent histology study demonstrated that application of capsaicin results in neuronal death.[106] Because it is a "natural substance," current formulations of capsaicin have not undergone the rigors of the FDA new drug application (NDA) approval process. Of note, a novel topical patch formulation of topical capsaicin is currently in Phase 2 trials for the treatment of PHN in the United States.

While there are clinical trials of varied designs (large and small, open-label or double-blind, placebo-controlled trials) evaluating capsaicin for the treatment of PHN, definitive evidence of benefit remains elusive.[107-109] Investigators have been hard pressed to design randomized, placebo-controlled trials to evaluate this agent due to the difficulty in masking the burning sensation associated with its application to intact skin. This can potentially unblind a study and poses a limitation for published trials, unraveling their strength.[107]

When a clinical trial of capsaicin is initiated, patients should apply the formulation to intact skin at the affected area four times daily. Patients must avoid contact with mucous membranes (e.g., eyes, mouth, nose) and should thoroughly wash their hands with soap and water immediately following application. Side effects include burning, stinging, or erythema on application. The degree of these side effects may be substantial enough to cause patients to discontinue use of capsaicin, even if they report pain relief.[107]

EMLA

EMLA (lidocaine 2.5% and prilocaine 2.5%) is available in a cream and "anesthetic disc" formulations. EMLA currently has an FDA-approved indication as a topical anesthetic for use on normal intact skin to produce local anesthesia (i.e., numbness). This lipophilic formulation permits the local anesthetic combination to penetrate the stratum corneum of intact skin in an amount sufficient to affect larger myelinated sensory neurons. EMLA does not, however, have an indication for the treatment of any type of chronic pain. For chronic pain patients, loss of sensory function is not sought, particularly if a patient is already experiencing sensory deficits due to the pain syndrome itself. Therefore, affecting sensory neurons in addition to pain fibers is not desirable and differs from the lidocaine patch 5%, whose delivery technology does not facilitate the penetration of enough lidocaine to affect these larger neurons. A controlled trial of EMLA used in the treatment of PHN neuropathic pain did not demonstrate superiority over placebo,[110] whereas smaller uncontrolled trials suggested some benefit.[111,112]

ADDITIONAL OPTIONS AND INVESTIGATIONAL AGENTS

Systemic Local Anesthetic Agents

Intravenously administered lidocaine has been shown to be effective for short-term relief (few hours) of PHN patients.[78] Authorities indicate it is safe to use in cardiac-healthy PHN patients and can be useful to predict whether patients will benefit from oral therapy with mexilitine, a structural analog of lidocaine.[101] Mexilitine has not been evaluated for PHN pain treatment despite its apparent utility for painful diabetic neuropathy.[113]

Miscellaneous Agents

The role of the sympathetic nervous system in the development and maintenance of PHN has not been fully established. Investigators continue to learn about the relationship of the sympathetic nervous system as it contributes and relates to pain. Long-standing PHN does not seem to be relieved with the use of sympathetic nerve blocks, generally. It is suggested that this type of procedure be held as a last resort to try to accomplish short-term pain relief.[114] Extensive reviews of the utility of sympathetic blockade to treat PHN have been published elsewhere.[115,116] While widespread use of sympathetic nerve blocks with local anesthetics occurs, clinical trials reporting positive results have lacked scientific rigor (nonrandomized, noncontrolled).[115] As in AZH, prospective, randomized controlled trials of sufficient size must be designed to determine the extent that this approach is beneficial.

A paucity of randomized controlled trials of surgical procedures for the management of PHN pain exists. Surgical procedure descriptions for refractory PHN pain have been captured primarily by case report and individual clinical experience. These media are inherently fraught with limitations, even if an observation is positive in nature. Some examples of surgical procedures used to treat resistant PHN include dorsal rhizotomy, spinal cord stimulation, excising skin and dorsal root entry zone lesions. Loeser extensively reviewed the utility of surgical procedures elsewhere.[117]

Rational Polypharmacy

Rational polypharmacy is a term used to describe the use of a combination of medications with different and perhaps complimentary mechanisms of action to target the complex underlying mechanisms of neuropathic pain. However, data is lacking to give clinicians a sequential pharmacotherapy roadmap and to indicate the additive or synergistic effect of combination therapy. Little information exists evaluating various agents against one another.[72,90] However, clinicians can introduce a well-designed plan to address this complex and debilitating condition by taking a mechanistic approach to pharmacologic treatment. The lidocaine patch 5% targets delivery of medication directly to the pathophysiologic site(s) in the peripheral nervous system while minimizing the absorption of the active ingredient into the bloodstream and makes a sound therapeutic first choice. If there is need to supplement lidocaine patch 5% monotherapy, a logical addition may be that of a systemic agent with a different mechanism of action such as gabapentin. Despite the fact that these medications are both well tolerated and pose minimal risk for the development of drug–drug interactions, the lidocaine patch 5% may offer advantages over gabapentin. Lidocaine patch 5% does not require titration or have the side effects associated with this period (e.g., dizziness, somnolence, or peripheral edema) or the requirement for dosage adjustment for renally impaired patients.

Patients may already be taking long- and short-acting opioid medications for around the clock (ATC) and rescue analgesia due to pain from the underlying cancer problem. The opioid dose may be increased to try to address the neuropathic pain of PHN but it might be better to introduce the lidocaine patch 5% and/or gabapentin to avoid opioid-induced, dose-limiting side effects, particularly if the current dose of opioid is adequately addressing nociceptive-type pain attributed to the cancer. It may be necessary, however, to titrate the opioid upward or to add a TCA to the regimen, if inadequate pain relief continues. Rational titration approaches should continue after the introduction of numerous agents to manage positive (efficacy) and negative (emergence of side effects) outcomes. Too many simultaneous changes would make it difficult to determine which agent to attribute the success or side effects to. Thorough documentation to capture the results of the analgesic plan is tantamount to the ongoing success of analgesic treatment.

CONCLUSION

PHN is not an uncommon development in cancer patients. The development of PHN in a cancer patient can add another layer of management complexity to an already challenging disease (primary malignancy) and symptom (pain from primary malignancy or its treatment) process. Current first-line treatment for PHN, according to authorities, includes topical lidocaine patch 5%, gabapentin, pregabalin, opioids, and tricyclic antidepressants. Rational polypharmacy, the need to use multiple medications with different mechanisms of action in a logical manner is typically required to manage PHN pain. It is prudent to initiate therapy with the least invasive, local treatments to avoid drug–drug interactions and systemic side effects, if possible. Aggressive treatment of PHN is required in order to assist cancer pain patients in an effort to improve lost functionality, restore dignity, and reduce further suffering.

REFERENCES

1. Foley KM: Supportive care and quality of life. In De Vita VT, Hellman S, Rosenberg SA (eds): Cancer Principles and Practice of Oncology, 5th ed. Philadelphia, Lippincott-Raven, 1997, pp 2807–2841.
2. Watson CP: A new treatment for postherpetic neuralgia. N Engl J Med 343: 1514–1519, 2000.
3. Dworkin RH, Schmader KE: The epidemiology and natural history of herpes zoster and postherpetic neuralgia. In Watson CPN, Gershon AA (eds): Herpes Zoster and PHN 2nd Revised and Enlarged Edition Vol 11. Amsterdam, Elsevier Science, 2001, pp 39–64.
4. Davies L, Cossins L, Bowsher D, et al: The cost of treatment for post-herpetic neuralgia in the UK. Pharmacoeconomics 6:142–148, 1994.
5. Kübler-Ross E: On Death and Dying. New York, Simon and Shuster, 1997.
6. Choo PW, Donahue JG, Manson JE, et al: The epidemiology of varicella and its complications. J Infect Dis 172:706–712, 1995.
7. Straus SE: Overview: The biology of varicella-zoster virus infection. Ann Neurol 35(suppl):4–8, 1994.
8. Schmader KE: Epidemiology and impact on quality of life of postherpetic neuralgia and painful diabetic neuropathy. Clin J Pain 18:350–354, 2002.
9. Schmader KE: Herpes zoster in older adults. Clin Infect Dis 32:1481–1486, 2001.
10. Ragozzino MW, Melton LJ III, Kurland LT: Population-based study of herpes zoster and its sequelae. Medicine 61:310–316, 1982.
11. Donahue JG, Choo PW, Manson JE, Platt R: The incidence of herpes zoster. Arch Intern Med. 155:1605–1609, 1995.
12. Schmader K: Herpes zoster epidemiology. In: Arvin A, Gershon A (eds): Varicella-Zoster Virus, Cambridge, Cambridge University Press, 2000, pp 2220–2246.

13. Dworkin RH, Schmader KE: Treatment and prevention of postherpetic neuralgia. Clin Infect Dis 36:877–882, 2003.
14. Dworkin RH, Perkins FM, Nagasako EM: Prospects for the prevention of postherpetic neuralgia in herpes zoster patients. Clin J Pain 2(suppl):S90–100, 2000.
15. U.S. Bureau of the Census. International database. Table 094. Midyear population, by age and sex. Available at http://www.census.gov/population/www/projections/natdet-D1A.html. Accessed May 28, 2003.
16. Rustover JJ, Ahlgren P, Elhakim T, et al: Varicella-zoster infection in adult cancer patients: A population study. Arch Intern Med 148:1561–1566, 1988.
17. Rustover JJ, Ahlgren P, Elhakim T, et al: Risk factors for varicella-zoster disseminated infection among adult cancer patients with localized zoster. Cancer 62:1641–1646, 1988.
18. Rustover JJ: The risk of varicella-zoster infections in different patient populations: A critical review. Transfusion Med Rev 8:96–116, 1994.
19. Watson CPN, Oaklander AL, Deck JH: The neuropathology of herpes zoster with particular reference to postherpetic neuralgia and its pathogenesis. In Watson CPN, Gershon AA (eds): Herpes Zoster and PHN 2nd Revised and Enlarged Edition Vol 11. Amsterdam, Elsevier Science, 2001, pp 167–182.
20. Watson CPN, Deck JH, Morshead C, et al: Post-herpetic neuralgia: Further postmortem studies of cases with and without pain. Pain 44:105–117, 1991.
21. Gilden DH, Dueland AN, Devlin ME, et al: Varicella-zoster virus reactivation without rash. J Infect Dis 166(suppl):S30–S34, 1992.
22. Gilden DH, Wright RR, Schneck SA, et al: Zoster sine herpete: A clinical variant. Ann Neurol 35:530–533, 1994.

23. Helgason S, Sigurdsson JA, Gudmundsson S: The clinical course of herpes zoster: A prospective study in primary care. Eur J Gen Pract 2:12–16, 1996.
24. Burgoon CR II, Burgoon JS, Baldridge GD: The natural history of herpes zoster. JAMA 164:265–269, 1957.
25. Brown GR: Herpes zoster: Correlation of age, sex, distribution, neuralgia and associated disorders. South Med J 69:576–578, 1976.
26. Rogers RS, Tindall JP: Geriatric herpes zoster. J Am Geriatr Soc 19:495–504, 1971.
27. Max MB, Schafer SC, Culnane M, et al: Association of pain relief with drug side effects in postherpetic neuralgia: A single-dose study of clonidine, codeine, ibuprofen, and placebo. Clin Pharmacol Ther 43:363–371, 1988.
28. Harding SP, Lipton JR, Wells JCD: Natural history of herpes zoster ophthalmicus: Predictors of postherpetic neuralgia and ocular involvement. Br J Ophthalmol 71:353–358, 1987.
29. Rowbotham MC, Davies PS, Fields HS: Topical lidocaine gel relieves postherpetic neuralgia. Ann Neurol 37:246–253, 1995.
30. Baron R, Saguer M: Postherpetic neuralgia: Are C-nociceptors involved in signaling and maintenance of tactile allodynia? Brain 116:1477–1496, 1993.
31. Dworkin RH, Portenoy RK: Pain and its persistence in herpes zoster. Pain 67: 241–251, 1996.
32. Watson CPN: The medical treatment of postherpetic neuralgia: Antidepressants, anticonvulsants, opioids and practical guidelines for management. In Watson CPN, Gershon AA (eds): Herpes Zoster and PHN 2nd Revised and Enlarged Edition Vol 11. Amsterdam, Elsevier Science, 2001, pp 243–254.

33. Bowsher D: The effects of pre-emptive treatment of postherpetic neuralgia with amitriptyline: A randomized, double-blind, placebo-controlled trial. J Pain Symptom Manage 13:327–331, 1997.

34. Wu CL, Marsh A, Dworkin RH: The role of sympathetic nerve blocks in herpes zoster and postherpetic neuralgia. Pain 87:121–129, 2000.

35. Levin MJ: Use of varicella vaccines to prevent herpes zoster in other individuals. Arch Virol Suppl 17:151–160, 2001.

36. deMorgas JM, Kierland RR: The outcome of patients with herpes zoster. Arch Dermatol 75:193–196, 1957.

37. Choo PW, Galil K, Donahue JG, et al: Risk factors for postherpetic neuralgia. Arch Intern Med 157:1217–1224, 1997.

38. Hope-Simpson, RE: Postherpetic neuralgia. J R Coll Gen Pract 25:571–575, 1975.

39. Schmader K: Postherpetic neuralgia in immunocompetent elderly people. Vaccine 16:1768–1770, 1998.

40. Dworkin RH, Boon RJ, Griffin DRG, et al: Postherpetic neuralgia: Impact of famciclovir, age, rash severity, and acute pain in herpes zoster patients. J Infect Dis 178(suppl 1):S76–S80, 1998.

41. Decroix J, Partsch H, Gonzalez R, et al: Factors influencing pain outcome in herpes zoster: An observational study with valacyclovir. J Eur Acad Dermatol Venereol 14:23–33, 2000.

42. Fields HL, Rowbotham M, Baron R: Postherpetic neuralgia: Irritable nociceptors and deafferentation. Neurobio Dis 5:209–227, 1998.

43. Rowbotham MC, Baron R, Petersen K, Fields HL: Spectrum of pain mechanisms contributing to PHN. In Watson CPN, Gershon AA (eds): Herpes Zoster and PHN 2nd Revised and Enlarged Edition Vol 11. Amsterdam, Elsevier Science, 2001, pp 183–195.

44. Galer BS, Jensen MP, Ma T, et al: The lidocaine patch 5% effectively treats all neuropathic pain qualities: Results of a randomized, double blind, vehicle-controlled, 3 week efficacy study with use of the neuropathic pain scale. Clin J Pain 18:297–301, 2002.

45. Kost RG, Straus SE: Postherpetic neuralgia–Pathogenesis, treatment and prevention. N Engl J Med 335:32–42, 1996.

46. Wallace MS, Oxman MN: Acute herpes zoster and postherpetic neuralgia. Anesthesiol Clin North Am 15:371–404, 1997.

47. Galer BS: Advances in the treatment of postherpetic neuralgia: The topical lidocaine patch. Today's Therapeutic Trends 18:1–20, 2000.

48. Lidoderm® Complete Prescribing Information. Chadds Ford, PA, Endo Pharmaceuticals Inc, 2002.

49. Rowbotham MC, Davies PJ, Verkempinck CM, Galer BS: Lidocaine patch: Double-blinded controlled study of a new treatment method for postherpetic neuralgia. Pain 65:39–45, 1996.

50. Galer BS, Rowbotham MC, Perander J, Friedman E: Topical lidocaine patch relieves postherpetic neuralgia more effectively than a vehicle topical patch: Results of an enriched enrollment study. Pain 80:533–538, 1999.

51. Dworkin RH: Advances in neuropathic pain: Diagnosis, mechanisms, and treatment recommendations. Arch Neurol 60:1524–1534, 2003.

52. Perkins FM: Coping with postherpetic neuralgia and painful diabetic neuropathy: Treatment similarities and differences. Consultant 42:2–8, 2002.

53. Galer BS, Dworkin RH (eds): A Clinical Guide to Neuropathic Pain. Minneapolis, Health Information Programs McGraw-Hill Healthcare Information, 2000.

54. Rowbotham MC, Davies PS, Galer BS: Multicenter, double-blind, vehicle-controlled trial of long term use of lidocaine patches for postherpetic neuralgia. In Abstracts of the 8th World Congress of the International Association for the Study of Pain. Vancouver, British Columbia, Canada (August 17–22, 1996a) Abstract 184, p 274.

55. Data on file. Endo Pharmaceuticals Inc Regulatory Affairs Department, July 2003.

56. Katz NP, Gammaitoni AR, Davis MW, et al: Lidocaine patch 5% reduces pain intensity and interference with quality of life in patients with postherpetic neuralgia: An effectiveness trial. Pain Med 3:1–10, 2002.

57. Gammaitoni AR, Davis MW: Pharmacokinetics and tolerability of lidocaine patch 5% with extended dosing. Ann Pharmacother 36:236–240, 2002.

58. Gammaitoni AR, Alvarez NA, Galer BS: Pharmacokinetics and safety of continuously applied lidocaine patches 5%. Am J Health Sys Pharm 59:2215–2220, 2002.

59. Gimbel J, Galer BS, Gammaitoni AR: Impact of the lidocaine patch 5% on quality of life when used in combination with gabapentin in three chronic pain states [abstract]. J Pain 4(suppl 1):882, 2003.

60. Bergouignan M: Cures heureuses de nevralgies faciales essentielles par diphenylhidantoinate de soude. Rev Laryngol Otol Rhinol (Bord) 63:34–41, 1942.

61. Blom S: Trigeminal neuralgia: Its treatment with a new anticonvulsant drug. Lancet 1:839–840, 1962.

62. Rowbotham M, Harden N, Stacey B, et al: Gabapentin for the treatment of postherpetic neuralgia: A randomized controlled trial. JAMA 280:1837–1842, 1998.

63. Rice ASC, Maton S, et al: Gabapentin in postherpetic neuralgia: A randomized, double blind, placebo controlled study. Pain 94:215–224, 2001.

64. McQuay HJ, Moore RA: An evidence-based resource for pain relief. Oxford, Oxford Press, 1999, pp 221–231.

65. Backonja MM: Anticonvulsants (Antineuropathics) for neuropathic pain syndromes. Clin J Pain 16:S67–S72, 2000.

66. Backonja M, Beydoun A, Edwards KR, et al: Gabapentin for the symptomatic treatment of painful neuropathy in patients with diabetes mellitus: A randomized controlled trial. JAMA. 280:1831–1836, 1998.

67. Morello CM, Leckband SG, Stoner CP, et.al: Randomized double-blind study comparing the efficacy of gabapentin with amitriptyline on diabetic peripheral neuropathy. Arch Intern Med 159:1931–1937, 1999.

68. Dworkin RH, Corbin AE, Young JP, et al: Pregabalin for the treatment of postherpetic neuralgia: A randomized, placebo-controlled trial. Neurology 60:1274–1283, 2003.

69. Neurontin® Complete Prescribing Information. New York, Parke Davis, a division of Pfizer, Inc, May 2002.

70. Gerson GR, Jones RB, Luscombe DK: Studies on the concomitant use of carbamazepine and clomipramine for the relief of post-herpetic neuralgia. Postgrad Med J 53:104–109, 1977.

71. Watson CP, Babul N: Efficacy of oxycodone in neuropathic pain: A randomized trial in postherpetic neuralgia. Neurology 50:1837–1841, 1998.

72. Raja S, Haythornthwaite J, Pappagallo M, et al: Opioids versus antidepressants in post herpetic neuralgia: A randomized, placebo-controlled trial. Neurology 59:1113–1126, 2002.

73. Rowbotham MC, Twilling L, Davies PS, et al: Oral opioid therapy for chronic peripheral and central neuropathic pain. N Engl J Med 348:1223–1232, 2003.

74. Gimbel JS, Richards P, Portenoy RK: Controlled-release oxycodone for pain in diabetic neuropathy: A randomized controlled trial. Neurology 60:927–934, 2003.

75. Cherny NI: Opioid analgesics: Comparative features and prescribing guidelines. Drugs 51:713–737, 1996.

76. Stein C: The control of pain in peripheral tissue by opioids. N Engl J Med 332:1685–1690, 1995.

77. Gutstein HB, Akil H: Opioid Analgesics. In Hardman JG, Limbird LE, Gilman AG (eds): Goodman and Gilman's The Pharmacological Basis of Therapeutics 10th ed. New York, McGraw Hill Medical Publishing Division, 2001, pp 569–619.

78. Rowbotham MC, Reinser-Keller LA, Fields H: Both intravenous lidocaine and morphine reduce the pain of postherpetic neuralgia. Neurology 41:1024–1028, 1991.

79. Galer BS, Coyle N, Pasternak GW, et al: Individual variability in the response to different opioids: Report of five cases. Pain 50:205–208, 1992.

80. Gammaitoni AR, Fine P, Alvarez NA, et al: Clinical application of opioid equianalgesic data. Clin J Pain 19:286–297, 2003.

81. Pereira J, Bruera E: Emerging neuropsychiatric toxicities of opioids. J Pharma Care Pain Symptom Control 5:3–27, 1997.

82. Consensus Statement: Definitions Related to the Use of Opioids in Pain Treatment. The American Academy of Pain Medicine. Glenview, IL: The American Pain Society and the American Society of Addiction Medicine, 2001.

83. Gobel H, Stadler T: Treatment of postherpes zoster pain with tramadol: Results of an open pilot study versus clomipramine with or without levomepromazine. Drugs 53(suppl 2):34–39, 1997.

84. Ultram® Complete Prescribing Information. Raritan, NJ: Ortho-McNeil Pharmaceutical, Inc., August 2001.

85. Fishbain D: Evidence-based data on pain relief with antidepressants. Ann Med 32:305–316, 2000.

86. Collins SL, Moore RA, McQuay HJ, et al: Antidepressants and anticonvulsants for diabetic neuropathy and postherpetic neuralgia: A quantitative systemic review. J Pain Symptom Manage 20:449–458, 2000.

87. Sindrup SH, Jensen TS: Efficacy of pharmacological treatments of neuropathic pain: An update and effect related to mechanism of drug action. Pain 83:389–400, 1999.

88. Watson CPN, Evans RJ, Reed K, et al: Amitriptyline versus placebo in post herpetic neuralgia. Neurology 32: 671–673, 1982.
89. Watson CP, Chipman M, Reed K, et al: Amitriptyline versus maprotiline in postherpetic neuralgia: A randomized, double-blind, crossover trial. Pain 48:29–36, 1992.
90. Watson CP, Vernich L, Chipman M, et al: Nortriptyline versus amitriptyline in postherpetic neuralgia: A randomized trial. Neurology 51:1166–1171, 1998.
91. Kishore-Kumar R, Max MB, Schafer SC, et al: Desipramine relieves postherpetic neuralgia. Clin Pharmacol Ther 47: 305–312, 1990.
92. Graf-Radford SB, Shaw LR, Naliboff BN: Amitriptyline and fluphenazine in the treatment of postherpetic neuralgia. Clin J Pain 16:188–192, 2000.
93. Max MB, Schafer SC, Culnane M, et al: Amitriptyline but not lorazepam relieves post herpetic neuralgia. Neurology 38:1427–1432, 1988.
94. Max MB, Kishore-Kumar R, Schafer SC, et al: Efficacy of desipramine in painful diabetic neuropathy: A placebo-controlled trial. Pain 45:3–9, 1991.
95. Max MB, Lynch SA, Muir J, et al: Effects of desipramine, amitriptyline and fluoxetine on pain in diabetic neuropathy. N Engl J Med 326:1250–1256, 1992.
96. Max MB: Thirteen consecutive well-designed randomized trials show that antidepressants reduce pain in diabetic neuropathy and postherpetic neuralgia. Pain Forum 4:248–253, 1995.
97. Basbaum AI, Fields HL: Endogenous pain control mechanisms: Review and hypothesis. Ann Neurol 4:451–462, 1978.
98. Brau ME, Dreimann M, Olschewski A, et al: Effects of drugs used for neuropathic pain management on tetrodotoxin-resistant Na(+) currents in rat sensory neurons. Anesthesiology 94:137–144, 2001.

99. Jacobson LO, Bley K, Hunter JC, et al: Anti-thermal hyperalgesic properties of antidepressants in a rat model of neuropathic pain. American Pain Society annual meeting, A-105 ([abstract]), 1995.
100. Watson CPN: Antidepressant drugs as adjuvant analgesics. J Pain Symptom Manage 9:392–405, 1994.
101. Galer BS, Argoff CE: Zoster and postherpetic neuralgia: Pain mechanisms and current management. In Arnoff GM: Evaluation and Treatment of Chronic Pain, 3rd ed. Baltimore, Williams and Wilkins, 1999.
102. Vestergaard K, Andersen G, Jensen TS: Treatment of central post-stroke pain with a selective serotonin reuptake inhibitor. Eur J Neurol 3(suppl 5):169, 1996.
103. Sindrup SH, Gram LF, Brosenk EO, et al: The selective serotonin reuptake inhibitor paroxetine is effective in the treatment of diabetic neuropathy symptoms. Pain 42:135–144, 1990.
104. Sindrup SH, Bjerre U, Degaard A: The selective serotonin reuptake inhibitor citalopram relieves the symptoms of diabetic neuropathy. Clin Pharmacol Ther 52:547–552, 1992.
105. Lacy CF, Armstrong LL, Goldman MP, Lance LL (eds): Drug Information Handbook, 11th ed. Hudson, Ohio, Lexi-Comp, 2003, pp 1156–1157.
106. Chard PS, Bleakman D, Savidge JR, et al: Capsaicin-induced neurotoxicity in cultured dorsal root ganglion neurons: Involvement of calcium-activated proteases. Neuroscience 65:1099–1108, 1995.
107. Rowbotham MC, Watson CPN: Topical agents for postherpetic neuralgia. In Watson CPN, Gershon AA (eds): Herpes Zoster and PHN 2nd Revised and Enlarged Edition Vol 11. Amsterdam, Elsevier Science, 2001, pp 231–242.
108. Drake HF, Harries AJ, Gamester GE, et al: Randomized double-blind study of topical capsaicin for treatment of post-herpetic

neuralgia [abstract]. Pain 5(suppl): S58, 1999.
109. Watson CPN, Evans RJ, Watt VR: Postherpetic neuralgia and topical capsaicin. Pain 33:333–340, 1988.
110. Lycka B, Watson CPN, Nevin K, et al: EMLA cream for treatment of pain caused by postherpetic neuralgia : A double-blind controlled study [abstract]. In Proceeding of American Pain Society meeting; November 14–17, 1996; Washington DC, 1996:A111 .
111. Attal N, Brasseur L, Chauvin M, et al: Effects of single and repeated applications of a eutectic mixture of local anaesthetics (EMLA) cream on spontaneous and evoked pain in post-herpetic neuralgia: Pain 81:203–209, 1999.
112. Stow PJ, Glynn CJ, Minor B: EMLA cream in the treatment of post-herpetic neuralgia: Efficacy and pharmacokinetic profile. Pain 39:301–305, 1989.
113. Dejgard A, Petersen P, Kastrup J: Mexiletine for treatment of chronic diabetic neuropathy. Lancet 2:9–11, 1988.
114. Dworkin RH, Johnson RW: A belt of roses from hell: Pain in herpes zoster and postherpetic neuralgia. In Block AR, Kremer EF, Fernandez E (eds): Handbook of Pain Syndromes: Biopsychosocial Perspectives. Hillsdale, NJ, Erlbaum, 1999, pp 371–402.
115. Wu CL, Marsh A, Dworkin RH: The role of sympathetic nerve blocks in herpes zoster and postherpetic neuralgia. Pain 87: 121–129, 2000.
116. Fine PG: Nerve blocks, herpes zoster, and postherpetic neuralgia. In Watson CPN, Gershon AA (eds): Herpes Zoster and PHN 2nd Revised and Enlarged Edition Vol 11. Amsterdam, Elsevier Science, 2001, pp 223–229.
117. Loeser JD: Surgery for postherpetic neuralgia. In Watson CPN, Gershon AA (eds): Herpes Zoster and PHN 2nd Revised and Enlarged Edition Vol 11. Amsterdam, Elsevier Science, 2001, pp 255–264.

Multidisciplinary Approach to the Patient with Cancer Pain

CHAPTER 13

Neuroradiologic Evaluation of the Patient with Cancer Pain

Ronald A. Alberico, MD, Ahmed Abdel-Halim, MD, and Syed Hamed S. Husain, DO

The development of technologic advances in imaging in recent decades has enabled physicians to obtain detailed information about the patient with relatively noninvasive techniques. Although the wide variety of advanced imaging techniques have resulted in increased diagnostic efficacy, they may also lead to confusion as to the most appropriate test for a given clinical situation. This chapter discusses the application of imaging modalities to the patient with cancer-related pain from the perspective of a neuroradiologist. It is intended as a clinical guide to selection of the most appropriate imaging study to evaluate the patient in the setting of oncologic pain that is related to the neural axis. Involvement of the radiologist in the selection of imaging modality and examination will result in a more directed and detailed evaluation of the patient. A detailed history on the radiologic request combined with a direct communication with the radiologist will allow the examination to be selected with the likely pathology in mind and enable the radiologist to tailor the examination such that the patient's suspected pathology is most conspicuous. Providing the radiologist with history and clinical feedback will not only improve patient care, but it is likely to improve the quality of the radiology service as well. Interaction with clinical services and feedback about the accuracy and utility of diagnostic imaging and interpretation will enable the radiologist to adapt to their needs and optimize imaging techniques.

IMAGING MODALITIES

The imaging modalities available for assessment of cancer pain in the neural axis include radionuclide bone scanning, computed tomography (CT), and magnetic resonance imaging (MRI). Other modalities such as fluoroscopy, myelography, and plain film radiography have taken on a secondary role in specific cases. Figure 13–1 illustrates the available imaging choices.

Diskography and other provocative tests have a more limited role in patients with cancer-related pain and are not discussed in this chapter.

Magnetic Resonance Imaging

MRI is by far the most important modality for evaluating the neural axis in patients with cancer-related pain. MRI provides the most detailed soft tissue discrimination possible, enabling visualization of the source of pain in many cases and allowing the differentiation of treatment-related pathology from neoplastic pathology in many cases.[1-3] The detection of perineural spread of disease in the head and neck is well described in the literature on MRI and CT but is typically more sensitively detected with MRI.[4-6] Epidural disease in the spine and leptomeningeal carcinomatosis is also identifiable with MRI. The detection of leptomeningeal disease in the spine is most sensitive with serial lumbar punctures; however, intracranial carcinomatosis is more sensitively detected with MRI. In one study 18% of autopsy proven cases had only epidural or subdural metastases as the manifestation of intracranial disease.[7]

Cancer patients also can suffer from non-neoplastic diseases, such as disk herniation and spondylosis, and inflammatory and vascular conditions. The clinical manifestation of any of these processes can involve pain. MRI is well known to be one of the most versatile methods for detecting and identifying those various pathologic processes. In many cases, MRI can distinguish vertebral compression fractures related to neoplastic infiltration from secondary osteoporosis or even osteomyelitis.[8]

The combination of MRI and gadolinium contrast agents is the most sensitive technique available for detecting brain metastases. Modern MRI sequences can distinguish acute stroke from abscess or tumor, allowing appropriate clinical treatments to be initiated. High-resolution studies of the orbit, skull base, and sinuses can detect neoplastic or inflammatory conditions that

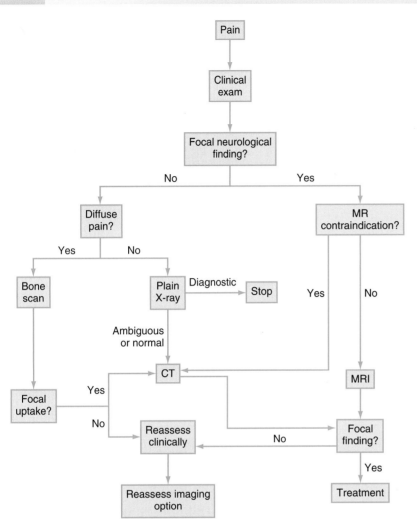

FIGURE 13-1 This flow diagram acts as a starting point for patients with oncologic pain related to the neural axis. Magnetic resonance imaging (MRI), the more expensive and less well-tolerated study, is reserved for patients with high clinical suspicion of anatomic disease. Computed tomography (CT) is the central screening tool for anatomic disease. Nuclear medicine bone scan and plain x-ray are used to focus cross-sectional imaging to specific body regions. In some cases (such as long bone fracture), plain x-rays are the only imaging modality required.

are inconspicuous on CT and invisible in nuclear medicine or radiographic studies.

MRI may be useful in assessing nonstructural information. Functional MRI (fMRI) has been shown to be possible using blood oxygen level dependent contrast. Functional MRI techniques involve repetitive tasks performed by the patient during active scanning. Complex processing of the image data acquired can reveal subtle differences in blood flow that occur during the stimulus and can lead to the identification of various functional centers within the brain.[9] Some fMRI studies have been performed that indicate differences between cutaneous and visceral pain centers in the brain, as well as areas of brain activation corresponding to expected pain centers. Specifically, subcortical areas have been identified in fMRI studies as being involved in pain processing.[10-12] Although much of this work is still experimental, it does hold promise for future evaluation of drug therapy, as well as potential functional surgical manipulation (such as gamma knife ablation of pain centers).

Other forms of fMRI include MR spectroscopy and perfusion imaging. MR spectroscopy is a method of detecting various metabolic compounds in the body and determining their relative concentration without

sampling the tissue.[13] This technique generates graphs, or spectra, for a specific area defined during the scanning process, and it is currently most useful in the brain and prostate gland. MR spectroscopy can distinguish tumor from radiation necrosis in the brain.[14,15] It is known that exogenous compounds such as alcohol and mannitol can be detected within the brain using these techniques (Figure 13–2). Although not yet determined, it is conceivable that other exogenous compounds may be detected with MR spectroscopy, potentially enabling the in vivo assessment of biodistribution. If correlated with fMRI data this could provide exciting avenues for future objective treatment assessment.

Another advantage of MRI over other modalities is the lack of ionizing radiation. MRI is accomplished using strong magnetic fields in combination with radio waves to create an image. The process is made possible by powerful computers in combination with radio waves tuned to specific frequencies. No negative effects have been demonstrated from exposure to the MR environment, including the use of MRI for fetal assessment.

Despite evident superiority of MRI over other imaging modalities in the evaluation of the neural axis in cancer pain patients, there are several reasons why alternatives

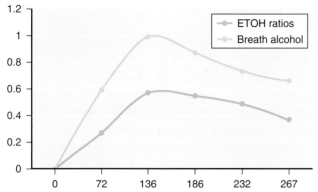

NORMALIZED
ETOH PEAK RATIOS VS BREATH ALCOHOL

FIGURE 13–2 This graph demonstrates the kinetics of ethanol metabolism in the brain as measured by magnetic resonance spectroscopy in two healthy volunteers. The top curve is breath alcohol (ETOH) level as measured over time by a Breathalyzer typically available to state police. The bottom curve is measured alcohol peak ratios from magnetic resonance spectroscopy over the same time intervals. This in vivo pharmacokinetic study of a drug in the brain offers initial support for the idea of using magnetic resonance spectroscopy to track drugs in the brain and potentially identify structurally mediated concentration differences.

to MRI continue to be important. The major reasons can be summed up as availability, tolerability, and expense. Because of the physical reality of acquiring an MR signal, imaging takes time. Typically, an MRI of the brain takes between 20 and 45 minutes, whereas a thorough evaluation of the cervical/thoracic and lumbar spine may take as long as 2 hours. The result is a limited number of time slots for scanning in a given day. Depending on the site, delays in scheduling MR examinations can be measured in weeks. MRI is also not well tolerated by many patients because of claustrophobia, implanted devices such as pacemakers or aneurysm clips, and because of an inability to lie flat. MRI is very sensitive to motion artifacts (even eyeball movement). Any discomfort that makes the patient move will seriously limit the scan. Some patients are also too large to fit in the MR bore. Opened MRI examinations can serve as alternatives for the claustrophobic or large patient, but these typically have lower image quality. Finally, MRI examinations are more expensive than the other modalities; the result is required pre-approval for most third-party payers and a drive to limit the number of MR examinations performed. The expense of the equipment alone ($1 million to $5 million) may limit the availability of more advanced techniques, which are dependent on high-end equipment, to major academic centers. Minor limitations to MRI include poor visualization of calcifications and bony cortices. This is where CT excels. MRI also suffers from a large number of artifacts that make interpretation more difficult than other modalities. A thorough knowledge and understanding of artifacts that occur in MRI

and at least a moderate degree of comfort with MRI physics is a requirement for proper image interpretation.[16] Lastly, MRI has a low positive predictive value in certain post-treatment situations, particularly after head and neck surgery/radiation.

Computed Tomography

Advances in CT technology have increased the role of CT in imaging once again. The modern CT scanner has an array of 4, 8, 16, or even 32 radiation detectors that rotate continuously around the patient during scanning. This array of detectors enables multiple sections to be obtained simultaneously and increases the speed of scanning proportionally. It also enables the use of thinner sections to cover large anatomic regions, providing higher resolution and more detail of small anatomic structures. Once acquired, the volume data sets generated by these machines can be sectioned into any plane and can be displayed in three-dimensional volume rendered formats. These displays can provide guidance for surgical procedures or can be transformed into detailed bony, arterial, or venous maps. Sources of arthritic pain can be investigated, as can details of metastatic disease. Tumor vessel relationships can be shown in three-dimensional models to guide procedures and define vascular pathology.

For the evaluation of cancer pain, CT can outperform MRI in some areas. Evaluation of perceived bony pathology on MRI can sometimes be more specific on CT images. Tumor calcification patterns in mesenchymal neoplasm can be important, as can subtle periosteal reactions. For some patients, the speed of CT is necessary to eliminate motion artifact. CT can also provide additional information about perceived bony abnormalities and is occasionally more specific than MRI. Although both CT and MRI can image vascular anatomy, CT is winning the race as a noninvasive alternative to conventional diagnostic angiography. CT has been shown to be almost as sensitive as catheter angiography in detecting intracranial aneurysms, and also has provided detailed representations of venous anatomy in adult and pediatric patients.[17-19] Catheters and epidural access devices are readily seen on CT images, whereas on MRI they are frequently inconspicuous. CT in combination with contrast agents can be used to confirm the position of various epidural or intrathecal catheters.

CT is a superb modality for image-guided procedures. The rapidity of imaging and simultaneous display of soft tissue, vascular, and bony anatomy makes CT the best choice for guiding difficult anatomic access. There is almost no space in the body that cannot be accurately targeted with CT guidance so that the safest procedure can be performed. CT can be used for biopsy, abscess drainage, and guidance of skull base procedures such as rhizotomy in patients suffering from trigeminal neuralgia.

Disadvantages of CT include the need for ionizing radiation, the use of iodinated contrast agents, and cost. In general, the risk of ionizing radiation exposure is acceptable given the information obtained. For those patients who are allergic to iodinated contrast, alternatives such as gadolinium may be used.[20] Although less expensive than MRI, CT examinations certainly are not cheap. When possible, less expensive alternatives such as fluoroscopy should be used.

Fluoroscopy

There are still some situations in which fluoroscopy outperforms CT and MRI. There is true real-time information provided during fluoroscopy that can be necessary for performing certain procedures safely, specifically vertebroplasty and kyphoplasty.[21,22] The large area of view provided in combination with continuous real-time visualization can also decrease the time needed to perform nerve blocks or other needle placements. Although CT fluoroscopy has provided an alternative in some cases, it is generally a higher radiation dose procedure and provides a smaller field of view.

Nuclear Medicine

Nuclear medicine remains the most sensitive technique for evaluating disease sites in the peripheral skeleton, but it can be nonspecific. MRI in the axial skeleton can be more sensitive than bone scan for some situations, particularly multiple myeloma and osteomyelitis.[23] It is a good method of screening for skeletal lesions and narrowing the scope of cross-sectional imaging evaluations to areas of specific abnormality. Conversely, isolated areas of abnormality that are detected in the neural axis on cross-sectional imaging may lead to nuclear medicine assessment (particularly bone scan) to evaluate possible other sites of disease. This can provide targets for biopsy that are less challenging than those originally detected on the cross-sectional images.

THE ROLE OF IMAGING

Diagnosis

Now that we have considered the various imaging modalities in detail, we should consider the reasons for neuroradiologic assessment of patients with oncologic pain. These can be summed up as diagnosis, guidance, and surveillance. Of primary importance in oncologic pain is the evaluation of the extent or existence of neoplastic involvement at the site of the pain and along the appropriate neural pathways. Most neoplastic processes that involve the neural axis are in a position to cause rapid decline in patient function and death and can result in a wide variety of pain syndromes.[24,25] Diagnosis and description of disease extent is, therefore, the first job at hand. The modality of choice for focal pain along well-defined neural pathways is always MRI. When MRI is contraindicated or intolerable, CT is the next alternative for focal disease assessment in the brain or spinal canal. More detail can be obtained in the spinal canal if the CT is combined with intrathecal contrast (CT myelography). If MRI is performed and no neoplastic disease is found in the neural structures, CT can be performed to broaden the scope of the study and include adjacent structures. It is important to remember that oncology patients can also have non-neoplastic sources of pain, some of which are more critical to diagnose than the oncology (Figure 13–3). For patients with regional complaints that are less specific to the neural axis and may be related to other areas of the body, CT can be the initial evaluation with focal MRI when and if disease is detected. For generalized complaints that are difficult to localize, CT again can take a primary role; however, nuclear medicine bone scan would be most appropriate for evaluating bone pain.

Guidance

Once the diagnosis is made, neuroradiology can aide in the guidance of pain procedures. Fluoroscopic guidance is most useful for guiding needle and catheter placements during facet block, nerve block, and epidural catheter placement.[26] Fluoroscopy is also required for more invasive procedures that require continuous monitoring of images in real time such as vertebroplasty and kyphoplasty. These procedures are detailed in Chapter 35. CT guidance can be used to target deep structures such as foramen ovale or the sacral roots. MRI can be used in combination with stereotactic frames to provide targeting guidance for gamma knife or other three-dimensional conformal radiosurgery techniques. This includes treatment for metastatic disease or for neoplastic processes that involve cranial nerves at the skull base. With special MR compatible equipment, MR-guided procedures can be performed but are usually less available than comparable CT-guided procedures.

Surveillance

After diagnosis and therapy guidance, imaging takes on a surveillance role. CT and MRI are useful in this regard. Catheter position can be assessed with CT, whereas actual disease status is best, if possible, with MRI. Complications can also be evaluated such as pneumothorax (CT or chest x-ray), epidural hematoma (MR), and epidural abscess (MR) (Figure 13–4).

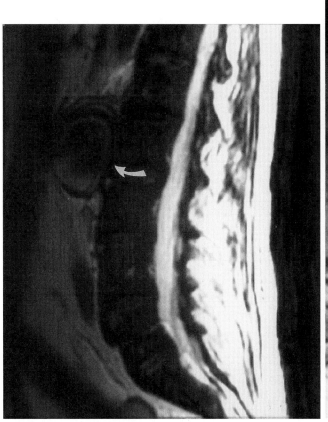

A

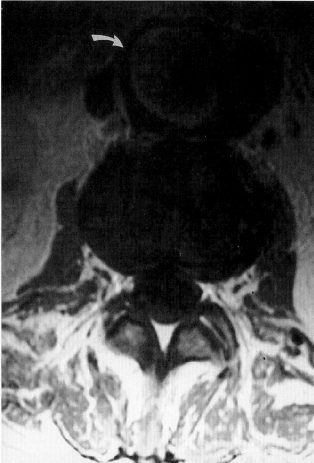

B

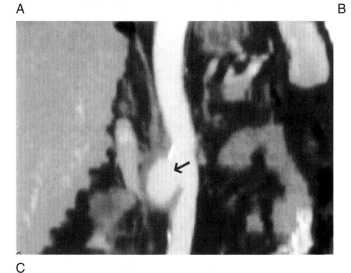

C

FIGURE 13–3   This 53-year-old patient had a history of prostate cancer and symptoms of sudden severe back pain. *A*, This sagittal T2 weighted MRI image reveals a round area of low intensity anterior to the spine (arrow). *B*, The axial T1 weighted MRI image confirmed the rounded mass anterior to the spine (arrow). *C*, This coronal image from a computed tomography angiogram (CTA) reveals the mass to be a contained rupture of an abdominal aortic aneurysm (arrow).

CONCLUSION

The neuroradiologic evaluation of the patient with cancer pain is a multistep process in a complex patient population. The questions addressed include diagnosis of the pain source, guidance of the pain interventions, and surveillance of the treated patient. Optimal results are obtained when the appropriate imaging modality is selected and the study is tailored to the needs of the patient. This is best accomplished with detailed history and clinical evaluation, in combination with communication between the clinical service and the neuroradiologist. Through our best efforts, excellent pain management can be a major factor in the quality of life and psychologic well-being of our patients.

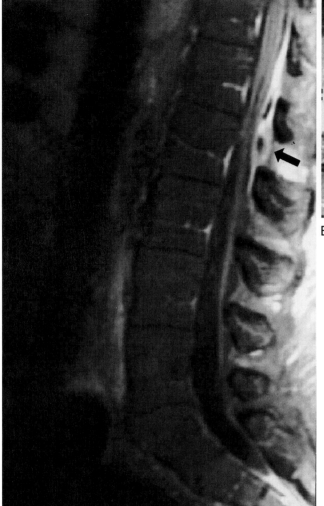

A

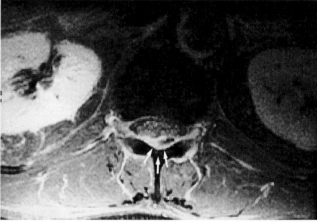

B

FIGURE 13–4 This 43-year-old man with a history of lung cancer developed severe back pain in combination with a low-grade fever. An epidural catheter had been in place for approximately 1 month in an effort to control pain from pleural involvement of the tumor. *A,* The sagittal T1 weighted MR image reveals a posterior epidural enhancing mass (arrow). *B,* The axial contrast enhanced T1 weighted image confirms the presence of the mass (arrows), which proved to be an epidural abscess at surgery.

REFERENCES

1. Greenspan JD, Winfield JA: Reversible pain and tactile deficits associated with a cerebral tumor compressing the posterior insula and parietal operculum. Pain 50:29–39, 1992.
2. Avdelidis D, Singounis E, Missir O, et al: Episodic pain associated with a tumor in the parietal operculum: A case report and literature review. Pain 72:201–208, 1997.
3. Ploner M, Freund HJ, Schnitzler FA: Pain affect without pain sensation in a patient with a postcentral lesion. Pain 81:211–214, 1999.
4. Nemzek W, Hecht S, Granour-Edwards R, et al: Perineural spread of head and neck tumors: How accurate is MR imaging? Am J Neuroradiol 19:701–706, 1998.
5. Woodruff W, Yeates A, McLendon R: Perineural tumor extension to the cavernous sinus from superficial facial carcinoma: CT manifestations. Radiology 161: 395–399, 1986.
6. Lain F, Braun I, Jensen M, et al: Perineural tumor extension through the foramen ovale: Evaluation with MR imaging. Radiology 174:65–71, 1990.

7. Posner JB, Chennik NL: Intracranial metastases from systemic cancer. Adv Neurol 19:579, 1978.
8. Yuh WTC, Zachar CK, Barloon TJ, et al: Vertebral compression fractures distinction between benign and malignant causes with MR imaging. Radiology 172:215–218, 1989.
9. Kurata J: Functional magnetic resonance imaging explained for pain research and medicine. Reg Anesth Pain Med 27: 68–71, 2002.
10. Bingel U, Quante M, Knab R, et al: Subcortical structures involved in pain processing: Evidence from a single trial of fMRI. Pain 99:313–321, 2002.
11. Rainville P, Bushnell K, Duncan GH: Representation of acute and persistent pain in the human CNS: Potential implications for pain intolerance. Ann NY Acad Sci 933:130–141, 2001.
12. Casey KL, Sandkuhler J, Bromm B, Gebhart GF: Concepts of pain mechanisms: The contribution of functional imaging of the human brain. Prog Brain Res 129:277–287, 2000.

13. Kwok L: Localized MR spectroscopy: Basic principles. Neuroimaging Clin N Am 8:713–732, 1998.
14. Castillo M, Kwok L, Drayer B: Proton MR spectroscopy of common brain tumors. Neuroimaging Clin N Am 8:733–752, 1998.
15. Taylor JS, Ogg JR, Langston JW: Proton MR spectroscopy of pediatric brain tumors. Neuroimaging Clin N Am 8:753–780, 1998.
16. Joseph PM, Atlas S: Magnetic Resonance Imaging of the Brain and Spine, 3rd ed. Philadelphia, Lippincott Williams and Wilkins, 2002, pp 239–275.
17. Alberico RA, Barnes P, Robertson R, et al: Helical CT angiography: Dynamic cerebrovascular imaging in children. Am J Neuroradiol 20:328–334, 1999.
18. Alberico RA, Patel M, Casey SO, et al: Evaluation of the circle of Willis with 3-D CT angiography in patients with suspected intracranial aneurysms. Am J Neuroradiol 16:1571–1578, 1995.
19. Casey SO, Alberico RA, Patel M, et al: Cerebral CT venography. Radiology 198:717–722, 1997.

20. Gupta AK, Alberico RA, Litwin A, et al: Gadopentetate dimeglumine is potentially an alternative contrast agent for three-dimensional computed tomography angiography with multidetector-row helical scanning. JCAT 26:869–874, 2002.

21. Murphy KJ, Deramond H, Jensen ME: Percutaneous vertebroplasty in benign and malignant disease. Neuroimaging Clin N Am 10:535–546, 2000.

22. Jensen ME, Dion JE: Percutaneous vertebroplasty in treatment of osteoporotic compression fractures. Neuroimaging Clin N Am 10:547–568, 2000.

23. Rosenthal D: Radiologic diagnosis of bone metastases. Cancer 80(suppl 8): 1595–1607, 1997.

24. Christiaans MH, Kelder JC, Arnoldus EP, et al: Prediction of intracranial metastases in cancer patients with headache. Cancer 94:2063–2068, 2002.

25. Forsyth PA, Posner JB: Headaches in patients with brain tumors.Neurol 43:1678–1683, 1993.

26. Schellhas K: Facet nerve blockade and radiofrequency neurotomy. Neuroimaging Clin N Am 10:493–502, 2000.

CHAPTER 14

Behavioral Assessment of the Patient with Cancer Pain

Michael A. Zevon, PhD, and Stephen D. Schwabish, PhD

When confronted by the complexity of assessing and treating cancer-related pain, it is tempting to respond much as the beleaguered Claude Raines did in the movie *Casablanca* and "round up the usual suspects." In this case, these include the typical comments regarding the multidimensional nature of pain-related behaviors and the significant challenges associated with understanding and changing such behaviors. Behavioral principles, often unjustly criticized as simplistic and reductionistic in their approach to understanding human behavior, are typically underrepresented in such "round ups" of useful approaches to pain assessment and management.

Our purpose is to present an alternative view that behavioral principles can and do make an important contribution to understanding and treating pain in cancer patients. Rather than oversimplifying the often-belabored complexity of pain assessment and treatment, we maintain that a behavioral perspective can function in the service of Occam's razor in understanding pain-related behaviors. We would argue that understanding and treating the patient through an ontologically parsimonious behavioral lens is an important component of any effective pain assessment and management program. Indeed, the integration of behavioral techniques within an overall self-management strategy emphasizing the patient's control and responsibility for active participation in managing their pain is a particularly powerful intervention, a theme that we will revisit later.

BACKGROUND

An understanding of the rich conceptual and empirical background of behaviorism facilitates understanding the use of behavioral principles in treating cancer pain. The evolution of behaviorism, from its earliest formulations to the more radical perspective most often associated with B.F. Skinner, covers a wide range of theory and

research. Smith,[1] for example, contends that a significant indirect influence on Skinner dates from the philosophical positions of Francis Bacon. Writing at the beginning of the Scientific Revolution, Bacon urged scientists to reject the sanctity of the past, arguing instead that only the inductive process would expand scientific knowledge.

The movement begun by Bacon influenced scientists of subsequent generations. Ernst Mach, for example, insisted that sensations form the basis of all science. He argued for a descriptive approach wherein unbiased observations facilitated the understanding of the interactions between individuals and scientific laws. Mach attempted to economize the inductive positivism begun by Bacon by urging simplicity and economy, basic principles of the behavioral position that parallel Darwin's conception of the laws of nature. Interestingly, Mach's work indirectly influenced that of Jacques Loeb, an animal psychologist whose major disciple was W.J. Crozier, a faculty member in whose laboratory Skinner worked at Harvard. Skinner has credited Crozier[2] with having had a direct influence on his thinking.

Loeb, in turn, influenced John B. Watson, founder of the objective system of psychology called behaviorism, as did John Dewey and James Angell.[3,4] Dewey,[5] in an 1896 paper that precipitated the functionalist movement, argued that behavior must be viewed on a macro rather than a micro level, and that its functions constitute the most important area of study. He further criticized the prevailing reflex arc framework that identified three discrete components of behavior: (1) an afferent sensory component initiated by the stimulus and mediated by sensory nerves; (2) a control or associative component, mediated by the spinal cord and the brain; and (3) an efferent, or motor, component moderated by motor nerves and resulting in a response. This molar perspective was augmented by Angell's[6] contention that functionalism was truly concerned with the relationship of the organism to the environment. The following tenets summarize Watson's contribution to behaviorism:

1. Behavior is composed of response elements that can be successfully analyzed by objective, natural scientific methods.
2. Behavior is reducible to physiochemical processes.
3. There is an immediate response to every effective stimulus; that is, every response has a preceding stimulus. There is, therefore, a strict cause and effect determinism in behavior.
4. Conscious processes, if indeed they exist at all, cannot be scientifically studied, and formulations based on consciousness represent "supernatural" tendencies that are hangovers from earlier prescientific thinking, and must, therefore, be ignored.

Between Watson's earliest writings and before Skinner's later work, other theorists argued for an expanded stimulus–organism–response (S-O-R) model. Edward C. Tolman,[7] for example, initiated the so-called neobehaviorist model by inserting the organism between the stimulus and response (S-R) constructs, the paradigm endorsed by the more conservative behaviorists. The organism was viewed as a mediating variable through which the evaluation of stimuli resulted in a selected response. Overall, these theorists promoted a perspective on behaviorism that described an active organism that was constantly involved in stimulus analysis and response selection. This view of the individual as an active agent in the evaluation of information from the environment, as well as in the selection of a behavioral response, was and remains the most significant variant in any comparison with "radical" behaviorism.

Against this backdrop, Skinner stressed an experimental method that he described as offering the most complete and quantitative description of individual behavior to date. This work represented years of laboratory research and Skinner's program for establishing behaviorism as a natural science alongside biology, chemistry, and physics. In this regard, he began the evolving process of distinguishing his work from the classical conditioning model stressed by Pavlov.

Skinner[8,9] argued that operant behaviors (behaviors that "operated" on the environment) were spontaneously emitted by the individual, unlike the elicited behaviors identified by Pavlov. New behaviors could be added to an individual's natural behavioral repertoire through the reinforcement of successive approximations of the desired end behavior. Thus, reinforcers, depending on the schedule by which they were supplied, always increased the probability of the behaviors with which they were paired.

During subsequent years, Skinner expanded the complexity and depth of his position, as well as emphasizing its relevance to understanding and changing behavior. Although he acknowledged that individuals have internal states such as feelings and desires, he argued that the most important causes of behavior are environmental, and it only confuses matters to talk about the organisms' inner drives. Skinner concentrated on operant behaviors and focused on the environmental responses that would serve to either increase or decrease the reoccurrence (probability) of a particular behavior. A reinforcing stimulus was defined as any stimulus that increased the probability of a response, whereas a punishment was any stimulus that decreased the probability of a response.

Reinforcement was further subdivided into two classes, positive and negative, with positive reinforcement increasing the frequency of behavior as a result of the delivery of a valued stimulus, and negative reinforcement increasing the frequency of a behavior as a result of the "elimination" of an aversive stimulus. Accordingly, if we wanted to increase the probability that a given behavior would reoccur, the individual would receive either positive reinforcement, presentation of a stimulus that the organism desired (e.g., food), or negative reinforcement, the removal of a stimulus that the organism would normally try to avoid (e.g., shock). The elimination of the aversive stimulus increases the probability that the behavior will reoccur.

While Skinner divided reinforcement into unlearned or primary (those that satisfy physiologic requirements such as food) and learned or secondary (initially neutral stimuli that gain reinforcing properties by being paired with primary reinforcement; eventually assume reinforcing value of their own, i.e. money), their strength is in large measure determined by their allocation schedules. Two basic types of reinforcement schedules were defined; the first is the continuous or nonintermittent type that provides reinforcement after each of the desired behaviors, thereby constantly reinforcing and thus strengthening the behavior. The second type is the intermittent schedule where reinforcement is delivered on a noncontinuous basis after a number of responses or the passage of time.

Typical intermittent schedules are the ratio, interval, and compound or mixed schedules. The ratio schedule requires that the individual emit a number of responses before reinforcement. Varieties of this schedule include the fixed ratio, during which the number of required behaviors are held constant, and the variable ratio under which the number of required behaviors vary according to a set pattern. The interval schedule provides reinforcement after a period of time.

Similar to the ratio schedule, the fixed interval schedule is based on the passage of a constant period of time before reinforcement, whereas the variable interval schedule delivers reinforcement after a varying time period. Compound or mixed schedules vary these four basic schedules in different combinations.

Although these schedules have all been shown to be effective in changing and controlling behavior, they vary in terms of the characteristics of the behavior that results from their use. For example, continuous reinforcement provides the most rapid method of establishing a new behavior, yet when reinforcement stops, the behavior is rapidly extinguished. Intermittent schedules, both response frequency and time based, produce more enduring behavior and slower extinction rates than do fixed schedules. Finally, through a process called shaping, these schedules can be used to produce, by reinforcing closer and closer approximations of the desired end behavior (the method of successive approximations), more complex patterns of behaviors.

APPLICATION TO PAIN-RELATED BEHAVIOR ASSESSMENT AND CHANGE

As described earlier, the behavioral perspective argues that the organism spontaneously emits behavior. The strength or probability that these operant behaviors would reoccur is a function of the reinforcement, or lack thereof, that follows them. Both types of reinforcement, positive and negative, are characterized by the fact that they increase the frequency of the preceding behavior. Conversely, punishment refers to procedures that decrease the frequency of a response. In the punishment paradigm, behavior decreases as a result of the delivery of a contingent aversive stimulus. Finally, the frequency of a behavior can be reduced through extinction, a process where reinforcement is suspended and the previously reinforced behavior is eliminated.

One of the first applications of the behavioral paradigm to the assessment and treatment of pain behavior was reported by Fordyce.[10,11] Fordyce described pain behavior in general and chronic-pain behavior specifically as essentially operant behaviors because they are controlled by environmental reinforcing consequences. His descriptions of the use of operant behavioral techniques in the treatment of chronic pain resulted in an increased interest in the use of operant behavioral approaches, although these early studies had small sample sizes and were limited in scope. Subsequent studies[12-15] with more extensive follow-up, however, further demonstrated that pain patients assessed and treated with a behavioral program achieved significant patient outcomes such as increased activity levels and decreased medication use.

An interesting early study by Block, Kremer, and Gaylor[16] broadened the use of the behavioral paradigm in pain studies by reporting an investigation of the severity of patient's pain reports as a function of their spouses reinforcement or lack of reinforcement of their pain complaints. In this study the spouses positively reinforced the patient pain reports by their expressions of support and empathic responding. Interestingly, for the patients with supportive (reinforcing) spouses,

patient pain complaints were higher in the presence of their spouses and lower when their spouses were not present, whereas for patients whose spouses were not supportive, pain reports were less severe when their spouses were present. Additional studies expanded the number of outcomes examined and reported a clear association between social reinforcement and pain patient behaviors such as verbal outbursts[17] and performance levels.[18]

As a group these studies stimulated interest in applying well-established behavioral principles to the management of pain-related behaviors. Obstacles to a more widespread acceptance existed, however, to a great extent on the basis of the fact that the rich empirical and theoretical history described herein had little exposure within medical, and specifically pain management, literature. Studies that did appear in the medical literature demonstrated effectiveness but were primarily case studies or included small patient samples examined in relation to limited patient outcomes.

ASSESSMENT AND INTERVENTION: FUNCTIONAL ANALYSIS AND THE INTERVENTION PLAN

An important advantage of the use of a behavioral perspective in the assessment and treatment of cancer-related pain is the efficiency of the transition from the assessment to the treatment framework. The primary aim of a behavioral assessment of cancer pain–related behavior is to conduct what is described as a functional analysis. A functional analysis is a detailed assessment of the person–environment interactions related to the patient's pain. This functional analysis should include evaluation of physiologic, social, emotional/attributional, and environmental factors that are acting, in isolation or in concert, to maintain the targeted pain-related behaviors. The goal of the assessment is to increase our understanding of pain-related behaviors, that is, to identify the reinforcing stimuli that are acting to maintain maladaptive pain-related behaviors or disability in excess of that which is clearly the result of the patients medically determined functional limitations.

The process of conducting a functional analysis consists of two components. First, the targeted behaviors are observed to identify antecedents and consequences (reinforcers), and second, a trial manipulation of the reinforcing stimuli is conducted to empirically evaluate their association with changes in the frequency of the targeted pain-related behaviors. This procedure is very much in the radical stimulus–response, Skinnerian operant behavioral framework in that its focus is exclusively on the contingencies of emitted behaviors. Data collected in this functional analysis would incorporate, for example, the careful description of the patient's pain-related behavior to include the settings in which it occurs, the intensity and duration of the pain-related behavior, changes in the patient's activities as a result of their pain, changes in the spouse and family members behavior in response to the patient's pain behavior, the temporal pattern of the pain behavior, and the identification of other environmental and social reinforcing contingencies.

A careful assessment is needed to ensure that negatively reinforcing contingencies that maintain maladaptive pain behaviors are also identified. These relationships can be more subtle because the increased frequency of the behavior in the case of negative reinforcement is based on the patients avoiding aversive activities or situations, rather than resulting from the contingent presentation of a primary or secondary positive reinforcer (e.g., financial gain or increased spousal attention and support). The functional assessment must, therefore, be multimodal, in the sense that both classes of reinforcing contingencies must be identified if an effective behavioral treatment is to be developed. Subsequent interventions will be most successful when multiple causes of behavior are simultaneously evaluated from both the positive and negative reinforcement perspectives.

At this point in the treatment process it is helpful to move into an educational framework and discuss the typical ways patients cope with pain and how these behavioral patterns serve to either amplify or reduce pain. This process can help structure the patient's identification of their behavioral responses to pain. The patient's responses can then be organized and common maladaptive responses can be better identified. These could include responses such as social withdrawal (being alone, not wanting to talk to anyone), sensory withdrawal (laying down, turning the lights off), and inactivity. These behavioral patterns should be interpreted to the patient as intuitive and understandable responses to their pain, yet not as effective as the strategies that will be developed during the current treatment.

In addition, the clinician should discuss how self-preoccupation and a focus on the patient's pain can be triggered by a variety of everyday environmental cues. Such questions as "How is your pain today?" or "Is your pain any better?" as well the mere act of entering the pain clinic may serve as cues to the patient to turn their attention inward and to become more aware of their pain. Although some of these environmental inward-focusing triggers are unavoidable (such as visits to the pain clinic), others are within the patient's control.

The main goal of this psycho-educational component is to impart the information the patient needs to initiate the process of self-management. More specifically, the goals are to aid the patient in identification and modification of current behavioral patterns that promote self-preoccupation and set the stage for excessive pain-related disability, and to help the patient develop a greater sense of control over their pain. The achievement of these goals can be measured formally and informally using the patients' verbalization of the understanding of the concepts, their homework completion, and self-reported statements of satisfaction, or more systematically with the help of perceived control over pain and pain intensity scales.

The intervention plan builds on the results of the functional analysis and the trial manipulation of reinforcement contingencies. An important component of the development of the plan is a clear behavioral description of the goals and expected outcomes of the intervention. The intervention plan should address the patient's specific maladaptive pain-related behavior and include reinforcers that have a demonstrated ability to affect the patient's behavior. Prior to the initiation of the plan the base rate for the targeted behaviors should be quantified. Precise base rate data is needed to accurately assess the behavioral impact of the intervention.

When designing the assessment and intervention plan, it is important to clearly prioritize the targeted behaviors. Maladaptive pain-related behaviors that cause the most significant and generalized excessive pain-related disability should be targeted first. Ideally, one or two of these behaviors should be addressed rather than attempting to modify a large number of targeted behaviors. A method for the in vivo collection of data will need to be developed that is computable with the environments in which the behavior is expressed.

AN EXPANDED FRAMEWORK

The functional analysis and associated intervention plan are excellent tools for identifying the reinforcers that maintain a patient's dysfunctional pain-related behaviors. They are, however, less effective in identifying internally predisposing factors, such as patient attributions, that can significantly contribute to the development and maintenance of problematic pain-related behavior. Although the more radical stimulus–response behavioral approach concentrates exclusively on modifying overt, observable actions, the most efficacious application of behavioral principles in cancer pain management results from the reintroduction of the organism into the expanded stimulus–organism–response paradigm described earlier. The more contemporary expression of this method is described as cognitive-behavioral in approach and employs techniques that focus on changing overt behavior by altering the individual's thoughts, interpretations, and assumptions about their pain-related behavior. The cognitive-behavioral perspective, therefore, reintroduces cognitions and patient attributions (processes internal to the organism) as appropriate therapeutic targets and postulates that cognitions have the ability to affect behavior acquisition and frequency.

This broader S-O-R perspective on "behavior" is to a great extent based on the belief that the overall goal of a behavioral pain assessment and treatment plan is to cause the patient to redefine their pain behavior as under their control rather than the helpless-in-the-face-of-pain response more characteristic of pain-related cognitions. This critical shift in the patient's perspective on their pain behavior is really a subset of the individual's broader orientation to solving problems, in this case their health and pain-related concerns. When a patient experiences a pain symptom, they respond to the experience by making a set of judgments or attributions regarding the causes of their symptom and the likely outcome of their management of the symptom. This search for an explanation also influences the individual's emotional response to their symptoms.

These important attributional processes have been extensively described in the psychologic literature. The paradigm we will draw on in analyzing the patient's pain-related attributions was first described in an extensive earlier body of work examining the judgments or attributions an individual makes in responding to life or health-related difficulties.[19,20] This model proposes that an important determinant of an individual's response to a health problem is the attributions they make in regard to two critical aspects of their illness: (1) Who is to blame for the problem; that is, who is responsible for the *cause* or origin of the problem; and (2) Who is to have control over the problem; that is, who or what is responsible for the *solution* to the problem.

Rather than the more typical one-dimensional view of responsibility for health-related problems, this perspective views responsibility for cause and solution as independent dimensions; individuals, therefore, can be viewed as having either high or low responsibility for the cause of their problems, as well as high or low responsibility for the solution to their problems. Crossing these two dimensions results in four attributional models, each specifying a particular combination of responsibility judgments for the cause of and solution to illness-related problems, and a particular role for the patient and their health care provider. These models, more fully described later, are labeled the medical, compensatory, moral, and enlightenment models.

Traditionally, responsibility for the cause of the problem and responsibility for the solution to the problem were assumed to be correlated (e.g., "You got yourself into this, now get yourself out" or "It's my fault, let me fix it"). Although responsibility for the problem's cause and solution may often vary, in many cases it is incorrect to think that knowing the solution to the problem implies knowing the cause, or that once the cause of the problem has been isolated, the solution to the problem has been identified. For many patients, the cause of the problem may be attributed to one set of conditions, whereas the solution to the problem is contingent on a different set entirely. In the following section, we describe the nature and implications of the four helping models. For a more complete description of these attributional models see Brickman, Rabinowitz, Karuza, and colleagues (1982).[19]

Medical Model

The helping model in which patients are not held responsible for either the cause of their health-related problem or its solution is called the medical model because the practice and orientation of modern medicine most clearly exemplify these attributional assumptions. In this model, patients see themselves, or are seen by their health care providers, as ill and the victims of forces that were and will be beyond their control. Neither the illness nor the treatment is regarded as being the patient's responsibility. Implicit in this model is a view of the patient and of human nature as essentially passive.

The health care provider is seen as the primary agent of change and is expected to take responsibility for problem solutions, applying their professional training to recognize the symptom and provide the necessary treatment. Ultimately, the responsibility for prescribing the solution and judging its effectiveness rests with the professional, not the patient.

The foremost advantage of this model is that it allows patients to seek and accept care without being blamed for their weakness. One significant drawback of this model is that it may foster needless and dysfunctional dependency. Patients may be taught to become overly passive as a result of the role expectations implicit in their care, or may be dissuaded from questioning the diagnosis or adequacy of the treatment because of the authority associated with their health care provider.

Compensatory Model

The model in which patients are not held responsible for the cause of their problems (their illness) but are still held responsible for finding a solution is described as the compensatory model. The term reflects the underlying rationale of the model; namely, that patients see themselves, or are seen by others, as having to personally compensate for the impact of their health care problems. Patients are assumed to be individuals who were not given the education or tools needed to participate in and manage their health-related problems.

Although the cause of the health problem is seen as beyond the control of the patient, the ultimate responsibility for its solution and return to wellness is regarded as within the patient's grasp. Patients are expected to adopt a problem-solving orientation in overcoming the difficulties they face. It is assumed that patients will take charge and find a solution to their pain problem by developing a partnership with their physician and learning new skills. The essential agent of change is the patient; the health care professional, therefore, assumes a supportive role. Within this model, pain management interventions are based on a redefinition of the health care problem in such a way as to allow the patient to feel a sense of control over the situation. As treatment progresses, the physician works with the patient by mobilizing resources and providing training.

The advantage of this model is that it permits patients to become actively involved in finding a solution to problems related to their pain. This engagement fosters a sense of control in the patient and works against the more passive stance associated with the adoption of the traditional medical model attributional perspective. At the same time, the model allows patients to discount past failures; and in so doing, feelings of guilt or incompetence are relieved. Further, the model permits patients to maintain their self-respect because they are not blamed for the problem and are given credit for developing an adaptive solution as one emerges.

Moral Model

The model in which patients are held responsible for both the cause of the problem and its solution is called the moral model. This term springs from the notion that individual's health problems are of their own making and that it is their moral duty to help themselves. In this model, patients see themselves, or are seen by others, as causing problems for themselves as a result of their misdirected efforts or lack of compliance. In addition, the model proposes that only patients can find a solution to their problems. Implicit in this model is the view that patients are basically strong and have the potential to reorient themselves and solve their problems. The essential agent or change is the patient, for it is assumed that no one else should (or can) effect a change. The activity of the health care provider in this model is limited to reminding patients of their responsibility for causing their problems and for finding a solution to them, and to exhorting patients, by coercion or praise, to change themselves.

The primary advantage of this model is that patients are able to assume total responsibility for their health-related problems and thereby are motivated to work harder, longer, and more effectively in dealing with their problems.[21] In addition, by taking responsibility for causes and solutions, patients may avoid the dependency and passivity associated with the medical model. The danger of this model is that patients may begin to adopt a view of the world in which everything is contingent on their own behavior, and medical problems are personally caused and solved only by the patient's force of will. Under these circumstances, patients may feel alone and separated from their caregivers because only they have the ability to effect cure. A number of the more popular alternative therapies operate from this attributional perspective. When problems are truly beyond the patient's control, however, their unrealistic notion of self-sufficiency may preclude the patient from drawing on more appropriate forms of treatment.

Enlightenment Model

The model in which patients are held responsible for the causes of their problems but not responsible for finding a solution is described as the enlightenment model. This term reflects the belief that patients must be enlightened about the true nature of their health problems and the difficult course of action that will be needed to deal with them. In this model, patients are seen as guilty, or at least culpable for their problems and suffering. Their lack of impulse control is the cause of the problem, and the flawed nature of the patient makes self-control of these impulses impossible.

Implicit in this model is the view of patients as out of control and unable to come to grips with their health problems or their habits. Patients are expected to accept this blame and submit to the knowledge, support, and discipline of legitimate medical authority. This submission to authority constitutes the solution to the patient's impulse control–based medical problems. Because the solution to the problem lies outside the patient's control, treatment and eventual cure requires patients to maintain a close tie to external authority.

Examples of the enlightenment model approach can be found in the treatment of addiction-related health problems such as alcoholism, drug addiction, and obesity. The advantage of the enlightenment model lies in the patient's admission that the solution to their pain or health problem is beyond their control. Coincident with this admission is a sense of relief based on relaxation of the patients' often fruitless striving for cure. Further, the support and structure that are offered by the health care system may engender in patients' feelings of comfort and the knowledge that control of the problem is possible.

APPLICATION TO PAIN MANAGEMENT

The first step in the selection of the most effective model to use in a particular pain management situation should be based on an extensive behavioral assessment of the patient's problematic pain-related behaviors. The clear description of the behavior that results from such an assessment can then be crafted into a behaviorally focused intervention couched in the attributional frameworks described earlier. In general, the medical and compensatory attributional models will have the greatest relevance to pain assessment and the management of dysfunctional pain-related behavior.

Indeed, Hanson and Gerber,[22] in their work on coping with pain, identify the medical model and the compensatory model (described as the self-management model in their work) as the two primary schemas for managing pain-related behaviors. They make the interesting suggestion that these models are complementary in the sense that each is appropriate under specific conditions and further that the medical model of care is best applied early in the treatment process. This echoes what has been described in the psychotherapeutic literature as "process redefined"[23]: the idea that different intervention models are appropriate at differing stages of treatment. Although the more directed medication or surgically based medical model intervention may prove reassuring to the patient early in the treatment process, the passivity

often associated with the long-term use of this model may interfere with long-term treatment.

The compensatory model, however, fosters a sense of control and active participation in medical care that is particularly important when patient's pain treatment assumes a more chronic framework. Holding the patient ultimately responsible for the management of his or her pain and pain-related behavior capitalizes on the documented beneficial impact of control in terms of the patient's avoidance of depression and improved compliance.

Employing a more fluid attributional approach tailored to the pain patient's presenting situation and stage of treatment allows the health care provider to capitalize on the powerful psychological impact associated with these models. This, in turn, can result in the development of a more comprehensive and effective pain management program. Rather than being antithetical to these goals, the use of the behavioral perspective and behavioral techniques in the treatment of cancer pain can provide an empirically derived and efficient method to monitor and alter maladaptive pain-related behaviors.

REFERENCES

1. Smith LD: Knowledge as power: The Baconian roots of Skinner's social meliorism. In Smith LD, Woodward WR (eds): B. F. Skinner and Behaviorism in American Culture. London, American University Press, 1995.
2. Skinner BF: The Behavior of Organisms: An Experimental Analysis. New York, Appleton-Century, 1938.
3. Watson JB: Psychology as the behaviorist views it. Psych Rev 20:158–177, 1913.
4. Watson JB: Behaviorism. New York, WW Norton, 1930.
5. Dewey J: The reflex arc concept in psychology. Psych Rev 3:357–370, 1896.
6. Angell JR: The province of functional psychology. Psych Rev 14:61–91, 1907.
7. Knapp TJ: A natural history of The Behavior of Organisms. In Todd JT, Morris EK (eds): Modern Perspectives on B. F. Skinner and Contemporary Behaviorism. Westport, Connecticut, Greenwood, 1995.
8. Skinner BF: Beyond Freedom and Dignity. New York, Knopf, 1971.
9. Skinner BF: Recent Issues in the Analysis of Behavior. Columbus, Ohio, Merrill Publishing Company, 1989.

10. Fordyce WE, Fowler RS, DeLateur B: An application of behavior modification technique to a problem of chronic pain. Beh Res Ther 6:105–107, 1968.
11. Fordyce WE, Fowler RS, Lehmann JF, et al: Some implications of learning in problems in chronic pain. J Chron Dis 21:179–190, 1968.
12. Anderson TP, Cole TM, Gullickson G, et al: Behavior modification of chronic pain: A treatment program by a multidisciplinary team. Clin Orthop Relat Res 129:96–100, 1977.
13. Cairns D, Thomas L, Mooney V, et al: A comprehensive treatment approach to chronic low back pain. Pain 2:301–308, 1976.
14. Fordyce WE, Fowler E, Lehmann J, et al: Operant conditioning in the treatment of chronic pain. Arch Phys Med Rehab 54:399–408, 1973.
15. Roberts AH, Reinhardt L: The behavioral management of chronic pain: Long-term follow-up with comparison groups. Pain 8:151–162, 1980.
16. Block A, Kremer E, Gaylor M: Behavioral treatment of chronic pain: The spouse as a discriminative cue for pain behavior. Pain 9:243–252, 1980.

17. Redd WH: Treatment of excessive crying in a terminal cancer patient: A time-series analysis. J Behav Med 5:225–236, 1982.
18. Varni J, Bessman C, Russo D, et al: Behavioral management of chronic pain in children: A case study. Arch Phys Med Rehab 61:375–379, 1980.
19. Brickman P, Rabinowitz VC, Karuza J, et al: Models of helping and coping. Am Psychol 37:368–384, 1982.
20. Zevon MA, Karuza J, Brickman P: Responsibility and the elderly: Implications for psychotherapy. Psychother-Theor Res Pract 19:405–411, 1982.
21. Janoff-Bulman R, Brickman P: Expectations and what people learn from failure. In Feather NT (ed): Expectations and Actions. Hillsdale, New Jersey, Erlbaum, 1982.
22. Hanson RW, Gerber KE: Coping with Chronic Pain: A Guide to Patient Self-Management. New York, Guilford Press, 1990.
23. Rabinowitz VC, Zevon MA, Karuza J: Psychotherapy as helping: An attributional analysis. In Abramson LY (ed): Social Cognition and Clinical Psychology: A Synthesis. New York, Guilford Press, 1988.

CHAPTER 15

Diagnosis and Treatment of Psychiatric Complications

Michael A. Weitzner, MD

As patients with cancer become progressively ill and enter the advanced stages of illness, the burden of both physical and psychologic symptoms becomes enormous.[1,2] In fact, physical symptoms such as pain, dyspnea, and constipation are not the most prevalent symptoms of patients with advanced cancer. Rather, psychologic symptoms such as worrying, nervousness, lack of energy, insomnia, and sadness are among the most prevalent and distressing symptoms encountered in this population.[2] Neuropsychiatric symptoms and syndromes, such as mood disorders (i.e., depression), cognitive impairment disorders (i.e., delirium), anxiety, insomnia, and suicidal ideation have a crucial role in symptom management in patients with advanced disease. They frequently coexist with other physical and psychologic symptoms, interacting with each other, and negatively affecting quality of life.

Pain and suffering are among the most feared consequences of a cancer illness. In fact, pain is a common problem for cancer patients, with approximately 70% of patients experiencing severe pain at some point in the course of their illness.[3] Nearly 75% of advanced cancer patients in the United States have pain and, despite the availability of treatments, 25% of cancer patients still die in severe pain.[4] Although aggressive medical management of cancer pain often leads to profound relief of pain, many patients continue to suffer pain because of unaddressed psychiatric complications of cancer. Psychiatric symptoms and disorders in the cancer pain patient require the same degree of aggressive attention and focus of care, particularly when they threaten compliance with treatments and patient and staff safety or interfere dramatically with quality of life.[5] This chapter reviews the most common psychiatric complications and issues encountered in the cancer patient with pain: delirium, major depression, and the specter of substance abuse and their interaction on the management of pain in the cancer population.

DELIRIUM AND COGNITIVE IMPAIRMENT DISORDERS

Delirium is extremely common in cancer patients, particularly those with advanced disease. Given its association with increased morbidity and mortality, delirium causes much distress for patients, family members, and staff.[6] Delirium can interfere significantly with the identification and control of other physical and psychologic symptoms, such as pain.[7,8] It is not uncommon for delirium to occur as a preterminal event, associated with significant physiologic disturbance. Most deliria involve multiple medical etiologies, including infection, organ failure, medication side effects, as well as extremely rare paraneoplastic syndromes.[9]

Delirium is one of the most prevalent mental disorders in the medical setting. At greater risk for delirium are the elderly, the postoperative, and cancer patients.[10] As many as 33% of hospitalized medically ill patients have serious cognitive impairments.[11] Approximately 30% to 40% of medically hospitalized patients develop delirium,[12] and as many as 65% to 80% develop some form of organic mental disorder.[13] In cancer inpatients, the prevalence of cognitive impairment is 44%,[10] with the prevalence rising to 62.1% just before death. Delirium also occurs in up to 51% of postoperative patients.[14]

The clinical features of delirium include a variety of neuropsychiatric symptoms that are also common to other psychiatric disorders such as depression, dementia, and psychosis (Table 15–1). Certain symptoms have been emphasized as pathognomonic of delirium: disordered attention and cognition, accompanied by disturbances of psychomotor behavior and the sleep–wake cycle.[14,15] Two subtypes of delirium have been described clinically based on psychomotor behavior and arousal levels.[14] The subtypes include the hyperactive (agitated or hyperalert) subtype and hypoactive (lethargic or hypoalert)

TABLE 15–1 Clinical Features of Delirium

Prodromal symptoms (restlessness, anxiety, sleep disturbance, irritability)
Rapidly fluctuating course
Reduced attention (i.e., distractibility)
Altered arousal
Increased or decreased psychomotor activity
Disturbance of sleep–wake cycle
Affective symptoms (emotional lability, sadness, anger, euphoria)
Altered perceptions (misperceptions [i.e., illusions], hallucinations)
Disorganized thinking (i.e., poorly formed delusions); incoherent speech
Disorientation to time, place, and/or person
Memory impairment (i.e., inability to register new information)

Modified from Trzepacz PT, Wise MG: Neuropsychiatric aspects of delirium. In Yudofsky SC, Hales RE (eds): Textbook of Neuropsychiatry, 3rd ed. Washington, DC, American Psychiatric Association, 1997, pp 447–470.

subtype (Table 15–2). Other researchers have proposed a "mixed" subtype,[16] with alternating features of each. Whereas the hyperactive form is most often characterized by hallucinations, delusions, agitation, and disorientation typical of withdrawal syndromes and anticholinergic-induced delirium, the hypoactive form is characterized by confusion and sedation but is rarely accompanied by hallucinations, delusions, or illusions. The hypoactive form is typical of hepatic or metabolic encephalopathies, acute intoxications from sedatives, or hypoxia.[17]

As part of diagnosing a delirium in the cancer patient, the clinician must formulate a differential diagnosis. Most often, the cause of the delirium is multifactorial or cannot be determined. A thorough diagnostic assessment should be pursued in an attempt to reverse the delirium, unless the patient is imminently terminal. One study found that 68% of delirious cancer patients could be improved, despite a 30-day mortality of 31%.[18] The diagnostic workup should include an assessment of potentially reversible causes of delirium. A full physical examination should assess for evidence of sepsis, dehydration, or major organic failure. Chemotherapeutic agents that could contribute to the delirium should be reviewed. A screen of laboratory parameters will allow assessment of the possible role of metabolic abnormalities, such as hypercalcemia, and other problems, such as hypoxia or disseminated intravascular coagulation. Imaging of the brain and assessment of the cerebrospinal fluid may be appropriate in some instances.[19]

TABLE 15–2 Contrasting Features of Subtypes of Delirium

	Hyperactive	Hypoactive
Type	Hyperalert Agitated	Hypoalert Lethargic
Symptoms	Hallucinations Delusions Hyperarousal	Sleepy Withdraw Slowed
Examples	Withdrawal syndromes (benzodiazepines, alcohol)	Encephalopathies (hepatic, metabolic) Benzodiazepine intoxication
Pathophysiology	Elevated or normal cerebral metabolism EEG: fast or normal Reduced GABA activity	Decreased global cerebral metabolism EEG: diffuse slowing Increased GABA activity

Modified from Breitbart W, Cohen K: Delirium in the terminally ill. In Chochinov HM, Breitbart W (eds): Handbook of Psychiatry in Palliative Medicine. New York, Oxford University Press, 2000, pp 75–90.

Although delirium may occasionally be due to the direct effect of cancer on the central nervous system, it is more common for delirium to be related to the indirect effects of cancer. Electrolyte imbalance, especially sodium, potassium, calcium, and magnesium, may constitute a metabolic cause of altered mental status.[20] Intentional and oftentimes needed polypharmacy, combined with a fragile physiologic state, can cause even routinely ordered hypnotics to precipitate an episode of delirium. Opiates may play a role in the development of a delirium, particularly in those patients who are elderly or have significant hepatic or renal dysfunction. The toxic accumulation of meperidine's metabolite, normeperidine, is associated with florid delirium accompanied by myoclonus and possible seizures.[21] It is extremely rare for stable regimens of oral or intravenous opioid analgesics for the control of cancer pain to induce an overt delirium or confusional state.[22,23] However, significant cognitive impairment, as well as delirium, is now commonly identified as a dose-limiting adverse effect during opioid dose titration, observed most commonly in older patients receiving intravenous opioid infusions.[21,24]

The approach to management of delirium in the medically ill cancer patient includes identifying and correcting the underlying cause, which is usually multifactorial. Although, this process may take some time, it is important to provide relief to the behavioral symptoms the patient may be experiencing as a result of the confusion. Simple measures that can be taken include environmental manipulations, such as keeping a dim light on in the patient's room, frequent reorientation of the patient by the nursing staff, observation by a one-to-one companion when the patient is agitated. Physical restraint, either by Posey vest or hand/ankle restraints should be avoided, as these tend to add to the patient's agitation. Instead, chemical restraint, with the use of a neuroleptic, will be more efficacious.

Haloperidol, a high-potency neuroleptic, is the drug of choice in this situation.[25] It can be given orally, subcutaneously, and intravenously. The dose and route of administration will depend on the type of delirium experienced by the patient. For the hypoalert delirious patient, low dosages of haloperidol are most often successful in relieving the confusion and may help to increase the patient's ability to focus and sustain his or her attention. If the patient can swallow and there is no concern regarding a potentially compromised airway, then oral haloperidol, 1 mg every 8 hours, may be used with additional as needed doses available every 2 to 4 hours. If there is concern about a potentially compromised airway or stomatitis related to chemotherapy, then the intravenous route is preferred. Haloperidol's bioavailability intravenously is twice that of the oral route.[26] Thus, a starting dose of 0.5 mg every 8 hours would be indicated for the hypoalert patient, whereas, for the hyperalert delirious patient, in which agitation and potential for self-harm is high, the usual starting dose is 1 mg every 4 hours around the clock, with additional doses available as needed every 30 to 60 minutes depending on the level of agitation. It is not uncommon for continuous intravenous infusions of haloperidol to be prescribed for the severely agitated, delirious patient. If intravenous access is unavailable, a subcutaneous infusion may be started until either intravenous access is available or the oral route becomes available as the patient's condition improves and the agitation lessens.

A common approach to management of confusion caused by opioid therapy is to lower the dose if the patient's pain is controlled, or to change to another opioid if there is still pain coincident with the confusion.[27] Another option that is becoming more widely used is the addition of a psychostimulant to offset the sedation and confusion that a patient may experience related to higher doses of opiates.[28] The most commonly used psychostimulant is methylphenidate, used in beginning doses of 5 mg orally twice per day (at 0800 and 1200) and increasing to 20 mg orally twice per day. A newer psychostimulant, modafanil, works by a totally different mechanism (i.e., the hypothalamus rather than the reticular activating system), allowing for the patient to have increased alertness without the increased energy and motivation.[29] This is helpful in the situation of the patient who is sedated and very confused, where it is less desirable to stimulate the patient while increasing alertness. Modafanil is started at 100 mg orally once per day, usually in the morning, and can be increased to 400 mg once daily. Doses have been given up to 1200 mg once daily without adverse effects.[29]

For the treatment of deliria caused by withdrawal states from alcohol, benzodiazepines, and barbiturates, the goal may be to stabilize the patient on a benzodiazepine. The concern for all three of these agents is that withdrawal can manifest with seizure activity. Thus, patients need to be placed on benzodiazepines quickly and titrated based on physiologic parameters. For withdrawal caused by any of these substances, the patient needs to be administered lorazepam orally or intravenously, starting with 1 mg every 4 hours around the clock with additional doses available every 30 to 60 minutes based on vital sign parameters (i.e., pulse >90 beats per minute, diastolic blood pressure >90 mmHg, tremulousness, and diaphoresis).[30] Vital signs need to be checked hourly and patients need to be vigorously hydrated, unless the patient has congestive heart failure, hepatic dysfunction as evidenced by decreased albumin or significant peripheral edema, or renal impairment, in which case hydration is administered judiciously. The additional as-needed lorazepam doses that are administered over a 24-hour period are, then, added to the scheduled doses for the next 24-hour period. The as-needed lorazepam doses are administered and added to the scheduled doses until the physiologic parameters normalize indicating that steady state has then been reached. After 24 hours, the total lorazepam dose can be decreased by 10% to 20% and then this is done daily until the lorazepam is discontinued. If the withdrawal is severe, it may be necessary to administer the lorazepam in a continuous intravenous infusion, ranging from 0.5 mg/hr to as much as 6 mg/hr based on physiologic parameters. The addition of scheduled haloperidol intravenously (i.e., 1 mg IV q4h) may help to keep the lorazepam dose requirements down.[31]

MAJOR DEPRESSIVE DISORDER

Given that the majority of patients with cancer have pain as part of their illness, the way they cope with stress will have an impact on their perception of pain intensity and, ultimately, their response to pain management. Severe and chronic stress related to a life-threatening illness, such as cancer, in the face of less effective coping strategies, can foster the development of major depressive disorder and anxiety disorders. Less effective coping is also associated with the abuse of alcohol and other substances, further complicating the treatment of pain. Recent evidence indicates that depression may amplify medical symptoms[32] and has been associated with role impairment and loss of function.[33,34] It is clear from the nonmalignant pain literature that patients with chronic pain are more likely to have a psychiatric disorder (i.e., major depressive disorder, general anxiety disorder, and substance use disorders) than patients without pain. In fact, one of the few studies to evaluate multiple Axis I comorbidities in chronic pain patients found 58% of men and 61% of women were likely to have more than one Axis I diagnosis.[35] A major goal of multidisciplinary pain programs is to treat pain and restore function. However, recent research has shown that psychiatric comorbidity often negatively impacts both these goals. Specifically, anxiety contributes to decreased pain thresholds and increased pain intensity ratings. Chronic pain patients with comorbid depression have been shown to have increased autonomic activity and are more sensitive to acute pain stimuli.[36,37]

Depression is the mood disorder most often observed among patients with chronic pain, in general, and among patients with cancer, in particular. An early study[38] reported that approximately 50% of patients with malignancies experience some kind of psychiatric disorder and that adjustment disorders and major depression are the most common psychiatric disorders in randomly selected patients with cancer. The majority of other research in the field suggests that the average incidence of current major depression in cancer patients is closer

to 28% and 43% for past episodes of depression.[39,40] To place these statistics in perspective, the 12-month prevalence of major depression in the general population in the United States is 5% and the lifetime prevalence is 17%.[41] Of particular interest are the results of another study that reanalyzed the data from Derogatis and colleagues.[38] Breitbart and Holland[42] found that the roughly 50% of patients who met criteria for a psychiatric diagnosis according to DSM-III were twice as likely to have significant pain as compared with those without a psychiatric diagnosis (39% vs. 19%).

Two other studies emphasize the relationship between depression and pain in cancer patients. One study[43] documented that, in a group of cancer patients with or without metastatic disease and with either high or low levels of pain, 33% of patients in the high-pain group versus 13% of patients in the low-pain group met criteria, based on a diagnostic interview, for current major depressive disorder. Similarly, another study[44] focused on the prevalence of desire for death in advanced cancer patients and its association with psychiatric disorders and pain. Although occasional wishes that death would come soon were common (44.5%), only 8.5% of patients acknowledged a serious and pervasive desire to die. Importantly, the desire for death was significantly correlated with ratings of pain and low family support and with measures of depression. The prevalence of diagnosed depressive syndromes was 58.8% among patients with a desire to die and 7.7% among patients without such a desire. Those patients with a current major depressive disorder were also more likely to have had previous episodes, suggesting that these patients are more vulnerable to depression when under stress. Moreover, 77% of those with a desire had moderate to severe pain and poor family support, whereas 46% of those without a desire had moderate to severe pain.

The diagnosis of major depression is based on specific diagnostic criteria. The DSM-IV[45] criteria are listed in Table 15–3. For major depression to be present, the patient must admit to at least a 2-week history of depressed mood and/or loss of interest in usual activities (i.e., anhedonia). Without at least one of these two symptoms present, the diagnosis of major depression cannot be made. The somatic symptoms of depression, such as anorexia, insomnia, fatigue, and weight loss, are unreliable and lack specificity in the cancer patient who may have no appetite because of chemotherapy; who sleeps poorly because of pain or hospitalization; and who is fatigued because of the cancer, radiation therapy, or chemotherapy.[46] Thus, the psychologic symptoms of depression can be substituted for greater diagnostic value. They include the following: dysphoric mood, hopelessness, worthlessness, guilt, and suicidal ideation.[47,48] Family history of depression and history of previous depressive episodes further suggest the reliability

TABLE 15–3   DSM-IV Criteria for Major Depressive Episode

A. Five (or more) of the following symptoms have been present during the same two-week period and represents a change from previous functioning; at least one of the symptoms is either (1) depressed mood or (2) loss of interest or pleasure.
Note: Do not include symptoms that are clearly due to a general medical condition or mood-incongruent delusions or hallucinations.
  1. Depressed mood most of the day, nearly every day, as indicated by either subjective report (e.g., feels sad or empty) or observation made by others (e.g., appears tearful).
  2. Markedly diminished interest or pleasure in all, or almost all, activities most of the day, nearly every day (as indicated by either subjective report or observations made by others).
  3. Significant weight loss when not dieting or weight gain (e.g., a change in more than 5% of body weight in one month), or decrease or increase in appetite nearly every day.
  4. Insomnia or hypersomnia nearly every day.
  5. Psychomotor agitation or retardation nearly every day (observable by others, not merely subjective feelings of restlessness or being slowed down).
  6. Fatigue or loss of energy nearly every day.
  7. Feelings of worthlessness or excessive or inappropriate guilt (which may be delusional) nearly every day (not merely self-reproach or guilt about being sick).
  8. Diminished ability to think or concentrate, or indecisiveness, nearly every day (either by subjective account or as observed by others).
  9. Recurrent thought of death (not just fear of dying), recurrent suicidal ideation without a specific plan, or a suicide attempt or a specific plan for committing suicide.

B. The symptoms do not meet criteria for a mixed episode.
C. The symptoms cause clinically significant distress or impairment in social, occupational, or other important areas of functioning.
D. The symptoms are not due to the direct physiological effects of a substance (e.g., a drug of abuse, a medication) or a general medical condition (e.g., hypothyroidism). The symptoms are not better accounted for by bereavement, i.e., after the loss of a loved one, the symptoms persist for longer than two months or are characterized by marked functional impairment, morbid preoccupation with worthlessness, suicidal ideation, psychotic symptoms, or psychomotor retardation.
Adapted from American Psychiatric Association: Diagnostic and Statistical Manual of Mental Disorders, 4th ed. Washington, DC, American Psychiatric Association, 1994.

of a diagnosis. The evaluation should consider organic factors that can precipitate or exacerbate depression, including uncontrolled pain, electrolyte imbalances, thyroid disease, steroids, beta-blockers, and interferon, among others.

As already mentioned, the issue of depression in cancer patients is important for many reasons, one of which has to do with the impact that depression can have on the amplification of medical symptoms such as the expression of pain. A recent study compared cancer outpatients with pain and without pain to determine the differential impact that depression would have on these two groups.[49] It was observed that 54% of the cancer patients had experienced pain in the prior month and these patients experienced a significant increase in mood disturbances compared with the patients who did not have pain. The patients with cancer-related pain reported higher levels of anxiety, depression, fear, anger, and confusion, all of which were associated with increases in both pain intensity and duration of the pain complaint. In addition, the cancer patients with pain were more fatigued, confirming other findings that cancer pain interferes moderately or greatly with activity,

walking, work, social relationships, and overall enjoyment of life.[50]

Another consideration regarding pain expression has been the influence of depression on the use of sensory and affective descriptors of pain. A recent study found that depressed pain patients scored higher on the affective pain intensity dimension than nondepressed pain patients and this was consistent in both cancer and noncancer patients.[51] Depressed pain patients are more likely to use terms including tiring, exhausting, fearful, frightening, punishing, grueling, and vicious to describe their pain. Greater pain intensity was found to be significantly correlated with higher levels of cognitive-affective depression, suggesting that the presence of pain, rather than the nature of the underlying medical condition, is the factor most closely associated with the intensity of depressive symptoms. A related study also showed a positive correlation between pain intensity and negative affect.[52] Moderate to high levels of frustration, anger, exhaustion, and helplessness were seen across gender, reinforcing the classification of frustration and anger as a significant contributor to the overall affective unpleasantness accompanying chronic pain.[53] Interestingly, fear and hopelessness were not found to be significantly associated with pain intensity.

It appears that this relationship between pain and depression is not gender-specific. Another study evaluated cancer patients with pain to determine if gender had an additional effect on pain expression over psychologic factors.[54] Men and women did not differ in regard to level of depression, pain severity, or functional limitations. However, both men and women who had a dysfunctional psychologic profile (i.e., high levels of pain, disability, functional limitation, psychologic distress, and low levels of activity and sense of control) had higher levels of depression. It was concluded that the patients' gender in chronic pain may be less important than their psychologic and behavioral responses. When compared with chronic noncancer pain patients, cancer patients reported comparable levels of pain severity but higher levels of perceived disability and lower degrees of activity.[55] Interestingly, cancer patients with pain had significantly higher levels of support and solicitous behaviors from significant others compared with the chronic, nonmalignant pain group.

Depression in cancer patients is optimally managed by using a combination of supportive psychotherapy, cognitive-behavioral techniques, and antidepressant medications.[47] Psychotherapy and cognitive-behavioral techniques are useful in the management of psychologic distress in cancer patients, and they have been applied to the treatment of depressive and anxious symptoms related to cancer and cancer pain. Psychotherapeutic interventions, either in the form of individual or group counseling, have been shown to effectively reduce psychologic distress and depressive symptoms in cancer patients.[56] Psychopharmacologic interventions are the mainstay of management in the treatment of cancer patients with severe depressive symptoms who meet criteria for major depressive episodes.[47] The efficacy of antidepressants in the treatment of depression in cancer patients has been well established.[57] The medications used in patients with cancer for depression are selective serotonin reuptake inhibitors (SSRIs), tricyclic antidepressants (TCAs), and psychostimulants. Today, SSRIs are used most commonly to treat major depressive disorder.[58] The choice of antidepressant is usually dictated by the symptoms that the patient is expressing and the opportunity that the clinician has to use the side effect profile of a particular medication to enhance overall symptom control of the major depression. For example, if a patient is having a significant sleep disturbance as part of his or her presentation of depression, the use of a sedating SSRI, such as paroxetine or citalopram, may be indicated. If the patient is having somatizing symptoms associated with the depression, such as nausea or diarrhea, paroxetine (20 mg to 40 mg nightly) and citalopram (20 mg to 40 mg nightly) may be the drugs of choice, given their

anticholinergic side effect profile. On the other hand, if the patient has no sleep disturbance but is acknowledging significant fatigue, than a more activating SSRI, such as sertraline (50 mg to 200 mg in the morning), may be in order.[59] It is important to point out that fluoxetine (10 mg to 20 mg in the morning), although a good antidepressant, has a rather limited usefulness in the cancer patient, unless the patient is in remission, not receiving any antineoplastic therapies, and has no other significant medical comorbidities. Simply put, fluoxetine is the most potent inhibitor of the cytochrome P450 IID6 microenzyme, potentially causing significant drug–drug interactions with other medications that are metabolized through that microenzyme (i.e., opiates, many antibiotics, antiarrhythmics).[60]

Typically, although the starting doses of antidepressants for patients with cancer are lower, they usually require the same doses as do healthy patients. Most antidepressants take 3 to 6 weeks to show efficacy. Therefore, it is usually not imperative to begin a medication immediately after recognition of depressive symptoms, so a medical workup of possible causes can take place. A patient's prior response to a particular medication, or a family member's experience with an antidepressant, are helpful predictors of response.[61] Patients who are unable to swallow pills may be able to take an antidepressant elixir (sertraline, paroxetine, citalopram), or immediate-release venlafaxine, mirtazapine, and nefazodone can be crushed and given in a liquid of choice.

SUBSTANCE ABUSE IN CANCER PATIENTS

Another consideration for the health care practitioner who cares for cancer patients with and without pain is the role that premorbid substance abuse problems (either past or current) play on the patient's symptom presentation and ability to cope with his or her disease. To place this in perspective, in the Epidemiological Catchment Area (ECA) study, a survey of mental health and substance disorders in almost 20,000 adult Americans, the lifetime prevalence of alcohol abuse/dependence was 13.5% in the general U.S. population in the 1980s.[62] In the 1990s, the Institute of Medicine (IOM) reported that approximately 6.4% of the U.S. population over the age of 12 years probably needed treatment for alcohol-use disorders.[63] During the same period, the lifetime incidence of alcohol and comorbid drug disorders affected approximately 20% of the population.[64] There is no evidence that these percentages have improved. Alcohol and drug use have a substantial economic impact when both direct and indirect costs such as crime and impact on mental health are considered, accounting for 25% of the national health care budget in 1995 and costing the U.S. economy $300 billion per year in 1994.[65] Thirty-four billion of these dollars are ascribed to direct health care costs. A small percentage of these dollars goes to prevention and treatment. In 1993, an estimated $20 billion was spent on the treatment of addictions and $5 billion was spent on prevention.[66] In 1998, alcoholism and comorbid drug addiction were associated with 25% to 50% of general medical admissions and 50% to 75% of psychiatric admissions and contributed to costs and medical complications of patients admitted to hospitals for other reasons.[62]

Considering the rather high incidence of alcohol and substance abuse disorders in the general population, it comes as no surprise that the comorbidity of substance use disorders and chronic pain has been shown to be high. In a review of studies focusing on this issue, it has been concluded that the prevalence percentages for the diagnoses of drug abuse, dependence, or addiction in chronic pain patients (including cancer pain) are in the range of 3% to 19%.[67] More recent studies have reported current drug dependence statistics of 20% and 34%, respectively.[68,69]

The recognition and management of alcohol and substance abuse in cancer patients, even those with advanced disease, is extremely important. Otherwise, there is the potential for significant deleterious effects, including increased patient suffering, increased stress and frustration for family members and caregivers, masking of symptoms important to the patient's care, family concern over misuse of medication, reluctance by providers to provide adequate pain medications, poor patient compliance with medical regimen, and decreased quality of life.[70,71] Substance use and misuse among cancer patients are frequent problems. One study showed that greater than 25% of patients admitted to an inpatient palliative care unit were found to have problems with alcohol abuse.[72]

In addition, risk factors including neuropathic and incidental pain, opioid tolerance, somatization or psychologic distress, and history of drug or alcohol abuse are important in the predisposition to opioid-induced cognitive dysfunction, which usually occurs in the form of delirium but may also manifest as a dementia when subclinical cognitive deficits were present before treatment.[73,74] For example, the incidence of cognitive changes after brain irradiation is fairly common. These cognitive changes may now cause the patient to have a narrow therapeutic window for the sedating adverse effects of medications, including analgesics. Therefore, the patient's sedation following administration of opioids or other sedating medication may reflect this narrow therapeutic window rather than the patient's use of analgesics to procure these psychic effects.[75,76]

Given the incidence and prevalence of substance abuse in the United States, it would be expected that 6% to 10% of cancer patients (with or without pain) would have problems with abuse of substances. Documentation in the cancer literature regarding the incidence of substance abuse is sparse and based on reports of referrals to psychiatric services in tertiary cancer hospitals, an inherently biased sample.[75] The low rates of substance abuse reported in the cancer literature relies on clinicians with little education and experience assessing substance use disorders and recognizing when a consult is indicated. In addition, these low numbers may reflect institutional biases or a tendency for patients to underreport in tertiary care hospitals. Social forces may also prevent patients from reporting drug use behavior. Many drug abusers feel alienated from the health care system and are of a lower socioeconomic standing and, consequently, may not seek care in tertiary care centers. Furthermore, those who are treated in these centers may be hesitant to acknowledge drug abuse because they fear stigmatization.[75-77]

To have a better sense regarding substance abuse in a cancer population, a recent study focused on drug-taking behaviors in an oncology and HIV/AIDS population.[78] A total of 83% of the cancer patients reported a prior history of alcohol use; 39% of these patients were currently using alcohol. Cocaine was used in the past by 18% of the cancer patients, while past marijuana use was present in 41% of the cancer patients and 8% of them were currently using. About 14% of the cancer patients had a past history of using nonprescribed downers, and 2% of them were continuing that practice. Finally, 10% of the cancer patients had a past history of hallucinogen use. These patients also had certain views regarding aberrant drug behavior. Approximately 25% to 50% of patients endorsed a willingness to use illicit drugs to relieve symptoms. Up to 31% experienced a willingness to use prescribed drugs for nonprescribed purposes. Patients also reported beliefs that their peers engaged in illicit drug use. Many cancer patients believed that getting "high" from pain medications (62%), using illicit drugs for medical purposes (77%), raising the dose on one's own (86%), and seeking multiple doctors (83%) are common behaviors.

For those clinicians who focus on psychosocial issues in cancer, it is clear that cancer patients who have used illicit drugs are being encountered more frequently in oncology settings. Cancer patients who use illicit drugs, misuse prescribed medications, or have substance abuse disorders are among the most difficult patients to treat because of problems with adherence to medical therapy and safety during treatment, adverse interactions between illicit drugs and medications that are prescribed as part of a patient's treatment, the undermining of the patient's social support network that can serve to buffer the chronic stressors associated with cancer and its treatment.[77,79] Issues that may confound the diagnosis of abuse or addiction when assessing drug-taking behaviors in cancer patients include pseudoaddiction, sociocultural influences on the definition of aberrancy in drug taking, and the importance of cancer-related variables. Research has shown and continues to show that pain is undertreated in cancer patients and this may be one motivation for aberrant drug-taking behaviors in an effort to self-medicate.[80,81]

Distinguishing aberrant drug-taking behaviors from abuse and addiction is difficult. These definitions are derived from social and cultural norms of drug taking. Although abuse is defined as the use of an illicit drug or prescription drug without medical indication, addiction refers to the continual use of either type of drug in a compulsive manner, regardless of harm to the user or others. However, when a drug is prescribed for a medically diagnosed purpose, it is unclear if the behaviors could be aberrant. In addition, the potential for a diagnosis of drug abuse or addiction increases. Recent literature supports the difficulties inherent in diagnosing addictive disease in chronic pain patients maintained on opioid analgesics.[82] The American Society of Addiction Medicine (ASAM) has recognized the limitations of other diagnostic criteria and developed separate recommendations for defining addiction in chronic pain patients treated with opioids (Table 15–4). Characteristics identified as central to diagnosing addiction in this population include the presence of adverse consequences associated with the use of opioids, loss of control over the use of opioids, and preoccupation with obtaining opioids despite the presence of adequate analgesia.[82] Although it is difficult to disagree with the aberrancy of certain behaviors, such as intravenous injection of oral formulations,

various other behaviors are less obvious (e.g., a patient who is experiencing unrelieved pain taking an extra dose of prescribed opioids) (Table 15–5).[75,76,78]

A recent study evaluated chronic opioid therapy for patients with nonmalignant pain and a history of substance abuse.[83] It was shown that those patients who did not abuse opioid therapy were more likely to have a history of alcohol abuse alone or a remote history of polysubstance abuse, to be active members of Alcoholics Anonymous (AA), and to have a stable family or other similar support system. In contrast, those who abused opioid therapy showed characteristic aberrant patterns of behavior in their management, which indicated a clear pattern of prescription abuse early in the course of therapy. Those patients were more likely to be recent polysubstance abusers and none was active in AA. Signing an opioid treatment agreement was not, in and of itself, a predictor of successful outcome. This study underscores the importance of conducting a comprehensive assessment for screening cancer patients for substance abuse or aberrant behaviors.

Evaluating and Treating the Cancer Patient with a History of Substance Abuse

Clinicians involved in caring for patients with chronic cancer pain with a comorbid substance abuse and addictive history are faced with the complex problem of managing the pain without adversely affecting the substance abuse problem. A majority of nonpain physicians are reluctant to use opioids or other controlled

---

TABLE 15–4   **American Society of Addiction Medicine Definitions Related to the Use of Opioids in Pain Treatment**
The Committee on Pain of the American Society of Addiction Medicine recognizes the following definitions as appropriate and clinically useful definitions and recommends their use when assessing the use of opioids in the context of pain treatment.
Physical Dependence Physical dependence on an opioid is a physiologic state in which abrupt cessation of the opioid or administration of an opioid antagonist result in a withdrawal syndrome. Physical dependency on opioids is an expected occurrence in all individuals in the presence of continuous use of opioids for therapeutic or for nontherapeutic purposes. It does not, in and of itself, imply addiction.
Tolerance Tolerance is a form of neuroadaptation to the effects of chronically administered opioids (or other medications), which is indicated by the need for increasing or more frequent doses of the medication to achieve the initial effects of the drug. Tolerance may occur both to the analgesic effects of opioids and to unwanted side effects such as respiratory depression, sedation, or nausea. The occurrence of tolerance is variable in occurrence, but it does not, in and of itself, imply addiction.
Addiction Addiction in the context of pain treatment with opioids is characterized by a persistent pattern of dysfunctional opioid use that may involve any or all of the following: • Adverse consequences associated with the use of opioids • Loss of control over the use of opioids • Preoccupation with obtaining opioids despite the presence of adequate analgesia

TABLE 15–5	Spectrum of Aberrant Behaviors Suggestive of Addiction
More Suggestive of Addiction	**Less Suggestive of Addiction**
Stealing drugs from others or obtaining drugs from nonmedical sources	Aggressive complaining about the need for more drugs
Prescription forgery	Drug hoarding during periods of reduced symptoms
Selling of prescription drugs	Requesting more drugs
Injecting oral formulations	Requesting specific drugs
Concurrent alcohol or illicit drug use	Intense expression of anxiety about recurrent symptoms
Repeated dose escalations or noncompliance despite multiple warnings	Occasional unsanctioned dose escalation or other noncompliance
Repeated resistance to changes in therapy despite evidence of adverse drug effects	Resistance to change in therapy associated with tolerable adverse effects
Repeated visits to other clinicians or emergency departments without informing prescriber	Openly acquiring similar drugs from other medical sources
Drug-related deterioration in function at work, in the family, or socially	Reporting psychic effects not intended by the physician

Modified from Passik SD, Portenoy RK: Substance abuse issues in palliative care. In Berger A (ed): Principles and Practice of Supportive Oncology. Philadelphia, Lippincott-Raven, 1998, pp 513–524.

substances with these patients; hence they are consistently undermedicated.[81,84,85] To that end, for these clinicians, the first hurdle is identifying the patient who has a current substance use problem, a remote substance abuse problem, or the patient who is at risk for misusing opiate medications. The identification of these at risk patients is best obtained through the comprehensive medical evaluation that occurs at the patient's first visit, specifically the psychologic and psychosocial history component of the evaluation. Whether the psychologic and psychosocial part of the history is obtained by the pain physician or through referral to a mental health practitioner, this portion of the history provides information that helps to determine the contribution of the affective and environmental factors to the patient's pain complaint, as well as the potential role of clinical depression.[86] A key consideration is that often what contributes to the patient's pain experience at the onset of the disease is not what is present when the patient is eventually seen by the physician. A history of prior psychologic disorders, substance abuse, vocational problems, family role models of chronic illness or pain, and recent stressors can enhance the understanding of the patient's current problem. This information is crucial for optimizing the possible treatment strategies for the patient.[87] Clearly, abuse of or dependence on alcohol or other substances can interfere with efforts to treat pain and disability and may require specialized treatment beyond that used for pain. Excessive alcohol, sedative-hypnotics, and opioid use may contribute to dysphoria, irritability, mood swings, decreased energy, sleep disturbance, cognitive impairment, and appetite and weight changes, which may not be recognized as substance- or medication-related.[88]

Although taking a detailed psychosocial history may not be possible for the busy physician, several screening questionnaires for alcohol and drug problems have been developed for clinical use, including the CAGE and T-ACE questions, as well as the RAFFT questions (Table 15–6).[89-91] The CAGE questionnaire is increasingly popular in clinical settings because it is easy to remember and administer. The CAGE has a cut-off score of 2 or more, indicating a positive test result. It has been shown that patients who screened positively with the CAGE questionnaire also reported a higher opioid intake.[72] The CAGE questionnaire may also be used in screening for other substances of abuse.[92,93] The T-ACE questionnaire has a higher sensitivity (70% to 81%) than an equivalent specificity to the CAGE questionnaire. Although the RAFFT has only been validated in an adolescent population, it has relevance in the adult population as well and may be used clinically. Patients who screen positively with one of these screening instruments can be referred on for more in-depth questioning by a mental health professional who has experience in evaluating and treatment patients with addictions. When the patient is reluctant to disclose alcohol and substance use or may underestimate consumption, a better source of information is the significant other or other family member, who usually accompanies that patient to the interview. Important information is also obtained by questioning significant others about the effects of medications on the patient's physical and cognitive functioning, mood, and behavior. Information confirming interference with any of these areas of functioning is suggestive of a significant problem with substance abuse or dependency. Referral to a chemical dependency treatment program may be necessary before the pain problem can be treated.[87,94]

TABLE 15–6   Screening Questionnaires for Substance Abuse

CAGE[89]		T-ACE[90]		RAFFT[91]	
C	Have you felt you needed to Cut down on drinking?	T	How many drinks does it take to make you feel high? (Tolerance)	R	Do you drink/drug to RELAX, feel better about yourself, or fit in?
A	Have you felt Annoyed by criticism of your drinking?	A	Have you felt Annoyed by criticisms of your drinking?	A	Do you ever drink/drug while you are by yourself, ALONE?
G	Have you felt Guilt about drinking?	C	Have you ever felt the need to Cut down on drinking?	F	Do any of your closest FRIENDS drink/drug?
E	Have you felt you needed a drink first thing in the morning (Eye-opener)?	E	Have you ever taken a drink first thing in the morning? (Eye-opener)	F	Does a close FAMILY member have a problem with alcohol/drugs?
				T	Have you ever gotten into TROUBLE from drinking/drugging?

These questions can be modified for any drug of abuse.

The three patterns of substance abuse encountered include: (1) chronic cancer pain patients with a remote history of substance abuse; (2) chronic cancer pain patients with a persistent substance abuse problem; and (3) chronic cancer pain patients with a remote history of substance abuse who are actively involved in a recovery program (psychotherapeutic or pharmacologic).[70] It is evident that persistent pain can place additional stress on patients who are already strained in their ability to cope, as evidenced by their chemical coping with substances. One can draw on the patient's significant social support network, if the substance abuse history is remote and the patient continues his or her recovery program. Similarly, the patient with a remote history of substance abuse who is not in recovery can be encouraged to enter a recovery program to increase the level of social support available to him or her.[70]

The patients with active substance abuse are the most difficult to treat because they are the most troubled, the most confused, have the most significant psychopathology, and are the most unwilling to accept therapeutic assistance. They tend to not have good social support systems and, because of their substance abuse, are less likely to be working, have worn their family supports thin, and lack the financial resources for treatment. Although these patients may be noncompliant, manipulative, and drug-seeking throughout treatment, they should still be treated with opiate medications for the pain related to their cancer. Managing these patients' pain can be successful with the implementation of several procedures. Although it is important to have all patients seeking treatment for cancer pain to sign a treatment agreement that details the respective responsibilities of the treating physician and the patient, it is essential for the treatment of the cancer pain patient with an ongoing substance abuse problem. The responsibilities of the patient include using only one pharmacy for filling prescriptions and providing consent for the pain physician to contact all other physicians providing care for the patient. This allows the pain physician to inform them that he or she is prescribing opiate medications for the patient and that they are not to prescribe these medications and to inform the pain physician should the patient attempt to get opiate prescriptions from them. Additional patient responsibilities include not canceling appointments without sufficient notice, not requesting refills before they are due, and following through on the treatment plan that the pain physician develops. Should the patient not remain compliant with treatment, the treatment agreement can stipulate that the patient must submit to random urine or serum toxicology screening and, if the patient remains noncompliant, that the patient–physician relationship will be terminated. Appropriate documentation in the patient's medical record should accompany this treatment agreement. The inclusion of mental health practitioners in this process will also provide additional resources for the pain physician in helping the patient to adhere to the treatment agreement.[70]

CONCLUSION

Delirium, depression, and problems with past or current substance abuse are among the most commonly occurring psychiatric complications encountered in cancer patients. When severe, these disorders require as urgent and aggressive attention as do other distressing physical symptoms, such as escalating pain. Increased awareness of these psychiatric conditions and complications can lead to earlier diagnosis and involvement of mental health practitioners, such as psychiatrists and psychologists, in the effective and successful management of these conditions.

REFERENCES

1. Breitbart W, Chochinov HM, Passik SD: Psychiatric aspects of palliative care. In Doyle D, Hanks GW, MacDonald N (eds): Oxford Textbook of Palliative medicine, 2nd ed. Oxford, Oxford University Press, 1997, pp 933–954.

2. Portenoy RK, Thaler HT, Kornblith AB, et al: The memorial symptom assessment scale: An instrument for evaluation of symptom prevalence, characteristics and distress. Eur J Cancer 30A:1326–1336, 1994.

3. Foley KM: The treatment of cancer pain. N Engl J Med 313:84–95, 1985.

4. Fitzgibbon DR, Chapman CR: Cancer pain: Assessment and diagnosis. In Loeser JD, Butler SH, Chapman CR, Turk DC (eds): Bonica's Management of Pain, 3rd ed. Philadelphia, Lippincott Williams & Wilkins, 2001, pp 623–658.

5. Strain JJ: Adjustment disorders. In Holland JC, Breitbart W, Jacobsen PB, et al (eds): Psychooncology. New York, Oxford University Press, 1998, pp 509–517.

6. Stiefel F, Holland J: Delirium in cancer patients. Int Psychogeriatr 3:333–336, 1991.

7. Coyle N, Breitbart W, Weaver S, et al: Delirium as a contributing factor to "crescendo" pain: Three case reports. J Pain Symptom Manage 9:44–47, 1994.

8. Breitbart W: Diagnosis and management of delirium in the terminally ill. In Bruera E, Portenoy RK (eds): Topics in Palliative Care, vol 5. New York, Oxford University Press, 2001, pp 303–321.

9. Inouye SK: Delirium and other mental status problems in the older patient. In Goldman L, Bennett JC (eds.): Cecil's Textbook of Medicine, 21st ed. St. Louis, WB Saunders, 1999, pp 18–22.

10. Pereira J, Hanson J, Bruera E: The frequency and clinical course of cognitive impairment in patients with terminal cancer. Cancer 79:835–842, 1997.

11. Knight EB, Folstein MF: Unsuspected emotional and cognitive disturbance in medical patients. Ann Internal Med 87: 723–724, 1977.

12. Hodkinson HM: Mental impairment in the elderly. J R Coll Physicians 7:305–317, 1973.

13. Lipowski ZJ: Delirium: Acute Brain Failure in Man. Springfield, IL, Charles C. Thomas, 1980.

14. Lipowski ZJ: Delirium: Acute Confusional States. New York, Oxford University Press, 1990.

15. American Psychiatric Association: Diagnostic and Statistical Manual of Mental Disorders (DSM-IV), 4th ed. Washington, DC, American Psychiatric Association, 1994.

16. Trzepacz PT, Wise MG: Neuropsychiatric aspects of delirium. In Yudofsky SC, Hales RE (eds): Textbook of Neuropsychiatry, 3rd ed. Washington, DC, American Psychiatric Press, 1997, pp 447–470.

17. Ross CA: CNS arousal systems: Possible role in delirium. Int Psychogeriatr 3: 353–371, 1991.

18. Bruera E, MacMillan K, Kuehn N, et al: The cognitive effects of the administration of narcotics. Pain 39:13–16, 1989.

19. Breitbart W, Cohen K: Delirium in the terminally ill. In Chochinov HM, Breitbart W (eds): Handbook of Psychiatry in Palliative Medicine. New York, Oxford University Press, 2000, pp 75–90.

20. Tuma R, DeAngelis L: Altered mental status in patients with cancer. Arch Neurol 57:1727–1731, 2000.

21. Bruera E, Fainsinger R, Miller MJ, et al: The assessment of pain intensity in patients with cognitive failure: A preliminary report. J Pain Symptom Manage 7:267–270, 1992.

22. Liepzig RM, Goodman H, Gray P, et al: Reversible narcotic-associated mental status impairment in patients with metastatic cancer. Pharmacology 53:47–57, 1987.

23. Jellema JG: Hallucinations during sustained-release opioid and methadone administration. Lancet 2:392, 1987.

24. Pereira J, Bruera E: Emerging neuropsychiatric toxicities of opioids. J Pharmaceut Care Pain Symptom Control 5:3, 1997.

25. Akechi T, Uchitomi Y, Okamura H, et al: Usage of haloperidol for delirium in cancer patients. Support Care Cancer 4:390–392, 1996.

26. Haloperidol prescribing information. Springhouse, McNeil Lab, 1998.

27. Kloke M, Rapp M, Bosse B, et al: Toxicity and/or insufficient analgesia by opioid therapy: Risk factors and impact of changing the opioid—A retrospective analysis of 273 patients observed at a single center. Support Care Cancer 8:479–486, 2000.

28. Wilwerding MB, Loprinzi CL, Mailliard JA, et al: A randomized, crossover evaluation of methylphenidate in cancer patients receiving strong narcotics. Support Care Cancer 3:135-8, 1995.

29. Modafinil prescribing information. Westchester, Cephalon, 1999.

30. D'Onofrio G, Rathlev NK, Ulrich AS, et al: Lorazepam for the prevention of recurrent seizures related to alcohol. N Engl J Med 340:915–919, 1999.

31. Palestine ML: Drug treatment of alcohol withdrawal syndrome with delirium tremens: A comparison of haloperidol with mesoridazine and hydroxyzine. Q J Stud Alcohol 34:185–193, 1973.

32. Katon WJ: Depression in patients with inflammatory bowel disease. J Clin Psychiatr 58(suppl 1):20–23, 1997.

33. Magee WJ, Eaton WW, Wittchen HU, et al: Agoraphobia, simple phobia, and social phobia in the national comorbidity survey. Arch Gen Psychiatry 53:159–168, 1996.

34. Mauskopf JA, Simeon GP, Miles MA, et al: Functional status in depressed patients: The relationship to disease severity and disease resolution. J Clin Psychiatr 77:588, 1996.

35. Fishbain DA, Goldberg M, Meagher BR, et al: Male and female chronic pain patients categorized by DSM-III psychiatric diagnostic criteria. Pain 26:181–197, 1986.

36. Weisberg JN, Gorin A, Drozd K, et al: The relationship between depression and psychophysiological reactivity in chronic pain patients. In International Association for the Study of Pain, 8th World Congress of Pain, Vancouver, Canada, 233:71, 1996.

37. Krass S, Gallagher RM, Myers P, et al: The effect of chronic pain and depression on pain perception in chronic pain patients. American Pain Society 15th Annual Meeting, Washington, DC, 685:71, 1996.

38. Derogatis LR, Morrow GR, Fetting J, et al: The prevalence of psychiatric disorders among cancer patients. J Am Med Assoc 249:751–757, 1983.

39. Ciaramella A, Poli P: Assessment of depression among cancer patients: The role of pain, cancer type, and treatment. Psycho-Oncology 10:156–165, 2001.

40. Akechi T, Okamura H, Nishiwaki Y, et al: Psychiatric disorders and associated and predictive factors in patients with unresectable nonsmall cell lung cancer: A longitudinal study. Cancer 92:2609–2622, 2001.

41. Kessler R, McGonagle K, Zhao S, et al: Lifetime and 12 month prevalence of DSM-III-R psychiatric disorders in the United States. Arch Gen Psychiatr 51:8–19, 1994.

42. Breitbart W, Holland J: Psychiatric aspects of cancer pain. Adv Pain Res Ther 16:73–87, 1990.

43. Spiegel D, Sands S, Koopman C: Pain and depression in patients with cancer. Cancer 74:2570–2578, 1994.

44. Chochinov HM, Wilson KG, Enns M, et al: Desire for death in the terminally ill. Am J Psychiatr 152:1185–1191, 1995.

45. American Psychiatric Association: Diagnostic and Statistical Manual of Mental Disorders, 4th ed. Washington, DC, American Psychiatric Press, 1994.

46. Breitbart W, Passik SD: Psychiatric aspects of palliative care. In Doyle D, Hanks GW, MacDonald N (eds): Oxford Textbook of Palliative Medicine. Oxford, Oxford University Press, 1993, pp 609–626.

47. Massie MJ, Holland JC: Depression and the cancer patient. J Clin Psychiatr 51:12–17, 1990.

48. Endicott J: Measurement of depression in patients with cancer. Cancer 53:2243–2248, 1983.

49. Glover J, Dibble SL, Dodd MJ, et al: Mood states of oncology outpatients: Does pain make a difference? J Pain Symptom Manage 10:120–128, 1995.

50. Portenoy RK, Miransky J, Hornung J, et al: Pain in ambulatory patients with lung or colon cancer: Prevalence, characteristics, and effect. Cancer 70:1616–1624, 1992.

51. Sist TC, Florio GA, Miner MF, et al: The relationship between depression and pain language in cancer and chronic non-cancer pain patients. J Pain Symptom Manage 15:350–358, 1998.

52. Sela RA, Bruera E, Conner-Spady B, et al: Sensory and affective dimensions of advanced cancer pain. Psycho-Oncology 11:23–34, 2002.

53. Fernandez E, Turk DC: The scope and significance of anger in the experience of chronic pain. Pain 61:165–175, 1995.

54. Turk DC, Okifuji A: Does sex make a difference in the prescription of treatments and the adaptation to chronic pain by cancer and non-cancer patients? Pain 82:139–148, 1999.

55. Turk DC, Sist TC, Okifuji A, et al: Adaptation to metastatic cancer pain, regional/local cancer pain and non-cancer pain: Role of psychological and behavioral factors. Pain 74:247–256, 1998.

56. Massie MJ, Holland JC, Straker N: Psychotherapeutic interventions. In Holland JC, Rowland JH (eds): Handbook of Psychooncology. New York, Oxford University Press, 1989, pp 455–469.

57. Massie MJ, Shakin EJ: Management of depression and anxiety. In Breitbart W, Holland JC, (eds): Psychiatric Aspects of Symptom Management in Cancer Patients. Washington, DC, American Psychiatric Press, 1994.

58. Peretti S, Judge R, Hindmarch I: Safety and tolerability considerations: Tricyclic antidepressants vs. selective serotonin reuptake inhibitors. Acta Psychiatr Scand Suppl 403:17–25, 2000.

59. Kando JC, Wells BG, Hayes PE: Depressive Disorders. In Dipiro JT et al (eds): Pharmacotherapy: A pathophysiologic approach, 4th ed. Stamford, CT, Appleton & Lange, 1999, pp 1141–1160.

60. Fluoxetine prescribing information. Indianapolis, Dista Products, 1995.

61. Roth AJ, Holland JH: Treatment of depression in cancer patients. Primary Care Cancer 14:23–29, 1994.

62. Swift RM, Miller NS, Lewis DC: Addictive disorders. In Goldman LS, Wise TN, Brody DS (eds): Psychiatry for Primary Care Physicians. Chicago: American Medical Association, 1998.

63. Institute of Medicine: Broadening the base of treatment for alcohol problems. Washington, DC, National Academy Press, 1990.

64. Institute of Medicine: A study of the evolution, effectiveness, and financing of public and private drug treatment systems.In Gerstein DR, Harwood HJ (eds): Treating Drug Problems. Vol 1. Washington, DC, National Academy Press, 1990.

65. Falco M: Drug abuse prevention makes a difference. Current Issues in Public Health 2:101–105, 1996.

66. McGinnis JM, Foege WH: Actual causes of death in the United States. J Am Med Assoc 270:2207–2212, 1993.

67. Fishbain DA, Steele-Rosomoff R, Rosomoff HL: Drug abuse, dependence, and addiction in chronic pain patients. Pain 8:77–85, 1992.

68. Hoffman NG, Olofsson O, Salen B, et al: Prevalence of abuse and dependency in chronic pain patients. Int J Addiction 30:919–927, 1995.

69. Chabal C, Erjavec MK, Jacobson L, et al: Prescription opiate abuse in chronic pain patients: Clinical criteria, incidence, and predictors. Clin J Pain 13:150–155, 1997.

70. Aronoff GM: Opioids in chronic pain management: Is there a significant risk of addiction. Curr Rev Pain 4:112–121, 2000.

71. Passik SD, Theobald DE: Managing addiction in advanced cancer patients: Why bother? J Pain Symptom Manage 19:229–234, 2000.

72. Bruera E, Moyano J, Seifert L, et al: The frequency of alcoholism among patients with pain due to terminal cancer. J Pain Symptom Manage 10:599, 1995.

73. Bruera E, Schoeller T, Wenk R, et al: A prospective multi-center assessment of the Edmonton Staging System for cancer pain. J Pain Symptom Manage 10:348–355, 1995.

74. Lawlor PG: The panorama of opioid-related cognitive dysfunction in patients with cancer: A critical literature appraisal. Cancer 94:1836–1853, 2002.

75. Passik SD, Portenoy RK, Ricketts PL: Substance abuse issues in cancer patients. Part 1: Prevalence and diagnosis. Oncology 12:517–521, 1998.

76. Passik SD, Portenoy RK: Substance abuse issues in palliative care. In Berger A, Portenoy R, Weissman D (eds): Principles and Practice of Supportive Oncology. Philadelphia, Lippincott-Raven, 1998, pp 513–524.

77. Whitcomb LA, Kirsh KL, Passik SD: Substance abuse issues in cancer pain. Curr Pain Headache Rep 6:183–190, 2002.

78. Passik SD, Kirsh KL, McDonald MV, et al: A pilot survey of aberrant drug-taking attitudes and behaviors in samples of cancer and AIDS patients. J Pain Symptom Manage 19:274–286, 2000.

79. Passik SD, Portenoy RK: Substance abuse disorders. In Holland JC (ed): Psycho-Oncology. New York, Oxford University Press, 1998, pp 576–586.

80. Glajchen M, Fitzmartin RD, Blum D, et al: Psyhosocial barriers to cancer pain relief. Cancer Pract 3:76–82, 1995.

81. Ward SE, Gordon D: Application of the American Pain Society quality assurance standards. Pain 56:299–306, 1994.

82. Compton P, Darakjian J, Miotto K: Screening for addiction in patients with chronic pain and "problematic" substance use: Evaluation of a pilot assessment tool.

J Pain Symptom Manage 16:355–363, 1998.

83. Dunbar SA, Katz NP: Chronic opioid therapy for nonmalignant pain in patients with a history of substance abuse: Report of 20 cases. J Pain Symptom Manage 11:163–171, 1996.

84. Vourakis C: Substance abuse concerns in the treatment of pain. Nurs Clin North Am 33:47–60, 1998.

85. Ferrell BR, Griffith H: Cost issues related to pain management: Report from the cancer pain panel of the agency for health care policy and research. J Pain Symptom Manage 9:221–234, 1994.

86. Bradley LA, Haile JM, Jaworsky TM: Assessment of psychological status using interviews and self-report instruments. In Turk DC, Melzack R (eds): Handbook of Pain Assessment. New York, Guilford Press, 1992, pp 193–213.

87. Loeser JD: Medical evaluation of the patient with pain. In Loeser JD, Butler SH, Chapman CR, Turk DC (eds): Bonica's Management of Pain, 3rd ed. Philadelphia, Lippincott Williams & Wilkins, 2001, pp 267–278.

88. Schofferman J: Long-term use of opioid analgesics for the treatment of pain of nonmalignant origin. J Pain Symptom Manage 8:279–288, 1993.

89. Mayfield DG, McLeod G, Hall P: The CAGE questionnaire: Validation of a new alcoholism screening instrument. Am J Psychiatr 131:1121–1123, 1974.

90. McQuade WH, Levy SM, Yanek LR, et al: Detecting symptoms of alcohol abuse in primary care settings. Arch Family Med 9:814–821, 2002.

91. Bastiaens L, Francis G, Lewis K: The RAFFT as a screening tool for adolescent substance use disorders. Am J Addict 9:10–16, 2000.

92. Hinkin CH, Castellon SA, Dickson-Fuhrman E, et al: Screening for drug and alcohol abuse among older adults using a modified version of the CAGE. Am J Addict 10:319–326, 2001.

93. Bradley KA, Kivlahan DR, Bush KR, et al: Variations on the CAGE alcohol screening questionnaire: Strengths and limitations in VA general medical patients. Alcohol Clin Exp Res 25:1472–1478, 2001.

94. Turner JA, Romano JM: Psychological and psychosocial evaluation. In Loeser JD, Butler SH, Chapman CR, Turk DC (eds): Bonica's Management of Pain, 3rd ed. Philadelphia, Lippincott Williams & Wilkins, 2001, pp 329–341.

Pharmacologic Management
of Cancer Pain

CHAPTER 16

Opioid Analgesics and Routes of Administration

Luis Vascello, MD, and Robert J. McQuillan, MD

The number of cancer patients in the world is increasing and the majority of the patients present with advanced disease requiring complex pain management and palliative care. Cancer pain has been defined as pain attributable to cancer or its therapies.[1] Approximately, 30% of cancer patients receiving active treatment for metastatic disease have significant cancer-related pain, and this percentage increases to 90% in those with advanced disease.[2-4] The pathophysiology of cancer pain may involve nociceptive (somatic and visceral) or neuropathic mechanisms, or both, and requires a comprehensive approach for treatment. The World Health Organization's (WHO) proposed method for relief of cancer pain was originally published in 1986[5] with an update in 1996.[6] The guidelines contain the WHO analgesic ladder, a simple yet effective method for controlling cancer pain, which, when used as described, can provide substantial relief of pain in 75% to 90% of cancer patients.[7-10] Unfortunately, approximately 25% of cancer patients die in significant pain despite the availability of appropriate tools for adequate pain control.[11,12] In an effort to mitigate this problem several organizations, including the American Society of Anesthesiologists[13] and the American Pain Society Quality of Care Committee, have issued statements or guidelines to improve cancer pain management.[14] Long-term opioid treatment is now the primary therapeutic approach to cancer pain, and improved use of current techniques for opioid therapy is one of the goals of the treatment guidelines for cancer pain published by the U.S. Agency for Health Care Policy and Research.[15]

Comprehensive cancer care includes adequate pain management and encompasses a continuum that progresses from disease-oriented, curative, and life-prolonging treatment through symptom-oriented, supportive, and palliative care extending to terminal hospice care.[16] Design of an effective pain control strategy for the individual cancer patient requires knowledge of the way in which cancer, cancer therapy, and pain therapy interact.

A model approach has been outlined by the WHO in their principles of pharmacotherapy, and the key concepts are outlined next.

The stepwise approach outlined in the WHO analgesic ladder still provides the standard of care. This approach emphasizes the intensity of the pain rather than its mechanism or the stage of the disease.

By Mouth: When possible, patients should take analgesic medications by mouth. Alternative routes can be used in patients with dysphagia, uncontrolled vomiting, gastrointestinal obstruction, and so on.

By the Clock: Patients with continuous pain should take analgesic medications at fixed intervals of time, administering the next dose before the effect of the previous dose has fully worn off. Some patients may need rescue doses for breakthrough pain.

By the Ladder:

Step 1 of the ladder involves the use of nonopioids.

Step 2 of the ladder involves the addition of a weak opioid if the pain is not relieved.

Step 3 of the ladder indicates the substitution of the weak opioid for an opioid for moderate to severe pain.

Use adjuvant drugs for specific indications.

For the Individual: The right dose is the dose that relieves the patient's pain with a minimum of side effects. Do not use the same opioid if patients had previous unsatisfactory experiences with that drug. Most drugs used for mild to moderate pain have a dose limit because of formulation (e.g., combined with acetylsalicylic acid or acetaminophen) or because of a disproportionate increase in adverse effects at higher doses (e.g., codeine).

With Attention to Detail: Carefully outline and monitor the patient's analgesic regimen. Select the appropriate analgesic drug, administer the drug by the appropriate route, and prescribe the appropriate dose and the appropriate dosing interval. Titrate the drug aggressively. Prevent persistent pain and treat breakthrough pain. Follow up regularly with the patient by monitoring compliance, drug efficacy, and side effects. Anticipate adverse effects and, in some situations, treat them preemptively.

The WHO ladder advocates the use of three classes of analgesics: nonopioid, adjuvant, and opioid. In the clinical arena, it is important to optimize the use of nonopioids and adjuvants along with the use of opioids, and consider the use of interventional and noninterventional techniques (i.e., biofeedback) to reduce opioid use. In some cases, a change in the route of administration may add significant benefit.

OPIOID-RELATED SIDE EFFECTS: PREVENTION AND TREATMENT

One of the most important aspects of opioid therapy is the anticipation, prevention, assessment, and treatment of side effects. Side effects are so common that most patients report more than one on initiation of opioid therapy and the risks or inconvenience, or both, imposed by them determines the upper limit or the rate of dose titration. Because marked interindividual differences exist among patients, the best predictor of patient response to an opioid is the patient's past experience with a particular drug. The occurrence of side effects depends in part on the individual response of the patient to the drug administered, the dose, and rate of dose increase. Large doses or rapid titration are associated with more severe and an increased incidence of side effects.[17]

Opioid-related side effects occur because of opioid receptor pharmacodynamics, the production of toxic metabolites, or both.[18,19] Stimulation at the sigma opioid receptor produces dysphoria, depersonalization, and psychotomimetic experiences,[20] and the standard opioid antagonists do not relieve these side effects because the sigma receptor is naloxone-inaccessible. The sigma receptor does, however, have high affinity for haloperidol, which can be useful in combating these side effects.[21] Some side effects result from the production of toxic metabolites (i.e., normeperidine and norpropoxyphene),[22,23] whereas the role of morphine-3-glucuronide (M3G), a metabolite of morphine, is less clear because it does not bind to opioid receptors and yet it seems to exert antagonist effects.[24,25] Some authors speculate that the antagonist effects of M3G are responsible for some of morphine's side effects, including myoclonus.[24]

Tolerance to various opioid effects develop at different rates; therefore, it is usually possible to titrate the dose for an individual patient without encountering any dose-limiting side effects. Fortunately, patients tend to develop tolerance to most side effects more rapidly than to pain relief; tolerance to respiratory depression develops rapidly, whereas the most common side effect, constipation, does not appear to be attenuated at all by prolonged opioid therapy. New peripheral opioid antagonists are under clinical investigation for the treatment of opioid-induced constipation (alvimopan). Tolerance to nausea, vomiting, or both, typically appears within 2 to 3 days and opioid-induced sedation is usually transient.[26] Less common side effects are dysphoria, cognitive impairment, pruritus, and clinically relevant respiratory depression, all of which are reduced with chronic therapy. Myoclonus is a rare side effect which is not relieved by chronic therapy and may require opioid rotation (see later), or palliative treatment with other drugs such as benzodiazepines.

Other opioid side effects include increased pressure in the biliary tract, urinary retention, and hypotension. Morphine causes histamine release, which can cause bronchoconstriction and vasodilatation and has the potential to precipitate or exacerbate asthmatic attacks. Other mu receptor agonists that do not release histamine (such as fentanyl derivatives) may be better choices for such patients. True allergic reactions are not common and are manifested as urticaria and skin rashes. Anaphylactoid reactions have been reported after intravenous administration of codeine and morphine but fortunately are rare.

There are several therapeutic strategies that can be used to prevent or treat opioid-related side effects. These include administration of symptomatic drugs, administration by alternative routes, and administration of a different opioid. For patients with constant pain, the early introduction of a long-acting opioid as soon as dose titration permits may help to attenuate side effects. If side effects are significant, the clinician should allow time for tolerance to develop. This may require a period of 3 to 7 days. Protecting the patient from severe side effects during this period is appropriate and does not prevent tolerance development. For example, a patient with nausea could benefit from a 1-week course of antiemetic medication at the outset of opioid therapy. Changing from one opioid to another may enhance pain relief and reduce opioid-related side effects, particularly if incomplete cross-tolerance to opioid effect is experienced.[27-31] In some cases, changing the route of administration for a particular drug (such as morphine) may eliminate certain difficult side effects.[32] It is possible to alleviate many of the most difficult side effects pharmacologically when necessary. For example, administering methylphenidate can help protect the cognitive functioning of patients using high doses of opioids.[33,34]

Opioid-induced gastrointestinal problems may manifest as nausea and vomiting, mild abdominal discomfort, constipation, gaseous abdominal distension, and functional colonic obstruction. Opioids may cause constipation in part by slowing colonic transit in the proximal colon and by inhibiting defecation.[35]

Opioids can cause or exacerbate confusion, and these effects may range from mild impairment in concentration to frank delirium with disorientation, disorganized thinking, perceptual distortions, and hallucinations.[36] Obviously, when this problem occurs it is important to consider other causes of altered mental status. When cognitive dysfunction is caused by opioids, it generally follows a recent increase in dose and usually resolves with tolerance or as the dose is reduced. Cognitive dysfunction occurs frequently in the advanced cancer population, typically within the context of the syndrome of delirium. Its recognition warrants objective cognitive monitoring, which in itself is often reassuring to patients with undue fear of opioid-induced cognitive dysfunction. The opioid contribution to this dysfunction is sometimes difficult to evaluate in the presence of multiple other cancer disease and treatment-related factors, highlighting the need for a multidimensional approach to patient assessment.[37]

INTERACTIONS WITH OTHER DRUGS

The depressant effects of some opioids may be potentiated by phenothiazines, monoamine oxidase inhibitors, and tricyclic antidepressants; the mechanisms of these interactions are not fully understood but may involve alterations in the rate of metabolic transformation of the opioid or alterations in neurotransmitters involved in the actions of opioids. Phenothiazines reduce the amount of opioid required to produce a given level of analgesia. Also, the respiratory-depressant effects seem to be enhanced, the degree of sedation is increased, and the hypotensive effects are more pronounced.

Small doses of amphetamine substantially increase the analgesic and euphoric effects of morphine and may decrease its sedative side effects. Some antihistamines exhibit modest analgesic actions and hydroxyzine enhances the analgesic effects of low doses of opioids. Antidepressants such as amitriptyline are used in the treatment of chronic neuropathic pain but have limited analgesic actions in acute pain. Antidepressants may enhance morphine-induced analgesia.[38]

SELECTION AND DOSING OF ORAL OPIOIDS

The distinction between weak and strong opioids for the treatment of mild to moderate and moderate to severe pain, respectively, is based on a ceiling effect and on the manner in which these drugs are usually prescribed.

The WHO considers codeine as the basic opioid for mild to moderate pain with dihydrocodeine, dextropropoxyphene, standardized opium, and tramadol as alternatives.[4] Low-dose (0.2 mg every 8 hours) buprenorphine, a partial agonist, is also considered an alternative drug. For moderate to severe pain, morphine is considered the basic opioid, with methadone, hydromorphone, oxycodone, levorphanol, meperidine, fentanyl, and buprenorphine (high dose up to 1 mg every 8 hours) as possible alternatives. Mixed agonist-antagonists and partial agonist drugs have predominantly agonist actions, but many also have a potentially significant antagonist action. The effect of the opioids on their receptors is shown in Table 16-1. Never change patients currently treated with pure agonists to either mixed agonist-antagonists or partial agonists because this may precipitate a withdrawal reaction. However, it is safe to change patients treated with mixed agonist-antagonists or partial agonists to pure agonists.

In the United States, it is common practice to initiate opioid therapy with a commercial product that contains an opioid combined with aspirin or acetaminophen. The dose of these products can be increased only until the safe maximum level of the nonopioid component is reached. Patients who fail to obtain adequate analgesia at the maximum doses of a combination product typically change to opioids commonly used for the management of moderate to severe pain, of which morphine is the opioid of first choice.

The mechanism of action of all opioids is similar and there is no clear scientific evidence supporting the use of multiple opioids simultaneously for the treatment of

TABLE 16–1 Action and Selectivity of Opioids at Different Opioid Receptors

Drug	Mu	Delta	Kappa
Methadone	+++		
Morphine	+++		+
Fentanyl	+++		
Sufentanil	+++	+	+
Nalbuphine	--		++
Pentazocine	Partial +		++
Butorphanol	Partial +		+++
Buprenorphine	Partial +		--
Naloxone	---	-	--
Naltrexone	---	-	---

Activity and affinity of drugs on receptors. Symbols: + = agonist, - = antagonist, Partial + = partial agonist.
Modified from Hardman JG, Limbird LE, Molinoff PB, et al: Goodman and Gilman's The pharmacological basis of therapeutics, 9th ed. New York, McGraw-Hill, 1996, pp 524.

cancer pain. In fact, the guidelines issued by the WHO suggested the use of one opioid at a time. Despite this, the use of multiple opioids simultaneously in the same patient is common in clinical practice and this probably originates from a reluctance to adjust the dose of a single opioid to an effective range. Most patients have constant or frequently recurring pain and respond best to around-the-clock dosing. In selected circumstances, as-needed dosing alone may prove helpful such as the start of opioid therapy in the opioid-naive patient or during periods of rapidly declining pain (i.e., following radiation treatment), and in the treatment of patients with intermittent pain.

Titration of the opioid dose usually is necessary at the start of therapy and repeatedly during the patient's course of treatment. The absolute dose is not important as long as therapy is not compromised by dose-limiting toxicity, cost, or excessive inconvenience produced by the number of pills. The rate of titration depends on the severity of pain, appearance of side effects, or both. Patients who present with severe pain may be best managed initially by repeated intravenous boluses of opioid until pain is partially relieved.

The development of physical dependence and tolerance occurs with chronic use of opioids. Patients with stable disease often remain on the same dose for weeks or months[39] unless tumor progression occurs and, as a consequence, opioid escalation is required.[40] Furthermore, wide clinical experience has shown that addiction does not usually occur in cancer patients receiving opioids for relief of pain.[4,41,42] The degree of pain relief that a given opioid provides varies both intraindividually and interindividually, and depends on the type and time aspects of the pain experienced, the drug and drug characteristics, and the route of administration.

Guidelines concerning the choice of opioids have been released by the European Association for Palliative Care (EAPC) indicating the evidence supporting each recommendation.[43] These include the following:

- Use of morphine as first choice for the treatment of moderate to severe pain.
- Use of the oral route with two formulations: normal release (for dose titration) and sustained release for maintenance.
- The simplest method for titration is with a dose of normal release morphine given every four hours and the same dose for breakthrough pain given as often as required (up to hourly). The regular dose can then be adjusted to take into account the total amount of rescue morphine.

Neuropathic pain and incident pain are among the poor prognostic factors for opioid treatment outcome. The treatment of incident pain is difficult because the doses of analgesics needed to control the incident pain are often so high that toxicity occurs when the incident pain is absent.

In terms of pharmacodynamic factors, the most relevant polymorphisms concern the cytochrome p450 enzymes CYP2D6, CYP2C19, and CYP2C9. Poor metabolizers of CYP2D6 will metabolize some opioids and antidepressants much more slowly than expected, causing either a much prolonged and pronounced action or toxicity (active drugs) or reduced efficacy of pro-drugs. In terms of opioid factors, some drugs, such as methadone, act at different receptors including mu agonist and N-methyl-D-aspartate (NMDA) receptor antagonist offering potential advantages such as incomplete cross-tolerance, treatment of neuropathic pain, and so on. Several factors must be considered if opioids are to be used effectively (Table 16–2).

A prospective study, based on the EAPC and the U.S. Agency for Health Care Policy and Research Guidelines for Management of Cancer Pain, investigated the use of sustained-release formulation for initial titration of morphine. It was found that the use of sustained-release formulation did not increase the time to find the correct dose or the intensity of opioid-induced adverse effects. Some advantages to this approach include convenience and no need for conversion once the controlled-release dose is effective.[44]

Morphine

Morphine is the standard opioid against which all new analgesics are measured, and it still remains the opioid of choice for the control of moderate to severe cancer pain. After oral administration of morphine solution or

TABLE 16–2   Relevant Factors Associated with Successful Opioid Therapy in Cancer Patients

Age and weight (pharmacokinetic/pharmacodynamic differences)
Psychological factors
History of addiction
Response to previous opioid therapy (patient's preference)
Allergies
Severity and pathophysiology of pain
Severity, nature, and extent of disease (cancer)
Coexisting disease (cardiovascular, pulmonary, gastrointestinal, etc.)
Renal and liver function altering opioid pharmacokinetics
Pharmacodynamic factors and pharmacologic interactions

TABLE 16–3 Available Oral/Rectal Preparations of Morphine in the United States			
Duration of Action	Preparation	Dosage	Comments
Immediate release	Tablet/capsule	15 mg, 30 mg	
	Soluble/sublingual	10 mg	
	Solution	10 mg/5 mL 10 mg/2.5 mL 20 mg/5 mL concentrate 20 mg/mL	Can be given by sublingual, oral, rectal
	Suppository	5, 10, 20, 30 mg	
Controlled/Sustained release	MS Contin	15, 30, 60, 100, 200 mg	
	Oramorph SR	15, 30, 60, 100 mg	
	Kadian	20, 30, 50, 60, 100 mg	Sprinkle*
	Avinza	30, 60, 90, 120 mg	Sprinkle*

*Content can be sprinkled in food without altering drug's sustained-release mechanism.

Modified from Loeser JD, Butler SH, Chapman CR, Turk DC: Bonica's management of pain, 3rd ed. Philadelphia, Lippincott Williams & Wilkins, 2001, pp 669.

immediate release tablets, peak plasma concentrations are reached within approximately 60 minutes.[45,46] These formulations have a rapid onset and the duration of the analgesia is approximately 4 hours. Controlled-release morphine tablets produce delayed peak plasma concentrations after 2 to 4 hours and analgesia usually lasts for 12 hours.[47-49] Controlled-release morphine is considered the gold standard for long-acting opioids, and four preparations are available in the United States (Table 16–3). Numerous studies demonstrate the efficacy and safety of MS Contin and Oramorph SR for patients with cancer pain. Controlled-release opioid medication facilitates pain relief on a regular, around-the-clock basis, allowing for a more stable plasma level of drug with less incidence of adverse effects or inadequate pain control in comparison with short-acting opioids. Other advantages include less frequent dosing, improved medication compliance, and the ability to relieve pain for long periods, especially through the night.[50-53]

MS Contin and Oramorph SR are manufactured in a resin matrix that slowly dissolves in the gastrointestinal tract, releasing morphine over approximately a 12-hour period. Although it is standard practice to prescribe MS Contin and Oramorph SR every 12 hours, it is sometimes necessary to prescribe these medications every 8 hours, particularly when higher doses are required. Food does not affect the oral bioavailability of MS Contin or Oramorph SR.[54,55] These preparations should not be crushed or chewed because it could cause the release of a potentially toxic dose. MS Contin and Oramorph SR tablets have different physical, pharmacokinetic, and clinical characteristics. Results of biopharmaceutical studies indicate that these two products are not bioequivalent.[56]

Kadian, an even longer-acting controlled-release morphine preparation, is intended for 24-hour administration. It is available in clear capsules containing small polymer-coated pellets of drug. Each capsule contains multiple pellets and this has the effect of providing more controlled and uniform release characteristics. Each pellet consists of a morphine sulfate–containing core that acts as a drug reservoir. Kadian's pharmacokinetic profile may offer some advantages over the other available controlled-release morphine preparations,[57] such as a more reliable and stable plasma morphine concentration. The use of Kadian has been shown to provide a significantly higher minimum (with less fluctuation) plasma morphine concentration, a longer time associated with the maximum morphine concentration, and a greater time that the plasma morphine concentration was greater than or equal to 75% of an index of the control the formulation exerts over the morphine release rate, compared with that of MS Contin.[58] Kadian offers a particular advantage for patients with swallowing difficulties because the capsule can be broken and the pellets sprinkled into liquids or soft foods without affect on the time-release mechanism. Patients favored the convenience of 24-hour administration of Kadian. Further trials are required to evaluate the 24-hour use of Kadian.[57]

Avinza, a new formulation of controlled-release morphine, also offers a once-daily dosing schedule. Its efficacy has been demonstrated in two clinical trials comparing it to MS Contin.[59] Avinza is similar to Kadian but may provide a more rapid onset (a potential therapeutic advantage over other controlled-release formulations) due to its spheroidal oral drug absorption system (SODAS) developed by Elan and Ligand. More trials are needed in cancer patients to determine if a true clinical advantage can be demonstrated.[60]

The amount of morphine absorbed following oral administration is essentially the same whether the source is morphine controlled-release or a conventional formulation. Because of presystemic elimination (i.e., metabolism in the gut wall and liver), only about 40% of the administered dose reaches the central compartment. Thirty percent of the morphine present in plasma is bound to proteins. The major pathway for the metabolism of morphine is conjugation with glucuronic acid. The two major metabolites are morphine-6-glucuronide and morphine-3-glucuronide. Small amounts of morphine-3, 6-diglucuronide are also formed. Morphine-6-glucuronide has pharmacologic actions indistinguishable from those of morphine. In animal models and in human beings, morphine-6-glucuronide is approximately twice as potent as morphine. With chronic administration, it accounts for a significant portion of morphine's analgesic actions, and in fact plasma levels exceed those of morphine.[61-63] At this time, no clear evidence exists in humans; however, it has been suggested that morphine-6-glucuronide is associated with less respiratory depression than morphine and, if this is true, it could become a primary analgesic agent with an improved safety profile.[64-67] More research is needed to determine the role of morphine-6-glucuronide, which is currently undergoing phase III clinical trials and will be marketed as an analgesic for postoperative and chronic pain. Morphine-6-glucuronide is excreted by the kidney. As a result, patients with renal failure present higher levels of morphine-6-glucuronide caused by accumulation, and therefore potency and duration of action are increased. Other considerations when dosing morphine include the extremes of age. Pediatric patients do not achieve adult renal function values by 6 months of age. In older patients, smaller doses are recommended on the basis of its smaller volume of distribution and the general decline in renal function.[38]

Morphine-3-glucuronide has little affinity for opioid receptors but may contribute to excitatory effects of morphine and could antagonize morphine-induced analgesia. Other metabolic pathways for morphine include N-demethylation and N-dealkylation, which are less important in humans. Small amounts of morphine are excreted unchanged in the urine. It is eliminated by glomerular filtration, primarily as morphine-3-glucuronide, 90% of the total excretion takes place during the first day. Enterohepatic circulation of morphine and its glucuronides occurs, which accounts for the presence of small amounts of morphine in the feces and in the urine for several days after the last dose.[38]

Long-term treatment with 10- to 20-fold increases of oral doses over a period of 6 to 8 months does not seem to change the kinetics of oral morphine.[45]

Dose requirements may vary 1000-fold, but relatively few patients need daily doses above 200 to 300 mg.[42]

Methadone

Although methadone, a synthetic opioid agonist, has been recommended as a second-line opioid for the treatment of pain in patients with cancer, the authors have used it as a first-line agent in patients with moderate to severe cancer pain. The effectiveness, cost, and side effect profile make this drug a very reasonable first-line agent. The analgesic activity of the racemic mixture is almost entirely the result of L-methadone, which is 8 to 50 times more potent than the D-isomer. D-methadone also lacks significant respiratory depressant action and addiction liability, but it does posses antitussive activity. Methadone binds preferentially to the mu opioid receptor and exerts noncompetitive antagonist activity at the NMDA receptor.[68] Activation of NMDA receptors within the spinal cord has been shown to play a crucial role in the development of tolerance to the analgesic effects of morphine and the generation and maintenance of spinal states of hypersensitivity.[69] The NMDA receptor appears to be involved in the process of central hypersensitization and may contribute to the development of neuropathic pain, allodynia, and other chronic pain states.[70] Methadone by possessing NMDA receptor antagonism properties may improve pain control by attenuating the development of tolerance to morphine.

Methadone is available as methadone hydrochloride powder that can be used for the preparation of oral, rectal, and parenteral solutions and is available commercially in a variety of preparations. Methadone presents outstanding features, including excellent absorption from the gastrointestinal tract (oral and rectal bioavailability varies from 41% to 99%), no known active metabolites, high potency, high lipid solubility, low cost, and longer administration intervals. Other advantages include possibly enhanced analgesia from incomplete cross-tolerance with the potential to control pain no longer responsive to other mu-opioid receptor agonist drugs.[71-74]

Methadone can be detected in plasma within 30 minutes after oral administration and reaches peak concentration at about 4 hours. The onset of analgesia occurs 10 to 20 minutes following parenteral administration and 30 to 60 minutes after oral medication. Approximately 90% of the circulating methadone is bound to plasma proteins. Methadone is characterized by a large interindividual variation in pharmacokinetics and by rapid and extensive distribution phases (half-life alpha = 2 to 3 hours; half-life beta = 15 to 60 hours). Some patients have considerably longer elimination half-lives, even extending to 120 hours.[75] Methadone undergoes extensive biotransformation in the liver, and inactive metabolites result from N-demethylation and cyclization. These are excreted in the urine and the bile along with small amounts of unchanged drug. The amount of methadone excreted in the urine is increased when the urine is acidified. After repeated administration there is gradual accumulation because methadone is firmly bound to protein in various tissues, including brain. When administration is discontinued, low concentrations are maintained in plasma by slow release from extravascular binding sites leading to the occurrence of a relatively mild but prolonged withdrawal syndrome. Tolerance develops more slowly to methadone than to morphine in some patients, especially with respect to the depressant effects. However, this may be related in part to cumulative effects of the drug or its metabolites. Tolerance to the constipating effects of methadone does not develop as fully as does tolerance to other effects.[38]

Depending on the severity of the pain and the response of the patient, oral methadone could be started at a dose between 2.5 and 15 mg, whereas the initial parenteral dose should be titrated (usually 2.5 to 10 mg). Despite its longer plasma half-life, the duration of the analgesic action of a single dose is similar to morphine. With repeated dosing over a period of several days, the drug will accumulate because of its prolonged half-life and either a lower dose or a longer interval between doses becomes possible. Schedules for initial oral dosing titration by patient-administered analgesia have been proposed.[76,77]

Patients treated with methadone for opioid addiction, who subsequently develop pain, are customarily treated with a second opioid while the methadone maintenance is continued. However, chronic exposure to methadone may have an effect on opioid tolerance via different mechanisms leading to relative refractoriness to opioid analgesia from opioids other than methadone. Discontinuation of methadone in these patients will end the NMDA antagonistic activity and potentially increase the analgesic tolerance to other opioids. Adjustment of the dose of methadone from the maintenance dose to analgesic dose has been performed and demonstrated to be effective.[78] The authors have used such an approach to treat acute pain, which can occur on top of chronic cancer pain. Examples include surgical interventions and traumatic injuries in cancer inpatients on methadone programs, and it is carried out by changing the route of administration to IV and adjusting the doses to achieve adequate analgesia.

Hydromorphone

Hydromorphone is a semisynthetic congener of morphine that has a short half-life requiring at least an every 4-hour dosing schedule to maintain adequate plasma levels for patients with chronic cancer pain. Hydromorphone is approximately five times as potent as morphine, and the usual oral adult dose is 2 to 4 mg every 4 to 6 hours. The usual parenteral dose is 0.5 to 2 mg every 4 to 6 hours.[38] There is a controlled-release preparation of hydromorphone, which is not currently available in the United States. The primary benefit from this preparation lies in the convenience of the capsule formulation, which allows the patient to sprinkle it onto liquids or food. Preliminary data indicate some benefits and efficacy for cancer pain management.[79]

Oxycodone

Oxycodone is a semisynthetic mu agonist with a pharmacokinetic profile resembling that of morphine.[80] The intrinsic antinociceptive effect of oxycodone could derive from its actions at kappa-opioid receptors, in contrast with morphine, which interacts primarily with mu-opioid receptors.[81] Oxycodone is rapidly absorbed by the oral route and produces an initial peak plasma concentration in approximately 2 hours,[82,83] and it has a higher oral bioavailability (60% to 87%)[84-86] than morphine (20% to 25%)[87,88] (most likely because of the methoxy group at carbon 3, not present in morphine, which protects it from extensive first-pass glucuronidation). These bioavailability values for oxycodone are in accord with the higher oral to parenteral efficacy ratio (0.5 to 0.75) compared with that of morphine (0.17).[89] Once peak plasma concentrations are reached, oxycodone concentrations rapidly decline, with an apparent terminal half-life ranging from 3.0 to 5.7 hours,[82,84] requiring frequent dosing to maintain plasma concentrations within the therapeutic analgesic range.

Oxycodone is extensively metabolized to noroxycodone and oxymorphone and their metabolites. Noroxycodone is considerably weaker than oxycodone, whereas oxymorphone (which possesses moderate analgesic activity) is present in the plasma only in low concentrations.[38] A controlled-release formulation of oxycodone (Oxycontin) is available in strengths of 10, 20, 40, and 80 mg. A significant advantage of this formulation compared with the immediate-release preparation is the relatively long duration of action of approximately 12 hours. The controlled-release dosage form has pharmacokinetic characteristics that permit 12-hour dosing. Oxycontin is characterized by a rapid absorption component (half-life absorption = 37 minutes) accounting for 38% of the available dose and a slow absorption component (half-life absorption = 6.2 hours) accounting for 62% of the available dose.[90] Controlled-release oxycodone is a useful alternative to controlled-release morphine.[91,92] Immediate-release oxycodone causes approximately twice as many adverse experiences, several of longer duration, than controlled-release oxycodone.[93] Oxycontin and MS Contin share a similar pharmacodynamic profile, their incidence of adverse effects is similar, and the two opioids provide comparable pain relief.[85]

Levorphanol

Levorphanol is a highly potent synthetic analgesic with properties and actions similar to those of morphine. The D-isomer (dextrorphan) is relatively devoid of analgesic action but may have inhibitory effects at NMDA receptors. The pharmacologic effects of levorphanol closely parallel those of morphine, and it may produce less nausea and vomiting. It is approximately five times more potent than morphine and has a long half-life of 12 to 16 hours.[38] Repeated administration at short intervals may lead to accumulation of the drug in plasma. Its duration of action ranges from 6 to 8 hours. It is recommended for the relief of moderate or severe pain and is available in oral and parenteral formulations; the normal starting dose is 2 mg every 6 hours orally, 1 mg every 6 hours parenterally.[38]

Sufentanil

Sufentanil citrate has been reported to be as much as 10 times more potent than fentanyl and 1000 times more potent than morphine. The drug is lipophilic and when used intrathecally or epidurally the risk of respiratory depression due to rostral spread is reduced (as compared with morphine).[94,95] The peak effect when administered intravenously is approximately 5 minutes. Recovery from analgesic effects also occurs quickly, however, with prolonged infusions or larger doses the effect becomes longer lasting. As with other mu opioids, nausea, vomiting, and itching can be observed. Respiratory depression is similar to that observed with other opioids, but the onset is more rapid.[96] Delayed respiratory depression could be seen after the use of fentanyl, sufentanil, or alfentanil, possibly caused by enterohepatic circulation. Sufentanil is highly lipophilic and rapidly crosses the blood–brain barrier. The half-life for equilibration between the plasma and cerebrospinal fluid (CSF) is approximately 5 minutes. The levels in plasma and CSF rapidly decline because of redistribution from highly perfused tissue groups to other tissues, such as muscle and fat. As saturation of less well-perfused tissue occurs, the duration of effect of sufentanil approaches the length of their elimination half lives of between 3 and 4 hours. Therefore, with the use of higher doses and prolonged infusions, sufentanil effectively becomes longer acting. Sufentanil is more often used as an anesthetic adjuvant, and the drug can be used intravenously, subcutaneously, epidurally, or intrathecally.[38,97]

Fentanyl

Fentanyl is a synthetic phenylpiperidine derivative characterized by high potency and lipid solubility. The drug is 100 times more potent than morphine. It has a short duration of action, 30 to 60 minutes after a single intravenous bolus of 100 µg, mainly because of its large volume of distribution and redistribution and uptake into fatty tissues. It is available in several preparations, including transdermal, transmucosal, and parenteral. Parenteral fentanyl is a short-acting analgesic at steady-state conditions, when half-life is primarily determined by redistribution.[38]

Transdermal Fentanyl

Because of its low molecular weight and high lipid solubility, fentanyl can be administered transdermally[98] and is available in a presentation (patch) that provides sustained release for 48 hours or more. Absorption is variable depending on skin conditions such as fever (increased absorption) and so on. Transdermal therapeutic system (TTS)-fentanyl may be considered a first-line treatment modality for moderate to severe cancer pain. It offers the advantage of continuous administration of a potent opioid in the absence of needles and expensive drug-infusion pumps for the treatment of cancer pain and is a good choice for patients when oral administration or compliance are a problem. Several studies have investigated and confirmed the successful management of cancer pain with TTS-fentanyl.[99-105] Fentanyl patches are rectangular transparent units and the amount of fentanyl released from each system per hour is proportional to the surface area (25 µg per hour per 10 cm²). The skin under the system absorbs fentanyl and creates a depot of the drug concentrated in the upper skin layers. Fentanyl then becomes available to the systemic circulation; however, a lag time of approximately 2 hours occurs before clinically useful systemic levels of drug are achieved after applying the patch.[106] Serum fentanyl concentrations increase gradually after application, generally leveling off between 12 and 24 hours. The system delivers fentanyl continuously for up to 72 hours. After sequential 48- or 72-hour applications, patients reach and maintain steady-state serum concentrations that are determined by individual variation in skin permeability and body clearance of fentanyl. A number of studies demonstrate that constant serum levels are maintained with the application of the second transdermal patch and that fluctuations of serum levels are small after the first 72 hours.[107,108] After patch removal, serum fentanyl concentrations decline gradually, falling approximately 50% in 17 hours (range 13 to 22). Because of the possibility of temperature-dependent increases in fentanyl release from the system, it is important to advise patients to avoid exposing the application site to direct external heat sources, such as heating pads and heated waterbeds.[38]

The common intravenous to transdermal conversion ratio of 1:1 is often considered too low.[109] Other authors have suggested a conversion ratio increase of 50% to a ratio of 1:1.5, yet experience has shown that in spite of these increases the conversion ratio is often still too low in the majority of patients, with most requiring an average increase of 100% at the end of the first week.[101] Pharmacokinetic studies indicate a relative steady state (pseudo steady state) 15 hours[110] and 16 to 20 hours after application of the patch,[111] suggesting the possibility of early titration with TTS-fentanyl at 24-hour intervals. Fentanyl patches are available in 25, 50, 75, and 100 µg/hour.

Oral Transmucosal Fentanyl

Fentanyl Oralet (lollipop) provides rapid absorption through the oral mucosa. Unfortunately, this presentation (initially indicated for opioid naive patients) was associated with a high incidence of side effects (nausea, vomiting, pruritus, and respiratory depression). Actiq, a similar product, is available in a higher strength and is used for breakthrough cancer pain.[38]

Oral transmucosal fentanyl citrate (OTFC) units consist of a lozenge and are available in a variety of strengths, from 200 to 1600 µg. In the mouth, the unit dissolves in saliva and a portion of the fentanyl diffuses across the oral mucosa; the patient swallows the remainder, which is partially absorbed in the stomach and intestine. Patients must smear the lozenge either on the buccal mucosa or under the tongue and avoid swallowing for a period of time to avoid first-pass metabolism in the liver. Onset of action is rapid (5 to 15 minutes). Peak analgesic effect is 20 to 30 minutes and duration is approximately 2 hours. Of the total available dose, 25% is absorbed transmucosally over a 15-minute period, and an additional 25% is absorbed through the gastric mucosa during the next 90 minutes.[112] Potential advantages of this drug delivery system include rapid-onset analgesia, transmucosal absorption (i.e., no need to swallow), ease of titration, and ease of use.

The effect of OTFC for breakthrough pain has been evaluated in a double-blind, randomized trial of 130 cancer patients.[113] The Food and Drug Administration has approved the use of transmucosal fentanyl for the management of procedure-associated pain and for the management of breakthrough pain in cancer patients. The main clinical application for this preparation may be for breakthrough and incident pain in the cancer patient,[114,115] but further clinical evaluation is underway.

The concurrent use of TTS-fentanyl patches with OTFC units appears attractive and merits future study.

Alfentanil and Remifentanil

Alfentanil and remifentanil are useful for short and painful procedures that require intense analgesia where rapid recovery is an issue (e.g., thoracocentesis, paracentesis). These drugs have a rapid onset (1 to 1.5 minutes) and, therefore, they can be easily and consistently titrated. Particularly the rapid offset makes them suitable for short surgical procedures. These drugs share pharmacologic properties of fentanyl including side effects. There are several pharmacologic differences between these drugs. The duration of action with alfentanil is dependent on both the dose and length of administration. Alfentanil is metabolized in the liver and has an elimination half-life of 1 to 2 hours. Remifentanil is metabolized by plasma esterases and has an elimination half-life of 8 to 20 minutes, which is independent of hepatic metabolism or renal excretion. The administration of remifentanil for maintenance of analgesia is better suited by using it as an infusion due to its short duration of action. There is no prolongation of effect with repeated dosing or prolonged infusion of remifentanil. Age and weight can affect clearance of remifentanil, requiring that dosage be reduced in the elderly and based on lean body mass. The primary metabolite of remifentanil is 3000 times less potent than remifentanil and is renally excreted. Peak respiratory depression after bolus doses occurs after 5 minutes.[38]

Meperidine

Meperidine is a predominant mu receptor agonist. It should not be used longer than 48 hours (toxic metabolite), in doses higher than 600 mg/24 hours, or in chronic pain. After oral administration, the analgesic effects are detectable in about 15 minutes. Fifty percent of the drug escapes first-pass metabolism to enter the circulation, and peak concentrations in plasma are usually observed in 1 to 2 hours. After subcutaneous or intramuscular administration, the onset and time to peak serum concentration is faster (10 minutes and 1 hour, respectively). The duration of effective analgesia is approximately 1.5 to 3 hours. Meperidine is hydrolyzed to meperidinic acid and N-demethylated to normeperidine, and a small amount is excreted unchanged. Meperidine is mainly metabolized in the liver (with a half-life of 3 hours), and in patients with liver failure, the bioavailability is increased to as much as 80%, and the half-lives of meperidine and normeperidine are prolonged. Approximately 60% of meperidine in plasma is protein bound.[38] In terms of equianalgesic ratio,

100 mg of meperidine given parenterally is approximately equivalent to 10 mg of morphine. At equianalgesic doses, meperidine produces the same side effects as morphine: sedation, respiratory depression, and euphoria. Meperidine is about one third as effective when given by mouth as when administered parenterally. Meperidine may cause tremors, muscle twitches, and seizures (caused by accumulation of normeperidine). As with other opioids, tolerance develops to some of these effects.[38,116]

Meperidine should not be used in patients taking monoamine oxidase inhibitors because of the ability of meperidine to block neural reuptake of serotonin and the resultant serotonergic hyperactivity (delirium, hyperthermia, headache, hypertension or hypotension, rigidity, convulsions, coma, and death). Dextromethorphan also inhibits neuronal serotonin uptake and should be avoided in these patients. Concomitant administration of promethazine or chlorpromazine may enhance meperidine-induced sedation.[38]

Codeine

Codeine is commonly prescribed for the management of mild to moderate pain. It is most often prescribed in combination with aspirin or acetaminophen. Codeine has a high oral to parenteral potency ratio because of less first-pass metabolism in the liver. Once absorbed, codeine is metabolized by the liver, and its metabolites are excreted chiefly in the urine, largely in inactive forms. Approximately 10% is O-demethylated to form morphine, and both free and conjugated morphine can be found in the urine after therapeutic doses of codeine. Codeine has an exceptionally low affinity for opioid receptors, and the analgesic effect of codeine is caused by its conversion to morphine. However, its antitussive actions appear to involve distinct receptors that bind codeine itself. The half-life of codeine in plasma is 2 to 4 hours. The usual adult dose ranges between 15 and 60 mg every 4 to 6 hours and in children 0.5 mg/kg. The conversion of codeine to morphine is affected by the cytochrome P450 enzyme CYP2D. Because of genetic polymorphism of this enzyme, 10% of the Caucasian population has an inability to convert codeine to morphine, thus making codeine ineffective as an analgesic. On the other hand, other polymorphism can lead to enhanced metabolism and thus increased sensitivity to codeine's effects. Chinese people produce less morphine from codeine than Caucasians and are also less sensitive to morphine's effects because of a decreased production of morphine-6-glucuronide. It is important to consider the possibility of polymorphism in any patient who does not receive adequate analgesia from codeine.[38] Patients with a deficiency of CYP2D6 enzymes or those taking inhibitors of CYP2D6, such as quinidine, cimetidine, or fluoxetine,

may not be able to convert codeine into morphine and, therefore, may get little or no analgesic effect from codeine.[117] Dihydrocodeine is an equianalgesic codeine analog. In the United States, it is available only in combination with acetaminophen or aspirin. The drug is available in injectable form 15 mg/mL and 30 mg/mL, compounding powder, oral solution 3 mg/mL, oral tablets 15 to 30 and 60 mg.

Hydrocodone

Hydrocodone is a derivative of codeine. The usefulness of hydrocodone has been limited by its common preparation in fixed combination with nonopioid analgesics (aspirin, acetaminophen, and ibuprofen). Combination hydrocodone is available in a variety of strengths (2.5, 5, 7.5, and 10 mg). The strength of the nonopioid component varies in these preparations, and it is important not to exceed toxic doses of the nonopioid analgesics when prescribing these medications for breakthrough pain, particularly when using acetaminophen combinations. Vicoprofen, consisting of hydrocodone bitartrate, 7.5 mg, and ibuprofen, 200 mg, may be useful as a short-acting opioid in limited doses for patients with preexisting liver disease.[38]

Propoxyphene

Propoxyphene is structurally related to methadone. Its analgesic effect resides in the dextro-isomer, D-propoxyphene (dextropropoxyphene). Levopropoxyphene seems to have some antitussive activity. Although slightly less selective than morphine, propoxyphene binds primarily to mu-opioid receptors and produces analgesia and other central nervous system (CNS) effects that are similar to those seen with morphine-like opioids. It is likely that at equianalgesic doses the incidence of side effects, such as nausea, anorexia, constipation, abdominal pain, and drowsiness, would be similar to those of codeine. Propoxyphene is about 50% to 70% as potent as codeine given orally and 90 to 120 mg of propoxyphene administered orally would equal the analgesic effects of 60 mg of codeine, a dose that usually produces about as much analgesia as 600 mg of aspirin.[38] Combinations of propoxyphene or codeine with aspirin afford a higher level of analgesia than either agent given alone. Following oral administration, concentrations of propoxyphene in plasma reach their highest value at 1 to 2 hours. There is great variability between subjects in the rate of clearance and the plasma concentrations that are achieved. The average half-life of propoxyphene in plasma after a single dose is from 6 to 12 hours, which is longer than that of codeine. In humans, the major route of metabolism is N-demethylation to yield norpropoxyphene. The half-life of norpropoxyphene is about 30 hours, and its accumulation with repeated doses may be responsible for some of the observed toxicity. Moderately toxic doses usually produce CNS and respiratory depression, but with still larger doses the clinical picture may be complicated by convulsions in addition to respiratory depression. Delusions, hallucinations, confusion, cardiotoxicity, and pulmonary edema also have been noted. Naloxone antagonizes the respiratory-depressant, convulsant, and some of the cardiotoxic effects of propoxyphene. Abrupt discontinuation of chronically administered propoxyphene (up to 800 mg per day, given for almost 2 months) results in mild abstinence phenomena.[38]

Tramadol

Tramadol hydrochloride is a centrally acting synthetic codeine analog. The drug exerts its analgesic actions involving a weak mu-receptor agonist activity and inhibition of uptake of norepinephrine and serotonin. Although its affinity for mu opioid receptors is 1/6000 of morphine, the primary O-demethylated metabolite (M1) of tramadol is 2 to 4 times as potent as the parent drug and may account for part of the analgesic effect. Tramadol is supplied as a racemic mixture, which is more effective than either enantiomer alone. The (+) enantiomer binds to the mu receptor and inhibits serotonin uptake. The (–) enantiomer inhibits norepinephrine uptake and stimulates alpha 2 adrenergic receptors. Racemic tramadol is rapidly and almost completely absorbed after oral administration with a bioavailability of approximately 75%. The mean peak plasma concentration of racemic tramadol and M1 occurs at 2 and 3 hours, respectively. Tramadol is only 20% bound to plasma proteins and the compound undergoes hepatic metabolism and renal excretion, with an elimination half-life of 6 hours for tramadol and 7.5 hours for its active metabolite. Analgesia begins within an hour of oral dosing, and the effect peaks within two to three hours. The duration of analgesia is about 6 hours and steady-state plasma concentrations of both tramadol and M1 are achieved within 2 days. Approximately 30% of the dose is excreted in the urine as unchanged drug, whereas 60% of the dose is excreted as metabolites.[38]

The maximum recommended daily dose of tramadol is 400 mg. Common side effects include nausea, vomiting, dizziness, dry mouth, sedation, and headache. Respiratory depression appears to be less than with equianalgesic doses of morphine, and the degree of constipation is less than seen after equivalent doses of codeine. Tramadol can cause or exacerbate seizures in patients with predisposing factor. Although tramadol-induced analgesia is not entirely reversible by naloxone, tramadol-induced respiratory depression can be reversed by naloxone. Physical dependence and abuse have been reported and withdrawal symptoms may occur if tramadol is discontinued abruptly. Because of its inhibitory effect on serotonin uptake, tramadol should not be used in patients taking monoamine oxidase (MAO) inhibitors.[118,119] Patients with cancer who are most likely to benefit from tramadol are those with mild to moderate pain not relieved by acetaminophen who cannot tolerate NSAIDs and wish to avoid taking other opioids.[120]

Opioids to Avoid in Cancer Pain Treatment

There are several opioids that are not recommended for routine use in patients suffering from moderate to severe cancer pain. Meperidine is a short-acting opioid and its metabolite, normeperidine, is toxic.[116] Partial agonists such as buprenorphine have a ceiling effect and at greater than a certain dose produce toxicity without additional analgesia. Mixed agonist-antagonists such as pentazocine, butorphanol, and nalbuphine are classified as kappa-receptor agonists and mu-receptor antagonists. However, they are more accurately described as partial agonists at both kappa and mu receptors. These agents have a ceiling effect and have the potential to reverse mu-receptor analgesia. When taken by patients already receiving full agonists they can precipitate a physical withdrawal syndrome.[38,121] Propoxyphene is a poor choice for routine use because of its long half-life and the risk of accumulation of norpropoxyphene, a toxic metabolite.[38,116]

New Preparations

There are a few commercial preparations available in Europe, which combine morphine with dextromethorphan (Morphidex) (ratio 1:1). This combination has been reported to provide satisfactory pain relief at a significantly lower daily dose when compared to immediate-release morphine. In addition, this combination appears to have a faster onset and longer duration of action.[122,123]

Buprenorphine is available in Europe in a transdermal delivery system, and on the basis of survey results, transdermal buprenorphine is considered an effective opioid treatment for patients with stable cancer pain; it may prove particularly useful in patients who have experienced side effects taking oral analgesic preparations, as well as in those who are taking extensive comedications.[124]

Coadministration of Opioid Agonists and Antagonists

The coadministration of morphine and very low doses of naloxone or naltrexone markedly enhances the intensity and duration of analgesia. Additionally, long-term treatment reduces tolerance and dependence through a direct competitive antagonism of Gs-coupled excitatory opioid receptor functions. Other clinical studies using low-dose naloxone plus pentazocine, codeine plus naltrexone, morphine plus nalmephene and other such combinations, have demonstrated similar results.[121] A review analyzes the complex phenomenon and the mechanisms underlying opioid-induced pain.[125]

Opioid Tolerance in Cancer Pain

Tolerance is a complex pharmacologic phenomenon characterized by either the need for higher opioid doses to maintain constant effects or the disappearance of opioid side effects. The central activation of NMDA receptors is involved in the development of morphine tolerance.[68] Noncompetitive NMDA receptor antagonists can attenuate the development of tolerance to the analgesic effect of morphine without affecting acute morphine analgesia.[126] Intracellular events (increase in Ca^{2+} concentration, production of nitric oxide, and possibly regulation of gene expression) initiated by NMDA receptor activation may initiate neuronal plastic changes in the CNS and thus mediate morphine tolerance.[69] With chronic morphine use, a functional uncoupling of opioid receptors from guanosine triphosphate–binding proteins (G proteins) occurs and the acute effects of the drug decrease. As a result, triggering the second messenger response requires higher doses of opioid.[127] Several authors believe that escalation of doses in cancer patients results most often from disease progression rather than from development of tolerance.[128,129]

Equianalgesic Ratios and Opioid Rotation in Cancer Pain

A successful conversion from one opioid to another requires an understanding of opioid pharmacokinetics and equianalgesic potency. Equianalgesic potency is defined as the ratio of the doses of two opioids required to produce the same degree of pain relief (Table 16–4).

TABLE 16–4   Equianalgesic Potency of Opioids

Drug	Oral (mg)	Parenteral (mg)
morphine	30	10
oxycodone	20-30	n/a
methadone	10	10
hydromorphone	6	2
levorphanol	2-3	2
codeine	130	75

Modified from Loeser JD, Butler SH, Chapman CR, Turk DC: Bonica's management of pain, 3rd ed. Philadelphia, Lippincott Williams & Wilkins, 2001, pp 675.

There is incomplete cross-tolerance among opioids, and tolerability and side effects can vary dramatically in individual patients. The mechanisms underlying these observations are not completely understood. Often sequential trials are necessary to identify the optimal drug. As a general rule, patients receiving regular opioid doses and switching to another opioid should receive 50% to 75% of the equianalgesic dose because cross-tolerance is incomplete. For the elderly or medically frail patient, it is wise to plan a further dose reduction of approximately 25%.

Opioid rotation has become an accepted strategy to address a poor response to a specific opioid. Other options include the use of alternative routes for administration of opioids such as parenteral or neuraxial administration. Opioid rotation is the most common way to address a poor response to an opioid, as well as when other issues arise such as neurotoxicity (delirium, myoclonus, and hyperalgesia), convenience, and cost/benefits. This approach derives from the observation that there are large interindividual variations in the pattern of adverse effects and analgesia produced by opioids. *When changing opioids, caution must be exercised because the equianalgesic dose ratios that are found on widely available published tables largely represent average data from controlled single-dose studies in selected populations. The ratios fail to account for the incomplete cross-tolerance, which would render the new drug more potent than anticipated.*[130] Equianalgesic tables propose a morphine–methadone ratio varying between 1:1 and 4:1 for the oral route and between 1:1 and 2.7:1 for the parenteral route.[6,7,14] However, methadone has been found to be more potent than previously recognized (particularly with repeated dose administration), and the dose ratio between methadone and morphine (and hydromorphone) is not a fixed number as proposed in the equianalgesic tables, but rather is related to the previous opioid dose.[27,73,74,131,132]

In situations in which morphine has ceased to be effective for the control of cancer pain, rotation to methadone could be performed using an initial dose of methadone that is one-tenth of the total daily morphine dose, but not greater than 100 mg.[133] Methadone is usually used as a second-line drug in the treatment of moderate to severe cancer pain. Use methadone if morphine causes intolerable side effects and the patient wishes to continue with noninterventional approaches or if a change in opioid may enhance analgesia because of incomplete cross-tolerance. Direct conversion from long-acting oral morphine to TTS-fentanyl has been suggested with a ratio of 100:1.[99]

Morphine's side effects, particularly sedation, cognitive impairment, and myoclonus at high doses, have provoked the use of opioid rotation to alternatives such as methadone and hydromorphone. The tables generally propose a dose ratio of 5:1 between morphine and hydromorphone.

In the case of a change from subcutaneous hydromorphone to methadone, the tables indicate dose ratios ranging from 1:6 to 1:10. Hydromorphone is five times more potent than morphine when given second, but it is only 3.7 times more potent when given first.[134] Hydromorphone to methadone ratio correlated with total opioid dose was 1.6 in patients receiving more than 330 mg of hydromorphone per day before the change versus 0.95 in patients receiving an average of 330 mg of hydromorphone per day.[27]

Rotation from a high-dose opioid agonist to methadone should only be performed by physicians with experience in cancer pain management. Occasionally, serious toxicity can occur during the administration of methadone[135] and curiously occurs more frequently in patients previously exposed to high doses of opioids. Guidelines for converting patients receiving high-dose oral opioids to oral methadone have been issued.[27]

Switching patients on methadone to another opioid also presents unique challenges. Patients engaged in methadone maintenance programs are likely to experience acute and chronic pain to the same degree and frequency as the general population. There are conflicting reports on the antinociceptive effects of additional opioids in these patients. It has been suggested that these patients are cross-tolerant to the antinociceptive effect of morphine and hyperalgesic to a cold pressor test.[136] In a prospective study, involving a small group of patients receiving methadone, opioid rotation was performed from methadone to a different opioid. The results of this study demonstrated that rotation from methadone to a different opioid is not as effective as the traditional rotation (from other opioid to methadone). Perhaps, gradual tapering of methadone while the other drug is started could enhance pain control and improve outcomes.[137]

ROUTES OF ADMINISTRATION

Several considerations must be taken into account when selecting one preparation or delivery system over another, including the therapeutic indication, the ability of the patient to use the system, the efficacy of the system, ease of use by the patient or caregiver, complications associated with the system, and the cost. Table 16-5 lists some of the routes and related bioavailability.

In general, opioids are well absorbed from the gastrointestinal tract, including the rectal mucosa. Lipophilic opioids are well absorbed through the nasal or buccal mucosa. Those with the greatest solubility can also be absorbed transdermally. Opioids are absorbed readily after subcutaneous or intramuscular injection and can adequately penetrate the spinal cord following epidural or intrathecal administration.

TABLE 16-5   Routes of Administration and Bioavailability

Route of Administration	Bioavailability
Intravenous	100% (all opioids)
Transdermal	90% (fentanyl)
Subcutaneous	80% (hydromorphone)
Transmucosal	30–60% (morphine-fentanyl)
Rectal	30–40% (morphine)
Oral	33% (morphine) and 60–80% (oxycodone)

Opioids should be delivered by the least invasive and safest route capable of providing adequate analgesia. The route of morphine administration may influence the morphine to metabolite ratio both in plasma and CSF due to the high first passage effect. Switching from oral to parenteral administration may reduce the metabolite–morphine relationship and thus toxicity caused by accumulation of metabolites.[138]

Nebulized Opioids

Dyspnea is relatively common in patients that have advanced cancer, affecting an estimated 50% to 70% of terminally ill patients during the final weeks of life. There are several reports from small studies indicating that nebulized morphine and other opioids could be an effective option in treating dyspnea. Although the mechanism of action has not been elucidated, there are multiple potential targets of action for opioids in the treatment of dyspnea. At least two possible peripheral mechanisms have been postulated. First, opioid agonists inhibit stimulus-evoked release of acetylcholine (ACh); and second, there may be activation of "J-receptors" on vagal C-fibers that are believed to be located within the alveolar wall.[139] The relatively low doses used for dyspnea in cancer patients, especially when effective in those already receiving much higher doses for pain relief, raise questions about whether the effect is central.[140] In fact, the bioavailability of morphine by this route is variable.

The effective use of nebulized morphine for postoperative analgesia has also been reported. Wide dosing ranges, concentrations, and volumes have been used. Doses from 5 to 10 mg of morphine every 4 hours have been suggested in opioid naive patients, and 10 to 20 mg in opioid tolerant patients. The bioavailability is only 5% to 30%.[140]

Nebulized fentanyl, 25 µg with 2 mL of normal saline via nebulizer, has been used for the treatment of dyspnea in patients with end-stage cancer. Several parameters were obtained, including oxygen saturation, respiratory rate, and subjective perception of their breathing difficulties reported by the patients. The majority of the patients reported improvement along with improved respiratory rates and oxygen saturation. The effects lasted for at least one hour. There were limitations of this study because it was not a placebo-controlled trial.[141] Use of fentanyl 25 μg with 2 mL of normal saline administered every 2 to 3 hours has been reported,[142] and in the case of its use for the treatment of breakthrough pain, the doses used (200 μg) are generally higher than the dose for dyspnea.[143]

Although conclusive evidence is still lacking, the use of nebulized opioids seems an attractive route of administration in select cases. This is based on the evidence suggesting a wide distribution of opioid receptors throughout the pulmonary system and a possible role in the palliation of such a devastating symptom as terminal dyspnea.

Intranasal Route

The nasal route of administration is potentially the most convenient alternative method for drug delivery. Nasal drug absorption is aided by a highly vascular epithelium, a large surface area, and the avoidance of first-pass metabolism. Morphine, a highly hydrosoluble agent, is poorly absorbed nasally. The combination of morphine with chitosan, a bioadhesive material that slows the mucociliary clearance of morphine, allows more time for absorption. Two concentrations have been tested (morphine-chitosan 5 mg/0.1 mL and 20 mg/0.1 mL) that allowed morphine doses in the range of 5 to 80 mg to be administered in 1 to 4 sprays from 0.1 mL unit dosing devices (maximum of two sprays per nostril). Twenty episodes of breakthrough pain using different doses were treated in 14 patients at a palliative care unit. The majority of the patients rated the treatment as at least "good." Improvements in pain intensity and relief were reported at 5 minutes and reached a maximum after 45 minutes. Nasal symptoms were minimal, but a bitter taste was reported 5 minutes after administration. The majority of the patients reported some degree of sedation. The addition of chitosan, a nontoxic, nonabsorbed, nonirritant, increases the bioavailability of morphine from 10% to 54%. Confirmation of these findings is necessary in large controlled-randomized studies.[144]

Oral Route

As a general rule, the oral route should be used unless contraindicated (e.g., swallowing or gastrointestinal problems, head and neck cancers) or ineffective for cancer patients because it is the easiest and least invasive route. Bioavailability after oral administration of opioids is variable because of significant first-pass metabolism in the liver (oxycodone 60% to 87%; methadone 50%, morphine 30% to 40%). Duration of action is often somewhat longer with the oral route.

Transdermal Route

Transdermal delivery of a drug is a noninvasive alternative to the oral route. The most widely used drug for this route of administration is fentanyl. The advantages of this route are that it is noninvasive and it has the capability of maintaining stable plasma concentrations for prolonged periods. Transdermal fentanyl is not suitable for rapid dose titration; it is most appropriate for patients with relatively stable pain syndromes. Also, it may provide an alternative option for patients who show poor compliance or dissatisfaction with their oral regimen. Some reports suggest improved bowel function, relief of nausea and vomiting, and so on. The route may be indicated in patients with dysphagia, nausea, vomiting, GI obstruction, and so forth. A general conversion ratio is 300 mg/day of morphine to 100 μg/hour fentanyl. Dermatologic reactions, such as contact dermatitis, have been described.

Iontophoresis is a method of transdermal administration of ionizable drugs in which the electrically charged components are propelled through the skin by an external electric field. Drugs such as morphine, fentanyl, and the like, can be delivered iontophoretically. The technique is not pain free and not used in clinical settings.

Rectal Route

Drugs administered by the rectal route are absorbed by passive diffusion and therefore drug solubility will be very important. The rectum has a surface area of 200 to 400 cm^2 compared to a small intestine surface area of 200 cm^2. It has no resting peristalsis, is usually empty of solid material, and contains a small amount of alkaline fluid (3 to 4 mL). Any absorbed drug will be taken up into the superior, middle, and inferior rectal veins. The superior rectal vein drains into the portal system, whereas the middle and inferior drain into the systemic circulation. Because of the presence of extensive anastomoses between these venous systems, the proportion of systemic and portal drainage will vary among individuals. As a consequence, it is impossible to predict what proportion of drug will avoid first-pass metabolism by the liver.

Advantages of this route include absorption (not affected by food, nausea, vomiting, poor GI motility, malabsorption, or opioid-induced delay in gastric emptying), no need for swallowing, no breakdown of molecules by acid or digestive enzymes, unpleasant taste will not matter, first-pass effect by the liver may be partly avoided, easily administered by an unskilled attendant (in comparison with parenteral administration), and availability of sustained-release formulations.

Disadvantages of this route include the possible interruption of drug administration by defecation or constipation, degradation of drug by microorganisms or rectal-wall enzymes, unwillingness of the patient or caregiver to use this form of administration, wide interindividual variation in absorption and response, which makes titration of the dose necessary, and it is not a viable route if a painful anal condition (rectal fistula) is present.[145]

There are several suppositories available in the United States (morphine 5-10-20 mg, hydromorphone 3 mg, oxymorphone 5 mg, methadone). In addition, any tablet of any opioid could be administered rectally, including controlled-release formulations. Oral and rectal routes are considered equipotent despite differences in pharmacokinetics and bioavailability. Some pharmacies can compound different formulations. Most suppositories are composed of drug particles suspended in cocoa butter or synthetic derivatives and molded into suppositories, which melt at body temperature and spread through the rectum to a variable extent. Hydrogels and osmotic minipumps have also been developed and have some potential therapeutic use. The rectal administration of methadone has been shown to provide rapid and extensive absorption and is comparable to the oral route. It is imperative to individualize the proper dose of methadone via the rectal route due to large interindividual variation in plasma methadone levels.[146,147]

Sublingual or Oral Transmucosal Route

In theory, any opioid could be administered sublingually to patients who lose the ability to swallow liquids or tablets because of dysphagia or nausea and vomiting. Bioavailability of hydrophilic drugs is poor (e.g., morphine). Highly lipophilic drugs, such as methadone, fentanyl, sufentanil, and buprenorphine, are better choices and present an alternative for patients that cannot swallow. Recent fentanyl formulations (Actiq) have demonstrated rapid onset with potential use for the treatment of breakthrough pain. Actiq is available in 200, 400, 600, 800, 1200, and 1600 μg doses. Almost 25% of the dose is absorbed rapidly from the oral mucosa and the remaining 75% is absorbed from the stomach and undergoes first pass, with a bioavailability of 33%. The overall bioavailability approaches 50%. Because sublingual venous drainage is systemic rather than portal, hepatic first pass can be avoided. The bioavailability of buprenorphine is 60%, fentanyl 51%, methadone 35%, and morphine 22%.

Patient-Controlled Analgesia

Patient-controlled analgesia (PCA) is a technique for drug administration at the patient's demand. The PCA device consists of a microprocessor-controlled infusion pump that allows the use of a continuous infusion, a demand dose, or both. It adjusts for variations in response to therapy that result from interpatient differences in pharmacokinetics and pharmacodynamics and allows patients considerable control. PCA produces an overall improvement in analgesia without adding significant risks. PCA use can alleviate the usual gaps between analgesic requirement and administration by nursing personnel.

Although most of the experience with PCA is derived from intravenous opioid administration in acute postoperative patients, the use of intravenous PCA in cancer patients has also been widespread. PCA can be used in almost any situation in which oral pain management is not possible. This technique can be used by several routes, such as intravenous, subcutaneous, epidural, and intrathecal, and the safety of this technique has been demonstrated in almost all age-groups, from pediatric to elderly patients. General principles of PCA use suggest that to achieve a uniformly high quality of pain management and optimal safety, all orders concerning PCA management should be written by a pain management consulting team. At the very least, expert consultants must be available to assist with problems.

Parenteral Route: Subcutaneous and Intravenous

Most patients can be adequately managed using oral opioids; however, a small percentage require alternative routes. In these situations, the parenteral route of administration is preferred for patients who require rapid onset of analgesia or doses of medication that cannot be delivered conveniently by other routes. Repetitive intramuscular administration should be avoided. If repeated administration is necessary, then the intravenous or subcutaneous (using a small butterfly needle that can be used for up to a week) routes are preferred.

Intravenous Opioid Therapy

Morphine, methadone, hydromorphone, fentanyl, and sufentanil can be used for intravenous therapy. Although the advantages of intravenous therapy have been reviewed, the major disadvantages include the need for continuous intravenous access (with its associated costs), which is a potential source of infection; increased costs of pharmaceutical preparation; need for personnel to administer the drug or an external pump/device; and home-health/skilled nurses when an outpatient. The intravenous route should be considered for patients who require rapid onset of analgesia and for highly tolerant patients who require doses that cannot otherwise be conveniently administered.[148] Ideally, patients with severe, uncontrolled pain who require intravenous therapy should start treatment in a monitored inpatient setting. Once pain is under control, it is possible to continue therapy safely at home with the aid of a home infusion service.[149-151]

Several studies comparing opioid-related side effects with the use of intravenous opioid therapy in postoperative pain models failed to show a difference between morphine and hydromorphone[152] and morphine, meperidine, and fentanyl.[153] Coda and colleagues[154] found differences in efficacy and side effects for morphine, hydromorphone, and sufentanil in bone marrow transplantation patients with severe oral mucositis pain. Table 16-6 lists systemic side effects of opioid therapy. The pain relief achieved in all three opioid groups was nearly equivalent, whereas measures of side effects, especially for the combination of sedation, sleep, and mood disturbances, were statistically lower in the morphine group than in the hydromorphone or sufentanil groups. After an intravenous bolus of hydromorphone, the onset of analgesia is rapid (within 5 minutes) the maximum analgesic effect occurs between 10 and 20 minutes, and the analgesic effect lasts approximately 2 hours. Hydromorphone is approximately three to five times as potent as morphine on a milligram basis.[155,156] Peak CNS effects of methadone coincide with peak plasma concentrations, thus corresponding well to the observed early onset of action of 3 to 5 minutes after intravenous administration.[157] Morphine, on the other hand, has a slower onset of action, probably related to its relatively poor lipid solubility. Experiments in dogs showed that following an intravenous bolus administration of morphine, peak concentrations in CSF did not occur for approximately 15 to 30 minutes.[158]

Intravenous fentanyl, a highly lipophilic opioid, has a rapid analgesic onset with a peak effect of less than 6 minutes.[159] Intermittent boluses of opioids (such as fentanyl) with rapid onset and early peak effect offer advantages for patients whose predominant pain stems from activity or weight-bearing and occurs intermittently. Patients with constant, severe, intractable cancer pain and large opioid requirements may benefit from the use of intravenous methadone by PCA and continuous infusion. This approach offers some advantages over the more hydrophobic drugs such as morphine and hydromorphone. The more rapid peak analgesic effect and longer elimination half-life of methadone offers earlier intense analgesia with prolonged analgesic effect, particularly after patients reach steady-state plasma levels with repeated administration.

Subcutaneous Opioid Therapy

This route is adequate for patients who do not have IV access. A continuous subcutaneous infusion (using a butterfly needle with a clear dressing changed weekly) offers a safe, simple, and cost-effective alternative to intravenous infusion when patients cannot take medications orally for the homebound or hospitalized patient.[151,163-165] The safety and efficacy of subcutaneous versus intravenous infusion of hydromorphone in cancer patients has been demonstrated. Pain intensity, pain relief, mood, and sedation did not differ between the two techniques.[166]

Opioids suitable for this route must be nonirritating and well absorbed. Morphine, hydromorphone, fentanyl, sufentanil, and methadone are commonly used by this route. Although hydromorphone has the highest bioavailability by this route (78%), methadone can produce irritation. The absorption of opioid from the subcutaneous compartment into the systemic circulation is relatively fast.[167] Subcutaneous administration is not recommended in patients with generalized edema, coagulation disorders, or poor peripheral circulation or in patients who develop erythema, soreness, or abscesses with subcutaneous administration. Several recommendations for this route of administration have been published.[91,164,166] In general, avoid subcutaneous rates larger than 2 mL/hour to allow comfort at the insertion site. PCA doses may equal 25% to 50% of the hourly infusion rate every 10 to 15 minutes as needed. Expect longer time to peak plasma levels after bolus injection and consequently set the

TABLE 16-6 Side Effects of Systemic Opioid Therapy

Side Effect	Cause	Treatment
Sedation, drowsiness	Dose-related	Dose limiting Consider alternative therapies (e.g., neuraxial)[160]
Myoclonus/grand mal seizures[24] Hyperalgesia[161] Hyperexcitability Confusion[161]	Neurotoxicity secondary to high-dose opioids Morphine-3-glucuronide (M3G) Intravenous hydromorphone (>60 mg/d), morphine (>60 mg/hr)	Dose reduction and/or opioid rotation[30] Clonazepam, phenobarbital[162]

lockout interval from 10 to 15 minutes versus the usual intravenous PCA lock out interval of 6 to 8 minutes.

Morphine has been successfully used by this route. The usual initial concentration is 5 mg/mL. Fentanyl and sufentanil have also been used and demonstrated effectively. Sufentanil seems particularly useful when a patient requires higher doses of a lipophilic opioid.[168]

Neuraxial Administration

Intraspinal (epidural or intrathecal) infusion of opioids has been well established for the treatment of cancer pain. Epidural or intrathecal infusions can involve externalized spinal catheters (tunneled), subcutaneous reservoirs for intermittent injection, or implanted infusion pumps, with either a constant rate or a programmable rate. Epidural or intrathecal morphine can produce profound analgesia that lasts for approximately 12 to 24 hours. Because of the hydrophilic nature of morphine, there is rostral spread of the drug in the CSF and respiratory depression can emerge up to 24 hours later as the opioid reaches supraspinal respiratory control centers. With highly lipophilic opioids such as fentanyl or hydromorphone, rapid absorption by spinal neural tissues produces a localized and largely segmental analgesic effect. The duration of action is shorter because of distribution of the drug in the systemic circulation, and thus the occurrence and severity of respiratory depression may be more directly related to plasma concentrations and to a lesser degree, rostral spread in the CSF.

It is difficult to determine the long-term benefits of epidural and intrathecal opioid therapy for cancer pain. In many centers, oncologists manage pain, and they may be more aggressive with systemic analgesics and more conservative with invasive measures than anesthesiologists. They tend to refer patients for neuraxial therapy late in the course of the illness, when metastases are widespread, nociceptive inputs are high, and tolerance is a substantial problem. Frequently, such patients require supplementary local anesthetics for pain control.

The goal of neuraxial administration is the delivery of small doses in the vicinity of the spinal opioid receptors to enhance analgesia and thus reduce systemic side effects. In some cases, this technique could be particularly beneficial. For instance, a "drug holiday" consists of interrupting therapy for a few weeks to resensitize the opioid receptors. Therefore, infusions of local anesthetics, alpha-2 agonists, and opioids or their mixture can be used to provide pain relief.

Epidural Administration

Long-term epidural administration can be safely accomplished through a percutaneous catheter (tunneled) or a totally implanted catheter connected to a subcutaneous

TABLE 16–7   Advantages and Disadvantages of the Epidural Route

Advantages	Disadvantages
Ease of placement Ambulatory management	Risk of infection (rare)[169]
External pump (ready access for dose adjustment, drug changes)	Technical problems: dislodgement, fibrosis around catheter tip, and pain with injection

injection port. The benefits and disadvantages of the epidural route are listed in Table 16–7.

The objective of epidural administration is to restrict the drug to analgesic sites in the spinal cord. Nonetheless, all epidurally administered drugs reach the systemic circulation to some extent. Morphine clearly produces analgesia by actions in the spinal cord,[170] and it is the standard of comparison for all other epidurally administered opioids. Several clinical studies of postoperative patients have clearly shown that little or no value exists in administering highly lipophilic drugs, such as fentanyl, sufentanil, or alfentanil, into the lumbar epidural space.[171-175] The plasma concentration is no different when the drug is given epidurally or intravenously. However, in combination with local anesthetics, these drugs are widely used and may provide benefit; in this setting, fentanyl is the most widely used agent.

Meperidine may yield greater efficacy with epidural versus intravenous administration. Patients using lumbar epidural meperidine PCA required less drug and generated lower plasma meperidine concentrations while reporting better pain relief, less sedation, and better satisfaction than others using intravenous PCA meperidine, indicating a spinal mu-receptor site of action for meperidine.[176] However, the drug's well-known local anesthetic effects could also explain the greater efficacy. Approximately 30 times more meperidine than morphine is required for epidural analgesia. Epidural methadone is only half as potent as epidural morphine.[177]

The safety and efficacy of long-term epidural bupivacaine-opioid infusion in patients with cancer pain refractory to epidural opioids has been demonstrated.[178] Epidural metastases may reduce the efficacy of epidural pain management.[179] Progression of disease may result in multiple sites of pain that may require supplementation by alternative routes, drugs, or strategies.

Intrathecal Administration

The intrathecal route is sometimes more efficient and less expensive than epidural delivery for the treatment of refractory cancer pain. Potential advantages of intrathecal administration include better distribution of medication to the target site and enhanced pain relief.[180,181] Despite this, the intrathecal route is less frequently used than the epidural route.[182]

Concerns about externalized intrathecal catheters are focused on the potential of increased risks for complications, particularly meningitis, than with epidural catheters. These concerns appear to be largely unfounded.[183] Implanted systems, especially if programmable, are the most convenient for long-term treatment with intrathecal opioids. Use of infusion technology is not without problems, and complication rates varying from 5% to 15% appear in the literature.[184-189] In addition, other disadvantages include the high cost of the devices, the low capacity of the infusion reservoir, limited choice of drugs, and so on. According to cost–benefit analysis, an implanted infusion pump is more favorable when survival times exceed 3 months.[190] The intrathecal use of opioids for cancer pain has been studied in numerous reports.[128,184,185,191-201] The true incidence of treatment failure with implantable intrathecal infusion systems is unknown. Patients with cancer pain of somatic origin had greater relief with intrathecal opioid infusions than patients with other types of pain. The average dose used by cancer patients escalated quickly and then stabilized.[128,199] The response to intrathecal opioid therapy may depend more on pain characteristics than on the specific opioid used.[186] Curiously, intrathecal methadone produces analgesia of inferior quality even in dosages 10 times higher than morphine.[202]

An expert panel issued guidelines to structure clinical decision-making based on the best available evidence. There is little information about long-term efficacy and safety of the numerous drugs that have been used intraspinally. Important information, such as pump–drug compatibility, drug–drug stability, and the effects of the pH and diluents on various outcomes, is lacking. The panel suggested that the overall approach to intraspinal infusion could be considered a hierarchy of therapeutic strategies. A four-line strategy has been issued to provide a stepwise approach based on scientific evidence. The first-line approach gains clear support from the available data and extensive clinical experience. The panel agreed that the first-line drug for long-term intrathecal infusion is morphine. The second line includes an alternative opioid (hydromorphone) or the combination of morphine with either clonidine or bupivacaine. The third line includes fentanyl or sufentanil, the combination of morphine with bupivacaine and clonidine or hydromorphone, or sufentanil or fentanyl with bupivacaine or clonidine. The fourth line includes three different categories: category one—meperidine, methadone, ropivacaine, or neostigmine; category two—baclofen; and category three—tetracaine, midazolam, and NMDA receptor antagonists.[203]

Side Effects of Neuraxial Opioid Therapy

Some side effects last for the first several days after initiation of therapy and resolve spontaneously. The most frequent side effects (affecting almost 50% of the patients) are constipation, disturbance of micturition, and nausea.[204] The frequency of occurrence is high early in the course of therapy and the response to appropriate treatments is usually positive. Some patients experience loss of libido or amenorrhea for the first 6 to 8 months of therapy, but these side effects prove self-limiting to most patients and disappear after 12 to 14 months. Escalating doses of intrathecal morphine may prove problematic because of increased risk for hyperalgesia and myoclonus, especially at doses higher than 15 mg/day.[197] Pain relief is excellent in 45% to 90% of patients with initiation of intraspinal opioid therapy. However, dose escalation and increased need for supplemental oral opioid therapy occur commonly over 2 to 4 months of therapy.[128,184,194,205,206]

Intrathecal Therapy with Bupivacaine and Morphine

The combination of intrathecal bupivacaine with morphine may be more efficacious than epidural administration when given for cancer pain relief. These two agents may act synergistically through different mechanisms at the spinal cord level.[181,207,208] In addition, this approach probably delays the occurrence of tolerance to intrathecal morphine because of the smaller doses and the added analgesic effects of bupivacaine.

Patient-Controlled Intrathecal Analgesia

A variety of medications, including morphine, bupivacaine, and clonidine, may be used intrathecally by PCA pumps for the control of cancer pain. One aspect of the efficacy and high acceptance of PCA is the higher degree of satisfaction of patients who are involved in self-administration of drugs and self-monitoring of pain and side effects.[209,210] The use of intrathecal PCA morphine for cancer pain has been reported.[211]

Intracerebroventricular Administration

This form of drug delivery is indicated for head and neck cancer pain and, rarely, for patients with a good initial response to intraspinal infusions of opioids and subsequent development of apparent tolerance who have limited (1 to 3 months) remaining survival time. An implanted ventricular catheter is connected by subcutaneous tubing to an implanted infusion pump (placed subcutaneously in the anterior abdominal wall). Morphine sulfate gains a marked increase in potency when delivered by this route, affecting supraspinal pathways for analgesia as compared with intrathecal or epidural infusion routes. Daily morphine doses range from 50 to 700 µg per day.[212,213]

Home Infusion Therapy

Advances in pain management technology, such as ambulatory PCA and the use of silicone subcutaneously tunneled neuraxial catheters, have expanded the success of interventional pain management beyond the hospital to the home. PCA therapy may be superior to oral analgesia, especially in the treatment of severe oscillating pain. Potential benefits of home infusion therapy include decreased health care costs, patient and caregiver convenience, and less time spent in hospital. A possible disadvantage to home infusion therapy may include the additional burden placed on the patient or caregiver in terms of role responsibilities and schedules. PCA is increasingly more commonly used in the home setting as an effective option in pain management. As discussed previously, the subcutaneous and intravenous routes are the primary methods of administration. The safety and efficacy of PCA opioid therapy has been extensively reported. The use of morphine PCA in the home environment was both safe and effective in the home environment, attaining excellent results in 66% patients and satisfactory pain relief in 30%. PCA was considered insufficient in 4% cases. Side effects, in general, were considered mild: the most common being constipation, fatigue, and nausea.[149] The experience of the authors is similar with home PCA.

CONCLUSION

Pain is the most common symptom experienced by cancer patients, and it requires aggressive treatment to maximize both quality and quantity of the patient's life. Comprehensive cancer care encompasses a continuum that progresses from disease-oriented, curative, life-prolonging treatment through symptom-oriented, supportive, and palliative care extending, for some patients, to terminal hospice care. Opioids are the mainstay of pharmacologic treatment of cancer pain and long-term opioid treatment through various routes of administration is the primary therapeutic approach to cancer pain at this time. Pain relief must be a priority in the care of cancer patients and design of an effective pain control strategy for the individual cancer patient requires knowledge of the way in which cancer, cancer therapy, and pain therapy interact. Most patients can attain adequate symptomatic relief of cancer pain using appropriate oral pharmacotherapy. The concurrent use of adjunctive or specialized therapies is sometimes necessary, however, and referral for specialized surgical, anesthetic, or psychological intervention benefits a significant number of patients. In addition, the growth of the home care industry has broadened the possibilities of extending interventional pain management strategies into the home.

REFERENCES

1. Principles of Analgesic Use in the Treatment of Acute Pain and Cancer Pain. Fourth Edition. Glenview, IL, American Pain Society 1999.
2. Foley KM: The treatment of cancer pain. N Engl J Med 313:84–95, 1985.
3. Daut RL, Cleeland CS: The prevalence and severity of pain in cancer. Cancer 50: 1913–1918, 1982.
4. Twycross R: Pain Relief in Advanced Cancer. London, Churchill Livingstone, 1994.
5. World Health Organization. Cancer Pain Relief. Geneva, Switzerland, World Health Organization, 1986.
6. World Health Organization. Cancer Pain Relief with a Guide to Opioid Availability. Geneva, Switzerland, World Health Organization, 1996.
7. Agency for Health Care Policy and Research. Management of Cancer Pain. A Clinical Practice Guideline. Rockville, MD, AHCPR, March 1994.
8. Hanks GW, Justins DM: Cancer pain: Management. Lancet 339:1031–1036, 1992.
9. Schug SA, Zech D, Don U: Cancer pain management according to WHO analgesic guidelines. J Pain Symptom Manage 5:27–32, 1990.
10. Grond S, Zech D, Schug SA, et al: Validation of World Health Organization guidelines for cancer pain relief during the last days and hours of life. J Pain Symptom Manage 6:411–422, 1991.

11. McCaffery M: Pain control. Barriers to the use of available information. World Health Organization Expert Committee on Cancer Pain Relief and Active Supportive Care. Cancer 70:1438–1449, 1992.
12. Zech DF, Grond S, Lynch J, et al: Validation of World Health Organization Guidelines for cancer pain relief: A 10-year prospective study. Pain 63:65–76, 1995.
13. Practice guidelines for cancer pain management. A report by the American Society of Anesthesiologists Task Force on Pain Management, Cancer Pain Section. Anesthesiology 84:1243–1257, 1996.
14. American Pain Society. Quality of Care Committee. Quality improvement guidelines for the treatment of acute pain and cancer pain. JAMA 274:1874–1880, 1995.
15. Jacox A, Carr DB, Payne R, et al: Management of Cancer Pain. Clinical Practice Guideline No. 9. AHCPR Publication No. 94-0592. Rockville, MD, Agency for Health Care Policy and Research, U.S. Department of Health and Human Services, Public Health Service, March 1994.
16. Levy MH: Supportive oncology: Forward. Semin Oncol 21:699–700, 1994.
17. Meuser T, Pietruck C, Radbruch L, et al: Symptoms during cancer pain treatment following WHO-guidelines: A longitudinal follow-up study of symptom prevalence, severity and etiology. Pain 93:247–257, 2001.

18. Poole SC, Sahr JS: Opiate receptors: A review of analgesic properties and pharmacological side effects. J La State Med Soc 144:106–108, 1992.
19. Goldstein DJ, Meador-Woodruff JH: Opiate receptors: Opioid agonist-antagonist effects. Pharmacotherapy 11:164–167, 1991.
20. Deutsch SI, Weizman A, Goldman ME, et al: The sigma receptor: A novel site implicated in psychosis and antipsychotic drug efficacy. Clin Neuropharmacol 11:105–119, 1988.
21. Musacchio SM: The psychotomimetic effects of opiates and the sigma receptor. Neuropsychopharmacology 3:191–200, 1990.
22. Davies G, Kingswood C, Street M: Pharmacokinetics of opioids in renal dysfunction. Clin Pharmacokinet 31: 410–422, 1996.
23. Kaiko RF, Foley KM, Grabinski PY, et al: Central nervous system excitatory effects of meperidine in cancer patients. Ann Neurol 13:180–185, 1983.
24. Christrup LL: Morphine metabolites. Acta Anaesthesiol Scand 41:116–122, 1997.
25. Smith MT, Watt JA, Cramond T: Morphine-3-glucuronide—a potent antagonist of morphine analgesia. Life Sci 47:579–585, 1990.
26. Bruera E, Macmillan K, Hanson J, et al: The cognitive effects of the administration of narcotic analgesics in patients with cancer pain. Pain 39:13–16, 1989.

27. Bruera E, Pereira S, Watanabe S, et al: Opioid rotation in patients with cancer pain. A retrospective comparison of dose ratios between methadone, hydromorphone, and morphine. Cancer 78:852–857, 1996.

28. de Stoutz ND, Bruera E, Suarez AM: Opioid rotation for toxicity reduction in terminal cancer patients. J Pain Symptom Manage 10:378–384, 1995.

29. Ripamonti C, Zecca E, Bruera E: An update on the clinical use of methadone for cancer pain. Pain 70:109–115, 1997.

30. Sjogren P, Jensen NH, Jensen TS: Disappearance of morphine-induced hyperalgesia after discontinuing or substituting morphine with other opioid agonists. Pain 59:313–316, 1994.

31. Thomas Z, Bruera E: Use of methadone in a highly tolerant patient receiving parenteral hydromorphone. J Pain Symptom Manage 10:315–317, 1995.

32. Walsh TD: Prevention of opioid side effects. J Pain Symptom Manage 5:362–367, 1990.

33. Bruera E, Miller MS, Macmillan K, et al: Neuropsychological effects of methylphenidate in patients receiving a continuous infusion of narcotics for cancer pain. Pain 48:163–166, 1992.

34. Bruera E, Brenneis C, Paterson AN, et al: Use of methylphenidate as an adjuvant to narcotic analgesics in patients with advanced cancer. J Pain Symptom Manage 4:3–6, 1989.

35. Kaufman PN, Krevsky B, Malmud LS, et al: Role of opiate receptors in the regulation of colonic transit. Gastroenterology 94:1351–1356, 1988.

36. Bruera E, Schoeller T, Montejo G: Organic hallucinosis in patients receiving high doses of opiates for cancer pain. Pain 48:397–399, 1992.

37. Lawlor PG: The Panorama of opioid-related cognitive dysfunction in patients with cancer: A critical literature appraisal. Cancer: 94:1836–1853, 2002.

38. Hardman JG, Limbird LE, Gilman AG: Goodman and Gilman's The Pharmacological Basis of Therapeutics, 10th ed. New York, McGraw-Hill, 2001.

39. Foley KM: Controversies in cancer pain. Medical perspectives. Cancer 63: 2257–2265, 1989.

40. Collin E, Poulain P, Gauvain-Piquard A, et al: Is disease progression the major factor in morphine 'tolerance' in cancer pain treatment? Pain 55:319–326, 1993.

41. Doyle D: Morphine: Myths, morality and economics. Postgrad Med J 67(Suppl 2): S70–73, 1991.

42. Schug SA, Zech D, Grond S, et al: A long-term survey of morphine in cancer pain patients. J Pain Symptom Manage 7:259–266, 1992.

43. Hanks GW, de Conno F, Cherny N, et al: Morphine and alternative opioids in cancer pain: The EAPC recommendations. Expert Working Group of the Research Network of the European Association for Palliative Care. Br J Cancer 84:587–593, 2001.

44. Klepstad P, Kaasa S, Jystad A, et al: Immediate- or sustained-release morphine for dose finding during start of morphine to cancer patients: A randomized, double-blind trial. Pain 101:193–198, 2003.

45. Sawe J: High-dose morphine and methadone in cancer patients. Clinical pharmacokinetic considerations of oral treatment. Clin Pharmacokinet 11:87–106, 1986.

46. Sawe S, Dahlstrom B, Rane A: Steady-state kinetics and analgesic effect of oral morphine in cancer patients. Eur J Clin Pharmacol 24:537–542, 1983.

47. Savarese JJ, Goldenheim PD, Thomas GB, et al: Steady-state pharmacokinetics of controlled release oral morphine sulfate in healthy subjects. Clin Pharmacokinet 11:505–510, 1986.

48. Poulain P, Hoskin PJ, Hanks GW, et al: Relative bioavailability of controlled release morphine tablets (MST continuous) in cancer patients. Br J Anaesth 61:569–574, 1988.

49. Hanks GW: Controlled-release morphine (MST Contin) in advanced cancer. The European experience. Cancer 63:2378–2382, 1989.

50. Warfield CA: Guidelines for the use of MS Contin tablets in the management of cancer pain. Postgrad Med J 67(Suppl 2):S9–12, 1991.

51. Thirlwell MP, Sloan PA, Maroun SA, et al: Pharmacokinetics and clinical efficacy of oral morphine solution and controlled-release morphine tablets in cancer patients. Cancer 63:2275–2283, 1989.

52. Kaiko RF, Grandy RP, Oshlack B, et al: The United States experience with oral controlled-release morphine (MS Contin tablets). Parts I and II. Review of nine dose titration studies and clinical pharmacology of 15-mg, 30-mg, 60-mg, and 100-mg tablet strengths in normal subjects. Cancer 63:2348–2354, 1989.

53. Finn SW, Walsh TD, MacDonald N, et al: Placebo-blinded study of morphine sulfate sustained-release tablets and immediate-release morphine sulfate solution in outpatients with chronic pain due to advanced cancer. J Clin Oncol 11: 967–972, 1993.

54. Bass S, Shepard KV, Lee SW, et al: An evaluation of the effect of food on the oral bioavailability of sustained-release morphine sulfate tablets (ORAMORPH SR) after multiple doses. J Clin Pharmacol 32:1003–1007, 1992.

55. Drake S, Kirkpatrick CT, Aliyar CA, et al: Effect of food on the comparative pharmacokinetics of modified-release morphine tablet formulations: Oramorph SR and MST Continuous. Br J Clin Pharmacol 41:417–420, 1996.

56. Hunt TL, Kaiko RF: Comparison of the pharmacokinetic profiles of two oral controlled-release morphine formulations in healthy young adults. Clin Ther 13: 482–488, 1991.

57. Broomhead A, Kerr R, Tester W, et al: Comparison of a once-a-day sustained-release morphine formulation with standard oral morphine treatment for cancer pain. J Pain Symptom Manage 14:63–73, 1997.

58. Gourlay GK, Cherry DA, Onley MM, et al: Pharmacokinetics and pharmacodynamics of twenty-four-hourly Kapanol compared to twelve-hourly MS Contin in the treatment of severe cancer pain. Pain 69:295–302, 1997.

59. Caldwell JR, Rapoport RJ, Davis JC, et al: Efficacy and safety of a once-daily morphine formulation in chronic, moderate-to-severe osteoarthritis pain: Results from a randomized, placebo-controlled, double-blind trial and an open-label extension trial. J Pain Symptom Manage 23:278–291, 2002.

60. Portenoy RK, Sciberras A, Eliot L, et al: Steady-state pharmacokinetic comparison of a new, extended-release, once-daily morphine formulation, Avinza, and a twice-daily controlled-release morphine formulation in patients with chronic moderate-to-severe pain. J Pain Symptom Manage 23:292–300, 2002.

61. Portenoy RK, Thaler HT, Inturrisi CE, et al: The metabolite morphine-6-glucuronide contributes to the analgesia produced by morphine infusion in patients with pain and normal renal function. Clin Pharmacol Ther 51:422–431, 1992.

62. Klepstad P, Kaasa S, Borchgrevink PC: Start of oral morphine to cancer patients: Effective serum morphine concentrations and contribution from morphine-6-glucuronide to the analgesia produced by morphine. Eur J Clin Pharmacol 55:713–779, 2000.

63. Paternak GW, Bodnar RJ, Clark JA, et al: Morphine-6-glucuronide, a potent mu agonist. Life Sci 41:2845–2849, 1987.

64. Sarton E, Teppema L, Nieuwenhuijs D, et al: Opioid effect on breathing frequency and thermogenesis in mice lacking exon 2 of the mu-opioid receptor gene. Adv Exp Med Biol 499:399–404, 2001.

65. Osborne R, Thompson P, Joel S, et al: The analgesic activity of morphine-6-glucuronide. Br J Clin Pharmacol 34:130–138, 1992.

66. Thompson PI, Joel SP, John L, et al: Respiratory depression following morphine and morphine-6-glucuronide in normal subjects. Br J Clin Pharmacol 40:145–152, 1995.

67. Romberg R, Olofsen E, Sarton E, et al: Pharmacodynamic effect of morphine-6-glucuronide versus morphine on hypoxic and hypercapnic breathing in healthy volunteers. Anesthesiology 99:788–799, 2003.

68. Gorman AL, Elliott KS, Inturrisi CE: The D- and L-isomers of methadone bind to the non-competitive site on the N-methyl-D-aspartate (NMDA) receptor in rat forebrain and spinal cord. Neurosci Lett 223:5–8, 1997.

69. Mao S, Price DD, Mayer DJ: Mechanisms of hyperalgesia and morphine tolerance: A current view of their possible interactions. Pain 62:259–274, 1995.

70. Dickenson AN: NIMDA receptor antagonists: interactions with opioids. Acta Anaesthesiol Scand 41:112–115, 1997.

71. Leng G, Finnegan MS: Successful use of methadone in nociceptive cancer pain unresponsive to morphine. Palliat Med 8:153–155, 1994.

72. Crews JC, Sweeney NJ, Denson DD: Clinical efficacy of methadone in patients refractory to other mu-opioid receptor agonist analgesics for management of terminal cancer pain. Case presentations and discussion of incomplete cross-tolerance among opioid agonist analgesics. Cancer 72:2266–2272, 1993.

73. Manfredi PL, Borsook D, Chandler SW, et al: Intravenous methadone for cancer pain unrelieved by morphine and hydromorphone: Clinical observations. Pain 70:99–101, 1997.

74. Fitzgibbon DR, Ready LB: Intravenous high-dose methadone administered by patient controlled analgesia and continuous infusion for the treatment of cancer pain refractory to high-dose morphine. Pain 73:259–261, 1997.

75. Plunmier JL, Gourlay GK, Cherry DA, et al: Estimation of methadone clearance: Application in the management of cancer pain. Pain 33:313–322, 1988.

76. Mercadante S, Sapio M, Serretta R, et al: Patient-controlled analgesia with oral methadone in cancer pain: preliminary report. Ann Oncol 7:613–617, 1996.

77. Sawe I, Hansen I, Ginman C, et al: Patient controlled dose regimen of methadone for chronic cancer pain. BMJ 282:771–773, 1981.

78. Manfredi PL, Gonzalez GR, Cheville AL, et al: Methadone analgesia in cancer patients on chronic methadone maintenance therapy. J Pain Symptom Manage 21:169–174, 2001.

79. Hays H, Hagen N, Thirlwell M, et al: Comparative clinical efficacy and safety of immediate release and controlled release hydromorphone for chronic severe cancer pain. Cancer 74:1808–1816, 1994.

80. Poyhia R, Vaiio A, Kalso E: A review of oxycodone's clinical pharmacokinetics and pharmacodynamics. J Pain Symptom Manage 8:63–67, 1993.

81. Ross FB, Smith MT: The intrinsic antinociceptive effects of oxycodone appear to be kappa-opioid receptor mediated. Pain 73:151–157, 1997.

82. Leow KP, Smith MT, Watt JA, et al: Comparative oxycodone pharmacokinetics in humans after intravenous, oral, and rectal administration. Ther Drug Monit 14:479–484, 1992.

83. Kalso E, Vaiio A, Mattila MI, et al: Morphine and oxycodone in the management of cancer pain: plasma levels determined by chemical and radioreceptor assays. Pharmacol Toxicol 67:322–328, 1990.

84. Leow KP, Smith MT, Williams B, et al: Single-dose and steady-state pharmacokinetics and pharmacodynamics of oxycodone in patients with cancer. Clin Pharmacol Ther 52:487–495, 1992.

85. Heiskanen T, Kalso E: Controlled-release oxycodone and morphine in cancer related pain. Pain 73:37–45, 1997.

86. Poyhia R, Seppala T, Olkkola KT, et al: The pharmacokinetics and metabolism of oxycodone after intramuscular and oral administration to healthy subjects. Br J Clin Pharmacol 33:617–621, 1992.

87. Hoskin PS, Hanks GW, Aherne GW, et al: The bioavailability and pharmacokinetics of morphine after intravenous, oral and buccal administration in healthy volunteers. Br J Clin Pharmacol 27:499–505, 1989.

88. Osborne R, Joel S, Trew D, et al: Morphine and metabolite behavior after different routes of morphine administration: demonstration of the importance of the active metabolite morphine-6-glucuronide. Clin Pharmacol Ther 47:12–19, 1990.

89. Beaver WT, Wallenstein SL, Rogers A, et al: Analgesic studies of codeine and oxycodone in patients with cancer. II. Comparisons of intramuscular oxycodone with intramuscular morphine and codeine. J Pharmacol Exp Ther 207:101–108, 1978.

90. Mandema SW, Kaiko RF, Oshlack B, et al: Characterization and validation of a pharmacokinetic model for controlled-release oxycodone. Br J Clin Pharmacol 42:747–756, 1996.

91. Roy SD, Flynn GL: Solubility and related physicochemical properties of narcotic analgesics. Pharm Res 5:580–586, 1988.

92. Kaiko R, Lacouture P, Hopf K, et al: Analgesic onset and potency of oral controlled-release (CR) oxycodone and CR morphine. Clin Pharmacol Ther 59:130(abst), 1996.

93. Reder RF, Oshlack B, Miotto SB, et al: Steady-state bioavailability of controlled-release oxycodone in normal subjects. Clin Ther 18:95–105, 1996.

94. Klepper ID, Sherrill DL, Boetger CL, et al: Analgesia and respiratory effects of extradural sufentanil in volunteers, and the influence of adrenaline as an adjuvant. Br J Anesth 59:1147–1155, 1987.

95. Hansdottir V, Hedner T, Woestenborghs R, et al: The CSF and plasma pharmacokinetics of sufentanil after intrathecal administration. Anesthesiology 74:264–270, 1992.

96. Yaksh TL: Spinal opiates: a review of their effect on spinal function with emphasis on pain processing. Acta Anaesthesiol Scand 31:25–37, 1987.

97. Yaksh TL, Noueihed R: The physiology and pharmacology of spinal opioids. Annu Rev Pharmacol Toxicol 25:433–445, 1985.

98. Roy SD, Flynn GL: Transdermal delivery of narcotic analgesics: pH, anatomical, and subject influences on cutaneous permeability of fentanyl and sufentanil. Pharm Res 7:842–847, 1990.

99. Dormer B, Zenz M, Tiyba M, et al: Direct conversion from oral morphine to transdermal fentanyl: A multicenter study in patients with cancer pain. Pain 64:527–534, 1996.

100. Dormer B, Zenz M, Strumpf M, et al: Long-term treatment of cancer pain with transdermal fentanyl. J Pain Symptom Manage 15:168–175, 1998.

101. Grond S, Zech D, Lehmann KA, et al: Transdermal fentanyl in the long-term treatment of cancer pain: A prospective study of 50 patients with advanced cancer of the gastrointestinal tract or the head and neck region. Pain 69:191–198, 1997.

102. Korte W, de Stoutz N, Morant R: Day-to-day titration to initiate transdermal fentanyl in patients with cancer pain: Short- and long-term experiences in a prospective study of 39 patients. J Pain Symptom Manage 11:139–146, 1996.

103. Payne R: Transdermal fentanyl: Suggested recommendations for clinical use. J Pain Symptom Manage 7:S40–44, 1992.

104. Payne R, Chandler S, Einhaus M: Guidelines for the clinical use of transdermal fentanyl. Anticancer Drugs 6(Suppl 3):50–53, 1995.

105. Payne R, Mathias SD, Pasta DI, et al: Quality of life and cancer pain: Satisfaction and side effects with transdermal fentanyl versus oral morphine. J Clin Oncol 16:1588–1593, 1998.

106. Plezia PM, Kramer TH, Linford J, et al: Transdermal fentanyl: Pharmacokinetics and preliminary clinical evaluation. Pharmacotherapy 9:2–9, 1989.

107. Portenoy RK, Southam MA, Gupta SK, et al: Transdermal fentanyl for cancer pain. Repeated dose pharmacokinetics. Anesthesiology 78:36–43, 1993.

108. Varvel JR, Shafer SL, Hwang SS, et al: Absorption characteristics of transdermally administered fentanyl. Anesthesiology 70:928–934, 1989.

109. Zech DF, Grond SU, Lynch J, et al: Transdermal fentanyl and initial dose-finding with patient-controlled analgesia in cancer pain. A pilot study with 20 terminally ill cancer patients. Pain 50:293–301, 1992.

110. Gourlay GK, Mather LE: Pharmacokinetics and pharmacodynamics. In: Lehmann KA, Zech D, eds: Transdermal fentanyl. Berlin, Springer-Verlag, 1991, pp 119–140.

111. Sandler AN, Baxter AD, Katz S, et al: A double-blind, placebo-controlled trial of transdermal fentanyl after abdominal hysterectomy. Analgesic, respiratory, and pharmacokinetic effects. Anesthesiology 81:1169–1180, 1994.

112. Streisand SB, Varvel JR, Stanski DR, et al: Absorption and bioavailability of oral transmucosal fentanyl citrate. Anesthesiology 75:223–229, 1991.

113. Farrar JT, Cleary S, Rauck R, et al: Oral transmucosal fentanyl citrate: randomized, double-blinded, placebo-controlled trial for treatment of breakthrough pain in cancer patients. J Natl Cancer Inst 90:611–616, 1998.

114. Christie JM, Simmonds M, Patt R, et al: Dose-titration, multicenter study of oral transmucosal fentanyl citrate for the treatment of breakthrough pain in cancer patients using transdermal fentanyl for persistent pain. J Clin Oncol 16:3238–3245, 1998.

115. Fine PG, Marcus M, DeBoer AL, et al: An open label study of oral transmucosal fentanyl citrate (OTFC) for the treatment of breakthrough cancer pain. Pain 45:149–153, 1991.

116. Inturrisi CE, Unams JG: Meperidine biotransformation and central nervous system toxicity in animals and humans. In Foley KM, Inturrisi CE, eds: Advances in Pain Research and Therapy, vol 8: Opioid Analgesics in the Management of Clinical Pain. New York, Raven Press, 1986, p 143.

117. Ereshefsky L, Riesenman C, Lam YW: Antidepressant drug interactions and the cytochrome P450 system. The role of cytochrome P450 2D6. Clin Pharmacokinet 29(Suppl 1):10–18, 1995.

118. Shipton EA: Tramadol: present and future. Anaesth Intens Care 28:363–374, 2000.

119. Wilder-Smith CH, Schimke J, Osterwalder B, et al: Oral tramadol, a mu-opioid agonist and monoamine reuptake-blocker, and morphine for strong cancer-related pain. Ann Oncol 5:141–146, 1994.

120. Grond S, Radbruch L, Meuser T, Loick G: High-dose tramadol in comparison to low-dose morphine for cancer pain relief. J Pain Symptom Manage 18:174–179, 1999.

121. Hoskin PS, Hanks GW: Opioid agonist-antagonist drugs in acute and chronic pain states. Drugs 41:326–344, 1991.

122. Caruso FS: Morphidex pharmacokinetic studies and single dose analgesic efficacy studies in patients with postoperative pain. J Pain Symptom Manage 19:S31–36, 2000.

123. Goldblum R: Long-term safety of morphi-dex. J Pain Symptom Manage 19(18):S50–56, 2000.

124. Radbruch L: Buprenorphine TDS: Use in daily practice, benefits for patients. Int J Clin Pract Suppl 133:19–22, 2003.

125. Ossipov MH, Laij, Vanderah TW, et al: Induction of pain facilitation by sustained opioid exposure: Relationship to opioid antinociceptive tolerance. Life Sci 73:783–800, 2003.

126. Trujillo KA, Akil H: Inhibition of morphine tolerance and dependence by the NMDA receptor antagonist MK-801. Science 251:85–87, 1991.

127. Trujillo KA, Akil H: Opiate tolerance and dependence: Recent findings and synthesis. New Biol 3:915–923, 1991.

128. Yaksh TL, Onofrio BM: Retrospective consideration of the doses of morphine given intrathecally by chronic infusion in 163 patients by 19 physicians. Pain 31:211–223, 1987.

129. Foley K: Changing concepts of tolerance to opioids: What the cancer patient has taught us. In: Chapman CR, Foley K (eds): Current and Emerging Issues in Cancer Pain: Research and Practice. New York, Raven, 1993, pp 331–350.

130. Enting RH, Oldenmenger WH, Van Der Rijt CCD, et al: A prospective study evaluating the response of patients with unrelieved cancer pain to parenteral opioids. Cancer 94:3049–3056, 2002.

131. Lawlor PG, Turner KS, Hanson S, et al: Dose ratio between morphine and methadone in patients with cancer pain: A retrospective study. Cancer 82:1167–1173, 1998.

132. Ripamonti C, DeConno F, Groff L, et al: Equianalgesic dose/ratio between methadone and other opioid agonists in cancer pain: comparison of two clinical experiences. Ann Oncol 9:79–83, 1998.

133. Morley JS, Watt SWG, Wells SC, et al: Methadone in pain uncontrolled by morphine [letter]. Lancet 342:1243, 1993.

134. Lawlor P, Turner K, Hanson S, et al: Dose ratio between morphine and hydromorphone in patients with cancer pain: a retrospective study. Pain 72:79–85, 1997.

135. Hunt G, Bruera E: Respiratory depression in a patient receiving oral methadone for cancer pain. J Pain Symptom Manage 10:401–404, 1995.

136. Doverty M, Somogyi AA, White JM, et al: Methadone maintenance patients are cross-tolerant to the antinociceptive effects of morphine. Pain 93:155–163, 2001.

137. Moryl N, Santiago-Palma J, Kornick C, et al: Pitfalls of opioid rotation: substituting another opioid for methadone in patients with cancer pain. Pain 96:325–328, 2002.

138. Mercadante S: Expert Rev. Anticancer Ther. 1(3), 487–494, 2001.

139. Zebraski SE, Kochenash SM, Raffa RB: Lung opioid receptors: pharmacology and possible target for nebulized morphine in dyspnea. Life Sciences 66(23):221–231, 2000.

140. Chandler S: Nebulized opioids to treat dyspnea. Am J Hosp Palliat Care 16:418–422, 1999.

141. Coyne PJ, Viswanathan R, Smith TJ: Nebulized fentanyl citrate improves patient's perception of breathing, respiratory rate, and oxygen saturation in dyspnea. J Pain Symptom Manage 23(2):157–160, 2002.

142. Coyne PJ: The use of nebulized fentanyl for the management of dyspnea. Clin J Oncol Nurs 7(3):334–335, 2003.

143. Zeppetella G: Nebulized and intranasal fentanyl in the management of cancer-related breakthrough pain. Palliat Med 14(1):57, 2000.

144. Pavis H, Wilcock A, Edgecombe J, et al: Pilot study of nasal morphine-chitosan for the relief of breakthrough pain in cancer patients. J Pain Symptom Manage 24:598–602, 2002.

145. Cole L, Hanning CD: Review of the rectal use of opioids. J Pain Symptom Manage 5:118–126, 1990.

146. Ripamonti C, Zecca E, Brunelli C, et al: Rectal custom made suppositories can be made by mixing methadone powder in a hydrogenated oil base and solidified in a refrigerator for 45 minutes. Methadone in cancer patients with pain. Ann Oncol 6:841–843, 1995.

147. Bruera E, Watanabe S, Faisinger RL, et al: Custom-made capsules and suppositories of methadone for patients on high-dose opioids for cancer pain. Pain 62:141–146, 1995.

148. Cherny NI, Portenoy RK: Cancer pain management. Current strategy. Cancer 72:3393–3415, 1993.

149. Meuret G, Socham H: Patient-controlled analgesia (PCA) in the domiciliary care of tumor patients. Cancer Treat Rev 22(Suppl A):137–140, 1996.

150. Patt RB: PCA: Prescribing analgesia for home management of severe pain. Geriatrics 47:69–72, 1992.

151. Swanson G, Smith S, Bulich R, et al: Patient-controlled analgesia for chronic cancer pain in the ambulatory setting: A report of 117 patients. J Clin Oncol 7:1903–1908, 1989.

152. Rapp SE, Egan KS, Ross BK, et al: A multidimensional comparison of morphine and hydromorphone patient-controlled analgesia. Anesth Analg 82:1043–1048, 1996.

153. Woodhouse A, Hobbes AF, Mather LE, et al: A comparison of morphine, pethidine and fentanyl in the postsurgical patient-controlled analgesia environment. Pain 64:115–121, 1996.

154. Coda BA, O'Sullivan B, Donaldson G, et al: Comparative efficacy of patient-controlled administration of morphine, hydromorphone, or sufentanil for the treatment of oral mucositis pain following bone marrow transplantation. Pain 72:333–346, 1997.

155. Coda B, Tanaka A, Jacobson RC, et al: Hydromorphone analgesia after intravenous bolus administration. Pain 71:41–48, 1997.

156. Dunbar PS, Chapman CR, Buckley FP, et al: Clinical analgesic equivalence for morphine and hydromorphone with prolonged PCA. Pain 68:265–270, 1996.

157. Inturrisi CE, Colbum WA, Kaiko RF, et al: Pharmacokinetics and pharmacodynamics of methadone in patients with chronic pain. Clin Pharmacol Ther 41:392–401, 1987.

158. Hug CC Jr, Murphy MR, Rigel EP, et al: Pharmacokinetics of morphine injected intravenously into the anesthetized dog. Anesthesiology 54:38–47, 1981.

159. Scholz S, Steinfath M, Schulz M: Clinical pharmacokinetics of alfentanil, fentanyl and sufentanil. An update. Clin Pharmacokinet 31:275–292, 1996.

160. Bruera E, Lawlor P: Cancer pain management. Acta Anaesthesiol Scand 41:146–153, 1997.

161. Sjogren P, Jonsson T, Jensen NH, et al: Hyperalgesia and myoclonus in terminal cancer patients treated with continuous intravenous morphine. Pain 55:93–97, 1993.

162. Eisele SH Jr, Grigsby EJ, Dea G: Clonazepam treatment of myoclonic contractions associated with high-dose opioids: Case report. Pain 49:231–232, 1992.

163. Drexel H, Dzien A, Spiegel RW, et al: Treatment of severe cancer pain by low-dose continuous subcutaneous morphine. Pain 36:169–176, 1989.

164. Bruera E, Brenneis C, Michaud M, et al: Use of the subcutaneous route for the administration of narcotics in patients with cancer pain. Cancer 62:407–411, 1988.

165. Kerr IG, Sone M, Deangelis C, et al: Continuous narcotic infusion with patient-controlled analgesia for chronic cancer pain in outpatients. Ann Intern Med 108:554–557, 1988.

166. Moulin DE, Kreeft JH, Murray Parsons N, et al: Comparison of continuous subcutaneous and intravenous hydromorphone infusions for management of cancer pain. Lancet 337:465–468, 1991.

167. Waldmann CS, Eason JR, Rambohul E, et al: Serum morphine levels. A comparison between continuous subcutaneous infusion and continuous intravenous infusion in postoperative patients. Anaesthesia 39:768–771, 1984.

168. Paix A, Coleman A, Lees S, et al: Subcutaneous fentanyl and sufentanil infusion substitution for morphine intolerance in cancer pain management. Pain 63:263–269, 1995.

169. DuPen SL, Peterson DG, Williams A, et al: Infection during chronic epidural catheterization: Diagnosis and treatment. Anesthesiology 73:905–909, 1990.

170. Inagaki Y, Mashimo T, Yoshiya I: Time-related differential effects of epidural morphine on the neuraxis. Anesth Analg 76:308–315, 1993.

171. Loper KA, Ready LB, Downey M, et al: Epidural and intravenous fentanyl infusions are clinically equivalent after knee surgery. Anesth Analg 70:72–75, 1990.

172. Glass PS, Estok P, Ginsberg B, et al: Use of patient-controlled analgesia to compare the efficacy of epidural to intravenous fentanyl administration. Anesth Analg 74:345–351, 1992.

173. Ellis DJ, Millar WL, Reisner LS: A randomized double-blind comparison of epidural versus intravenous fentanyl infusion for analgesia after cesarean section. Anesthesiology 72:981–986, 1990.

174. Miguel R, Barlow I, Morrell M, et al: A prospective, randomized, double-blind comparison of epidural and intravenous sufentanil infusions. Anesthesiology 81:346–352, 1994.

175. Coda BA, Brown MC, Schaffer RL, et al: A pharmacokinetic approach to resolving spinal and systemic contributions to epidural alfentanil analgesia and side-effects. Pain 62:329–337, 1995.

176. Paech MJ, Moore JS, Evans SF: Meperidine for patient-controlled analgesia after cesarean section. Intravenous versus epidural administration. Anesthesiology 80:1268–1276, 1994.

177. Chrubasik J, Chrubasik S, Martin E: The ideal epidural opioid—fact or fantasy? Eur J Anaesthesiol 10:79–100, 1993.

178. DuPen SL, Kharasch ED, Williams A, et al: Chronic epidural bupivacaine-opioid infusion in intractable cancer pain. Pain 49:293–300, 1992.

179. Appelgren L, Nordborg C, Sjoberg M, et al: Spinal epidural metastasis: Implications for spinal analgesia to treat 'refractory' cancer pain. J Pain Symptom Manage 13:25–42, 1997.

180. Nitescu P, Appelgren L, Linder LE, et al: Epidural versus intrathecal morphine-bupivacaine: assessment of consecutive treatments in advanced cancer pain. J Pain Symptom Manage 5:18–26, 1990.

181. Sjoberg M, Appelgren L, Einarsson S, et al: Long-term intrathecal morphine and bupivacaine in 'refractory' cancer pain. I. Results from the first series of 52 patients. Acta Anaesthesiol Scand 35:30–43, 1991.

182. Amer S, Rawal N, Gustafsson LL: Clinical experience of long-term treatment with epidural and intrathecal opioids—a nationwide survey. Acta Anaesthesiol Scand 32:253–259, 1988.

183. Nitescu P, Sjoberg M, Appelgren L, et al: Complications of intrathecal opioids and bupivacaine in the treatment of "refractory" cancer pain. Clin J Pain 11:45–62, 1995.

184. Ventafridda V, Spoldi E, Caraceni A, et al: Intraspinal morphine for cancer pain. Acta Anaesthesiol Scand Suppl 85:47–53, 1987.

185. Brazenor GA: Long term intrathecal administration of morphine: A comparison of bolus injection via reservoir with continuous infusion by implanted pump. Neurosurgery 21:484–491, 1987.

186. Plummer JL, Cherry DA, Cousins MJ, et al: Long-term spinal administration of morphine in cancer and non-cancer pain: a retrospective study. Pain 44:215–220, 1991.

187. Crul BJ, Delhaas EM: Technical complications during long-term subarachnoid or epidural administration of morphine in terminally ill cancer patients: A review of 140 cases. Reg Anesth 16:209–213, 1991.

188. Devulder I, Ghys L, Dhondt W, et al: Spinal analgesia in terminal care: Risk versus benefit. J Pain Symptom Manage 9:75–81, 1994.

189. Paice JA, Winkelmuller W, Burchiel K, et al: Clinical realities and economic considerations: Efficacy of intrathecal pain therapy. J Pain Symptom Manage 14:S14–26, 1997.

190. Bedder MD, Burchiel K, Larson A: Cost analysis of two implantable narcotic delivery systems. J Pain Symptom Manage 6:368–373, 1991.

191. Greenberg HS, Taren S, Ensminger WD, et al: Benefit from and tolerance to continuous intrathecal infusion of morphine for intractable cancer pain. J Neurosurg 57:360–364, 1982.

192. Penn RD, Paice JA: Chronic intrathecal morphine for intractable pain. J Neurosurg 67:182–186, 1987.

193. Hassenbusch SJ, Pillay PK, Magdinec M, et al: Constant infusion of morphine for intractable cancer pain using an implanted pump. J Neurosurg 73:405–409, 1990.

194. Onofrio BM, Yaksh TL: Long-term pain relief produced by intrathecal morphine infusion in 53 patients. J Neurosurg 72:200–209, 1990.

195. Abram SE: Continuous spinal anesthesia for cancer and chronic pain. Reg Anesth 18:406–413, 1993.

196. Cousins MJ, Mather LE: Intrathecal and epidural administration of opioids. Anesthesiology 61:276–310, 1984.

197. De Conno F, Caracem A, Martini C, et al: Hyperalgesia and myoclonus with intrathecal infusion of high-dose morphine. Pain 47:337–339, 1991.

198. Follett KA, Hitchon PW, Piper S, et al: Response of intractable pain to continuous intrathecal morphine: A retrospective study. Pain 49:21–25, 1992.

199. Paice SA, Penn RD, Shott S: Intraspinal morphine for chronic pain: a retrospective, multicenter study. J Pain Symptom Manage 11:71–80, 1996.

200. Schultheiss R, Schramm S, Neidhardt S: Dose changes in long- and medium-term intrathecal morphine therapy of cancer pain. Neurosurgery 31:664–669, 1992.

201. Wagemans MF, Bakker EN, Zuurmond WW, et al: Intrathecal administration of high-dose morphine solutions decreases the pH of cerebrospinal fluid. Pain 61:55–59, 1995.

202. Jacobson L, Chabal C, Brody MC, et al: Intrathecal methadone and morphine for postoperative analgesia: A comparison of the efficacy, duration, and side effects. Anesthesiology 70:742–746, 1989.

203. Bennett G, Burchiel K, Buchser E, et al: Clinical guidelines for intraspinal infusion: Report of an expert panel. J Pain Symptom Manage 20:S37–S43, 2000.

204. Winkelmuller M, Winkelmuller W: Long-term effects of continuous intrathecal opioid treatment in chronic pain of nonmalignant etiology. J Neurosurg 85:458–467, 1996.

205. Amer S, Amer B: Differential effects of epidural morphine in the treatment of cancer-related pain. Acta Anaesthesiol Scand 29:32–36, 1985.

206. Shetter AG, Hadley MN, Wilkinson E: Administration of intraspinal morphine sulfate for the treatment of intractable cancer pain. Neurosurgery 18:740–747, 1986.

207. Penning JP, Yaksh U: Interaction of intrathecal morphine with bupivacaine and lidocaine in the rat. Anesthesiology 77:1186–2000, 1992.

208. Fink BR: Mechanisms of differential axial blockade in epidural and subarachnoid anesthesia. Anesthesiology 70:851–858, 1989.

209. Jamison RN, Taft K, O'Hara SP, et al: Psychosocial and pharmacologic predictors of satisfaction with intravenous patient-controlled analgesia. Anesth Analg 77:121–125, 1993.

210. Chapman CR: Psychological aspects of postoperative pain control. Acta Anaesthesiol Belg 43:41–52, 1992.

211. Hardy PA, Wells SC: Patient-controlled intrathecal morphine for cancer pain. A method used to assess morphine requirements and bolus doses. Clin J Pain 6:57–59, 1990.

212. Lazorthes Y: Intracerebroventricular administration of morphine for control of irreducible cancer pain. Ann NY Acad Sci 531:123–132, 1988.

213. Dennis GC, DeWitty RL: Long-term intraventricular infusion of morphine for intractable pain in cancer of the head and neck. Neurosurgery 26:404–407; discussion 407–408, 1990.

CHAPTER 17

Immunologic Effects of Acute and Chronic Opiate Administration

Ricardo Vallejo, MD

Evidence of the use of opium for medicinal and recreational purposes dates back to 4000 BC.[1] The most important property of opium is pain relief. Few drugs have had greater acceptance and use as analgesics. Opium is obtained from the unripe seeds of the capsules of the commonly known poppy plant *Papaver somniferum*.

The first breakthrough in our understanding of the pharmacologic effects of opium was in 1803 when a German apothecary called Serturner isolated the alkaloid morphine from opium. Serturner named the alkaloid morphine after Morpheus, the god of dreams.[2] Morphine is the primary derivative of the opium poppy and is the standard for other analgesics.[3]

By the 19th century, another dozen derivatives of opium were discovered and in use. This includes codeine, which is actively used today. It was not until 1874 that diacetylmorphine (diamorphine), commonly known as heroin, was discovered. Heroin, a semisynthetic derivative of morphine, was initially used to treat morphine addiction.

In the beginning, morphine's analgesic effects were thought to be secondary to its ability to affect emotional responses to pain, rather than to act directly on the transmission of pain as a sensory modality.[4] In 1973, Pers and Snyder characterized the opioid receptors in the brain.[5] Opioids exert their pharmacologic effects by binding these receptors. Initial evidence confirmed the presence of these receptors in multiple areas of the central nervous system (CNS). The general consensus is that the antinociceptive effects of opioids are mediated by opioid receptors within the CNS.

There are three major types of opioid receptors: the μ-(mu), κ-(kappa), and Δ-(delta) opioid receptors (MOR, KOR, and DOR). Early studies identified these receptors on cell bodies in the dorsal root ganglion (DRG) and on central terminals of primary afferent neurons within the dorsal horn of the spinal cord.[6] In the early 1990s, the opioid receptors were cloned.[7] This made it possible to demonstrate mRNA for all the receptors in the DRG and small diameter primary afferent neurons. MOR, DOR, and KOR are members of the Gi (inhibitory) protein-coupled seven transmembrane receptor (GPCR) super family. The major endogenous ligands for these receptors are endomorphin 1 and 2 (MOR agonist), leu- and met-enkephalin (DOR), and dynorphin (KOR). β-Endorphin is an additional endogenous opioid that interacts with MOR and DOR. Further investigations led to the conclusion that the endogenous opiates are synthesized as precursors. These are proenkephalin A, prodynorphine (or proenkephalin B), and propiomelancortin.[8-10]

The first opioid antagonist, naloxone, and its congener, naltrexone, were synthesized in 1940. The first two endogenous peptide ligands for the opioid receptor were isolated in 1975.[11-13] Until a few years ago, the main medicinal property of opiates was pain relief, one of the four cardinal signs of inflammation defined by Cornelius Celsus (53 BC to 7 AD). Since 1995, reports describing the presence of opioid receptors outside the CNS and the generation of analgesia by these peripheral receptors are accumulating. Such analgesic effects are more evident during states of inflammation.[14] The relationship between inflammation and pain is pervasive in medicine. Neuroimmunologists, studying inflammatory illness response, and pain researchers realized the similarities of their work in the early 1990s. The description by Wall of the chronic phases of pain is strikingly similar to illness response.[15] It is typified by decreased activity, lack of eating and drinking, increased sleep, decreased social interaction, and enhanced pain. Inflammation is a local response to tissue injury, infection, or irritants. This leads to the activation of immune cells that release substances which signal the brain, triggering a constellation of coordinated responses designed to enhance survival.[16] Recently, an appreciation of the broad effects of opioids on the inflammatory response has emerged.

The idea that opioids may modulate the immune response is not new. In the late 19th century, Canta-cuzene demonstrated that opium suppressed cellular immunity and lowered resistance of guinea pigs to bacterial infection. There is growing evidence that opioid receptors are expressed by cells of the immune system and that opioids may modulate immune response by central and peripheral mechanisms. Increased incidence of infection in heroin addicts was originally attributed to the use of nonsterile and contaminated needles or by impurities in street heroin. More recently, opiates have been implicated as cofactors in the pathogenesis of the human immunodeficiency virus (HIV). The role of morphine, an active metabolite of heroin, in the modulation of immune function in multiple ways has gained significant interest.[17,18]

Although exogenous opioids mediate immunosuppression, endogenous opiates exert opposite actions. The addition of beta-endorphin or met-enkephalin (MET) to ^{51}Cr-release microcytotoxicity assays has been shown to augment natural killer (NK) cell activity. This effect is antagonized by the injection of naloxone.[19]

BRIEF OVERVIEW OF THE IMMUNE SYSTEM

To understand the natural involvement of pain in immune activation, it is necessary to understand a few basic aspects about the function of the immune system. Traditionally, the immune system is considered in terms of the cells and molecules responsible for coordinating and executing a host reaction in response to the introduction of a foreign substance in the organism. However, multiple noninfectious substances can initiate an immune response. The immune system, once activated by foreign infectious or noninfectious substances, can elicit a reaction that is capable of causing tissue injury and disease. During illness, infection and injury activated immune cells release substances that signal the brain, initiating a collection of coordinated responses designed to strengthen survival. One of the most important functions of the immune system is the recognition of foreign cells (virus, bacteria, protozoa, etc.) or other nonself entities (tumors, endotoxins, senescent red blood cells, damaged cells, etc.). The immune response to one of these phenomena is classically divided into innate and adaptive immunity. The innate response, also called natural immunity, consists of cellular and biochemical defense mechanisms that are in place even before infection and are able to respond rapidly to infections. The principal components of the innate immune system include physical and chemical barriers (skin, tears, acid in the stomach, etc.), phagocytic cells (neutrophils, macrophages), NK cells, blood proteins (complement system

and other inflammatory mediators), and cytokines. Cytokines are proteins released by cells in response to a variety of stimuli.

The other form of immunity is called adaptive or acquired because it is activated by an invader organism and adapts to increase the magnitude of response with successive exposure. The response is specific, as it is capable of distinguishing different microbes and molecules. Other than specificity, the cardinal features of the adaptive response include diversity (allows response to a variety of antigens), memory (leads enhanced responses with repeated exposure), specialization (generates optimal responses to different types of microbes), self-limitation (responds to newly encountered antigens), and nonreactivity (prevents injury to the host during responses to foreign antigens). The adaptive immune response is mediated by lymphocytes and their products. There are two types of adaptive immune response: (1) Humoral immunity, which is mediated by antibodies that are secreted by B lymphocytes. Antibodies recognize foreign molecules, neutralize them, and target them for elimination by various effector mechanisms. Antibodies are specialized and activate different effects including phagocytosis and the release of inflammatory mediators from different cells. (2) Cellular immunity is mediated by T lymphocytes and is targeted against intracellular viruses or bacteria that are not accessible to circulating antibodies.

The ontogeny of the immune response begins in the yolk sac of the developing embryo. The cell progenitor populations start their journey to the fetal liver and then migrate to their primary residence in the adult life, bone marrow. All lymphocytes go through a complex process of maturation mediated by growth factors and cytokines, during which they express antigen receptors and acquire the functional and phenotypic characteristics of mature cell. B lymphocytes become fully mature in the bone marrow, whereas T lymphocytes mature in the thymus. After cell maturation, lymphocytes are released into circulation and populate peripheral lymphoid organs. These mature cells are called naïve lymphocytes.

Cytokines are low molecular weight proteins that are released in response to microbes or other antigens and stimulate diverse cells involved in immunity and inflammation. Cytokines are usually not stored as preformed molecules, and their synthesis is transient as a result of gene transcription. One cytokine may act in different cell types, whereas multiple cytokines may exert the same functional effects. These actions are referred to as pleiotropy and redundancy, respectively.

The ability of one cytokine to mediate the synthesis of other may lead to a cascade of events in which one of the cytokines produced as a result of the activation by another cytokine may exert multiple functions, even antagonizing the effect of the first cytokine. The binding of one cytokine with its specific receptor, which is also expressed by stimulation from external signals, will activate multiple intracellular messengers that will generate the transcription of DNA with the resultant synthesis of proteins. This will exert specific biologic functions. Cytokines, therefore, mediate and regulate innate and adaptive immunity and stimulate the growth and differentiation of cells in the immune system. One particular group of cytokines that are of interest for the purpose of this chapter is the chemokines, which are a large family of structurally homologous cytokines that regulate movement and migration of inflammatory cells. More than 50 different types of chemokines have been identified and are classified on the basis of the number and location of the N-terminal cysteine residues. The two major families are the CC chemokines, with the cysteine residues adjacent, and the CXC chemokines, with the cysteine residues separated by one amino acid. Both types of chemokines are produced by leukocytes and other cell types, including endothelial cells, epithelial cells, and fibroblasts. Their secretion may be induced by other cytokines, mainly tumor necrosis factor (TNF) and interleukin-1 (IL-1). Multiple subtypes of receptors have been identified for chemokine families (CCR 1 to CCR11 and CXCR1 to CXCR6). Certain chemokine receptors, specifically CCR5 and CXCR4, act as co-receptors for HIV. Some activated T lymphocytes secrete chemokines that bind to CCR5 and block infection with HIV by competition with the virus.

The relationship between the immune system and the development and maintenance of chronic pain has only gained attention in the last two decades, when researchers in both areas realized that the clinical findings in both entities had striking similarities. Peripheral injury is followed by inflammation, which is associated with migration of leukocytes and other immune cells. Some of the substances released in the area of injury include K^+, H^+, bradykinin, substance P (sP), prostanoids, and cytokines including neurotrophic growth factor and chemokines. Cytokines, by promoting different transcriptional factors in the nucleus of the cell, mediate the synthesis and release of active substances like prostaglandin E2 and sP, and play a significant role in the sensitization of the dorsal horn neurons in the spinal cord. In animal models of chronic neuropathic pain, the use of specific antibodies against certain cytokines, such as IL-1 and TNF, consistently prevent the development of neuropathic pain behavior.[20]

Endogenous opioids administered in vitro to human peripheral blood mononuclear cells augment NK activity in a naloxone sensitive manner. This immunomodulation occurs rapidly (4 to 6 hours). This rules out the involvement of cytokines, such as interferon gamma and interleukin 2, known to augment NK cytotoxic activity. Opioid peptides increase Ca^{2+} influx or uptake rapidly by murine T lymphocytes. Ca^{2+} is required for the release and execution of perforin and granzyme A during the lytic process elicited by most cytolytic effector cells.[21]

Acute and chronic administration of opioids is known to have inhibitory effects on antibody and cellular immune responses, NK cell activity, cytokine expression, and phagocytic activity. Consistent with these findings, opioid administration has been associated with increased susceptibility of animals to bacterial and viral infections, and with decreased survival in tumor-bearing animals.

The effects of exogenous opioids on the immune system may be mediated through central and peripheral mechanisms. The potential mechanisms by which central opioid receptors modulate these peripheral immune functions may involve both the hypothalamic–pituitary–adrenal (HPA) axis and the autonomic nervous system. Acute administration of morphine or related compounds appears to primarily alter peripheral immune function through the sympathetic nervous system, whereas more prolonged exposure to opioids alters the immune system predominantly by activation of the HPA axis. On the other hand, immune cells in the periphery, under the influence of cytokines, release endogenous opioids and modulate analgesia and inflammation at the site of injury. Also, exogenous opioids may modulate the secretion and receptor expression of inflammatory cytokines, creating a bidirectional system in which opioids and immune cells and mediators dynamically interact.

NATURAL KILLER CELL ACTIVITY AND OPIOID INTERACTION

Several in vivo and in vitro studies suggest that morphine induces suppression of NK cell activity primarily, if not exclusively, by binding opioid receptors in the CNS. The central and peripheral effects of opioids on NK cell activity were evaluated by morphine administration in the right lateral ventricle of male Fisher rats. As previously observed, when morphine was given systemically, the intracerebroventricular injection produced a significant decrease in NK cell cytolytic activity. In both cases, the simultaneous administration of naltrexone, an opioid antagonist that is able to cross the blood–brain barrier, inhibited the immunosuppressive effect. To determine if the mechanism behind this effect involved opioid receptors in the periphery or the CNS, N-methyl-morphine (an active quaternary derivative of morphine that does not cross the blood–brain barrier) was injected systemically, with failure to produce any changes in the NK cell cytolytic activity.[22-24]

On the basis of these studies, several investigators began the search for the specific areas in the brain where the interaction of exogenous opioids and their receptors exerted such phenomena. The suppression of splenic NK cell cytolytic activity seems to occur specifically in an area of the brain closed to the periaqueductal gray (PAG). Microinjection of morphine into different areas of the brain in Fisher rats, specifically the anterior hypothalamus, arcuate nucleus–ventro medial hypothalamus, medial thalamus, medial amygdala, dorsal hippocampus, and PAG, demonstrates that the PAG was the only area of opioid receptors that produces suppression of NK cell activity. When morphine was injected into the lateral ventricle, it induced pronounced dose-dependent depression of lymphocyte proliferation to T- and B-cell mitogens, NK cell cytotoxicity, and the cytokine production (interleukin-2 and interferon-gamma). In contrast, microinjection of morphine into the caudal aspect of the PAG induced dose-dependent alterations in NK cell cytotoxicity but had no effect on lymphocyte proliferation or cytokine production. These results indicate that opioid receptors in the PAG are involved in the regulation of NK cell activity but are not associated with morphine's effects on T-lymphocyte proliferation or cytokine production. A subsequent study showed that the effect of morphine in the PAG is restricted to the more caudal aspects of the PAG because microinjections of morphine into the rostral aspects did not result in any alteration of immune status. Activation of opioid receptors in the PAG is required for morphine's effects on NK cell activity. The administration of N-methylnaltrexone directly into the PAG antagonized morphine's effect on NK cell activity, which indicates that activation of opioid receptors within the PAG are required for morphine to alter NK cell activity. Therefore, activation of opioid receptors within the more caudal aspects of the PAG is required for morphine to induce alterations in splenic NK cell activity. The results also suggest that other brain regions are responsible for morphine's effect on lymphocyte proliferation and cytokine production. Even further, it seems that inside of the PAG the caudal area mediates these effects.[23-25]

Morphine at large doses loses its specificity for the MOR and is capable of binding to and acting on DOR and KOR. Studies with the more selective MOR agonist D-Ala, N-MePhe, Gly-enkephalin (DAMGO) have shown that deactivation of these receptors lead to the suppression of splenic NK cell activity, whereas the administration of a specific DOR agonist produces a significant increase in NK cell activity. This suggests a complex central opioid regulation of this immune parameter.[26]

When endogenous opioids, like beta-endorphins and MET were injected in the cisterna magna (CM), a significant enhancement of NK cell activity was noted. This response is not seen when dynorphin, the other endogenous opioid, is injected in the same location. The observation that a central mechanism is involved in the triggering of the elevation of NK cell activity

when beta-endorphin and met-enkephalin are injected in the CM is supported by antagonization of this effect with the systemic administration of naltrexone (which can cross the blood–brain barrier), but not with quaternary naltrexone (which only produces peripheral effects).[27,28]

CENTRAL EFFECTS OF OPIOIDS ON T-LYMPHOCYTE PROLIFERATION

Another parameter of the immune response that decreases after the administration of exogenous opioids is the T-lymphocyte proliferation. Systemic injection of morphine suppresses mitogen-induced proliferation of blood lymphocytes by a receptor-mediated, dose-dependent mechanism. Associated with the inhibition of T-lymphocyte proliferation, rats exposed to systemic morphine, showed a 2- to 4-fold increase in corticosterone concentration. The decrease in T-lymphocyte proliferation seems to be independent of the high corticosterone concentration, as the use of a glucocorticosteroid antagonism did not change the response to systemic morphine. When morphine or N-methyl morphine was injected in the anterior hypothalamus, lymphocyte proliferation decreased by 50%, without producing analgesia or increasing the levels of corticosteroid, suggesting a supraspinal mechanism for immunosuppression, distinct from those mediating opioid analgesia and adrenal activation.[29]

Central mechanisms involved in the modulation of T-lymphocyte proliferative responses and phenotypic expression of lymphocyte cell surface markers in rats has been investigated by the injection of equianalgesic doses of subcutaneous and intrathecal morphine. Mitogen-induced T-lymphocyte proliferation was evaluated with phytohemagglutinin, concanavalin A, pokeweed, and lipopolysaccharide, whereas phenotypic expression was documented by the use of monoclonal antibody for cell surface markers (T cell, B cell, CD4+, CD8+). Subcutaneous morphine acutely suppressed lymphocyte proliferation to the mitogens phytohemagglutinin, pokeweed, and concanavalin A; however, proliferative responses returned to baseline within 24 hours. Morphine treatment did not alter the response to lipopolysaccharide. The number of splenic lymphocytes also decreased, whereas the percentage of lymphocytes expressing the CD4+ marker (T helper/inducer cells) increased moderately. Intrathecal morphine did not alter lymphocyte proliferative responses, nor did it change phenotypic expression of cell surface markers.

In contrast, the administration of systemic morphine produces a suppression of mitogen-stimulated lymphocyte proliferation, whereas the administration of systemic

N-methyl morphine did not produce this suppression. The lack of T-lymphocyte proliferation to the *N*-methyl morphine, a quaternary derivative that does not readily penetrate the blood–brain barrier, supports the central mechanism for the innovation of lymphocyte proliferation. The location of the opioid receptor that mediates the previously mentioned effect seems to be located supraspinally, as intrathecal administration of morphine does not alter peripheral lymphocyte function.[30,31]

Other experiments that support the central mechanisms involved in the suppression of lymphocyte proliferation include studies done with Lewis and Wistar rats. The effects of systemic administration of morphine on lymphocyte proliferation were antagonized by injecting the lateral ventricle with the opioid antagonist *N*-methyl naltrexone. In contrast with the location of the opioid receptors that modulate the NK cell activity, receptors that modulate lymphocyte proliferation seem to be located in a different area. Administration of morphine into the anterior hypothalamus of Sprague-Dawley rats inhibited blood lymphocyte proliferation without changing either the tail flick latency or the plasma corticosterone levels.[31]

Morphine injected in the PAG region did not cause the same effects on blood or spleen lymphocyte proliferation. Therefore, effects of exogenous opioids on NK cell activity and the lymphocyte proliferation response seem to be mediated by distinct neuronal structures. The specific type of receptor that mediates the inhibition of lymphocyte proliferation was investigated using mu-opioid receptor knockout mice (MOR-KO). Morphine modulation of several immune functions, including macrophage phagocytosis and macrophage secretion of TNF-alpha, was not observed in the MOR-KO animals, suggesting that these functions are mediated by the classical mu-opioid receptor. In contrast, morphine reduction of splenic and thymic cell number and mitogen-induced proliferation were unaffected in MOR-KO mice, as was morphine inhibition of IL-1 and IL-6 secretion by macrophages. These latter results are consistent with morphine action on a naloxone insensitive morphine receptor. This conclusion is supported by previous studies characterizing a nonopioid morphine binding site on immune cells. Alternatively, morphine may act either directly or indirectly on these cells, by a mechanism mediated by either delta or kappa opioid receptors.[32]

In contrast with these observations, intracerebroventricular administration of [D-Ala(2),*N*-Me-Phe(4), Gly-ol(5)] enkephalin (DAMGO), a mu-receptor selective agonist, [D-Pen(2,5)] enkephalin (DPDPE), a delta-opioid receptor agonist, or U69,593, a kappa-receptor agonist to Lewis rats, showed that the mu-receptor selective agonist DAMGO produced a dose-dependent decrease in NK cell activity and T-lymphocyte proliferation to the mitogen concanavalin-A, whereas no immunologic changes were found following DPDPE or U69,593 treatment. Administration of the opioid antagonist *N*-methyl naltrexone before DAMGO treatment attenuated the DAMGO-induced changes in immune status, supporting a partial involvement of the mu-opioid receptors in the inhibition of T-lymphocyte proliferation.

Despite most of the evidence pointing to a central mechanism in the depression lymphocyte proliferation, the final target for these effects may involve other peripheral mechanisms. In vivo administration of morphine to rats suppresses concanavalin-A (Con A)-stimulated proliferation of splenic lymphocytes in a dose-dependent, naltrexone-reversible manner. The possible mechanism involved in morphine-induced suppression of Con A–stimulated proliferation of lymphocytes is an increase in macrophage production of NO. The addition of hemoglobin, a scavenger of extracellular NO, to Con A–stimulated splenocyte cultures dose-dependently attenuates the suppressive effect of morphine on proliferation, whereas the addition of superoxide dismutase, a scavenger of superoxide anions, does not antagonize the suppressive effect of morphine on Con A–stimulated proliferation. The dose-dependent addition to splenocyte cultures of either methylene blue or 6-anilino-5,8-quinolinedione (LY 83583), two inhibitors of soluble guanylate cyclase, antagonizes the suppressive effect of morphine on Con A–stimulated proliferation. These results suggest that in vivo administration of morphine increases the synthesis and extracellular release of NO from macrophages in Con A–stimulated splenocyte cultures. The activation of soluble guanylate cyclase by NO in target cells, most likely the lymphocytes, accounts more completely for the morphine-induced suppression of lymphocyte proliferation.[33]

EFFECTS OF CENTRAL OPIOIDS ON CELLULAR AND HUMERAL IMMUNE RESPONSES

Central opioid receptors have also been implicated in the modulation of more complex in vivo immune responses, including the delayed-type hypersensitivity reactions and humoral immune responses. These reactions are significantly more complex than those previously described, as they involve different cell types. The role of brain delta-opioid and kappa-opioid receptors in the regulation of plaque-forming cells (PFC) response, Arthus hypersensitivity reactions, and delayed hypersensitivity reactions was studied by intracerebroventricular administration of DOR agonist methionine-enkephalin (Met-Enk), DOR antagonist ICI 174864, KOR agonist MR 2034, and KOR antagonist MR 2266. The DOR agonist and the KOR antagonist stimulated and suppressed PFC response, Arthus and delayed skin reactions respectively. At the same time, the DOR antagonist decreased the number of PFC and intensity of hypersensitivity skin reactions. Whereas the antagonism of KOR led to an increased number of PFC, it did not affect hypersensitivity reactions to a greater extent. Stimulation of PFC produced by Met-Enk was completely blocked by DOR antagonism, whereas the KOR agonist-induced suppression was antagonized by MR 2266. The present results suggest that brain opioid receptors differentially affect humoral and cell-mediated immune responses. The injection of the endogenous opioid Met-Enk decreases humoral immune responses in a dose-dependent manner. The central application of leucine-enkephalin (Leu-Enk) elicits potentiation and suppression of humoral immune responses through DOR and KOR receptors, respectively. Interestingly, both effects were found to be additionally dependent on MOR receptor function as they were antagonized by the injection of the MOR receptor antagonist beta-funaltrexamine (beta-FNA). On the basis of these findings, it may be concluded that central MOR receptors are permissive for the central immunomodulatory action of endogenous opioid peptides and Leu-Enk. In contrast, the central immunoenhancing effect of Met-Enk appears to be mediated through MOR-independent DOR-receptors.[34-36]

Therefore, brain opioid receptors differentially affect humoral and cell-mediated immune responses. The effects of centrally applied Met-Enk were antagonized by centrally administered quaternary naltrexone (QNtx) but not when this compound was administered systemically. This suggests a dominant central opioid component in the regulation of the humeral immune response. On the other hand, there is evidence that the delayed-type hypersensitivity is also dose dependent, with high doses suppressing the effect of Met-Enk and low doses enhancing this immune response. The effects of the low doses, which mediate both humoral and cellular immune-enhanced activation, seem to be mediated by the DOR, as it is specifically antagonized by the delta-receptor antagonist ICI174864.

The pronounced suppression of humoral immunity, seen with KOR agonist, seems to be mediated mainly by kappa opioid receptors and to a lesser extent by mu opioid receptors. Intracerebroventricular administration of QNtx moderately attenuated the suppressive effect of MR 2034, whereas intraperitoneal QNtx completely prevented it, suggesting a peripheral mechanism of action, with only minor involvement of brain opioid receptors. Peripheral kappa opioid receptors down-regulate primary humoral immune response in the rat. This effect may be produced by direct interference with plasma cell activity.[34,37,38]

It is clear that the delta opioid receptors mediate the immunomodulatory effect of low doses of endogenous opioids in the CNS. However, the effect of other opioid receptors is not well understood. The central administration of a specific opioid agonist for MOR and KORs has been shown to suppress both the humeral and delayed-type hypersensitivity reactions. The suppression of the humeral response mediated by MR2034 was not antagonized by QNtx administered into the ventricles of the rat.[37]

These data suggest that DOR receptors appear to mediate the low dose effects of delayed-type hypersensitivity response, whereas other opioid receptors may be involved in the effects observed at higher doses. The effects of the DOR modulation in the immune response appear to be mostly central, whereas effects of the activation of MOR and KOR may have both central and peripheral components. An important consideration regarding the interpretation of physiologic responses following the intraventricular administration of any particular drug is that the drug can activate different opioid receptors at different doses. Therefore, the results of these injections may reflect the activation of multiple opioid receptors. For that reason, future studies should focus on the identification of a specific neuroimmune modulatory pathway within the CNS.[25]

As described earlier, the effects of activation of opioid receptors in the CNS seem to modulate peripheral immune responses. How the central opioid receptor activation translates this modulation in the immune response is an area of controversy. The CNS communicates with the periphery via two major systems: (1) the neuroendocrine system and (2) the sympathetic system.

The Neuroendocrine System

Although there is no evidence that endogenous corticosteroids produce changes in immunologic parameters, it is believed that they do, on the basis of the assumption that the immune system may respond in the same way as it does when potent exogenous corticosteroids are administered systemically. Corticosteroids have the potential to lead to changes in many parameters of the immune function, including lymphocyte redistribution. Acute and chronic morphine administration can activate the HPA axis, and prolonged morphine exposure may alter lymphocyte proliferation responses to the mitogen Con A. This change in lymphocyte proliferation is associated with atrophy of the spleen and thymus, as well as adrenal hypertrophy, suggesting elevated corticosteroid production. The fact that adrenalectomy suppresses the spleen and thymus atrophy supports the concept that the T-lymphocyte proliferation is decreased by activation of the hypothalamus pituitary access.

In vitro experiments in murine leukocytes exposed to corticotropin-releasing hormone (CRH) and arginine vasopressin enhanced NK cell activity. The use of naloxone, a MOR antagonist, or naltrindole, a DOR antagonist, can block this effect. The increased NK cell activity of murine leukocytes to CRH is both dose- and time-dependent. Beta-endorphin also enhances NK cell activity in a naloxone-reversible manner, while adrenocorticotropic hormone (ACTH) has a negligible effect. Macrophage depletion before incubation with CRH blocks the CRH-induced NK cell augmentation. These results suggest hypothalamic-releasing hormones such as CRH may modulate the immune system cells either directly or indirectly through the induction of neuropeptide hormones known to have immunomodulatory capabilities.

There is also evidence that activation of the HPA axis by morphine injection in mice produces decreased NK cell activity, which was antagonized by the steroid antagonist RU486. In this particular model there is also splenic and thymic atrophy, but in contrast with the decrease of lymphocyte proliferation, it is not completely antagonized by adrenalectomy, which suggests that mechanisms other than the HPA axis are involved in this depression of NK cell activity.[39-43]

Experiments on Sprague-Dawley rats showed that morphine and naltrexone increased the plasma level of corticosteroids. Despite that naltrexone had no effect on lymphocyte proliferation or NK cell activity by itself, which suggests that immunosuppression is unlikely to be only secondary to activation of the HPA axis.

The effects of acute or chronic morphine administration seem to alter the immune response in a different way. The effects of acute morphine administration appear to be largely independent of the HPA axis response as seen on experiments done on the Sprague-Dawley and Lewis rats. On the other hand, the chronic administration of morphine may modify the MOR via different mechanisms that include the activation of the HPA axis. This produces a decrease in lymphocyte proliferation and NK cell activity.

The Sympathetic System

The effects of the sympathetic system on lymphocyte function are complex. Primary and secondary lymphoid organs are innervated by the sympathetic nervous system. The evidence for parasympathetic innervations is scarce. Direct administration of opioids into the CNS produces systemic elevation of epinephrine, norepinephrine, and dopamine from the adrenal medulla, as well as from sympathetic nerve terminals.[44]

There is significant evidence that injection of opioids in the CNS produces systemic elevation of epinephrine, norepinephrine, and dopamine. These are released from the adrenal medulla, as well as from the sympathic nerve terminals.[25,45,46]

Morphine effects on murine splenic NK cell activity involve alpha 1 adrenergic pathways. Pretreatment with the broad-acting alpha-adrenoceptor antagonist phentolamine before the systemic injection of morphine showed a modest suppression of splenic NK activity, whereas pretreatment with the peripheral-acting alpha-adrenoceptor antagonist doxazosin showed a significant decrease in splenic NK activity following morphine administration. Morphine also significantly increases splenic serotonin levels relative to saline-treated controls. Both phentolamine and doxazosin pretreatment completely or partially blocked morphine-mediated elevation of splenic serotonin levels, respectively. This seems to modulate the ability of morphine to decrease the ability of NK cells to form conjugates with target (YAC-1 lymphoma) cells and decreased the number of active killer cells within the conjugate population. These results suggest a central alpha-adrenergic mechanism following acute morphine administration in suppressing splenic NK activity indirectly through a reduction in the number of effector-target conjugates and active cytolytic effector cells.[47,48]

The involvement of the beta-adrenergic system in the immunomodulatory effects of morphine was investigated in male Lewis rats. The rats received either the nonselective beta-adrenergic antagonist nadolol, the beta 1-selective adrenergic antagonist atenolol, or the beta 2-selective adrenergic antagonist erythro-DL-1-(7-methylindan-4-yloxy)-3-isopropylaminobuta n-2-ol (ICI-118,551) at different doses, before the administration of 15 mg/kg morphine. Pretreatment with all three beta-adrenergic antagonists completely antagonized the suppressive effects of morphine on the proliferative responses of splenic leukocytes to Con A), phytohemagglutinin (PHA), lipopolysaccharide (LPS), and the combination of ionomycin and phorbol myristate acetate (PMA). None of the antagonists blocked the suppressive effects of morphine on the proliferative responses of blood leukocytes to Con A or phytohemagglutinin, splenic NK cell activity, total splenic leukocyte counts, and blood leukocyte counts per milliliter. The involvement of beta-adrenergic receptors in certain morphine's immunosuppressive effects seem to be exerted in the periphery, as nadolol and atenolol peripheral-acting compounds.[49,50]

The suppressive effect of acute morphine administration on the immune cell activity may be adrenal independent as suppression was reported on NK cell activity after acute morphine treatment in adrenalectomized Lewis rats. Therefore, it may be concluded that acute and chronic exposure to morphine may alter the immune system via different mechanisms. The effects of acute morphine administration seem to be independent of either pituitary or adrenal activation, implicating different mechanisms for the morphine-inducing immunosuppression. The prolonged morphine administration leads to the decreased lymphocyte perforation and NK cell activity by the modulation of the HPA axis.[25]

Cytotoxic T lymphocytes, another important population of effector cells that monitor tumor and viral pathogenesis, are activated when exposed to beta-endorphin. This activation seems to be at least partially dependent on the release of IL-2.

OPIOIDS AND CYTOKINES

Opioids share many properties of cytokines, the principal mediators of the immune function. As previously described, exogenous opiates and endogenous opioid peptides have diverse effects on the immune system. This immunosuppression is mediated indirectly via the CNS or through direct interaction with immunocytes. The precise cellular mechanism that mediates these immunomodulatory effects is largely unknown, although, as previously described, may involve central and peripheral complex interactions, not only with opioid receptors, but also with the HPA axis.

Some of the properties that opioids share with cytokines include the production by immune cells with paracrine, autocrine, and endocrine sides of action; functional redundancy; and pleiotropy effects that are both dose and time dependent. Like cytokines, endogenous opioids are low molecular weight proteins that are widely distributed throughout the nervous system. They function as communicating signals, neurotransmitters, or modulators of neuronal activity. As it has already been pointed out, opioids can alter the function of all types of immunocytes (T, B, NK, peripheral lymphocytes, monocytes, macrophages, and neutrophils).[17,51]

Peripheral administration of morphine is followed by a rapid and significant increase in the level of the proinflammatory cytokine, interleukin-6 (IL-6). Central injection of morphine mimics the effects of peripherally administered morphine. Coadministration of a ganglionic blocker, chlorisondamine, blocked the elevation of IL-6, suggesting a role of the autonomic nervous system. Activation of the adrenal cortex seems to be required for the elevation of IL-6 levels, as adrenalectomized animals did not respond with increased IL-6 levels after morphine injection, and the effects remain intact in adrenal demedullated animals.[52]

Another example of the interaction between the opioids and the cytokine system is the stimulation of opioid receptors of the hypothalamic neurons by interferon alpha and beta-endorphin synthesized in the brain or by stress. This causes the opioid-dependent inhibition of NK cytotoxicity, an important component of immunosurveillance, through an activation of the hypothalamic CRF-sympathetic nervous system.

As discussed earlier, some of the in vivo effects of the immune cells appear to be indirectly mediated via the CNS through the activation of the HPA axis or the autonomic nervous system. There is also considerable evidence that supports the potential for direct effects of the opioids on immune cells. Lymphocytes and mononuclear-phagocytes have been demonstrated to express MOR, DOR, and KOR.[17,53-55]

The relation between immune cells and opium peptides goes even further because immunocytes are able to produce opioid peptides. Expression of mRNA for β–endorphin and other proopiomelanocortin-derived peptides by peripheral blood splenic cells, lymphocytes, and macrophages has been demonstrated.[17,56,57] Endogenously produced opioids like preproenkephalin and Met-Enk are expressed by T-helper cells in an autocrine and paracrine manner. Memory type T cells within inflamed tissue are capable of synthesizing and releasing beta-endorphin.[58-60]

Local analgesic effects of exogenous opioid agonists are particularly prominent in painful, inflammatory conditions and are mediated by opioid receptors on peripheral sensory nerves. In a rat model of inflammatory pain, animals are injected in the hind paw with Freund's adjuvant, IL-1, and CRF, which stimulates the release of Met-Enk and dynorphin (DYN) from peripheral lymphocytes in a dose-dependent manner. Injection of CRF into the hind paw may exert analgesia that is blocked by administration of specific antibodies against Met-Enk and DYN. These experiments support the role of the immune system in the control of inflammatory pain. Cytokines and opioid interaction within the CNS includes modulation of cytokines' effect on the CNS by endogenous opiates and the modulation of neural effects of opioids by cytokines.[17,61-63]

Once considered merely as a physical support system for neurons, the glial cells constitute over 70% of the total cell population in the brain and spinal cord. Recently, glial cells (microglia, astrocytes, and oligodendrocytes) have been under intense scrutiny as key modulatory neurotropic and neuroimmune elements in the CNS. Microglia cells of monocyte origin are the macrophages of the brain and perform multiple immune-related duties. Microglial activation involves proliferation, increase expression of immune molecules, recruitment to the site of injury, and functional changes, including the release of cytokines or inflammatory mediators, or both. Proenkephalin mRNA and proenkephalin peptides have been shown to be expressed by astrocytes. The expression of DOR by astrocytes appeared to be regulated by cytokines whereas met-proenkephalin has been shown to suppress the growth of astroglia.[64,65] Astrocytes and microglial cells, which produce a variety of cytokines, have also recently been reported to express KORs. All these studies suggest that opioids and classical cytokines participate in glial-to-glial as well as glial-to-neuron communication.[17]

Opioid and chemokine receptors are members of the G-inhibitory protein-linked seven-transmembrane receptor family, which are widely distributed in brain tissues and in the periphery. Pretreatment with opioids, including morphine, heroin, Met-enk, DAMGO, or the selective DOR agonist [D-Pen, D-Pen] enkephalin (DPDPE), leads to the inhibition of the chemotactic response of leukocytes to complement-derived chemotactic factors, and to the chemokine macrophage inflammatory protein. The activation of MOR and DORs produce desensitization of the CC chemokine receptor 2, and the CXC subtype chemokine receptors CXCR1 and CXCR2. In fact, the latter two receptors become phosphorylated by prior administration of opioids. Other chemokine receptors affected by pretreatment include CCL3 and CCL5. This receptor crosstalk resulting in heterologous desensitization and phosphorylation of some chemokine receptors may contribute to the suppressive effects of the opioids. Opiates acting through DOR and MORs expressed on human monocytes and neutrophils are capable of inhibiting subsequent migratory responses to chemokines.

Conversely, the chemotactic activities of MOR and DOR were desensitized following activation of different chemokine receptors.[66] For this reason, the process should be considered bidirectional, with desensitization of opioid receptors by chemotactic factors, as well as desensitization of chemotactic receptors by the use of MOR and DOR receptor agonists. Therefore, in episodes of acute inflammation and tissue injury, elevated levels of chemokines in the brain would result in altered neuronal function and reduce MOR-mediated analgesia. On the other hand, the immunomodulatory role of endogenous opiates may be modulation of the leukocyte recruitment at the site of inflammation. The precise mechanisms for the development of the desensitization of chemokine receptors are not well understood. It seems that the forceful relation of the G-inhibitory transmembrane receptor that has been previously observed does not translate into protein C forceful relation in the intracellular portion of the receptor, which leads to a lack of indenization chemokine-induced CA^2 class flux and absence of chemokine receptor indenization by opioids. It is also known that the chemokine receptor desensitization is not mediated by NO as other effects of morphine on leukocytes are. It is also not well understood what the role of the KOR receptor is, as the KOR agonist does not have chemokines effects. On the other hand, KOR activation in heated replication of HIV-1 microglial cells suggests a divergence between blood monocytes and tissue macrophage in opioid receptor expression or responsiveness.[67,68]

Recent evidence suggests that morphine-induced modulation of chemokines may facilitate encephalopathy, which is a governed manifestation of many retroviolent infections and is one of the AIDS-defining conditions associated with HIV-1 infection. Patients infected with HIV-1 expressed an elevated level of IL-8 that may be responsible for some of the clinical features of AIDS.[69] HIV-derived viral proteins activate endothelial cells in the CNS to produce IL-8, which acts as a stimulator and chemoattractant for neutrophils and lymphocytes.

Both microglia and astrocytes produce alpha and beta chemokines.[70] Seven members of the chemokine receptor family, including CCR 3, CCR 5, CXCR 2, and CXCR 4, which have been detected in human brain cells, including microglia, astrocytes, neurons, and vascular endothelial cells, have also been identified as HIV-1 core receptors, that, in conjunction with the $C4^+$ receptor, mediate the entry of the virus into target cells.[71,72] Using cell cultures for astrocytoma cell line U87 on primary normal human astrocyte (NHA), it has been demonstrated that in vitro cultured cells exposed to progressively higher concentrations of morphine decreased their IL-8 gene expression, while increasing the expression of the CXCR 2 receptor gene. It was also found that morphine could induce the expression of the genes of the chemokines receptor. HIV coreceptors CCR5 and CCR3 concomitantly inhibit both the expression of the genes of the HIV-protected chemokines IL-8 and macrophage inflammatory protein-1 beta and the synthesis of both proteins by natural human astrocytes.[71] The alpha and beta chemokines, which are expressed during the subacute, acute, and chronic stages of HIV-1 infection, may play an important role in trafficking mononuclear pyocytes within the brain. The mechanism by which morphine decreases the secretion of alpha and beta chemokines (important inhibitory cytokines for the expression of HIV), and at the same time increases the expression of chemokine receptors CCR 5 and CCR 3 (coreceptors for HIV) seems to be mediated by the MOR, as those effects were completely blocked by the additional of β-funaprexamine (a selected MOR antagonist). Therefore, MOR is pivotal in mediating the immunomodulatory effects of opioids on astroglia cells of the CNS.[71] This morphine regulation of the expression of both CCR 5 and CCR 4, which are the two major HIV-1 core receptors, might also be seen in the periphery, including the expression of CCR 5 in monocytes and T-cells. This significantly increases the susceptibility to HIV infection. As previously described, KOR antagonist decreased the susceptibility to HIV by inhibiting the expression of CXCR 4 by CD-4 cells, which is associated with decreased susceptibility to infection with X4-strain of HIV-1.[43,73,74]

Miscellaneous Topics

Heroin (diacetylmorphine) administration has been shown to alter the induction of nitric oxide, a molecule known to play a critical role in the regulation of immune responses and resistance to infectious challenges.

Another area of interest in the relationship of exogenous opiates and the immune system is the activation of angiogenesis and endothelial microvascular proliferation observed in vivo and in vitro after morphine injection. Morphine in clinically relevant doses promotes tumor neovascularization in a human breast tumor xenograft model in mice, leading to increased tumor progression. Despite all the in vivo evidence of morphine-mediated immunosuppression, analgesic doses of morphine significantly reduce the tumor-promoting effects from surgery. Binding sites for opioids in lymphocytes, astrocytes, microglia, and endothelial cells (normal and cancer cells), and (possibly) the peripheral nerves, have been referred as mu 3 receptors. Some opiates, such as morphine and methadone, interact with mu 3 receptors, while others such as fentanyl do not. The activation of mu 3 opioid receptors induces the release of NO. Thus, morphine or methadone may down-regulate the inflammatory response related to surgery by increase of NO release from endothelial cells and decrease granulocyte adherence. Methadone and morphine have also been found to be potent inducers of apoptosis in several types of human cancer cells, resulting in the inhibition of tumor growth.[75,76] In human lung cancer cells, treatment with methadone or morphine produced morphologic and cleavage changes of DNA, which are characteristic of apoptosis. These changes were blocked by naloxone, which also blocks mu-3 receptor. The apoptotic effect appears to be partially mediated by down-regulation of protein kinase C activity and by the antisomatostatin effects of morphine.[76]

The somatostatin receptor is part of the seven-transmembrane spanning G protein-coupled receptors that include opioid and bombesin receptor. Methadone's inhibition of MAP kinase activity and of *bcl-2* oncogene may also be explained through a nonopioid mechanism involving the bombesin receptor. This receptor is known to play a central role in the early events of pulmonary carcinogenesis.[77] Some opioids may induce immunosuppression and cause tumor growth, whereas others, such as methadone and possibly morphine may have a more favorable profile, by favoring apoptosis of tumor cells.

CONCLUSION

Opiates behave like cytokines. Their similarity to cytokines, including pleiotropy and redundancy, implicate complex interactions with multiple cell types and unpredictable biologic effects. While endogenous opioids enhance some immune functions, exogenous opiates do the opposite. Direct and indirect effects, mediated by the interaction of the opioid receptors with their endogenous or exogenous ligands determine activation or inhibition of cellular mediated immune function, respectively. Opioid receptors that mediate immunosuppression are located in the CNS, peripheral sensory neurons, and immune cells.

Clinically, the interaction of opioids with other cytokines, including chemokines and their receptors, and associated inhibition of the cellular response, predispose to the propagation of HIV infection in heroin addicts. The effects of acute and chronic opioid therapy after surgery or in patients with chronic pain need to be elucidated. The fact that surgery and pain create a state of immunosuppression and the complex interaction between opioids and the immune system makes it difficult to weigh the impact of each one of these factors in the perioperative immunosuppression.

Another clinically relevant question is whether or not this immunosuppression has positive or negative consequences in the development of cancer. Evidence of the apoptotic effects exerted by certain opioids make this question even more difficult to answer. It is possible that the route of opioid administration, may affect the immune system differently. Theoretically, the intrathecal route may avoid central (PAG) and peripheral opioid receptors, thus being less likely to induce immunosuppression. Long-term, randomized control studies in patients exposed to chronic opioid therapy are warranted in order to determine the clinical implications of such therapies.

ACKNOWLEDGMENTS

I would like to acknowledge the assistance of Gail Livingston, Stephanie Oliver, Jennifer Johns, and Kristine Dennis in the manuscript preparation and editing of this chapter.

REFERENCES

1. Rogers TJ, Peterson PK: Opioid G protein-coupled receptors: Signals of the crossroads of inflammation. Trends Immunol 24(3):116–121, 2003.
2. Pilowsky I: Illness behavior and sociocultural aspects of pain. In: Kosterlitzs HW, Terenius LY (eds): Pain and Society. Weinheim, Germany, Verlag Chemie, 1980, pp 445–460.
3. Schmitz R: Friedrich Wilhelm Serturner and the discovery of morphine. Pharm Hist 27(2):61–74, 1985.
4. O'Callaghan JP: Evolution of a rational use of opioids in chronic pain. Eur J Pain 5(suppl A):21–26, 2001.
5. Pert CB, Snyder SH: Properties of opiate-receptor binding in rat brain. Proc Natl Acad Sci USA 70(8):2243–2247, 1973.
6. Stein C: The control of pain in peripheral tissue by opioids. N Engl J Med 332(25):1685–1690, 1995.
7. Kieffer BL: Recent advances in molecular recognition and signal transduction of active peptides: Receptor for opioid peptides. Cell Mol Neurobiol 15(6):615–635, 1995.
8. Noda M, Furutani Y, Takahasi H, et al: Cloning and sequence analysis of cDNA

for bovine adrenal proenkephalin. Nature 295(5846):202–206, 1982.

9. Kakidani H, Furutani Y, Takahashi H, et al: Cloning and sequence analysis of cDNA for porcine β-neo-endorphin/dynorphin precursor. Nature 298(5871):245–249, 1982.

10. Nakanishi S, Inoue A, Kita T, et al: Nucleotide sequence of cloned cDNA for bovine corticotropin-beta-lipotropin precursor. Nature 278(5703):423–427, 1979.

11. Hughes J, Smith TW, Kosterlitz HW, et al: Identification of two related pentapeptides from the brain with potent opioid agonist activity. Nature 285(5536):577–580, 1975.

12. Li CH, Chung D: Isolation and structure of an untriakontapeptide with opiate activity from camel pituitary glands. Proc Natl Acad Sci USA 73(4):1145–1148, 1976.

13. Pasternak GW, Simantov R, Snyder SH: Characterization of and endogenous morphine-like factor (enkephalin) in mammalian brain. Mol Pharmacol 12(3):504–513, 1976.

14. Stein C, Machelska H, Schafer M: Peripheral analgesic and anti-inflammatory effects of opioids. Z Rheumatol 60(6):416–424, 2001.

15. Wall PD: On the relation of injury to pain. The John T. Bonica lecture. Pain 6:253–264, 1979.

16. Walkins LR, Maier SF (eds): Illness-induced hyperalgesia: Mediators, mechanisms and implications. In: Cytokines and Pain. Basel, Switzerland, Birkhauser, 1999, pp 39–57.

17. Peterson PK, Molitor TW, Chao CC: The opioid-cytokine connection. J Neuroimmunol 83(1–2):63–69, 1998.

18. Patel K, Bhaskaran M, Dani D, et al: Role of heme oxygenase-1 in morphine-modulated apoptosis and migration of macrophages. J Infect Dis 187(1):47–54, 2003.

19. Mathews PM, Froelich CJ, Sibbitt WL Jr, Bankhurst AD: Enhancement of natural cytotoxicity by beta-endorphin. J Immunol 130(4):1658–1662, 1983.

20. Sacerdote P, Bianchi M, Gaspani L, et al: The effects of tramadol and morphine on immune responses and pain after surgery in cancer patients. Anesth Analg 90(6):1411–1414, 2000.

21. Carr DJ, Serou M: Exogenous and endogenous opioids as biological response modifiers. Immunopharmacology 31(1):59–71, 1995.

22. Shavit Y, Depaulis A, Martin FC, et al: Involvement of brain opiate receptors in the immune-suppressive effect of morphine. Proc Natl Acad Sci USA 83(18):7114–7117, 1986.

23. Hoffman KE, Maslonek KA, Dykstra LA, Lysle DT: Effects of central administration of morphine on immune status in Lewis and Wistar rats. Adv Exp Med Biol 373:155–159, 1995.

24. Lysle DT, Hoffman KE, Dykstra LA: Evidence for the involvement of the caudal region of the periaqueductal gray in a subset of morphine-induced alterations of immune status. J Pharmacol Exp Ther 277(3):1533–1540, 1996.

25. Mellon RD, Bayer BM: Evidence for central opioid receptors in the immunomodulatory effects of morphine: Review of potential mechanism(s) of action. J Neuroimmunol 83(1–2):19–28, 1998.

26. Band LC, Pert A, Williams W, et al: Central opioid receptors mediate suppression of NK cell activity in vivo. Prog Neurol Endocrinol Immunol 5:95–101, 1992.

27. Hsueh CM, Chen SF, Ghanta VK, Hiramoto RN: Expression of the conditioned NK cell activity is beta-endorphin dependent. Brain Res 678(1–2):76–82, 1995.

28. Hsueh CM, Hiramoto RN, Ghanta VK: The central effect of methionine-enkephalin on NK cell activity. Brain Res 578(1–2):142–148, 1992.

29. Flores LR, Hernandez MC, Bayer BM: Acute immunosuppressive effects of morphine: Lack of involvement of pituitary and adrenal factors. J Pharmacol Exp Ther 268(3):1129–1134, 1994.

30. Hamra JG, Yaksh TL: Equianalgesic doses of subcutaneous but not intrathecal morphine alter phenotypic expression of cell surface markers and mitogen-induced proliferation in rat lymphocytes. Anesthesiology 85(2):355–365, 1996.

31. Hernandez MC, Flores LR, Bayer BM: Immunosuppression by morphine is mediated by central pathways. J Pharmacol Exp Ther 267(3):1336–1341, 1993.

32. Roy S, Barke RA, Loh HH: MU-opioid receptor-knockout mice: Role of mu-opioid receptor in morphine mediated immune functions. Brain Res Mol Brain Res 61(1–2):190–194, 1998.

33. Fecho K, Maslonek KA, Dykstra LA, Lysle DT: Mechanisms whereby macrophage-derived nitric oxide is involved in morphine-induced suppression of splenic lymphocyte proliferation. J Pharmacol Exp Ther 272(2):477–483, 1995.

34. Radulovic J, Jankovic BD: Opposing activities of brain opioid receptors in the regulation of humoral and cell-mediated immune responses in the rat. Brain Res 661(1–2):189–195, 1994.

35. Dimitrijevic M, Stanojevic S, Kovacevic-Jovanovic V, et al: Modulation of humoral immune responses in the rat by centrally applied Met-Enk and opioid receptor antagonists: Functional interactions of brain OP1, OP2 and OP3 receptors. Immunopharmacology 49(3):255–262, 2000.

36. Jankovic BD, Veljic J, Pesic G, Maric D: Enkephalinase-inhibiters modulate immune responses. Int J Neurosci 59(1–3):45–51, 1991.

37. Radulovic J, Miljevic C, Djergovic D, et al: Opioid receptor-mediated suppression of humoral immune response in vivo and in vitro: Involvement of kappa opioid receptors. J Neuroimmunol 57(1–2):55–62, 1995.

38. Veljic J, Ranin J, Maric D, Jankovic BD: Modulation of cutaneous immune reactions by centrally applied methionine-enkephalin. Ann N Y Acad Sci 650:51–55, 1992.

39. Roy S, Loh HH: Effects of opioids on the immune system. Neurochem Res 21(11):1375–1386, 1996.

40. Bryant HU, Bernton EW, Holaday JW: Immunosuppressive effects of chronic morphine treatment in mice. Life Sci 41(14):1731–1738, 1987.

41. Bryant HU, Bernton EW, Kenner JR, Holaday JW: Role of adrenal cortical activation in the immunosuppressive effects of chronic morphine treatment. Endocrinology 128(6):3253–3258, 1991.

42. Freier DO, Fuchs BA: A mechanism of action for morphine-induced immunosuppression: Corticosteroid mediates morphine-induced suppression of natural killer cell activity. J Pharmacol Exp Ther 270(3):1127–1133, 1994.

43. Bryant HU, Roudebush RE: Suppressive effects of morphine pellet implants on in vivo parameters of immune function. J Pharmacol Exp Ther 255(2):410–414, 1990.

44. Bryant HU, Bernton EW, Holaday JW: Immunomodulatory effects of chronic morphine treatment: Pharmacologic and mechanistic studies. NIDA Res Monogr 96:131–149, 1990.

45. Gomes C, Svensson TH, Trolin G: Effects of morphine on systemic catecholamine turn over, blood pressure and heart rate in the rat. Naunyn Schmiedebergs Arch Pharmacol 294:141–147, 1996.

46. Vogel WH, Miller J, DeTurck KH, Routzahn BK Jr: Effects of psychoactive drugs on plasma catecholamines during stress in rats. Neuropharmocology 23(9):1105–1108, 1984.

47. Carr DJ, Gebhardt BM, Paul D: Alpha adrenergic and mu-2 opioid receptors are involved in morphine-induced suppression of splenocyte natural killer activity. J Pharmacol Exp Ther 264(3):1179–1186, 1993.

48. Carr DJ, Mayo S, Gebhardt BM, Porter J: Central alpha-adrenergic involvement in morphine-mediated suppression of splenic natural killer activity. J Neuroimmunol 53(1):53–63, 1994.

49. Fecho K, Dykstra LA, Lysle DT: Evidence for beta adrenergic receptor involvement in the immunomodulatory effects of morphine. J Pharmacol Exp Ther 265(3):1079–1087, 1993.

50. Fecho K, Maslonek KA, Dykstra LA, Lysle DT: Assessment of the involvement of central nervous system and peripheral opioid receptors in the immunomodulatory effects of acute morphine treatment in rats. J Pharmacol Exp Ther 276(2):626–636, 1996.

51. Eisenstein PK, Hilburger ME, Laewrence DMP: Immunomodulation by morphine and other opioids. In: Friedman H, Klein TW, Specter S (eds): (SVES) Drugs of Abuse, Immunity and Infection. Boca Raton, Fla, CRC Press, 1996, pp 103–120.

52. Houghtling RA, Bayer BM: Rapid elevation of plasma interleukin-6 by morphine is dependent on autonomic stimulation of adrenal gland. J Phamacol Exp Ther 300(1):213–219, 2002.

53. Carr DJ, DeCosta BR, Kim CH, et al: Opioid receptors on cells of the immune system: Evidence for delta- and kappa-classes. J Endocrinol 122(1):161–168, 1989.

54. Makman MH: Morphine receptors in immunocytes and neurons. Adv Neuroimmunol 4(2):69–82, 1994.

55. Chuang TK, Killam KF Jr, Chuang LF, et al: Mu opioid receptor gene expression in immune cells. Biochem Biophys Res Commun 216(3):923–930, 1995.

56. Stephanou A, Fitzharris P, Knight RA, Lightman SL: Characteristics and kinetics of proopiomelanocortin mRNA expression by human leukocytes. Brain Behav Immun 5(4):319–327, 1991.

57. Westley HJ, Kleiss AJ, Kelley KW, et al: New Castle disease virus-infected splenocytes express the proopiomelanocortin gene. J Exp Med 163:1589–1594, 1986.

58. Zurawski G, Benedik M, Kamb BJ, et al: Activation of mouse T-helper cells induces abundant preproenkephalin mRNA synthesis. Science 232(4751):772–775, 1986.

59. Linner KM, Quist HE, Sharp BM: Met-enkephalin-containing peptides encoded by proenkephalin A mRNA expressed in activated murine thymocytes inhibit thymocyte proliferation. J Immunol 154(10):5049–5060, 1995.

60. Cabot PJ, Carter L, Schafer M, Stein C: Methionine-enkephalin- and dynorphin A-release from immune cells and control of inflammatory pain. Pain 93(3):207–212, 2001.

61. Hori T, Nakashima T, Take S, et al: Immune cytokines and regulation of body temperature, food intake, and cellular immunity. Brain Res Bull 27(3-4):309–313, 1991.

62. Ahmed MS, Llanos QJ, Dinarello CA, Blatteis CM: Interleukin 1 reduces opioid binding in guinea pig brain. Peptides 6(6):1149–1154, 1985.

63. Jeanjean AP, Moussaoui SM, Maloteaux JM, Laduron PM: Interleukin-1β induces long-term increase of axonally transported opiate receptors and substance P. Neuroscience 68(1):151–157, 1995.

64. Low KG, Allen RG, Melner MH: Differential regulation of proenkephalin expression in astrocytes by cytokines. Endocrinology 131(4):1908–1914, 1992.

65. Steine-Martin A, Hauser KF: Opioid-dependent growth glial cultures: Suppression of astrocyte DNA synthesis by met-enkephalin. Life Sci 46(2):91–98, 1990.

66. Szabo A, Xiaiao-Hong, Szabo I, et al: Heterologous desensitization of opioid receptors by chemokines inhibits chemotactics and enhances the perception of pain. PNAS 99(16):10276–10281, 2002.

67. Grimm MC, Ben-Baruch A, Taub DD, et al: Opiates transdeactivate chemokine receptors: Delta and mu opiate receptor-mediated heterologous desensitization. J Exp Med 188(2): 317–325, 1998.

68. Magazine HI, Liu Y, Bilfinger TV, et al: Morphine-induced conformational changes in human monocytes, granulocytes, and endothelial cells and in invertebrate immunocytes and microglia are mediated by nitric oxide. J Immunol 156(12): 4845–4850, 1996.

69. Hofman FM, Chen P, Incardona F, et al: HIV-1 tat protein induces the production of interleukin-8 by human brain-derived endothelial cells. J Neuroimmunol 94(1-2):28–39, 1999.

70. Nitta T, Allegretta M, Okumura K, et al: Neoplastic and reactive astrocytes express interleukin-8 gene. Neurosurg Rev 15(3):203–207, 1992.

71. Mahajan SD, Schwartz SA, Shanahan TC, et al: Morphine regulates gene expression of alpha- and beta-chemokines and their receptors on astroglial cells via the opioid mu receptor. J Immunol 169(7): 3589–3599, 2002.

72. Mukakami T, Yamamoto N: Role of chemokines on chemokine receptors in HIV-1 infection. J Hematol 72:412, 2000.

73. Steele AD, Henderson EE, Rogers TJ: Mu-opioid modulation of HIV-1 coreceptor expression and HIV-1 replication. Virology 24(3):116–121, 2003.

74. Lokensgard JR, Gekker G, Peterson PK: Kappa-opioid receptor agonist inhibition of HIV-1 envelope glycoprotein-mediated membrane fusion and CXCR4 expression on CD4(+) lymphocytes. Biochem Pharmacol 63(6):1037–1041, 2002.

75. Page GG, Blakely WP, Ben-Eliyahu S: Evidence that postoperative pain is a mediator of the tumor-promoting effects of surgery in rats. Pain 90(1-2):191–199, 2001.

76. Maneckjee R: Anticancer effects of therapeutic opioids. Pain Forum 8:213–215, 1999.

77. Maneckjee R, Minna JD: Opioids induce while nicotine suppresses apoptosis in human lung cancer cells. Cell Growth Diff 5:1033–1040, 1994.

CHAPTER 18

Management of Opioid-Related Side Effects

JUAN-DIEGO HARRIS, MD, CCFP, AND FAYEZ KOTOB, MD

The use of opioids for the management of cancer pain has increased significantly over the past two decades.[1,2] This has resulted in improved pain management and quality of life for cancer patients, but it has also resulted in increased reports of opioid side effects (Table 18–1), in particular neurotoxicity. Up to 30% of patients receiving opioids for cancer pain have unacceptable side effects, poor analgesia, or both.[3] Thus, the effective management of opioid-related side effects cannot be understated. Some patients can even under-report pain because they are fearful of potential opioid side effects. This chapter provides a brief overview of the etiology of opioid-related side effects, but its focus is on strategies that can be used to prevent and manage them.

GENERAL STRATEGIES TO MANAGE OPIOID SIDE EFFECTS

There are different therapeutic strategies that can be used to manage opioid-related side effects.[4] Figure 18–1 provides a useful guide to manage opioid side effects based on the review of the literature and clinical experience. It is important to carefully evaluate the patient to rule out other causes for the adverse effects. Biochemical imbalances such as hypercalcemia, dehydration, infection, brain metastasis, and other medications, such as tricyclic antidepressants, corticosteroids, and benzodiazepines, can be responsible for similar side effects.[3]

Decreasing Opioid Dose

If a patient's pain is well controlled but side effects are intolerable, gradual reduction of the dose by 25% to 50% can result in diminished side effects while retaining adequate pain control.[3] If the pain is not well controlled, it is important to optimize the use of adjuvant analgesics or consider regional anesthetic blocks. In addition,

palliative radiation, chemotherapy, or surgery that targets the cause of the pain are alternative strategies.

Changing the Route of Administration

There is evidence suggesting that parenteral (intravenous or subcutaneous) administration of opioids causes less accumulation of toxic metabolites as compared with oral administration.[3] This can lead to decreased toxicity and may be of particular importance in patients with renal or advanced hepatic impairment, in which toxic metabolites have a greater propensity to accumulate.[5] This strategy can be attractive in a setting in which there may not be other opioids available. Other alternative routes include rectal, transdermal, and transmucosal administration. Epidural and intrathecal administration may also lead to decreased side effects.[6]

Pharmacologic Management of Side Effects

The use of medications to manage opioid-related side effects is common. Even though this is the case, only a few studies have evaluated prospectively the efficacy of these approaches, and there are no data evaluating the potential toxicity over the long term.[3] In addition, the use of multiple medications can lead to complications from lack of compliance and drug interactions,[3] as well as increased costs.

Opioid Rotation

Switching from one opioid to another has been performed with increasing frequency over the past decade. In some cancer centers, more than 40% of patients receiving opioids for pain management require at least one opioid rotation.[7,8] Switching the administered opioid allows for the clearance of toxic opioid metabolites and of the

TABLE 18–1 Opioid-Related Side Effects

Neurologic
Delirium
Hallucinations
Sedation
Myoclonus
Hyperalgesia
Muscle rigidity
Seizures
Headaches
Cardiopulmonary
Respiratory depression
Non-cardiogenic pulmonary edema
Bradycardia
Hypotension
Cardiac dysrhythmias
Gastrointestinal
Nausea and Vomiting
Constipation
Xerostomia
Gastroesophageal reflux disease
Obstruction of the common bile duct
Urologic
Altered kidney function
Urinary retention
Peripheral edema
Endocrinologic
Hypogonadism/Sexual dysfunction
Osteoporosis
Dermatologic
Pruritus
Diaphoresis
Immunologic
Immune Suppression

opioid itself, resulting in a decrease in opioid adverse effects and improved pain relief.[6] It is an important strategy to consider because clinical studies have shown that patients who do not tolerate one opioid will frequently tolerate others with diminished side effects or increased analgesia, or both. This is because each opioid interacts in a unique manner at the mu-opioid receptors (the main opioid receptors). In addition, there is likely variability in the amount and types of receptors among different individuals.[9,10]

In recent years, methadone has become an attractive alternative for opioid rotation. It has no known neuro-active metabolites, has excellent oral and rectal bioavailability, potential additional benefit for neuropathic pain, minimal renal clearance (and thus it does not accumulate in renal failure), and an extremely low cost.[4,11,12] Guidelines on how to implement an opioid rotation are given in Chapter 16.

MANAGEMENT OF SPECIFIC OPIOID-RELATED SIDE EFFECTS

Table 18-1 provides a comprehensive list of the opioid-related side effects that are discussed in this chapter. It is important to note that the degree of severity of these side effects is variable from person to person. In addition, they can occur with any of the opioids (i.e., they are not limited to morphine). Some of these side effects are experienced more commonly than others (e.g., nausea and vomiting, constipation, and sedation); some more often with chronic opioid therapy (e.g., hypogonadism and sexual dysfunction); others more commonly with higher opioid doses (e.g., hyperalgesia); and others are just starting to be described in the literature (e.g., osteoporosis and immune suppression).

GASTROINTESTINAL SIDE EFFECTS

Nausea and Vomiting

More than 50% of patients with advanced malignancies suffer nausea and vomiting (NV) during their illness,[13] with increasing frequency during the last weeks of life.[14] Up to 40% of the time it can be secondary to opioid use.[15] Inadequate management can worsen quality of life and lead to increased length of stays in hospitals.[16]

Opioid-induced NV involves various mechanisms of action. Nausea results from stimulation of the chemoreceptor trigger zone (CTZ), the vestibular apparatus, the gastrointestinal tract, and the cerebral cortex. Vomiting is a neuromuscular reflex caused by stimulation of these areas. This process is coordinated by the vomiting center (Figure 18-2), which is a nucleus of cells located in the medulla oblongata that receives afferent input from the previously listed areas. There are multiple emetogenic receptors in the central nervous system (CNS): dopaminergic, muscarinic, cholinergic, histaminic, and serotonergic. Blocking of these receptors is the basis of the antiemetic medications.[17]

The CTZ is located in the area postrema of the brainstem and is exposed to the systemic circulation. Opioids can exert a strong emetic effect by direct

FIGURE 18-1   General guide for the
management of opioid-related side effects.

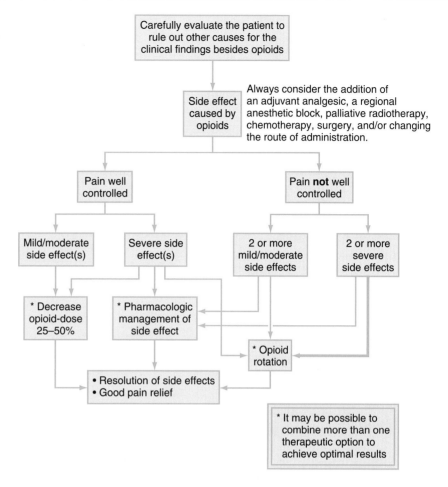

FIGURE 18-1   General guide for the management of opioid-related side effects.

stimulation of the CTZ. In the vestibular system, opioids increase vestibular sensitivity to movement.[18] In the gastrointestinal tract, opioids cause delayed gastric emptying[6] and decreased propulsion and motility. This can contribute to NV by stimulating mechanoreceptors and chemoreceptors, which send ascending signals to the vomiting center via the vagus nerve.[17] Stimulation of

the cerebral cortex can also lead to NV. This action does not appear to be mediated by specific neurotransmitters, but rather learned responses. For example, this stimulus can result from a patient remembering nausea associated with past opioid therapy.[19]

Tolerance to NV tends to develop after a few days.[6] But in some patients it becomes a chronic problem

FIGURE 18-2   Mechanisms of opioid-induced nausea and vomiting and sites of mechanism of action of commonly used antiemetics. (Modified from Herndon CM, Jackson KC, 2nd, Hallin PA: Management of opioid-induced gastrointestinal effects in patients receiving pallative care. Pharmacotherapy 22:240-250, 2002.)

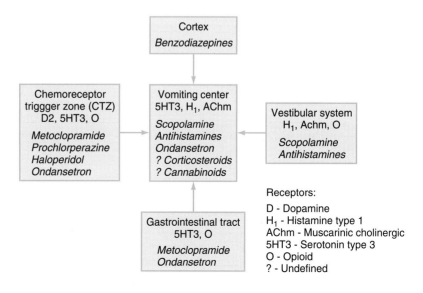

(15% to 30% on oral morphine).[3] Other causes of NV include accumulation of opioid metabolites (e.g., morphine-6-glucuronide [M6G]), particularly in chronic cases.[20] The presence of uncontrolled pain can also be a stimulus for vomiting.[21]

Management

Before instituting antiemetic therapy, it is important to rule out a bowel obstruction and severe constipation or impaction as the cause. Other causes include autonomic failure, metabolic abnormalities, chemotherapy, radiotherapy, infection, cachexia, and other medications.[14]

The various antiemetics used (Table 18–2) have limited randomized, placebo-controlled studies in the cancer population not receiving radiation or chemotherapy. Thus, treatment decisions result mainly from extrapolated data from studies dealing with management of postoperative opioid-induced NV, chemotherapy and radiation-induced NV, and from expert opinion.

There is no convincing evidence indicating that prophylactic antiemetic treatment should be given routinely to prevent opioid-induced NV. Suggested guidelines are presented in Figure 18–3. Dopamine receptor antagonists are often used as first-line therapy because of their strong action in the CTZ, an area with high concentration of opioid receptors. For intractable NV, a multimodal approach combining antiemetics targeting different receptors is recommended.

Dopamine Receptor Antagonists

These are commonly used as first-line antiemetics for opioid-induced NV because of their direct action in the CTZ. Potential adverse effects include dry mouth, sedation, and extrapyramidal symptoms (akathesia, dystonic effects, pseudo-parkinsonism, and tardive dyskinesia).[17] These are further divided into benzamides, butyrophenones, and phenothiazines. Dopamine (D) receptor antagonists commonly used in the management of opioid-induced NV are metoclopramide, haloperidol, and prochlorperazine.

Metoclopramide. Metoclopramide is a benzamide commonly used in cancer patients. It is a strong D_2 receptor antagonist and weak serotonin receptor antagonist and has both a peripheral and a central action. In the periphery, it increases lower esophageal sphincter tone and promotes gastrointestinal motility, thus preventing the delayed gastric emptying caused by opioids.[17] Centrally, it acts mainly at the CTZ. In low doses (10 mg) it has relatively few side effects.

Haloperidol. Haloperidol is a butyrophenone commonly used as an antiemetic in the palliative care setting.[22] It has strong D_2 receptor antagonistic activity at the CTZ and no gastrointestinal effect. Its duration of action can last up to 12 hours.[17] Older individuals are potentially more prone to its anticholinergic and parkinsonian side effects because of decreases in cholinergic and dopaminergic neurons with age.[19]

Prochlorperazine. Prochlorperazine is a phenothiazine with direct D_2 antagonistic effect at the CTZ, plus moderate antihistamine and anticholinergic action.[17] Their dopaminergic antagonistic effect is less potent than haloperidol, but it is often preferred because of its lower incidence of extrapyramidal symptoms, even though it is more sedating.[17] Prochlorperazine is only slightly effective against motion sickness and has no gastrointestinal effect.[23]

TABLE 18–2 Management of Opioid-Induced Nausea and Vomiting

Drug	Dose	Route
Dopamine Receptor Antagonists		
Metoclopramide	10–20 mg q4–6h	PO/SC/IV
Haloperidol	0.5–2 mg q6–12h	PO/SC/IV/PR
Prochlorperazine	10–20 mg q6h	PO/IV
	25 mg q6h	PR
Anticholinergics		
Scopolamine	1–3 patches q72h	Transdermal
	0.1–0.4 mg q4–6h	SC/IV
Antihistamines		
Dimenhydrinate	50–100 mg q4–6h	PO/IV
Diphenhydramine	25–50 mg q4–6h	PO/IV
Hydroxyzine	25–50 mg q6h	PO
Meclizine	25–50 mg q6h	PO
Benzodiazepines		
Lorazepam	0.5–2 mg q4–6h	PO/SC/IV/PR
Serotonin Receptor Antagonists		
Ondansetron	4–8 mg BID–TID	PO/IV
Granisetron	1 mg daily–BID	PO/IV
Dolasetron	100 mg daily	PO/IV
Corticosteroids		
Dexamethasone	4–20 mg/day divided BID–QID	PO/IV
Cannabinoids		
Dronabinol	2.5–5 mg TID	PO

BID, twice daily; *IV*, intravenously; *PO*, per os; *PR*, per rectum; *QID*, four times a day; *qxh*, every x hours; *SC*, subcutaneously; *TID*, three times a day.

FIGURE 18-3 Guidelines for the management of opioid-induced nausea and vomiting.

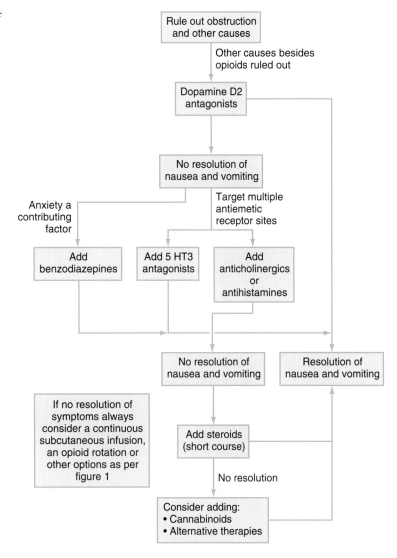

FIGURE 18-3 Guidelines for the management of opioid-induced nausea and vomiting.

Anticholinergics

Anticholinergics (e.g., scopolamine) are potent inhibitors of muscarinic and cholinergic CNS emetic receptors.[17] They exert their antiemetic action at the vestibular apparatus and the vomiting center. Scopolamine is commonly used in this category and has been shown to be effective.[17,24] The main disadvantages are the anticholinergic side effects (e.g., dry mouth, sedation, blurred vision, urinary retention, and confusion), but these tend to occur infrequently at the doses used.[19]

Antihistamines

Antihistamines (e.g., diphenhydramine, dimenhydrinate, hydroxyzine, meclizine) block acetylcholine and histamine H_1 receptors in the vestibular apparatus and the vomiting center,[17,19] and have little action in the CTZ. Sedation is a frequent limiting side effect. Other side effects include dry mouth, blurred vision, and urinary retention.[17]

Benzodiazepines

Benzodiazepines (e.g., lorazepam, midazolam, diazepam) do not appear to show true antiemetic receptor binding affinity, but decrease anxiety by decreasing the production of catecholamines.[17] Thus, they may be beneficial in the treatment of opioid-induced nausea of anticipatory origin.[19]

Serotonin Receptor Antagonists

These 5-hydroxytryptamine type 3 ($5HT_3$) receptor antagonists (e.g., ondansetron, granisetron, tropisetron, dolasetron) are effective in the control of opioid-induced NV[25] and do not have the side effects of the older traditional antiemetics discussed earlier. In general, they are very well tolerated. Headache and dizziness are their main side effects.[17] They should not be considered first-line therapy because they are expensive and have not been shown to be superior to other antiemetics in this setting. They are usually reserved for refractory cases, often used in combination with other antiemetics.[26] $5HT_3$ receptors are located in the CTZ, the vomiting center, and peripherally on vagal nerve terminals.[21]

Corticosteroids

The antiemetic effect of corticosteroids is not completely understood, but may be via an anti-inflammatory component or an antiprostaglandin effect.[17] They are a useful adjunct for NV and have been used effectively in combinations with metoclopramide[14] and serotonin receptor antagonists.[23,27] Because of the side effect profile of steroids, if used on a long-term basis, it is important to use the minimal effective dose possible. Dexamethasone is commonly used. Its duration of action is greater than 24 hours.[28]

Cannabinoids

Dronabinol is the major active ingredient in marijuana (delta-9-tetrahydrocannabinol). It is clinically indicated for the use of chemotherapy-induced NV.[29] Animal studies have shown that cannabinoid receptor agonists' activity at CB_1 receptors (the main cannabinoid receptor subtypes identified) prevent opioid-induced vomiting by inhibiting the action of the vomiting center.[30] However, there are no controlled studies showing its benefit in opioid-induced NV in humans. A trial of dronabinol may be useful in refractory cases.

Nonpharmacologic Management

Acupressure at the P6 (Nei-Kuan) point in the wrist via an elastic pressure band with spherical beads or through transcutaneous acupoint electrical stimulation (TAES) has been used effectively for postoperative NV[17] and may be an alternative to conventional antiemetic treatment in opioid-induced NV; more research in nonpharmacological approaches is needed.

Constipation

Constipation is defined as infrequent or difficult bowel movements.[31] Objectively, patients who have less than three bowel movements per week may be considered to be constipated.[32] Constipation is the most frequent opioid side effect associated with long-term therapy, reported in 40% to 90% of advanced cancer patients receiving opioids.[33-35] Even though it is so common, assessment is often neglected when an opioid is started. A full assessment should include a history of bowel movements (before and after opioid therapy) and a physical examination, including a digital rectal examination.[35] If the diagnosis is unclear, an abdominal x-ray may help confirm the diagnosis.[31]

Constipation is caused mainly by a direct action of the opioid in the gastrointestinal tract on opioid receptors present in the gastrointestinal smooth muscle. In addition, direct action in the central nervous system (CNS) may also affect gut motility.[31,36] This results in decreased gastric motility; decreased propulsive peristalsis of both the small and large intestine (leading to decreased absorption of medications, straining, incomplete evacuation, abdominal distension); increased nonpropulsive contractions (leading to cramps and pain and increased oral–cecal transit time); increased anal sphincter tone (leading to difficulty evacuating); decreased gastrointestinal secretions (leading to hard stools); and increased fluid absorption, which also leads to hard stools.[31,36] Although other opioid-related side effects tend to be present more commonly at the initiation of therapy and diminish with time, the constipation effect is dose related, and most patients do not develop tolerance to this side effect, needing to take laxatives on a regular basis. As a result, prophylaxis is an essential step in its management. It can prevent serious complications such as fecal impaction with overflow diarrhea and bowel (pseudo)obstruction.[31,33]

Management

The choice of pharmacologic treatment (Table 18–3) is controversial because of a lack of well-controlled studies in the long-term management of opioid-induced constipation.[31] In addition, laxatives can account for a large number of the oral medications taken, making compliance difficult.[31]

Before instituting laxative therapy, it is important to rule out bowel obstruction, fecal impaction, and other factors besides opioids that are a common cause of constipation in cancer patients. These include biochemical abnormalities (e.g., hypercalcemia, hypokalemia), dehydration, lack of physical activity, and other medications (e.g., antihistamines, nonsteroidal anti-inflammatory drugs [NSAIDs], phenothiazines, tricyclic antidepressants, anticonvulsants, and diuretics).[31]

Figure 18–4 shows recommended guidelines for the management of opioid-induced constipation. Standard prophylactic regimen includes a stool softener and a bowel stimulant. Gradual increase in the doses before adding other laxatives is recommended if constipation is not controlled. For refractory cases, consider changing the route of opioid administration to avoid the oral route. Opioid rotation may also be a useful strategy for the management of constipation. It has been reported in the literature that patients on methadone and fentanyl require fewer laxatives than with other opioids.[35,37] Both are lipophilic and therefore reach the CNS faster than morphine; they may have less affinity for the opioid receptors in the gastrointestinal tract[35,37]; and the

TABLE 18–3 Management of Opioid-Induced Constipation

Drug	Dose	Route
Stimulants		
Senna	2 tabs (1 tab = 8.6 mg) at bedtime up to 3 tabs BID	PO
	1 suppository (30 mg) q2–3 days	PR
Bisacodyl	5 mg at bedtime up to 15 mg BID	PO
	10 mg suppository q2–3 days	PR
Prune juice	120 mL daily up to 240 mL BID	PO
Casanthranol	2 tabs at bedtime up to 8 tabs BID	PO
Stool Softeners		
Docusate sodium	100 mg BID up to 300 mg BID	PO
Osmotic Agents		
Lactulose	15 mL daily up to 30 mL QID	PO
Milk of magnesia	15 mL daily up to 30 mL QID	PO
Magnesium citrate	125 to 250 mL × 1—may repeat in 24 h (for acute short-term management)	PO
Polyethylene glycol	1 tsp in 240 mL of water × 1—may repeat in 24 hr (for acute short-term management)	PO
Lubricant Laxatives		
Mineral oil	15–45 mL daily	PO
	120 mL as an enema	PR
Glycerine suppositories	1 suppository q2–3 days	PR
Enemas		
Various preparations (see text)	1 q3 days prn (for acute short-term management)	PR
Prokinetic Agents		
Metoclopramide	10–20 mg q6h	PO/SC/IV
Domperidone	10–40 mg QID	PO
Erythromycin (see text)		
Opioid Antagonists (see text)		

BID, twice daily; *IV,* intravenously; *PO,* per os; *PR,* per rectum; *QID,* four times a day; *SC,* subcutaneously.

transdermal route of the fentanyl patch directly bypasses the opioid receptors in the gastrointestinal tract.[37]

Nonpharmacologic approaches include increasing fluid intake and level of activity, but these interventions may not always be possible in advanced cancer patients.

Bulk Agents

These (e.g., cellulose, psyllium seeds) agents generally are not recommended in the management of opioid-induced constipation in cancer patients. These supplement the fiber in the diet but require much fluid consumption (>1200 mL/day),[36] which is not always possible for advanced cancer patients. As a result they may worsen symptoms, causing distension, bloating, and abdominal pain.[31] Bulk production may also aggravate a partial bowel obstruction.

Stimulants

These are the most commonly administered laxatives for opioid-induced constipation. They act by increasing peristalsis via direct action in the myenteric plexus and by decreasing water absorption. Short-term use is safe, but long-term complications include damage to the myenteric plexus leading to dependency on the stimulant to produce laxation, as well as dehydration.[31,38] Other side effects include cramps and bloating. The most commonly used are senna, derived from the senna plant, and bisacodyl. They usually exert an effect within 12 to 24 hours. Other stimulants include casanthranol, cascara, danthron, phenolphthalein, oxyphenisatin, and prune juice. Castor oil is also a stimulant with a fast onset of action, but chronic use may lead to nutrient malabsorption, limiting its use for management of acute constipation.[31]

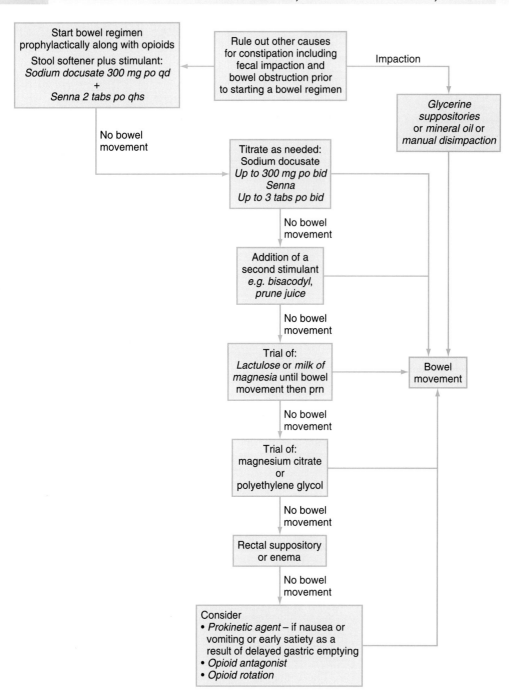

Stool Softeners

They act as surfactants, allowing water to penetrate the stool mass. Docusate is the most commonly used and it is well tolerated. It is considered a stool softener rather than a stimulant, but dosages above 400 mg/day may produce an increase in peristalsis.[19] A systematic review of the literature[39] has questioned its efficacy, even though a combination of a stool softener and a stimulant is standard practice for the prophylactic management of opioid-induced constipation. In addition, there have been some safety concerns regarding hepatotoxicity.[39]

Osmotic Agents

These agents osmotically draw fluids into the bowel, distending it, and inducing peristalsis. Results are usually achieved within 6 hours.[38] It is not a physiologic action, and long-term use should be avoided. Use can lead to electrolyte imbalance, excessive gas, cramps, and dehydration. Special care should be used in patients with cardiac or renal failure.[31] These can be further subdivided into: (1) Saline laxatives, which include magnesium citrate, milk of magnesia, and sodium phosphates. (2) Lactulose and sorbitol, which in addition to an osmotic action, breakdown of its sugars may lower the intestinal pH and further stimulate peristalsis.[19,31] Sorbitol is not used as often, even though it is less expensive, has fewer side effects, and is as efficacious.[19] (3) Polyethylene glycol, which does not cause significant changes in fluid and electrolyte balance.[38]

Lubricant Laxatives

Lubricant laxatives, such as mineral oil and glycerin suppositories, lubricate and soften the stool surface, allowing for easier passage. In addition, they irritate the bowel, increasing peristalsis. Glycerin suppositories, in addition, draw fluid into the rectum.[31] Lubricant laxatives may be useful in the management of fecal impaction and transient acute constipation. Chronic use can lead to malabsorption of fat-soluble vitamins and perianal irritation. Effect may take up to 3 days.[31]

Prokinetic Agents

Prokinetic agents can be considered as options in the management of constipation that has not responded to more conventional treatment. It includes agents such as metoclopramide, domperidone, erythromycin, and cisapride.

Metoclopramide action in the periphery increases lower esophageal sphincter tone and promotes gastrointestinal motility. It is discussed in more detail in the Nausea and Vomiting section. Domperidone (Motilium) has a dopamine antagonist effect in the upper gastrointestinal tract, which causes increased peristalsis. It does not have anticholinergic activity and has poor penetration into the CNS, causing fewer potential dystonic and extrapyramidal reactions than metoclopramide.[31] Domperidone is commonly available in Europe and Canada, but it has been removed from the market in some countries including the United States because of its association with QT-interval prolongation.[40,41] Cisapride has beneficial effects for constipation management[31] and has a more potent prokinetic effect than metoclopramide,[42,43] but its use has been restricted in the United States because of drug interactions that can cause potentially fatal cardiac arrhythmias.[44] Erythromycin stimulates gastrointestinal motility by acting at motilin receptors localized in the gastric and duodenal smooth muscle and enteric nerves (motilin is a hormone released from endocrine cells in the duodenal mucosa).[45] This results in accelerated gastric emptying[46] and shortened oro-cecal transit time.

Enemas

Enemas can be useful for the acute management of constipation. They soften the stool by increasing its water content. They also distend the colon and induce peristalsis. Various preparations are available. Microenemas may be less distressing for patients.[31] Other preparations include sodium phosphate (Fleet) enemas, soap and water enemas, saline enemas, and oil enemas. Fluid and electrolyte imbalance are possible complications of enemas.[31]

Opioid Antagonists

Naloxone is a competitive opioid antagonist that reverses central and peripheral opioid effects. Only 2% has the potential of reaching the CNS after oral administration because of the extensive first-pass metabolism.[38] Even though it may reverse opioid-induced constipation, the therapeutic window appears to be very narrow and can potentially induce opioid withdrawal symptoms. There are no consistent dosing recommendations in the literature.[47] As a result, it is recommended to start low (0.6–1 mg PO three times a day) and titrate upward as needed up to 5 mg PO three times a day.

Opioid antagonists that do not have central effects have a potentially important role in managing opioid-induced constipation in cancer patients. These include methylnaltrexone, which is a quaternary opioid receptor antagonist that does not cross the blood–brain barrier,[48,49] and ADL 8-2698 (Alvimopan), a peripherally restricted mu-opioid receptor antagonist that has low systemic absorption and limited ability to enter the CNS (200 times more potent at blocking peripheral vs. central mu receptors).[50] Both have been shown to be effective in reversing opioid-induced constipation without affecting analgesia or causing withdrawal symptoms via intravenous and oral administration.

Xerostomia

Opioids are among commonly used medications that can cause dry mouth in cancer patients. Other such medications include cytotoxic agents (e.g., cisplatin, cyclophosphamide, and methotrexate), antihistamines, antiemetics, anxiolytics and antidepressants.[51,52] This frequent side effect can worsen if any combination of these medications is used. Other common causes of this condition include radiation of the head and neck, mucositis, and dehydration. Fortunately, it lessens or disappears when the responsible agents are stopped. Although xerostomia is not a serious side effect, it can deteriorate the patient's quality of life by worsening chewing, swallowing, and talking. In addition, xerostomia is also known to reduce or even block the oral transmucosal absorption of medications (e.g., nitroglycerin and fentanyl).[53, 54]

Management

Symptomatic treatment includes the use of alcohol-free mouthwash or saltwater solutions, frequent sipping on water, eating small amounts of tart and moist food, chewing sugar-free gum, sucking on sugar-free candies or ice chips, and squirting a fine mist of water in the mouth. Alcohol; tobacco; acidic, salty, spicy, dry, sticky foods; and glycerin swabs should be avoided because they have a drying effect. The use of lip moisturizers might prevent or relieve lip drying and chapping.[52] If the patient is complaining of a dry mouth, avoiding oral transmucosal fentanyl (OTF, Actiq) for the management of breakthrough pain and switching to another short-acting opioid is suggested. If OTF use is therapeutically crucial, then it is essential to synchronize this therapy with measures to ameliorate preexisting or resultant xerostomia.[54]

Severe cases of dry mouth could respond to parasympathomimetic drugs, such as oral pilocarpine (Salagen), 5 mg four times a day, or cevimeline (Evoxac) 30 mg three times a day.[55,56] Oral pilocarpine and intravenous (IV) amifostine (Ethyol) can be used during radiation therapy of the head or the neck for the prevention of radiation-induced hyposalivation.[55,57] Bethanechol (Urecholine) is a parasympathomimetic drug with an indication for the treatment of urinary retention and chronic gastroesophageal reflux disease (GERD). However, it has been used experimentally with success at 25 mg three times a day in the management of drug- and radiation-induced xerostomia, with an added observation of fewer adverse effects compared to other parasympathomimetic drugs.[54] Refractory xerostomia may satisfactorily respond to acupuncture.[58]

Gastroesophageal Reflux Disease

GERD has been described as part of a constellation of adverse gastrointestinal effects termed opioid bowel dysfunction.[36] It is thought to be secondary to decreased gastric motility and emptying, as well as decreased lower esophageal sphincter tone resulting from opioid administration.[36,59] Prokinetic agents as described previously,

as well as the use of Histamine-2 (H2) receptor antagonists or proton pump inhibitors can provide adequate relief.

Obstruction of the Common Bile Duct

Opioids can increase common bile duct and sphincter of Oddi pressure, but the clinical consequences are usually minimal.[60] If abdominal or epigastric pain is suspected to be secondary to the opioid, opioid rotation is suggested. Ultrasonographic studies have indicated that although morphine can cause a significant reduction in the diameter of the common bile duct, fentanyl and sufentanil have no significant effect on the common bile duct.[61,62]

NEUROLOGIC SIDE EFFECTS

Opioid-induced neurologic side effects generally occur because of one or more of the following reasons: At low doses they most likely represent an idiosyncratic hypersensitivity reaction; this, though, is relatively rare. They can also be secondary to the accumulation of opioid toxic metabolites[3,6,12,52,63]; and finally, very large concentrations of the opioid itself can lead to neurotoxicity.[52] Knowledge of the pharmacology of opioid receptors and metabolites is essential to achieving a better understanding of the mechanisms related to opioid neurotoxicity (see Chapter 17). Opioid rotation in particular plays a very important role (see Chapter 16). Table 18–4 presents the common symptoms caused by opioid metabolite toxicity, and Table 18–5 summarizes the pharmacologic management of the most common CNS side effects of opioids.

Delirium and Hallucinations

There are many potential causes of delirium and hallucinations in patients with advanced cancer, including

---

TABLE 18–4 Common Symptoms Caused by Opioid Metabolite Toxicity

Opioid	Known Active Metabolites	Metabolite Toxicity
Morphine	Morphine-6-glucuronide (M6G) Morphine-3-glucuronide (M3G) Normorphine	Drowsiness, nausea and vomiting, respiratory depression Delirium, hallucinations, myoclonus, seizures, hyperalgesia Neurotoxicity similar to M3G
Hydromorphone	Hydromorphone-6-glucuronide Hydromorphone-3-glucuronide	Neurotoxicity similar to M6G Neurotoxicity similar to M3G
Oxycodone	Noroxycodone Oxymorphone	Main metabolite, but it is not clinically significant Potent mu agonist but not present in significant amounts
Fentanyl	No known active metabolites	—
Methadone	No known active metabolites	—

TABLE 18-5 Management of the Most Common Neurologic Opioid-Related Side Effects			
Symptom	**Drug**	**Dose**	**Route**
Delirium and Hallucinations	*Neuroleptics*		
	Haloperidol	0.5–5 mg BID & q4h as necessary	PO/SC/IV/PR
	Chlorpromazine	15–50 mg BID as necessary	PO/IV
	Risperidone	0.5–4 mg BID	PO
	Olanzepine	2.5 mg at bedtime — 10 mg BID	PO
	Benzodiazepines		
	Lorazepam	0.5–2 mg BID & q1h as necessary	PO/SC/IV/PR
	Midazolam	10–60 mg/24 h (as continuous infusion)	SC/IV
Sedation	*"Traditional" Psychostimulants*		
	Methylphenidate	2.5–30 mg BID (e.g., 8 AM and 1 PM or as necessary)	PO
	Dextroamphetamine	2.5–30 mg BID (e.g., 8 AM and 1 PM or as necessary)	PO
	Caffeine	100–200 mg q4h as necessary (1 cup of coffee ~ 75–100 mg of caffeine)	PO
	"New" Psychostimulants		
	Modafinil	100–600 mg daily	PO
	Donepezil	2.5–15 mg daily	PO
Myoclonus	Clonazepam	0.5–2 mg QID as necessary	PO
	Baclofen	5–20 mg TID as necessary	PO
	Valproic acid	125–500 mg TID	PO

BID, twice daily; *IV*, intravenously; *PO*, per os; *PR*, per rectum; *qxh*, every x hours; *SC*, subcutaneously; *TID*, three times a day.

opioids. It is common to experience mild cognitive changes after initiating an opioid or escalating the dose. These symptoms may disappear after a few days of stable dosing.

Management

Pharmacologic management includes the use of neuroleptics and benzodiazepines. Opioid rotation is suggested for cases that do not respond to the addition of neuroleptics or benzodiazepines, or the side effects of these are not tolerable.

Neuroleptics

If the symptoms persist or become severe, addition of a neuroleptic is the first pharmacologic choice. Haloperidol is commonly used.[6] For cases of severe agitation, a more sedating neuroleptic such as chlorpromazine may be more effective. The newer atypical antipsychotics such as risperidone and olanzapine can also be used effectively and offer the advantage of less anticholinergic side effects.

Benzodiazepines

Benzodiazepines, such as lorazepam or midazolam, can also be used in severe cases. They must be used with caution, though, as they may exacerbate sedation and acute confusional states.

Sedation

Sedation is commonly cited as one of the main reasons for the inability to titrate an opioid to the point of achieving adequate analgesia.[64] It is a common side effect of opioids (20%–60% of cancer patients receiving oral morphine[3]), occurring more often in opioid-naive patients and following a dose escalation. The mechanism of action causing opioid-induced sedation is uncertain. It is known that cholinergic pathways are important in modulating cortical arousal and information processing,[65] and that opioids can decrease intracerebral acetylcholine activity.[66] This decrease can result in decreased arousal and attention, decreased ventilatory drive (via decreased sensitivity of chemoreceptors to carbon dioxide), and sleep cycle alterations (e.g., decreased REM sleep).[65,67] Sedation, particularly severe sedation, can also be a sign of opioid neurotoxicity.[11] In a study in which the serum morphine-6-glucuronide (M6G) concentration was measured in cancer patients receiving morphine, 7 out of 9 episodes of critical adverse effects, specifically respiratory depression and severe sedation, were found to have very elevated plasma concentrations of M6G.[68]

Management

Opioid-induced sedation most often improves within 7 days without any therapeutic intervention. If sedation persists and is affecting significantly the quality of life of the patient, pharmacologic treatment is appropriate (Table 18-5). The resulting improvement in cognitive alertness from the management of opioid-induced sedation can allow the use of greater quantities of opioids, which at times is necessary to achieve optimal analgesia.[68]

"Traditional" Psychostimulants

Methylphenidate is the most widely studied agent for opioid-induced sedation.[64,70,71,72,73] Methylphenidate and dextroamphetamine have been shown to decrease sedation, increase cognitive abilities and potentiate analgesia.[69] They may also be useful as fast-acting antidepressants.[74] The mechanism of action is unknown.[75] Other agents include caffeine and pemoline. The mentioned psychostimulants can produce side effects such as agitation, confusion, hallucinations, decreased appetite, tremor and tachycardia. Pemoline has less sympathomimetic activity,[75] but its use has fallen out of favor because of concerns regarding an increased risk of acute liver failure.

"New" Psychostimulants

This category includes modafinil and acetylcholinesterase inhibitors:

Modafinil: Modafinil, which is approved for the management of narcolepsy and shift work sleep disorder, shows promise for management of opioid-induced sedation.[76] Modafinil may exert its effect by inhibiting GABA (gamma aminobutyric acid—an inhibitory neurotransmitter important for sleep) transmission in the cerebral cortex.[76] Modafinil is generally well tolerated,[77] but expensive.[78]

Acetylcholinesterase inhibitors: Acetylcholinesterase inhibitors are approved for the management of Alzheimer's disease. Recent studies of their use (donezepil) for the management of opioid-induced sedation have shown encouraging results.[65,67,79] By acting centrally, they lead to an increase in central acetylcholinesterase activity, resulting in improved arousal and attention, improved ventilatory drive (as central cholinergic activity is essential in regulating respiratory function), and improved sleep cycle (e.g., improved REM sleep).[65] Donezepil does not have sympathomimetic activity and it is in general well tolerated.[79] Side effects are mainly gastrointestinal, and include nausea and vomiting, abdominal cramps, bloating and loose bowel movements[79] (the latter may be an advantage if the patient is suffering from opioid-induced constipation). Some patients may experience anorexia secondary to the gastrointestinal effects.

Corticosteroids

Corticosteroids can be useful in the management of opioid-induced sedation because they can be associated with a feeling of well-being and a sensation of increased energy.[80] In addition, they are analgesic[81] and decrease opioid analgesic tolerance.[82] This can result in the use of a lower amount of opioid to achieve adequate analgesia, which can in itself result in less sedation.

Myoclonus

It is defined as sudden, brief, involuntary muscle contractions arising from the CNS, which can occur in different areas of the body. Active opioid metabolites have been attributed as a cause.[6] The effect appears to be dose related, but in an unpredictable manner. A conservative estimate of the incidence as a side effect of opioid therapy is 3% to 4%.[83]

Management

Lowering the opioid dose and opioid rotation are useful strategies in managing myoclonus. Pharmacologic management includes:

Benzodiazepines

Initial management with a benzodiazepine, such as clonazepam,[3,84] starting at 0.5 mg PO at bedtime and titrating as needed up to 2 mg four times a day is recommended.

Muscle Relaxants

Baclofen and other antispasmodics are also useful in the management of myoclonus.[3]

Anticonvulsants

Valproic acid has also been shown to be effective.[3,84]

Hyperalgesia

Hyperalgesia is defined as an increased response to a stimulus that is normally painful.[85] Evidence suggests that opioids intended to abolish pain can unexpectedly produce hyperalgesia.[86] Studies have also established a close link between tolerance and hyperalgesia. Thus, even though the diminished opioid analgesic efficacy during a course of opioid therapy is often first thought of as the result of the development of analgesic tolerance, it may in fact be the first sign of opioid-induced hyperalgesia. This may explain why opioid tolerant cancer patients, particularly those on high-dose opioids, methadone maintenance programs, or active abuse (e.g., heroin) appear to be "more sensitive" to pain and have higher perioperative opioid requirements. In addition it may help explain why some patients receiving rapidly escalating opioid doses experience no relief or worsening pain. In these patients, an opioid dose reduction or rotation rather than an opioid dose escalation may be warranted.

The development of hyperalgesia is mediated through complex neural mechanisms. These include the transmission of nociceptive input to the spinal cord from the rostral ventromedial medulla (RVM),[87] increased activity of cholecystokinin (CCK) in the RVM,[88] the activation of the central glutaminergic system via the N-methyl-D-aspartate (NMDA) receptors,[89,90] increased spinal dynorphin levels,[89-91] and increased activity of excitatory neuropeptides such as substance P and calcitonin gene related peptide (CGRP).[89] In addition, opioid neurotoxic metabolites (e.g., morphine-3-glucuronide [M3G] and hydromorphone-3-glucuronide [H3G]),[63,92] the presence of different opioid receptor subtypes[9,10,89] and variability in receptor affinity to different opioids play a role in the development of hyperalgesia.

Management

A growing body of evidence suggests the development of tolerance and the development of hyperalgesia share common cellular and molecular mechanisms. Hence, "treating" one may "take care" of the other. It is often difficult, however, to distinguish between the actual preexisting pain and opioid-induced pain. The following are features that can help us make this distinction.[89] With opioid-induced hyperalgesia:

1. The patient is experiencing greater pain than the "baseline" pain, even though there is absence of disease progression. If there is only tolerance development, there is a return to baseline despite gradually incrementing opioids.
2. The pain would tend to be diffuse rather than localized to the original site of pain. This is generally the situation but not always so.
3. An increase in opioids would be accompanied by an increase in pain. Thus a trial of opioid dose escalation can help differentiate between opioid-induced pain and preexisting pain.

To date there are no established standards for the management of opioid-induced hyperalgesia. The following are guidelines that can be used in the management of opioid-induced hyperalgesia based on the review of the literature and clinical experience:

1. **Decreasing the opioid dose.** This will diminish toxicity caused by the opioid itself and/or its metabolites.
2. **Opioid rotation.** As mentioned previously in this chapter, this is an effective strategy for the management of opioid side effects, including hyperalgesia. Methadone has also been shown to have NMDA antagonistic properties.[93,94] Thus, opioid rotation to methadone may provide additional advantages as compared to rotation to other opioids.
3. **NMDA antagonists.** Ketamine has been increasingly used as an adjuvant in the management of cancer pain.[95] Intravenous ketamine at subanesthetic doses (e.g., 0.5 mg/kg bolus and 0.25 mg/kg/h),[96] potentially can be helpful in the management of opioid-induced hyperalgesia.
4. **Alpha-2 adrenergic agonists.** Clonidine is an alpha-2 adrenergic agonist with an established role in pain management.[97] Epidural clonidine administration (4 µg/kg in 10 mL NS × 20 minutes followed by 2 µg/kg/h for 12 hours) has been efficacious for the management of opioid-induced hyperalgesia.[98] Intravenous, oral, and transdermal formulations potentially will be of benefit in this setting, but further studies are needed. Hypotension is the most significant side effect.
5. **Lidocaine.** Because morphine elicited hyperalgesia has been shown to be abolished by injecting lidocaine into the RVM,[99] lidocaine may also play an important role in the management of hyperalgesia. Lidocaine IV at 1 to 3 mg/kg over 20 to 30 minutes, followed by a continuous infusion SC or IV at 0.5 to 2 mg/kg/h have been shown to be effective in the management of severe intractable cancer pain.[100] Similar doses can potentially be helpful in the management of opioid-induced hyperalgesia.
6. **Low dose naloxone.** Low doses of naloxone have been shown to selectively block excitatory activity mediated by the µ opioid receptor.[101,102] Trials using low dose naloxone for postoperative pain[103,104] and case reports for management of opioid central side effects[105] are described in the literature. Slow infusions of 0.05 mg/h have been used,[105] but further clinical trials are needed to further verify its safety and efficacy for the management of opioid-induced hyperalgesia and pain in opioid tolerant patients.

Muscle Rigidity

Rapid intravenous administration of opioids is associated with an increase in muscle tone, which can cause chest wall rigidity and occasionally severe truncal stiffness.[106,107] This side effect is more significant intraoperatively. However, it is of clinical relevance if intravenous opioids are used in the hospital, nursing home, or hospice setting. Mechanisms for opioid-induced muscle rigidity are not due to direct effect on muscle fibers but probably due to opioid activation of central µ-receptors in the CNS.[106,107] Slow administration of opioid boluses would significantly avoid this undesired effect. Management of severe cases consists of either administration of naloxone or neuromuscular blockers.[106]

Seizures

Seizures have been described as a neuroexcitatory side effect of opioids.[107] Opioid neurotoxic metabolite accumulation, such as M3G for morphine, H3G for hydromorphone, and normeperidine for meperidine, have been implicated in the etiology of seizures.[63,108,109] They are certainly not the only cause of opioid-induced seizures as opioids devoid of known neurotoxic metabolites (e.g., fentanyl and remifentanil) have also been implicated as causing seizures.[107]

In cancer patients, seizures have generally been documented in cases when extremely high doses are used and there is rapid opioid escalation, particularly in association with other neurotoxic phenomena such as myoclonus and hyperalgesia.[108,110] It should be noted that rapid narcotic withdrawal can also cause seizures, and this has been reported up to 4 days after stopping the medication.[111] In order to avoid seizures from narcotic withdrawal, gradual tapering of the opioids is recommended prior to withdrawing a patient from opioids.

Management

It is important to rule out other causes for the seizures besides opioids, such as brain metastasis, stroke, or metabolic abnormalities. Initially, it is essential to stabilize the patient and attend to airway, breathing, and circulation, as well as to obtain intravenous access, monitor vital signs, and arrange for routine and special laboratory tests.[110] Combination therapy with standard anticonvulsants (e.g., phenytoin) and a benzodiazepine (e.g., midazolam, diazepam) is recommended first-line therapy for seizures.[110] However, for opioid-induced seizures, the use of benzodiazepines only should suffice because non-benzodiazepine anticonvulsants are not as effective in this setting.[108] Opioid rotation is also recommended.[108] This will allow for the clearance of the opioid associated with the seizure as well as its metabolites.

Headaches

Opioid-induced headaches are a rare complication of opioid therapy.[112] Opioids may trigger vascular headaches, especially migraines, as well as tension headaches.[113] In addition, opioids can cause medication overuse chronic daily headaches (also known as drug-induced rebound headaches),[114] particularly in patients who do not adhere to their opioid regimen and tend to overuse short-acting opioids.[115]

Management

Careful clinical evaluation is essential to rule out more common causes of headaches, especially among cancer patients, such as intracranial metastasis. Patient education and emphasis on adherence to therapy compliance is essential. The implementation of an opioid agreement might become necessary. Headaches associated with neuraxial opioid administration requires the exclusion of postdural puncture as the cause. If prolonged opioid therapy is to be discontinued, slow titration is recommended to avoid withdrawal symptoms, which include headaches. Opioid rotation may play a role but further research is needed to use this modality as a treatment option for opioid-induced headaches.

CARDIOPULMONARY SIDE EFFECTS

Respiratory Depression

Opioid-induced respiratory depression is a potentially life-threatening side effect. Opioids act on the respiratory center in the medulla oblongata and can depress respiratory activity.[83] Accumulation of opioid toxic metabolites has also been linked as a contributing factor leading to respiratory depression.[83] Usually, though, tolerance to this side effect tends to develop within a few days. Pain also appears to play a role in the development of tolerance,[84] making respiratory depression a rare occurrence in cancer patients taking opioids for pain management.

Management

It is important to first rule out other causes of respiratory depression such as metabolic encephalopathy, sepsis, brain metastasis, and stroke.[116] Proper evaluation of the respiratory status and level of consciousness is necessary, since clinically significant respiratory depression from opioid overdose does not occur when the patient is arousable. Reduction in the opioid dose or temporarily stopping the dose is usually all that is required. But if the patient is becoming progressively bradypneic and more difficult to arouse, naloxone is indicated. Naloxone is an opioid antagonist that acts centrally and peripherally. It is indicated for the reversal of opioid-induced respiratory depression and overdose and has a rapid onset of action (<2 minutes). But too often, naloxone is administered precipitously, leading to acute withdrawal symptoms (e.g., nausea and vomiting, sweating, tachycardia, pulmonary edema) and severe pain.[116] Patients on chronic opioids are extremely sensitive to naloxone. Diluted naloxone should be given with the exception of a true respiratory arrest. Recommended naloxone doses for the management of respiratory depression are shown in Table 18–6.[117]

Non-Cardiogenic Pulmonary Edema

Morphine has an established therapeutic role in the treatment of acute cardiogenic pulmonary edema, especially when associated with myocardial infarction, left

TABLE 18–6 Management of Opioid-Induced Respiratory Depression

Symptom	Naloxone Dosing
Opioid-induced respiratory depression and obtundation	Dilute 0.4 mg of naloxone in 9 mL NS (0.04 mg/mL) Administer 1 mL intravenous push over 15 seconds every 1–3 min as needed
Respiratory arrest (code status)	Administer 1 mL intravenous push of naloxone (**NOT diluted**: 0.4 mg/mL). May repeat in 1–3 minutes as needed up to 3 doses
NOTE: A continuous infusion to be given for a few hours may be necessary due to the short duration of action of naloxone (~45 min). Consider especially when long-acting opioid preparations, fentanyl patch, and methadone are involved	2 mg (5 × 0.4 mg/mL ampules) of naloxone diluted in 500 mL of NS or D5W (= 0.004 mg/mL = 4 µg/mL). The rate to be given is determined by the patient's response

Modified from Intravenous Medication Guidelines: Naloxone. Pharmacy Therapeutics Committee. Memorial Sloan-Kettering Cancer Center, New York, 1994.

ventricular failure, or distressing dyspnea in patients with advanced cancer.[118] However, high doses of opioids might cause non-cardiogenic pulmonary edema. Non-cardiogenic pulmonary edema is seen in 50% to 80% of hospital admissions from heroin overdose; however, only in less than 3% of inhouse patients therapeutically treated with opioids.[119] The precise etiology is unknown. Proposed mechanisms include ventilatory compromise secondary to hypoxia, and perhaps more significantly to hypercapnia,[120] which results in precapillary pulmonary hypertension with enhanced permeability of the pulmonary capillary and thus, fluid leak.[119] Other hypothesized mechanisms include hypersensitivity reaction to opioids, direct toxicity to the alveolar membrane, central neurogenic effects in response to increased intracranial pressure, and increased capillary permeability secondary to opioid-mediated release of leukotrienes and histamine.[119] The time interval between exposure and symptom onset is usually less than 2 hours for heroin-related cases and less than 6 to 12 hours for those caused by methadone. Clinical presentation usually reveals an opioid-overdosed stuporous or comatose patient with pink, frothy bronchial secretions and cyanosis. Respiratory depression and miotic pupils are typical.[119]

Management

Emergent airway management is essential. Naloxone for the reversal of opioid overdose is generally indicated. Although naloxone administration is generally safe in patients with suspected opioid toxicity, pulmonary edema remains a rare, but reported, side effect of naloxone administration. Thus, careful and intermittent parenteral injection of naloxone is advised. It is suggested that, in the presence of opioid-induced non-cardiogenic pulmonary edema, hypercapnia is corrected prior to the administration of naloxone,[120] in contrast to a non-complicated opioid overdose. Arterial blood gases and serum glucose levels should be evaluated immediately

by bedside testing, and thiamine should be administered to all patients with altered levels of consciousness.[119] Mechanical ventilation, pulmonary support, and admission to an intensive care setting might be necessary. Pharmacologic intervention would include diuretics, nitroglycerin, angiotensin converting enzyme inhibitors, vasodilators, and other vasoactive agents. This should be conducted under the supervision of or with the collaboration of an intensivist, cardiologist, or both.

Bradycardia and Hypotension

In general, opioids have no direct effect on the myocardial contractility or output.[107] Therefore, they do not produce severe hemodynamic instability. However, most opioids can cause dose-dependent, asymptomatic bradycardia. Meperidine, on the other hand, may produce tachycardia. In either case, lowering the opioid dose would be beneficial.[107]

Histamine-releasing opioids (particularly morphine) cause vasodilation, which could lead to hypotension, particularly among hypovolemic or dehydrated cancer patients. Morphine should be used with great care in patients with cor pulmonale because deaths after ordinary therapeutic doses have been reported. Hypotension is more prominent when opioids are used parenterally, especially intraoperatively or postoperatively. The hypotensive effects of the opioids can be minimized by providing slow opioid infusions, keeping patients supine, and maintaining an adequate intravascular volume.[107]

Cardiac Dysrhythmias

Reports in the literature suggest that methadone has been associated with QTc interval prolongation.[121,122] Kornick and colleagues[123] identified all patients over a 20-month period at a cancer center who were receiving methadone or morphine intravenously via continuous infusion. The mean difference in QTc intervals on and off methadone among 42 patients with EKGs was 41.7 (±7.8) ms ($P < 0.0001$). In addition, a linear relationship between the QTc interval and the methadone dose was present, suggesting that patients receiving higher doses of methadone are especially at risk. Krantz and colleagues[124] conducted a retrospective case series analysis of 17 patients on methadone who developed torsades des pointes. The mean QTc interval was 615 ms and the QTc prolongation appeared to be dose-related. In pain management, methadone is often prescribed with tricyclic antidepressants, further increasing the risk of QTc interval prolongation. In the palliative setting, it may also be combined with other QTc prolonging drugs such as haloperidol and selective serotonin reuptake inhibitors.

If used with proper precautions, methadone will continue to be an excellent opioid analgesic because of its efficacy, lack of active metabolites, N-methyl-D-aspartate (NMDA) receptor antagonism, and low cost.[12] Safety precautions, such as obtaining a baseline EKG before starting methadone and repeating the EKG in 4 weeks and every 3 months afterward when doses greater than 120 mg/day of methadone are used and discontinuing the medication if there is any evidence of QTc prolongation have been instituted at some cancer centers.[125]

UROLOGIC SIDE EFFECTS

Altered Kidney Function

It is believed that opioids can depress kidney function by decreasing renal plasma blood flow through two mechanisms: directly affecting glomerular filtration and decreasing systemic blood pressure. Additionally, opioids increase the sodium reabsorption in the renal tubules, and may stimulate the release of antidiuretic hormone (ADH).[118] The influence that opioids have on the renal system is directly related to the opioid agonist receptor. For example, mu-opioid receptor activity has an antidiuretic effect, whereas kappa agonist activity might promote diuresis.[118,126] Oxycodone can cause direct granulomatous glomerulonephritis if injected intravenously, which might lead to acute renal failure.[127] Also, severe chronic renal failure caused by non-IgA fibrillary nephropathy was witnessed in two oral oxycodone addicts.[128]

Although mainly metabolized in the liver, most opioids have active metabolites that are excreted in the urine. An existing renal insufficiency could cause an accumulation of these active metabolites in the plasma with resulting excessive therapeutic effect or the appearance of adverse effects. Seizures are a serious side effect that is caused by an unadjusted opioid dosage (particularly with the use of codeine and meperidine[121,122]) in end-stage renal

disease (ESRD), which is not uncommon in cancer patients.

Management

Opioid rotation, particularly to methadone, may prove beneficial. Opioid rotation will allow for clearance of neurotoxic metabolites, and as mentioned previously in this chapter, methadone has minimal renal clearance and thus it does not tend to accumulate in renal failure. Fentanyl also appears to be safe to use in this setting.[129]

A good understanding of the relationship between opioids and the renal system is essential for any opioid-prescribing practitioner. Certain doses might need to be altered and some opioids avoided (e.g., morphine and codeine),[129] particularly in cases of compromised renal function to prevent further worsening of renal function or undesired opioid effects, or both.

Urinary Retention

Urinary retention occurs infrequently with opioid administration[130] and it is usually a self-limited side effect. It is particularly prominent with neuraxial opioid administration.[131,132] It results from increased sphincter spasm and decreased detrusor tone.[59]

Management

If urinary retention is persistent, manipulations such as running water, pouring warm water over the perineum, or gentle bladder massage could help resolve the retention. Discontinuing other pharmacologic agents (e.g., diphenhydramine or tricyclic antidepressants) that enhance the problem is helpful. The administration of a direct cholinomimetic agent, such as bethanecol, might become necessary.[130] Opioid rotation can also play a therapeutic role. Naloxone can be reserved for only severe refractory cases.

Peripheral Edema

Opioids should be included in the differential diagnosis of peripheral edema (PEd) in cancer patients receiving opioid therapy. PEd has been reported as an opioid side effect following oral and intrathecal administration.[133-135]

The mechanisms of opioid-induced PEd remain unclear and controversial. Animal models clearly indicate a role of the kidney in PEd during prolonged morphine administration,[136] and it has been shown that mu-opioid receptor activity on the renal system has an antidiuretic effect.[118] However, current research points to the role of peripheral mu receptors in the pathology of pain associated with acute inflammation and argue against the involvement of these receptors in edema formation.[137] In addition, PEd associated with prolonged opioid therapy can be a response to increased fluid intake to relieve a chronically dry mouth caused by opioids,[138] particularly in compromised patients.

Management

Opioid-induced PEd is usually mild and self-limiting, unless a coexistent cardiac, hepatic, or renal comorbidity exists. Management of PEd starts with simple measures such as leg raising, elastic stockings, compressive air pumps, and salt and fluid restriction. Diuretics may be used if needed.[135] Opioid rotation should be attempted if PEd is significant or intractable.

ENDOCRINOLOGIC SIDE EFFECTS

Hypogonadism and Sexual Dysfunction

Historically, opioid therapy has been implicated as a cause of hypogonadism, manifested by male impotence, decreased libido and anorgasmia in both genders, and other sexual abnormalities.[139,140] It is now believed that opioid-induced hypogonadism affects mostly male patients on chronic opioid therapy.[141] The connection between excessive use of opioids and hypogonadism has long been made with the observation in the 1970s of irregular menstrual cycle, amenorrhea, decreased sexual desire and performance, and male erectile dysfunction in heroin addicts and in methadone-therapy rehabilitation patients.[142-146] These observations are supported by studies indicating that opioids affect sexual behavior adversely.[147] Although hypogonadism is an uncommon side effect of opioid therapy, it is a severely distressing one, especially among male patients.[148] It is believed that even relatively low doses of opioids can impair normal gonadal function and such risk remains present even when opioid doses are reduced.[149] On the other hand, some clinicians noted improvement of sexual function in cancer survivors following the reduction of chronic high-dose opioid therapy.[150] Currently, there is an increased concern about opioid-induced hypogonadism caused by the increased rate of opioid therapy in general and the extensive use of long-term intraspinal opioid for the management of chronic malignant and non-malignant pain. Several studies have shown evidence of patients receiving intrathecal opioids who have developed hypogonadotropic hypogonadism manifested by sexual dysfunction; in addition, some have developed central hypocorticoidism or growth hormone (GH) deficiency.[151-154] Although it has not been reported yet as a result of intraspinal opioid-induced hypogonadism, osteoporosis remains a serious consequence of hypogonadism that warrants careful assessment should it become a problem (Table 18–7).[154]

Opioids cause hypogonadism by alteration of the hypothalamic–pituitary–gonadal (HPG) axis that controls the reproductive and sexual function of the body.

TABLE 18–7 Summary of Opioid-Induced Hypogonadism

Symptoms	Diagnosis

General:
• Fatigue
• Muscle wasting
• Osteoporosis and resulting fractures
• Increased pain
• Reduced opioid effectiveness
Gonadal:
• Loss of libido
• Erectile dysfunction
• Infertility
• Menstrual disturbances
	• Detect symptoms
	• Rule-out other cause of hypogonadism
	• Check laboratory tests:
	  • Testosterone, LH, FSH, estradiol
	  • Consider GH and morning cortisol levels
	• Consider bone densitometry
	• Consider testosterone trial therapy as a diagnostic measure

Management	Follow-Up
• Consider opioid-dose reduction • Consider adding a non-opioid • Hormone replacement therapy (HRT) (see text) • Endocrinology consultation • Non-pharmacological therapy (see text)	• Continue to optimize pain therapy • Continue to watch for hypogonadism • Monitor testosterone levels, if HRT initiated • Monitor PSA levels • Consider regular rectal examination • Monitor laboratory results (e.g., lipid profile and complete blood count) if indicated • Patient counseling

Modified from Katz N: The impact of opioids on the endocrine system. Pain Management Rounds 1, 2004.
FSH, follicle stimulating hormone; *GH,* growth hormone; *LH,* luteinizing hormone; *PSA,* prostate specific antigen.

We know that opioid analgesics stimulate the release of antidiuretic hormone (ADH), prolactin, and somatotropin and inhibit the release of luteinizing hormone (LH) and follicle-stimulating hormone (FSH). These effects suggest that endogenous opioid peptides, through effects in the hypothalamus, play regulatory roles in these systems.[118] Since opioid receptors are found in the hypothalamus,[155] one feasible theory to the disruption of the HPG axis is that when exogenous opioids bind to the opioid receptors in the hypothalamus (Figure 18–5), they inhibit the release of the gonadotropic-releasing hormone (GnRH), which in turn reduces the secretion of the LH and FSH from the pituitary gland, leading to a total reduction in sex hormone secretion from the gonads in both genders and atrophy of the uterus in women.[139] One can hypothesize a similar mechanism for growth hormone releasing hormone (GHRH) suppression (see Figure 18–5). Because opioid receptors have been found in the human posterior pituitary gland[156] and in the anterior pituitary gland of laboratory animals,[157] the assumption that opioids act only indirectly on the pituitary gland to inhibit LH and FSH can be challenged. It is also possible that opioids act directly in the periphery to reduce the quantities of circulating plasma testosterone. Researchers have found that testosterone-binding globulin is elevated among male heroin addicts and plasma levels of free testosterone are chronically reduced.[158]

Castration-produced hypotestosteronism in rats significantly lowered their pain threshold. Their previous pain threshold was reinstated by treatment with testosterone.[159] This has not been demonstrated in humans; however, it has been indirectly observed in a study on females with AIDS wasting.[160] Such observation raises a challenging consideration that opioid-induced hypogonadism increases pain sensitivity in chronic pain patients[141] and might explain the need for dose escalation in those patients.

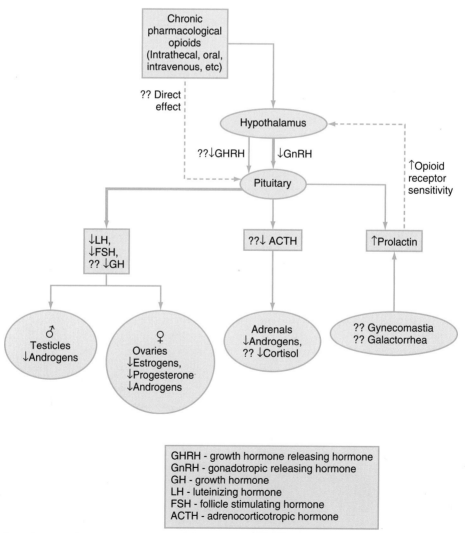

FIGURE 18–5 Schematic diagram of proposed opioid-induced hypogonadism by alteration of the hypothalamic-pituitary-gonadal (HPG) axis.

For cancer patients who are not debilitated and for cancer survivors with chronic pain issues, it is recommended to discuss the possibility of HPG axis disruption at the initiation of chronic opioid therapy. This is particularly important in younger patients and in those receiving intraspinal opioids. Issues such as potential sexual dysfunction, infertility, and possible bone demineralization should be discussed.[152] Any sign of hypogonadism, whether nonspecific (such as fatigue, anxiety, or depression) or specific (such as erectile dysfunction or irregular menstrual changes) should be taken seriously and prompt clinical assessment and, if needed, laboratory workup. In male patients, testosterone level needs to be verified.[148]

Management

It is essential to address other causes of hypogonadism in a cancer patient that could be contributing to sexual dysfunction, including the cancer itself (e.g., genitourinary) and treatments (e.g., orchiectomy, breast cancer chemotherapy).[161] To date, there are no established standards for management of presumptive opioid-induced hypogonadism and sexual dysfunction. Reduction of the opioid dose, if tolerated, may be beneficial in the treatment of opioid-induced hypogonadism. Opioid rotation has been recommended,[141] although no studies to support such an approach have been conducted yet. Hormone-replacement therapy (HRT) and phosphodiesterase-5 inhibitors also play an important role. Opioids, though, may need to be withdrawn, if the side effects are intolerable or unacceptable.[140]

Hormone-Replacement Therapy

Prior to instituting HRT, a proper endocrinologic consultation is warranted. For males, testosterone gel, 5 g per day topically, could be beneficial. Alternatively, 200 mg of intramuscular injection of testosterone every 2 weeks can be used. It is important to monitor testosterone levels every week for the first month, then every 6 months alongside the treatment course with testosterone. Potential risks include benign prostatic hypertrophy (BPH) and prostate cancer. Monitoring of prostate-specific antigen is important to detect any neoplastic activity caused by testosterone replacement therapy.[141]

Premenopausal females can be provided with estrogen pills. Estrogen replacement therapy provides good relief for symptoms of coital pain and lubrication complaints. Other female sexual symptoms including clitoral insensitivity, decreased sexual desire, and other nonspecific hypotestosteronemic symptoms caused by severe ovarian or adrenal failure would require testosterone replacement. Low-dose estrogen/testosterone treatment would be beneficial in such circumstances.[162] Female patients should be made aware of the potential risks and side effects of HRT, such as virilizing effects (e.g., acne, unwanted hair, deepening voice) with testosterone and thromboembolism with estrogens.

Phosphodiesterase-5 (PDE-5) Inhibitors

Oral PDE-5 inhibitors are recognized as the first-line of therapy for men with erectile dysfunction after radical prostatectomy[163]; however, this group of medication can also be used for the management of sexual dysfunction in both genders.[162,164] These include sildenafil, tadalafil, and vardenafil.

Nonpharmacologic Approaches

Men with erectile dysfunction might benefit from commercially available penile suction devices. Counseling for patients and their partners can be valuable. Applying the PLISSIT (**P**—permission giving; **LI**—limited information; **SS**—specific suggestions; **IT**—intensive therapy) model in cancer patients with sexual dysfunction is very useful.[165] It is a proven behavioral technique to address sexual difficulties in the general population. Patients might benefit from being provided with published informative literature. Such materials are available at the web sites of the National Cancer Institute, the American Cancer Society, and the American Pain Society.

Osteoporosis

As the population ages, concerns about increased incidence of osteoporosis-induced fractures is reflected in the medical practice.[166] Hypogonadism is the leading cause of secondary osteoporosis in men. As discussed previously, chronic opioid therapy is associated with hypogonadism and, thus, it potentially can cause secondary osteoporosis.[166]

Management

Patients receiving prolonged opioid therapy who present with clinical or laboratory evidence of hypogonadism, or who are considered high risk for osteoporosis in general, should be considered for bone mineral density (BMD) measurement to rule out and/or diagnose osteoporosis.[166] Additional workup would include, as necessary: serum levels of phosphorus, magnesium, alkaline phosphatase, vitamin D, parathyroid hormone (PTH), and thyroid function. If opioids were implicated in causing osteoporosis, then treatment would target iatrogenic hypogonadism as outlined in Table 18–7. In general, osteoporosis management would include smoking cessation, reduced alcohol consumption, and a balanced diet and exercise program.[167] Pharmacologic agents include calcium, vitamin D, bisphosphonates (particularly alendronate and risedronate, which have proven benefit in protecting vertebral as well as extravertebral bone structure), calcitonin, hormone replacement therapy (HRT), selective estrogen receptor modulators (SERMs), and PTH.[167] It is suggested that the management of osteoporosis be conducted with the consultation of an endocrinologist.

DERMATOLOGIC SIDE EFFECTS

Pruritus

The etiology of opioid-induced pruritus is uncertain. It almost certainly involves histamine release (opioids release histamine from mast cells[168] in the periphery), but the high incidence of pruritus following administration of neuroaxial analgesia[169] suggests a direct central nervous system effect. Endogenous opioid peptides and the mu-opioid receptors likely play a role in the pathogenesis of pruritus.[170] Opioids may enhance the disinhibition of itch-specific neurons.[171] In addition, morphine may activate serotonin, which may also play a role in pruritus. There is also the observation that pain suppresses pruritus; thus suppressing pain may disinhibit pruritus.[168] Patients may state they are "allergic" to an opioid after having developed "itching" following its administration. It is important to note that pruritus without a rash is considered an opioid side effect rather than a true allergic reaction.

Management

Pharmacologic management is included in the following section. Opioid rotation can also play a therapeutic role. Oxycodone and fentanyl may cause less histamine release,[172-174] and rotation to fentanyl has been observed to be effective in diminishing opioid-induced pruritus in children (Harris JD, Santiago-Palma JC, et al, unpublished data). In addition, rotation to hydromorphone from morphine has been successful in the management of opioid-induced pruritus.[175]

Topical Treatment

Application of cold compresses, medicated baths (oatmeal, baking soda), lotions containing menthol, anesthetic creams, and antihistamine creams can diminish pruritus.

Antihistamines

Traditional antihistamines can be effective[3] but have anticholinergic side effects (see Antihistamines under Management of Nausea and Vomiting).

Opioid Agonists–Antagonists

There are reports indicating that low-dose nalbuphine (e.g., 5 mg IV q4h prn) and intranasal butorphanol may reverse pruritus without compromising anesthesia[168]; but this may play a role more in the acute setting rather than in the chronic opioid setting.

Opioid Antagonists

Naloxone can be used in the management of opioid-induced pruritus in the postoperative setting, particularly in patients receiving neuraxial analgesia. The effect, though, is short lasting. At Roswell Park Cancer Institute, we use the following regimen, which has shown effectiveness in treating opioid-induced itching while preserving pain relief: Dilute 0.4 mg of naloxone in 9 mL of normal saline (NS). Administer 1 mL every 2 minutes until symptoms are relieved up to a maximum dose of 0.4 mg of naloxone (10 mL of 0.4 mg diluted with 9 mL NS). Methylnaltrexone (discussed in more detail previously in this chapter) has also been demonstrated to be effective in the treatment of opioid-induced pruritus in an acute setting.[170]

Paroxetine

There are case reports indicating its efficacy in the management of pruritus in advanced cancer patients.[176] It is a selective serotonin reuptake inhibitor, and the effect may be partly caused by the down-regulation of serotonin 5HT3 receptors.

Ondansetron

Ondansetron is a specific 5HT3 receptor antagonist. Several studies at doses of 4 mg to 8 mg have shown its efficacy in diminishing opioid-induced pruritus.[177]

Diaphoresis

Mild self-resolving sweating at the initiation of opioid therapy in opioid-naive patients is acceptable. Excessive sweating is commonly a sign of opioid withdrawal or another systemic illness with enhanced sympathetic firing, such as hyperthyroidism or anxiety. If it becomes suspected that the opioid is responsible for troublesome diaphoresis, opioid rotation is warranted.[178]

IMMUNOLOGIC SIDE EFFECTS

Chronic opioid administration may be associated with immune suppression. Increased rates of infection have been observed in heroin addicts and in patients with human immunodeficiency virus (HIV) and acquired immune deficiency syndrome (AIDS) who are receiving chronic opioids.[179,180] Although some point to confounding factors such as nutrition, lifestyle, and access to health care that may also play a role in these findings,[181] animal and clinical studies have supported this phenomenon.[182] Opioids have been found to inhibit lymphocyte proliferation, decrease natural killer (NK) cell activity, and affect antibody production.[182] In addition, they may increase the viral load in HIV infected patients.[180] The exact mechanisms involved in opioid-induced immunosuppression are not completely understood, and both central and peripheral pathways may be involved.[182]

In cancer patients who may already possess a suppressed immune system, the risk of further suppression by chronic opioid administration may become more problematic. However, to ascertain if opioid therapy has a significant clinical effect on these patients or not, more clinical studies are required. For a detailed account on this topic, see Chapter 17.

Management

To date, there are no established standards for the management of presumptive opioid-induced immunosuppression.

If immune suppression is diagnosed, opioid rotation may play an important role in its management because different opioids have exhibited different immunologic responses in some studies.[183,184] This, however, has not been adequately substantiated. Regardless, adequate personal hygiene and preventive vaccinations are recommended, and clearly, the detection of an infection dictates that management should focus on treating its cause.

CONCLUSION

Increasing use of opioids and in larger doses has led to increased reports of side effects. Management should be directed with the goal of decreasing or eliminating these side effects, while ensuring optimal pain control. Decreasing the opioid dose, if possible, should be the first alternative. Other alternatives include changing the route of administration, adding adjuvant analgesics, analgesic blocks, use of medications to treat the side effects, and opioid rotation. Opioid rotation is an attractive alternative because it decreases polypharmacy and can often result in achievement of optimal pain control with diminished side effects.

REFERENCES

1. International Narcotics Control Board: United Nations Demographic Yearbook. Pain and Policy Studies Group, University of Wisconsin/WHO Collaborating Center, 2005.
2. Gilson AM, Ryan KM, Joranson DE, Dahl JL: A reassessment of trends in the medical use and abuse of opioid analgesics and implications for diversion control: 1997-2002. J Pain Symptom Manage 28:176–188, 2004.
3. Cherny N, Ripamonti C, Pereira J, et al: Strategies to manage the adverse effects of oral morphine: An evidence-based report. J Clin Oncol 19:2542–2554, 2001.
4. Mercadante S, Casuccio A, Fulfaro F, et al: Switching from morphine to methadone to improve analgesia and tolerability in cancer patients: A prospective study. J Clin Oncol 19:2898–2904, 2001.
5. Mercadante S, Portenoy RK: Opioid poorly-responsive cancer pain. Part 1. Clinical considerations. J Pain Symptom Manage 21:144–150, 2001.
6. Mercadante S, Portenoy RK: Opioid poorly-responsive cancer pain. Part 3. Clinical strategies to improve opioid responsiveness. J Pain Symptom Manage 21:338–354, 2001.
7. Foley KM, Houde RW: Methadone in cancer pain management: Individualize dose and titrate to effect. J Clin Oncol 16:3213–3215, 1998.

8. Bruera E, Franco JJ, Maltoni M, et al: Changing pattern of agitated impaired mental status in patients with advanced cancer: Association with cognitive monitoring, hydration, and opioid rotation. J Pain Symptom Manage 10:287–291, 1995.
9. Pasternak GW: Incomplete cross tolerance and multiple mu opioid peptide receptors. Trends Pharmacol Sci 22:67–70, 2001.
10. Pasternak GW: Insights into mu opioid pharmacology the role of mu opioid receptor subtypes. Life Sci 68:2213–2219, 2001.
11. Bruera E, Neumann CM: Role of methadone in the management of pain in cancer patients. Oncology (Williston Park) 13:1275–1282; discussion 1285–1288, 1291, 1999.
12. Bruera E, Pereira J, Watanabe S, et al: Opioid rotation in patients with cancer pain. A retrospective comparison of dose ratios between methadone, hydromorphone, and morphine. Cancer 78:852–857, 1996.
13. Mannix KA: Palliation of nausea and vomiting. In Doyle D, Hanks GWC, MacDonald N (eds): Oxford Textbook of Palliative Medicine, 2nd ed. New York, Oxford University Press 1998, pp 489–499.
14. Bruera E, Seifert L, Watanabe S, et al: Chronic nausea in advanced cancer patients: A retrospective assessment of a metoclopramide-based antiemetic regimen. J Pain Symptom Manage 11:147–153, 1996.

15. Campora E, Merlini L, Pace M, et al: The incidence of narcotic-induced emesis. J Pain Symptom Manage 6:428–430, 1991.
16. Aparasu R, McCoy RA, Weber C, et al: Opioid-induced emesis among hospitalized nonsurgical patients: Effect on pain and quality of life. J Pain Symptom Manage 18:280–288, 1999.
17. Kovac AL: Prevention and treatment of postoperative nausea and vomiting. Drugs 59:213–243, 2000.
18. Ross DD, Alexander CS: Management of common symptoms in terminally ill patients: Part I. Fatigue, anorexia, cachexia, nausea and vomiting. Am Fam Physician 64:807–814, 2001.
19. Herndon CM, Jackson KC 2nd, Hallin PA: Management of opioid-induced gastrointestinal effects in patients receiving palliative care. Pharmacotherapy 22:240–250, 2002.
20. Hagen NA, Foley KM, Cerbone DJ, et al: Chronic nausea and morphine-6-glucuronide. J Pain Symptom Manage 6:125–128, 1991.
21. Hardy J, Daly S, McQuade B, et al: A double-blind, randomised, parallel group, multinational, multicentre study comparing a single dose of ondansetron 24 mg p.o. with placebo and metoclopramide 10 mg t.d.s. p.o. in the treatment of opioid-induced nausea and emesis in cancer patients. Support Care Cancer 10:231–236, 2002.

22. Critchley P, Plach N, Grantham M, et al: Efficacy of haloperidol in the treatment of nausea and vomiting in the palliative patient: A systematic review. J Pain Symptom Manage 22:631–634, 2001.
23. Gregory RE, Ettinger DS: 5-HT3 receptor antagonists for the prevention of chemotherapy-induced nausea and vomiting. A comparison of their pharmacology and clinical efficacy. Drugs 55:173–189, 1998.
24. Tarkkila P, Torn K, Tuominen M, et al: Premedication with promethazine and transdermal scopolamine reduces the incidence of nausea and vomiting after intrathecal morphine. Acta Anaesthesiol Scand 39:983–986, 1995.
25. Sussman G, Shurman J, Creed MR, et al: Intravenous ondansetron for the control of opioid-induced nausea and vomiting. International S3AA3013 Study Group. Clin Ther 21:1216–1227, 1999.
26. Thomas R, Jones N: Prospective randomized, double-blind comparative study of dexamethasone, ondansetron, and ondansetron plus dexamethasone as prophylactic antiemetic therapy in patients undergoing day-case gynaecological surgery. Br J Anaesth 87:588–592, 2001.
27. Ioannidis JP, Hesketh PJ, Lau J: Contribution of dexamethasone to control of chemotherapy-induced nausea and vomiting: A meta-analysis of randomized evidence. J Clin Oncol 18:3409–3422, 2000.
28. Tzeng JI, Hsing CH, Chu CC, et al: Low-dose dexamethasone reduces nausea and vomiting after epidural morphine: A comparison of metoclopramide with saline. J Clin Anesth 14:19–23, 2002.
29. Voth EA, Schwartz RH: Medicinal applications of delta-9-tetrahydrocannabinol and marijuana. Ann Intern Med 126:791–798, 1997.
30. Simoneau II, Hamza MS, Mata HP, et al: The cannabinoid agonist WIN55,212-2 suppresses opioid-induced emesis in ferrets. Anesthesiology 94:882–887, 2001.
31. Mancini I, Bruera E: Constipation in advanced cancer patients. Support Care Cancer 6:356–364, 1998.
32. Davies A, Prentice W: Re: Fentanyl, morphine, and constipation. J Pain Symptom Manage 16:141–144, 1998.
33. Glare P, Lickiss JN: Unrecognized constipation in patients with advanced cancer: A recipe for therapeutic disaster. J Pain Symptom Manage 7:369–371, 1992.
34. Yuan CS, Foss JF, O'Connor M, et al: Gut motility and transit changes in patients receiving long-term methadone maintenance. J Clin Pharmacol 38:931–935, 1998.
35. Daeninck PJ, Bruera E: Reduction in constipation and laxative requirements following opioid rotation to methadone: A report of four cases. J Pain Symptom Manage 18:303–309, 1999.
36. Pappagallo M: Incidence, prevalence, and management of opioid bowel dysfunction. Am J Surg 182(5A suppl):11S–18S, 2001.
37. Radbruch L, Sabatowski R, Loick G, et al: Constipation and the use of laxatives: A comparison between transdermal fentanyl and oral morphine. Palliat Med 14:111–119, 2000.
38. Liu M, Wittbrodt E: Low-dose oral naloxone reverses opioid-induced constipation and analgesia. J Pain Symptom Manage 23:48–53, 2002.

39. Hurdon V, Viola R, Schroder C: How useful is docusate in patients at risk for constipation? A systematic review of the evidence in the chronically ill. J Pain Symptom Manage 19:130–136, 2000.
40. Tamayo AC, Diaz-Zuluaga PA: Management of opioid-induced bowel dysfunction in cancer patients. Support Care Cancer 12:613–618, 2004.
41. Drolet B, Rousseau G, Daleau P, et al: Domperidone should not be considered a no-risk alternative to cisapride in the treatment of gastrointestinal motility disorders. Circulation 102:1883–1885, 2000.
42. Dickerson ED, Benedetti C, Davis, MP, et al: Palliative Care Pocket Consultant: AIMS, Oxford International Centre for Palliative Care, 1999.
43. Rowbotham DJ, Bamber PA, Nimmo WS: Comparison of the effect of cisapride and metoclopramide on morphine-induced delay in gastric emptying. Br J Clin Pharmacol 26:741–746, 1988.
44. Green SM (ed). Tarascon Pocket Pharmacopoeia. Tarascon Press, Loma Linda, CA, 2001, p 56.
45. Galligan JJ, Vanner S: Basic and clinical pharmacology of new motility promoting agents. Neurogastroenterol Motil 17:643–653, 2005.
46. Leung WK, Chan FK, Fung SS, et al: Effect of oral ethromycin on gastric and small bowel transit time of capsule endoscopy. World J Gastroenterol 11:4865–4868, 2005.
47. Meissner W, Schmidt U, Hartmann M, et al: Oral naloxone reverses opioid-associated constipation. Pain 84:104–109, 2000.
48. Yuan CS, Foss JF: Oral methylnaltrexone for opioid-induced constipation. JAMA 284:1383–1384, 2000.
49. Foss JF: A review of the potential role of methylnaltrexone in opioid bowel dysfunction. Am J Surg 182(5A suppl): 19S–26S, 2001.
50. Schmidt WK: Alvimopan* (ADL 8-2698) is a novel peripheral opioid antagonist. Am J Surg 182(5A suppl):27S–38S, 2001.
51. Andersen G, Sjogren P, Hansen SH, et al: Pharmacological consequences of long-term morphine treatment in patients with cancer and chronic non-malignant pain. Eur J Pain 8:263–271, 2004.
52. Mercadante S: Opioid rotation for cancer pain: Rationale and clinical aspects. Cancer 86:1856–1866, 1999.
53. Robbins J: Dry mouth and delayed dissolution of sublingual nitroglycerin, N Engl J Med 309:985, 1983.
54. Davies AN, Vriens J: Oral Transmucosal Fentanyl Citrate and Xerostomia. J Pain Symptom Manage 30:496–497, 2005.
55. Gotrick B, Akerman S, Ericson D, et al: Oral pilocarpine for treatment of opioid-induced oral dryness in healthy adults. J. Dent Res 83: 393–397, 2004.
56. Fox PC: Salivary enhancement therapies. Caries Res 38:241–246, 2004.
57. Koukourakis MI, Danielidis V: Preventing radiation-induced xerostomia. Cancer Treat Rev 31:546–554, 2005.
58. Johnstone PA, Peng YP, May BC, et al: Acupuncture for pilocarpine-resistant xerostomia following radiotherapy for head and neck malignancies. Int J Radiat Oncol Biol Phys 50:353–357, 2001.

59. Schug SA, Garrett WR, Gillespie G. Opioid and non-opioid analgesics. Best Prac Res Clin Anaesthesiol 17:91–110, 2003.
60. Fakuda K: Intravenous opioid anesthetics. In Miller RD (ed): Anesthesia, 6th ed. Philadelphia, Elsevier, 2005, pp 379–437.
61. Zsigmond EK, Vieira ZE, Duarte B, et al: Double-blind placebo-controlled ultrasonographic confirmation of constriction of the common bile duct by morphine. Int J Clin Pharm Ther Tox, 31:506–509, 1993.
62. Vieira ZE, Zsigmond EK, Duarte B, et al: Evaluation of fentanyl and sufentanil on the diameter of the common bile duct by ultrasonography in man: A double blind, placebo controlled study. Int J Clin Pharm Ther Tox 32:274–277, 1994.
63. Smith MT: Neuroexcitatory effects of morphine and hydromorphone: Evidence implicating the 3-glucuronide metabolites. Clin Exp Pharmacol Physiol 27:524–528, 2000.
64. Bruera E, Faisinger R, MacEachern T, et al: The use of methylphenidate in patients with incident cancer pain receiving regular opiates: Preliminary report. Pain 50:75–77, 1992.
65. Slatkin NE, Rhiner M: A retrospective chart review of 40 patients. Treatment of opiate-related sedation: Utility of the cholinesterase inhibitors. J Support Oncol 1:53–63, 2003.
66. Jones BE: The organization of central cholinergic systems and their functional importance in sleep-waking states. Prog Brain Res 98:61–71, 1993.
67. Slatkin NE, Rhiner M, Maluso Bolton T: Donepezil in the treatment of opioid-induced sedation: Report of six cases.
68. Tiseo PJ, Thaler HT, Lapin J, et al: Morphine-6-glucuronide concentrations and opioid-related side effects: A survey in cancer patients. Pain 61:47–54, 1995.
69. Dalal S, Melzack R: Potentiation of opioid analgesia by psychostimulant drugs: A review. J Pain Symptom Manage 16:245–253, 1998.
70. Bruera E, Chadwick S, Brenneis, et al: Methylphenidate associated with narcotics for the treatment of cancer pain. Cancer Treatment Rep 71:67–70, 1987.
71. Yee JD, Berde CB: Methylphenidate or dextroamphetamine as adjuvants in opioid analgesia [abstract]. J Pain Symptom Manage 6:162, 1991.
72. Bruera E, Miller MJ, Macmillan K, et al: Neuropsychological effects of methylphenidate in patients receiving a continuous infusion of narcotics for cancer pain. Pain 48:163–166, 1992.
73. Wilwerding MB, Loprinzi CL, Mailliard JA, et al: A randomized crossover evaluation of methylphenidate in cancer patients receiving strong narcotics. Support Care Cancer 3:135–138, 1995.
74. Katon W, Raskind M: Treatment of depression in the medically ill elderly with methylphenidate. Am J Psychiatry 137:963–965, 1980.
75. Homsi J, Walsh D, Nelson KA: Psychostimulants in supportive care. Support Care Cancer 8:385–397, 2000.
76. Webster L, Andrews M, Stoddard G: Modafinil treatment of opioid-induced sedation. Pain Medicine 4:135–140, 2003.
77. Mitler MM, Harsh J, Hirshkowitz M, et al: Long-term efficacy and safety of modafinil (Provigil(R)) for the treatment of

excessive daytime sleepiness associated with narcolepsy. Sleep Med 1:231–243, 2000.

78. www.drugstore.com. Approximate retail price of modafinil. Accessed January 22, 2005.

79. Bruera E, Strasser F, Shen L, et al: The effect of donepezil on sedation and other symptoms in patients receiving opioids for cancer pain: A pilot study. J Pain Symptom Management 26:1049–1054, 2003.

80. Ettinger AB, Portenoy RK: The use of corticosteroids in the treatment of symptoms associated with cancer. J Pain Symptom Manage 3:99–103, 1988.

81. Watanabe S, Bruera E: Corticosteroids as adjuvant analgesics. J Pain Symptom Manage 9:442–445, 1994.

82. Vaccarino AL, Couret LC Jr: Relationship between hypothalamic-pituitary-adrenal activity and blockade of tolerance to morphine analgesia by pain: A strain comparison. Pain 63:385–389, 1995.

83. Potter JM, Reid DB, Shaw RJ, et al: Myoclonus associated with treatment with high doses of morphine: The role of supplemental drugs. BMJ 299:150–153, 1989.

84. Hanks G, Cherny N: Opioid analgesic therapy. In: Doyle D, Hanks GWC, MacDonald N (eds): Oxford Textbook of Palliative Medicine, 2nd ed. New York, Oxford University Press 1998, pp 331–355.

85. International Association for the Study of Pain Subcommittee on Taxonomy: Classification of chronic pain. Descriptions of chronic pain syndromes and definitions of pain terms. Pain. 3 (suppl.):217–219, 1986.

86. Mercadante S, Ferrera P, Villari P, et al: Hyperalgesia: An emerging iatrogenic syndrome. J Pain Symptom Manage 26:769–775, 2003.

87. Porreca F, Ossipov MH, Gebhart GF: Chronic pain and medullary descending facilitation. Trends Neurosci. 25:319–325, 2002.

88. Ossipov MH, Lai J, King T, et al: Underlying mechanisms of pronociceptive consequences of prolonged morphine exposure. Biopolymers (Peptide Science) 80:319–324, 2005.

89. Mao J: Opioid-induced abnormal pain sensitivity: Implications in clinical opioid therapy. Pain. 100:213–217, 2002.

90. Mao J, Sung B, Ji RR, et al: Chronic morphine induces downregulation of spinal glutamate transporters: Implications in morphine tolerance and abnormal pain sensitivity. J Neurosci 22:8312–8323, 2002.

91. Vanderah TW, Gardell LR, Burgess SE, et al: Dynorphin promotes abnormal pain and spinal opioid antinociceptive tolerance. J Neurosci 20:7074–7079, 2000.

92. Sjogren P, Jonsson T, Jensen NH, et al: Hyperalgesia and myoclonus in terminal cancer patients treated with continuous intravenous morphine. Pain 55:93–97, 1993.

93. Davis AM, Inturrisi CE: d-Methadone blocks morphine tolerance and N-methyl-D-aspartate-induced hyperalgesia. J Pharmacol Exp Ther 289:1048–1053, 1999.

94. Inturrisi CE: Pharmacology of methadone and its isomers. Minerva Anestesiol 71:435–437, 2005.

95. Bell RF, Eccleston C, Kalso E: Ketamine as adjuvant to opioids for cancer pain: A qualitative systematic review. J Pain Symptom Manage 26:867–875, 2003.

96. De Kock M, Lavand'homme P, Waterloos H: "Balanced analgesia" in the perioperative period: Is there a place for ketamine? Pain 92:373–380, 2001.

97. Quan DB, Wandres DL, Schroeder DJ: Clonidine in pain management. Ann Pharmacother 27:313–315, 1993.

98. De Kock M, Crochet B, Morimont C, et al: Intravenous or epidural clonidine for intra- and postoperative analgesia. Anesthesiology 79:525–531, 1993.

99. Vanderah TW, Suenaga NM, Ossipov MH, et al: Tonic descending facilitation from the rostral ventromedial medulla mediates opioid-induced abnormal pain and antinociceptive tolerance. J Neurosci 21:279–286, 2001.

100. Ferrini R, Paice JA: How to initiate and monitor infusional lidocaine for severe and/or neuropathic pain. J Support Oncol 2:90–94, 2004.

101. Crain SM, Shen KF: Ultra-low concentrations of naloxone selectively antagonize excitatory effects of morphine on sensory neurons, thereby increasing its antinociceptive potency and attenuating tolerance/dependence during chronic cotreatment. Proc Natl Acad Sci USA 92:10540–10544. 1995.

102. Crain SM, Shen KF: Acute thermal hypealgesia elicited by low-dose morphine in normal mice is blocked by ultra-low-dose naltrexone, unmasking potent analgesia. Brain Res 888:75–82, 2001.

103. Cepeda MS, Alvarez H, Morales O, et al: Addition of ultralow dose naloxone to postoperative morphine PCA: Unchanged analgesia and opioid requirement but decreased incidence of opioid side effects. Pain 107:41–46, 2004.

104. Gan TJ, Ginsberg B, Glass PS, et al: Opioid-sparing effects of low-dose infusion of naloxone in patient administered morphine sulfate. Anesthesiology 87:1075–1081, 1997.

105. Mercadante S, Villari P, Ferrera P: Naloxone in treating central adverse effects during opioid titration for cancer pain. J Pain Symptom Manage 26:691–693, 2003.

106. Haas DA: Opioids, Analgesics, and Antagonists. In: Dionne RA, Phero JC, Becker DE (eds): Management of Pain and Anxiety in the Dental Office, 1st ed., Philadelphia, WB Saunders, pp 114–128, 2002.

107. Fukuda K: Intravenous Opioid Anesthetics. In Miller RD (ed): Miller's Anesthesia, 6th ed., New York, Churchill Livingstone, pp 379–438, 2005.

108. Hagen N, Swanson R: Strychnine-lie multifocal myoclonus and seizures in extremely high-dose opioid administration: Treatment strategies. J Pain Symptom Manage 15:143, 1998.

109. Latta K, Ginsberg B, Barkin R: Meperidine: A critical review. Am J Therapeut 9:53–68, 2002.

110. Twycross R: Re: Opioid-induced myoclonus and seizures. J Pain Symptom Manage 15:143, 1998.

111. Delanty N, Vaughan CJ, French JA: Medical causes of seizures. Lancet 352:383–90, 1998.

112. Hanks G, Charny NI, Fallon M: Opioid analgesic therapy. In Doyle D, Hanks G, Cherny NI, et al (eds): Oxford Textbook of Palliative Medicine, 3rd ed, New York, Oxford University Press, pp 316–40, 2004.

113. Symon DN: Twelve cases of analgesic headache. Arch Dis Child 78:555–556, 1998.

114. Couch JR: Rebound-withdrawal headache (medication overuse headache). Curr Treat Options Neurol. 8:11–19, 2006.

115. Gilani A: A case of opioid induced headaches. News Can Pain Soc No volume listed:3–4, 2004.

116. Manfredi PL, Ribeiro S, Chandler SW, et al: Inappropriate use of naloxone in cancer patients with pain. J Pain Symptom Manage 11:131–134, 1996.

117. Pharmacy Therapeutics Committee. Intravenous Medication Guidelines: Naloxone. New York, Memorial Sloan-Kettering Cancer Center, 1994.

118. Schumacher MA, Basbaum AI, Way WL: Opioid analgesics & antagonists. In Katzung BG (ed): Basic & Clinical Pharmacology, 9th ed. New York, The McGraw-Hill Co., 2003, pp 497–516.

119. Kleinschmidt KC, Wainscott M, Ford MD: Opioids. In Ford MD, Delaney KA, Ling LJ, et al (eds): Clinical Toxicology, 1st ed, Philadelphia, WB Saunders, pp 627–639, 2001.

120. Mills CA, Flacke JW, Miller JD, et al: Cardiovascular effects of fentanyl reversal by naloxone at varying arterial carbon dioxide tensions in dogs. Anesth Analg 67:730–736, 1988.

121. Kuo SC, Lin YC, Kao SM, et al: Probable codeine phosphate-induced seizures. Ann Pharmacother 38:1848–1851, 2004.

122. Seifert CF, Kennedy S: Meperidine is alive and well in the new millennium: Evaluation of meperidine usage patterns and frequency of adverse drug reactions. Pharmacotherapy 24:776–783, 2004.

123. Kornick CA, Kilborn MJ, Santiago-Palma J, et al: QTc interval prolongation associated with intravenous methadone. Pain 105:499–506, 2003.

124. Krantz MJ, Kutinsky IB, Robertson AD, et al: Dose-related effects of methadone on QT prolongation in a series of patients with torsade de pointes. Pharmacotherapy 23:802–805, 2003.

125. Harris JD, de Leon-Casasola OA: Methadone and QTc prolongation. In: Oral erythromycin and the risk of sudden death (Letter to the editor). N Engl J Med 352:302, 2005.

126. Mercadante S, Arcuri E: Opioids and renal function. J Pain 5:2–19, 2004.

127. Segal A, Dowling JP, Ireton HJ, et al: Granulomatous glomerulonephritis in intravenous drug users: A report of three cases in oxycodone addicts. Hum Pathol 29:1246–1249, 1998.

128. Hill P, Dwyer K, Kay T, et al: Severe chronic renal failure in association with oxycodone addiction: A new form of fibrillary glomerulopathy. Hum Pathol 33:783–787, 2002.

129. Dean M: Opioids in renal failure and dialysis patients. J Pain Symptom Manage 28:497–504, 2004.

130. Practice guidelines for cancer pain management: A report by the American Society of Anesthesiologists Task Force on Pain Management, Cancer Pain Section. Anesthesiology 84:1243–1257, 1996.

131. Dray A: Epidural opiates and urinary retention: New models provide new insights. Anesthesiology 68:323–324, 1988.

132. Dray A, Metsch R: Spinal opioid receptors and inhibition of urinary bladder motility in vivo. Neurosci Lett 47:81–84, 1984.

133. Gardner-Nix J: Opioids causing peripheral edema. J Pain Symptom Manage 23: 453–455, 2002.

134. Mahe I, Chassany O, Grenard AS, et al: Methadone and edema: A case-report and literature review. Eur J Clin Pharmacol 59:923–924, 2004.

135. Aldrete JA, Couto da Silva JM: Leg edema from intrathecal opiate infusions. Eur J Pain 4:361–365, 2000.

136. Supanz S, Likar R, Liebmann PM, et al: On the role of the kidneys in the pathogenesis of edema formation during permanent morphine application: An experimental study in rats. Arzneimittelforschung 54:259–264, 2004.

137. Whiteside GT, Boulet JM, Walker K: The role of central and peripheral mu opioid receptors in inflammatory pain and edema: A study using morphine and DiPOA ([8-(3,3-diphenyl-propyl)-4-oxo-1-phenyl-1,3,8-triaza-spiro[4.5] dec-3-yl]-acetic acid). J Pharmacol Exp Ther 314:1234–1240, 2005.

138. Morita T, Hyodo I, Yoshimi T, et al: Association between hydration volume and symptoms in terminally ill cancer patients with abdominal malignancies. Ann Oncol 16:640–647, 2005.

139. Thomas DR: Medications and sexual function. Clin Geriatr Med 19:553–562, 2003.

140. Christo PJ: Opioid effectiveness and side effects in chronic pain. Anesthesiol Clin North Am 21:699–713, 2003.

141. Katz N: The impact of opioids on the endocrine system. Pain Manage Rounds 1, 2005.

142. Pelosi MA, Sama JC, Caterini H, et al: Galactorrhea-amenorrhea syndrome associated with heroin addiction. Am J Obstet Gynecol 118:966–970, 1974.

143. De Leon G, Wexler HK: Heroin addiction: its relation to sexual behavior and sexual experience. J Abnorm Psychol 81:36–38, 1973.

144. Hanbury R, Cohen M, Stimmel B: Adequacy of sexual performance in men maintained on methadone. Am J Drug Alcohol Abuse 4:13–20, 1977.

145. Smith DE, Moser C, Wesson DR, et al: A clinical guide to the diagnosis and treatment of heroin-related sexual dysfunction. J Psychoactive Drugs. 14:91–99, 1982.

146. Crowley TJ, Simpson R: Methadone dose and human sexual behavior. Int J Addict 13:285–295, 1978.

147. Palha AP, Esteves M: A study of the sexuality of opiate addicts. J Sex Marital Ther 28:427–437, 2002.

148. Lussier D, Pappagallo M: 10 most commonly asked questions about the use of opioids for chronic pain. Neurologist 10:221–224, 2004.

149. Lenahan PM: Sexual health and chronic illness. Clin Fam Pract 6:955–973, 2004.

150. Rajagopal A, Bruera ED: Improvement in sexual function after reduction of chronic high-dose opioid medication in a cancer survivor. Pain Med 4:379–383, 2003.

151. Paice JA, Penn RD, Ryan WG: Altered sexual function and decreased testosterone in patients receiving intraspinal opioids. J Pain Symptom Manage 9:126–131, 1994.

152. Abs R, Verhelst J, Maeyaert J, et al: Endocrine consequences of long-term intrathecal administration of opioids. J Clin Endocrinol Metab 85:2215–2222, 2000.

153. Finch PM, Roberts LJ, Price L, et al: Hypogonadism in patients treated with intrathecal morphine. Clin J Pain 16:251–254, 2000.

154. Roberts LJ, Finch PM, Pullan PT, et al: Sex hormone suppression by intrathecal opioids: A prospective study. Clin J Pain 18:144–148, 2002.

155. Coolen LM, Fitzgerald ME, Yu L, et al: Activation of mu opioid receptors in the medial preoptic area following copulation in male rats. Neuroscience 124:11–21, 2004.

156. Jordan D, Tafani JA, Ries C, et al: Evidence for multiple opioid receptors in the human posterior pituitary. J Neuroendocrinol 8:883–887, 1996.

157. Carretero J, Bodego P, Rodriguez RE, et al: Expression of the mu-opioid receptor in the anterior pituitary gland is influenced by age and sex. Neuropeptides 38:63–68, 2004.

158. Lafisca S, Bolelli G, Franceschetti F, et al: Free and bound testosterone in male heroin addicts. Arch Toxicol Suppl 8:394–397, 1985.

159. Forman LJ, Tingle V, Estilow S, et al: The response to analgesia testing is affected by gonadal steroids in the rat. Life Sci 45:447–454, 1989.

160. Miller K, Corcoran C, Armstrong C, et al: Transdermal testosterone administration in women with acquired immunodeficiency syndrome wasting: A pilot study. J Clin Endocrinol Metab 83:2717–2725, 1998.

161. Bellati U, Noia G, Conte M, et al: Amenorrhea in drug dependence. Minerva Med 74:865–868, 1983.

162. Bachmann GA, Avci D: Evaluation and management of female sexual dysfunction. Endocrinologist 14:337–345, 2004.

163. Kendirci M, Hellstrom WJ: Current concepts in the management of erectile dysfunction in men with prostate cancer. Clin Prostate Cancer 3:87–92, 2004.

164. Cremers B, Bohm M: Non erectile dysfunction application of sildenafil. Herz 28:325–333, 2003.

165. Stausmire JM: Sexuality at the end of life. Am J Hosp Palliat Car 21:33–39, 2004.

166. Hajjar RR, Kamel HK: Osteoporosis for the home care physician. Part 1: Etiology and current diagnostic strategies. J Am Med Dir Assoc 5:192–196, 2004.

167. Kamel HK, Hajjar RR: Osteoporosis for the home care physician. Part 2: Management. J Am Med Dir Assoc 5:259–262, 2004.

168. Krajnik M, Zylicz Z: Understanding pruritus in systemic disease. J Pain Symptom Manage 21:151–168, 2001.

169. Chaney MA: Side effects of intrathecal and epidural opioids. Can J Anesthesia 42:891–903, 1995.

170. Friedman JD, Dello Buono FA: Opioid antagonists in the treatment of opioid-induced constipation and pruritus. Ann Pharmacother 35:85–91, 2001.

171. Schmelz M: Itch: Mediators and mechanisms. J Dermatol Sci. 28:91–96, 2002.

172. Mucci-LoRusso P, Berman BS, Silberstein PT, et al: Controlled-release oxycodone compared with controlled-release morphine in the treatment of cancer pain: A randomized, double-blind, parallel-group study. Eur J Pain 2:239–249, 1998.

173. Woodhouse A, Hobbes AF, Mather LE, et al: A comparison of morphine, pethidine and fentanyl in the post-surgical patient-controlled analgesia environment. Pain 64:115–121, 1996.

174. Flacke JW, Flacke WE, Bloor BC, et al: Histamine release by four narcotics: A double-blind study in humans. Anesth Analg 66:723–730, 1987.

175. Katcher J, Walsh D: Opioid-induced itching: morphine sulfate and hydromorphone hydrochloride. J Pain Symptom Manage 17:70–72, 1999.

176. Zylicz Z, Smits C, Krajnik M: Paroxetine for pruritus in advanced cancer. J Pain Symptom Manage 16:121–124, 1998.

177. Charuluxananan S, Somboonviboon W, Kyokong O, et al: Ondansetron for treatment of intrathecal morphine-induced pruritus after cesarean delivery. Reg Anesth Pain Med 25:535–539, 2000.

178. Winn PA, Dentino AN: Effective pain management in the long-term care setting. J Am Med Dir Assoc 5:342–352, 2004.

179. Haverkos HW, Lange WR: From the alcohol, drug abuse, and mental health administration. Serious infections other than human immunodeficiency virus among intravenous drug abusers. J Infect Dis. 161:894–902, 1990.

180. Carr DJ, Serou M: Exogenous and endogenous opioids as biological response modifiers. Immunopharmacology 31:59–71, 1995.

181. McLachlan C, Crofts N, Wodak A, et al: The effects of methadone on immune function among injecting drug users: A review. Addiction 88:257–63, 1993.

182. Wei G, Moss J, Yuan CS: Opioid-induced immunosuppression: Is it centrally mediated or peripherally mediated? Biochemi Pharmacol 65:1761–1766, 2003.

183. Yeager MP, Colacchio TA, Yu CT: Morphine inhibits spontaneous and cytokine-enhanced natural killer cell cytotoxicity in volunteers. Anesthesiology 83:500–508, 1995.

184. Yeager MP, Procopio MA, DeLeo JA, et al: Intravenous fentanyl increases natural killer cell cytotoxicity and circulating CD16 lymphocytes in humans. Anesth Analg 94:94–99, 2002.

CHAPTER 19

Cancer Pain Management in the Opioid-Tolerant Patient

OSCAR A. DE LEON-CASASOLA, MD

The number of patients receiving opioid therapy for the treatment of nonmalignant and malignant conditions has increased in recent years. Likewise, the estimated prevalence of illicit drug use is estimated to be between 3 and 8 per 1000 habitants in the European Union,[1] and about 1.8% of the population actively abuses opiates in the United States.[A] Moreover, the abuse of pain medications is on the rise: 22% of the population age 18 to 22 years old reported abusing opiates in 2002, in contrast to 7% in 1992.[A] When these patients undergo surgical procedures, they may present a significant problem for the management of postoperative pain because patients who have received or self-administered opioids for as little as 2 weeks before surgery may exhibit signs of opioid tolerance.[2] Thus, perioperative requirements may be higher.[2] Yet, their increased postoperative opioid requirement may be interpreted as opioid craving and their requirements may be met with inadequate pain control following as a result of this attitude. Moreover, the risk for physiologic withdrawal will also be present. This may occur if their daily drug requirements are abruptly decreased either because they do not report their usage pattern or due to reluctance of health providers to meet their preoperative requirements. This is particularly important in those patients who abuse opiates, because their daily opiate intake may be significantly greater than patients taking opiates for therapeutic purposes. Moreover, the former may also take other illicit drugs that may have effects on the N-methyl-D-aspartate (NMDA) receptor (e.g., phencyclidine [also known as angel dust, ozone, wack, and rocket fuel]. Killer joints and crystal supergrass are names that refer to PCP combined with marijuana).

Recent studies have helped to understand the cellular mechanisms of opioid tolerance. This information has been useful in defining protocols for the management of patients with a history of high opioid intake so that these patients may also experience adequate postoperative pain control.

CELLULAR MECHANISMS OF TOLERANCE

Tolerance occurs as a result of progressive loss of active receptor sites from prolonged agonist exposure. Desensitization or uncoupling of the receptor from the guanosine triphosphate (GTP)-binding subunit decreases agonist-binding affinity.[3-5] Loss of receptors from the cell surface may also result in less binding sites and decreased action.[3-5] Thus, the desensitization (a qualitative phenomenon) to agonist binding and the loss in the number of opioid receptors (a quantitative phenomenon) result in higher opioid requirements.

Trujillo and Akil[6] and Elliot and colleagues[7] have also implicated the NMDA receptor in the development of acute tolerance. Moreover, Mayer and collaborators[8] reported that opioid tolerance was associated with an increase in the second-messenger protein kinase C (PKC),[8] the production of nitric oxide (NO), and NO-activated poly(ADP) ribose synthetase (PARS)[9] activation within the superficial laminae of the dorsal horn. Because PKC has been shown to regulate the NMDA receptor (its phosphorylation results in removal of a blocking magnesium ion[10]), it is also possible that the development of acute tolerance reflects a PKC-mediated increase in opioid regulation of the NMDA receptor. In fact, opioid tolerance in rodents can be inhibited by noncompetitive NMDA receptor antagonists such as MK801, dextromethorphan, ketamine, and phencyclidine, and competitive NMDA receptor antagonists such as LY274614, NPC 17742, and LY235959.[11] Success has also been achieved with the use of partial glycine agonists (ACPC), glycine antagonists (ACEA-1328), and nitric oxide synthase

---

[A]National Survey on Drug Use and Health, 2002.

inhibitors (L-NNA, L-NMMA, and methylene blue.[11] A recent case report provides further support to the role of the NMDA receptor in opioid tolerance in humans.[12] The authors documented not only pain relief but also a decrease in opioid requirements in a young patient with a history of heroin abuse after a suicide attempt that resulted in multiple trauma. The potential use of ketamine in this setting is an important finding as it has been shown that either a single dose or repeated administration of opioids may lead to activation of the NMDA receptor just as effectively as repeated C-fiber stimulation.[13,14] Thus, ketamine, as well as other NMDA receptor antagonists, could be useful in the treatment of acute postoperative pain in patients with opioid tolerance as it not only reverses morphine tolerance and restores morphine effectiveness,[15] but it may also prevent the development of acute tolerance to opioids. An alternative exciting strategy is the use of benzamide, a selective PARS inhibitor that has been shown to reduce or even prevent the development of opioid analgesic tolerance and the resultant formation of dark neurons in adult male Sprague-Dawley rats.[9]

Acute administration of opioids also inhibits adenyl cyclase, cAMP, and PKA via Gi protein, which decreases the synthesis of cAMP and causes a reduction in protein kinase A (PKA)-mediated phosphorylation of intracellular proteins.[16] The level of cAMP returns to control levels and may even increase beyond control levels when opioid tolerance develops. These changes have been interpreted as an uncoupling of the opioid receptor from the inhibitory Gi protein.[17]

Because uncontrolled pain produces morphologic changes in the receptive field zone of the spinal cord, allowing chronic pain patients to experience acute pain for even short periods of time may result in higher requirements of opioids postoperatively or uncontrolled pain even in the face of increasing doses of opioids, or both.[18] Thus, blockade of afferent pain signals before the visceral stimulus starts may be even more important in the chronic opioid user patient than in the opioid naive patient.[19]

BACKGROUND ON CLINICAL STUDIES

Clinical studies in opioid-tolerant patients are scarce. Moreover, the phenomenon of cross-tolerance between systemic and intraspinal opioids is a controversial issue because of the design of the studies that have evaluated this phenomenon. Although this author and collaborators,[20-22] as well as others,[23] have published data that suggest that humans experience cross-tolerance between the oral and epidural route, others have not shown the same results.[24,25] In the studies by Pfeifer and colleagues[24] and Kossmann and colleagues,[25] patients received 5 to 10 mg of epidural morphine and were followed for only 24 hours. Pharmacokinetic data demonstrate that high

concentrations of morphine result in both the lumbar and cervical CSF of patients receiving similar doses of morphine as those used in the studies by Pfeifer and Kossman 6 to 8 hours after lumbar epidural injection.[26] These high concentrations may saturate the opioid receptors acutely, masking any down-regulation. Thus, cross-tolerance may not be evident after large epidural morphine doses particularly when pain evaluation and opioid utilization analysis is limited to a 24-hour period. As we have documented in our studies,[20-23] patients with a history of opioid use will not only require higher doses of opioids but also more days of therapy as compared with opioid naive patients.

PROTOCOLS FOR PATIENT CARE IN THE POSTOPERATIVE PERIOD

The Pain Service at Roswell Park Cancer Institute has used four different protocols. If there is a contraindication to the insertion of an epidural catheter or the site of surgery is not amenable for this type of therapy, intravenous (IV) patient-controlled analgesia (PCA) is utilized. We convert the patients' daily utilization of oral opioid to IV sufentanil and provide that dosage as a basal infusion over a 24-hour period. For this purpose, we assume that a daily dose of 90 mg of oral morphine, 60 mg of oral methadone, 45 mg of oral oxycodone, 12 mg of oral hydromorphone, or 25 µg/hour every 72 hours of transdermal fentanyl is equivalent to 2 to 4 µg/hour of IV sufentanil. Intravenous breakthrough doses of 2 µg/hour are also given every 6 minutes. The patient is evaluated every 6 hours after the PCA pump has been started, and the doses of sufentanil are adjusted to limit the number of breakthrough boluses to 2 to 3 per hour. If adequate pain control is not achieved despite increasing doses of sufentanil, a continuous infusion of ketamine is started at 10 µg/kg/minute and then titrated down to 2.5 µg/kg/minute as improved analgesia is experienced by the patient.

Patients treated with epidural anesthesia and analgesia receive a bolus dose of 5 to 15 mL of 0.5% ropivacaine 10 to 15 minutes before the surgical incision is made. A continuous infusion of 0.5% ropivacaine and 0.013% MS (4 mg of morphine in 30 mL of ropivacaine) is then started at 4 to 6 mL/hour and titrated according to hemodynamic responses. Postoperatively, patients receive a continuous epidural infusion of 0.2% ropivacaine + 0.02% MS at 4 to 6 mL/hour. Breakthrough doses of 2 to 3 mL every 10 minutes are provided. If dynamic pain control (VAPS <4/10 during movement) is not achieved within 1 hour, the infusion rate is increased by 1 mL every hour. The majority of patients can be managed this way but will require 8 to 10 days of therapy if infusions are only decreased by 1 mL/hour when the VAPS have remained below 4/10 for 6 consecutive hours.[22] Conversely, if pain control is not achieved despite adjustments in the basal infusion up to 8 mL/hour, 50 μg of sufentanil in 5 mL of normal saline are administered epidurally and morphine is replaced by sufentanil. The new solution (0.2% ropivacaine + 0.0002% [2 μg/mL] sufentanil) is infused at 4 to 6 mL/hour and breakthrough doses of 2 to 3 mL every 10 minutes are provided. The basal infusion is titrated every hour to maintain a dynamic VAPS less than 4/10. In this way, patients with severe opioid dependency have been managed successfully at our institution.[20,21]

Drug tolerance at the spinal level is characterized as being time-dependent[27] and dose-dependent.[28] Thus, in cancer patients the use of continuous infusion with small adjustments during the treatment period will result in more effective analgesia at lower doses as compared with intermittent bolus injections of opioids.

Finally, in our experience the use of epidural opioid analgesia not only was associated with excellent pain control in opioid-tolerant patients, but the appearance of physiologic withdrawal was also curtailed.[20-22] This phenomenon is probably due to relatively high concentrations of opioids in the cisterna magna and the limbic system, thus halting the development of withdrawal, despite significant vascular uptake and supraspinal redistribution seen with sufentanil following epidural administration.[20]

CONCLUSION

The high prevalence of opioid use for recreational purposes in the United States and the European Union, as well as the use of opioids for the treatment of chronic nonmalignant pain, has resulted in an increased number of opioid-tolerant patients who undergo surgery and require postoperative pain management. The approach to postoperative pain control in these patients is significantly different from the strategies used in opioid-naive patients. Improved understanding of the cellular mechanisms of opioid tolerance in animals has resulted in the transfer of concepts from the "bench" to the clinical arena. In the future, we may see that patients with opioid tolerance will be managed with anesthetic strategies that result in blockade of afferent signals followed by postoperative administration of opioids with high intrinsic efficacy; NMDA receptor antagonists; and PKC, NO, and PARS inhibitors.

CLINICAL PRACTICE POINTS

1. Opioid tolerance may occur as early as 2 weeks after therapy is started with opioids.
2. Patients who have received high doses of opioids preoperatively will respond better to therapy with opioids with high intrinsic efficacy, such as sufentanil.
3. Evidence supporting the role of the NMDA receptor in the development of tolerance suggests the use of NMDA receptor antagonists, such as ketamine, for the management of patients who are not responding to increasing doses of opioids.
4. Epidural techniques with a local anesthetic and higher doses of morphine or sufentanil are effective in the management of postoperative pain in patients with opioid tolerance.

SUGGESTED FURTHER READING

A. Carroll IR, Angst MS, Clark D: Management of perioperative pain in patients chronically consuming opioids. Reg Anesth Pain Manage 29:576–591, 2004.

REFERENCES

1. European Monitoring Center for Drugs and Drug Addiction: Extended annual report on the state of the drugs problem in the European Union. Luxembourg, Office for Official Publications of the European Community, 2000.
2. Twycross RG: Choice of strong analgesic in terminal cancer: Diamorphine or morphine? Pain 3:93–104, 1977.
3. Chavkin C, Goldstein A: Reduction in opiate receptor reserve in morphine-tolerant guinea pig ilea. Life Sci 31:1687–1690, 1982.
4. Chavkin C, Goldstein A: Opioid receptor reserve in normal and morphine-tolerant

guinea pig ileum myenteric plexus. Proc Natl Acad Sci USA 81:7253–7257, 1984.
5. Rogers NF, El-Fakahany EE: Morphine-induced opioid receptor down regulation detected in intact adult brain cells. Eur J Pharmacol 24:221–230, 1986.
6. Trujillo KA, Akil H: Inhibition of morphine tolerance and dependence by the NMDA receptor antagonist MK-801. Science 251:85–87, 1991.
7. Elliott K, Minami N, Kolesnikov YA, et al: The NMDA receptor antagonists, LY274614 and MK-801, and the nitric oxide synthase inhibitor, NG-nitro-L-arginine, attenuate analgesic

tolerance to the mu-opioid morphine but not to kappa opioids, Pain 56:69–75, 1994.
8. Mayer DJ, Mao J, Price DD: The development of morphine tolerance and dependence is associated with translocation of protein kinase C. Pain 61:365–374, 1995.
9. Mayer DJ, Mao J, Holt J, Price DD: Cellular mechanisms of neuropathic pain, morphine tolerance, and their interactions. Proc Natl Acad Sci 96:7731–7736, 1999.
10. Chen L, Huang LY: Protein kinase C reduces Mg++ block of NMDA-receptor channels as a mechanism of modulation. Nature 356:521–523, 1992.

11. Herman BH, Vocci F, Bridge P: The effects of NMDA receptor antagonists and nitric oxide synthetase inhibitors on opioid tolerance and withdrawal. Medication development issues for opiate addiction. Neuropsychopharmacology 13:269–293, 1995.

12. Haller G, Waeber J-L, Kooger-Infante N, Clergue F: Ketamine combined with morphine for the management of pain in an opioid addict. Anesthesiology 96:1265–1266, 2002.

13. Mao J, Price DD, Mayer DJ: Mechanisms of hyperalgesia and morphine tolerance: A current view of their possible interactions. Pain 62:259–274, 1995.

14. Larcher A, Laulin JP, Celerier E, et al: Acute tolerance associated with a single opiate administration: Involvement of N-methyl-D-aspartate-dependant pain facilitatory system. Neuroscience 84:583–589, 1998.

15. Schimoyama N, Schimoyama M, Inturrisi CE, Elliot KJ: Ketamine attenuates and reverses morphine tolerance in rodents. Anesthesiology 85:1357–1366, 1996.

16. Nestler EJ, Tallman JF: Chronic morphine treatment increase cyclic AMO-dependent protein kinase activity in the rat locus ceruleus. Mol Pharmacol 33:127–132, 1988.

17. Cox BM: Molecular and cellular mechanisms in opioid tolerance. In Basbaum AI, Beeson JM (eds): Towards a New Pharmacotherapy of Pain. Chichester, UK, Wiley, 1991.

18. Dubner R: Pain and hyperalgesia following tissue injury: New mechanisms and new treatments. Pain 44:213–214, 1991.

19. Woolf CJ: Recent advances in the pathophysiology of acute pain. Br J Anaesth 63:139–146, 1989.

20. de Leon-Casasola OA, Lema MJ: Epidural sufentanil provides superior analgesia for opioid tolerant patients unresponsive to epidural morphine. Anesthesiology 80:303–309, 1994.

21. de Leon-Casasola OA, Lema MJ: Epidural sufentanil for acute pain control in a patient with extreme opioid dependency. Anesthesiology 76:853–856, 1992.

22. de Leon-Casasola OA, Myers DP, Donaparthi S, et al: A comparison of postoperative epidural analgesia between chronic cancer patients taking high doses of oral opioids and opioid naive patients. Anesth Analg 76:302–307, 1993.

23. Muller H, Stoyanov M, Borner U: Epidural opiates for relief of cancer pain. In: Yaksh TL, Muller H, Engquist A (eds): Spinal Opiate Analgesia. Berlin, Springer, 1982, pp 125–137.

24. Pfeifer BL, Sernaker HL, Ter Horst Un, et al: Cross tolerance between systemic and epidural morphine in cancer patients. Pain 39:181–187, 1989.

25. Kossmann B, Dick W, Bowdler I: Modern aspects of morphine therapy. In Wilkes E, Levy J (eds): Advances in Morphine Therapy. London, Oxford University Press, 1984, pp 49–57.

26. Brose WG, Tanelian DL, Brodsky JB, et al: CSF and blood pharmacokinetics of hydromorphone and morphine following lumbar epidural administration. Pain 45:11–15, 1991.

27. Wisenfeld Z, Gustafson LL: Continuous intrathecal administration of morphine via an osmotic minipump in the rat. Brain Res 247:195–197, 1982.

28. Stevens CG, Monasky MS, Yaksh TL: Spinal infusion of opiate and alpha-2 agonists in rats: Tolerance and cross tolerance studies. J Pharmacol Exp Ther 244:63–70, 1988.

CHAPTER 20

Cancer Pain Management in the Patient with a History of Opiate Abuse

JOSEPH MOLEA, MD

Pain is a more terrible lord of mankind than even death itself.

Albert Schweitzer

In 1962 Oliver Cope, a Boston surgeon, was elected president of the American Surgical Association and on April 3, 1963, he delivered his presidential address entitled "On Balance." In it, he warned against always relying on radical surgery in the treatment of cancer and called attention to surgery's "fifth dimension": the idea that social factors play a part in formulating a patient's care. He became an activist in emphasizing the behavioral aspects of illness and care and reemphasizing the need to consider the psychologic and emotional aspects of illness in medical education.[1] Many in attendance thought that Cope abandoned his grounding in scientific discipline and a dedication to the quantitative assessment of disease in favor of an intuitive sense of social idealism.[2] Yet, Dr. Cope, in two influential conferences concerning the emotional basis of illness, continued to put forth his ideas.[3] Now, 40 years later, it is evident that Cope's concerns have been almost universally acknowledged. Today, the use of limited surgery with multimodality treatment has become the rule in the care of patients with malignancies. Sadly, though, the awareness of his so-called "fifth dimension," the idea currently known as the psychosocial aspect of illness, is still only marginally accepted outside the fields of psychiatry and addiction medicine.[4]

Although often destructive and disabling, conditions that manifest themselves with pain, anxiety, or sadness are often construed as less real than other medical conditions. The marginalization of such subjective and behavioral aspects of disease contributes to the widespread lack of physicians who take such disorders into consideration before developing treatment plans. To most physicians these problems are nuisances. To patients, however, they can mean real suffering gone unrecognized, uncredited, or ignored. In the cancer patient, when treating pain can

be the sole focus of the therapy, such lapses can mean the difference between the success or failure of the treatment.[4]

The central points are:

1. Pain alters human behavior.
2. Human behavior alters the perception of pain.

Like other instincts and emotions, the experience of pain is the sentinel of a survival mechanism. This mechanism, designed to alert an organism to life-threatening situations, is the subjective reflection of a system of dopamine and serotonin metabolism known to neuroanatomists as limbic, and is reflective of amphibian function.[5]

The French philosopher René Descartes, who imagined the human mind as distinct from the human body, has been dead for 350 years. Modern neuroscience has all but obliterated this so called "mind–body dichotomy." Yet, were Descartes to return, he would find most physicians willing to consider his perspective anew.[6] This "Cartesian dualism" polarizes the biologic and the psychosocial aspects of medicine. This misperception places clinicians on the fault line that, among other things, separates modern concepts of addiction from current pain medicine practice. Our goal of relieving pain and suffering under the heraldic admonition *to primum no nocare* (first do no harm) is more than challenging. The test we face of wrestling this clinical Cerberus from the threshold of the underworld of our patient's suffering, dogged as they are, by her three snarling heads: (1) exquisite pain, (2) irresistible medications urges, and (3) the ceaseless march of drug tolerance. Our success holds the promise of a human experience free from the living hell that ensues when acute pain, our natural ally, becomes chronic. At present, we lumber through the difficult reality of occasional success and regular complications that include worsening pain, warped personalities, and significant mental illness.

For now, here is what we know:

- Mental function arises from the electrochemical phenomenon of the brain.
- The subjective reality of thoughts and feelings we call "the mind" must be understood as the activity of the organ called the brain.
- Environment can and does alter the neurochemical landscape of the brain.
- Direct intervention with medication or by experiential maneuvers alters the patient's subjective experience of pain.

We now know, for example, that cortical development may be retarded by experiences of neglect and deprivation early in life. Fear as well, even in adults, limits cortical modulation of limbic, brainstem, and midbrain, leading to stereotypic responses in individuals.[7] Along the same lines, specific environmental, stressors (e.g., loss of status, loss of employment, divorce, loss of a loved one, or even the loss of a beloved pet) may trigger genetic vulnerabilities and illness. Behavioral changes are associated with serotonergic and noradrenergic alterations. Evidence is mounting that distraction and anxiety are not only environmentally and relationally determined but are centrally mediated as well.[8] Stated another way, medications have as much of a psychologic effect as they do a physiologic one. So too do psychotherapeutic interventions, which affect the brain at a neurochemical level to effect a psychologic impact.

The advances in neurobiology after the "decade of the brain" initiatives of the 1990s provided much needed knowledge of this biology/behavior relationship. Genes, it has been determined, activated by cellular developmental processes, have their expression regulated, to a large degree, by environmental signals. Environmental influences act through the alteration of gene expression to affect brain plasticity. Neural connections between the cortex, the limbic system, and the autonomic nervous system form circuits in the developing nervous system in accordance with these experiences. Emotion and memory circuits are linked together by consistent patterns of stimuli in the environment. In short, the brain possesses more plasticity than previously believed. It is just such brain plasticity, operating through environmental and developmental factors and acting on specific genes, that produces much mental illness. For the purposes of our discussion, the literature is clear in regard to chemical dependency: genetics, environment, and exposure to an activating agent (e.g., opiates) produce drug addiction. The implications of such a dynamic "new" homeostatic mechanism of neurologic function hold great promise for the treatment of "disorder of perception" of which addictions and chronic pain are but a few.

There is perhaps no phenomenon that better illustrates the disastrous implications of separating mind and body than the way our society has treated patients with severe addictions. Research has demonstrated that the conditions and disorders we are discussing here (pain, chemical dependency, and addiction) are real medical disorders of one particular organ of the body, the brain. The next urgent challenge is to succeed in communicating to front-line health care providers what we know through research: that disorders that affect and express themselves through pain and compulsive behavior are real neurophysiologic disorders. Learning how words, thoughts, and insights can change the physical workings of the brain and with what therapeutic effects and what side effects is one of the great challenges before us.

Provocative research on cancer patients now suggests that psychotherapy and meaningful supportive relationships can influence overall brain function with far-flung implications. Survivors of metastatic breast cancer live an average of 18 months longer than the controls when in group psychotherapy. Death rates in melanoma patients were lower and remissions were longer than controls in those who attended support groups that were a mere 6 weeks long.[9] Despite such breakthrough research little of the information is evident in clinical practice.

Patients suffering from cancer pain can benefit from this growing body of knowledge about the interaction between genes, medication, the environment, and the possibility of addiction. These developments point the way toward a new era of practice in which specific modes of therapy can be designed to target specific sites of brain functioning. We stand on the threshold of a sophisticated understanding of the interaction between the brain and the environment that may lead to truly integrative treatment strategies. This chapter attempts to help the clinician identify just such therapies in the hopes of lessening the impact of addictive disorders on the patient suffering cancer-related pain.

NEUROBIOLOGY OF ADDICTIVE DISORDERS

Scientific information about the neurobiology of addictive disorders provides important information impacting the rationale for opioid agonist pharmacotherapy in the field of pain management. The hypothesis underlying that research in the early 1960s was to determine if heroin addiction in and of itself was a disease given that the evidence for heroin addiction before that time was based on clinical anecdotes and the natural history of opiate addiction.[10,11] Both clinical and laboratory-based research, using a variety of appropriate animal models, as well as in vitro techniques, has shown that drugs of abuse in general, and specifically the short-acting opiates, may alter molecular and neurochemical indices, and thus physiologic functions.[12,13] After chronic exposure to a short-acting opiate, these alterations may be persistent or even permanent and may contribute directly to the perpetuation of self-administration of opiates or return to opiate use after achieving a drug-free and medication-free state. There is ample evidence that disruption of several components of the endogenous opioid system, ranging from changes in gene expression to changes in behavior, may occur during cycles of short-acting opiate abuse.[14] Also, there are convincing studies that suggest that stress is altered by chronic abuse of short-acting opiates, including documentation of atypical hyporesponsiveness to stressors during cycles of opiate addiction; evidence of sustained hyper-responsiveness to stressors in the medication-free, illicit-opiate-free state; and in contrast, normalization of stress responsiveness, as reflected by the hypothalamic–pituitary–adrenal axis function in long-term, methadone-maintained patients.[13] Thus, both laboratory and clinical research studies provide firm documentation that the disruption of physiologic, as well as behavioral, functions occurs during chronic administration of short-acting opiates. Also, there is research evidence of an epidemiologic and, more recently of a molecular genetics type, that a genetic vulnerability to develop addictions in general, and opiate addiction specifically, may exist, and that early environmental factors may alter physiology to enhance vulnerability to develop opiate addiction when self-exposed.[14,15]

The inappropriate use of mood-altering drugs transcends the medical arena, and the health costs associated with such use are enormous. According to the National Council on Patient Information and Education, more than 50% of all prescriptions are used incorrectly. Misuse or noncompliance is a major health problem in the United States, resulting in 218,000 deaths and the hospitalization of 1 million people annually. The total cost to the economy is approximately $177 billion annually.[15] Most importantly, it is the physician who is often the first person to have an opportunity to identify individuals who either have the potential to become drug-dependent or are currently using mood-altering substances. Unfortunately, the conclusion often made by those devoted to the study of addictive behaviors is that physicians, who have been trained to be critical thinkers, lose this ability when dealing with patients who are addicted. Too many physicians share the perception that drug dependence, once developed, is primarily a character defect associated with criminal behavior, which might be best managed outside of the medical realm. In short, drug dependency is often perceived as a socioeconomic or psychosocial, rather than a medical, problem.[4]

There is no question that the sociologic, economic, and psychologic factors leading to inappropriate use of mood-altering drugs are important, as is the need for increased funding to develop cost-effective screening instruments to identify patients who may be at risk of developing dependence upon exposure to mood-altering drugs. However, recent evidence establishes the existence of neurobiologic determinants of both initial and especially continuing drug use.

The initiation of drug use is a voluntary, self-willed action (or so it would seem). Nonetheless, once this use continues, depending on the specific drug, considerable change occurs in the brain that, unless understood and addressed, makes it quite difficult to provide effective pain management without the development of iatrogenic dependence in certain patients.[4] With the exception of hallucinogens, laboratory animals will voluntarily self-administer mood-altering substances commonly used inappropriately by humans.[1] Although there are distinct differences between euphoria-producing and dependence-producing drugs (Table 20–1), with the inability of drugs within one group to adequately relieve withdrawal or "craving" for drugs in other groups, all of these agents do have one thing in common: they enhance the activity of specific neurobiologic circuits. These circuits are commonly described as the "brain reward system."

It is generally believed that the more efficacious a drug is at producing its pharmacologic actions at these sites, the greater its potential for addiction. The actual molecular sites of action of many of these drugs have been well categorized. Through imaging, microdialysis, and quantitative autoradiography, as well as other techniques, including genetic cloning, many of these initial sites of drug action have been well established, as have the involved neurotransmitters or neuropeptides. The effects of these substances of abuse on the reward system of the brain have been able to explain, in part, the clinical phenomena of the pleasure often associated with the use of these drugs; the persistent craving that causes the chronic drug user to continue taking the drug; and some of the reasons for both early and late physiologic syndromes of withdrawal when specific drugs, such as opiates or alcohol, are abruptly discontinued.

TABLE 20–1   Different Classes of Psychoactive Drugs

Opiates	Antipsychotics
Muscle relaxants	Stimulants (e.g., cocaine)
Barbiturates	Hypnotics (e.g., benzodiazepines)
Hallucinogens	Phencyclidine
Alcohol	Marijuana
Antidepressant	Antiseizure (e.g., gabapentin)
Nicotine	Mood stabilizers (e.g., lithium)

Neurotransmitter and Opioid Receptor Pathology in Addiction

Dopamine neurons in the dopamine system that originate in the ventral tegmental area and project to the nucleus accumbens, olfactory tubercle, and frontal cortex have long been implicated in reward and motivational processes. The accumulation of substantial neuropharmacologic data and recent data from electrophysiologic recording studies in primates and recent theoretical modeling studies provide significant new insights into the function of these mesolimbic dopamine neurons that have important implications for addiction medicine. Appetitive events, it seems, and not aversive events activate dopamine neurons in the mesolimbic dopamine system of primates. Dopamine neurons may be responsible for initiating action associated with significant changes in the value of incentives in the environment, and neuropharmacologic data show that the activation associated with approach to incentives is abolished by removal to the mesolimbic dopamine system. On the basis of these three lines of research it is hypothesized that the function of the mesolimbic dopamine system is to allow or actually release species-specific approach responses or modifications in direction toward changes in positive incentives. These results have implications for our understanding of the role of dopamine in specific aspects of drug dependence. Thus, multiple mechanisms of adaptation to kappa opioid exposure occur in mesocorticolimbic neurons. These data support the idea that the administration of kappa opioids might facilitate drug rehabilitation.

Excessive mesolimbic dopaminergic neurotransmission is closely related to the psychotic symptoms of mental illness, especially delusions. Increased firing rates in mesolimbic reward pathways could produce delusions and superstitious conditioning of the type seen in reinforcement addiction. Though difficult to test in animals, the hypothesis is testable as an explanation for the preoccupation and craving seen in individuals addicted to drugs and alcohol. Drug abuse (i.e., mere exposure to a mood or mind-altering substance), in and of itself does not cause such altered thinking. This type of thought disorder results, in great part, from persistent feelings of restlessness, irritability, and discontent that are normally reserved for instinctual drives. Obsession aimed at meeting a survival need is hardly pathologic (i.e., obsessing about food when hungry, or confronting a threat to safety or security). It is the preoccupation, rationalization, and justification of the bizarre behavior seen in drug seeking, for example, that defines the neuropsychiatric pathology seen in substance use disorders.[4]

The most prominent neurotransmitters and neuropeptides in mediating this process are dopamine, serotonin, glutamate, gamma-aminobutyric acid, and the endorphins.[16,17] Dopamine is credited with playing the primary role in producing most of the euphoria seen with cocaine, nicotine, alcohol, and other stimulants and is known to contribute to the positive reinforcing effects of opiates.[18] The mu receptors have been shown to be responsible for the primary action of opiate drugs, including the euphoria experienced by many, but not all, persons.[19] Opiate analgesia, tolerance, and addiction are mediated by drug-induced activation of the mu opioid receptor. A fundamental question in addiction biology is why exogenous opiate drugs have a high liability for inducing tolerance and addiction whereas native ligands do not. Studies indicate that highly addictive opiate drugs such as morphine are deficient in their ability to induce the desensitization and endocytosis of receptors. This regulatory mechanism reveals an independent functional property of opiate drugs that can be distinguished from established agonist properties. This property correlates with agonist propensity to promote physiologic tolerance, suggesting a fundamental revision of our understanding of the role of receptor endocytosis in the biology of opiate drug action and addiction.[20] The kappa opioid receptor is responsible for dysphoria, rather than euphoria, and may play a role in opioid withdrawal, although recent studies have shown that natural kappa receptor–directed ligands, the dynorphins, do not cause dysphoria and may augment, not oppose, mu receptor–directed events.[21]

Craving and Withdrawal

This phenomenon may explain the observed benefit of naltrexone in decreasing craving. Cells in the locus ceruleus that secrete norepinephrine have been demonstrated to be responsible for part of the withdrawal phenomena seen with sudden discontinuation of opioids, which results in an outpouring of norepinephrine. However, this "noradrenergic cascade" does not explain many of the acute and subacute phenomena of withdrawal or any of the signs and symptoms of protracted abstinences. Similarly, serotonin (5-HT) has been related not only to impulsiveness and appetite but also to dependence and craving. With respect to signal transduction, although opiates acutely inhibit the cyclic adenosine 3'5'-monophosphate pathway at time of administration, chronic use results in an up-regulation of the cAMP pathway. Abrupt cessation of opiate use leaves an up-regulated, unopposed pathway, which in the locus ceruleus results in an increased firing of these cells and withdrawal.[22] There is no question that as neuroscience continues to advance, additional neurotransmitters and receptor sites will be identified, and the understanding of molecular and cellular bases of addiction will become increasingly clear.

Physiologic Dependence and Addiction: What's the Difference?

Not all drug dependence is addiction. Physiologic dependence, which is often confused with addiction, is a result of the body's adaptation to a drug used over a period of time to treat a medical disorder. Physical dependence is, in essence, a withdrawal syndrome that occurs when a drug is suddenly discontinued or an antagonist is administered. Many patients on chronic opioids become physically dependent (estimates run as high as 80%), its presence cannot be used to differentiate the pain patient from the addict. So-called psychologic dependence (addiction) occurs in approximately 28% of patients on chronic opioid therapy and manifests as an overwhelming preoccupation and involvement with the acquisition and use of a drug. For example, a patient taking pain medication for several weeks would likely develop some degree of tolerance to the drug; he or she would become physically dependent and would have withdrawal symptoms if the drug were stopped abruptly. This type of dependence, however, is not addiction. A patient with a physiologic dependence can quit the drug, usually by being tapered off it, with medical supervision and without admission into a drug treatment program.

ADDICTION

Biopsychosocial Aspects: Host/User Variables

In general, the effects of drugs vary among individuals. Even blood levels show wide variation when the same dose of a drug on a milligram per kilogram basis is given to different people. Genes determine enzymes that may influence absorption, metabolism, excretion, receptor sensitivity, and so on. One of the results of these differences is that the degree of reinforcement or euphoria varies among individuals. The mechanisms are unclear at present, but the genetic influences on the development of alcohol dependence, for example, have received the most attention. Studies of babies adopted at birth and raised without contact with their biologic parents have permitted the separation of environmental from genetic influences.[23] Children of alcoholics show an increased likelihood of developing alcoholism even when adopted at birth by nonalcoholic parents. Also, the concordance rate for identical twins is much higher than that of fraternal twins. One biologic trait that recent data suggest may influence the development of alcoholism (alcohol addiction) is innate tolerance to alcohol. Having an innate tolerance to alcohol does not make a person an alcohol addict (alcoholic), but it seems to increase the probability significantly. Conversely, the probability

of becoming alcohol dependent is reduced in people by heredity, but the risk is not eliminated. No single factor is determinant. Those who inherit a tolerance to alcohol may remain abstinent. However, drugs may produce immediate subjective effects that relieve preexisting symptoms. People with anxiety, depression, insomnia, or even subtle symptoms such as shyness may find, on experimentation or by accident, that certain drugs give them relief. However, the apparent beneficial effects are transient. Although psychiatric symptoms are commonly seen in drug abusers presenting for treatment, most of these symptoms started after the person began abusing drugs. Thus, drugs of abuse appear to produce more psychiatric symptoms than they relieve. With repeated use of the drug, the person may develop tolerance and eventually compulsive, uncontrolled drug use. The process of self-medication is believed to be one mechanism whereby drug users become ensnared. The proportion of addicts who begin by a self-medication mechanism is unclear.

The Role of Pharmacokinetics: Agent/Drug Variables

Parallel to the advances in neurobiology, continued work on the pharmacokinetics of drugs of abuse has helped explain the clinical phenomenon with respect to choice of drugs of abuse. The goal of the drug user is to increase the rate of delivery of the drug to the brain.[15] This explains why opiate users may progress from pills to snorting and then to injecting opiates intravenously. An understanding of the pharmacokinetics of the euphoria produced by such drugs with a rapid onset and short duration of action is essential when discussing the concept of maintenance pain management and in understanding the appropriate drugs to use in choice of the pharmacologic therapy in patients with a history of addictions.[24] The quintessential "recovery pill," which does not exist today, would normalize brain function, specifically limbic discharge, limiting it to circumstances where the organism was confronted with a true or culturally perceived survival need.[4] Once resolved, obsessive preoccupation with meeting the need would melt away, leaving the individual with a sense of satiety. Baseline emotional discharge would be one of alert repose. Evidence would indicate that such an agent almost certainly would affect N-methyl-D-aspartate (NMDA) receptor metabolism, as discussed later.

Drugs vary in their ability to produce immediate good feelings in the user. Those drugs that reliably produce intensely pleasant feelings (euphoria) are more likely to be taken repeatedly. Animal models would seem to indicate that medications can be screened for their abuse potential in humans.[16] Unfortunately, animal models only measure the reinforcing properties of drugs on the basis of their ability to increase levels of the neurotransmitter dopamine in critical brain areas, particularly the nucleus accumbens (NAC) and a newer anatomic conception called the extended amygdala. All mood-altering drugs have been hypothesized to produce their rewarding effects by neuropharmacologic actions such as these. A common brain reward circuit called the extended amygdala involves the mesolimbic dopamine system and specific subregions of the basal forebrain, such as the shell of the nucleus accumbens, the bed nucleus of the stria terminalis, and the central nucleus of the amygdala.[25,26] Cocaine, amphetamine, ethanol, opioids, and nicotine all reliably increase extracellular fluid dopamine levels in the NAC region and the extended amygdala.[27] Drugs of abuse activate this system via specific pathways including:

1. Ethanol activation of gamma-aminobutyric acid receptors
2. Cocaine and methamphetamine activation dopamine receptors
3. Sedative hypnotic activation of the serotonergic system
4. Ethanol activation of the glutamate pathways

Nicotine and tetrahydrocannabinol (THC) both activate mesolimbic dopamine function and possibly opioid peptide systems in this circuitry via anandamide receptors in the VTA, nucleus accumbens, caudate nucleus, hippocampus, and cerebellum.[28,29] The binding of THC to these "THC receptors" in the hippocampus explains that its ability to interfere with memory and actions in the cerebellum are responsible for its ability to cause incoordination and loss of balance.

Repeated and prolonged drug abuse leads to compulsive use, and the mechanism for this transition involves, at the behavioral level, a progressive dysregulation of brain reward circuitry and a recruitment of brain stress systems such as corticotropin-releasing factor.[30] The molecular mechanisms of signal transduction in these systems are a likely target for residual changes in that they convey allostatic changes in reward set point, which lead to vulnerability to relapse. Such selective responsiveness to these abused drugs implies a special role for areas like the nucleus accumbens in mechanisms of drug reinforcement and suggests that some features of the drug-dependent state (e.g., tolerance) might be related to inhibition of G (alpha) 1-linked receptor activity.[15,31] Addictive drugs and natural rewards share the property of stimulating dopamine transmission preferentially in the nucleus accumbens shell. Similar increases in dopamine in this brain structure are also observed when an organism is presented with sweet foods or a sexual partner. In contrast, drugs that block dopamine receptors generally produce bad feelings (e.g., dysphoric effects).

Neither animals nor humans will spontaneously take such drugs. A causal relationship between dopamine and euphoria/dysphoria has not been established, but the data are reasonably consistent across different drugs with different mechanisms for increasing dopamine levels. The abuse liability of a drug is certainly enhanced by rapidity of onset. Effects that occur soon after administration are more likely to initiate the chain of neurochemical events that may lead to loss of control over drug taking.[32] The time that it takes for the drug to reach critical receptor sites in the brain and the concentrations achieved can be influenced by the form of the drug, route of administration, and rate of absorption and metabolism. What is not controlled for are baseline levels of these neurotransmitters and whatever subjective dysphoria may predate exposure to the mood-altering substance. Addiction can be understood as the expression of the excessive control over behavior acquired by drug-related stimuli as a result of abnormal associative learning after repeated stimulation of dopamine transmission in the nucleus accumbens shell.[25,33]

OPIOID ADDICTION: THE NEUROBIOLOGY OF "CHASING THE DRAGON"

Opiates activate opioid peptide receptors within the extended amygdala independent of the endogenous mechanisms active in the mesolimbic dopamine system via opioid peptides. Opioids, both endogenous peptides and exogenous alkaloids, affect the functioning of the central nervous system by interacting with membrane receptors.[27] Alterations at the receptor and transduction level have been the focus of many studies of opiate tolerance and dependence.[34,35] Pharmacologic studies suggest the presence of three major types of opioid receptors in the brain and spinal cord: mu, delta, and kappa. Each of the receptor types is further divided into multiple subtypes. These receptors are widely known to be coupled to G-proteins of the Gi and Go subtypes, but an increasing body of results suggests coupling to other G-proteins, such as Gs. Protein Gs, in particular, has implications for tolerance and dependence. Opioid receptor activation has been shown to mediate the inhibition of neuronal firing and neurotransmitter release in a variety of brain areas, including both locus ceruleus and hippocampus neurons.[7] Neurotransmitters modulate the excitability of neurons by affecting ion channel conductance, leading to membrane hyperpolarization and a decrease in neuronal firing rate.[36]

Environmental Variables

Initiating and continuing illicit drug use appears to be significantly influenced by societal norms and peer pressure.[37,38] Taking drugs may be seen initially as a form of rebellion against authority. In some communities, drug users and drug dealers are role models who seem to be successful and respected; young people emulate them.[38] There may also be a paucity of other options for pleasure or diversion. These factors are particularly important in communities where educational levels are low and job opportunities are scarce.[39] Of course, these environmental factors do not operate alone. They interact with the agent and host variables described earlier. One of the most remarkable observations about acute pain is that it can be suppressed, at least transiently, depending on the context in which it occurs.[40] That the perception of pain could be altered by environment was documented by observation of men with serious shrapnel wounds who often refused morphine, something almost never seen in civilian populations.[41]

The nervous system appears to be organized such that in circumstances that produce the greatest stress or fear, circumstances in which the survival value of running or fighting far outweighs the risk of using already damaged limbs, pain can be completely suppressed.[40]

The Tolerance Threshold

Equally important is an understanding of the clinical phenomena of euphoria, tolerance, and withdrawal with respect to the opioids.[42] In clinical practice, significant opioid tolerance is more common in clinical practice than animal models might at first indicate.[43] Tolerance may be present in the pain patient or the addict; by itself it is not diagnostic of addiction. It has been demonstrated repeatedly that an individual dependent on an opioid to which he/she has become tolerant has developed a tolerance threshold that, if exceeded too rapidly or too far, can produce euphoria and, if very rapidly and very far, an overdose.[44] Correspondingly, if this tolerance threshold is diminished too rapidly, withdrawal can occur. However, when an individual is at his/her "tolerance threshold" to an opioid, normal cognitive and motor functions are maintained and, unless an opioid antagonist is administered to produce withdrawal, it is quite difficult, if not impossible, to determine that the individual is taking an opioid.[45] This phenomenon explains why addicted individuals, as well as individuals suffering chronic pain syndromes, when maintained on opioids just greater than the tolerance threshold that relieves the pain but does not cause euphoria, function quite normally, and why individuals on long-acting opioid agonist maintenance therapy for opiate addiction with an appropriate agent (e.g., methadone or l-alpha-acetylmethadol) can lead productive and fruitful lives without any long-term risks. Even individuals with a history of chemical dependency can be managed safely

if the problem is known and the clinician has a plan in place for dealing with alternative measures, close monitoring and the possibility of runaway tolerance, drug seeking, and the possibility of intoxication.[30,46] Failure to understand this has resulted in the concept of pain management and maintenance therapy rejected by many in the health care industry, resulting in patients in chronic pain suffering needlessly.

Drug Use, Abuse, and Dependence: A Rose by Any Other Name

Use

We live in a culture that uses mood-altering substances. One third of the U.S. population has tried marijuana at least once in their lifetimes. Marijuana is the most commonly used illicit drug, with 10 million current users. Two million Americans use cocaine.[47,48] Statistics from the Substance Abuse and Mental Health Services Administration show that 30% to 50% of those drugs listed by patients treated for misuse or overdose in hospital emergency rooms are prescription drugs.[43] It is estimated that as much as 28% of all prescribed controlled substances are abused.[49] That estimate translates to tens of millions of drug doses being diverted annually for the purpose of abuse. Diversion refers to the redirecting of drugs from legitimate use into illicit channels. Fourteen of the top twenty most abused mood-altering substances in the United States are prescription drugs. Opioids are the second most abused substance after benzodiazepines.

When the DSM-IV addresses "substance use disorder," it implies the possibility of substance use that is, as it were, not disordered.[50,51] Simple use, of course, does not rise to the level of a disorder. It is behavior engaged in like any other and is no more or less noteworthy or problematic to the individual than any other enjoyable activity. There are patterns of use, however, that do rise to the level of dysfunction. The 2002 National Survey on Substance Use and Health (NSSUH) estimated that 27% of Americans will experience problems with alcohol and drug abuse and dependence at some point in their lives.

Drug Abuse

As mentioned earlier, drug abuse can be defined as the self-administration of any drug in a manner that deviates from the approved medical use or social patterns within a given culture.[42] The term conveys the notion of social disapproval, and it is not necessarily descriptive of any particular pattern of drug use or its potential adverse consequences. Drug abuse may include using a medication recreationally, using it for reasons other than those intended, or using the drug more frequently than indicated by the prescriber. Abuse may or may not involve addiction.[30]

Drug Dependency

Drug or alcohol addiction is characterized by compulsive use, loss of control over its use, and continued use despite adverse consequences. The state of addiction includes psychologic dependence (when the desire or need grows to a desperate craving for the drug) and physical dependence (when distinct withdrawal symptoms appear shortly after the drug abuser stops taking the drug and there is a need to take the drug again).[42] Recent surveys estimate 17% of Americans use illegal drugs such as marijuana, cocaine, and opiates. The statistics are roughly the same for those addicted to alcohol. When the incidence of "cross addiction" is considered in concert with figures for the prevalence of alcoholism, the overall statistics suggest that a staggering 30% of the population will have a drug or alcohol problem significant enough to need treatment during their lifetime.[52]

Addiction

Addictions and related disorders represent the perversion of the survival circuits that underlie fear. Emotional circuits decide whether what we perceive is a danger to be escaped or, alternatively, something positive to be approached.[4,53] Individuals with damage to such emotional circuits are unable to make appropriate choices in life, to plan, or to exhibit normal motivation. Despite normal intelligence and cognitive function, their lives fall apart. Individuals suffering addictive disorders often exhibit the same confounding behavior as those who suffer damage to such centers.[54] Addiction becomes a pattern of compulsive drug use characterized by a continued craving for drugs when, after exposure, the need to use these drugs for psychologic effects or mood alterations takes hold. It is characterized by the repeated, compulsive use of a substance despite adverse social, psychologic, or physical consequences. The key element is that the use of a drug or drugs is given priority over other aspects of a person's life. Addictive substances may be obtained through legal or illegal channels. The American Society of Addiction Medicine considers addiction "a disease process characterized by the continued use of a specific psychoactive substance despite physical, psychological, or social harm."[42] Addiction, then, is a chronic disease that is progressive: it worsens over time because of the interactions between a living organism and a drug, which are characterized by behavioral and other responses that always include a compulsion to take the drug on a continuous or periodic basis to experience its psychic effects and sometimes to avoid the discomfort of its absence. It can be diagnosed and treated, but without treatment it is often fatal. Data suggest that this is less a psychiatric syndrome than a neurologic one, although advances in the new psychodynamic psychiatry are blurring such distinctions.[55]

Misunderstanding of addiction and mislabeling of patients as addicts leads to one of two scenarios, both of which are agonizing from the patient's point of view: 1) The physician unnecessarily witholds opioid medications, or, 2) the opioids used to treat the pain are administered without adequate monitoring, leading to (iatrogenic) catastrophic psychological dependency. Unless the potential for this complication is recognized and protective measures are put in place, the likelihood that an addictive disorder can become active is very high. Yet, experience has shown that known addicts can benefit from the carefully supervised, judicious use of opioids for the treatment of pain due to cancer, surgery, or recurrent painful illnesses such as sickle cell disease.[39,46,56] So clear is the neurobiologic evidence on this matter that it is sure to be explored in the courts by aggressive trial lawyers who will be asking those unfortunates among us to explain how such a predictable syndrome, so easily recognizable and so amenable to treatment, is so readily ignored with such catastrophic consequences.

Risk Factors for the Development of Opioid Addiction

The sharpest increase of users of prescription drugs for nonmedical purposes occurs in the 12 to17 and 18 to 25 age-groups.[43,57] Other groups at increased risk for abusing opioids are medical professionals, abusers of other drugs, recovering people, alcoholics, and smokers. Additionally, extreme stress such as family tragedy, death, or divorce may precipitate abusive drug use and increase the risk of activating an occult dependency.

The "Unwitting" Opiate Addict

Many individuals who become dependent on prescription drugs are referred to as unwitting addicts.[58] Initially, many of these individuals do not realize the drug they are taking had addiction potential. But, whether they knew, individuals who have a prior history of drug abuse or addiction should be wary of any medication. However, many addicts first start using a prescribed drug for a legitimate medical problem, physical or emotional. At some point, these individuals start increasing the dosage of these medications on their own because the drug made them feel better or gave them some relief from physical or emotional distress. The nature of the drug required that they continue escalating the dosages to get the desired effect. Gradually, the abuse became full-blown addiction.

Risk of Iatrogenic Opioid Addiction

Pain and addiction problems are most likely to coexist in patients who have risk factors for drug abuse and addiction such as previous drug or alcohol problems. The risk of developing tolerance or addiction-related problems in patients treated with long-term opiate therapy for chronic malignant pain, then, should equal the prevalence of addictive disorders in the general population, a figure generally agreed to be between 18% and 28%.[39,59]

Addiction Treatment

Alcohol and drug addiction are treated similarly. Most frequently, withdrawal conditions require institutional management, support, and initiation of a recovery program.[60] This may occur in an inpatient or outpatient (ambulatory) setting. The failure of outpatient management is frequent. The addicted person receives medical care and is carefully monitored through the withdrawal process. This usually takes 4 to 7 days and often requires the use of tranquilizers and sedatives prescribed by a physician. Some alcoholics and drug addicts need treatment for depression during the withdrawal period. Continuing behavior modification, psychotherapy, and a 12-step program are also needed.[55]

Detoxification of Drug-Dependent Patients

Detoxification refers to the elimination of the drug from the body. This may be accomplished naturally without any medication, or depending on the situation, it may require transferring the patient to a drug that has cross-tolerance to the drug of dependence and gradually reducing the dose so as to prevent severe withdrawal symptoms.

Treatment of Withdrawal Symptoms

Persons dependent on alcohol or other drugs rarely use their drug according to a constant steady pattern. Stops and starts and attempts at reductions are typical. When the drug of dependence is stopped or significantly reduced, the withdrawal symptoms are generally opposite to the effects of the drug that they have been taking. Most of the early withdrawal symptoms occur without the user seeking medical help. For opiates, these symptoms are a "flu-like" syndrome characterized by mainly subjective discomfort, anxiety, nausea, diarrhea, muscle aches. The withdrawal is not life threatening. When the user presents for treatment, he can be given an opioid such as methadone in gradually decreasing doses. An alternative treatment is a drug that blocks the autonomic hyperactivity seen in many types of drug withdrawal. Clonidine (alpha-2-adrenergic agonist) when given orally activates auto-receptors of central nervous system (CNS) neurons (locus coeruleus) involved in the control of adrenergic activity. This action results in a reduction in blood pressure and for opioid addicts in withdrawal, a turning off of adrenergic hyperactivity. This antihypertensive medication is sometimes used in opioid withdrawal treatment; however, not all of the withdrawal symptoms are relieved by clonidine.

Sedative withdrawal, such as that from alcohol, barbiturates, or benzodiazepines, is potentially more dangerous than opioid withdrawal. Patients who are severely dependent should be treated in the hospital. Delirium tremens is a syndrome of severe alcoholic withdrawal marked by visual hallucinations, marked tremors, and severe autonomic hyperactivity. Fatalities can occur in complicated cases.

Relapse Prevention

This is the most important aspect of the treatment of addiction because it focuses on the essence of the drug dependence syndrome: the compulsion to relapse. Each case is different, but all require some form of psychological approach that may entail group support systems such as Alcoholics Anonymous; psychotherapy (including individual, family therapy, or group therapy); behavior therapy, including extinction of conditioned responses developed during drug use; and vocational therapy, which may involve job retraining or schooling.

Pharmacological Adjunctive Treatments

Although relapse prevention is primarily a psychological approach, many patients are unable or unwilling to undergo therapy without the support of medication. Patients with coexisting psychiatric disorders are particularly prone to drop out of drug-free therapy. Maintenance treatment is available for opioid dependence (e.g., heroin) on a long-term basis, and it has had an important positive impact on this national problem. Methadone is a long-acting opioid that maintains a person in a physiologically stable state if taken once daily. Thus, the dependence is transferred from the short-acting drug, such as heroin, to the long-acting maintenance drug. Methadone prevents opioid craving and withdrawal and permits the patient to engage in rehabilitation programs.

Maintenance Treatment

Overall, methadone treatment is the most effective modality for the large numbers of persons dependent on street opioids. The typical street heroin addict would refuse to even enter a drug-free treatment program, but these individuals readily accept methadone. About 125,000 persons are currently receiving this treatment in the United States, with good results for about 60% of patients.

Antagonist Treatment

Drugs that act at a specific receptor present the possibility of finding a specific antagonist that blocks or reverses the action of that specific drug. The antagonist can compete with the drug for the receptor-binding site and thus diminish or block the effects of the drug. Naloxone is a specific antagonist that has high affinity for opiate receptors, but it does not produce the consequences of receptor activation as do opiate agonists.[61] Naloxone can also displace opioid drugs from opiate receptors, thus potentially reversing an overdose or precipitating withdrawal symptoms in a dependent person. However, naloxone has a half-life of only about 25 minutes. This is convenient for reversing an overdose; however, the naloxone must be given repeatedly when the overdose is due to a long-acting opioid. The half-life of naloxone is too short to use a means of preventing relapse in formerly opioid-dependent persons.[27]

Naltrexone is similar to naloxone, but it has a longer half-life. Thus, naltrexone is practical to use in a treatment program to assist in preventing relapse.[62] For up to 72 hours after an oral dose, naltrexone and its active metabolites can antagonize the effects of opioids. This prevents relapse to opioid dependence as long as the antagonist continues to be taken. Naltrexone together with a comprehensive rehabilitation program has been effective with well-motivated street addicts,[63] many middle-class addicts, and members of the medical profession suffering from opioid dependence. Naltrexone treatment requires a structured rehabilitation program and a system to ensure that the patient continues to take naltrexone, which by itself has minimal, if any subjective effects.[37,64]

Naltrexone has also been reported to reduce craving for alcohol in alcoholics and to reduce relapse to alcoholism. We postulate that alcohol stimulates the release of endogenous opioids and that by blocking opiate receptors, naltrexone reduces some of the rewarding effects of alcohol.[65]

A new medication being considered for FDA approval is buprenorphine. This drug is a partial mu agonist and an antagonist at kappa receptors. Studies so far indicate that it can maintain opiate addicts comparable to a moderate dose of methadone, and it also has antagonist properties that block injected opiates.[61,62]

Rapid Opioid Detoxification During General Anesthesia

Opioid addiction therapy includes successful detoxification, rehabilitation, and sometimes methadone maintenance. However, the patient may have physical, mental, and emotional pain while trying to achieve abstinence. A new detoxification technique that incorporates general anesthesia uses a high-dose opioid antagonist to compress detoxification to within 6 hours while avoiding the withdrawal.[66] Although most patients have been successfully detoxified with no adverse anesthetic events and exhibiting no signs of withdrawal or hemodynamic changes during post-treatment challenge test doses of 0.4 mg naloxone, most patients are lost to follow-up, whereas only about one fourth of patients remained abstinent from opioids after treatment. Therefore, anesthesia-assisted opioid detoxification may be an alternative to conventional detoxification, although the wisdom of taking what is essentially a zero mortality procedure (deter) and increasing that to 1% or 2% simply to save time is questionable.

PAIN: PSYCHOSOCIAL FACTORS

Pain is a complex, highly individual experience that often has multiple components. The presence of addictive disease in a patient with pain must be considered in both the evaluation and treatment plan. The evaluation of pain must include careful identification of the nociceptive components of pain and have associated distresses such as sleep disturbance, anxiety, depression, alterations in usual roles, and drug dependence.[67] Successful treatment of pain in the addicted person must address each of the nociceptive components of pain, as well as distressing associated symptoms that may serve to perpetuate the pain.[39,42] Effective management of acute pain, chronic nonmalignant pain, and cancer pain can be achieved in persons with addictive disease if both physician and patient recognize the presence of the addictive disease process and address the issues it raises. Clear and honest communication with the patient is important.[68] The treatment plan must be specifically tailored to the type of pain and the nature and stage of the patient's addictive disease.[44] A team approach that involves an addiction medicine specialist, a primary care physician, and a pain medicine specialist often is valuable in successful treatment of pain in the patient with concurrent addictive disease.[42]

Pain-related behaviors may meet a person's coping needs in a way they are not completely aware of. In situations such as these, the pain a person is feeling brings with it secondary, and not always conscious, benefits.[69,70] These secondary benefits enable a person to cope in the absence of other coping strategies.[71] The identification of such issues are essential to the understanding of a person's pain and its effective treatment. If treatment fails, psychological consequences for the patient can be significant, including:

- Depression (about persisting discomfort and physical disability)
- Anxiety
- Anger (sometimes directed at the medical profession)

- Sleep disturbance
- Family and marital discord
- Social consequences, such as job loss, isolation due to physical restrictions, or financial difficulties[36]

People can then lose control in their lives and rely more heavily on medication. This can lead to dependence on medication and the seeking of relief from almost all of life's problems through the medication.[71,72]

NEUROBIOLOGY OF PAIN MANAGEMENT

Classes of Pain

In discussing general management principles, pain often is viewed in three broad categories: acute pain, chronic pain of nonmalignant origin, and cancer pain or pain related to other chronic and severely painful medical conditions. All pain—whether acute, chronic nonmalignant or cancer-related—has three experiential components: the physical or nociceptive component, the affective or mood component, and the functional component.[73] Like addictive disease, chronic pain is a complex disorder with biologic, psychological, and spiritual components.[74] Independent of each other, chronic pain and addictive disease may present quite similar pictures. When they occur concurrently, chronic pain and addictive disease may synergistically act to exacerbate or reinforce each other.[35]

Physical Mechanisms of Pain

Pain physiology is a complex subject. The neospinothalamic tract, which relays information about the precise localization and nature of the pain to those brain regions that analyze bodily sensations, orients the organism to the injury. A number of classification systems have been devised for the purpose of assessing clinical pain and designing effective treatment.[75] This is the experience that most lay people consider when they discuss pain. For the purposes of this discussion, it is helpful to examine the following three basic types of pain mechanisms.

Nociception, Neuropathic Pain, and Sympathetically Maintained Pain

Nociception refers to pain generated by nociceptors and conducted along the neurophysiologic pathways that normally act to warn the body of actual or impending harm.[76] Increased concentrations of prostaglandins, H^+ ion, norepinephrine, and bradykinins are thought to reduce the threshold of activation of nociceptors by a variety of mechanisms. Thus, medications that inhibit prostaglandins or attenuate inflammatory responses may reduce pain by elevating receptor thresholds.[77]

Substance P is the neurotransmitter best described in transmission of pain from peripheral fibers to secondary neurons at the spinal level.[78] Sympathetically mediated pain is classically represented by causalgia or reflex sympathetic dystrophy (RSD). Sustained pain syndromes in cancer patients are most often of neuropathic origin.

Pain-Sustaining Mechanism of Addiction

Some addiction medicine specialists and pain clinicians have described a "syndrome of pain facilitation or disinhibition" as occurring in the presence of a chronic pain syndrome and concurrent active addictive disease.[79] This putative syndrome is characterized by a diffuse anatomic pattern of pain, a relatively constant level of pain, and a lack of response to any intervention other than the administration of the chemical on which the individual is dependent (or sometimes other psychoactive and potentially dependence-producing medications).[80]

Addiction medicine specialists working in drug and alcohol treatment centers note that patients with active addiction and concurrent pain often believe that they are using alcohol, benzodiazepines, opiates, or other drugs at least partially to reduce their pain.[74,79] Patients often fear increased pain when the use of such chemicals is discontinued. After addiction treatment, however, patients usually report that pain is unchanged or even reduced. Occasionally, pain actually is resolved; only rarely does it increase.[39,81] Physicians who specialize in pain management have observed similar improvement after detoxification from addictive drugs.[44] In addition to general reduction in pain, observed changes may include the emergence of a clearer anatomic focus or pattern of pain, more variability in the intensity of pain, and an improvement in therapeutic responses to no pharmacologic approaches to pain treatment.[35]

On the other hand, alcohol and other drug intoxication may mask pain that otherwise would appropriately signal irritation or injury, thus allowing an individual to overuse his or her body in a way that perpetuates an underlying physical problem associated with the persistent pain problem.[82] The functional changes associated with addiction may augment the general distress of chronic pain. Individuals with active addictive disease often cannot fulfill their usual work and domestic roles, frequently have dysfunctional relationships, suffer financial losses, and may develop secondary physical discomforts and illnesses.[80] These all may feed into the cycle of chronic pain, causing escalation of pain, distress, and disability. Finally, individuals who are addicted may simply be unable to comply with prescribed regimens for treatment of their pain syndrome because of periods of intoxication or recovery from intoxication, or both.[45] Evaluation of pain in the individual with addictive disease must include careful delineation of each of the physical or nociceptive components of the pain syndrome, as well as identification of associated distresses that may act as perpetuating factors for pain. Treatment should address each of the identified physical causes of pain and each of the perpetuating factors.[83]

PHARMACOLOGIC PRINCIPLES INVOLVED IN PAIN TREATMENT

Tolerance Control: Role of the NMDA Receptor

A way of reducing tolerance would be of great benefit because it would allow doctors to use lower doses over longer periods and still control pain effectively. Like dopamine systems, the glutamatergic pathway has often been implicated in drug abuse and addiction, specifically NMDA channel receptors.

Given that NMDA antagonists interfere with sensitization, tolerance, and dependence related to stimulant, alcohol, benzodiazepine, barbiturate, and opiate use,[84,85] an NMDA antagonist is any agent that competitively or noncompetitively prevents glutamate from triggering neuronal excitability. This action should, theoretically, inhibit or blunt c-fiber induced nociceptic or neuropathic pain.[86,87] Furthermore, blockers of NDMA receptors have been shown to reduce naloxone-induced jumping in morphine-dependent mice.[88] NMDA antagonists act by occupying a binding site within a calcium channel, which is normally gated by glutamate, the brain's principle excitatory neurotransmitter. The use of NMDA antagonists seems promising in preventing or reversing tolerance to opioid analgesia.

Endocytosis and Tolerance

Morphine acts by binding a receptor (the mu opioid receptor) on the surface of nerve cells and signaling from it. When this receptor binds to its normal signaling molecule, it is activated and then becomes desensitized.[7] The receptor then moves into the cell by a process called endocytosis. Once in the cell, it can then be reactivated and transferred back to the cell surface, ready to bind to a new signaling molecule and signal again. Morphine, however, is not able to cause the desensitization and recycling, so morphine-bound receptors stay on the cell surface. Until quite recently, most researchers assumed that endocytosis of the receptors contributed to tolerance because it would reduce the number of receptors available on the cell surface for binding to morphine.[85] Endocytosis is associated with reduced tolerance in cultured cells. Morphine-bound receptors can still cluster, but they do not normally move into the cell interior. However, recent studies have led to an alternative view; in which endocytosis might in fact help to reduce

tolerance by recycling the receptors so they can become active again. Binding of certain compounds to a small number of receptors in a group can cause the whole group to be taken up. This should cause receptor endocytosis and thus a reduction in tolerance. A drug that acts in the same way to promote receptor endocytosis could be used with morphine to reduce tolerance, and thus increase the effectiveness of treatment. Until now, many drug discovery programs have thrown away candidate drugs that cause desensitization and endocytosis of morphine receptors because they were working on the assumption that they would increase tolerance.[89] These new results show that, in fact, the opposite seems to be true, which gives new hope for pain relief.

NMDA Receptor Agonists

Allodynia and hyperalgesia are thought to result from CNS hyperexcitability associated with prolonged or aberrant c-fiber afferent activity.[90] An NMDA antagonist that decreases allodynic responses or the level of hyperalgesia should, theoretically, attenuate neuropathic or chronic pain.[91] The following agents have been studied to determine if clinical evidence of this could be documented.

Ketamine

Ketamine is a dissociative general anesthetic agent used clinically for more than 30 years. The NMDA receptor antagonist properties of ketamine are well documented in both animal and human models. Collectively, studies involving ketamine provide convincing evidence that the NMDA receptor contributes to a range of pain syndromes.[92] Studies that examine ketamine's ability to modulate intractable neuropathic pain and evaluate ketamine's ability to decrease opioid dosage regimens in acute or nociceptive pain have shown the ability of subhypnotic doses of ketamine to improve neuropathic pain.[93] Ketamine significantly reduced pain scores in opioid-resistant neuropathic pain compared with saline in almost all patients. Ketamine is known to block NMDA receptors, and this is the likely mechanism by which neuropathic pain is reduced. The psychomimetic side effects associated with higher (anesthetic) doses of ketamine are well documented and probably contribute to the side effects experienced at lower doses.[92]

Ketamine also seems to have the ability to reduce opioid dosage requirements in acute or nociceptic type pain.[94] Ketamine resulted in a 50% morphine-sparing effect compared with placebo (saline) for the first 48 hours after surgery. When such studies are considered in a broad context, a nexus of addiction medicine and pain management can be imagined where the mu-opioid receptor activation leading to such sustained increase in glutamate synaptic effectiveness at the NMDA receptor level is found to be associated with central hypersensitivity to pain even in certain opiate naive patients. Were this to be true and if an accurate screening test for this predisposition were developed, problems with tolerance, drug seeking, and refractory pain might be mitigated by early intervention and an interdisciplinary approach.

Another example of the confounding nature of preexistent addictive physiology is the recent finding that fentanyl administration, normally associated with a marked increase in nociceptive threshold (analgesia), can be associated with a later response associated with sustained lowering of the nociceptive threshold below the basal value indicative of hyperalgesia on pain scales.[95] The higher the fentanyl dose used, the more pronounced was the fentanyl-induced hyperalgesia. In this case, ketamine pretreatment enhanced the earlier response (analgesia) and prevented the development of long-lasting hyperalgesia, making it appear as if fentanyl activates NMDA pain facilitatory processes, which oppose analgesia and lead to long-lasting enhancement in pain sensitivity.[96] Such "sensitization" is the bane of any physician faced with the dramatic escalation of tolerance and confounding clinical picture seen in some patients with or without a history of opiate exposure who, on more detailed questioning, may reveal an alcoholic drinking pattern, a history of "anxiety disorder," or a family history of vague mental illness.

Dextromethorphan

Dextromethorphan (DM) was originally synthesized more than 40 years ago and is a D-isomer of the codeine analog levorphanol. DM has an established safety record as an oral antitussive agent. It does not directly affect opioid receptors and is devoid of major opioid-like side effects such as respiratory or hemodynamic depression. The effect of preoperative DM administration on acute postoperative pain has been examined by a number of investigators.[97-99] DM reduced morphine requirements in this sample and a modest (but nonsignificant) reduction in pain scores was found. Thematic of the controversy surrounding the role of DM in acute pain management is the failure to demonstrate the specific opioid sparing effect expected with DM administration. The investigators concluded that DM does not improve acute pain scores even at high doses. Dextromethorphan is known to have an NMDA receptor antagonistic effect. The blood levels of dextromethorphan are raised by the concurrent administration of a selective serotonin reuptake inhibitor (SSRI) and tramadol (Ultram®). Side effects such as ataxia, dizziness, memory difficulty, and drowsiness can occur.

Magnesium

The importance of magnesium in the cardiac conduction system is well documented. It has also been used as a tocolytic for more than 20 years and is well tolerated clinically when administered orally or intravenously.[100-103] Recently, magnesium has been studied for its ability to block the NMDA receptor.[100] In human models, magnesium's ability to mediate the NMDA receptor is not always translated into pain reduction.

Methadone

Methadone is a synthetic opioid that has been available for more than 50 years. It has traditionally been used to treat addiction but has recently reemerged as a useful agent in the treatment of chronic nonmalignant and malignant pain. Methadone's pharmacokinetics are poorly understood but it is known to be an opioid receptor agonist that has an extended half-life. Some authors suggest that methadone's utility in treating pain is related to its ability to block the NMDA receptor.[93] Methadone's ability to attenuate pain in patients not responsive to mu opioid agonists makes it an intuitive choice for a drug that has NMDA blocking ability.

BEHAVIORAL EFFECT OF OPIOIDS: WHEN DR. JEKYLL BECOMES MR. HYDE

Inappropriate use of any drug can be either intentional or inadvertent.[43] Drugs that affect behavior are particularly likely to be taken in excess when the behavioral effects are considered pleasurable. The same pharmacologic principles apply to legal prescription drugs as to illegal drugs. The colloquial term, addiction, is used to describe the behavioral manifestations of the disease known by various, more descriptive terms including the DSM-IV designations of substance use disorder, substance dependence, chemical dependency, and alcoholism (Table 20–2).

Recent clinical observations and psychiatric diagnostic findings of drug-dependent individuals suggest that they are predisposed to other addictions because they suffer with painful affect states, which pre-date drug exposure or suffer related psychiatric disorders.[42] The drugs that addicts select are not chosen randomly.[104] Their drug of choice is the result of an interaction between the psychopharmacologic action of the drug and the dominant painful feelings with which they struggle.[105] Narcotic addicts prefer opiates because of their powerful muting action on the disorganizing and threatening affects of rage and aggression.[37,106,107] It should not be a concern for the acute postoperative patient receiving opioids for a short, determinable period, although precautions ought be taken with any patient who reports a history of drug abuse, alcoholism, or has a medical history significant for high risk

TABLE 20–2   Definitions of Addiction, Physical Dependence, and Tolerance
I. Addiction Addiction is a primary, chronic, neurobiologic disease, with genetic, psychosocial, and environmental factors influencing its development and manifestations. It is characterized by behaviors that include one or more of the following: impaired control over drug use, compulsive use, continued use despite harm, and craving
II. Physical Dependence Physical dependence is a state of adaptation that is manifested by a drug class–specific withdrawal syndrome that can be produced by abrupt cessation, rapid dose reduction, decreasing blood level of the drug, and/or administration of an antagonist
III. Tolerance Tolerance is a state of adaptation in which exposure to a drug induces changes that result in a diminution of one or more of the drug's effects over time
The American Academy of Pain Medicine, the American Pain Society, and the American Society of Addiction Medicine recognize the following definitions and recommend their use.

of developing an addictive syndrome. However, the implications for the prolonged use of opiate medications in the patient with a history of opiate abuse are significant.[39]

Addiction versus Pseudoaddiction

There is a subset of individuals who, while receiving pain management services, will exhibit drug-seeking–like behavior. In these individuals pain is not adequately controlled.[108] The syndrome is called pseudoaddiction and may be quite difficult to distinguish from true addiction, as they present quite similarly, including "doctor-shopping," using friends' or relatives' prescriptions, and even obtaining medication illegally. True addiction can be differentiated from pseudoaddiction by documenting the cessation of typical drug-seeking behavior when a patient's physical pain is controlled. On the other hand, a person with true addiction would continue such behaviors despite adequate pain control.

ASSESSMENT OF PATIENTS SEEKING OPIATE ANALGESIA FOR PAIN

The assessment of patients with pain requesting opiate analgesia should occur over a series of consultations.[109] The assessment should include an assessment of addiction—either potential or current. This will enable the doctor to get to know the patient adequately, establish a therapeutic relationship with the patient, conduct appropriate investigations, have reviews by specialists, and corroborate the patient's history. Often any inconsistencies in a patient's history become clearer over time.

Components of the Assessment

The assessment should include family history of alcohol or drug abuse and screening with "CAGE" questionnaire.[110]

CAGE questionnaire:

Cut (Have you ever felt you ought to cut down on your drinking?)

Annoyed (Have people annoyed you by criticizing your drinking?)

Guilt (Have you ever felt bad or guilty about your drinking?)

Eye opener (Have you ever had an eye-opener to steady nerves in the morning?)

Interpretation of CAGE questions:

Answering yes to 2 questions: Strong indication for alcoholism

Answering yes to 3 questions: Confirms alcoholism

Abbreviated CAGE questions: Conjoint screening test

Questions:

1. Have you used substances more than intended this year?
2. Have you ever felt the need to cut down?

Efficacy:

Personal history of alcohol or drug abuse

Yes to both is 80% sensitive and predictive.

Ask about previous alcohol problems, prior treatment for detoxification, or participation in a rehabilitation program. Check for any history of DWI (driving while intoxicated) or history of legal complications that may be associated with the use of drugs and alcohol. On physical examination, look for "stigmata" of drug or alcohol abuse, or both: icterus, track marks, spider angioma, hepatomegaly, tremor, or mild peripheral neuropathy. Laboratory tests should include blood alcohol level, complete blood cell count (CBC), liver enzymes, PT/PTT, and blood/urine toxicology.[111] Significant findings include:

- Evidence of the etiology and severity of the pain
- Evidence of IM and IV injections and track marks

- Evidence of other drug or alcohol use
- Evidence of intoxication and withdrawal from opiates and other drugs or alcohol (unexplained trauma, poor hygiene, neglected illness).[74,112]

If opiates seem the appropriate treatment, only a sufficient quantity should be supplied to allow the patient pain relief for the period until the history can be verified—normally one or two days worth of medication only.

Management of Chronic Cancer Pain in the Addicted Patient

Treatment of cancer-related pain in the patient with addictive disease is similar to that in the person without addictive disease. The comfort of the patient should be the primary goal. Opioids should never be withheld when they are needed to achieve pain relief because of concerns regarding the development or perpetuation of addiction.[44] Cancer patients may be in an acute, curative-therapy phase, in remission, tumor free, or apparently cured but with severe pain as complications of antitumor therapy.[113] In any of these phases they may suffer from acute and chronic somatic and visceral pain, which may be nociceptive, inflammatory, and neuropathic pain.[7] The tumor directly impinging on or infiltrating nervous tissue causes neuropathic pain. Treatment-induced neuropathic pain is especially problematic as it may persist in patients apparently cured of their cancer. This includes neuropathic pain from surgical damage of nervous tissue, scar after surgery or irradiation encroaching on nerves, and neurotoxic effects of radiotherapy and chemotherapy. Opioids remain the cornerstone of pharmacotherapy for cancer pain.[34] In addition to severity of pain, coexisting disease, response to previous therapy, and the drug's pharmacokinetics and available formulations influence the choice of an opioid agent.[24] Neuropathic pain may require treatment with sodium blocking, antiepileptic, or antidepressive drugs; neuro-modulating techniques; and psychosocial interventions from a multimodal pain relief facility. Successful pharmacologic cancer pain management with opioids is ideally used in an integrated way with disease-modifying therapy and palliative non-pharmacologic measures.[68]

Even in the hands of experienced palliative care physicians, opioids occasionally fail to relieve the extreme pain and suffering of certain dying patients. This may be caused by a generalized allodynic, hyperpathic pain induced by complex neurobiologic reactions to tissue damage and neuro-psychiatric side effects of complex polypharmacy, including morphine and its metabolites.[7] These are superimposed on the biochemical disturbances from advanced disease and organ failure, dehydration and a failing cardiovascular system, interference with pharmacodynamics and pharmacokinetics of analgesic and

anxiolytic drugs, and the complex psychosocial interactions among the suffering patient, desperate family members, and caregivers.[114]

Family or previous personal history of alcoholism or other addictive disorders are primary risk factors for developing difficult problems during opioid analgesic treatment for chronic pain.[39] They are relatively strong, but not absolute contraindications for starting a trial of opioid treatment for chronic noncancer pain.[83] Individual variations in response to opioid analgesics make selection of an optimal drug and dosing a matter of sequential trials of available opioids and individual titration of doses to find the optimal balance between analgesia and adverse effects. About 1 in 10 patients develop challenging compliance problems, even for an experienced pain clinician.[36]

It is sometimes difficult for patients with addictive disorders and for their physicians to distinguish which aspect of the patient's distress represents pain and which represent opioid craving.[42] Many former illicit drug users may be fearful of losing control and thus refuse any analgesia.[39] First and foremost their request for no pain medication should be respected. Eventually, pain may overcome this fear and a request for pain medication will be forthcoming. On the other hand, some patients with pain and co-existing addictive disease initially believe their chemical dependence is a product of their pain.[74] Indeed, most patients find that their pain and associated symptoms are improved or at least unchanged after treatment of addiction. The sequelae of addiction often include perpetuating factors for pain, such as sleep disturbance, anxiety, or depressive symptoms; changes in muscle and sympathetic tone; and dysfunction in usual life roles.[39] When treatment of addiction produces improvement in these factors, pain often resolves or improves.[115]

Long-term opiate medication, if deemed necessary, should be prescribed in a long-acting orally taken form. Monitoring of treatment progress, compliance and symptoms should be undertaken frequently early in treatment, becoming less frequent with good progress over time. Vigilance for evidence of drug abuse should continue throughout the process.[24,34] The question of whether the patient is in real need of an escalation of the opioid dose or is developing an iatrogenically induced psychological dependence may be illusive and best resolved by the expertise of an addiction medicine specialist.[35] If no history of addiction is present and the history is suggestive or the patient is thought to be drug seeking (i.e., asking for drugs by name, reporting allergies to non-narcotic medication, or voicing resistance to alternative treatments), addictive disease should be identified and addressed early in the treatment of chronic pain. A team approach and a highly structured program are recommended.[116] Ideally, the team should include an addiction medicine specialist, the patient's primary care physician, and a pain specialist. A written contract should be developed with the patient that specifies the prescriber, the pharmacy to be used, the dose and schedule of medications, recovery activities expected, and the circumstances under which treatment will be continued or discontinued.[35,45,117]

The following behaviors provide some indication that drug abuse may be occurring:

- Increased medical practitioner attendance
- Demanding increased doses
- Supplementation with other drugs
- Drug use taking priority over other activities
- Use of the opiates for "emotional stress"
- All problems increasingly related to "insufficient analgesia"
- Surreptitious use
- Seeing other doctors
- Lost doses[39]

If there is any evidence of drug abuse and pseudo-addiction has been excluded, a change to frequent dispensing of small amounts with clear dose limits and only one prescriber should be considered followed by referral for evaluation by an addiction specialist. It should be understood that it is never in the patient's best interest to have no limits placed on pathologic behaviors.[106] Familiarity with individuals in recovery from chemical dependency allows addiction medicine physicians to guide the patient to recovery systems such as 12-step programs and sponsors and meetings that can provide meaningful support.[35,109,118]

The Methadone-Dependent Person and Pain

Some clinicians incorrectly assume that the methadone-maintained patient has no need for pain relief.[119] The methadone-maintained patient is easily treated for pain. Patients maintained on methadone have developed a tolerance or resistance to the narcotic, analgesic (pain killing), and tranquilizing properties of methadone.[120] Consequently, they feel pain to the same degree as persons who are not maintained on methadone and need adequate doses of morphine or other narcotics to relieve acute and chronic episodes of pain.[119] The concern of the physician should be to achieve satisfactory analgesia. Physicians need not be concerned with those methadone patients maintained on a blockade dose of 80 mg/day or greater because methadone patients at a blockade dose are protected from respiratory depression.[119] It must be remembered that methadone patients or opiate-dependent individuals should never be given mixed opiate agonist/antagonist drugs until detoxification had been achieved, as this will precipitate the abstinence syndrome.[61]

Breakthrough Pain

This is transient flares of more intense pain occurring in a patient with a background pain that is otherwise well controlled and tolerated. Breakthrough pain has traditionally been managed by a "rescue" analgesic, usually a rapidly acting opioid taken by mouth as needed. Given the subjective nature of pain, such episodes should be taken at face value and treated. If after review of pertinent clinical data the episode appears consistent with drug-seeking, this should be reported to the addiction medicine physician for further consideration.[43,121]

CONCLUSION

Drug and alcohol dependence disorders are the product of multiple causative factors. Clinicians must understand the pharmacologic principles, such as tolerance, cross-tolerance, physiologic dependence, and withdrawal, to safely prescribe mood-altering substances such as opiates. It is necessary to apply such principles in prescribing medication for all patients and especially in properly prescribing medications to patients with a family history or personal history of abuse or dependence. Physicians must understand the difference between normal reactions to medications, such as tolerance, physiologic dependence or peudoaddiction, and problematic drug use that includes denial, drug seeking, drug abuse, and addiction.

Understanding the pharmacologic factors alone is not sufficient. Addiction is not solely a function of the drug's ability to cause habituation. It is also necessary to understand the social, psychological, and genetic factors that influence the development of substance dependence disorders.

Ketamine, dextromethorphan, magnesium, methadone, amantadine, and memantine are all agents that are promising NMDA antagonists. Each agent produces relatively few side effects at doses used to treat pain. Much like methadone, however, a dearth of literature related to the specific NMDA antagonism properties currently exists. What information does exist reports confounding, inconsistent information.[92] It appears that regardless of its exact pharmacologic actions, methadone will be increasingly used as an analgesic agent in selected populations. However, further study into the NMDA blocking properties of each of these agents is warranted given their potential to provide not only improved methods of controlling pathologic pain, but also because of the insight they may provide into the addictive process on a molecular level. Such insights leave this author with the hope that out of the suffering of the many who die painful deaths from cancer despite our best efforts may come a ray of hope: a solution for those who suffer and die horrible deaths from addictive disorders.

REFERENCES

1. Cope O: On balance. Ann Surg 158: 321–332, 1963.

2. Cope Z: What have I learned from medicine? Med World 99:347–351, 1963.

3. Gazzette THU: Memorial Minute. Harvard University Gazzette. Cambridge, Harvard University Press, 1997.

4. Molea J: The Neurobiology of Addiction and Recovery: The Science Behind the Twelve Steps, vol 1. Springfield, Illinois, Charles C. Thomas, 2004, p 400.

5. Andreasen NC: Linking mind and brain in the study of mental illnesses: A project for a scientific psychopathology. Science 275:1586–1593, 1997.

6. Gabbard GO: A neurobiologically informed perspective on psychotherapy. Br J Psychiatry 177:117–122, 2000.

7. Mayer DJ, et al: Cellular mechanisms of neuropathic pain, morphine tolerance, and their interactions. Proc Natl Acad Sci USA 96:7731–7736, 1999.

8. Paradiso S, et al: Emotional activation of limbic circuitry in elderly normal subjects in a PET study. Am J Psychiatry 154:384–389, 1997.

9. Fawzy FI, Fawzy NW: A structured psycho-educational intervention for cancer patients. Gen Hosp Psychiatry 16:149–192, 1994.

10. Vaillant GE: A 20-year follow-up of New York narcotic addicts. Arch Gen Psychiatry 29:237–241, 1973.

11. Stimmel B: Heroin addiction: A communicable disease or a sociological phenomena? [editorial] Am J Drug Alcohol Abuse 1:445–447, 1974.

12. Garry MG, et al: Knock down of spinal NMDA receptors reduces NMDA and formalin evoked behaviors in rat. Neuroreport 11:49–55, 2000.

13. Stimmel B, Kreek MJ: Neurobiology of addictive behaviors and its relationship to methadone maintenance. Mt Sinai J Med 67:375–380, 2000.

14. Ling W, Wesson DR: Drugs of abuse: Opiates. West J Med 152:565–572, 1990.

15. Leshner AI, Koob GF: Drugs of abuse and the brain. Proc Assoc Am Physicians 111:99–108, 1999.

16. Jackson A, et al: AMPA receptors and motivation for drug: Effect of the selective antagonist NBQX on behavioral sensitization and on self-administration in mice. Behav Pharmacol 9:457–467, 1998.

17. Burst J: Substance abuse, neurobiology and ideology. Arch Neurol 56:12, 1999.

18. Jones EA, et al: The role of dorsal striatal GABA(a) receptors in dopamine agonist-induced behavior and neuropeptide gene expression. Brain Res 836:99–109, 1999.

19. Kreek MJ, Koob GF: Drug dependence: Stress and dysregulation of brain reward pathways. Drug Alcohol Depend 51:23–47, 1998.

20. Bohn LM, Belcheva MM, Coscia CJ: Mu-opioid agonist inhibition of kappa-opioid receptor-stimulated extracellular signal-regulated kinase phosphorylation is dynamin-dependent in c6 glioma cells. J Neurochem 74:574–581, 2000.

21. King A: Acute subjective effects of dynorphin a (1-13) infusion in normal healthy subjects. Drug Alcohol Depend 54:87–90, 1999.

22. Nestler EJ, AG, et al: Molecular and cellular basis of addiction. Science 278:58–65, 1997.

23. Schuckit M, Irwin M, Brown S: The history of anxiety symptoms among primary alcoholics. J Studies Alcohol 51:31–41, 1989.

24. Pappagallo M: Aggressive pharmacologic treatment of pain. Rheum Dis Clin North Am 25:193–213, vii, 1999.

25. Heimer L: A new anatomical framework for neuropsychiatric disorders and drug abuse. Am J Psychiatry 160:1726–1739, 2003.

26. Koob GF: Neuroadaptive mechanisms of addiction: Studies on the extended amygdala. Eur Neuropsychopharmacol 13:442–452, 2003.

27. Greenwald MK, et al: Comparative clinical pharmacology of short-acting mu opioids in drug abusers. J Pharmacol Exp Ther 277:1228–1236, 1996.

28. Castellano C, et al: Cannabinoids and memory: Animal studies. Curr Drug Target CNS Neurol Disord 2:389–402, 2003.

29. Mao J, et al: Two distinctive antinociceptive systems in rats with pathological pain. Neurosci Lett 280:13–16, 2000.

30. Lowinson JH, Stimmel B: Clinical relevance of basic concepts in substance abuse. Adv Alcohol Subst Abuse 3:1–4, 1984.

31. Fudge JL, Emiliano AB: The extended amygdala and the dopamine system: Another piece of the dopamine puzzle. J Neuropsychiatry Clin Neurosci 15: 306–316, 2003.

32. Blum K: A commentary on the neurotransmitter restoration as common mode of treatment of alcohol, cocaine, and opiate abuse. Integrative Psychiatry 6:199–204, 1989.

33. Alheid GF: Extended amygdala and basal forebrain. Ann NY Acad Sci 985:185–205, 2003.

34. Halpern LM: Analgesic drugs in the management of pain. Arch Surg 112:861–869, 1977.

35. Enck RE: Understanding tolerance, physical dependence and addiction in the use of opioid analgesics. Am J Hosp Palliat Care 8:9–11, 1991.

36. Sosnowski M: Pain management: Physiopathology, future research and endpoints. Support Care Cancer 1:79–88, 1993.

37. Stimmel B: Alcoholism and drug abuse in the affluent: Is there a difference? Adv Alcohol Subst Abuse 4:1–10, 1984.

38. Morrison MA, et al: At war in the fields of play: Current perspectives on the nature and treatment of adolescent chemical dependency. J Psychoactive Drugs 25: 321–330, 1993.

39. Savage SR: Addiction in the treatment of pain: Significance, recognition and treatment. J Pain Symptom Manage 8:265–278, 1993.

40. Beecher HK: Relationship of significance of wound to pain experienced. JAMA 161:1609–1613, 1956.

41. Beecher HK: A method for quantifying the intensity of pain. Science 118:322–324, 1953.

42. Heit HA: Addiction, physical dependence, and tolerance: Precise definitions to help clinicians evaluate and treat chronic pain patients. J Pain Palliat Care Pharmacother 17:15–29, 2003.

43. Wilford BB: Abuse of prescription drugs. West J Med 152:609–612, 1990.

44. Foley KM: Current issues in the management of cancer pain: Memorial Sloan-Kettering Cancer Center. NIDA Res Monogr 36: 169–181, 1981.

45. Bressler LR, Geraci MC, Schatz BS: Misperceptions and inadequate pain management in cancer patients. DICP 25:1225–1230, 1991.

46. Dunbar SA, Katz NP: Chronic opioid therapy for nonmalignant pain in patients with a history of substance abuse: Report of 20 cases. J Pain Symptom Manage 11:163–171, 1996.

47. Morral AR, McCaffrey DF, Chien S: Measurement of adolescent drug use. J Psychoactive Drugs 35:301–309, 2003.

48. Wesson DR, Washburn P: Current patterns of drug abuse that involve smoking. NIDA Res Monogr 99:5–11, 1990.

49. Wilford BB, et al: An overview of prescription drug misuse and abuse: Defining the problem and seeking solutions. J Law Med Ethics 22:197–203, 1994.

50. Mason BJ, et al: Psychiatric comorbidity in methadone maintained patients. J Addict Dis 17:75–89, 1998.

51. Vaillant GE: Mental health. Am J Psychiatry 160:1373–1384, 2003.

52. Cherpitel CJ: Changes in substance use associated with emergency room and primary care services utilization in the United States general population: 1995–2000. Am J Drug Alcohol Abuse 29:789–802, 2003.

53. Leshner AI: Science-based views of drug addiction and its treatment. JAMA 282:1314–1316, 1999.

54. Leshner AI: Science is revolutionizing our view of addiction—and what to do about it. Am J Psychiatry 156:1–3, 1999.

55. Gabbard GO: Dynamic therapy in the decade of the brain. Conn Med 61:537–542, 1997.

56. Kim KS, Glajchen M, Portenoy RK: Unwillingness to fill opioid analgesic prescriptions by local pharmacies. J Pain Symptom Manage 20:160–162, 2000.

57. Clark DB, et al: Clinical practices in the pharmacological treatment of comorbid psychopathology in adolescents with alcohol use disorders. J Subst Abuse Treat 25:293–295, 2003.

58. Baker JP: A new series of oral medications for chronic (cancer) pain relief. Compr Ther 10:48–54, 1984.

59. Vaillant G: Cultural factors in the etiology of alcoholism: A prospective study. Ann NY Acad Sci 472:142–148, 1986.

60. Breitfeld C, et al: Opioid "holiday" following antagonist supported detoxification during general anesthesia improves opioid agonist response in a cancer patient with opioid addiction. Anesthesiology 98: 571–573, 2003.

61. Eissenberg T, et al: Buprenorphine's physical dependence potential: Antagonist-precipitated withdrawal in humans. J Pharmacol Exp Ther 276:449–459, 1996.

62. Stimmel B: Maintenance therapy for opioid addiction with methadone, LAAM and buprenorphine: The emperor's new clothes phenomenon. J Addict Dis 20:1–5, 2001.

63. Tedeschi M: Naltrexone for opioid dependence: An additional tool for general practitioners. Aust Fam Physician 31:18–20, 2002.

64. Petersen-Crair P, et al: An impaired physician with complex comorbidity. Am J Psychiatry 160:850–854, 2003.

65. Swift RM: Medications and alcohol craving. Alcohol Res Health 23:207–213, 1999.

66. McCabe S, Rapid detox: Understanding new treatment approaches for the addicted patient. Perspect Psychiatr Care 36: 113–120, 2000.

67. Weissman DE, et al: Educational role of cancer pain rounds. J Cancer Educ 4:113–116, 1989.

68. Barbuto JP: Beyond narcotics for effective pain management. J Manage Care Pharm 9:175–176, 2003.

69. Keefe FJ, et al: Changing face of pain: Evolution of pain research in psychosomatic medicine. Psychosom Med 64:921–938, 2002.

70. Pud D, et al: The tridimensional personality theory and pain: Harm avoidance and reward dependence traits correlate with pain perception in healthy volunteers. Eur J Pain 8:31–8, 2004.

71. Price DD: Psychological and neural mechanisms of the affective dimension of pain. Science 288:1769–1772, 2000.

72. McWilliams LA, Cox BJ, Enns MW: Mood and anxiety disorders associated with chronic pain: An examination in a nationally representative sample. Pain 106: 127–133, 2003.

73. Farrar JT, et al: Defining the clinically important difference in pain outcome measures. Pain 88:287–294, 2000.

74. Jones EM, Knutson D, Haines D: Common problems in patients recovering from chemical dependency. Am Fam Physician 68:1971–1978, 2003.

75. Wesson DR, Ling W: The clinical opiate withdrawal scale (COWS). J Psychoactive Drugs 35:253–259, 2003.

76. Kim D, et al: Thalamic control of visceral nociception mediated by T-type Ca^{2+} channels. Science 302:117–119, 2003.

77. Hart I, Sawyer R: A guide to pain medicine. Anaesthesia 59:209, 2004.

78. Fras C, et al: Substance P-containing nerves within the human vertebral body: An immunohistochemical study of the basivertebral nerve. Spine J 3:63–67, 2003.

79. Trafton JA, et al: Treatment needs associated with pain in substance use disorder patients: Implications for concurrent treatment. Drug Alcohol Depend 73:23–31, 2004.

80. Cohen MJ, et al: Ethical perspectives: Opioid treatment of chronic pain in the context of addiction. Clin J Pain 18:99–107, 2002.

81. Passik SD, et al: A pilot survey of aberrant drug-taking attitudes and behaviors in samples of cancer and AIDS patients. J Pain Symptom Manage 19:274–286, 2000.

82. Twycross RG: Opioid analgesics in cancer pain: Current practice and controversies. Cancer Surv 7:29–53, 1988.

83. Scimeca MM, et al: Treatment of pain in methadone-maintained patients. Mt Sinai J Med 67:412–422, 2000.

84. Bisaga A, et al: The NMDA antagonist memantine attenuates the expression of opioid physical dependence in humans. Psychopharmacology (Berl.) 157:1–10, 2001.

85. Popik P, Kozela E: Clinically available NMDA antagonist, memantine, attenuates tolerance to analgesic effects of morphine in a mouse tail flick test. Pol J Pharmacol 51:223–231, 1999.

86. Bennett DA, Amrick CL: 2-Amino-7-phosphonoheptanoic acid (AP7) produces discriminative stimuli and anticonflict effects similar to diazepam. Life Sci 39:2455–2461, 1986.

87. Bennett G, et al: Evidence-based review of the literature on intrathecal delivery of pain medication. J Pain Symptom Manage 20:12–36, 2000.

88. Popik P, Kozela E, Pilc A: Selective agonist of group II glutamate metabotropic receptors, ly354740, inhibits tolerance to analgesic effects of morphine in mice. Br J Pharmacol 130:1425–1431, 2000.

89. Finn AK, Whistler J: Endocytosis of the mu opioid receptor reduces tolerance and a cellular hallmark of opiate withdrawal. Neuron 32:829–839, 2001.

90. Dickenson AH: Neurophysiology of opioid poorly responsive pain. Cancer Surv 21:5–16, 1994.

91. Mercadante S, et al: Analgesic effect of intravenous ketamine in cancer patients on morphine therapy: A randomized, controlled, double-blind, crossover, double-dose study. J Pain Symptom Manage 20:246–252, 2000.

92. Fisher K, Coderre TJ, Hagen NA: Targeting the N-methyl-D-aspartate receptor for chronic pain management: Preclinical animal studies, recent clinical experience and future research directions. J Pain Symptom Manage 20:358–373, 2000.

93. Gagnon B, Bruera E: Differences in the ratios of morphine to methadone in patients with neuropathic pain versus non-neuropathic pain. J Pain Symptom Manage 18:120–125, 1999.

94. Suzuki M, et al: Small-dose ketamine enhances morphine-induced analgesia after outpatient surgery. Anesth Analg 89:98–103, 1999.

95. Celerier E, et al: Long-lasting hyperalgesia induced by fentanyl in rats: Preventive effect of ketamine. Anesthesiology 92:465–472, 2000.

96. Celerier E, et al: Progressive enhancement of delayed hyperalgesia induced by repeated heroin administration: A sensitization process. J Neurosci 21:4074–4080, 2001.

97. Wu CT, et al: Preincisional dextromethorphan treatment decreases postoperative pain and opioid requirement after laparoscopic cholecystectomy. Anesth Analg 88:1331–1334, 1999.

98. Wong CS, et al: Preincisional dextromethorphan decreases postoperative pain and opioid requirement after modified radical mastectomy. Can J Anaesth 46:1122–1126, 1999.

99. Weinbroum AA, et al: Dextromethorphan for the reduction of immediate and late postoperative pain and morphine consumption in orthopedic oncology patients: A randomized, placebo-controlled, double-blind study. Cancer 95: 1164–1170, 2002.

100. Jaitly V: Efficacy of intravenous magnesium in neuropathic pain. Br J Anaesth 91:302, 2003.

101. Marshall J, et al: Calcium channel and NMDA receptor activities differentially regulate nuclear C/EBP beta levels to control neuronal survival. Neuron 39:625–639, 2003.

102. Kohr G, et al: Intracellular domains of NMDA receptor subtypes are determinants for long-term potentiation induction. J Neurosci 23:10791–10799, 2003.

103. Brill S, et al: Efficacy of intravenous magnesium in neuropathic pain. Br J Anaesth 89:711–714, 2002.

104. Bie B, Pan ZZ: Presynaptic mechanism for anti-analgesic and anti-hyperalgesic actions of kappa-opioid receptors. J Neurosci 23:7262–7268, 2003.

105. Compton P, Geschwind DH, Alarcon M: Association between human mu-opioid receptor gene polymorphism, pain tolerance, and opioid addiction. Am J Med Genet 121:76–82, 2003.

106. Vaillant GE: Adaptive mental mechanisms. Their role in a positive psychology. Am Psychol 55:89–98, 2000.

107. Cui XJ, Vaillant GE: Antecedents and consequences of negative life events in adulthood: A longitudinal study. Am J Psychiatry 153:21–26, 1996.

108. Weissman DE, Haddox JD: Opioid pseudoaddiction: An iatrogenic syndrome. Pain 36:363–366, 1989.

109. Vaillant GE: What can long-term follow-up teach us about relapse and prevention of relapse in addiction? Br J Addict 83:1147–1157, 1988.

110. Mayfield D, McLeod G, Hall P: CAGE questions for alcoholism screening. Am J Psychiatry 131:1121–1123, 1974.

111. Cohen A, et al: The use of an alcoholism screening test to identify the potential for alcoholism in persons on methadone maintenance. Am J Drug Alcohol Abuse 4:257–266, 1977.

112. Walker RD, et al: Practice guidelines in the addictions. Recent developments. J Subst Abuse Treat 12:63–73, 1995.

113. Mercadante S, Casuccio A, Fulfaro F: The course of symptom frequency and intensity in advanced cancer patients followed at home. J Pain Symptom Manage 20: 104–112, 2000.

114. Mercadante S, et al: Factors influencing the opioid response in advanced cancer patients with pain followed at home: The effects of age and gender. Support Care Cancer 8:123–130, 2000.

115. Savage SR: Opioid therapy of chronic pain: Assessment of consequences. Acta Anaesthesiol Scand 43:909–917, 1999.

116. Savage SR: Opioid use in the management of chronic pain. Med Clin North Am 83:761–786, 1999.

117. Aronoff GM: Opioids in chronic pain management: Is there a significant risk of addiction? Curr Rev Pain 4:112–121, 2000.

118. Lovejoy M, et al: Patients' perspective on the process of change in substance abuse treatment. J Subst Abuse Treat 12:69–282, 1995.

119. Manfredi PL, et al: Methadone analgesia in cancer pain patients on chronic methadone maintenance therapy. J Pain Symptom Manage 21:169–174, 2001.

120. McCaffery M, Pasero C: The merits of methadone. Am J Nurs 100:22–23, 2000.

121. Wilford B: Doctor: Are you being duped? Mich Hosp 23:41–42, 1987.

CHAPTER 21

Nonopioid Analgesics

FAYEZ KOTOB, MD, AND MARK J. LEMA, MD, PHD

Pain relief can be achieved by using medications that act on the nervous system either by modifying the sensory response and the emotional experience as in using opioids or by interfering, in various tissues, with the metabolism of pain-producing peripheral substances, such as prostaglandins and kinins. Peripheral analgesia can be accomplished by using various drugs. Some are primarily indicated for pain relief; for example aspirin. Others are not principally indicated for analgesia, such as vasodilators to relieve ischemic pain and antacids to neutralize the effect of gastric acid caused by a peptic ulcer and subsequently achieving relief of ulcer pain.

Care providers are faced with the challenge of balancing providing their patients with adequate analgesia while avoiding or lessening the undesired side effects that surface as a result of using various analgesic agents. Analgesics are defined as drugs that relieve pain without blocking the conduction of neural impulse or markedly altering sensory function.[1] Analgesics do not cure the cause of the pain, but they provide temporary relief, facilitate tolerance or acceptance to chronic pain states, and improve quality of life for chronic pain sufferers.

"True analgesics" are medications that are primarily indicated and used to reduce or eliminate the experience of pain. Drugs with a primary indication other than pain relief can be used for alleviating pain of any type and are called "adjuvant analgesic."[2,3] Drugs in this group comprise medications that will be discussed in other chapters of this book, and include, but are not limited to, antidepressants, anticonvulsants, local anesthetics, α_2 adrenergic agonists, N-methyl-D-aspartate (NMDA) receptor antagonists, and steroids. In cancer patients, adjuvant analgesics should be distinguished from "adjuvant drugs."[2] The latter are medications usually used for symptom management, either to alleviate the side effects of cancer treatment or the side effects of cancer pain treatment. Examples of adjuvant drugs are antiemetics, laxatives, gastric acid antagonists, hypnotics, appetite-enhancing drugs, psychostimulants, anxiolytics, and antidepressants when used to treat associated depression, not in the capacity of adjuvant analgesics.

In the world of true analgesics, there are opioids and nonopioids.[1] Almost all nonopioid analgesics are nonsteroidal anti-inflammatory drugs (NSAIDs).[4] NSAIDs hold in variation the three major clinical effects of being antipyretic, analgesic, and antiinflammatory. Acetaminophen is the only nonopioid antipyretic that is analgesic but does not have antiinflammatory qualities, and therefore is not considered a true NSAID. Tramadol is a synthetic analgesic that is chemically related to codeine, and similar to opioids, it binds centrally to μ receptors and is considered a semi-opioid.[5] For the purpose of this chapter, it will be discussed as a nonopioid. Ziconotide is a nonopioid, nonlocal anesthetic, with a relation to calcium channel blockers that was approved by the Food and Drug Administration (FDA) of the United States for the intrathecal treatment of severe refractory chronic pain.[6] It will be presented at the end of the chapter.

THE ANALGESIC LADDER

Therapeutic approaches for cancer pain are variable, from drugs to surgery to alternative options. Treatments vary from individual to individual, depending on the type and severity of pain, risk factors involved with using a particular treatment, and personal preference. Analgesic drug therapy is the main pain relief system used for most cancer patients. Between 70% and 90% of a cancer patient's pain can be controlled using a combination of nonopioid, opioid, and adjuvant drugs, usually following the Analgesic Ladder. In 1986, the World Health Organization (WHO) published three-level guidelines for the treatment of cancer pain.[7] These guidelines are known as the WHO Analgesic Ladder (Figure 21–1). This ladder became the gold standard for the pharmacologic approach to almost all types of chronic pain, not exclusively to cancer pain. The ladder correlates the use of analgesics with severity of pain.

The first step in the ladder is the use of nonopioids for mild to moderate pain. Adjuvant drugs to enhance

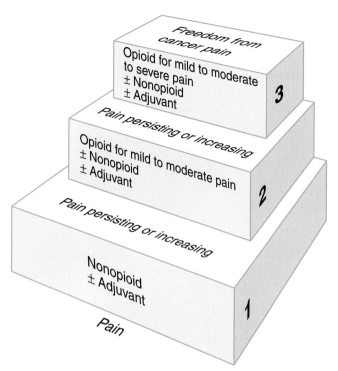

FIGURE 21–1 The WHO analgesic ladder. (Reproduced with permission of the WHO.)

analgesic efficacy, treat concurrent symptoms that exacerbate pain, and provide independent analgesic activity for specific types of pain may be used at any step. When pain persists or increases, a mild opioid, such as codeine or hydrocodone, could be added to (not substituted for) the nonopioid. Opioids at this step are often administered in fixed-dose combinations with acetaminophen or aspirin because this combination provides additive analgesia.[8] The use of fixed-combination products may become limited in observation of the dose-related toxicity of acetaminophen, aspirin, or ibuprofen that is usually found in these compounds. When higher doses of opioid are necessary, the third step is used. At this step, separate dosage forms of the opioid and nonopioid analgesic should be used to avoid exceeding maximum recommended doses of acetaminophen or the NSAID. Pain that is persistent or moderate to severe at the outset should be treated by increasing opioid potency or using higher dosages. Drugs such as codeine or hydrocodone are replaced with more potent opioids, as described in Chapter 16.

The WHO Analgesic Ladder had a significant effect on pain management around the world. Multiple studies have reported the durability and efficacy of this approach.[9,10] It is reported to be effective in relieving pain for 69% to 100% of patients with cancer[11-13]; as well as in 75% of terminally ill patients.[14] It even showed success in the treatment of different neuropathic cancer pain entities.[15] Following the WHO guidelines of cancer pain treatment was complemented with reduction of associated symptoms, such as nausea and anorexia, and was shown to

be safe with low rate of treatment complication occurrences.[16] Since its launch in the late 1980s, the WHO Analgesic Ladder serves as the fundamental algorithm to recognize, implement, and adhere to its principles in clinical pain management practice.[17,18] Multiple critiques, however, have been offered to challenge, modify, or amend the three-step ladder. Although some advocated the need for flexibility and the value of skipping steps in particular patients,[19,20] others proposed adding more steps to the ladder, so it would address the procedural aspect of cancer pain treatment in specific and the chronic pain in general when conventional pharmacologic analgesia is optimized.[21,22] The development of low-dose preparation of potent opioids has blurred the distinction between steps 2 and 3 of the ladder. It is generally agreed among experts that two therapeutic principles are to be learned from the WHO Analgesic Ladder. These are that treatment is to be based on the severity of pain and adjuvant analgesics are to be added when determined to be necessary by the clinician.[23]

Nonopioid therapy is recommended by the WHO for use at all three steps on the analgesic ladder, either alone or in combination with an opioid or adjuvant medication, or both. When evaluated in a retrospective study, adequate differentiation between the therapeutic effects of nonopioids, opioids, and adjuvant drugs was not possible. However, adequate combination of these drugs was effective and safe in the treatment of cancer pain.[24] There is support in favor of eliminating nonopioids in selected patients, such as the American Geriatric Society's call for opioids to be substituted for NSAIDs for mild to moderate pain.[25]

In their attempt to define an optimal pharmacologic regimen for the treatment of cancer pain, the group from the Netherlands Cancer Institute in Amsterdam and associated centers and hospitals managed to formulate a minimal comparative equianalgesic dose of common nonopioids and opioids.[26] The study they conducted evaluating patients with pain resulted from a comprehensive list of causes, including various types of malignancies, cancer spreading, and therapies for cancer. As in opioid equianalgesic scales, the group adopted morphine as the gold standard default measurement. As shown in Table 21–1, a dose of 2000 mg acetaminophen, 1200 mg ibuprofen, 100 mg diclofenac, 500 mg naproxen, or 200 mg tramadol given orally is equianalgesic to 30 mg oral morphine.

CANCER PAIN OVERVIEW

Implementing management strategy for cancer pain involves identification of the nature and type of the presenting pain syndrome, as well as recognition of the therapeutic aspects of this management.

TABLE 21–1	Comparative Equianalgesic Dose of Nonopioids and Opioids		
Drug		**Oral (mg)**	**Parenteral (mg)**
Nonpioids[a]	Acetaminophen	2000	—
	Ibuprofen	1200	—
	Diclofenac	100	—
	Naproxen	500	—
	Tramadol	200	—
Opioids[b]	Morphine	30	10
	Codeine	200	—
	Meperidine	300	75
	Dextropropoxyphene	—	300
	Nicomorphine	—	45
	Piritramide	—	15

[a]One-day of nonopioid was considered equivalent to one-day dose of 2000 mg acetaminophen.
[b]Amount of opioid was converted to oral morphine.

Clinical Presentations

Almost 65% of cancer pain patients suffer from pain caused by the primary or secondary (metastatic) tumor.[27] Another 25% complain of pain related to cancer therapy, such as procedures, surgery, chemotherapy and radiation therapy, or to cancer complication such as infections or fractures.[27] About 10% of patients with malignancy suffer from a pain complaint that is not related to the tumor or its therapy. However, they will be managed as cancer pain patients, as long as their pain course is occurring while they are undergoing treatment or follow-up of a malignant tumor.[28,29]

As with nonmalignant pain, cancer pain could be **acute** or **chronic** (Table 21–2).[21,29] The cause of acute pain is generally known, usually short-lasting, and responds to the treatment of the offending disease. In contrast, chronic pain is long-lasting with a frequently unknown cause and may appear or persist long after the conclusion or

TABLE 21–2	Comparison of Different Types of Pain	
Variable		
	Acute	*Chronic*
Time		
Causative factor(s)	Usually known	Usually unknown
Style	Usually well characterized	Usually vague or mixed
		Often multiple
		Episodes of exacerbation (breakthrough)
Duration	Brief	Ongoing
	Concludes with healing or resolution of offending element	On-and-off
Treatment	Usually satisfactory	Symptomatic
	Curative if offending factor removed	Results vary
Example	Postoperative pain	Postchemotherapy pain
	Traumatic bone pain	Cancer bone pain
	Headache	Headache
	Nociceptive	*Neuropathic*
Mechanism		
Causative factor(s)	Damage to body tissues	Abnormal neural activity secondary to disease or injury affecting the nervous system
Style	Somatic: well localized but variable in description and experience	Nonsympathetically maintained: arising from damage to a peripheral nerve without autonomic changes
	Visceral: poorly localized, deep, dull, and cramping	Sympathetically maintained: arising from a peripheral nerve lesion and associated with autonomic changes
		Central: arises from abnormal CNS activity
Duration	Resolves following disappearance of pathology	Could remain persistent without ongoing disease
	Can be chronic	
Treatment	Results vary	Difficult to achieve sustained relief
	Responds well to pathology resection or correction	Irresponsive to opioids
Example	Postoperative pain	Postherpetic neuralgia
	Bone pain (mostly)	Complex regional pain syndrome
	Pleurisy	Phantom limb pain

recovery from the offending disease or agent. "Breakthrough pain" is often an incidental pain that occurs with sudden movement or other activity in about 65% of cancer patients with therapeutically-controlled pain.[30,31]

Classification

Because pain results from various dynamic and complex mechanisms, classification of pain can assist in the planning of treatment. Clinically, cancer pain can be divided into **nociceptive** and **neuropathic** or a combination of both (see Table 21–2).[29,31-33] Nociceptive pain has two subtypes, *somatic* or *visceral*.[21,29,31] Somatic pain occurs as a result of the activation of nociceptors following an insult or injury to cutaneous or deeper tissues. Somatic pain is typically constant and well localized and is frequently described as aching, throbbing, or gnawing.[32] Both bone metastasis and dermal or muscular injury produce somatic pain. Visceral pain originates from injury to sympathetically innervated organs.[32] Causes of visceral pain include serosal or mucosal irritation, necrosis, ischemia of visceral muscle, or abnormal distension or contraction of smooth muscle walls within a hollow viscus. The pain is characterized as deep, dull, and aching or it can be paroxysmal and colicky. Both subtypes of nociceptive pain respond well to treatment by NSAIDs.[34]

Neuropathic pain usually involves a process of neural tissue damage or dysfunction resulting from tumor invasion or cancer treatment.[35,36] In cancer patients, neuropathic pain can occur following surgery, radiation therapy, or chemotherapy with certain agents, such as paclitaxel and vincristine,[37] or as a direct effect of tumor itself. This pain is characterized by burning, tingling, and numbing sensations. Compared to somatic and visceral pain, neuropathic pain responds less predictably to true analgesics and has a better response to adjuvant analgesics.[35,36] **Mixed** nociceptive and neuropathic pain frequently exists, particularly in cancer patients.[36,38]

Cancer Bone Pain

The initial symptom of the most common malignancies, such as lung, breast, and prostate cancers, is almost always bone pain.[39] Bone pain results from metastasis from these primary common tumors, multiple myeloma, as well as other types of metastatic tumors to the bone.[40] Additionally, bone pain is the most common chronic type of cancer pain, which can be severe and difficult to fully control.[40,41] It, traditionally, is presented as the classical example of nociceptive pain. However, this understanding has been challenged by the discovery of neural arborization in the bone marrow and trabecular bone next to the periosteum in animal models.[42]

Furthermore, a recent report that the membrane-stabilizing agent *gabapentin* normalizes cancer-induced bone pain and attenuates pain behavior in laboratory rats,[43] points to a neuropathic component of bone pain. Clinically, bone pain has two presentations: one is in the form of ongoing pain and the other one is pain stimulated by activity such as ambulation. Pharmacologically, bone pain responds well to opioids, NSAIDs, and adjuvant therapy, such as steroids and bisphosphonate.[33,41,44,45]

Pathophysiology

Pain is not a homogeneous experience. Several distinct forms of pain exist, and an enormous body of literature has been produced discussing pain mechanisms. Of particular interest, the various works attempt to explain the molecular basis of pain transformation from a brief physiologic event into a morbid status. **Nociceptive** pain can be normal or pathologic pain.[46] It also can be divided according to length of time to acute, subchronic, and chronic.[47] Nociceptive pain is thought to be the adaptive and protective response of the human body to an injury.[48] It frequently involves an inflammatory process.[48,49] **Neuropathic** pain results from neural damage either in the peripheral nervous system (PNS), as in postherpetic neuralgia and chemotherapy-induced neuropathic pain syndromes, or in the central nervous system (CNS), as in pain caused by cord compression from epidural metastasis or brain tumors.[47-51]

Primary Afferent Sensory Neuron

The primary afferent sensory neuron refers to a nerve cell (neurons) that has a cell body in the dorsal root ganglion (DRG).[A] This neuron has an axon that extends to the periphery to collect nociceptive information and another axon that extends to the spinal cord or to the brainstem to deliver this information. **Nociceptors** are free nerve endings found throughout the human body. In general, they are of Aδ and C type. Activation of these receptors by a noxious stimulant results in depolarization of membranous proteins, which is followed by transmission of action potential from the peripheral tissue to dorsal horn and termination in the brain. This is facilitated by the action of voltage-gated sodium channels. In the brain, this action potential is interpreted as a sensation of pain as well as danger.[49,52-54]

Nociception

External or deep structures of the human body that encounter a pain-producing element (noxious stimulus) such as mechanical force, heat, and chemicals report a

---

[A]Or the trigeminal ganglia for head and neck peripheral information.

TABLE 21–3 **Physiologic Stations of Nociception Journey**

Station	Definition
Transduction	Conversion of energy from a noxious stimulus (mechanical, thermal, or chemical) into nerve impulses by sensory receptors (nociceptors)
Transmission	Transference of neural signals from the site of transduction (periphery) to the central nervous system (spinal cord and brain)
Modulation	Alterations of ascending signals initially in the dorsal horn and continues throughout the central nervous system. This includes descending inhibitory and facilitatory input from the brain that influences (modulates) nociceptive transmission at the level of the spinal cord
Perception	Receipt and appreciation of signals arriving at higher central nervous system structures as pain

noxious stimulus to the CNS via nerve fibers, particularly fast, myelinated Aδ and slow, unmyelinated C fibers, to the DRG and through a series of complex electrochemical events, which conclude in the feeling of pain.[47,52,55,56] Nociception is the pain journey from the peripheral tissue to the brain through *transduction, transmission, modulation*, and *perception* and passing through the following stations: nociceptors, second-order neurons, central processing unit (composed of the thalamus and midbrain) and arriving at the brain (Table 21-3, Figure 21-2).[52-54]

Nociceptors detect noxious stimuli by various molecular sensors that are specific to certain offending elements. For example, the *vanilloid receptor* TRPV1, which is expressed by most nociceptors, detects heat, protons (H$^+$), and lipids. *Prostaglandin receptor* (EP) detects prostaglandin E$_2$ (PGE$_2$) that is produced by cancer and inflammatory cells. Nerve growth factor (NGF) released by macrophages

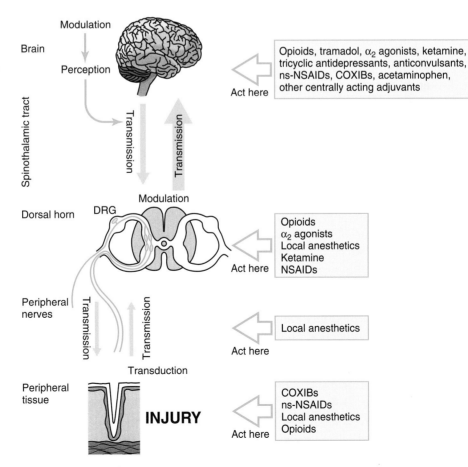

FIGURE 21–2 Anatomic scheme of nociception route coupled with the antinociceptive sites of various analgesics. COXIBs, selective cyclooxygenase-2 inhibitors; DRG, dorsal horn ganglion; NSAIDs, nonsteroidal anti-inflammatory drugs; ns-NSAIDS, nonspecific NSAIDs.

binds to the *tyrosine kinase receptor* TrkA, whereas extracellular adenosine triphosphate (ATP) that increases as a result of mechanical insults binds to the *purinergic* P_2X_3 *receptor*. Activation of these receptors increases the excitability of the nociceptors by inducing the phosphorylation of sodium channels. Mechanical stimuli are detected by the *dorsal-root acid-sensing ion channel* (DRASIC), as in the case of sensory fiber distension by tumor growth.[50,53,54]

Primarily a functional defense mechanism, pain becomes pathologic when it persists longer than the time needed for warning the patient to the potential insult, or when it occurs without an existing or persisting nociception.[57] Nociceptors do not respond to nonnoxious stimuli[58]; and unlike other sensory receptors, they do not adapt to noxious stimuli.[58-59] In cancer pain, nociceptors behave in a way similar to general pain, as became evident with cancer pain developed in animal models.[53-54] Pain in neoplastic diseases is still a subjective experience because pain-eliciting stimuli are modified by genetics, past experiences, mood, expectation, and social environment (culture, religious belief, profession, and so on), just as it is for those with nonmalignant pain.[60]

Inflammatory Response to Nociception

Although pain is one of the four cardinal signs[B] of inflammation, it is important to recognize that not all painful states are caused by inflammation. Inflammatory pain is also a physiologic or pathologic response of the body to overwhelming tissue damage following a bodily injury, an inflammatory process, or both.[48,49] A good example of such pain is postoperative pain or pain generated by pressure from expanding tumor mass. These events cause a series of neurochemical signals, which could exaggerate the pain response. At this level, distinguishing between nociceptive pain and neuropathic pain becomes hazy due to shared features; and they are only differentiated by identifying neural damage that raises neuropathic pain.

Following tissue damage, chemicals are released from injured cells. Inflammatory cells surround the area and release an assortment of cytokines and chemokines. Released agents are referred to as the "inflammatory soup," which includes, but is not limited to, tumor necrosis factor-α (TNFα), interleukins 1 and 6 (IL-1 and IL-6), protons, leukotrienes (LTs), norepinephrine, bradykinin, histamine, potassium, substance P, glutamate, serotonin, endothelins, platelet-activating factor (PAF), and calcitonin gene-related peptide (CGRP). These chemicals are chiefly meant to mediate the process of healing and promote tissue regeneration. However, they act as irritants in the damaged tissue and change the properties of the local primary sensory neurons, which in turn

---

[B]*Rubor, tumor, calor,* and *dolor*

activate a cascade of biologic enzymes. Particularly, cyclooxygenase type-2 (COX-2), which after neural injury gets up-regulated in peripheral tissue and spinal cord. This up-regulation is TNFα-dependent in the periphery.[50] COX-2 synthesizes prostaglandins (PGs), especially PGE_2.[46-48,52-54,61,62] PGs and other inflammatory mediators, such as kinins and NGF,[61-62] activate protein kinases A and C.[48] These enzymes regulate the activity and level of both intracellular signaling messengers and ion channels in the cellular membrane of the nociceptor. Phosphorylation of these enzymes lowers the threshold of the primary sensory neurons producing a state of pain hypersensitivity, leading to the clinical phenomena of increased nociception known as hyperalgesia and allodynia.[48,49,53,60,61] The analgesic effect of NSAIDs is primarily a result of interrupting the production of PGs by blocking COX activity.[48,53,63]

Nitric oxide (NO) is a gaseous signaling molecule that readily diffuses across cell membranes and regulates a wide range of physiologic and pathophysiologic processes, including inflammatory, immunologic, cardiovascular, and neuronal functions.[64] NO plays a role in both acute and chronic inflammation and therefore in nociception. In acute inflammation, NO promotes the synthesis of inflammatory PGs by activating COX-2. NO is synthesized by nitric oxide synthase (NOS). Three isoforms of NOS have been identified. Whereas NOS-1 and NOS-3 are constitutive, NOS-2 is inducible (also known as iNOS). NO proinflammatory effects include edema and vascular permeability vasodilation, cytotoxicity, and the mediation of cytokine-dependent processes that can lead to tissue destruction.[65] On the contrary, NO acts as a protective mediator when secreted by the endothelial cell. NOS may serve as an anti-inflammatory agent as well. Both functions are achieved by preventing the adhesion and release of oxidants by activated neutrophils in the microvasculature.[64,65]

On the nuclear level, nuclear factor-κB (NF-κB) plays a key role in the regulation of cellular responses to tissue injury. NF-κB is a rapid response transcription factor in cells involved in immune and inflammatory reactions. NF-κB contributes to immunologically mediated diseases, such as allograft rejection, rheumatoid arthritis, and bronchial asthma, by transcripting the genes for inflammatory mediators such as cytokines, chemokines, cell adhesion molecules, growth factors, and immunoreceptors.[66] Spinal COX-2 up-regulation and pain hypersensitivity after peripheral inflammation are mediated through the activation of the NF-κB-associated pathways.[67]

Tissue Acidosis in Nociception

Tissue acidosis, which occurs in various physiologic and pathologic states, including neoplastic disorders, has an important role in initiating and maintaining the picture of inflammatory pain. The postinjury release of protons lowers local pH, leading to direct sensitization of nociceptors, as well as the activation of the local inflammatory mediators.[54,55,68,69] Protons excite nociceptors via activation of potential $TRPV_1$ receptor and the acid-sensing ion channel (ASIC) family.[53,54,70]

Cancer causes a decrease in tissue pH. This occurs predominantly through the release of protons from inflammatory cells as they invade the neoplastic tissue. Tumors, in general, spur large amount of apoptosis, which releases intracellular ions to create an acidic environment, dropping the local pH. On the other hand, some types of cancer secrete protons or at the least promote an acidic environment for its continued growth or action, and accordingly, pain. This last phenomenon is particularly prominent in bony metastatic pain because it is extremely important for osteoclastic activity on bone resorption.[53,54]

As an added bonus to their primary analgesic action by COX blockade, NSAIDs induce pain relief by inhibiting both inflammation-induced expression and activity of ASICs.[69,71]

Cancer Involvement in Nociception

Direct tumor expansion might cause nerve entrapment, signaling direct nociception that would be complemented by the two mechanisms discussed earlier. Nerve entrapment could result in nerve compression, ischemia, or proteolysis and paves the road for neuropathic pain syndromes. Furthermore, tumor destruction of regional normal tissue promotes a surge in the level of local growth factors, such as NGF and glial-derived neurotrophic factor (GDNF), which in turn increase provoked nociception.[53,54]

Additionally, certain tumor cells secrete a variety of chemical agents that can independently stimulate nociception. Many of these agents are common secretory chemicals of normal cells, such as endothelins, proteolytic enzymes, protons, catecholamines, and serotonin.[52,53]

The Role of Lipids in Pain Regulation

Several categories of lipid molecules including, but not limited to, arachidonic acid metabolites, phosphatidyl inositol bisphosphate, ceramide, fatty acyl dopamines, and acetylethanolamides are shown to influence and control important systems in the regulation of pain responses.[52-54,72] These molecules exert their actions by interacting with a variety of receptor systems and signaling pathways, by activating specific prostanoid receptors, or by enhancing the action of other agents such as TRPV1 receptors and the NGF.[51,53,66] There is both in vivo and in vitro evidence for the participation of

these chemicals in the regulation of pain responses.[51,52,66] Acylethanolamides appears to inhibit pain responses, whereas the rest of the lipid products seem to enhance pain responses.[66]

PAF is a phospholipid released from leukocytes and mast cells during inflammation and causes platelets to aggregate, release arachidonic acid metabolites and lysosomal enzymes, and generate superoxide (i.e., release reactive oxygen radicals).[73] PAF exerts proinflammatory effects, including increased vascular permeability, hyperalgesia, edema, and infiltration of neutrophils.[73] PAF also produces effects that suggest its importance in asthma and other inflammatory diseases.[73] These effects are thought to be the result of PAF-stimulated increase in PGE_2. This function is mediated by COX-2, and perhaps the use of NSAIDs would be of help in this clinical situation.[74] Furthermore, it was shown in human subjects that PAF is capable of producing hyperalgesia on its own and is 50 times more potent than PGE_2.[75] In laboratory animals, PAF was a potent inducer of tactile allodynia and thermal hyperalgesia at the level of the spinal cord.[76]

Neural Plasticity

This physiologic action represents the property of the nervous system that enables it to produce cellular changes in response to a stimulus.[77] The following are major examples of pain neural plasticity.

Peripheral Sensitization

Following tissue damage and the development of inflammation in the injured tissue, intense, repetitive, or prolonged noxious stimulation as well as inflammatory mediators, particularly PGE_2, IL-1 and IL-6, can lower the threshold for activation and increase the rate of firing from nociceptors.[48,53-55]

Phenotypic Switch

Chronically inflamed nociceptors release CGRP, substance-P, and ATP in the periphery and recruit touch receptors and normally nonpain-transmitting, large-diameter, highly myelinated Aβ mechanoreceptors to rapidly transmit pain to the spinal cord.[48,54,78]

Central Sensitization

A state of CNS neuronal hyperexcitability results from continued afferent input. It describes the progression of nociceptors' hyperexcitability from peripheral levels to central levels. When C-fibers are discharged by a sustained stimulus at a high frequency; the dorsal horn is activated and a cascade of hyperexcitable events occur in the nervous system throughout the duration of the stimulus. "Wind-up" becomes potentiated along the peripheral nerves and culminates in a hypersensitivity response from the dorsal horn of spinal cord and, consequently, the brain.[79] It is believed that the "wind-up" phenomenon can be prevented by controlling nociceptive inputs to the dorsal horn using early and aggressive pain management. Such a belief raised the concept of implementing preemptive analgesia.

Exogenous (e.g., frequent surgical operations) or endogenous (e.g., tumor expansion) repetitive noxious stimulation causes "wind-up," which in turn increases the levels of neurotransmitters in the CNS and consequently causes changes in the brain's electrical signals. The role of prostaglandins in generating central sensitization, directly or indirectly, has become common knowledge. Clinically, central sensitization is believed to trigger the development of many chronic pain syndromes.[46-48,69,80]

Hyperalgesia and Allodynia

Hyperalgesia is a state of an exaggerated or prolonged perception of pain produced by a noxious stimulus. *Primary hyperalgesia* is caused by sensitization of neuronal C fibers (peripheral sensitization) and occurs immediately within the area of the injury. It is characterized by hypersensitivity to both mechanical and thermal stimuli.[56] This type of hyperalgesia is believed to be directly mediated by the effect of bradykinin, PGs, NGF, and CGRP.[55,61,62] *Secondary hyperalgesia* is caused by sensitization of dorsal horn neurons (central sensitization) and is observed in areas beyond the region of injury, frequently adjacent to the injured tissue.[56,79,81,82] This type of hyperalgesia is chiefly the result of the actions of substance P, TNFα, and CGRP[55,61,62] that lead to massive release of IL-1$_\beta$ in the CNS, which in turn up-regulates the expression of COX-2 and subsequently produces a significant increase of PGE$_2$ in the CNS.[83] An example of secondary hyperalgesia is abdominal wall tenderness during an intra-abdominal inflammatory process. **Allodynia** refers to pain that is produced by innocuous stimulus.[79-81]

EICOSANOIDS

The role of lipid products in the generation and regulation of inflammation and pain is well established. Eicosanoids are the largest family of lipid mediators.[83-86] They are derivatives of the oxygenation of the polyunsaturated 20-carbon chain fatty acid arachidonic (AA). Ubiquitously found in animals and humans, as well as some plants, eicosanoids include a considerable selection of compounds that control a wide variety of biologic functions. Prostanoids and hydroperoxyeicosatetraenoic

acids (HPETEs) are the two major groups of eicosanoids, and both have a role in inflammation. Prostanoids include prostaglandins (PGs), prostacyclin, and thromboxanes (TXs), which are casually bundled under the label prostaglandins. HPETEs include LTs, hydroxyeicosatetraenoic acids (HETEs), lipoxins (LXs), and epoxides.[83-86] Prostanoids, LTs, and epoxides are proinflammatory, while LXs are anti-inflammatory.[85] All of these agents have an indirect role in pain regulation; however, prostaglandins, and in particular PGE$_2$, have a direct and major role in pain generation and maintenance (Figure 21-3).[48,53,54,72,82,83]

Eicosanoids serve several physiologic bodily functions and are implicated in a number of clinical conditions, including acute and chronic inflammation, postischemic injury, aging, degenerative diseases, and cancer as summarized in Figure 21-3.[83-85,87,88] Eicosanoids facilitate and modulate cellular communications and cellular growth in states that involve tissue injury.[89] This role can be beneficial in promoting postoperative tissue recovery, as in the case of tissue removal.[89] This same role can be harmful in other situations, particularly in cellular death following massive injuries (e.g., third-degree burns), or the use of cytotoxic chemicals (e.g., smoking or postchemotherapy).[89] One explanation for this dichotomous role is the condition of the remaining cells in the damaged tissue.[89] If the surviving cells are healthy and completely functional, then eicosanoid-induced regeneration and recovery is expected.[89] On the other hand, if the surplus cells are weakened or partially damaged, then pathologic states may occur, including inept cellular communications, as in neuropathic pain syndromes, or abnormal growth, as in malignancies.[88]

As shown in Figure 21-3, oxygenation of AA is achieved by one of three major pathways: the COX pathway, the lipoxygenase (LOX) pathway, and the epoxygenase (P$_{450}$) pathway.[67,84,85] Eicosanoids are expressed in all human cells; however, they are essentially observed in mast cells, leukocytes, platelets, endothelial cells, and epithelial cells, where end-product mediators (e.g., PGs) are secreted in amounts sufficient to generate inflammatory reactions. All three pathways require the availability of AA. In most cases, the latter becomes offered in response to a physiologic or pathologic stimulus, by hydrolysis of the phospholipids found in the bilipid cellular membrane. This biologic action is catalyzed by a variety of phospholipases (PLs) but is chiefly the work of PLA-2, and to a lesser extent the work of PLC and PLD. Inflammatory cytokines such as IL-1, IL-6, and TNFα induce PLA-2. It is long known that **glucocorticosteroids** express their analgesic and anti-inflammatory action by interdicting the PL pathway by means of activating lipocortins, which are a group of enzymes that inhibit PL.[90-92] Lipocortin are also referred to as calpactins or annexins.[93] The precise mechanism is still not fully

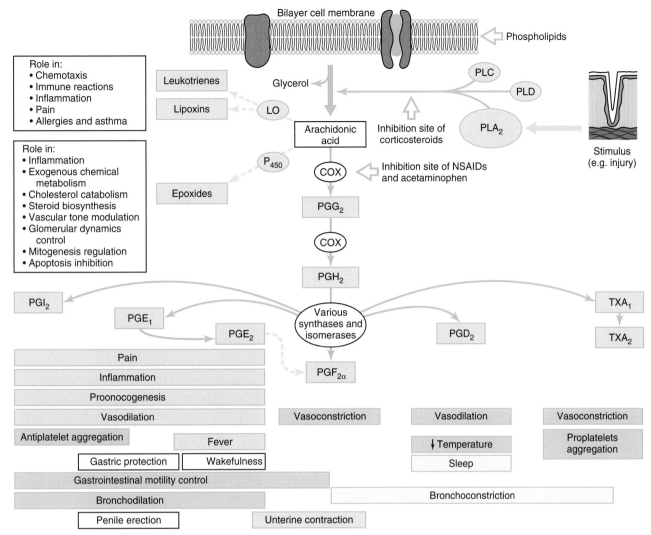

FIGURE 21–3 The arachidonic acid cascade, summarizing various effects of eicosanoids. COX, cyclooxygenase; LO, lipooxygenase; P_{450}, cytochrome P_{450}; PG, prostaglandine; PL, phospholipase; TX, thromboxane.

understood, and the increased synthesis of lipocortin cannot completely account for the inhibition of prostaglandin synthesis brought about by glucocorticosteroid.[94] PLA-blockade by glucocorticosteroids cannot completely explain the paradoxical behavior of glucocorticosteroids as carcinogenesis enhancers and inhibitors.[95] The end-products of the PLA-metabolism of AA are considered tumor growth regulators.[96] Perhaps their variable action toward neoplasm can explain the various effects of glucocorticosteroids on mitogenesis.

Although AA is the major product resulting from the PLs' actions on membrane phospholipids, other mediators are produced by PLs that have important roles in inflammation. Diacylglycerol is a precursor of AA, yet it serves a critical role in cellular transduction in the inflammatory process. Another important PL end-product is lysophosphatidic acid (LPA). This mediator serves as a growth factor in the repair phase of the inflammatory process, and it is gaining interest in current molecular research. Its role in pain regulation, if any, is yet to be determined.[72,85]

Prostanoids

Prostaglandin endoperoxide synthase or COX is bifunctionally composed of *bis*-cyclooxygenase activity directed at both C-11 and C-15 of AA and hydroperoxidase activity directed to the peroxide adduct at C-15 of PGG_2 to produce PGH_2.

COX-2 and COX-1 (and possibly its variation COX-3)[c] execute the transformation of AA to PGs and TXs. The term PG is liberally used to include TX. COX-1 is constantly produced in most body tissues to maintain "housekeeping" biologic bodily functions. COX-1 titers

---

[c]COX-3 was discovered in canine cerebral cortex, but not identified in humans yet.

increase two- to fourfold following an injury. COX-2 is expressed constitutively in the kidney[84,97] and plays a major role in renal physiology and pathophysiology.[98] Developmentally, it plays a significant role in nephrogenesis during gestational age 15 to 24 weeks.[99,100] NSAID use during the third trimester by pregnant females may contribute to fetal renal syndromes.[100] In humans, COX-2–produced substances modulate renal hemodynamics by controlling vasomotor activity and regulating sodium–potassium excretion and plasma levels.[101] COX-2 is inducibly expressed in other parts of the body with a titer increase of 10- to 20-fold following an insult. COX-2 is also expressed constitutively in the spinal cord, and it plays a major role in the initiation of tissue injury–induced hyperalgesia that follows peripheral tissue injury.[102] Compared to COX-1, COX-2 appears, to a lesser degree, to be involved in safeguarding gastric mucosa. More accurately, COX-2 expresses larger participation in the healing process of the gastric mucosa when gastric ulcer and *Helicobacter pylori (H. pylori)* gastritis are present.[103,104] Whereas Figure 21–3 shows details of arachidonic acid metabolism, as well as the corresponding biologic functions of the end-products, Figure 21–4 shows the most likely functional results for the action of specific COX isozymes.

Histologically, prostanoids generate their action by binding to cellular receptors.[105] These receptors are specific to each PG or TX and labeled according to the correlating prostanoids. For example, all PGE_2 receptors are prefixed with the letter E and suffixed with

a number correlating the sequence of their discovery: EP_1, EP_2, EP_3, and EP_4. Following the binding of the prostanoid to its specific receptor, a series of molecular processes occur such as activation of various enzymes or mobilization of electrolytes via the nuclear or cytoplasmic membranes. These actions generate other processes and eventually wrap up with a final action, such as smooth muscle contraction or dilation.[84–86,105]

Molecular and pharmacologic research provided evidence consistent with a role for both COX-1 and COX-2 in inflammation. Even though COX-2 is the predominant source, COX-1 also contributes to the marked increase in the PG formation that is evoked by offending factors.[106] By contrast, neither COX isozyme is an important source of lipid peroxidation in this human model of inflammation. Therefore, it is a sensible idea to investigate the value of combined antioxidant and COX inhibitor therapy in clinical situations where COX activation and oxidant stress are concurrent.[107]

The expression and action of COX isozymes is inhibited endogenously and exogenously. Endogenously, high levels of circulating corticosteroids (gluco- and mineralo-) seem to selectively inhibit COX-2 predominantly in the kidney[108] and in inflammatory cells, especially monocytes.[109] However, there is no evidence of COX-1 inhibition by these agents. Epoxyeicosatrienoic acids (EETs) inhibit the expression of COX-2 and inducible nitric oxide synthase (iNOS).[110] Exogenously, corticosteroids and NSAIDs differ in their selectivity of inhibiting the various forms of COX.[111,112]

In a state of health, PGs carry out a variety of physiologic functions. Most prominently, all PGs have a role in maintaining vascular homeostasis. PGE_2 and PGI_2 (also known as prostacyclin) particularly contribute the most to the renal homeostasis. PGD_2 regulates the sleep cycle and performs an opposing act to PGE_2 to keep the body temperature stable. PGE_2 plays a clear role in the regulation of cellular and humoral immune responses.[113] Increased production of PGE or increased sensitivity to PGE causes depressed cellular immunity.[113] PGE_1 and PGE_2 have a mucosal gastroprotective function. PGE_1, PGE_2, PGI_2, and $PGF_{2\alpha}$ control the gastrointestinal motility in various ways by acting on the digestive smooth muscles. $PGF_{2\alpha}$ with assistance from PGE_2 facilitates the contraction of the laboring uterine. The ability of NSAIDs to prolong gestation has been used by obstetricians to inhibit premature delivery.[114] PGE_1 contributes to male erection by its effect on the penile smooth muscles.

In pathologic states, PGE_2 and to a lesser extent PGI_2 and PGE_1 mediates hyperalgesia after a painful event or in chronic pain conditions. This was thought to be the work of COX-2; however, mounting evidence points to a larger role for COX-1 in this activity, particularly in chronic conditions.[106,115]

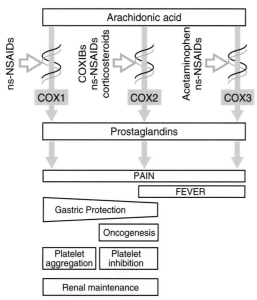

FIGURE 21–4 Major effects of arachidonic acid metabolites by various cyclooxygenase isozymes, showing the site and selectivity of various COX inhibitors. COX, cyclooxygenase; COXIBs, COX2 inhibitors; ns-NSAIDs, nonspecific nonsteroidal anti-inflammatory drugs.

Fever is the result of disturbance to the temperature regulation center in the hypothalamus, which maintains equilibrium between heat production and heat loss by using a thermostat-like neurochemical system that keeps the human body at a preset temperature.[83-85] The mechanism of such disturbance occurs as a part of a local inflammatory process in the hypothalamus after bodily exposure to a pyrogenic stimulus such as bacterial endotoxins. Pyrogenic stimuli release IL-1 in the hypothalamus, which, through the action of COX, in turn generates the degradation of AA into PGE_1 that transform to PGE_2. Both of these PGs cause the preset point of temperature to increase by acting on PG receptors particularly EP_3. Although COX-2 is primarily involved in the fever response to endotoxins, source components of this response are dependent on COX-1.[83,84] The revelation that acetaminophen inhibits COX-1 variation in canine brains, COX-3, might indicate a larger involvement of COX-3 in the synthesis of the pyretic PGEs.[116] That is, providing it becomes identified in humans.

Thromboxane-A_2 (TXA_2) plays a life-saving role by promoting platelet aggregation and enhancing vasoconstriction to stop a leaking vessel.[84,85] This action is normally opposed by the act of PGI_2 on inhibiting inappropriate platelet aggregation and vasodilation.[84,85]

In acute ischemic vascular events, this opposition is absent. This has led to the conclusion that production of PGI_2, which antagonizes inappropriate platelet aggregation, is the product of continuously induced COX-2, based on the observation of a higher incidence of cardiac events with patients on chronic therapy with a selective COX-2 inhibitor (COX2I).[117]

$PGF_{2\alpha}$ seems to be present in many chronic pathologic states of the body such as diabetes[118] and chronic cigarette smoking.[119] Actual $PGF_{2\alpha}$ contribution is still elusive; however, these findings might indicate a larger role for inflammation in these diseases. Interestingly, the long-term use of low-dose aspirin lowers these elevated $PGF_{2\alpha}$ levels.[118,120,121] Table 21–4 has an itemized list of PGs' functions.[120]

Pharmaceutical analogs for various PG with therapeutic use have been developed. Of particular interest to us is **misoprostol** (Cytotec), which is indicated for the prevention of NSAID-induced GI ulceration.[84,85,121]

The Role of COX in Chronic Pain

Strong laboratory evidence suggests that during the initial several months after nociception, peripherally over-produced PGs play an important role in the maintenance of neuropathic pain.[122]

TABLE 21–4 Major Prostanoids and Their Functions

Prostanoid	Primarily Found in	Major Biologic Action
TXA_2	Platelets Monocytes	Platelet aggregation Vasoconstriction Bronchoconstriction Cellular proliferation
PGI_2 (Prostacyclin)	Vascular endothelium Vascular subendothelium	Inhibition of inappropriate platelet aggregation Vasodilation Vascular permeability Bronchodilation Inflammation Cholesterol efflux from arteries
PGE_2	Renal medulla Gastric lining Platelets Microvascular endothelium	Vasodilation Inflammation Fever Na^+-K^+ excretion/reabsorption Bronchodilation Presynaptic adrenergic activity Cardioprotection
$PGF_{2\alpha}$	Brain Uterus	Vasoconstriction Bronchoconstriction Uterine constriction
PGD_2	Mast cells Brain	Sleep regulation Bronchoconstriction Temperature control Vasodilation

The Role of COX in Cancer

There is ample evidence that the COX pathway of AA catabolism, and mostly COX-2 division, is involved in carcinogenesis, as in activation of tobacco smoke carcinogen, increasing angiogenesis, and mediating resistance to apoptosis.[40,84,86,123,124] COX-2 is now associated with at least one type of cancer in each of the body's major tissues including, but not limited to, small and large intestines, lungs, breasts, brain, with added evidence that many of these cancers occur at a lesser rate among NSAIDs regular users.[84,86] Increased expression of COX-2 has been documented in biopsies from colorectal adenomas and from carcinomas of the colon, stomach, esophagus, pancreas, bladder, and skin.[40,84,86,125,126] COX-2's overexpression has been reported in most gynecologic neoplasms, including breast, cervix, endometrial, and epithelial ovarian cancers.[127,128] Moreover, COX-2 may be involved in the resistance of tumors to chemotherapeutic drugs.[126]

The Role of COX in Alzheimer's Disease

Neuropathologic features of Alzheimer's disease (AD) include the accumulation of microglia around plaques, a local cytokine-mediated acute-phase response, and activation of the complement cascade. This inflammatory response may damage neurons and exacerbate the underlying pathology. Microglia express COX-1, whereas neurons express COX-2. Although nonspecific NSAIDs (ns-NSAIDs) block both COX-1 and COX-2, the beneficial effects could be primarily attributed to inhibition of COX-1 in the microglia.[123,129]

On the other hand, evidence suggests that COX-2 is important in AD prophylaxis. COX-2 is clearly induced after various neurotoxic stimuli in the brain.[40,84] Furthermore, elevated COX-2 is also found in other neurodegenerative diseases like amyotrophic lateral sclerosis.[84]

Leukotrienes

LTs are the end-products of the LOX pathway of AA catabolism. 5-LOX converts AA to 5-HETE, which becomes leukotriene A_4 (LTA_4).[83,85,86] The latter can convert, by the act of other lipoxygenases, to other LTs, including LTB_4, LTC_4, LTD_4, LTE_4, and LTF_4 or to lipoxins. Pharmacologically, LOX is inhibited by various drugs, such as glucocorticosteroid, which, besides blocking PLs, seem to directly inhibit certain LOXs,[83,85,131] as well as selective LOX inhibitors like *zileuton* (Zyflo) that are useful in the treatment of asthma, and cysteinyl leukotriene receptor antagonists, such as *zafirlukast* (Accolate) and montelukast (Singulair).[83,131]

LTs have an important physiologic role in inflammatory and immune reactions, primarily by enhancing chemotaxis, increasing vascular permeability, smooth muscle contraction, bronchoconstriction and mucus production, and promoting vasoconstriction.[83,85,131] These functions, in inflammation-associated diseases, become pathologic and present an important role in asthma, chronic bronchitis, osteoarthritis, and various cancer states. LTs play an important cytoprotective role particularly during radiation insult, whether unintentional or therapeutic.[83,85,130]

The role of LTs in pain mechanisms is subtle and seems to be complementary to PGs. Whereas some LTs, particularly LTB_4 and other LOX-pathway intermediate chemicals, produce hyperalgesia at inflammatory site, other intermediate LOX-pathway products, such as dihydroxyeicosatrienoic acids (diHETEs), can produce hypoalgesia to counteract the work of algesic LTs.[131] LTB_4 also indirectly produces hyperalgesia by recruiting polymorphonuclear leukocytes, sparing direct effect on the pain receptors.[132,133] Furthermore, there is evidence that suggests a significant role for LTs, as well as PGs, in hyperalgesia produced by intervertebral disc herniation in laboratory animals.[134] LTs, particularly LTB_4, facilitate the work of PAF in hyperalgesia and inflammatory polymorphonucleocytes aggregation.[135,136]

Lipoxins

LXs are another end-product of the LOX pathway.[85,137-140] They oppose the work of LTs, particularly LTB_4 and LTD_4, in what has become known as the stop-signal phenomenon in the inflammatory process.[139-141] In this regard, they are considered endogenous anti-inflammatory agents. LXs down-regulate inflammation by antagonizing the effects of TNFα.[141,142] LXs counteract the effect of LTs in asthmatics and are observed to have higher bronchial concentration in mild asthmatics compared with severe asthmatics.[143]

The relationship between the generation of LXs and the pharmacology of NSAIDs is becoming more clear. It is now thought that one of the anti-inflammatory mechanisms of aspirin, besides inhibiting COX, is to mediate the production of endogenous agents, which display anti-inflammatory activity that resembles or potentiates lipoxins. These agents are two distinguished groups: *aspirin-triggered lipoxins* (ATLs)[137,144] and *resolvin*.[140,145] Both agents are thought to exert a potential for greater therapeutic use in inflammatory, cardiovascular, and malignant syndromes.[137,140,144,145]

Epoxides

Epoxides are agents caused by the metabolism of AA by cytochrome P_{450} epoxygenases. This category includes various biologically active eicosanoids such as EETs, HETEs, and diHETEs.[87,146,147]

Epoxides' main biologic function is exerted on epithelial ion transport and vascular smooth muscle fibers.[148] Epoxides are predominantly mediators of vascular tone modulation, including coronary and cerebral arteries.[146,148,149] EETs are potent vasorelaxants, whereas 20-HETEs are renal vasoconstrictors.[150] EETs increase coronary blood flow and protect the myocardium from ischemia-reperfusion injury. EETs participate in local regulation of cerebral blood flow by dilating cerebral arteries through a mechanism that involves activation of K^+ channels.[151] Specific cytochrome P_{450} enzymes that synthesize EETs in human vascular endothelial cells remain unidentified.

HISTORY OF PAIN KILLERS

Analgesics are commonly called *pain killers*.[83,86,105] The use of these medicinal agents to relieve pain and fever dates back to the decoction of dried leaves of myrtle in ancient Egypt, which were applied to the back and abdomen of laboring parturient women.

Aspirin and Aspirin-Like Drugs

The Greeks and Arabs chewed extracts of the willow bark (*Salix alba*) to reduce fever and to alleviate labor pain.[86,122] The first published report of the benefits of the willow bark was in England in 1763. Afterward, *salicin* was identified as the active component of willow bark. In the body, salicin is metabolized to salicylate.[86,123]

In 1860 *salicylic acid* was synthesized in Germany. The successful oral use of salicylic acid to reduce fever and rheumatic pain was complicated by indigestion and bitter taste. This led, in 1875, to the modification of the drug into a more acceptable form: *acetylsalicylic acid*. Later on, in 1899, this new compound acquired the name Aspirin; the "A" referring to the acetyl grouping and the "spirin" recalling the botanical genus *Spiraea*, from which salicylates could be extracted.[86,123]

In early 20th century, *aspirin* was recognized as an analgesic, antipyretic, and anti-inflammatory drug. It also became a first-line drug in the treatment of acute migraine attacks. More than 130 years after its discovery, aspirin is still the most globally recognized medication for the treatment of the same indicated ailments it was used for in the 18th century! Because of its popularity and common use in the United States, aspirin lost its trademark status, and "aspirin" became the scientific and generic name in place of acetylsalicylic acid. However, Bayer currently still retains the trademark status in a few countries around the world. Aspirin gastrotoxicity was noticed as soon as the drug went on sale. The first clinical documentation of this serious side effect was published in 1938.[86,122] This drove the pharmaceutical field into ongoing research for an aspirin-like drug with fewer side effects, particularly gastrointestinal.

The idiom "nonsteroidal anti-inflammatory drug" (NSAID) was initially used for *phenylbutazone* after its launch in 1949, three years following the exhibition of the antiinflammatory properties of glucocorticoids. The development of *phenylbutazone* and then *indomethacin* in 1963, both of which exerted clinical effects similar to aspirin, stirred scientists to look for a common mechanism. In 1960, it was suggested that aspirin-like medication acts by inhibiting an underlying cellular mechanism that was mediated by endogenous substances.[152] This turned the attention to prostaglandins that were discovered earlier in 1930. It was not until 1969 that the first association between prostaglandins and the actions of aspirin-like drugs was made. In 1971, it was demonstrated that aspirin and similar drugs cause a dose-dependent reduction in prostaglandin synthesis. This was the main trigger to the continuing cascade of laboratory work and discoveries based on associating the work of aspirin-like drugs with the interference with prostaglandin functions. By 1996, there were about 20 NSAIDs available in the United States and even more worldwide.[153] The discovery of COX's second isozyme in early 1990s made the discovery of a new NSAID class possible. The new drugs expressed higher selectivity to COX-2 inhibition and became known as COX-2 inhibitors (COX2Is) or COXIBs. Celecoxib and rofecoxib were introduced to the market in 1998 and 1999, respectively. More COXIBs evolved at the turn of the century including those in Table 21–5. The GI tolerability of COXIBs was found to be superior to that of ns-NSAIDs, and therefore had a favorable effect on patient quality of life. Enthusiasm for COXIBs' encouraging GI profile led into a major shift in NSAID prescribing habits among practitioners, especially primary care providers, favoring COXIBs over ns-NSAIDs. This shift was mostly undiscerning and frequently irresponsible.[154]

In 1995, scientists in the Rotterdam Study[D] concluded that an unknown mechanism allowed NSAIDs to delay the onset and slow the progression of AD in clinical trials.[155] This opened a new venue of medical research, and since then, others have observed the amelioration of AD in patients using NSAIDs.[156] Most prominent was the Baltimore Longitudinal Study on Aging (BLSA), which showed a significant drop in the overall risk of developing AD by using a nonaspirin NSAID, but not acetaminophen, over a 2 year or greater period.[40] Less benefit was observed with the use of low-dose aspirin. On December 20, 2004, the National Institutes of

---

[D]A study from 1990 to 1993 to investigate the prevalence and incidence of risk factors for chronic diseases in the elderly conducted in the suburbs of Rotterdam, the Netherlands.

TABLE 21-5 Overview of Nonopioid Analgesics

Name	Discovery (yr)	Trade Name (USA)	COX-1:COX-2 Selectivity	Half-Life (hr)	Renal Excretion (%)	Dosing Schedule	Starting Analgesic Dose (mg)	Maximum Dose (mg/d)	Pediatric Dose (mg/kg)	Average Monthly Cost (US$ 2001)	Additional Notes
Para-aminophenol derivatives											
Acetaminophen[a]	1893	Tylenol	4:1	2-3	85	q4-6 hr	650	4000	10-15	39-268	Selective COX-2/COX-3 inhibitor?
Salicylates											
Aspirin[ab]	1875	Aspirin	2:1	1/4	100	BID-QID	325	4000	10-15	3-15	Noncompetitive COX inhibitor (acetylation)
Diflunisal[ab]	1978	Dolobid	5:1	7-15	90	q8-12 hr	500	1500	N/A	62-87	Weak COX inhibitor. High doses are needed
Choline Magnesium Trisalicylate[b]	?	Trilisate		9-17	100	BID-TID	500	3000	N/A	63	No effects on platelets. Hardly any GI toxicity
Salsalate[b]	1955	Disalcid		1	100	BID-QID	500	3000	N/A	7-36	Gentle on stomach
Arylpropionic acids											
Ibuprofen[ab]	1960	Motrin	1:1	2	50-75	BID-QID	300	3200	4-10	4-43	Gentle on stomach
Naproxen[ab]	1967	Naprosyn	1.5:1	14	95	q8-12 hr	200	600	as adults	46-82	May cause arousal disturbance
Fenoprofen[ab]	1971	Nalfon		3	98	TID-QID	300	3200	N/A	40-46	Rare association with interstitial nephritis
Ketoprofen[ab]	1972	Oruvail	2:1	1	50-90	q6-8 hr	25	75	N/A	14-64	
Flurbiprofen[ab]	1966	Ansaid	3:1	4	65-85	BID-TID	50	500	N/A	49-53	
Oxaprozin[ab]	1971	Daypro	1.5:1	50-60	60	QID	1200	1800	10-12		
Arylacetic acids											
Indomethacin[abc]	1963	Indocin	10:1	4	60	QD-TID	25	200	N/A for pain	31-64; IV formula is available for PDA Rx and obstetric use	Most selective COX-1 inhibitor. Excellent analgesia in migrainous headaches. Best results in ankylosing spondylitis

Drug	Year	Ratio								Comments
Tolmetin[b]	1971	1:0.5	100	1	QD-TID	200	1800	N/A	102–142	Ineffective in gout
Sulindac[b]	1975	1.5:1	50	8	BID	150	400	N/A	58–72	↑ LFTs common; Active metabolite induces apoptosis in tumor cells
Diclofenac[b]	1988	3:1	50–70	2	BID-TID	50	150	N/A	95–106	↑ LFTs common
Ketorolac[ab]	1982	1:1	90	IM/IV: 2.5–9 PO: 3.5–9	q6–8 hr q4–6 hr	30 10	120 40	0.5–1 0.5		Oral doses are indicated only for those who received the drug parenterally. Rx should not exceed 5 days. Can combine PO/IM/IV. High GI and renal toxicity
Etodolac[abc]	1974	10:1	60	7	QD/q6–8 hr	200	1200	N/A for pain	132–151	Extended formula indication for juvenile RA
Bromfenac[b]	1987		100	1.3	BID	1 gtt OD/OS				Only ophthalmic solution in USA
Nabumetone	1974	1:1	80	22	QD	500	2000	N/A	109	Less gastrotoxicity than ns-NSAIDs
Anthranilates										
Mefenamic acid[ab]	1961	1:2	52	3–6	q4–6 hr	50	400	N/A	400	
Meclofenamic acid[ab]	1961	1:1	70	4–6	q4–6 hr	50	400	N/A	38–294	
Enolic acids										
Piroxicam	1971	3:1	95	45	QD	20	20	N/A	53–63	
Meloxicam	1979	1:11	50	20	QD	7.5	15	N/A	97	Less gastrotoxicity than ns-NSAIDs
COXIBs										
Celecoxib[a]	1991	1:8	27	10	BID	100	400	N/A	134	Contraindicated in sulfa allergy
Rofecoxib	1998	1:11	72	17	QD	12.5	25	N/A	118	Withdrawn from market in September 2004

Continued

TABLE 21–5   Overview of Nonopioid Analgesics—cont'd

Name	Discovery (yr)	Trade Name (USA)	COX-1:COX-2 Selectivity	Half-Life (hr)	Renal Excretion (%)	Dosing Schedule	Starting Analgesic Dose (mg)	Maximum Dose (mg/d)	Pediatric Dose (mg/kg)	Average Monthly Cost (US$ 2001)	Additional Notes
Valdecoxib[b]	2000	Bextra	1:30	8–11	70	QD	10	20	N/A	N/A	Withdrawn from market in April 2005
Etoricoxib	1998	Arcoxia	1:105	15	71						FDA approved for acute pain, but production is on hold for further studying
Parecoxib	1996	Dynastat	1:30	15	70	These three medications are available in some countries. Their future in the USA is pending further investigation into their long-term safety					Prodrug for valdecoxib, planned for IV injection only. Not yet approved by FDA
Lumiracoxib	2002	Prexige	54	3–6							Promising gastric and cardiovascular profile. Not yet approved by the FDA
Other nonopioids											
Tramadol	1962	Ultram	N/A	6–7	90	q4–6 hr	50	400	N/A	About 68	μ receptor agonist and serotonin and norepinephrine spinal reuptake inhibitor

The table reflects information of these drugs in the United States. Different names, doses, and indications may exist in other countries.

Trade names used in this table represent the most known ones, which may not be necessarily the first patended name. Also, some of the trade names are not available on the market anymore.

Year of discovery usually does not correlate with year of FDA approval or launch.

COX selectivity is based on the result of whole blood assays, rather than cellular assays. In case of more than one whole blood assay is available, the result of the one that agrees with cellular assays and/or clinical experience is chosen.

[a]FDA indication for pain treatment.

[b]When higher doses are used, regular periodic check up including stool for occult blood, liver and kidney basic function tests.

[c]Extended-release formula is available.

COX, cyclooxygenase; FDA, Food and Drug Administration; GI, gastrointestinal; IM, intramuscular; IV, intravenous; LFTs, liver function tests; PDA, patent ductus arteriosus; PO, by mouth.

Health (NIH) suspended the AD antiinflammatory prevention trial (ADAPT) over worries of increased cardiovascular and cerebrovascular events.[157] ADAPT was designed to assess the potential benefit of long-term use of naproxen, an ns-NSAID, and celecoxib for decreasing the risk of developing AD in people older than 70 years who were considered to be at increased risk because of family history, but did not have symptoms of the disease.

In 2001, it was suggested that rofecoxib could be linked to an increased incidence of stroke and serious cardiac events.[158] The FDA issued a warning letter to Merck, the pharmaceutical manufacturer of rofecoxib, for misrepresenting the safety of their drug. Initially, the manufacturer responded that the VIGOR study's data falsely inflated the cardiovascular risk of rofecoxib because it was compared to naproxen, which has antiplatelet properties similar to aspirin. Accumulating data emphasized those observations. Eventually, on September 30, 2004, Merck announced voluntary withdrawal of the drug from the worldwide market. The FDA convened an advisory panel on COXIBs in early 2005. After 3 days deliberation, the panel decided on February 18, 2005, that all market-available COX2Is carry serious risks of heart attack and stroke and recommended that the FDA demand that the drugs carry "black box" warnings of the potential cardiovascular risk. However, the panel did not recommend that the drugs be withdrawn from the market.[159] Additionally, they requested that all inserts of prescription NSAIDs and the package labeling for over-the-counter (OTC) NSAIDs be revised to provide a better explanation of the potential GI and CV risk from using NSAIDs.[160] In April 7, 2005, based on FDA advice, the maker of valdecoxib withdrew the drug from the markets because of evidence of serious dermatologic side effects of the drug. However, this was overshadowed by multiple reports of cardiodepressive effects of valdecoxib. Etoricoxib, a promising COX2I, which is already approved by the European regulatory authority and is available in some countries outside the United States has received an initial approval from the FDA. However, its introduction to the U.S. market was put on hold upon pending further studies. Parecoxib, lumiracoxib, and other COX2Is are not approved by the FDA.[161]

They Call It Panadol, We Say Tylenol

Although discovered in 1893, acetaminophen was not recognized as an analgesic and antipyretic until 1948. It was approved for sale by the FDA in 1955 and went on sale in Britain in 1956 under the generic name *paracetamol*. Extended-release acetaminophen was launched in 1998. The mechanism of acetaminophen's clinical effect has been a mystery until a recent revelation that it does not act differently from NSAIDs. In the 21st century, acetaminophen is the most sold analgesic in the United States and in most industrial nations. In 2002, acetaminophen, which has been considered for many years as a non-antiinflammatory analgesic and antipyretic, was found to block the action of a variation of the enzyme COX-1 that was found in the canine brain[123,162] and therefore gained tentative recognition among the NSAIDs, at least at the molecular level. The excitement of this revelation rushed some authors into prematurely nominating an NSAID subgroup called "COX-3 inhibitors" that included only acetaminophen.[163] Most authorities are still using the broader term of "para-aminophenol derivative" as the analgesic subgroup that has acetaminophen as its member.

The Story of COX

Prostaglandin endoperoxide synthase was isolated in 1976 from ovine and bovine vesicular glands. This enzyme became known as cyclooxygenase (COX).[86,123] The discovery of COX explained the missing link of NSAIDs' principal pharmacologic effect of inhibiting prostaglandin synthesis. In 1990, the possible existence of two different cyclooxygenase enzymes was suggested by observing that glucocorticoids inhibit the increase in COX activity induced by bacterial lipopolysaccharides in macrophages but not the basal production of prostaglandins or leukotrienes. In 1992, COX-2 was cloned in animals and humans. Its expression was shown to be increased by inflammatory and proliferative conditions and decreased by glucocorticoids. Thus, it earned the description "inducible." The older COX became known as COX-1 and labeled "constitutive" because it is thought to mediate regular physiologic functions, including cytoprotection of the stomach and platelet aggregation. However, the theory of inducible versus constitutive is still being updated. COX-2 is found to be constitutively expressed in various tissues for physiologic functions, On the other hand, COX-1 levels were also induced during tissue injury.[86,123]

Whereas COX-2–produced prostaglandins are called "inflammatory" prostaglandins, prostaglandins produced as a result of the catalytic action of COX-1 on AA are called "housekeeping" prostaglandins and are believed to be primarily responsible for gastroprotection, autocrine response to circulating hormones, and platelet aggregation. In the 1990s, COX-1 received credit mistakenly for the production of PGI_2, which is believed to be in charge of vasodilation and inhibition of inappropriate platelet aggregation.[164] Current research strongly suggests that PGI_2 is produced by COX-2 that is constantly induced in the cells.[164]

The search for medications that would selectively block the work of COX-2 without intervening with COX-1 became the target of perhaps the most extensive pharmaceutical work in history. This was preceded by comparing the selectivity of existing NSAIDs between the two COXs. Although this concept seemed simple, practice proved it to be more difficult than thought. Inhibition of COX can be quantified in recombinant or natural enzyme preparations, cellular systems, isolated human cell populations, such as platelets for COX-1 and white blood cells for COX-2, or in vitro stimulated whole blood samples. The closer the experimental system to physiologic state, the lower the selectivity of the COXIB.[86] The human whole blood assay and its modifications proved to be the most reliable detectors of such selectivity because it mimics in vivo conditions such as plasma binding.[86] Unfortunately, several variations were observed among different testing laboratories (Table 21–5) and they were based on the result of whole blood assays, rather than cellular assays.[86] Should more than one whole blood assay be available, the result of the one that agrees with cellular assays, clinical experience, or both, is chosen. The earlier concept that COX-2 is solely responsible for generating nociception has been challenged, and evidence that COX-1 could play a role in pain and inflammation has been surfacing (see Table 21–5).[165]

Following COX-2 discovery, the genetic structures of both COX isozymes were characterized. COX-1 was encoded on chromosome 9 and COX-2 on chromosome 1. It was found that COX-2 gene contains regions characteristic of early response genes, allowing a rapid up-regulation in response to inflammatory stimuli.[84,86] With the exception of minor differences in amino acid sequence, both COX-1 and COX-2 were found to be homologous. Yet, the binding site of COX-2 is 25% larger than that of COX-1. These differences lead to the distinct inhibition profiles between traditional NSAIDs and COXIBs. Researchers continued to look for variations of the existing COXs. Several COX-1 variants were discovered during the 1990s, some in association with an inflammatory process and others linked to oncogenesis, however, all without an identifiable specific biologic function in humans. In 2002, a distinct variant of COX-1 was identified and labeled COX-3. COX-3 was found to be selectively inhibited by acetaminophen in a dog's brain. Some scientists refused the title COX-3, and they renamed it COX-1v, where v stands for variant.[115] At the time of COX-3 discovery, it was revealed that recently identified COX-1 splice variants encoding partial COX-1 (PCOX-1) proteins were isolated. However, no biologic function was identified. Recently, it has been reported that this COX-1 variant is not expressed in humans.[166]

Recognized Studies in Analgesia

The following reports are major US or international studies that involved one or more NSAIDs and had an impact on the practice of pain medicine. They are listed in chronologic order. Table 21–6 lists in alphabetical order most of major NSAIDs studies regardless of their bearing on the practice of pain medicine.

MUCOSA

Misoprostol Ulcer Complication Outcomes Safety Assessment (MUCOSA) (July 1991 to August 1993) was a multicenter, randomized, double-blinded, placebo-controlled trial that validated positive therapeutic effects of misoprostol in reducing serious NSAID-induced upper gastrointestinal complications by 40% compared with placebo.[167]

OMNIUM

Omeprazole versus Misoprostol for NSAID-induced Ulcer Management (OMNIUM) (April 1992 to April 1995) was a multicenter, double-blinded, randomized study. The goal was to compare the efficacy of omeprazole and misoprostol in healing and preventing ulcers associated with NSAIDs treatment. The study concluded both drugs were equally efficient in healing ulcers and erosions caused by NSAIDs. On the other hand, maintenance therapy with omeprazole was associated with a lower rate of relapse than misoprostol. Additionally, omeprazole was tolerated by patients better than misoprostol.[168]

ASTRONAUT

Acid Suppression Trial: Ranitidine versus Omeprazole for NSAID-Associated Ulcer Treatment (ASTRONAUT) (August 1992 to April 1995). A multicenter, randomized, double-blinded study to compare the efficacy of omeprazole, representing proton pump inhibitors (PPIs) and ranitidine, representing histamine receptor-2 blockers (H_2 blockers) in patients with gastroduodenal ulcers and erosions associated with continuous NSAID treatment. The study concluded that daily omeprazole is superior to ranitidine with respect to healing and preventing gastroduodenal ulcers and erosions, as well as controlling dyspeptic symptoms. The comparison on the NSAID-induced ulcer complication was not studied.[169]

VIGOR

Vioxx Gastrointestinal Outcomes Research (VIGOR) (January to July 1999) was a multicenter, randomized, double-blinded, active comparator-controlled, parallel-group trial that did not have a placebo group because to do so would have meant patients with rheumatoid arthritis would have been randomized to receive no pain relief. The trial was intended to prove that rofecoxib, representing selective COX2Is, is associated with

TABLE 21–6 Alphabetical List of Famous Acronyms for NSAIDs Clinical Trials

Acronym	Trial Full Name	Dates	Comments
ADAPT	Alzheimer Disease Anti-inflammatory Prevention Trial	2001–2004	See text
ADONIS	Aspirin Dose Optimized in Noncardioembolic Ischemic Stroke	Ongoing	Double-blind, randomized, multicenter study. To determine the optimal dose of aspirin that would minimize both the recurrence of noncardioembolic ischemic stroke and the risk of drug-related adverse events
APC	Adenoma Prevention with Celecoxib	2002–2004	On December 12, 2004 NIH stopped the trial due to observation of 2.5-fold increased risk of major fatal and nonfatal cardiovascular events for articipants on celecoxib vs. those on a placebo
APPROVe	Adenomatous Polyp Prevention on Vioxx	2003–2004	See text
ASAAC	Acetylsalicylic acid Versus Anticoagulants Study	1990	Study concluded that a combination of low-dose aspirin and anticoagulation should be investigated to reduce graft occlusion rates
ASTRONAUT	Acid Suppression Trial: Ranitidine Versus Omeprazole for NSAID-Associated Ulcer Treatment	1992–1995	See text
AVASIS	Aspirin Versus Anticoagulants in Symptomatic Intracranial Stenosis	Stopped in June 2004 to slow enrollment	Randomized, comparative, multicenter, parallel, open trial to compare safety and efficacy of aspirin and oral anticoagulants in the 2° prevention of vascular events in patients with symptomatic stenosis of the middle cerebral artery
BLSA	Baltimore Longitudinal Study on Aging	1958–ongoing (of interest reports from 1990–1994)	America's longest-running scientific study of human aging. It found that the use of NSAIDs was associated with reduced risk of Alzheimer's disease
CLASS	Celecoxib Long-term Arthritis Safety Study	1998–2000	See text
CRESCENT	Celecoxib Rofecoxib Efficacy and Safety in Comorbidities Evaluation Trial	2004–2005	12-week, double-blind trial, patients with type 2 diabetes, hypertension, and osteoarthritis were randomized to treatment with 200 mg of celecoxib once daily ($n = 136$), 25 mg of rofecoxib once daily ($n = 138$), or 500 mg of naproxen twice daily ($n = 130$) for 12 weeks
EDGE	Etoricoxib Versus Diclofenac Sodium Gastrointestinal Tolerability and Effectiveness	2002	6-week double-blind, active comparator controlled, parallel-group study eligible osteoarthritis patients were randomized to receive either etoricoxib 60 mg once daily or diclofenac 50 mg three times daily
HOPE	Heart Outcomes Prevention Evaluation Study	1993–1999	970 patients on aspirin who were enrolled in this 5-year follow up international, randomized, placebo-controlled, 2×2 factorial trial, were evaluated for aspirin resistance
MASH	Magnesium and Acetylsalicylic Acid in Subarachnoid Hemorrhage	2004–2005	Randomized, placebo-controlled, multicenter, factorial trial to determine whether magnesium and/or aspirin reduce frequency of delayed cerebral ischemia in patients with acute aneurysmal subarachnoid hemorrhage

Continued

TABLE 21–6   Alphabetical List of Famous Acronyms for NSAIDs Clinical Trials—cont'd

Acronym	Trial Full Name	Dates	Comments
MELISSA	Meloxicam Large-Scale International Study Safety Assessment		Large-scale, prospective, double-blind, double-dummy, randomized, international trial of 9323 patients to evaluate meloxicam versus diclofenac GI tolerability over 28 days. It concluded that meloxicam has better profile
MUCOSA	Misoprostol Ulcer Complication Outcomes Safety Assessment	1991–1993	See text
NHANES III	3rd National Health and Nutrition Examination Survey	1988–1994	Nationally representative sample of people aged 17 and older found an estimated 147 adults used NSAIDs in one month. 76% were OTC and 9% prescribed. Females more likely to use than males
OMNIUM	Omeprazole Versus Misoprostol for NSAID-Induced Ulcer Management	1992–1995	See text
TARGET	Therapeutic Arthritis Research and Gastrointestinal Event Trial of Lumiracoxib	2003–2004	See text
VICOXX	Valoración del Impacto de los COXIB	2003	6 month prospective study to compare the efficacy of rofecoxib and ns-NSAIDs in the treatment of osteoarthritis. It concluded that rofecoxib has a superior therapeutic profile
VIGOR	Vioxx Gastrointestinal Outcomes Research	1999	See text
WARCEF	Warfarin-Aspirin Reduced Cardiac Ejection Fraction	2003–ongoing	Two-arm, double-blinded, randomized, multicenter trial to compare efficacies of warfarin and aspirin in preventing death, ischemic stroke, and intracerebral hemorrhage in patients with heart failure
WARIS-II	Warfarin-Aspirin Reinfarction Study	2002	Warfarin, alone or in combination therapy, was found more effective than aspirin alone in preventing subsequent cardiovascular events in patients with MI but was associated with a greater risk of bleeding
WARSS	Warfarin Aspirin Recurrent Stroke Study	1995–2001	7-year double-blind, randomized largest clinical trial in history comparing aspirin to warfarin for recurrent stroke prevention. No difference between aspirin and warfarin in the prevention of recurrent ischemic stroke or death or in the rate of major hemorrhage
WASID	Warfarin-Aspirin Symptomatic Intracranial Disease Study	Ended 2004	Prospective, double-blind, randomized, multicenter trial to compare prophylactic efficacies of warfarin and aspirin against stroke and vascular death in patients with symptomatic stenosis of a major intracranial artery. No clear difference between the two drugs and the study authors concluded that aspirin should be used instead of warfarin for patients with intracranial arterial stenosis

significantly fewer clinically important upper gastrointestinal (UGI) events than treatment with naproxen, representing ns-NSAIDs, which was successfully proven. However, VIGOR had instigated a new concern that rofecoxib showed higher incidence of unexpected cardiovascular effects, which were not observed with the use of naproxen. This led to further investigation, controversy, and the ultimate withdrawal of the drug.[168]

CLASS

Celecoxib Long-term Arthritis Safety Study (CLASS) (September 1998 to March 2000) was a double-blinded, randomized, comparator-controlled prospective trial intended to determine if celecoxib, representing COX2Is, is associated with a lower incidence of serious UGI ulcer complications compared with ibuprofen or diclofenac, representing ns-NSAIDs. The study determined that celecoxib, when used for 6 months in a dosage 2 to 4 times the maximum therapeutic dosage, is associated with a lower incidence of combined clinical UGI events than comparator ibuprofen and diclofenac used at standard therapeutic dosages. Patients who took ibuprofen or diclofenac had significantly higher rates of symptomatic ulcers or ulcer complications than did patients who took celecoxib, but the rate for ulcer complications did not differ. Patients who were on concomitant use of low-dose aspirin for cardiovascular prophylaxis had higher ulcer

complication rate with the use of any of the three NSAIDs. Neither drug had a higher incidence of undesired cardiovascular events, irrespective of aspirin use.[171,172] Table 21-7 provides an easy comparative pinpoint scale between VIGOR and CLASS.

APPROVe

Adenomatous Polyp Prevention on Vioxx (APPROVe) (2003-2004) was a multicenter, randomized, placebo-controlled prospective, double-blind clinical trial to determine the effect of 156 weeks (3 years) of treatment with rofecoxib on the recurrence of neoplastic polyps of the large bowel in patients with a history of colorectal adenoma. The trial was stopped by Merck because of the observation of a twofold increased relative risk for confirmed cardiovascular events, such as heart attack and stroke, beginning after 18 months of treatment in the patients taking rofecoxib compared with those taking placebo. This complemented earlier observation from VIGOR.[173] Vioxx (rofecoxib) was voluntarily withdrawn from the worldwide market by the manufacturer on September 28, 2004.

TARGET

Therapeutic Arthritis Research & Gastrointestinal Event Trial of lumiracoxib (TARGET) (2003-2004). This was

TABLE 21-7 Comparative Analysis between the CLASS and VIGOR Trials

Element	VIGOR	CLASS
Study type	Randomized, double-blinded, and comparator-controlled	Randomized, double-blinded and comparator-controlled
Indication for NSAID	Rheumatoid arthritis	Osteoarthritis/rheumatoid arthritis
Sample number	8076	7968
COXIB	Rofecoxib 50 daily	Celecoxib 400 mg BID
Control NSAID	Naproxen 500 mg BID	Ibuprofen 800 mg TID Diclofenac 75 mg BID
Patient on low-dose aspirin?	No	Yes: 21%
Primary endpoint	Clinical UGI event	Complicated peptic ulcers
Secondary endpoint	Complicated UGI events	Symptomatic peptic ulcers
Length of trial	Median = 9 months Maximum = 13 months	Median = 9 months Maximum = 13 months
Length reported	6 months	13 months
Clinical observation	No significant reduction in new ulcer complications Rofecoxib has better GI profile Raised concern of cardiovascular toxicity	Aspirin users: no advantage for celecoxib over ns-NSAIDs 13-Month analysis: as above vs. 9 months celecoxib is better

an international double-blind study and the largest COXIB trial to date, enrolling 18,325 patients with osteoarthritis who received treatment with lumiracoxib 400 mg once daily (two or four times the recommended chronic dose for osteoarthritis), naproxen 500 mg twice daily (maximum therapeutic dose), or ibuprofen 800 mg three times daily (maximum therapeutic dose) for 52 weeks. In this trial, lumiracoxib was compared with ibuprofen or naproxen, which helped to dissect the potential of naproxen's putative antithrombotic effect. Furthermore, patients were stratified on the basis of their taking low-dose aspirin. The researchers concluded that lumiracoxib is the first COX-2 selective inhibitor to significantly reduce gastrointestinal events without compromising cardiovascular safety compared to naproxen and ibuprofen. However, these conclusions were met with sound criticism that TARGET quantifies lumiracoxib's narrow benefit over two NSAIDs with a trade-off. The absolute reduction in ulcer complications was only 0.72% with a surplus of 2.0% of liver function test abnormalities for patients not taking aspirin. The alleged benefit is further compromised if naproxen is the NSAID, with a 0.17% excess of myocardial infarction (MI). For patients taking low-dose aspirin, it is hard to justify this COXIB because there is no benefit in ulcer complication reduction and the risk of MI and hepatotoxicity persists.[174,175]

An Opioid Imitation

Tramadol was first synthesized in 1962 in Germany and been in therapeutic use there since 1977 and marketed under the trade name Tramal.[176] On March 3, 1995, the FDA approved an oral form of the drug, which was marketed in the United States under the trade name Ultram. In March 1996, the manufacturer issued a warning of the possibility of drug abuse, seizures, and anaphylactoid reactions associated with tramadol use. In 2001, Ultram reached sales of $662 million.[177] The FDA issued an approvable letter for Ralivia ER (extended-release tramadol HCl tablets, Biovail Corporation) in December 2004, following the February 2004 new drug application (NDA) filing.[177] The proposed indication for the once-daily oral extended-release drug is for the treatment of moderate to moderately severe pain. An orally disintegrating tablet (Ralivia FlashDose) was approved by the FDA in May 2005, but the date of commercial availability in the United States is currently unknown.

A ZESTful Analgesic

Ziconotide, a synthetic form of the cone snail peptide *w*-conotoxin M-VII-A and an N-type calcium channel blocker,[178] was patented in the United States in 1998 under the name Prialt. In December 2004, and in view of analyzing the results of phase III of the intrathecal ziconotide effectiveness and safety trial (ZEST), the drug was approved by the FDA for the management of refractory intractable chronic pain when delivered as an infusion into the cerebrospinal fluid using an intrathecal pump system.[6,178]

NONSTEROIDAL ANTI-INFLAMMATORY DRUGS

Nonsteroidal anti-inflammatory drugs (NSAIDs) are a tremendously diverse group of drugs that is currently composed of two main categories: nonspecific NSAIDs (ns-NSAIDs) and specific COX-2 inhibitors (COX2Is). A list of current NSAIDs is available in Table 21–5.

Classification

NSAIDs are grouped in various chemical classes as shown in Table 21–5. The diversity of these classes generates a broad range of pharmacokinetic characteristics. All ns-NSAIDs are weak acids except for nabumetone, which is a ketone prodrug that becomes metabolized into an acidic active agent. The chemical structure of an NSAID facilitates easily remembered classification.[86] Classification of NSAIDs can also be based on clinical observation based on their efficacy and elimination half-life.

Pharmacokinetics

In most cases, NSAIDs are completely absorbed in the GI tract to the systemic circulation. Food changes their bioavailability only trivially. Increase of gastric pH reduces NSAIDs absorption. Antacids reduce the bioavailability of salicylates and indomethacin but not diflunisal.[179-181] NSAIDs tend not to undergo the first-pass elimination step, and they are highly bound to plasma proteins, usually albumin. Some NSAIDs are metabolized by phase I followed by phase II (glucuronidation) mechanisms and other NSAIDs are metabolized by direct phase II alone. Most NSAIDs by-products are degraded partially in the liver by enzymes from the P_{450} family.

Most NSAIDs go through enterohepatic circulation by enduring different levels of biliary excretion and then reabsorption. Moreover, the extent of irritation that is induced by NSAID in lower gastrointestinal (LGI) tract is linked to the sum of enterohepatic circulation. Renal excretion remains the most important course for NSAIDs' final removal from the body.[86]

The elimination half-life of an NSAID does not reflect automatically its duration of action. Following recurring doses, all NSAIDs can be found in synovial fluid. Drugs with short half-lives remain in the joints longer than would be predicted from their half-lives, whereas drugs with longer half-lives disappear from the synovial fluid at a rate proportionate to their half-lives.

Mechanisms of Action

The main effect of NSAIDs is doubtlessly accomplished via the reduction of PG synthesis by inhibiting the COX enzyme.[47,52,61] Prostaglandins are key mediators that sensitize primary afferent nerves in response to noxious stimuli in the periphery, and they facilitate the inflammatory response following the activation of immunologically competent cells by a foreign organism or antigenic substance. Although inhibition of these peripheral processes clarifies both the analgesic and antiinflammatory effects of NSAIDs, PG inhibition in the CNS also contributes to the analgesia produced by these drugs. The inequality between the antiinflammatory and the analgesic potencies is seemingly a reflection of the central effects of each NSAID. Presumably, ns-NSAIDs inhibit PG synthesis by blocking all COX isozymes, whereas COX2Is selectively exercise their main effect on COX-2.

Whereas most ns-NSAIDs are reversible COX inhibitors, aspirin irreversibly acetylates and blocks COX. This has significant clinical implications on the work of TX_2 produced by platelet COX. Selectivity for COX-1 versus COX-2 is uneven among older NSAIDs; however, COXIBs are highly selective inhibitors of COX-2, and they do not influence platelet function at their standard doses. Table 21–5 compares each NSAID COX-1 to COX-2 selectivity.[86] As listed, COX selectivity is based on the result of whole blood assays, rather than cellular assays. When more than one whole blood assay is available, the result of the one that agrees with cellular assays or clinical experience, or both, is chosen. In testing using human whole blood, aspirin, indomethacin, piroxicam, and sulindac were rather effective in inhibiting COX-1, whereas ibuprofen and meclofenamic acid inhibited the two isozymes nearly evenly. The therapeutic effectiveness of COXIBs amounts to that of ns-NSAIDs, whereas GI damage may decrease. In contrast, COX2Is might upsurge the incidence of edema, hypertension, and other cardiovascular events.

Although it was originally thought that NSAIDs have minimal inhibitory effect on LOX pathway of AA metabolism, there is existing evidence of reduced LT production by certain NSAIDs, such as diclofenac and indomethacin.[181,182] On the other hand, it is theorized that NSAIDs may potentiate LT formation by rechanneling their substrate from the cyclooxygenase cascade. This might provide a partial explanation for the asthmatic and hypersensitivity reactions seen following the use of NSAIDs.[184]

Another possible NSAID mechanism of action is superoxide radical production and superoxide scavenging, including inhibition of chemotaxis, down-regulation of IL-1 production, and decreased production of free radicals and superoxide, which are produced by neutrophils and macrophages and may contribute to tissue damage.

As previously mentioned, other mechanisms of action include:

1. Antinociception by inhibiting both inflammation-induced expression and activity of ASICs.[69,71]
2. Individual NSAIDs include inhibition of neutrophils activation by inflammatory mediators, such as C5-derived peptides and LTB_4.[184]
3. Interference with G-protein–mediated signal transduction on the cellular level.[185,186]
4. Interference with calcium-mediated intracellular events.[187]
5. Inhibition of cytokines production and cartilage metabolism.[188]
6. Interference with the action of glutamate and substance P in the central nervous system when cyclooxygenase is inhibited.[189]

In the decades before the discovery of COX-2's role in central sensitization, scattered but valid evidence suggested other potential central antinociceptive mechanisms for traditional NSAIDs.[190] These included opioid-like mechanisms,[190,191] activation of descending serotonin pathways,[190,192] and reducing NMDA-induced messenger RNA.[190,192] Enthusiasm for these mechanisms has faded with the extensive work on developing newer generations of highly selective COX2Is. The recent revelations of the undesired link between COX-2 inhibition and cardiovascular events may bring these abandoned theories back to the stage.

Studies have shown that salicylates, ibuprofen, flurbiprofen, sulindac, and perhaps other ns-NSAIDs, but not COXIBs, inhibit the expression of factor NF-κB.[193] NF-κB is also inhibited by glucocorticoids and antioxidants.[66] Yet, salicylates themselves act as antioxidants by trapping hydroxyl radicals, the most damaging reactive oxygen species.[194] Recently, it has been shown that salicylates inhibit molecular transcription mediated by the nuclear factor of activated T cells (NFAT),[195] and interfere with intracellular signaling mechanisms such as kinases, including the mitogen-activated protein-kinases (MAPK) cascade.[193,194] These last three actions are achieved via a much more COX-independent molecular complex event and, thus far, it appears that they are not shared by all NSAIDs. To the contrary, celecoxib, and perhaps other COXIBs, activates NF-κB, a mechanism that could explain the anticarcinogenic quality of celecoxib in colon cancer.[193] Aspirin and other salicylates exert antiinflammatory effects by inducing the release of large quantities of adenosine into the extracellular fluid by uncoupling intracellular oxidative phosphorylation.[194]

Studies indicate that ibuprofen, indomethacin, and flurbiprofen, independent of COX inhibition, lower A^β, a pathologic hallmark of AD,[196,197] but neither naproxen nor aspirin lower A^β, yet both have protective effects against AD.

Finally, aspirin inhibits endogenous AA derivative anti-inflammatory lipoxins, which are called ATLs and resolvins.[137,140,144,145,194]

Pharmacodynamics

To varying degrees, all NSAIDs have analgesic, anti-inflammatory, and antipyretic properties. NSAIDs do not reduce normal body temperature or elevated temperatures in heat stroke, which is caused by hypothalamic malfunction.[4] All NSAIDs (except COX2Is and the non-acetylated salicylates) inhibit platelet aggregation. Through their various mechanisms, NSAIDs decrease the sensitivity of blood vessels to bradykinin and histamine, affect lymphokine production from T lymphocytes, and reverse vasodilation. NSAIDs are gastric irritants, though the newer NSAIDs appear to exhibit less gastric cytotoxicity when compared with aspirin. Nephrotoxicity has been observed for all NSAIDs for which extensive experience has been reported, and hepatotoxicity can also occur with any NSAID. PGs are necessary for the renal excretion of several electrolytes, toxins, and drug metabolites. By inhibiting the synthesis of PGs, NSAIDs decrease the renal clearance of these materials. NSAIDs show a direct dose response relationship in terms of desired effects and both gastrointestinal and renal adverse effects.[198-200] NSAIDs' high affinity for plasma proteins disposes them to displace other drugs from binding sites. This clinically could mean increasing the other drugs pharmacologic effect as in the case of warfarin and naproxen, ibuprofen, and other NSAIDs.[201]

NSAID Statistics

NSAIDs are the most commonly used drugs around the world. In the United States, four of the drugs in this category are available OTC (Table 21–8). In the mid-1980s, it was evident that more than 15 million Americans use these agents on a daily basis for pain relief.[202] Currently, approximately 111.4 million prescriptions for NSAIDs are filled in the United States annually—at a cost of $4.8 billion[203] in comparison with 60 million NSAIDs prescriptions that were written annually in 1990s.[204] In Canada, where health care is nationalized, it is estimated that one Canadian dollar is added to the cost for each patient using NSAIDs while on the medication.[205] The global market for COX-2 inhibitors surpassed $6 billion in sales in 2002.[206] In 2004, worldwide sales of celecoxib and valdecoxib approximated $3.3 and $1.3 billion respectively.[207] Between 1999, when Vioxx was launched,

and 2004 when it was removed from the market, an estimated 20 million Americans had used the drug.[208] This is about 7% of the U.S. population. Most reports showed that COX2Is were prescribed to patients who were not in the GI risk categories.

There is an estimated 16,500 NSAID-related deaths and about 75,000 NSAID-complication admissions annually in the United States.[4] Ten years ago, the estimated annual NSAID-gastric ulceration was around 12,000 in the United Kingdom, resulting in 1200 deaths annually.[209] NSAID-gastroenteropathy causes a large economic burden. Medicaid data from the U.S. federal government for 1981 to 1983 showed that 31% of the total cost of care for patients with an arthritic diagnosis was for management of GI adverse events.[210] GI complications attributed to NSAIDs increase the bill of a single patient in Canada by 70% compared with a standard patient.[205]

Therapeutic Benefits

NSAIDs, in general, have three common therapeutic effects: analgesic, antipyretic, and antiinflammatory. Other applications for individual NSAIDs, such as aspirin, include anticoagulation prophylaxis during an ongoing heart attack. All these practices can be relevant to patients with a malignant disease or to cancer survivors. The chapter briefly discusses all these usages and discusses in detail the analgesic aspect.

Analgesic Use

When employed as analgesics, NSAIDs are effective for the treatment of pain with low-to-moderate intensity. Although their maximal effects are much lower than opioids, they lack the undesired opioid effects on the CNS, such as respiratory depression, constipation, and the potential of developing physical dependence. Unlike opioids, NSAIDs do not alter the perception of sensory modalities except for pain. Acute postoperative pain or pain arising from an inflammatory process is particularly well controlled by NSAIDs, whereas visceral pain is only partially relieved (Table 21–9).

NSAID Efficacy in Cancer Pain

The role of NSAIDs in cancer pain has been well established for the treatment of mild pain and in association with opioids in the treatment of moderate-to-severe pain. The use of NSAIDs reduces the need for an opioid dose escalation or allows the use of lower doses. Their use is associated with a more intense gastric discomfort but results in less opioid-related constipation. The eventual additive cost for NSAIDs therapy is negligible, especially in patients taking high doses of morphine.[211]

TABLE 21–8   Pros and Cons of NSAIDs and Acetaminophen

Category	Drugs			
	Aspirin	*ns-NSAIDs*	*COX2Is*	*Acetaminophen*
Price[a]	Cheap	Cheap to inexpensive	Expensive	Cheap
Dispencity[b]	OTC/Script	Script only (except for ibuprofen and ketoprofen)	Script only	OTC/Script
Preparations[b]				
Generic formula?	Yes	Yes	No	Yes
Combination with other analgesics?	Yes	Only ibuprofen	No	Yes
Enteric-coated formula?	Yes	Only diclofenac and naproxen[c]	No	Yes
Extended time-release formula?	Yes	Only etodolac, indomethacin, ketoprofen and naproxen[d]	No	Yes
Combination with nonanalgesics?	Yes	Some yes		Yes
Parenteral formula?	No	Only ketorolac	Only parecoxib	No
Duration of action[e]	Short acting	Short acting	Long acting	Short acting
Medical experience[f]	Extensive	Broad	Growing	Extensive
Systemic toxicity				
Gastric[a]	Probable	Unlikely to probable[g]	Unlikely	Unusual
Hepatic[h]	Unlikely	Unlikely	Unlikely	Possible
Renal[a]	Possible	Possible	Possible	Unlikely
Cardiac[i]	Unusual	Unusual	Possible	Unusual
Coagulopathic	Blood thinning—irreversible effect[j]	Blood thinning—reversible effect	No effect	No effect

COX2I, cyclooxygenase 2 inhibitors; *ns-NSAIDs*, nonspecific nonsteroidal anti-inflammatory drugs; *OTC/Script*, available over the counter or by prescription; *Script only*, available only by prescription.

[a]For other than aspirin: Compared with aspirin.
[b]In the United States market.
[c]In Canada, ketoprofen is available in enteric-coated tablets.
[d]In Canada, also diclofenac, flurbiprofen and tiaprofenic acid are available in extended-release formula, but not etodolac.
[e]In standardized doses and commercial formulas.
[f]Compared to valdecoxib.
[g]Check text for details.
[h]For other than acetaminophen: Compared with acetaminophen toxic doses.
[i]For other than rofecoxib: Compared with rofecoxib.
[j]This is also used therapeutically for the prevention of cardiovascular occlusive diseases.

According to a meta-analysis report of 25 studies of NSAIDs for treatment of cancer pain published in 1994,[19] it can be concluded that an NSAID alone can be effective to ease mild cancer pain. For more intense pain, notably bone pain, an NSAID can enhance the relief provided by an opioid. The studies probing the use of a single-dose NSAID found superior analgesia than with placebo, reaching the effect of an intramuscular injection of 5 to 10 mg morphine. Pain scores between aspirin and three other NSAIDs did not differ. NSAIDs were 1.5 to 2 times more beneficial than placebo, but no convincing dose–response relationship was found for these drugs. This study also confirmed a **ceiling analgesic effect** with NSAIDs.[19] Since then the number of randomized, controlled trials evaluating analgesic drugs for cancer pain relief remains small. Direct interclass comparisons of efficacy are possible between opioids and NSAIDs. The included trials do not differentiate the relative efficacy of these two types of agents administered through various routes to patients with mild, moderate, or severe cancer pain. Studies have demonstrated an opioid dose-sparing effect from coadministration of an NSAID but no consistent reduction in side effects from coadministration.[212] These findings should not discourage clinicians from using NSAIDs for postoperative analgesia, but it should prompt them to monitor the adverse effects of both types of agents, if used concurrently, and address these side effects promptly.[213]

TABLE 21–9   Comparison of Opioids and NSAIDs

	Opioids	NSAIDs
Mechanism	Mainly central	Mainly peripheral
Availability	Controlled substances	Noncontrolled/ Some available OTC
Therapeutic ceiling	No	Yes
Tolerance	Yes	No
Addiction	Possible	Not possible
GI side effects 　N/V 　Constipation 　Gastric ulceration 　GI bleeding	 More frequent Frequent No No	 Less frequent No Possible Possible
Respiratory side effects	Depression	Infrequently asthma
Pupillary changes	Yes	No
Cognitive impairment	Yes	No
Depressive sensory effects (other than pain)	Yes	No

NSAIDs, nonsteroidal anti-inflammatory drugs; *OTC*, over the counter; *GI*, gastrointestinal; *N/V*, nausea and vomiting.

Placebo controls, particularly in analgesic trials, are valuable to prevent overestimation of treatment effects; yet, for ethical reasons such controls are rare in cancer pain trials. The heterogeneity of existing trials precludes meta-analyses to address most sub-questions. Some trials comparing the efficacy of NSAIDs with "weak" opioids (i.e., opioids commonly prescribed for mild to mild-moderate pain) reveal no difference in analgesic efficacy between these two classes of agents, even when the latter are coadministered with the same NSAID tested in the former arm.[212] Yet, when comparing NSAIDs with acetaminophen or opioids, regardless of the opioid potency, NSAIDs have continually shown superior quality of analgesia in cancer patients.[214]

Researchers demonstrated that mechanical hyperalgesia associated with intratibial injection of cancer cells was attenuated by the repeated administration of lumiracoxib, a novel COX2I.[215] A similar reduction in mechanical hyperalgesia, as determined by measuring the weight-bearing threshold, was observed following administration of valdecoxib. The reduction in weight bearing in this model is reminiscent of hyperalgesia in cancer patients, and its reversal by lumiracoxib and valdecoxib could therefore be predictive of clinical efficacy.[215]

NSAIDs are the first line of therapy in malignant bone pain and should be used in any cancer pain if no contraindication exists as recommended by the WHO Analgesic Ladder.[30] Cancer sufferers or survivors may have pain issues not related to cancer and could benefit from NSAIDs as in arthritic pain or myofascial pain.

The Role of NSAIDs in Postoperative Analgesia

Cancer patients undergo all types of operative diagnostic, prognostic, and therapeutic procedures. Many of those patients could be suffering from some type of pain and already on a short- or long-term pain treatment regimen. Either way, postoperative analgesic requirements must be addressed efficiently.[38] Independently, NSAIDs provide adequate analgesia for mild-to-moderate pain, although some recent data suggest that NSAIDs may be more effective as analgesics than previously recognized. Thus, for an anticipated mild-to-moderate postoperative pain, an NSAID, if not contraindicated, is very effective. When used as an adjunct to opioids, NSAIDs **may** improve postoperative analgesia, reduce opioid requirements, facilitate resumption of gastrointestinal function, reduce nausea, decrease respiratory depression, and improve patient satisfaction.[216] Decreased hemostasis, renal dysfunction, gastrointestinal hemorrhage, and adverse effects on bone healing are of specific concern when an NSAID is used perioperatively. Patients with hypovolemia, abnormal renal function, or serum electrolytes imbalance may be at higher risk for developing NSAID-induced renal dysfunction.[216] The negative effect on platelets aggregation makes NSAIDs an undesirable analgesic option to avoid postoperative bleeding in certain circumstances (e.g., in existing coagulopathy). However, NSAIDs are probably safe postoperatively if there is no concomitant factor to promote bleeding.

A large observational study of perioperative ketorolac did not demonstrate any significant increase in bleeding at the operative site.[217] In general, the risk of adverse events with ketorolac is increased with high doses, prolonged use (over 5 days), and in vulnerable patients such as the elderly or active cancer patients undergoing aggressive chemotherapy.[218] Current recommended dosing for postoperative analgesia is 10 to 30 mg per injection with daily maximum of 90 mg (60 mg for greater than 65 years) up to five days.[218] Our practice at Roswell Park Cancer Institute is to administer ketorolac, if not contraindicated, to all patients whose preoperative serum creatinine level is less than 1 mg/dL, parenterally for postoperative in-patients, 30 mg every 8 hours, up to seven doses. Dose is usually reduced by 50% for elderly patients.

A recent report from Italy compared the analgesic efficacy of combined tramadol-ketorolac-ranitidine-ondansetron via IV continuous infusion with local anesthetic (ropivacaine)-opioid (fentanyl) epidural continuous infusion for postpulmonary thoracic surgery in two patient-randomized groups. They found almost equally sufficient analgesic results for both techniques, with negligible side effects for both (excluding itching) observed in some patients who received the epidural infusion, but not the systemic infusion.[219] The analgesia achieved for breakthrough pain was slightly faster with the epidural technique. However, those patients who received the epidural infusion showed less acceptance of this technique compared with the other group.[219] Despite the limitation of this study, it is still in line with common clinical observation and brings an insight for future exploration of the continuous, systemic use of nonopioids analgesic for postoperative pain management.

A Spanish double-blind, randomized trial found that when ketorolac and tramadol are given separately every 6 hours intravenously after abdominal surgery, tramadol has superior pain relief over ketorolac; however, there is also an increased incidence of severe nausea or vomiting.[220] The observation that postoperative systemic administration of NSAIDs causes less nausea and vomiting than tramadol has been cited in other studies.[221] In the United States, tramadol is yet to be approved for parenteral use, and ketorolac is the only NSAID approved for parenteral administration. Ketoprofen and metamizol are available in other countries in parenteral formulation and seem to offer effective postoperative analgesia with a tolerable GI profile.[222] Furthermore, ketorolac and metamizol tend to potentiate the antinociceptive effects of morphine,[223,224] the most common opioid used postoperatively. Parecoxib, a pro-drug of valdecoxib that was licensed in Europe and Canada for perioperative parenteral analgesia, was a promising alternative. However, the recent withdrawal of valdecoxib from the international market has reduced, if not eliminated, the chance of introducing this drug, and perhaps other COXIBs, in the United States. In contrast, current research is revealing more than we knew before about the involvement of COX-1 in perioperative nociceptive events on the molecular level. The new findings suggest that preoperative administration of specific COX-1 inhibitors directly to the CNS may be more useful to treat postoperative pain.[225] What is surprising is the call of some authors to abandon the whole group of NSAIDs for perioperative pain management and solely use opioids in light of these developments.[226]

In the outpatient surgery setting, oral NSAIDs can be prescribed for minor procedures or surgeries, such as dental extraction or bone marrow biopsy. NSAIDs with rapidly dissolving formulas, such as naproxen, diclofenac, and ketorolac, may be preferred for postoperative breakthrough pain. NSAIDs combined with mild or short-acting opioids present a superior alternative for the management of outpatient or short-stay postoperative pain.[214] In the U.S. market, only aspirin, ibuprofen, and ketoprofen are available with an opioid in one combination (Table 21–10).

The Role of NSAIDs in Preemptive Analgesia

Despite supporting studies in laboratory animals, rising interest in the concept and practice of preemptive analgesia faded because of contradictory clinical data.[226] For NSAIDs, few trials, including one that used acetaminophen to explore the role of these agents in preemptive analgesia for oral surgery, demonstrated measurable differences between the same doses given preoperatively and postoperatively.

In 2002, an extensive meta-analysis concluded that there was a lack of evidence for preemptive treatment with NSAIDs, IV opioids, IV ketamine, peripheral local anesthetics, and caudal analgesia.[227] However, in the same year, a study of rofecoxib (50 mg) taken 1 hour before ambulatory arthroscopic knee surgery was compared with the same dose following surgery in a placebo-controlled study. The researchers found that the patients who took rofecoxib 1 hour before surgery had a longer duration of pain relief, decreased opioid use, and lower pain scores compared with the same dose taken after surgery.[228] This finding, and in light of newer reports of the suppressive action of COXIBs to central sensitization to nociception, ignited that abandoned enthusiasm for preemptive analgesia with COX2Is, particularly with rofecoxib. The introduction in Europe of parecoxib with indication of pre- and postoperative analgesia enhanced the passion to use COXIBs preemptively. The withdrawal of rofecoxib and valdecoxib from the markets almost killed this practice. The withdrawal of valdecoxib hopefully will not delay the pharmaceutical makers of parecoxib from pursuing an FDA approval for a limited indication of strict perioperative use of no more than a preauthorized number of injections within a certain period of time. Conversely, the introduction of a limited indication would discourage off-label use of the drug.

TABLE 21–10   NSAID-Opioid Commercial Drug Combinations

Combination	Trade Name	Strength mg	Dose by pill PRN (max #/d)	Indication	Comments
Aspirin + caffeine + dihydrocodeine	Synalgos	356.4+30+16	1–2 q4 hr	Moderate to moderate severe pain	Good for postoperative and breakthrough pain. Also, headaches and migraine attacks
Aspirin + carisoprodol + codeine	Soma Compound w/codeine	325+200+16	1–2 TID-QID (6)	Painful muscle spasm	Good for postoperative and breakthrough pain, especially pain associated w/spasm
Aspirin + codeine	Empirin w/codeine #3 Empirin w/codeine #4	325+30 325+60	1–2 q4 hr 1 q4 hr	Mild to moderate pain	Good for postoperative and breakthrough pain
Aspirin + hydrocodone	LortabASA	500+5	1 q4 hr	Moderate severe acute pain	Good for postoperative and breakthrough pain. No longer available in the United States
Aspirin + oxycodone	Percodan-Demi Percodan	325+2.25 325+4.5	1 q6 hr	Moderate pain	Good for postoperative and breakthrough pain
Ibuprofen + oxycodone	Combunox	400+5	1 daily–QID	Moderate pain	Good for postoperative and breakthrough pain
Ketoprofen + hydrocodone	Vicoprofen Darvon Compound -65	200+7.5 389+32.4+65	1 q4–6 hr (5)	Acute pain	Good for postoperative and breakthrough pain

Leaders in pain management feel that COXIBs are a vanishing class of drugs.[229] In fact, these beliefs arise from the fact that the decision to keep or remove a medication from the market is a corporate, not a clinical, one. However, limited studies have shown that celecoxib and ibuprofen (IV or PO) exert preemptive qualities, which, if methodologically probed, could rekindle the practitioners' interest in NSAIDs use for preemptive analgesia.[230-232] Therefore, preemptive analgesia continues to have promise for the effective treatment of postoperative pain. Evaluation of the true importance of preemptive analgesia will have to await further research with new, more comprehensive approaches.[226]

NSAIDs as Analgesic for Pediatric Cancer Patients

The WHO analgesic guidelines are appropriate to use in the treatment of children with cancer pain. However, the clinician must be vigilant to the fact that pediatric pain in general is a concealed problem. The age and developmental level of the child, emotional factors, stage of the disease, and parental influence are some of the many factors that give rise to this predicament. It is easy to underdose or overdose various analgesics in children with cancer if a careful clinical evaluation is not conducted.

As in adults, opioids remain the first choice for the management of severe pain. NSAIDs as analgesics can be used at any level of pain with young patients, providing no contraindication exists. Specific adverse reactions arise in children with cancer from the administration of NSAIDs. For example, frequent NSAID suppository usage can result in mucous membrane injury of the rectum and the descending colon, which in turn may lead to a fatal disorder in severely ill pediatric cancer patients.[233] Other unusual side effects of NSAIDs, like platelet dysfunction and Stevens-Johnson syndrome, could become exacerbated in children who are immunocompromised either from the cancer itself or because of the many variations of cancer treatment (e.g., children receiving bone marrow transplant therapy). Ibuprofen is available as a syrup, which makes it a first choice medication in most children. In children, salicylates should be avoided unless there is no other choice to avoid the risk of Reye's syndrome. As for COX2Is, there are only a few limited studies of their pediatric use,[234] and their role in pediatric cancer pain is certainly unidentified.

NSAIDs as Analgesic for Geriatric Cancer Patients

The elderly, in general, are susceptible to the harmful effects from NSAIDs. Those elderly patients taking NSAIDs should be monitored attentively for GI bleeding, declining renal function, congestive heart failure, or edema. In patients older than 65 years, NSAIDs should be considered only if opioid reduction is desired and other nonopioid or adjuvant analgesics are not satisfactory. Many of the elderly with cancer pain suffer from preexisting arthritic pain. If acetaminophen is inadequate, prescribing ibuprofen, meloxicam, or nabumetone with gastroprotective prophylaxis, such as PPIs, is a good choice. Ibuprofen *may need* to be avoided if the patient is already on cardioprophylactic low-dose aspirin. Choline magnesium trisalicylate and salsalate cause minimal GI toxicity and have no effect on platelet function, despite their potent anti-inflammatory effect.[21] Choline magnesium trisalicylate is available as a syrup, which makes it popular in a palliative care setting. Diclofenac is another good choice and it is available combined with misoprostol in one tablet (Arthrotec). The use of celecoxib should be reserved for those elderly who have no cardiac risk, good kidney function, at least an additional GI risk factor, and are not using low-dose aspirin daily.[172,173] Following clinical evaluation, careful consideration of the costs of these agents before choosing one over another is effective, as well as safe, in the elderly population. This is particularly important when resources are limited, such as in hospice settings. Because many of the elderly are usually on antihypertensive therapy, regular monitoring of blood pressure is a necessity because all NSAIDs cause sodium retention, enhance vasoconstrictor responses to pressor hormones, and antagonize the effects of antihypertensive agents, with the possible exception of calcium channel blockers.[235]

NSAIDs as Analgesic in Headaches and Migraine

NSAIDs are valuable for both prophylaxis and relief of migraine, as well as treatment of various types of headaches.[236,237] Naproxen has been used effectively for prophylaxis of migraine; however, all NSAIDs show high prophylactic efficacy comparable to naproxen. Ketorolac (parenterally or orally) is excellent in treating acute migraine attacks.[238] The addition of an antiemetic seems to enhance the effect of any analgesic in the treatment of migraine attacks.[237,238]

Topical NSAIDs

Topical NSAIDs for pain relief remain one of the more controversial subjects in analgesia practice. Although not approved in the United States, in some parts of the world their use is regarded as sensible, and is supported by evidence for this mode of delivery. In other parts of the world, NSAIDs are regarded as little more than placebo, with any effect caused by the application of the salve. A reliable placebo-controlled study from Britain

demonstrated that the preemptive application of topical ibuprofen 5% cream, 2 hours before elective cardioversion reduced pain and inflammation. The study recommended considering the use of prophylactic application of topical ibuprofen as routine treatment for chest wall pain resulting from elective cardioversion.[239]

The experience with topical NSAIDs in cancer patients is limited to the treatment of coexisting joint aches from associated rheumatoid arthritis or osteoarthritis, and perhaps perioperatively for those patients undergoing minor procedures (e.g., bone marrow biopsy or interventional pain management procedures).

Antipyretic Use

It is thought that NSAIDs and acetaminophen largely, but not exclusively, exhibit their antipyretic activity via the blockage of PG synthesis with COX. Besides acetaminophen, aspirin and ibuprofen are the most common NSAIDs used for the sole purpose of reducing fever. Aspirin's adult dose for fever indication is 325 to 650 mg PO q4 hours PRN, and ibuprofen's adult dose for fever indication is 200–400 PO q4 hours PRN. As for children, analgesic doses apply (check Table 21–5).

Anti-inflammatory Use

NSAIDs are the first line of therapy and subsequent maintenance treatment in many chronic inflammatory diseases. Examples include chronic musculoskeletal conditions, rheumatic fever, pericarditis, irritable bowel syndrome, most arthritic conditions, such as osteoarthritis, rheumatoid arthritis, juvenile idiopathic arthritis, ankylosing spondylitis, and the other autoimmune types of arthritis. Although, in this capacity, NSAIDs are used for their potential to reduce or terminate the inflammatory process and accordingly the advancement of the disease, the high doses of NSAIDs that could be given in these conditions will exert sufficient analgesic effects, as well as increase the possibility of adverse effects.

In rheumatoid arthritis, NSAIDs offer mainly symptomatic relief by reducing inflammation and subsequent pain, as well as preserving joint function, but they have little effect on the progression of bone and cartilage destruction. Topical NSAIDs might offer analgesic benefits when applied to aching joints, although there is not enough evidence to make a definitive statement in favor of this application.

Aspirin Use for Thromboprophylaxis Therapy

Platelets, platelet products, and clotting factors participate in the occurrence of occlusive vascular events. By irreversibly inhibiting platelet-dependent COX activity, aspirin decreases its ability to aggregate for the life of the platelet, and therefore aspirin is used for the prophylaxis and treatment of intra-arterial thrombosis that may cause or complicate MI, thrombotic stroke, and peripheral vascular disease. A small daily dose (81 to 162 mg) of aspirin is used for the prevention of MI and thrombotic stroke.[240] Aspirin decreases the incidence of transient ischemic attacks, unstable angina, coronary artery thrombosis with MI, and thrombosis after coronary artery bypass grafting.[86] Failure to suppress TX generation by aspirin (a phenomenon known as *aspirin resistance*) has been documented. Patients who are relatively resistant to the effects of aspirin and require thromboprophylaxis therapy may benefit from additional antiplatelet therapies.[241] A recent report suggests that a 100 mg (or less) daily dose of aspirin, which may have lower side effects, is associated with a higher incidence of aspirin resistance in patients with coronary artery disease. Prospective randomized studies are warranted to elucidate the optimal aspirin dosage for preventing ischemic complications of atherothrombotic disease.[242]

Ibuprofen has been assumed to negate the clinical benefit of aspirin in cardiovascular disease.[243-245] Although this phenomenon was not observed with diclofenac,[246] it still raised concerns that the simultaneous use of low-dose aspirin and long-term use of other ns-NSAIDs could reduce the cardioprotective effect of aspirin.[229] Based upon the *limited* evidence available, ibuprofen may have a clinically relevant, unfavorable interaction. The mechanism of this interference is not clear yet; however, it is thought to be caused by receptor-binding competition from the therapeutically dosed ibuprofen against the low-dosed aspirin. Under these circumstances, it is rational to avoid chronic ibuprofen administration in patients using low-dose aspirin for cardiovascular protection and perhaps select another NSAID if long-term therapy with these agents is needed.[229]

In 2004, one study could not demonstrate an increased risk of MI among patients simultaneously consuming aspirin and ibuprofen compared with aspirin alone,[247] suggesting that the cardiac events seen in the earlier studies could be independent from the effect of ibuprofen. Additionally, a large retrospective case-controlled analysis from Switzerland and Britain that enlisted 8688 patients with a new onset of acute MI and almost 34,000 control subjects examined the concurrent use of ibuprofen, naproxen, or diclofenac with aspirin in 650 patients and 2339 control subjects and concluded that no existing evidence for a reduced cardioprotective effect of aspirin with concomitant NSAID use existed.[248] For the time being and until a clear consensus emerges, avoiding ns-NSAIDs other than ibuprofen is not necessary. Acetaminophen can also be a reasonable alternative in these situations.

Obstetric and Gynecologic Therapeutic Uses

Benefiting from its inhibition of PG synthesis, indomethacin is used by obstetricians to prolong gestation or suppress uterine contraction in preterm labor. Indomethacin and sulindac are used in the treatment of polyhydromnias. Indomethacin is administered to newborns that have patent ductus arteriosus to facilitate closure and avoid surgical intervention. NSAIDs, especially mefenamic acid, are used in the treatment of dysmenorrhea.

Treatment of Bartter Syndrome

Bartter syndrome is a triad of hypokalemia, hyperreninemia, and hyperaldosteronism. Pathologically it is characterized by juxtaglomerular hyperplasia, normal blood pressure, and resistance to the pressor effect of angiotensin II. Excessive production of renal PGs has been implicated in the pathogenesis of some of the metabolic abnormalities in this syndrome, and NSAIDs, via their COX inhibitory effects, have been found to be useful in the treatment of this disorder.

Potential Anticarcinogenic Use

NSAIDs have been shown to reduce cancer incidence and evoke tumor regression in the GI tract.[40,84] The mechanism is multifactorial, but the induction of apoptosis is essential for these drugs to cause tumor regression and to prevent tumor growth.[40,84] Apoptosis induction by NSAIDs in tumors of the GI tract, and perhaps elsewhere, is largely unknown.[84] One hypothesized explanation of NSAIDs' anticarcinogenic effect is their inhibition of PG-induced angiogenesis,[40,249] which is the same theory for their negative effects on gastric ulceration healing. NSAIDs might block tumor progression by inhibiting fibroblast hyaluronic acid and could lead to a novel indication of minimizing or stopping metastasis of existing carcinomas.[250] The continuous use of ns-NSAID is not only associated with decreased colonic adenoma incidence but also with a lower colorectal cancer incidence and cancer-associated mortality.[251] In a randomized trial of aspirin for the prevention of colorectal adenomas, low-dose aspirin had a moderate chemopreventive effect on adenomas in the large bowel, but no dose–response relationship was found. The lowest dose (81 mg/day) was more effective than the highest dose (325 mg/day).[252] If ns-NSAIDs are to be used in cancer prevention, this has to be weighed against their adverse effects, principally gastroenteropathy.

Potential Use in Alzheimer's Disease Prevention

NSAIDs seem to be more effective in *preventing* than in *treating* AD. Epidemiologic studies suggest that NSAIDs can delay the onset and slow the progression of Alzheimer's disease.[40,84,86,155,196] Further understanding of the mechanism involved in the NSAID-induced interdiction of AD may provide new therapeutic possibilities for diseases involving oxidative stress.[84,196]

Adverse Effects

All NSAIDs (including COX2Is) manifest some common side effects. The difference is in the frequency of occurrence. This forms the basis of the art of choosing an NSAID for therapy. Most adverse events are preventable, a fact that raises hope for improved future application of these drugs if proper education of NSAID use is implemented.[253]

Common Side Effects

The most common side effects include nonspecific complaints such as headache, drowsiness, indigestion (stomach upset), easy bruising, high blood pressure, and fluid retention. Less common side effects are gastritis and heartburn. These symptoms are usually mild and transient, but if severe, the medicine may need to be stopped, and symptomatic treatment should be applied.

Serious Side Effects

Gastrointestinal Toxicity

All NSAIDs can cause mucosal damage of the GI tract. Because cytoprotective PGs are produced by COX-1, NSAIDs higher in selectivity to COX-2 make them gentler on the GI tract. Long-term use of ns-NSAIDs carries three times greater relative risk for serious adverse GI events. The ns-NSAIDs differ noticeably in their propensity to produce GI erosions. One in five chronic ns-NSAIDs users will have gastric damage.[254] Two distinct mechanisms are involved in gastropathy caused by these drugs. Orally administered NSAIDs allow back diffusion of acid into the gastric mucosa and induce tissue damage and local irritation. On the other hand, parenteral administration may also cause damage and bleeding, correlated with inhibition of the biosynthesis of gastric PGs, especially PGE_1 and PGE_2, which serve as cytoprotective agents in the gastric mucosa, as discussed previously. The use of COX2Is in the CLASS and VIGOR studies resulted in less GI mucosal damage compared to ns-NSAIDs.[170,172] NSAID enteropathy is often unnoticed until the occurrence of small or large bowel ulceration, intestinal strictures, or perforations.[255] A comprehensive list of NSAID-GI toxicities is available in Table 21–11.

One way to minimize NSAIDs' gastric toxicity is the use of enteric-coated preparations that are designed to resist disintegration in the stomach and dissolve in the more neutral-to-alkaline environment of the duodenum. Clinical practice has shown that enteric-coated

aspirin may reduce erosions on endoscopy, but it does not protect against clinically relevant GI bleeding. This finding is not surprising, because injury that is severe enough to induce bleeding is thought to reflect the systemic rather than the topical effects of NSAIDs.[255] Economic analyses indicate that NSAID-associated GI side effects markedly increase health care costs. Medications given to prevent GI events or to treat dyspepsia may represent the greatest cost, adding as much as 31% to the cost of the NSAID therapy. Although the infrequent, expensive hospitalizations for GI complications can also contribute to the higher cost of NSAID therapy.[203]

Risk factors for clinical NSAIDs gastroenteropathy include: a history of ulcers or GI complications, advanced age (over 65), concomitant anticoagulation therapy, concurrent corticosteroid use, long duration of NSAID therapy, high-dose NSAIDs or multiple NSAIDs use (including an NSAID plus low-dose aspirin).[153,203] Concurrent illness (e.g., severe rheumatoid arthritis, heart disease) has also been reported to increase the risk of GI events.

Although the effect of H. pylori on NSAID-induced ulcers and ulcer complications is controversial, many specialists believe that H. pylori infection does not potentiate the risk of NSAID-associated ulcer or ulcer complications.[203] Moreover, some believe that, paradoxically, H. pylori infection promotes gastric, but not duodenal, ulcer healing in patients on NSAIDs therapy.[257] In Asia, physicians believe that the data presented by the earlier group are invalid. They surmise that the protective effect of H. pylori in long-term NSAID users reported in earlier group studies was related to weeding out of susceptible patients who were intolerant to NSAIDs.[258] The latter group believes that there is no convincing evidence that eradication of H. pylori has any clinically important adverse effect on the healing and prevention of ulcers in NSAID users.[258] Moreover, the presence of H. pylori infection increases the risk of upper gastrointestinal complications in NSAIDs users by two- to fourfold suggesting that all patients requiring regular NSAIDs therapy be tested for H. pylori, and if positive, considered for eradication therapy before the administration of chronic therapy with NSAIDs. H. pylori eradication is probably desirable in patients who are able to stop taking NSAIDs entirely but may be useless or harmful in those who have to continue, particularly if they have had gastric ulcers. Moreover, acid suppression is more effective in the healing and prevention of ulcers in patients who are H. pylori positive.[257]

The most agreeable stand on H. pylori versus NSAIDs, nowadays, is to implement H. pylori eradication for patients that will undergo prolonged NSAID treatment (e.g., low-dose aspirin) who happen to be H. pylori positive; have another GI risk factor, such as dyspepsia

TABLE 21–11   Summary of NSAID-Related Gastrointestinal Problems

1. Risk Factors for NSAID-Induced Ulcers and Upper Gastrointestinal Complications

		Estimated Increased Risk
Established	Prior clinical GI event (ulcer or complication)	2.5–4×
	Advanced age (over 65 years)	2–3.5×
	Concomitant anticoagulation therapy	3×
	Concurrent corticosteroid use	2×
	High-dose NSAID or multiple NSAIDs use	2–4× (compared to low-dose aspirin alone)
	Major comorbidity (e.g., severe rheumatoid arthritis, heart disease)	
Probable	Long-term NSAID use	
	Coexisting *H. pylori* infection	
	Dyspepsia caused by an NSAID	
Possible	Cigarette smoking	
	Alcohol consumption	

2. Serious Gastrointestinal Complications Associated with NSAID Use
Bleeding
Perforation
Obstruction
Recurrent ulceration

3. Possible Mechanisms of NSAID-Induced Gastropathy

Topical   Reverse H^+ diffusion → gastric mucosa → tissue damage → local irritation → erosions → gastritis

Systemic

4. Pharmacologic Agents for Prophylaxis and Treatment of NSAID Gastroenteropathy

Group	Drug		Prophylaxis	Treatment
	Generic name	*Brand name*		
Proton pump inhibitors (PPI)	Omeprazole	Prilosec	20–40 mg daily	20–40 mg daily
	Lansoprazole	PrevAcid	15–30 mg daily	30 mg daily (available IV)
	Rabeprazole	AcipHex	20 mg daily	20 mg daily
	Pantoprazole	Protonix	40 mg daily	40 mg daily BID (available IV)
	Esomeprazole	Nexium	20 mg daily	20–40 mg daily (available IV)
PG analog	Misoprostol	Cytotec	100–200 µg QID	300 mg qid PO/IV/IM
H_2 blockers	Cimetidine	Tagamet		150 mg bid PO
	Ranitidine	Zantac		50 mg q18–24 hr IV/IM
	Famotidine	Pepcid		40 mg qHs
	Nizatidine	Axid		300 mg qHs
Mucosal sealant	Sucralfate	Carafate	1 g BID PO	1 g BID PO

BID, twice daily; *GI*, gastrointestinal; *H_2 blockers*, histamine receptor 2 blockers; *IM*, intramuscularly; *IV*, intravenously; *NSAID*, nonsteroidal anti-inflammatory drug; *PO*, per os; *qHs*, for every hour of sleep; *QID*, four times a day.

from NSAIDs; or previous history of peptic ulcer disease (PUD). This intervention should take place **before** the commencement of NSAID therapy to make it effective.[258,260] Various eradication regimens are available.[260] In the United States, a cocktail of two antibiotics (e.g., clarithromycin + amoxicillin or clarithromycin + metronidazole) with an acid reducer, such as a PPI or bismuth, for 7 days, seems to deliver a successful eradication rate of more than 84%. This should be followed by an adjuvant acid reducer while the patient is on NSAID for the length of the therapy in patients with GI high risk or those who become symptomatic and the NSAID cannot be stopped.[261]

Sucralfate, H$_2$ blockers, and antacids are useful for treating dyspepsia, but may not prevent ulcer formation or bleeding caused by NSAIDs.[262-264] Sucralfate and H$_2$ blockers will successfully treat an NSAID-induced peptic ulcer only if the patient completely stops using the NSAID,[253,257] but their role in gastroprotection is limited compared to PPIs. Yet, sucralfate has an FDA-approved indication for NSAID gastroprotection. Identifying candidates who have GI risk factors for therapy with NSAID facilitates the implementation of prophylaxis with a PPI.

Controlled studies show that the incidence of recurrent bleeding from peptic ulcer can be substantially reduced by coadministration of PPIs.[265] Recent data show that PPIs and COX2Is can play complementary roles in the management of patients with moderate to severe dyspepsia and at high risk of ulcer complications.[265] The risk reduction seen with COXIBs does not make up for their increased costs compared with ns-NSAIDs in patients who are not at high risk for gastroenteropathy, particularly in light of the reports of their potential cardiovascular compromise. Nevertheless, COXIBs may be more pharmacoeconomic in patients with a history of bleeding ulcers.[266] The use of COXIBs would become unjustified, if the patient, regardless of his GI or cardiac risk factors, uses and would continue to use cardioprophylactic low-dose

aspirin. The risk for upper GI complications from low-dose aspirin used concomitantly with a COXIB appears to be similar to that from an ns-NSAID alone.[267]

Both PPIs and misoprostol are effective; however, PPIs are better tolerated among patients while decreasing heartburn and dyspepsia as well.[261] If diclofenac is to be used, it makes sense to use it in its commercially available combination with misoprostol formula (Arthrotec). Otherwise a PPI is a reasonable choice to start with if gastric protection is desired. All of the studies that addressed the upper GI risk from long-term NSAID therapy were conducted in patients with arthritis. For the cancer population, there are no large studies to address most of the issues discussed in this section. However, the previously listed guidelines can be implemented in cancer pain patients. Fragile, debilitated, geriatric, terminally ill, and pediatric cancer patients require meticulous assessment in establishing a therapeutic approach with respect to their unique issues (Table 21–12).

Cardiovascular Toxicity

COX2Is causes unopposed TXA$_2$ production in atherosclerotic vessels, increasing the likelihood for thrombotic events, resulting in myocardial ischemia.[268] Furthermore, following cardiac ischemia, COX-2-produced PG mediates late ischemic preconditioning by collaborating with the NOS system.[269] Thus, inhibiting COX-2 would block this physiologic rescue mechanism and cause

TABLE 21–12 Current Suggested Strategy for NSAID Therapy in Relation to Cardioprophylaxic Low-Dose Aspirin^a

		Patient has no gastrointestinal risk		Patient has gastrointestinal risk	
		Positive GI side effects?		Positive GI side effects?	
		No	Yes	No	Yes
Not on low-dose aspirin	Positive cardiac risk? No	ns-NSAID alone	**Transient:** add antacid or H$_2$ Blocker **Moderate:** add PPI or switch to COX2I **Persistent:** treat as +ve GI risk ⇒	COX2I alone	Add PPI + consider acetaminophen or tramadol
	Positive cardiac risk? Yes	ns-NSAID alone	**Transient:** add antacid or H$_2$ blocker **Moderate:** add PPI **Persistent:** treat as +ve GI risk ⇒	ns-NSAID + PPI	Stop NSAID + consider acetaminophen or tramadol
On low-dose aspirin	Positive cardiac risk? No	↑ aspirin dose or use another ns-NSAID	**Transient:** add antacid or H$_2$ blocker Consider to hold aspirin temporarily **Moderate:** add PPI and consider holding aspirin **Persistent:** treat as +ve GI risk ⇒	ns-NSAID + PPI	Stop NSAID + consider acetaminophen or tramadol Consider to stop aspirin
	Positive cardiac risk? Yes	↑ aspirin dose or use another ns- NSAID	**Transient:** add PPI **Moderate:** add PPI + consider stopping NSAID **Persistent:** treat as +ve GI risk ⇒	ns-NSAID + PPI	Do not use any NSAID + consider acetaminophen or tramadol Cardiology consult to stop aspirin & consider clopidogrel

^{a}Consider *H. pylori* eradication prior to administering long-term NSAID therapy, if patient is NSAID-naive, *H. pylori* positive, and if time allows.

further escalation of myocardial ischemia. A novel theory of the COX2I-produced disruption of the COX-2/NOS collaborative work in the myocardium is that after the reduction of PGs produced by COX-2, the myocardial COX-1 attempts to partially replenish those lost PGs.[269] If this proves to be true, then ns-NSAIDs (excluding aspirin) would possibly have a negative effect on the heart comparable to or even worse than the effect of COX2Is because the previous agents block both COX enzymes. This hypothetical view could explain the findings in a study that looked at the risk of acute MI in 650,590 patients over 18 years old who were diagnosed with arthritis and treated with ns-NSAIDs or selective COX2Is between January 1999 and June 2004.[270] The researchers concluded that many, but not all, of the NSAIDs increased the probability of heart attacks: indomethacin by 71%, sulindac by 41%, and ibuprofen by 11%. Among COXIBs, rofecoxib increased the risk by 32% and celecoxib by 9%. As a class, ns-NSAIDs increased the risk of acute MI by 12%, whereas rofecoxib was the only COX2I having a drastically increased risk of cardiac events compared with ns-NSAIDs. The risk of MI appeared, in this study, to be dose-dependent. For example, rofecoxib increased the risk from 16% at daily doses of 12.5 mg to 240% at daily doses over 50 mg. Interestingly, it has been known for a long time that high doses of aspirin (over 4 g daily) increase the frequency of anginal attacks in sick hearts. Arrhythmias of all kinds are reported with salicylates overdose.[271]

NSAIDs could be associated with a slight increase in risk for hypertension or edema, or both.[272] This effect appears to be present equally in both ns-NSAIDs and COX2Is. Although the average degree of increase in blood pressure may be minimal, there may be a small population of patients who are at a significantly greater risk.[272] NSAIDs also can antagonize antihypertensive medication.[270] The CRESCENT study found that rofecoxib causes hypertension more than celecoxib and naproxen.[273]

In light of the different adverse effects caused by NSAIDs, the long-term treatment with any NSAID should be evaluated in light of the preexisting cardiac risks.[271] Additionally, because the linear relation between systolic blood pressure and the risk of cardiovascular disease may be consistent at all levels of blood pressure, any small change in blood pressure for patients on prolonged treatment with NSAIDs might represent an increase in those risks. Therefore, any new elevation in blood pressure (BP) caused by treatment with NSAIDs should be closely monitored and treated if necessary.[272]

Renal Toxicity

All NSAIDs have the propensity to alter kidney function. In healthy adults, NSAIDs cause minor effects on renal function, since PGs have an insignificant vasodilatory role in normovolemic persons. Nevertheless, NSAIDs reduce renal blood flow and, thus, the rate of glomerular filtration in hypovolemic individuals or in patients suffering from chronic renal disease, hepatic cirrhosis with ascites, diabetes, or congestive heart failure. Renal perfusion in patients with such conditions is more reliant on PGs' vasodilatory effects than in healthy individuals. Acute renal failure can be precipitated in such circumstances.[269] NSAIDs affect the kidneys by promoting salt and fluid retention (causing edema), commonly observed in some patients on NSAID therapy. This is usually mild unless other comorbidities exist. NSAIDs promote hyperkalemia by several mechanisms, a side effect that can be therapeutically advantageous in the treatment of Bartter syndrome.[269] NSAIDs cause a clinically insignificant transient reduction in renal function in the early postoperative period in patients with normal preoperative renal function. However, NSAIDs should not be withheld from adults with normal preoperative renal function because of concerns about postoperative renal impairment.[274]

Although acute interstitial nephritis is a rare complication of NSAIDs therapy, NSAID-induced nephropathy (i.e., analgesic nephropathy) is typically linked to long-term use of high-dose NSAIDs or the ingestion of large quantities of analgesic cocktails. This type of nephropathy is characterized by papillary necrosis, chronic interstitial nephritis and reduced tubular function and concentrating ability. The injury is often insidious in onset and may evolve into irreversible renal insufficiency, especially if misuse of NSAIDs continues. Females are more affected than are males, and frequently, there is a history of recurrent urinary tract infection. Emotional disturbances and psychiatric disorders commonly coexist, and other drugs may also be concurrently abused. NSAID-induced nephropathy is associated with pelvic carcinoma of the urinary tract, including the kidneys, ureters, and bladder.

Hematologic Toxicity

Rarely, spontaneous bleeding outside the GI tract results from the use of ns-NSAIDs in individuals with normal hemostasis. In general, significant bleeding in patients taking NSAIDs does not complicate most types of surgery. In fact, it is unnecessary to discontinue them or delay surgery for the purpose of restoring normal hemostasis.[275] Preoperative discontinuation of aspirin (7 to 14 days) and other ns-NSAIDs (3 to 5 days) should be considered, however, in patients undergoing surgery at sites where optimal hemostasis is critical (e.g., when surgical manipulation of the head, neck, spine, and genitourinary tract or when neuraxial anesthesia is planned). Most important bleeding problems that occur with the use of ns-NSAIDs are encountered in patients with coexisting coagulation abnormalities, particularly inherited coagulopathies, severe thrombocytopenia, liver disease, or in those who are simultaneously using alcohol or anticoagulants.[275]

Hepatotoxicity

Although hepatotoxicity is listed as a class warning for NSAIDs, and practically every NSAID has been reported to cause an asymptomatic elevation in aminotransferases, it is often not a clinically relevant side effect. Aspirin, diclofenac, and sulindac are most commonly associated with this problem.[276] The clinical presentation of hepatic injury is variable, ranging from mild cholestasis to severe hepatocellular injury, with the latter being uncommon. The most common cause of hepatotoxicity is an idiosyncratic reaction associated with an immunologic response. Management consists of discontinuation of the offending NSAID and symptomatic treatment.

Other Systemic Toxicity

Systemic toxicities can include respiratory, metabolic, reproductive, nervous, and psychiatric derangement. These side effects are unusual and occur, in most cases, with individual drugs rather than the whole group. Table 21-13 shows an extensive listing of most documented NSAID adverse effects.

Drug Interactions

Warfarin

NSAIDs and warfarin have synergistic effects on GI bleeding. Aspirin competes with warfarin (both are highly protein-bound drugs) for the same binding site in plasma, increasing levels of free warfarin and potentiating its therapeutic effect to an undesirable level.

Antihypertensives

The antagonistic action of NSAIDs with these medications, excluding Ca^{++} channel blockers, might make the patient's hypertension refractory if they are used concomitantly. Hypertensive crisis is unusual.

Digoxin

Elevated digoxin levels have been reported in patients receiving NSAIDs. In those patients, digoxin levels need to be monitored.

Oral Hypoglycemics

There have been rare reports of abnormal blood glucose levels, in patients on concurrent therapy with both a hypoglycemic agent and an NSAID. Those patients were either normoglycemic or had a controlled blood glucose level. Diabetics who are on NSAID therapy need to consider periodic glucose measurements (e.g., weekly finger stick), if that is not part of their regimen.

Methotrexate and Cyclosporine

Suppressing the production of renal PGs increases the toxicity of these two medications. The concurrent use of NSAIDs with methotrexate and cyclosporine worsen major side effects of these two drugs, such as gastric irritation and ulceration, potassium retention, and patients may end up with GI ulceration or bleeding and nephrotoxicity. Cancer patients receiving these agents with an NSAID should have periodic renal function check up and perhaps occult fecal detection.

Lithium

By worsening renal function, NSAIDs reduce renal lithium clearance and elevate plasma lithium levels, making patients susceptible to lithium toxicity.

Antacids

Antacids may delay NSAID absorption, and the bioavailability of misoprostol if coadministered. Mg^{++} containing antacids can also exacerbate misoprostol-induced diarrhea. Patients receiving misoprostol gastroprotection with their NSAID therapy should avoid antacids, particularly those that contain Mg^{++}.

Diuretics

NSAIDs may inhibit the activity of diuretics. Concurrent NSAID-therapy with K^+-sparing diuretics may be associated with hyperkalemia.

Steroids

Steroids alone rarely irritate the GI system; however, if used concurrently with all NSAIDs, this could produce or exacerbate side effects as discussed earlier.

Sertraline

A Polish study found that sertraline, a potent selective serotonin reuptake inhibitor (SSRI), enhances the antinociceptive effects of indomethacin and metamizol in laboratory animals.[277] If further investigation into these data supports the study's findings, it could be an important discovery in multimodal pain management.

Aspirin and Other ns-NSAIDs

Aspirin may displace other NSAIDs from their binding sites, producing lower plasma levels of the other drug. Until the debate over the assumed antagonism of ibuprofen with low-dose aspirin's cardioprophylactic effect is resolved, it is prudent not to combine these two agents until a consensus is achieved.

TABLE 21–13 Summary of NSAIDs' Adverse Effects

System	Adverse Effect	Risk Factor	Management	Prevention
Gastrointestinal	Nausea and vomiting; dyspepsia; PUD and UGIB; esophagitis and esophageal stricture; NSAID enteropathy; NSAID colitis	Age > 65; history of PUD/UGIB; anticoagulation Rx; corticosteroid Rx; ↑ dose NSAIDs; multiple NSAID use; prolonged NSAID use; major comorbidity; *H. pylori* infection; NSAID dyspepsia; cigarette smoking; alcohol consumption	Stop, switch and/or treat adverse effect See Figure 21–5 for roadmap	Use stomach-friendly drug Advice patient to take medicine with food and plenty of liquid and not to crush enteric-coated pills Consider *H. pylori* eradication prior to starting Rx Consider gastroprotection Rx
Cardiovascular	Hypertension; thrombotic events; coronary spasm; arrhythmias	Cardiovascular disease; hypertension; diabetes; dyslipidemia; cigarette smoking; alcohol consumption; ↑ coagulopathy; age > 65	Stop, switch and/or treat Consider cardiology consult	Do not initiate Rx in high-risk patients Cardiology consult for clopidogrel prophylaxis Stop smoking Address cardiac risks
Renal	Na⁺ retention; edema; hyperkalemia; acute renal failure; interstitial nephritis; NSAID-induced nephropathy	Preexisting renal disease; hypovolemia; elderly; major comorbidity; diuretic therapy; malignancy; history of drug abuse and/or emotional disturbances	Stop, switch and/or treat accordingly; Rehydrate if needed; Nephrology consult	Avoid hypovolemia; correct electrolyte imbalance; educate patient of the risks of NSAID abuse; identify high-risk patients
Hematological	Bleeding, especially UGIB/LGIB Hemorrhagic stroke (uncommon but serious)	Warfarin therapy; coagulopathy; thrombocytopenia; malignancy; perioperative (especially cardiac)	Stop, switch and/or treat accordingly	Good H&P; communicate with other physicians; try acetaminophen for pain
Hepatic	Hepatic dysfunction Reye's syndrome	Rheumatic disorders; autoimmune disease; alcoholism; hepatic disease Children on aspirin; acute viral prodrome	Stop, switch and/or treat	Periodic LFTs monitoring in high-risk patients. Avoid alcohol Avoid aspirin in children altogether
Dermatologic	Urticaria/rash; Stevens-Johnson syndrome; exfoliative dermatitis; erythema multiforme	Children; history of drug reactions; history of angioedema	Stop, switch and/or treat	Good H&P
Respiratory	Bronchospasm; status asthmaticus; Rhinitis; nasal polyps	Asthma; history of multiple allergies	Stop, switch and/or treat accordingly; Polyps regress on stopping the drug	Good H&P

Metabolic	Reduced bone formation	Elderly, postmenopausal, malignancy, osteoporosis	Stop, switch and/or treat accordingly	Identify patient at risk; Bone density scan
Immunologic	Hypersensitivity reaction; increased sulfa allergy; skin reaction	History of reactions to one NSAID or cross-reactions with another; multiple allergies; history of sulfa allergy	Stop, switch and/or treat accordingly	Good H & P
Reproductive	Infertility; Delayed ovulation, fertilization, or implantation	No specific population	Stop drug	Uncommon; Avoid in pregnancy (cause premature closure of DA)
Nervous	Headaches; tinnitus; blurred vision; memory deficit	Elderly; other CNS suppressants; drug overdose	Stop, switch, lower the dose, and/or treat accordingly	Start with lowest analgesic possible dose
Psychiatric	Delirium; cognitive disturbances; mood disturbances; depression	History of psychiatric illness	Stop, switch, lower the dose, and/or treat accordingly	Identify patients with psychiatric pathology and treat aggressively; psychiatric consult; avoid indomethacin and COX2Is
Sexual	Orgasm disturbances (reported only with naproxen)	Concomitant use of antidepressants, antipsychotics and some antihypertensives; history of drug abuse; previous sexual problems	Stop, switch, lower the dose, and/or treat accordingly	Choose a different NSAID

COX2Is, cyclooxygenase 2 inhibitors; DA, ductus arteriosus; H & P, history and physical examination; LFTs, liver function tests; LGIB, lower gastrointestinal bleeding; NSAID, nonsteroidal anti-inflammatory drug; PUD, peptic ulcer disease; Rx, therapy; UGIB, upper gastrointestinal bleeding.

ALTERNATIVE NSAIDS

The ongoing controversy over COX2Is and their potential cardiovascular adverse effects has led many nutritional merchants and alternative medicine clinics around the world to escalate promoting the sales of herbal medicines that claim to be natural NSAIDs or natural COX2Is.[278,279] These supplements are often compounded and include products such as boswellia, bromelain, grape seeds extract, and rosemary leaf extract. Although some clinical observations and nonclinical investigations have been conducted on a few of these agents,[280,281] these "natural formulations" have neither been studied in standardized trials for their stated purposes nor been approved or controlled by the FDA. These supplements are mentioned for the purpose of raising awareness that such products exist and their true efficacy is still unknown. The authors and the editor do not recommend or discourage their use.

Evidence of NSAID characteristics of a naturally occurring chemical, named *oleocanthal* by the researchers, was recently discovered in newly pressed extra-virgin olive oil.[282] The scientists were led to the discovery by the serendipitous observation that fresh extra-virgin olive oil irritates the throat in a manner similarly caused by solutions containing ibuprofen, which in turn led them to investigate potential common pharmacologic properties of these solutions. They found that although structurally dissimilar, both ibuprofen and oleocanthal molecules inhibit COX isozymes in the PG-biosynthesis pathway. Additionally, the researchers completed a de novo synthesis of oleocanthal, and studied the COX-inhibiting properties of both enantiomers of oleocanthal.[282] Their results showed that oleocanthal caused, in vitro, dose-dependent inhibition of COX-1 and COX-2, with potency similar to that of ibuprofen, but had no effect on LOX. This revelation might explain the health-related effects of the Mediterranean diet, which is rich in olive oil and is believed to confer various health benefits, some of which may be due to the natural anti-COX activity of oleocanthal from premium olive oils. The pioneering study also makes the case for pharmacologic activity based on irritation and furthers the concept, proposed in 1965 but never followed up on, that a compound's orosensory qualities might reflect its pharmacologic potency.[283]

EXPERIMENTAL NSAIDS

The relentless search for the analgesic that relieves pain without causing side effects continues. The pharmaceutical community received a massive blow with the COX2Is failure to deliver this promise. Yet, two promising mechanisms for pain relief are currently under investigation.

LOX/COX Bi-Inhibitors

The hypothesis behind these investigational medications purports that the exclusive inhibition of COXs by available NSAIDs disables only one pathway of the AA metabolism cascade, leaving large quantities of substrate for LOXs to continue producing more non-PG inflammatory agents, chiefly LTs. The excess of LT production facilitates the continuation of the inflammatory process, which could mean repetitive nociception and chronic pain, as well as unintentional and undesirable tissue damage such as gastric irritation seen in NSAID toxicity.[284,285] Furthermore, studies suggest a larger initial role for LOXs in triggering hyperalgesia.[131-136,285,286] Additionally, both the gastric and renal toxicities induced by traditional NSAIDs and COX2Is seem to be related to inhibition of prostaglandin, but not leukotriene synthesis. Maintaining the correct balance between PGs and LTs is perhaps essential for continuing good health, and a balanced inhibition of both enzyme families might produce safer analgesics and anti-inflammatory agents.[287]

Licofelone is currently in phase III trials and is the first agent of this new class, LOX/COX bi-inhibitors. Preliminary data on this drug seem promising, but further well-designed clinical trials of this agent in the elderly will be necessary before a final evaluation is possible.[286,287]

NO-NSAIDs

Under physiologic conditions, minor quantities of nitric oxide (NO) contribute to gastric mucosal gastroprotection. Similar to PGs, NO increases mucus and bicarbonate secretion in the microcirculation and decreases neutrophils–endothelial adherence—a key pathogenic element in NSAID gastropathy.[288] The recognition of NO's important role in gastroprotection has led to the development of a new class of drugs: nitric oxide–releasing NSAIDs (NO-NSAIDs). These drugs consist of a conventional NSAID esterified to a NO-releasing moiety. Animal studies demonstrated NO-NSAID gastric mucosal sparing on both acute and chronic administration.[289] In the laboratory, NO-NSAIDs do not produce detectable mucosal injury, in contrast with the administration of the parent NSAID (aspirin, naproxen, and indomethacin), when given in equimolar dosages to the laboratory animals.[289] In experimental models, NO-NSAIDs even protected gastric mucosa against damage induced by other deleterious stimuli and maintained gastric mucosal blood flow. Additionally, NO-NSAIDs improve anti-inflammatory and antinociceptive efficacy. Moreover, NO-aspirin has demonstrated an increased antithrombotic potency compared with conventional aspirin.[289] The broad biologic effects of slowly released NO combined with COX inhibition are likely to extend the inflammation and pain indications of NO-NSAIDs to the treatment and prevention of other diseases such as cancer or cardiovascular disorders. A study involving a total of 31 volunteers supported the data obtained in animal studies showing significantly reduced GI toxicity associated with NO-naproxen compared with conventional naproxen in humans.[290] NO-NSAIDs represent a promising therapeutic alternative to conventional NSAIDs with not only a reduced GI side effect profile but also a powerful therapeutic effect. Large, randomized studies are needed to definitively evaluate the clinical benefit of NO-NSAIDs in humans.[289]

ACETAMINOPHEN

Acetaminophen (known in Europe as paracetamol) remains the analgesic of choice for general pain. As the only member of its class, it has a key position on the WHO ladder as one of the first choices to treat cancer pain. For many years, acetaminophen has been available OTC, a fact that strengthened acetaminophen's acceptance as a safe and effective medication and a good self-administered analgesic and antipyretic. Therefore, acetaminophen is often the first drug used for control of mild to moderate pain. It is also useful for more severe pain, particularly when combined with an opioid analgesic.

Notwithstanding its seniority among analgesics, acetaminophen's mechanism of action has not been fully elucidated. Some authors have considered a peripheral local action, but this possibility was not supported by other studies.[291] Scientific data are more in favor of a central effect because acetaminophen:

1. crosses the blood–brain barrier[292];
2. induces an antinociceptive effect after central administration[293]; and
3. inhibits responses in noninflammatory pain models after systemic administration.[294]

Some of the suggested central mechanisms include:

1. activating the descending serotonergic pathways[294];
2. inhibition of NO synthases (NOSs)[295];
3. inhibiting L-arginine-nitiric oxide (L-Arg-NO) system, where L-Arg is a natural donor of NO[296]; and
4. inhibition of prostaglandin synthesis, probably through selective inhibition of one or more of the COXs.[297]

A spliced variant of the canine COX-1, or so-called COX-3 or COX-1v, that is selectively inhibited by acetaminophen in the brain of the canine species has been suggested as the site of action.[162] However, more studies on intact cells have also indicated that acetaminophen appears to be a selective inhibitor of COX-2.[297-300] The data from these studies support the hypothesis that acetaminophen produces its analgesic and antipyretic actions by blocking prostaglandin synthesis through the inhibition of COX-2; yet, its site of action on the COX-2 pathway remain unknown. Many scientists still believe that the work of acetaminophen is largely dependent on selective inhibition of both COX-2 and COX-1. The COX-3 theory was well accepted in the scientific field because it was easy to digest and analyze. Unfortunately, an acetaminophen-sensitive COX-3 has not yet been identified in humans. Nonetheless, acetaminophen behaves in a manner comparable to COX2Is, excluding their anti-inflammatory effects. Acetaminophen, contrary to aspirin and similar to celecoxib, is gentle on the stomach and does not interfere with platelet aggregation.

Clinically, acetaminophen is comparable to NSAIDs in its analgesic effects but is less effective for treating pain associated with inflammatory conditions. It can be administered to patients who are allergic to aspirin, and it appears to be safe at therapeutic dose levels during all stages of pregnancy and breast feeding. Unlike aspirin, it has not been associated with Reye's syndrome and can be used in children with varicella or influenza. It, also, does not inhibit platelet aggregation or affect prothrombin time and can be used in patients with bleeding disorders and for surgical procedures.

Acetaminophen is commercially available on its own or in combination with a wide range of nonprescription agents, such as aspirin, caffeine, diphenhydramine, other antihistamines, decongestants, and cough suppressants. It also is commercially available in combination with short-acting opioids. A complete list of these drug combinations can be found in Table 21–14.

The adult dosage range is 325 to 1000 mg q4–6h. The recommended daily dose should not exceed 4 g. Acetaminophen is administered orally (pills, syrup) or rectally (suppository). After oral administration, acetaminophen is rapidly and almost completely absorbed from the GI tract. Peak plasma concentrations are attained within 30 to 60 minutes, although serum concentrations and analgesia are not necessarily correlated. Binding to serum protein is about 25% after normal therapeutic dosages. In Europe, but not in the United States, the availability of an injectable form of acetaminophen and its pro-drug *propacetamol* has expanded its use in the perioperative period because of its predictable onset and duration of action.[301] A recent Scandinavian randomized, placebo-controlled, double-blind, parallel

TABLE 21–14 Acetaminophen Drug Combinations

Combination acetaminophen	Brand Name	Strength (mg)	Dose by pill PRN (max #/d)	Usual Use	Comments
+ aspirin + caffeine	Excedrin Extra-Strength Excedrin Migraine	250+250+65	1 q12–24 hr (2)	Tension headaches, migraine attacks	In Canada, no aspirin OTC
+ butalbital + caffeine above w/codeine	Fioricet Fioricet with codeine	325+50+40 325+50+40+30	1 q4 hr pRN(6) 1–2 q4 hr (6)	Tension headaches, pain following minor procedures/ surgeries	
+ caffeine + dihydrocodeine	Panlor DC Panlor SS	356.4+30+16 712.8+60+32	1–2 q4hr (10) 1 q4 hr (5)	Moderate to moderately severe pain	Good for postoperative and breakthrough pain
+ codeine	Tylenol#2 Tylenol#3 Tylenol#4	300+15 300+30 300+60	1–2 q4 hr (6)	Moderate to moderately severe pain	Good for postoperative and breakthrough pain Available in liquid. 2.5 mg codeine per mL
+ dichloraphenazone + isometheptene	Midrin	325+100+65	1 q1 hr (12)	Migraine attacks	Lost popularity with evolvement of Triptans
+ hydrocodone	Lorcet, Lortab Maxidone Norco Vicodine Zydone	500+2.5, 500+5, 500+7.5, 500+10,650+7.5, 650+10 750+10 325+5, 325+7.5 500+5, 660+10, 750+7.5 400+(5/7.5/10)	1–2 q4 hr (6)	Moderate to moderately severe pain	Good for postoperative and breakthrough pain Available in liquid. 0.5 mg hydrocodone per mL Most popular item of diversion in the US
+ oxycodone	Endocet Percocet Roxicet Tylox	325+(5/7.5/10), 650+10 325+(2.5/5/7.5), 650+10 325+5, 500+5 500+5	1–2 q6 hr (8–10)	Moderate to moderately severe pain	Good for postoperative and breakthrough pain Available in liquid. 1 mg oxycodone per mL. Second-most popular item of diversion in the US
+ pentazocine	Talacen	650/25	1 q4 hr (6)	Moderate pain	Good for postoperative and breakthrough pain
+ propoxyphen	Wygesic Darvocet	650+65 325+50, 325+100, 650+100	1 q4 hr (6)	Mild to moderate pain Mild pain	Good for postoperative and breakthrough pain
+ tramadol	Ultracet	325+37.5	1–2 q4–6 hr (8)	Acute pain	Good for postoperative and breakthrough pain

group trial has found that 1 g IV acetaminophen or 2 g IV propacetamol provided efficient analgesia following dental procedures.[302] The initial dose of injectable acetaminophen may be administered intraoperatively followed by an oral administration after being discharged home. Importantly, patients should be warned that commonly used opioid combinations consist of acetaminophen. Injectable acetaminophen is in preparation to be presented for an FDA approval in the United States.

At therapeutic dosage levels, acetaminophen is well tolerated, does not produce gastric irritation, or affect kidney or liver function. Side effects are rare and nonspecific or idiosyncratic in general.

Acetaminophen is effective in the relief of both acute and chronic pain. Acetaminophen may be preferred in elderly patients with osteoarthritis over other NSAIDs because of fewer GI and renal side effects. The American Geriatrics Society recommends acetaminophen as the analgesic of choice for minor aches and pains in patients older than 50 years. In cancer pain, acetaminophen can be added to a mild or strong opioid regimen to improve the balance between analgesia and side effects by either increasing analgesia without adding side effects or by maintaining analgesia with less side effects from opioids, NSAIDs, or other drugs. Such interventions have been successful in reducing pain and improving well-being without major side effects in patients with cancer and suffering from persistent pain despite a strong opioid regimen.[303]

Acute acetaminophen overdose will lead to dose-dependent hepatotoxicity and possibly acute renal failure. In addition, chronic ingestion of acetaminophen may also lead to hepatotoxicity or chronic analgesic nephropathy. Acetaminophen-induced hepatotoxicity and nephrotoxicity are caused by the formation of the oxidative metabolite, N-acetyl-para-benzoquinoneimine (NAPQI), in the liver and to a lesser degree in the kidney. NAPQI binds covalently to sulfhydryl groups on tissue macromolecules, leading to cell necrosis. Depletion of glutathione reserves leads to hepatotoxicity. Administration of N-acetylcysteine or methionine may reduce hepatotoxicity by binding to NAPQI. However, these agents do not prevent renal toxicity. Other toxic glutathione metabolites such as aminophenol-S-conjugates may play a role in acetaminophen-induced acute renal toxicity. Chronic analgesic nephropathy is characterized by interstitial nephritis and papillary necrosis. The mechanism of chronic analgesic necrosis is caused by reactive metabolites or other products that inhibit renal COX-1 and COX-2.

Indications for acetaminophen's use are arthralgia, fever, dental pain, dysmenorrhea, headache and migraine, and muscle ache. However, it can be used for any painful complaint. The only absolute contraindication for acetaminophen is hypersensitivity to the drug. It should be used with caution in chronic alcoholics, G6PD deficient patients, or patients with preexisting liver impairment because serious damage can occur, even at therapeutic dosage levels. Patients taking barbiturates, phenytoin, and zidovudine, which are known to induce hepatic microsomal enzymes, may also be at risk for acetaminophen toxicity. Tobacco smoking induces the cytochrome P_{450} isozyme CYP1A2 and may potentially increase the risk for acetaminophen-induced hepatotoxicity during overdose via enhanced generation of acetaminophen's hepatotoxic metabolite, NAPQI.[304] In one study, current tobacco smoking was found to be very frequent in patients admitted with acetaminophen poisoning. Tobacco smoking appears to be an independent risk factor of severe hepatotoxicity, acute liver failure, and death following acetaminophen overdose.[305]

TRAMADOL

Tramadol is a synthetic analog of codeine with a lower affinity to μ receptors.[5] Its main analgesic effect is produced by inhibition of norepinephrine and serotonin reuptake.[5] Tramadol's major metabolite, M_1, has a stronger μ-opioid effect. Tramadol has less potential for abuse or respiratory depression than other opiate agonists, but both may occur.[5] Tramadol has been effective in the control of postoperative pain when given intravenously, but may not be suitable as an adjunct to anesthesia because of low sedative properties and a high incidence of postoperative respiratory depression.[5]

Tramadol has been widely used in Europe since the late 1970s, where it is available in intravenous, rectal, and oral formulations. However, only the oral formula is available in the United States. Absorption is rapid and bioavailability is 68% after single doses and approaches 100% after multiple doses. The increase in bioavailability with multiple doses is thought to be caused by saturable first-pass metabolism. Bioavailability increases with age and decreased liver or renal function. Following intramuscular or rectal administration, the bioavailability of tramadol is 100% and 78%, respectively.[5] The rate and extent of oral absorption are not significantly affected by food. Tramadol is detected in plasma within 15 to 45 minutes of oral dosing. Peak plasma concentrations of tramadol occur about 2 hours post-dose. Peak plasma concentrations of the active metabolite M_1 occur about 3 hours after an oral dose. The time to analgesia onset is within 1 hour of administration, with a peak effect around 2 to 3 hours. Analgesia lasts about 6 hours. Steady-state concentrations are achieved after 2 days of multiple dosing. Tramadol has a high tissue affinity. Minimum protein binding occurs (about 20%).

Tramadol crosses the placenta and about 0.1% is distributed into breast milk.[5]

Tramadol has less potential for abuse or respiratory depression than other opiate agonists, but both may occur. Comparative studies with other analgesics for the treatment of postoperative pain indicate that tramadol is equivalent in analgesic relief to codeine but is less potent than acetaminophen–codeine and acetaminophen–hydrocodone combinations for the treatment of dental and acute musculoskeletal pain. Tramadol has been shown to be effective as an adjuvant to NSAID therapy in patients with osteoarthritis who experience breakthrough pain.[5] A randomized, double-blind study found that tramadol, at an average dose of 210 mg/day, was more effective than placebo for relieving pain, without any important effects on sleep.[306] The most frequent adverse effects in that study were nausea, constipation, headache, and somnolence.

The daily dose of tramadol should not exceed 400 mg because, like tricyclic antidepressants, it lowers seizure threshold.[307] It is prudent to avoid tramadol in patients predisposed to epileptic activity, such as those with brain tumors. Tramadol is less likely to cause respiratory depression and constipation than equianalgesic doses of pure opioids, but causes dizziness, nausea, dry mouth, and sedation.[5,306] Other randomized controlled trials have yielded positive results in painful diabetic neuropathy,[306] different neuropathic pain states,[308] and PHN.[309] The main side effects are constipation and drowsiness. A history of seizures and a previous history of drug abuse are relative contraindications for tramadol.

The use of tramadol as a preemptive analgesic in day-case arthroscopy patients does not significantly reduce postoperative pain scores or requirements for analgesia. In addition, the higher incidence of perioperative bradycardia, especially if associated with nausea and vomiting, suggests that tramadol's use in this group of patients is of questionable benefit. It is conceivable that using a larger study population might identify an improvement in pain scores.[310]

Tramadol has a role in neuropathic pain. It was suggested among neuropathic pain agents to be used as a first-line treatment for neuropathic pain by the review of the evidence-based literature on neuropathic pain treatment.[51] Other first-line agents included gabapentin, 5% lidocaine patch, opioids, and TCAs. It should be noted that these recommendations were made before the FDA approval of duloxetine and pregabalin. It was also suggested that a maximum dose of tramadol should not exceed 400 mg/day. Efficacy is usually evident at 250 mg/day in divided doses.

In patients with creatinine clearance less than 80 mL/minute, tramadol's half-life increases 1.5 to 2 times as compared with patients with normal renal function. Therefore, dose adjustments of tramadol are required in patients with renal dysfunction. Even if the patient is on hemodialysis, tramadol and M_1 are removed from the body by dialysis to a limited degree. The half-life of tramadol and M_1 in liver cirrhosis or significant liver dysfunction increases 2 to 3 times because of decreased liver clearance. Hence, tramadol's dose should be lowered by at least 50% in patients with hepatic dysfunction. Elderly patients may require lower doses as they may have an underlying renal or hepatic impairment.

Tramadol in Cancer Pain

The World Health Organization guidelines for cancer pain management classify tramadol as a step 2 agent. For patients with severe cancer pain, morphine is superior and most patients treated with tramadol require a change to a more potent opioid after a few weeks of treatment. The lack of significant cardiac effects and no association with peptic ulcer disease make tramadol an alternative in some patients who may not tolerate NSAIDs. The efficacy of tramadol was assessed in a double-blind, randomized, crossover comparison of tramadol and morphine in 20 patients with "strong" cancer pain.[311] By titrating doses over 4 days, equivalent pain ratings were achieved with both drugs. More patients and nurses preferred morphine, although constipation and nausea were less severe and total side effects were fewer with tramadol. Another study compared tramadol with buprenorphine in 131 patients with moderate cancer pain.[311] The trial was planned to last 6 months, but the average patient withdrew within 2 months because of inadequate analgesia. Efficacy, tolerability, and quality of life were better in the tramadol group.

Slow titration of tramadol to the effective analgesic dose (i.e., increase by 50 mg PO every 3 days) may decrease the incidence of nausea and vomiting. Tramadol does not need to be taken with food. Although the maximum recommended daily dose is 400 mg, the cancer pain patient might respond better to doses up to 600 mg/day. The dosing for the FDA-approved extended-release formula of tramadol will depend on the available strength. However, European trial for this formula in cancer pain patients revealed that up to 650 mg per day of extended-release tramadol may provide good analgesia without any severe side effects. Tramadol should be used in patients with mild to moderate pain and as an adjunct to opioid therapy in high levels of pain, those intolerant to typical opioids because of its potential to cause seizures at high doses, and because of its higher costs.[313] Treatment with tramadol ER results in statistically significant and clinically important sustained improvements in pain, stiffness, physical function, global status, and sleep in patients with chronic pain. A once-a-day formulation of tramadol has the potential to provide patients with increased control over the management of their pain, fewer interruptions in sleep and improved compliance.[314] Figure 21-5 provides a road map to plan the administration of an oral nonopioid for the symptomatic management of cancer pain, whether as the sole analgesic or as a complementary agent to opioids or any of the various therapeutic procedures.

ZICONOTIDE

Ziconotide, similar to other calcium channel modulators (such as oxcarbazepine and gabapentin) inhibits ectopic firing and attenuates neuronal responses, which occur following postinjury up-regulation of $a_{2\delta}$ subunits

FIGURE 21–5 Roadmap for using a nonopioid analgesic for cancer pain.

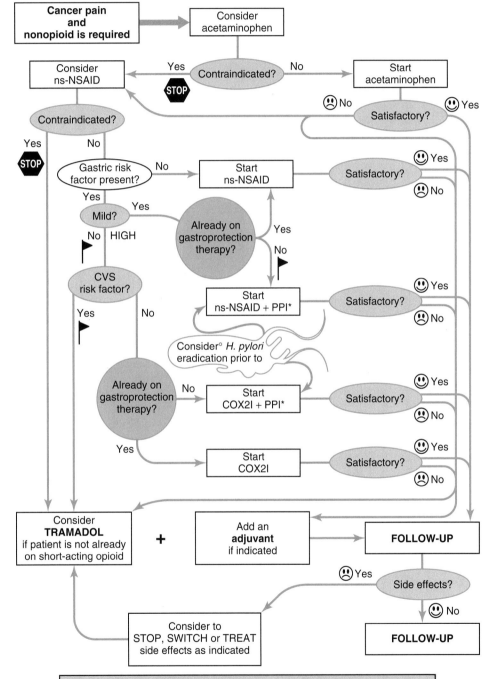

of voltage-activated calcium channels in both the DRG and spinal cord dorsal horn neurons.[314,315] These medications alleviate tactile allodynia commonly observed in postinjury neural states. Because it is administered directly into the CNS, ziconotide is not expected to modulate sodium channels of peripheral nerves—a mechanism thought to be manifested in other calcium channel modulators. Ziconotide has not been studied in pediatric patients.

Therapeutic Benefits

In the ZEST study, patients treated with intrathecal ziconotide showed significant improvement from baseline at all monthly assessments from week 4 through month 12 of treatment.[317] Stable mean dose requirements in conjunction with sustained Visual Analog Scale of Pain Intensity (VASPI) reductions suggest the potential for long-term analgesic benefit.[317] Reduction in oral opioid administration was also observed.[318]

Side Effects

The most frequently reported adverse effects of ziconotide in the ZEST study are understandably CNS related. They include, in descending order of occurrence, dizziness, nystagmus, confusion, memory impairment, abnormal gait, nausea and vomiting, urinary retention, stupor, urinary retention, meningitis, dysmetria, ataxia, agitation, hallucination, and coma.[315,319-321] Non-CNS adverse effects include skin rash, abnormal liver function tests, dose-dependent orthostatic hypotension, and bradycardia.[321] No data are available on the effect of renal or hepatic impairment on the pharmacokinetics of ziconotide. Patients with a preexisting history of psychosis should not be treated with ziconotide. Severe psychiatric symptoms and neurologic impairment may occur during treatment with the medication. All patients should be monitored frequently for evidence of cognitive impairment, hallucinations, or changes in mood or consciousness.[322]

Efficacy of Ziconotide in Cancer Pain

The initial reports of ziconotide's usefulness as a potent analgesic for refractory pain when administered intrathecally were in cancer and AIDS patients.[323] Both groups whose pain was unrelieved with opioids demonstrated analgesic efficacy. The drug is currently approved for clinical use, and research corroborates the effectiveness in relieving both malignant and nonmalignant pain of various causes.[323,324] Additionally, it appears to be well tolerated, with primarily mild to moderate adverse effects and low discontinuation rates.[323,324]

CONCLUSION

The role of nonopioids analgesics in the management of cancer pain is undoubtedly important. Nonopioid analgesics can and should be used at any level of cancer pain treatment. Besides analgesia, NSAIDs and acetaminophen have additional therapeutic effects, yet they retain dangerous qualities that are essential for the clinician to become aware of before treatment initiation. NSAIDs, in particular, manifest a vast number of physiologic and pathologic effects. Potential nonconventional uses of NSAID in the prevention of serious diseases, such as cancer and Alzheimer's disease, are under investigation and may add valuable benefit to this class of drugs. Scientific research to produce more effective NSAIDs with fewer side effects remains ongoing. NO-NSAIDs and LOX/COX bi-inhibitors are two potential classes that demonstrated promising outcomes. Furthermore, research to uncover better means and drugs to palliate or prevent analgesic side effects continues to thrive. New formulations of older drugs, such as the introduction of parenteral forms of ketoprofen, tramodal, and acetaminophen, as well as the launch of the extended-release formula of tramadol will expand the options for treating pain with nonopioid agents.

Ziconotide is a modern innovation in the field of nonopioid analgesics because it is centrally acting and directly infused into the CNS when opioid-induced hyperalgesia is suspected. This development, combined with improved understanding of pain pharmacology, provides possibilities to discover additional neuraxially administered drugs that are alternatives to opioids.

Care providers must have adequate understanding of the pathophysiology and clinical presentation of cancer pain. Adaptation of proven treatment guidelines, such as the WHO Analgesic Ladder, coupled with updated awareness of the various analgesics, their therapeutic strengths, and adverse effect profiles make treatment approaches more effective, better tolerated, and safer. If a combination opioid–nonopioid agent (e.g., Percocet) is used, vigilance is warranted to avoid abuse or diversion (see Chapter 20 for guidelines on prescribing controlled substances). Ultimately, an improved understanding of nonopioid analgesics combined with focused evaluations and careful applications will enhance their usefulness, efficacy, and safety.

REFERENCES

1. No author listed: "A" In The New Encyclopædia Britannica MICROPÆDIA Ready Reference, Vol 1, 15th ed. 1998. Chicago, Encyclopædia Britannica, Inc. 1998, p 366.
2. Lussier D, Huskey AG, Portenoy RK: Adjuvant analgesics in cancer pain management. Oncologist 9:571-591, 2004.
3. Ripamonti C, Bruera E: Pain and symptom management in palliative care. Cancer Control 3:204-213, 1996.
4. Buschmann H: What is pain? In: Buschmann H, Christoph T, Friderichs E, et al (eds): Analgesics from chemistry and pharmacology to clinical practice. Weinheim, Germany Wiley-VCH, 2002, pp 1-11.
5. Grond S, Sablotzki A: Clinical pharmacology of tramadol. Clin Pharmacokinet 43:879-923, 2004.
6. Meyer RJ: NDA 21-060 (an approval letter to Elan Pharmaceuticals), the FDA web site, http://www.fda.gov/cder/foi/appletter/2004/021060ltr.pdf. Accessed on February 6, 2005.
7. World Health Organization: Cancer Pain Relief and Palliative Care. Geneva, Switzerland, 1990.
8. Weingart WA, Sorkness CA, Earhart RH: Analgesia with oral narcotics and added ibuprofen in cancer patients. Clin Pharm 4:53-58, 1985.
9. Ventafridda V, Tamburini M, Caraceni A, et al: A validation study of the WHO method for cancer pain relief. Cancer 59:850-856, 1987.
10. Takeda F: Results of field-testing in Japan of the WHO Draft Interim Guideline on Relief of Cancer Pain. The Pain Clinic 1:83-90, 1986.
11. Jadad AR, Browman GP: The WHO analgesic ladder for cancer pain management: Stepping up the quality of its evaluation. JAMA 274:1870-1873, 1995.
12. Ventafridda V, Bianchi M, Ripamonti C, et al: Studies on the effects of antidepressant drugs on the antinociceptive action of morphine and on plasma morphine in rat and man. Pain 43:155-162, 1990.
13. Grond S, Zech D, Lynch J, et al: Validation of World Health Organization guidelines for pain relief in head and neck cancer: A prospective study. Ann Otol Rhinol Laryngol 102:342-348, 1993.
14. Grond S, Zech D, Schug SA, et al: Validation of World Health Organization guidelines for cancer pain relief during the last days and hours of life. J Pain Symptom Manage 6:411-422, 1991.
15. Grond S, Radbruch L, Meuser T, et al: Assessment and treatment of neuropathic cancer pain following WHO guidelines. Pain 79:15-20, 1999.
16. Zech DF, Grond S, Lynch J, et al: Validation of World Health Organization Guidelines for cancer pain relief: A 10-year prospective study. Pain 63:65-76, 1995.
17. Ahmedzai S: New approaches to pain control in patients with cancer. Eur J Cancer suppl 6:S8-14, 1997.
18. Parrott T: Using opioid analgesics to manage chronic noncancer pain in primary care. J Am Board Fam Pract 12:293-306, 1999.
19. Eisenberg E, Berkey CS, Carr DB, et al: Efficacy and safety of nonsteroidal antiinflammatory drugs for cancer pain: A meta-analysis. J Clin Oncol 12:2756-1265, 1994.
20. Portenoy RK: Three-step analgesic ladder for management of cancer pain. Anesthesiology News 30, pmn 10-14, 2004.
21. Plancarte R, Alvarez J, Arrieta MC: Interventional treatment of cancer pain. Semin Pain Med 1:34-42, 2003.
22. Slavin KV, Tesoro EP, Mucksavage JJ: The treatment of cancer pain. Drugs Today (Barc) 40:235-245, 2004.
23. Cherny NI: The management of cancer pain. CA Cancer J Clin 50:70-116, 2000.
24. Grond S, Zech D, Schug SA, et al: The importance of non-opioid analgesics for cancer pain relief according to the guidelines of the World Health Organization. Int J Clin Pharmacol Res 11:253-260, 1991.
25. AGS Panel on Chronic Pain in Older Persons, American Geriatrics Society: The management of chronic pain in older persons. Geriatrics 53:S8-S24, 1998.
26. de Wit R, van Dam F, Vielvoye-Kerkmeer A, et al: The treatment of chronic cancer pain in a cancer hospital in The Netherlands. J Pain Symptom Manage 17:333-350, 1999.
27. Bruera E, Kim HN: Cancer pain. JAMA 290:2476-2479, 2003.
28. Foley KM: Advances in cancer pain. Arch Neurol 56:413-417, 1999.
29. Kocoglu H, Pirbudak L, Pence S, et al: Cancer pain, pathophysiology, characteristics and syndromes. Eur J Gynaecol Oncol 23:527-532, 2002.
30. World Health Organization: Cancer Pain Relief and Palliative Care. Geneva, Switzerland, 1996.
31. Portenoy RK, Hagen NA: Breakthrough pain: Definition, prevalence and characteristics. Pain 41:273-281, 1990.
32. Patt RB: Classification of cancer pain and cancer pain syndromes. In Patt RB (ed): Cancer pain. Philadelphia, Lippincott, 1993, pp 3-22.
33. Hall EJ, Sykes NP: Analgesia for patients with advanced disease. I. Postgrad Med J 80:148-154, 2004.
34. Mercadante S, Casuccio A, Agnello A, et al: Analgesic effects of nonsteroidal anti-inflammatory drugs in cancer pain due to somatic or visceral mechanisms. J Pain Symptom Manage 17:351-356, 1999.
35. Vielhaber A, Portenoy RK: Advances in cancer pain management. Hematol Oncol Clin North Am 16:527-541, 2002.
36. Friedman LL, Rodgers PE: Pain management in palliative care. Clin Fam Pract 6:371, 2004.
37. Forman A: Peripheral neuropathy in cancer patients: Clinical types, etiology, and presentation. Part 2. Oncology (Huntingt) 4:85-89, 1990.
38. Caraceni A, Portenoy RK: An international survey of cancer pain characteristics and syndromes. IASP Task Force on Cancer Pain. International Association for the Study of Pain. Pain 82:263-274, 1999.
39. Mundy GR: Mechanisms of bone metastasis. Cancer 80(8 Suppl):1546-1556, 1997.
40. Lema MJ: Emerging options with coxib therapy. Cleve Clin J Med 69 Suppl 1: SI76-SI84, 2002.
41. Mercadante S: Malignant bone pain: Pathophysiology and treatment. Pain 69:1-18, 1997.
42. Mach DB, Rogers SD, Sabino MC, et al: Origins of skeletal pain: sensory and sympathetic innervation of the mouse femur. Neuroscience 113:155-166, 2002.
43. Donovan-Rodriguez T, Dickenson AH, Urch CE: Gabapentin normalizes spinal neuronal responses that correlate with behavior in a rat model of cancer-induced bone pain. Anesthesiology 102:132-140, 2005.
44. Brown JA, Von Roenn JH: Symptom management in the older adult. Clin Geriatr Med 20:621-640, v-vi, 2004.
45. Smith MR: Bisphosphonates to prevent skeletal complications in men with metastatic prostate cancer. J Urol 170:S55-S57, 2003.
46. Bolay H, Moskowitz MA: Mechanisms of pain modulation in chronic syndromes. Neurology 59(5: Suppl 2):S2-S7, 2002.
47. Millan MJ: The induction of pain: An integrative review. Prog Neurobiol 57:1-164, 1999.
48. Samad T: New understandings of the link between acute pain and chronic pain: Can we prevent long-term sequelae? In Carr DB, Novak G, Rathmell JP, et al (eds): The Spectrum of Pain. New York, McMahon Publishing Group, 2004, pp 16-27.
49. Scholz J, Woolf CJ: Can we conquer pain? Nat Neurosci 5(Suppl):1062-1067, 2002.
50. Schafers M, Marziniak M, Sorkin LS, et al: Cyclooxygenase inhibition in nerve-injury- and TNF-induced hyperalgesia in the rat. Exp Neurol 185:160-168, 2004.
51. Dworkin RH, Backonja M, Rowbotham MC, et al: Advances in neuropathic pain: Diagnosis, mechanisms, and treatment recommendations. Arch Neurol 60:1524-1534, 2003.
52. Julius D, Basbaum AI: Molecular mechanisms of nociception. Nature 413:203-210, 2001.
53. Mantyh PW, Nelson CD, Sevcik MA, et al: Molecular mechanisms that generate and maintain cancer pain. In Dostrovsky JO, Carr DB, Koltzenburg M (eds): Proceedings of the 10th World Congress on Pain, Progress in Pain Research and Management, Vol 24. Seattle, IASP Press, 2003, pp 663-681.
54. Mantyh PW, Clohisy DR, Koltzenburg M, et al: Molecular mechanisms of cancer pain. Nat Rev Cancer 2:201-209, 2002.
55. Markenson JA: Mechanisms of chronic pain. Am J Med 101:6S-18S, 1996.
56. Barry WC: Sensory transduction. In: Boron WF, Boulpaep EL (eds): Medical Physiology. Philadelphia, Saunders, 2005, pp 325-358.
57. McCleskey EW: Neurobiology: New player in pain. Nature 424:729-730, 2003.
58. de Leon-Casasola OA: Pain perception, translation and modulation. In Program Book, the American Academy of Pain Medicine 20th Annual Meeting, 2004, pp 93-99.
59. Sendil-Keskin D, Altunay H, Wise DL, et al: In vivo pain relief effectiveness of an

analgesic-anesthetic carrying biodegradable controlled release rod systems. J Biomater Sci Polym Educ 14:497–514, 2003.

60. Turk DC: Remember the distinction between malignant and benign pain? Well, forget it. Clin J Pain 18:75–76, 2002.

61. Farquhar-Smith WP, Jaggar SI, Rice AS: Attenuation of nerve growth factor-induced visceral hyperalgesia via cannabinoid CB(1) and CB(2)-like receptors. Pain 97:11–21, 2002.

62. Sommer C, Schäfers M: Mechanisms of neuropathic pain: The role of cytokines. Drug Discov Today 1:441–448, 2004.

63. Walker JS: NSAID: An update on their analgesic effects. Clin Exp Pharmacol Physiol 22:855–860, 1995.

64. Napoli C, Ignarro LJ: Nitric oxide-releasing drugs. Annu Rev Pharmacol Toxicol 43:97–123, 2003.

65. Abramson SB, Amin AR, Clancy RM, et al: The role of nitric oxide in tissue destruction. Best Pract Res Clin Rheumatol 15:831–845, 2001.

66. Lee JI, Burckart GJ: Nuclear factor kappa B: important transcription factor and therapeutic target. J Clin Pharmacol 38:981–993, 1998.

67. Lee KM, Kang BS, Lee HL, et al: Spinal NF-kB activation induces COX-2 upregulation and contributes to inflammatory pain hypersensitivity. Eur J Neurosci 19:3375–3381, 2004.

68. Issberner U, Reeh PW, Steen KH: Pain due to tissue acidosis: A mechanism for inflammatory and ischemic myalgia? Neurosci Lett 208:191–194, 1996.

69. Jones NG, Slater R, Cadiou H, et al: Acid-induced pain and its modulation in humans. J Neurosci 24:10974–10979, 2004.

70. Mamet J, Baron A, Lazdunski M, Voilley N: Proinflammatory mediators, stimulators of sensory neuron excitability via the expression of acid-sensing ion channels. J Neurosci 22:10662–10670, 2002.

71. Voilley N, de Weille J, Mamet J, et al: Nonsteroid anti-inflammatory drugs inhibit both the activity and the inflammation-induced expression of acid-sensing ion channels in nociceptors. J Neurosci 21:8026–8033, 2001.

72. Malan TP Jr, Porreca F: Lipid mediators regulating pain sensitivity. Prostaglandins Other Lipid Mediat 77:123–130, 2005.

73. Peplow PV: Regulation of platelet-activating factor (PAF) activity in human diseases by phospholipase A2 inhibitors, PAF acetylhydrolases, PAF receptor antagonists and free radical scavengers. Prostaglandins Leukot Essent Fatty Acids 61:65–82, 1999.

74. Teather LA, Wurtman RJ: Cyclooxygenase-2 mediates platelet-activating factor-induced prostaglandin E2 release from rat primary astrocytes. Neurosci Lett 340:177–180, 2003.

75. Sciberras DG, Goldenberg MM, Bolognese JA, et al: Inflammatory responses to intradermal injection of platelet activating factor, histamine and prostaglandin E2 in healthy volunteers: A double blind investigation. Br J Clin Pharmacol 24:753–761, 1987.

76. Morita K, Morioka N, Abdin J: Development of tactile allodynia and thermal hyperalgesia by intrathecally administered platelet-activating factor in mice. Pain 11:351–359, 2004.

77. Woolf CJ, Salter MW: Neuronal plasticity: Increasing the gain in pain. Science 288:1765–1769, 2000.

78. Neumann S, Doubell TP, Leslie T, et al: Inflammatory pain hypersensitivity mediated by phenotypic switch in myelinated primary sensory neurons. Nature 384:360–364, 1996.

79. Siddall PJ, Cousins MJ: Spinal pain mechanisms. Spine 22:98–104, 1997.

80. Siddall PJ, Cousins MJ: Persistent pain as a disease entity: Implications for clinical management. Anesth Analg 99:510–520, 2004.

81. Koltzenburg M: Neural mechanisms of cutaneous nociceptive pain. Clin J Pain 16(3 Suppl):S131–S138, 2000.

82. Samad TA, Moore KA, Sapirstein A, et al: Interleukin-1β-mediated induction of Cox-2 in the CNS contributes to inflammatory pain hypersensitivity. Nature 410:471–475, 2001.

83. Funk CD: Prostaglandins and leukotrienes: Advances in eicosanoid biology. Science 294:1871–1875, 2001.

84. Simmons DL, Botting RM, Hla T: Cyclooxygenase isozymes: The biology of prostaglandin synthesis and inhibition. Pharmacol Rev 56:387–437, 2004.

85. Foegh ML, Ramwell PW: The eicosanoids: Prostaglandins, thromboxanes, leukotrienes, & related compounds. In Katzung BG (ed): Basic & Clinical Pharmacology, 9th ed. New York, McGraw-Hill, 2003, pp 298–312.

86. Christoph T, Buschmann H: Cyclooxygenase inhibition: From NSAIDs to selective COX-2 inhibitors. In: Buschmann H, Christoph T, Friderichs E, et al (eds): Analgesics from chemistry and pharmacology to clinical practice. Weinheim: WILEY-VCH, 2002, pp 13–126.

87. Capdevila JH, Falck JR, Estabrook RW: Cytochrome P450 and the arachidonate cascade. FASEB J 6:731–736, 1992.

88. Poot M, Esterbauer H, Rabinovitch PS, et al: Disturbance of cell proliferation by two model compounds of lipid peroxidation contradicts causative role in proliferative senescence. J Cell Physiol 137:421–429, 1988.

89. Trosko JE, Madhukar BV, Hasler C, et al: Modulated intercellular communication: Consequence of extracellular molecules triggering intracellular changes. In Honn KV, Marnett LJ, Nigam S, et al (eds): Eicosanoids and Other Bioactive Lipids in Cancer and Radiation Injury. Boston, Kluwer Academic Publishers, 1991, pp 285–295.

90. Bockman RS: Prostaglandins in cancer: a review. Cancer Invest 1:485–493, 1983.

91. Wallner BP, Mattaliano RJ, Hession C, et al: Cloning and expression of human lipocortin, a phospholipase A2 inhibitor with potential anti-inflammatory activity. Nature 320:77–81, 1986.

92. Hirata F, Stracke ML, Schiffmann E: Regulation of prostaglandin formation by glucocorticoids and their second messenger, lipocortins. J Steroid Biochem 27:1053–1056, 1987.

93. Yao XL, Cowan MJ, Gladwin MT, et al: Dexamethasone alters arachidonate release from human epithelial cells by induction of p11 protein synthesis and inhibition of phospholipase A2 activity. J Biol Chem 274:17202–17208, 1999.

94. Hullin F, Raynal P, Ragab-Thomas JM, et al: Effect of dexamethasone on prostaglandin synthesis and on lipocortin status in human endothelial cells: Inhibition of prostaglandin I2 synthesis occurring without alteration of arachidonic acid liberation and of lipocortin synthesis. J Biol Chem 264:3506–3513, 1989.

95. Kennedy AR: Radiation injury and carcinogenesis. In Honn KV, Marnett LJ, Nigam S, et al (eds): Eicosanoids and Other Bioactive Lipids in Cancer and Radiation Injury. Boston, Kluwer Academic Publishers, 1991, pp 51–59.

96. Glasgow WC, Afshari CA, Barrett JC, et al: Modulation of the epidermal growth factor mitogenic response by metabolites of linoleic and arachidonic acid in Syrian hamster embryo fibroblasts: Differential effects in tumor suppressor gene (+) and (−) phenotypes. J Biol Chem 267:10771–10779, 1992.

97. Cheng HF, Harris RC: Cyclooxygenases, the kidney, and hypertension. Hypertension 43:525–530, 2004.

98. Kramer BK, Kammerl MC, Komhoff M: Renal cyclooxygenase-2 (COX-2): Physiological, pathophysiological, and clinical implications. Kidney Blood Press Res 27:43–62, 2004.

99. Madsen K, Stubbe J, Yang T, et al: Low endogenous glucocorticoid allows induction of kidney cortical cyclooxygenase-2 during postnatal rat development. Am J Physiol Renal Physiol 286:F26–37, 2004.

100. Khan KN, Stanfield KM, Dannenberg A, et al: Cyclooxygenase-2 expression in the developing human kidney. Pediatr Dev Pathol 4:461–466, 2001.

101. Roig F, Llinas MT, Lopez R, et al: Role of cyclooxygenase-2 in the prolonged regulation of renal function. Hypertension 40:721–728, 2002.

102. Ghilardi JR, Svensson CI, Rogers SD, et al: Constitutive spinal cyclooxygenase-2 participates in the initiation of tissue injury-induced hyperalgesia. J Neurosci 24:2727–2732, 2004.

103. Peskar BM: Role of cyclooxygenase isoforms in gastric mucosal defence. J Physiol (Paris) 95:3–9, 2001.

104. Tatsuguchi A, Sakamoto C, Wada K, et al: Localisation of cyclooxygenase 1 and cyclooxygenase 2 in Helicobacter pylori related gastritis and gastric ulcer tissues in humans. Gut 46:782–789, 2000.

105. Gerritsen ME: Physiological and pathophysiological roles of eicosanoids in the microcirculation. Cardiovasc Res 32:720–732, 1996.

106. Zhu X, Conklin D, Eisenach JC: Cyclooxygenase-1 in the spinal cord plays an important role in postoperative pain. Pain 104:15–23, 2003.

107. McAdam BF, Mardini IA, Habib A: Effect of regulated expression of human cyclooxygenase isoforms on eicosanoid and isoeicosanoid production in inflammation. J Clin Invest 105:1473–1482, 2000.

108. Schaefers HJ, Goppelt-Struebe M: Interference of corticosteroids with prostaglandin E2 synthesis at the level of cyclooxygenase-2 mRNA expression in kidney cells. Biochem Pharmacol 52:1415–1421, 1996.

109. Ristimaki A, Narko K, Hla T: Down-regulation of cytokine-induced cyclooxygenase-2 transcript isoforms by dexamethasone: Evidence for post-transcriptional regulation. Biochem J 318:325–331, 1996.

110. Campbell WB: New role for epoxyeicosatri-enoic acids as anti-inflammatory mediators. Trends Pharmacol Sci 21:125–127, 2000.

111. Croxtall JD, van Hal PT, Choudhury Q, et al: Different glucocorticoids vary in their genomic and non-genomic mechanism of action in A549 cells. Br J Pharmacol 135:511–519, 2002.

112. Sano H, Hla T, Maier A, et al: In vivo cyclooxygenase expression in synovial tissues of patients with rheumatoid arthritis and osteoarthritis and rats with adjuvant and streptococcal cell wall arthritis. J Clin Invest 89:97–108, 1992.

113. Goodwin JS, Ceuppens J: Regulation of the immune response by prostaglandins. J Clin Immunol 3:295–315, 1983.

114. Ostensen ME, Skomsvoll JF: Anti-inflammatory pharmacotherapy during pregnancy. Expert Opin Pharmacother 5:571–580, 2004.

115. Dou W, Jiao Y, Goorha S, et al: Nociception and the differential expression of cyclooxygenase-1 (COX-1), the COX-1 variant retaining intron-1 (COX-1v), and COX-2 in mouse dorsal root ganglia (DRG). Prostaglandins Other Lipid Mediat 74:29–43, 2004.

116. Botting R: COX-1 and COX-3 inhibitors. Thromb Res 110:269–272, 2003.

117. Caughey GE, Cleland LG, Penglis PS, et al: Roles of cyclooxygenase (COX)-1 and COX-2 in prostanoid production by human endothelial cells: Selective up-regulation of prostacyclin synthesis by COX-2. J Immunol 167:2831–2838, 2001.

118. Helmersson J, Vessby B, Larsson A, et al: Cyclooxygenase-mediated prosta-glandin F2a is decreased in an elderly population treated with low-dose aspirin. Prostaglandins Leukot Essent Fatty Acids 72:227–233, 2005.

119. Helmersson J, Larsson A, Vessby B, et al: Active smoking and a history of smoking are associated with enhanced prostaglan-din F(2-alpha), interleukin-6 and F(2)-isoprostane formation in elderly men. Atherosclerosis 181:201–207, 2005.

120. Mardini IA, FitzGerald GA: Selective inhibitors of cyclooxygenase-2: A growing class of antiinflammatory drugs. Mol Interv 1:30–38, 2001.

121. Stupnicki T, Dietrich K, Gonzalez-Carro P, et al: Efficacy and tolerability of pantopra-zole compared with misoprostol for the prevention of NSAID-related gastrointesti-nal lesions and symptoms in rheumatic patients. Digestion 68:198–208, 2003.

122. Ma W, Eisenach JC: Cyclooxygenase 2 in infiltrating inflammatory cells in injured nerve is universally up-regulated following various types of peripheral nerve injury. Neuroscience 121:691–704, 2003.

123. Botting RM, Botting JH: The discovery of COX-2. In Pairet M, van Ryn J (eds): COX-2 Inhibitors. Basel, Birkhäuser Verlag, 2004, pp 1–13.

124. Zha S, Yegnasubramanian V, Nelson WG, et al: Cyclooxygenases in cancer: Progress and perspective. Cancer Lett 215:1–20, 2004.

125. Thun MJ, Henley SJ, Gansler T: Inflammation and cancer: an epidemiological perspective. Novartis Found Symp 256:6–21, 2004.

126. Sorokin A: Cyclooxygenase-2: Potential role in regulation of drug efflux and multidrug resistance phenotype. Curr Pharm Des 10:647–657, 2004.

127. Munkarah A, Ali-Fehmi R: COX-2: A protein with an active role in gynecological cancers. Curr Opin Obstet Gynecol 17:49–53, 2005.

128. Jacobs EJ, Thun MJ, Connell CJ, et al: Aspirin and other nonsteroidal anti-inflammatory drugs and breast cancer incidence in a large U.S. cohort. Cancer Epidemiol Biomarkers Prev 14:261–264, 2005.

129. Hoozemans JJ, Veerhuis R, Janssen I, et al: The role of cyclo-oxygenase 1 and 2 activity in prostaglandin E(2) secretion by cultured human adult microglia: Implications for Alzheimer's disease. Brain Res 951:218–226, 2002.

130. Goodwin JS, Atluru D, Sierakowski S, Lianos EA: Mechanism of action of glucocorticosteroids. Inhibition of T cell proliferation and interleukin 2 production by hydrocortisone is reversed by leukotri-ene B4. J Clin Invest 77:1244–1250, 1986.

131. Levine JD, Lam D, Taiwo YO, et al: Hyperalgesic properties of 15-lipoxygenase products of arachidonic acid. Proc Natl Acad Sci USA 83:5331–5334, 1986.

132. Bisgaard H, Kristensen JK: Leukotriene B4 produces hyperalgesia in humans. Prostaglandins 30:791–797, 1985.

133. Roszkowski MT, Swift JQ, Hargreaves KM: Effect of NSAID administration on tissue levels of immunoreactive prostaglandin E2, leukotriene B4, and (S)-flurbiprofen following extraction of impacted third molars. Pain 73:339–345, 1997.

134. Singh VP, Patil CS, Kulkarni SK: Effect of zileuton in radicular pain induced by herniated nucleus pulposus in rats. Inflammopharmacology 12:189–195, 2004.

135. Dallob A, Guindon Y, Goldenberg MM: Pharmacological evidence for a role of lipoxygenase products in platelet-activating factor (PAF)-induced hyper-algesia. Biochem Pharmacol 36:3201–3204, 1987.

136. Moodley I, Stuttle A: Evidence for a dual pathway in platelet activating factor-induced aggregation of rat polymorpho-nuclear leucocytes. Prostaglandins 33:253–264, 1987.

137. McMahon B, Godson C: Lipoxins: Endogenous regulators of inflammation. Am J Physiol Renal Physiol 286:F189–201, 2004.

138. Serhan CN: Lipoxins and aspirin-triggered 15-epi-lipoxin biosynthesis: An update and role in anti-inflammation and pro-resolution. Prostaglandins Other Lipid Mediat 68-69:433–455, 2002.

139. Serhan CN, Chiang N: Lipid-derived mediators in endogenous anti-inflammation and resolution: Lipoxins and aspirin-triggered 15-epi-lipoxins. Sci World J 2:169–204, 2002.

140. Serhan CN, Chiang N: Novel endogenous small molecules as the checkpoint controllers in inflammation and resolution: Entree for resoleomics. Rheum Dis Clin North Am 30:69–95, 2004.

141. Serhan CN, Drazen JM: Antiinflammatory potential of lipoxygenase-derived eicosanoids: A molecular switch at 5 and 15 positions? J Clin Invest 99:1147–1148, 1997.

142. Ferrante JV, Ferrante A: Novel role of lipoxygenases in the inflammatory response: Promotion of TNF mRNA decay by 15-hydroperoxyeicosatetraenoic acid in a monocytic cell line. J Immunol 174:3169–3172, 2005.

143. Bonnans C, Chanez P, Chavis C: Lipoxins in asthma: potential therapeutic mediators on bronchial inflammation? Allergy 59:1027–1041, 2004.

144. McMahon B, Mitchell S, Brady HR, et al: Lipoxins: Revelations on resolution. Trends Pharmacol Sci 22:391–395, 2001.

145. Serhan CN, Hong S, Gronert K, et al: Resolvins: A family of bioactive products of omega-3 fatty acid transformation circuits initiated by aspirin treatment that counter proinflammation signals. J Exp Med 196:1025–1037, 2002.

146. Node K, Huo Y, Ruan X, et al: Anti-inflammatory properties of cytochrome P450 epoxygenase-derived eicosanoids. Science 285:1276–1279, 1999.

147. Spector AA, Fang X, Snyder GD, et al: Epoxyeicosatrienoic acids (EETs): Metabolism and biochemical function. Prog Lipid Res 43:55–90, 2004.

148. Imig JD: Eicosanoid regulation of the renal vasculature. Am J Physiol Renal Physiol 279:F965–F981, 2000.

149. Roman RJ: P-450 metabolites of arachidonic acid in the control of cardiovascular function. Physiol Rev 82:131–185, 2002.

150. Zhu Y, Schieber EB, McGiff JC, et al: Identification of arachidonate P-450 metabolites in human platelet phospholip-ids. Hypertension 25:854–859, 1995.

151. Gebremedhin D, Ma YH, Falck JR, et al: Mechanism of action of cerebral epoxyeicosatrienoic acids on cerebral arterial smooth muscle. Am J Physiol 263:H519–H525, 1992.

152. Collier HO: A pharmacological analysis of aspirin. Adv Pharmacol Chemother 7:333–405, 1969.

153. Polisson R: Nonsteroidal anti-inflamma-tory drugs: Practical and theoretical considerations in their selection. Am J Med 100:31S–36S, 1996.

154. Florentinus SR, Nielsen MW, van Dijk L, et al: Patient characteristics associated with prescribing of a newly introduced drug: The case of rofecoxib. Eur J Clin Pharmacol 61:157–159, 2005.

155. Andersen K, Launer LJ, Ott A, et al: Do nonsteroidal anti-inflammatory drugs decrease the risk for Alzheimer's disease? The Rotterdam Study. Neurology 45:1441–1445, 1995.

156. Breitner JC, Welsh KA, Helms MJ, et al: Delayed onset of Alzheimer's disease with nonsteroidal anti-inflammatory and histamine H2 blocking drugs. Neurobiol Aging 16:523–530, 1995.

157. National Institutes of Health: http://www.nih.gov, accessed on January 30, 2005.

158. Josefson D: FDA warns Merck over its promotion of rofecoxib. BMJ 323:767, 2001.

159. Lenzer J: FDA advisers warn: COX 2 inhibitors increase risk of heart attack and stroke. BMJ 330:440, 2005.

160. FDA website: http://www.fda.gov. Accessed on February 25, 2005.

161. FDA website: http://www.fda.gov. Accessed on April 8, 2005.

162. Chandrasekharan NV, Dai H, Roos KL, et al: COX-3, a cyclooxygenase-1 variant inhibited by acetaminophen and other analgesic/antipyretic drugs: cloning, structure, and expression. Proc Natl Acad Sci USA 99:13926–13931, 2002.

163. Dershwitz M: Analgesic cyclooxygenase inhibitors for ambulatory anesthesia. In Stele SM, Nielsen KC, Klein SM (eds): Ambulatory Anesthesia & Perioperative Analgesia. New York, McGraw-Hill, 2005, pp 215–221.

164. Mitchell JA, Stanford SJ: Cyclooxygenase-2 and the cardiovascular system. In Vane JR, Botting RM (eds): Therapeutic Roles of Selective COX-2 Inhibitors. London, William Harvey Press, 2001, pp 274–287.

165. Mazario J, Gaitan G, Herrero JF: Cyclooxygenase-1 vs. cyclooxygenase-2 inhibitors in the induction of antinociception in rodent withdrawal reflexes. Neuropharmacology 40:937–946, 2001.

166. Dinchuk JE, Liu RQ, Trzaskos JM: COX-3: In the wrong frame in mind. Immunol Lett 86:121, 2003.

167. Silverstein FE, Graham DY, Senior JR, et al: Misoprostol reduces serious gastrointestinal complications in patients with rheumatoid arthritis receiving nonsteroidal anti-inflammatory drugs: A randomized, double-blind, placebo-controlled trial. Ann Intern Med 123:241–249, 1995.

168. Hawkey CJ, Karrasch JA, Szczepanski L, et al: Omeprazole compared with misoprostol for ulcers associated with nonsteroidal antiinflammatory drugs. Omeprazole versus Misoprostol for NSAID-induced Ulcer Management (OMNIUM) Study Group. N Engl J Med 338:727–734, 1998.

169. Yeomans ND, Tulassay Z, Juhasz L, et al: A comparison of omeprazole with ranitidine for ulcers associated with nonsteroidal antiinflammatory drugs. Acid Suppression Trial: Ranitidine versus Omeprazole for NSAID-associated Ulcer Treatment (ASTRONAUT) Study Group. N Engl J Med 338:719–726, 1998.

170. Bombardier C, Laine L, Reicin A, et al: Comparison of upper gastrointestinal toxicity of rofecoxib and naproxen in patients with rheumatoid arthritis. VIGOR Study Group. N Engl J Med 343:1520–1528, 2002.

171. Boers M: NSAIDS and selective COX-2 inhibitors: Competition between gastroprotection and cardioprotection. Lancet 357:1222–1223, 2001.

172. Silverstein FE, Faich G, Goldstein JL, et al: Gastrointestinal toxicity with celecoxib vs nonsteroidal anti-inflammatory drugs for osteoarthritis and rheumatoid arthritis: The CLASS study—A randomized controlled trial. Celecoxib Long-term Arthritis Safety Study. JAMA 284:1247–1255, 2000.

173. Bresalier RS, Sandler RS, Quan H, et al: Cardiovascular events associated with rofecoxib in a colorectal adenoma chemoprevention trial. N Engl J Med 352:1092–1102, 2005.

174. Farkouh ME, Kirshner H, Harrington RA, et al: Comparison of lumiracoxib with naproxen and ibuprofen in the Therapeutic Arthritis Research and Gastrointestinal Event Trial (TARGET), cardiovascular outcomes: Randomised controlled trial. Lancet 364:675–684, 2004.

175. Topol EJ, Falk GW: A coxib a day won't keep the doctor away. Lancet 364:639–640, 2004.

176. Schenck EG, Arend I: The effect of tramadol in an open clinical trial. Arzneimittelforschung 28:209–212, 1978.

177. Biovail Corporation. Tramadol. Drugs R D 5:182–183, 2004.

178. Staats PS, Yearwood T, Charapata SG, et al: Intrathecal ziconotide in the treatment of refractory pain in patients with cancer or AIDS: A randomized controlled trial. JAMA 291:63–70, 2004.

179. Shastri RA: Effect of antacids on salicylate kinetics. Int J Clin Pharmacol Ther Toxicol 23:480–484, 1985.

180. Galeazzi RL: The effect of an antacid on the bioavailability of indomethacin. Eur J Clin Pharmacol 12:65–68, 1977.

181. Tobert JA, DeSchepper P, Tjandramaga TB, et al: Effect of antacids on the bioavailability of diflunisal in the fasting and postprandial states. Clin Pharmacol Ther 30:385–389, 1981.

182. Kothari HV, Lee WH, Ku EC: An alternate mechanism for regulation of leukotriene production in leukocytes: Studies with an anti-inflammatory drug, sodium diclofenac. Biochim Biophys Acta 921:502–511, 1987.

183. O'Neill LA, Lewis GP: Inhibitory effects of diclofenac and indomethacin on interleukin-1-induced changes in PGE2 release: A novel effect on free arachidonic acid levels in human synovial cells. Biochem Pharmacol 38:3707–3711, 1989.

184. Brune K: Safety of anti-inflammatory treatment: New ways of thinking. Rheumatology (Oxford) 43(Suppl 1):i16–20, 2004.

185. Abramson S, Weissmann G: The mechanisms of action of nonsteroidal anti-inflammatory drugs. Clin Exp Rheumatol 7(Suppl 3):S163–170, 1989.

186. Brune K, Beck WS, Geisslinger G, et al: Aspirin-like drugs may block pain independently of prostaglandin synthesis inhibition. Experientia 47:257–261, 1991.

187. Abramson S, Korchak H, Ludewig R, et al: Modes of action of aspirin-like drugs. Proc Natl Acad Sci USA 82:7227–7231, 1985.

188. Yoon JB, Kim SJ, Hwang SG, et al: Nonsteroidal anti-inflammatory drugs inhibit nitric oxide-induced apoptosis and dedifferentiation of articular chondrocytes independent of cyclooxygenase activity. J Biol Chem 278:15319–15325, 2003.

189. Malmberg AB, Yaksh TL: Hyperalgesia mediated by spinal glutamate or substance P receptor blocked by spinal cyclooxygenase inhibition. Science 257:1276–1279, 1992.

190. Bjorkman R: Central antinociceptive effects of non-steroidal anti-inflammatory drugs and paracetamol. Experimental studies in the rat. Acta Anaesthesiol Scand Suppl 103:1–44, 1995.

191. Domer F: Characterization of the analgesic activity of ketorolac in mice. Eur J Pharmacol 177:127–135, 1990.

192. McCormack K: Non-steroidal anti-inflammatory drugs and spinal nociceptive processing. Pain 59:9–43, 1994.

193. Tegeder I, Pfeilschifter J, Geisslinger G: Cyclooxygenase-independent actions of cyclooxygenase inhibitors. FASEB J 15:2057–2072, 2001.

194. Amann R, Peskar BA: Anti-inflammatory effects of aspirin and sodium salicylate. Eur J Pharmacol 447:1–9, 2002.

195. Aceves M, Duenas A, Gomez C, et al: A new pharmacological effect of salicylates: Inhibition of NFAT-dependent transcription. J Immunol 173:5721–5729, 2004.

196. Pratico D: Alzheimer's disease and non-steroidal anti-inflammatory drugs: Old therapeutic tools with novel mechanisms of action? Curr Med Chem CNS Agents 5:111–117, 2005.

197. Weggen S, Eriksen JL, Das P, et al: A subset of NSAIDs lower amyloidogenic Abeta42 independently of cyclooxygenase activity. Nature 414:212–216, 2001.

198. Garcia Rodriguez LA, Jick H: Risk of upper gastrointestinal bleeding and perforation associated with individual non-steroidal anti-inflammatory drugs. Lancet 343:769–772, 1994.

199. Langman MJ, Weil J, Wainwright P, et al: Risks of bleeding peptic ulcer associated with individual non-steroidal anti-inflammatory drugs. Lancet 343:1075–1078, 1994.

200. Perez Gutthann S, Garcia Rodriguez LA, Raiford DS, Duque Oliart A, Ris Romeu J: Nonsteroidal anti-inflammatory drugs and the risk of hospitalization for acute renal failure. Arch Intern Med 156:2433–2439, 1996.

201. Diana FJ, Veronich K, Kapoor AL: Binding of nonsteroidal anti-inflammatory agents and their effect on binding of racemic warfarin and its enantiomers to human serum albumin. J Pharm Sci 78:195–199, 1989.

202. Baum C, Kennedy DL, Forbes MB: Utilization of nonsteroidal antiinflammatory drugs. Arthritis Rheum 28:686–692, 1985.

203. Laine L: Gastrointestinal effects of NSAIDs and coxibs. J Pain Symptom Manage 25(2 Suppl):S32–40, 2003.

204. Phillips AC, Polisson RP, Simon LS: NSAIDs and the elderly: Toxicity and economic implications. Drugs Aging 10:119–130, 1997.

205. Rahme E, Joseph L, Kong SX, et al: Cost of prescribing NSAID-related gastrointestinal adverse events in elderly patients. Br J Clin Pharmacol 52:185–192, 2001.

206. Fox A, Medhurst S, Courade JP, et al: Anti-hyperalgesic activity of the cox-2 inhibitor lumiracoxib in a model of bone cancer pain in the rat. Pain 107:33–40, 2004.

207. Barrett A: Pfizer's funk. Bus Week pp. 72–82, February 28, 2005.

208. Hammond Jr WF: Merck faces flood of Vioxx lawsuits after drug recall. The New York Sun, New York section, October 27, 2004.

209. Hawkey CJ: Quality of life in users of non-steroidal anti-inflammatory drugs. Scand J Gastroenterol Suppl 221:23–24, 1996.

210. Bloom BS: Direct medical costs of disease and gastrointestinal side effects during treatment for arthritis. Am J Med 84:20–24, 1998.

211. Mercadante S, Fulfaro F, Casuccio A: A randomised controlled study on the use of anti-inflammatory drugs in patients with cancer pain on morphine therapy: Effects on dose-escalation and a pharmacoeconomic analysis. Eur J Cancer 38:1358–1363, 2002.

212. Goudas L, Carr DB, Bloch R, et al: Management of cancer pain. Evid Rep Technol Assess (Summ) 35:1–5, 2001.

213. Mercadente S: The use of anti-inflammatory drugs in cancer pain. Cancer Treat Rev 27:51–61, 2001.

214. Curatolo M, Sveticic G: Drug combinations in pain treatment: A review of the published evidence and a method for finding the optimal combination. Best Pract Res Clin Anaesthesiol 16:507–519, 2002.

215. Mangold JB, Gu H, Rodriguez LC, et al: Pharmacokinetics and metabolism of lumiracoxib in healthy male subjects. Drug Metab Dispos 32:566–571, 2004.

216. Brown AK, Christo PJ, Wu CL: Strategies for postoperative pain management. Best Pract Res Clin Anaesthesiol 18:703–717, 2004.

217. Strom BL, Berlin JA, Kinman JL, et al: Parenteral ketorolac and risk of gastrointestinal and operative site bleeding: A postmarketing surveillance study. JAMA 275:376–382, 1996.

218. Macario A, Lipman AG: Ketorolac in the era of cyclooxygenase-2 selective nonsteroidal anti-inflammatory drugs: A systematic review of efficacy, side effects, and regulatory issues. Pain Med 2:336–351, 2001.

219. Palermo S, Gastaldo P, Malerbi P, et al: Perioperative analgesia in pulmonary surgery. Minerva Anestesiol 71:137–146, 2005.

220. Olle Fortuny G, Opisso Julia L, Oferil Riera F, et al: Ketorolac versus tramadol: Comparative study of analgesic efficacy in the postoperative pain in abdominal hysterectomy. Rev Esp Anestesiol Reanim 47:162–167, 2000.

221. Kissin I: Preemptive analgesia. Anesthesiology 93:1138–1143.

222. Oberhofer D, Skok J, Nesek-Adam V: Intravenous ketoprofen in postoperative pain treatment after major abdominal surgery. World J Surg 29:446–449, 2005.

223. Hernandez-Delgadillo GP, Ventura Martinez R, Diaz Reval MI, et al: Metamizol potentiates morphine antinociception but not constipation after chronic treatment. Eur J Pharmacol 441:177–183, 2002.

224. Maves TJ, Pechman PS, Meller ST, et al: Ketorolac potentiates morphine antinociception during visceral nociception in the rat. Anesthesiology 80:1094–1101, 1994.

225. Zhu X, Conklin DR, Eisenach JC: Preoperative inhibition of cyclooxygenase-1 in the spinal cord reduces postoperative pain. Anesth Analg 100:1390–1393, 2005.

226. Ng A, Swanevelder J: Does the opioid-sparing effect of NSAIDs benefit the patient in the postoperative period? J Opioid Manage 1:67–69, 2005.

227. Moiniche S, Kehlet H, Dahl JB: A qualitative and quantitative systematic review of preemptive analgesia for postoperative pain relief: The role of timing of analgesia. Anesthesiology 96:725–741, 2002.

228. Reuben SS, Bhopatkar S, Maciolek H, et al: The preemptive analgesic effect of rofecoxib after ambulatory arthroscopic knee surgery. Anesth Analg 94:55–59, 2002.

229. Rathmell JP (moderator), de Leon-Casasola OA, Viscusi ER: Introducing a new drug into practice: Clinical considerations. A CME Dinner Symposium held during the American Society of Regional Anesthesia (ASRA) 30th Annual Spring Meeting on April 21, 2005.

230. Issioui T, Klein KW, White PF, et al: The efficacy of premedication with celecoxib and acetaminophen in preventing pain after otolaryngologic surgery. Anesth Analg 94:1188–1193, 2002.

231. Brinkmann A, Seeling W, Wolf CF: The impact of prostanoids on pulmonary gas exchange during abdominal surgery with mesenteric traction. Anesth Analg 85:274–280, 1997.

232. Kedek A, Derbent A, Uyar M, et al: Pre-emptive effects of ibuprofen syrup and lidocaine infiltration on post-operative analgesia in children undergoing adenotonsillectomy. J Int Med Res 33:188–195, 2005.

233. Kasai H, Sasaki K, Tsujinaga H: Pain management in advanced pediatric cancer patients: A proposal of the two-step analgesic ladder. Masui 44:885–889, 1995.

234. Pickering AE, Bridge HS, Nolan J, et al: Double-blind, placebo-controlled analgesic study of ibuprofen or rofecoxib in combination with paracetamol for tonsillectomy in children. Br J Anaesth 88:72–77, 2002.

235. MacFarlane LL, Orak DJ, Simpson WM: NSAIDs, antihypertensive agents and loss of blood pressure control. Am Fam Physician 51:849–856, 1995.

236. Pradalier A, Vincent D: Migraine and non-steroidal anti-inflammatory agents. Pathol Biol (Paris) 40:397–405, 1992.

237. Pfaffenrath V, Scherzer S: Analgesics and NSAIDs in the treatment of the acute migraine attack. Cephalalgia 15(Suppl 15):14–20, 1995.

238. Morgenstern LB, Huber JC, Luna-Gonzales H, et al: Headache in the emergency department. Headache 41:537–541, 2001.

239. Ambler JJ, Zideman DA, Deakin CD: The effect of topical non-steroidal anti-inflammatory cream on the incidence and severity of cutaneous burns following external DC cardioversion. Resuscitation 65:179–184, 2005.

240. Vane JR: Inhibition of prostaglandin synthesis as a mechanism of action for aspirin-like drugs. Nat New Biol 231:232, 1971.

241. Eikelboom JW, Hirsh J, Weitz JI, et al: Aspirin-resistant TX biosynthesis and the risk of MI, stroke, or cardiovascular death in patients at high risk for cardiovascular events. Circulation 105:1650–1655, 2002.

242. Lee PY, Chen WH, Ng W, et al: Low-dose aspirin increases aspirin resistance in patients with coronary artery disease. Am J Med 118:723–727, 2005.

243. MacDonald TM, Wei L: Effect of ibuprofen on cardioprotective effect of aspirin. Lancet 361:573–574, 2003.

244. No author listed: Do NSAIDs interfere with the cardioprotective effects of aspirin? Med Lett Drugs Ther 46:61–62, 2004.

245. Gottlieb S: Cardioprotective effects of aspirin compromised by other NSAIDs. BMJ 327:520, 2003.

246. Catella-Lawson F, Reilly MP, Kapoor SC, et al: Cyclooxygenase inhibitors and the antiplatelet effects of aspirin. N Engl J Med 345:1809–1817, 2001.

247. Patel TN, Goldberg KC: Use of aspirin and ibuprofen compared with aspirin alone and the risk of MI. Arch Intern Med 164:852–856, 2004.

248. Fischer LM, Schlienger RG, Matter CM, et al: Current use of nonsteroidal antiinflammatory drugs and the risk of acute myocardial infarction. Pharmacotherapy 25:503–510, 2005.

249. Shiff SJ, Rigas B: Aspirin for cancer. Nat Med 5:1348–1349, 1999.

250. August EM, Nguyen T, Malinowski NM, et al: Non-steroidal anti-inflammatory drugs and tumor progression: Inhibition of fibroblast hyaluronic acid production by indomethacin and mefenamic acid. Cancer Lett 82:49–54, 1994.

251. Hawk ET, Limburg PJ, Viner JL: Epidemiology and prevention of colorectal cancer. Surg Clin North Am 82:905–941, 2002.

252. Baron JA, Cole BF, Sandler RS, et al: A randomized trial of aspirin to prevent colorectal adenomas. N Engl J Med 348:891–899, 2003.

253. Verrico MM, Weber RJ, McKaveney TP, et al: Adverse drug events involving COX-2 inhibitors. Ann Pharmacother 37:1203–1213, 2003.

254. Hawkey CJ: COX-2 inhibitors. Lancet 353:307–314, 1999.

255. Byrne MF, McGuinness J, Smyth CM, et al: Nonsteroidal anti-inflammatory drug-induced diaphragms and ulceration in the colon. Eur J Gastroenterol Hepatol 14:1265–1269, 2002.

256. Bjorkman DJ: Nonsteroidal antinflammatory drug-induced gastrointestinal injury. Am J Med 101:25S–32S, 1996.

257. Hawkey CJ, Naesdal J, Wilson I, et al: Relative contribution of mucosal injury and Helicobacter pylori in the development of gastroduodenal lesions in patients taking non-steroidal anti-inflammatory drugs. Gut 51:336–343, 2002.

258. Chan FK: Should we eradicate Helicobacter pylori infection in patients receiving nonsteroidal anti-inflammatory drugs or low-dose aspirin? Chin J Dig Dis 6:1–5, 2005.

259. Chan FK, To KF, Wu JC, et al: Eradication of Helicobacter pylori and risk of peptic

ulcers in patients starting long-term treatment with non-steroidal anti-inflammatory drugs: A randomised trial. Lancet 359:9–13, 2002.

260. Labenz J, Blum AL, Bolten WW, et al: Primary prevention of diclofenac associated ulcers and dyspepsia by omeprazole or triple therapy in Helicobacter pylori positive patients: A randomised, double blind, placebo controlled, clinical trial. Gut 51:329–335, 2002.

261. Laine L: Proton pump inhibitor co-therapy with nonsteroidal anti-inflammatory drugs: Nice or necessary? Rev Gastroenterol Disord 4(Suppl 4):S33–41, 2004.

262. Roth SH: Efficacy of antacid therapy for NSAID-induced symptomatic gastropathy. Practical Gastroenterol 18:14–20, 1994.

263. Agrawal NM, Roth S, Graham DY, et al: Misoprostol compared with sucralfate in the prevention of non-steroidal anti-inflammatory drug induced gastric-ulcer: A randomized, controlled trial. Ann Intern Med 115:195–200, 1991.

264. Robinson MG, Griffin JW, Bowers J, et al: Effect on ranitidine on gastro-duodenal mucosal damage induced by non-steroidal anti-inflammatory drugs. Dig Dis Sci 34:424–428, 1989.

265. Hawkey CJ: Non-steroidal anti-inflammatory drugs: Who should receive prophylaxis? Aliment Pharmacol Ther 20 Suppl 2:59–64, 2004.

266. Spiegel BM, Targownik L, Dulai GS, et al: The cost-effectiveness of cyclooxygenase-2 selective inhibitors in the management of chronic arthritis. Ann Intern Med 138:795–806, 2003.

267. Hayden M, Pignone M, Phillips C, et al: Aspirin for the primary prevention of cardiovascular events: A summary of the evidence for the U.S. Preventive Services Task Force. Ann Intern Med 136:161–172, 2002.

268. Barnes EV, Edwards NL: Treatment of osteoarthritis. South Med J 98:205–209, 2005.

269. Birnbaum Y, Ye Y, Rosanio S, et al: Prostaglandins mediate the cardioprotective effects of atorvastatin against ischemia-reperfusion injury. Cardiovasc Res 65:345–355, 2005.

270. Lowey MA: High dose COXIBs and NSAIDs increase heart attack risk. Reuters Health Information, 2005. Available at www.medscape.com, accessed on June 14, 2005.

271. Schug SA, Garrett WR, Gillespie G: Opioid and non-opioid analgesics. Best Pract Res Clin Anaesthesiol 17:91–110, 2003.

272. Frishman WH: Effects of nonsteroidal anti-inflammatory drug therapy on blood pressure and peripheral edema. Am J Cardiol 89:18D–25D, 2002.

273. Sowers JR, White WB, Pitt B, et al: The effects of cyclooxygenase-2 inhibitors and nonsteroidal anti-inflammatory therapy on 24-hour blood pressure in patients with hypertension, osteoarthritis, and type 2 diabetes mellitus. Arch Intern Med 165:161–168, 2005.

274. Lee A, Cooper MC, Craig JC, et al: Effects of nonsteroidal anti-inflammatory drugs on postoperative renal function in adults with normal renal function. Cochrane Database Syst Rev (2):CD002765, 2004.

275. Schafer AI: Effects of nonsteroidal anti-inflammatory therapy on platelets. Am J Med 106:25S–36S, 1999.

276. Bjorkman D: Nonsteroidal anti-inflammatory drug-associated toxicity of the liver, lower gastrointestinal tract, and esophagus. Am J Med 105:17S–21S, 1998.

277. Pakulska W: Influence of sertraline on the antinociceptive effect of morphine, metamizol and indomethacin in mice. Acta Pol Pharm 61:157–163, 2004.

278. http://www.nsaids.com, accessed on November 10, 2004.

279. http://www.health-marketplace.com, accessed on March 8, 2005.

280. Chevrier MR, Ryan AE, Lee DY, et al: Boswellia carterii extract inhibits TH1 cytokines and promotes TH2 cytokines in vitro. Clin Diagn Lab Immunol 12:575–580, 2005.

281. Brien S, Lewith G, Walker A, et al: Bromelain as a treatment for osteoarthritis: A review of clinical studies. Evid Based Complement Alternat Med 1:251–257, 2004.

282. Beauchamp GK, Keast RS, Morel D, et al: Ibuprofen-like activity in extra-virgin olive oil. Nature 437:45–46, 2005.

283. Fischer R, Griffin F, Archer RC, et al: Weber ratio in gustatory chemoreception: An indicator of systemic (drug) reactivity. Nature 207:1049–1053, 1965.

284. Hudson N, Balsitis M, Everitt S: Enhanced gastric mucosal leukotriene B4 synthesis in patients taking non-steroidal anti-inflammatory drugs. Gut 34:742–747, 1993.

285. Martel-Pelletier J, Lajeunesse D, Reboul P, et al: Therapeutic role of dual inhibitors of 5-LOX and COX, selective and non-selective non-steroidal anti-inflammatory drugs. Ann Rheum Dis 62:501–509, 2003.

286. Singh VP, Patil CS, Kulkarni SK: Effect of licofelone against mechanical hyperalgesia and cold allodynia in the rat model of incisional pain. Pharmacol Rep 57:380–384, 2005.

287. Cicero AF, Derosa G, Gaddi A: Combined lipoxygenase/cyclo-oxygenase inhibition in the elderly: The example of licofelone. Drugs Aging 22:393–403, 2005.

288. Wallace JL, Miller MJ: Nitric oxide in mucosal defense: A little goes a long way. Gastroenterology 119:512–520, 2000.

289. Becker JC, Domschke W, Pohle T: Current approaches to prevent NSAID-induced gastropathy: COX selectivity and beyond. Br J Clin Pharmacol 58:587–600, 2004.

290. Hawkey CJ, Jones JI, Atherton CT, et al: Gastrointestinal safety of AZD3582, a cyclooxygenase inhibiting nitric oxide donor: Proof of concept study in humans. Gut 52:1537–1542, 2003.

291. Bonnefont J, Courade JP, Alloui A, et al: Mechanism of the antinociceptive effect of paracetamol. Drugs 63:1–4, 2003.

292. Bannwarth B, Netter P, Lapicque F, et al: Plasma and cerebrospinal fluid concentrations of paracetamol after a single intravenous dose of propacetamol. Br J Clin Pharmacol 34:79–81, 1992.

293. Pélissier T, Alloui A, Caussade F, et al: Paracetamol exerts a spinal antinociceptive effect involving an indirect interaction with 5-hydroxytryptamine3 receptors: In vivo and in vitro evidence. J Pharmacol Exp Ther 278:8–14, 1996.

294. Pélissier et al. 1996 + Hunskaar S, Fasmer OB, Hole K: Acetylsalicylic acid, paracetamol and morphine inhibit behavioral responses to intrathecally administered substance P or capsaicin. Life Sci 37:1835–1841, 1985.

295. Bujalska M: Effect of cyclooxygenase and NO synthase inhibitors administered centrally on antinociceptive action of acetaminophen: II. Pol J Pharmacol 55:1001–1011, 2003.

296. Bjorkman R, Hallman KM, Hedner J, et al: Acetaminophen blocks spinal hyperalgesia induced by NMDA and substance P. Pain 57:259–264, 1994.

297. Lucas R, Warner TD, Vojnovic I, et al: Cellular mechanisms of acetaminophen: role of cyclooxygenase. FASEB J 19:635–637, 2005.

298. Graham GG, Scott KF: Mechanism of action of paracetamol. Am J Ther 12:46–55, 2005.

299. Lee Y, Brahim J, Carmona G, et al: Acetaminophen inhibition of COX-2 function in a clinical model of tissue injury. Paper session 324: pain mechanisms: human studies, American Pain Society 2005 meeting. J Pain 6(3, Suppl 1): S6, 2005.

300. Kis B, Snipes JA, Simandle SA, et al: Acetaminophen-sensitive prostaglandin production in rat cerebral endothelial cells. Am J Physiol Regul Integr Comp Physiol 288:R897–902, 2005.

301. Holmer Pettersson P, Owall A, Jakobsson J: Early bioavailability of paracetamol after oral or intravenous administration. Acta Anaesthesiol Scand 48:867–870, 2004.

302. Moller PL, Juhl GI, Payen-Champenois C, et al: Intravenous acetaminophen (paracetamol): comparable analgesic efficacy, but better local safety than its prodrug, propacetamol, for postoperative pain after third molar surgery. Anesth Analg 101:90–96, 2005.

303. Stockler M, Vardy J, Pillai A, et al: Acetaminophen (paracetamol) improves pain and well-being in people with advanced cancer already receiving a strong opioid regimen: A randomized, double-blind, placebo-controlled cross-over trial. J Clin Oncol 22:3389–3394, 2004.

304. Hansten PD, Horn JR: Cytochrome P450 enzymes and drug interactions, table of cytochrome P450 substrates, inhibitors, inducers and P-glycoprotein and footnotes. In: The Top 100 Drug Interactions: A Guide to Patient Management. H&H Publications, Freeland, WA, 2005, pp 157–170.

305. Schmidt LE, Dalhoff K: The impact of current tobacco use on the outcome of paracetamol poisoning. Aliment Pharmacol Ther 18:979–985, 2003.

306. Harati Y, Gooch C, Swenson M, et al: Double-blind randomized, trial of tramadol for the treatment of the pain of diabetic neuropathy. Neurology 50:1842–1846, 1998.

307. Lewis KS, Han NH: Tramadol: A new centrally acting analgesic. Am J Health Syst Pharm 54:643–652, 1997.

308. Sindrup SH, Anderson G, Madsen C, et al: Tramadol relieves pain and allodynia in polyneuropathy: A randomized, double-blind, controlled trial. Pain 83:85–90, 1999.

309. Boureau F, Legallicier P, Kabir-Ahmadi M: Tramadol in post-herpetic neuralgia: A randomized, double-blind, placebo-controlled trial. Pain 104:323–331, 2003.

310. Jackson S, Sweeney BP: The efficacy of pre-emptive tramadol in orthopaedic day-surgery. Ambul Surg 11:7–9, 2004.

311. Wilder-Smith CH, Schimke J, Osterwalder B, et al: Oral tramadol, a mu-opioid agonist and monoamine reuptake-blocker, and morphine for strong cancer-related pain. Ann Oncol 5:141–146, 1994.

312. Brema F, Pastorino G, Martini MC, et al: Oral tramadol and buprenorphine in tumour pain: An Italian multicentre trial. Int J Clin Pharmacol Res 16:109–116, 1996.

313. Petzke F, Radbruch L, Sabatowski R, et al: Slow-release tramadol for treatment of chronic malignant pain: An open multicenter trial. Support Care Cancer 9:48–54, 2001.

314. Babul N, Noveck R, Chipman H, et al: Efficacy and safety of extended-release, once-daily tramadol in chronic pain: A randomized 12-week clinical trial in osteoarthritis of the knee. J Pain Symptom Manage 28:59–71, 2004.

315. Miljanich GP: Ziconotide: Neuronal calcium channel blocker for treating severe chronic pain. Curr Med Chem 11:3029–3040, 2004.

316. Rogawski MA, Loscher W: The neurobiology of antiepileptic drugs for the treatment of nonepileptic conditions. Nature Med 10:685–692, 2004.

317. Staats P, Wallace M, Presley R, et al: Non-opioid analgesics: Other long-term intrathecal ziconotide effectiveness in chronic malignant and nonmalignant pain. J pain 5(Supp 1): S55, 2004.

318. Atanassoff PG, Hartmannsgruber MW, Thrasher J, et al: Ziconotide, a new N-type calcium channel blocker, administered intrathecally for acute postoperative pain. Reg Anesth Pain Med 25:274–278, 2000.

319. Wallace M, Staats P, Presley R, et al: Non-opioid analgesics: Other safety assessment of intrathecal ziconotide treatment for chronic malignant and nonmalignant pain. J pain 5(Supp 1): S55, 2004.

320. Hayek SM, Joseph PN, Mekhail NA: Pharmacology of intrathecally administered agents for treatment of spasticity and pain. Semin Pain Med 1:238–253, 2003.

321. No author listed: Treatment for severe chronic pain. Nurse Pract 30:70, 2005.

322. Penn RD, Paice JA: Adverse effects associated with the intrathecal administration of ziconotide. Pain 85:291–296, 2000.

323. Collins R, Lieberburg I, Ludington E, et al: Effectiveness of intrathecal ziconotide in multiple pain etiologies: A meta-analysis of three controlled trials. In AAPM Annual Meeting Abstracts. Pain Med 6:165–197, 2005.

324. Webster L: Efficacy of intrathecal ziconotide for the treatment of severe chronic pain in adults. In AAPM Annual Meeting Abstracts. Pain Med 6:165–197, 2005.

CHAPTER 22

Tricyclic Antidepressants

THERESA A. MAYS, PHARMD, BCOP

Fifty-five to eighty-five percent of cancer patients will experience pain at some point in their illness. Severity of pain is related to the type and location of the malignancy and the extent of the disease.[1] Over 800,000 Americans and 18 million people worldwide are affected by cancer pain. The undertreatment of pain still exists, with greater than 50% of patients in developed countries suffering from unrelieved cancer pain. The use of adjuvant analgesics, in addition to other appropriate measures to manage pain, should improve the overall experience of patients worldwide experiencing cancer pain.

Tricyclic antidepressants (TCAs) are the most studied agents used as adjuvants in the management of pain. Published studies have examined their effects in diabetic neuropathy, postherpetic neuralgia, atypical facial pain, central pain, and low back pain. These agents are useful in cancer patients on opioid agents who have persistent neuropathic pain, pain with depression, and pain causing insomnia. Pain relief may be noted after several doses and definitely occurs before any antidepressant effect of the agents. The addition of a TCA to an existing opioid regimen may cause an "opioid sparing" effect resulting in the ability to lower the opioid dose.

This chapter discusses the clinical evidence for the use of TCAs in pain management and palliative care. Unfortunately, few clinical trials have been performed in oncology patients; however, the existing trials will be reviewed and presented. In addition, this chapter presents extensive information on dosing, adverse effects, and drug interactions to guide you in selecting appropriate TCAs for specific patients. Table 22–1 lists the TCAs and their available dosage forms and strengths. Table 22–2 includes initial dosing recommendations and dose ranges for both adults and elderly patients.

MECHANISM OF ACTION

One of the simplest ways to visualize the mechanism of action of TCAs is as five drugs in one. These agents act as serotonin reuptake inhibitors, norepinephrine reuptake inhibitors, anticholinergic–antimuscarinic drugs, alpha-1 adrenergic antagonists, and antihistamines.[2-4] The binding affinity for these receptors vary from agent to agent and should be considered when deciding which medication to use in an individual patient. Side effects such as constipation, dry mouth, ocular changes, and urinary hesitancy are associated with muscarinic receptor antagonism. Sedation is caused by blockade of the histamine type-1 receptor, whereas orthostatic hypotension is related to peripheral alpha-adrenoreceptor blockade.[5-7]

When TCAs are first administered to a patient, dopamine, noradrenaline, and serotonin levels are increased and continual dosing appears to stabilize these receptors. Various chemicals have been implicated in mediating or facilitating the pain process, including platelet-activating factor, bradykinin, serotonin, histamine, substance P, and prostaglandins. Stimulation or activation, or both, of these nociceptors by these chemicals leads to transmission of pain signals via the afferent nerve fibers to the central nervous system.[8]

Various antidepressant agents are thought to be analgesic through a number of mechanisms, including potentiation or enhancement of opioid analgesia, direct analgesic effects, and their antidepressant activity.[7,9] The underlying pathophysiology that causes pain is still being discovered; however, both norepinephrine and serotonin play an important role in this process.[6] Norepinephrine is an inhibitory transmitter that activates descending inhibitory pathways and has been associated with hyperalgesia in patients. Serotonin can activate the primary afferent nerve fibers via 5-HT$_3$ receptors. In addition, serotonin can cause mechanical hyperalgesia, most likely by effects on the 5-HT$_{1A}$-receptor subtype. Other authors have hypothesized that antidepressant agents effects at histamine receptors and direct neuronal activity may also contribute to their ability to provide pain relief.[9] Experiments indicate that excitation and sensitization of afferents are mediated by H$_1$ and not by H$_2$ or H$_3$ receptors.

TABLE 22–1 Tricyclic Antidepressants

Generic Name	Trade Name	Generic Available?	Available Dosage Forms and Strengths
Tertiary Amines			
Amitriptyline	Elavil, Enovil	Yes	Tablet: 10 mg, 25 mg, 50 mg, 75 mg, 100 mg, 150 mg Injection: 10 mg/mL (10 mL)
Clomipramine	Anafranil	Yes	Capsule: 25 mg, 50 mg, 75 mg
Doxepin	Adapin, Sinequan	Yes (capsule, solution)	Capsule: 10 mg, 25 mg, 50 mg, 75 mg, 100 mg, 150 mg Cream: 5%, 30 g, 45 g (contains benzyl alcohol) Solution: 10 mg/mL, 120 mL
Imipramine	Tofranil-PM, Tofranil	Yes (tablet)	Capsule (pamoate): 75 mg, 100 mg, 125 mg, 150 mg Tablet: 10 mg, 25 mg, 50 mg
Secondary Amines			
Amoxapine	Asendin	Yes	Tablet: 25 mg, 50 mg, 100 mg, 150 mg
Desipramine	Norpramin	Yes	Tablet: 10 mg, 25 mg, 50 mg, 75 mg, 100 mg, 150 mg
Nortriptyline	Aventyl, Pamelor	Yes	Capsule: 10 mg, 25 mg, 50 mg, 75 mg Solution: 10 mg/5mL (473 mL)
Protriptyline	Vivactil	No	Tablet: 5 mg, 10 mg
Trimipramine	Surmontil	No	Capsule: 25 mg, 50 mg, 100 mg

Modified from Lexi-Comp: Lexi-Comp clinical reference library online. November 15, 2003.

Studies have shown that opioids can be displaced from their binding sites with initial administration of antidepressants. Chronic administration of antidepressant medications can lead to modifications in opioid receptor densities leading to increased endogenous opioid levels. In addition, antidepressant medications can bind to the N-methyl-D-aspartate (NMDA) receptor complex, which reduces intracellular calcium accumulations acutely. Longer term administration alters the receptor binding of NMDA. Finally, antidepressants can inhibit potassium, calcium, and sodium channel activity. Other adjuvant agents, such as anticonvulsants or local anesthetics, are thought to work via effects on the sodium channel.[6] Table 22–3 lists the receptor binding properties of TCAs, their half-lives, and their onset of action.

PHARMACOKINETICS

To date, several studies have examined the pharmacokinetic differences between men and women receiving TCAs. Studies have shown higher plasma concentrations in women than in men for amitriptyline, nortriptyline, imipramine, and clomipramine.[10] The clinical significance of these higher plasma concentrations in women is currently unknown.

There is conflicting information regarding the appropriate dose of TCAs in pain management. Some authors have advocated using doses significantly lower than used for depression. However, other authors have shown poor outcomes with low doses and recommend higher doses. Little data exist to correlate a specific plasma drug concentration to relief of pain in patients receiving TCAs. Two studies have examined the concentration–response relationship between TCAs and pain relief.

Sindrup and colleagues[11] performed a single-blind dose-titration study of imipramine in 15 patients with diabetic peripheral neuropathy. Doses were individually adjusted until plasma concentrations of imipramine and desipramine were well above 400 nmol/L or until all neuropathy symptoms disappeared. Fourteen of the fifteen patients noted excellent symptom relief at or below 400 nmol/L. The plasma concentrations in the 14 patients were below 100 nmol/L when pain was relieved. The authors noted that there was considerable variation and concentrations of 400 to 500 nmol/L were required to ensure a maximum analgesic response in all patients.

McQuay and colleagues[12] performed a randomized, double-blind, crossover study evaluating the analgesic efficacy of amitriptyline in 29 patients with chronic pain. The treatment phases were 3 weeks in length and

TABLE 22-2   Dosing of Tricyclic Antidepressants[a] [14,38-41]

Generic Name	Initial Dose (Adult)	Dose Range (Adult)	Initial Dose (Elderly)[b]	Dose Range (Elderly [mg/day])	Comments
Amitriptyline	25 mg QHS	25–100 mg/day (pain) 50–300 mg/day (depression)	10–25 mg QHS	25–150 mg/day	Increase dose by 25 to 50 mg every week as tolerated Do not administer IV
Amoxapine	25 mg BID to TID	50–300 mg/day Maximum dose: 400 mg (outpatient) 600 mg (inpatient)	25 mg QHS	50–150 mg/day	Increase dose by 25 mg every week as tolerated May be given as a single bedtime dose when <300 mg/day
Clomipramine	25 mg QD	25–250 mg/day	25 mg QD	–	May increase to 100 mg/day during first 2 weeks
Desipramine	75 mg QD	150–200 mg/day, but may require doses up to 300 mg	10–25 mg QD	75–100 mg/day, but may require doses up to 300 mg	Increase dose by 10–25 mg every 3 days for inpatients and every week for outpatients
Doxepin	30–150 mg QHS or in 2–3 divided doses	50–300 mg/day	10–25 mg QHS	10–75 mg/day	Increase dose by 10–25 mg every 3 days for inpatients and every week for outpatients Single doses should not exceed 150 mg Topical: apply QID (at least 3–4 hr apart)
Imipramine	25 mg TID to QID	Maximum dose: 300 mg/day	10–25 mg QHS	50–150 mg/day	Increase dose by 10–25 mg every 3 days for inpatients and every week for outpatients May give total dose QHS
Nortriptyline	25 mg TID to QID	Maximum dose: 150 mg/day	10–25 mg QHS	75 mg QHS (average)	Increase dose by 10–25 mg every 3 days for inpatients and every week for outpatients One of the best tolerated TCAs in elderly patients
Protriptyline	15 mg TID to QID	15–60 mg TID to QID	5–10 mg/day	15–20 mg/day	Increase dose every 3–7 days by 5–10 mg
Trimipramine	50 mg QHS	Maximum dose: 200 mg/day (outpatient) 300 mg/day (inpatient)	25 mg QHS	Maximum: 100 mg/day	Increase dose by 25 mg every 3 days for inpatients and every week for outpatients

[a]Administer all TCAs with caution in patients with hepatic or renal dysfunction.
[b]Start at lower doses and adjust gradually on elderly.
BID, twice a day; QD, daily; QHS, at bedtime; QID, four times a day; TID, three times a day.

TABLE 22–3   Receptor-Binding Properties of TCAs[14,38-42]

Generic Name	Half-Life (hr)	Onset of Therapeutic Effect (days)[a]	Reuptake Antagonism Norepinephrine	Reuptake Antagonism Serotonin	Important Metabolites/ Comments
					Potency/selectivity of TCA for inhibition of NE and 5-HT vary significantly
Amitriptyline	9–25 22–88 (metabolite)	7–21	2+	4+	Nortriptyline (active); 10-Hydroxy-nortripyline, 10-Hydroxy-amitriptyline, demethylnortriptyline
Amoxapine	11–16 (parent) 30 (metabolite)	7–14	3+	2+	7-OH-amoxapine has significant dopamine receptor blocking activity similar to haloperidol 8-Hydroxy-amoxapine (active)
Clomipramine	30–150	14	2+	3–5+	Desmethylclomipramine (active)
Desipramine	7–60	7–21	4+	1–2+	
Doxepin	6–8	14	1–2+	2+	Desmethyldoxepin (active) 2-Hydroxyimipramine Desipramine 2-Hydroxydesipramine
Imipramine	6–18	14	2–3+	3–4+	Desipramine (active) 2-hydroxynortriptyline
Nortriptyline	28–31	7–21	2–3+	2–3+	8-Hydroxyamoxapine; 10-Hydroxynoriptyline Blocks cholinergic receptors
Protriptyline	54–92	14	3–4+	2+	
Trimipramine	20–26	7–21	1–2+	1–2+	2-Hydroxydesipramine

Symbols: 4+ = high, 3+ = moderate, 2+ = low, 1+ = very low, 0 = none.
[a]Based on antidepressant literature.

various doses of amitriptyline were evaluated (25 mg, 50 mg, and 75 mg/day). The 75 mg/day dose had greater analgesic efficacy in patients without significant difference in depression scores. Not surprisingly, side effects were greater with the 75 mg dose versus the lower doses.

On the basis of this information, obtaining plasma drug concentrations may be useful in patients who are not responding to therapy. Low levels may reveal patients who are poor absorbers or rapid metabolizers of these drugs and dose escalation is appropriate. Conversely, if the level is in the upper limit of the antidepressant range, further dose escalation is not warranted and the patient should be switched to another adjuvant analgesic.[13] Studies have shown up to a 30-fold variation in absorption for amitriptyline and patient's ability to tolerate

these agents may vary significantly.[5] Whether this effect was due to drug interactions, ability to absorb the agent, or rapid metabolism is unknown.

DRUG METABOLISM-CYTOCHROME P40 SYSTEM

The TCAs are mainly absorbed through the small intestine via passive diffusion, which continues even in the presence of malabsorption. These agents are lipophilic and have a high affinity for binding to plasma proteins and extensive distribution into fat. However, these drugs undergo a significant hepatic first-pass effect that results in approximately a 50% reduction in bioavailability.

These agents should be used with caution in patients with hepatic impairment. TCAs are primarily metabolized (55% to 85%) via the liver by the cytochrome P-450 system with renal elimination not having a significant role in primary elimination. However, the majority of metabolites are eliminated renally and may require decreased doses in patients with renal dysfunction.[7]

The cytochrome P-450 (CYP) system is involved in phase I metabolism and is estimated to be responsible for the metabolism of about 75% of medications currently on the market. The key enzymes for drug metabolism in humans, in decreasing order of magnitude, include CYP3A4 (50%), CYP2D6 (25%), CYP2C8/9 (15%), then CYP1A2, CYP2C19, CYP2A6, and CYP2E1. Certain CYP isoenzymes exhibit genetic polymorphisms, including CYP2B6 (3% to 4% Caucasians), CYP2C9 (1% to 3% Caucasians), CYP2C19 (3% to 5% Caucasian, 15% to 20% Asians), and CYP2D6 (5% to 10% Caucasians). These polymorphisms can result in either slow metabolizers or rapid metabolizers. This can result in slower metabolism and elimination of these agents, leading to increased toxicity. In addition, these people have a decreased conversion of codeine, hydrocodone, and oxycodone to morphine leading to decreased pain relief. If patients are on these agents, caution should be exercised when adding a medication also metabolized via the CYP2D6 pathway. Rapid metabolizers require increased doses of medications to achieve effect.[7,14-16]

CYP isoenzymes can also be induced (leading to decreased serum concentrations) or inhibited (leading to increased serum concentrations) by other medications. Isoenzyme induction may take several days to reach peak activity and can take several days to months to return to normal once medication is stopped. Inhibition can occur by several mechanisms, including reversible competition for the enzyme site or changing the functionality or structure of the enzyme. To further complicate the issue, a medication may affect a variety of CYP isoenzymes as a substrate, inducer or inhibitor, but only one or two of these interactions will be significant. This makes determination of the significance of CYP drug interactions difficult.[14]

When evaluating medications metabolized via the CYP system, one must evaluate the CYP isoenzymes that contribute to the metabolism of the substrate and the relative effectiveness of the inhibiting or inducting agent on this same isoenzyme. Other considerations include additional metabolic pathways, such as glucuronidation and P-glycoprotein.[14] Table 22–4 contains the CYP isoenzymes involved in the metabolism of

---

TABLE 22–4 Tricyclic Antidepressant Inhibitory Potential on the Cytochrome P450 Enzyme[14-16,38-41,43]

Generic Name	Receptors						
	CYP1A2	CYP2B6	CYP2C8/9	CYP2C19	CYP2D6	CYP2E1	CYP3A4
Amitriptyline	Substrate Inhibitor	Substrate	Substrate Inhibitor	Substrate Inhibitor	**Substrate** Inhibitor	Inhibitor	Substrate
Amoxapine		Substrate			**Substrate**		
Clomipramine	**Substrate**			**Substrate**	**Substrate** **Inhibitor**		Substrate
Desipramine	Substrate				Substrate Inhibitor	Inhibitor	
Doxepin	**Substrate**				**Substrate**		**Substrate**
Imipramine	Substrate Inhibitor	Substrate		**Substrate** Inhibitor	**Substrate** Inhibitor	Inhibitor	Substrate
Nortriptyline	Substrate			Substrate	**Substrate** Inhibitor	Inhibitor	Substrate
Protriptyline					Substrate		
Trimipramine				**Substrate**	**Substrate**		**Substrate**

Bolded text = enzyme appears to play a clinically significant role in drug's metabolism.
- Grapefruit juice may inhibit the metabolism of some TCAs and clinical toxicity may result.
- Avoid concurrent use of valerian, St. John's wort, SAMe, and kava kava with TCA.
- All TCAs are highly protein bound.
- ↑ Plasma concentrations of TCA: Cimetidine, diltiazem, SSRIs, haloperidol, methylphenidate, oral contraceptives, phenothiazines, verapamil.
- ↓ Plasma concentrations of TCA: Barbiturates, carbamazepine, phenytoin.
- TCA ↑ plasma concentrations of oral anticoagulants and hydantoins and ↓ plasma concentrations of levodopa.
TCA, tricyclic antidepressant; SAMe, S-Adenosylmethionine; SSRI, selective serotonin reuptake inhibitor.

the TCAs. When adding one of the agents to existing medications, it is very important to screen for relevant drug interactions.

CLINICAL TRIALS IN PAIN MANAGEMENT

There are over 125 trials published in the literature evaluating the use of TCAs in the management of pain. Forty one of these trials are placebo-controlled and all of these trials support the use of TCAs in the management of pain. Thirteen trials have examined these agents in the management of neuropathic pain. Amitriptyline is the most studied agent in this class, but data also exist for desipramine, imipramine, nortriptyline, clomipramine, and doxepin.[9,17] None of these trials were performed in oncology patients; however, we will review some of the pertinent trials in neuropathic pain and other pain syndromes and extrapolate this data to the oncology population.

Meta-Analyses in Nononcology Pain

In 1996 McQuay and colleagues[18] published a meta-analysis of randomized controlled trials of antidepressants in neuropathic pain. The authors reported their findings using odds ratios and the number needed to treat (NNT), which provides the number of patients needing to be treated for one patient to receive a positive outcome with the agents studied. A trial was considered to have a positive outcome if pain was relieved by >50%. A total of 18 trials met the inclusion criteria and several of these trials contained multiple treatment arms. This resulted in 21 placebo-controlled treatment arms and 11 active control arms. Four hundred patients were treated with 10 different antidepressants and 373 patients received placebo. Thirteen trials were in patients with diabetic peripheral neuropathy and in six of these trials the odds ratios showed significant benefit versus placebo. For all 13 trials the odds ratio was 3.6 (95% CI 2.5–5.2) and the overall NNT was 3 (95% CI 2.4–4), which included 9 different antidepressant agents. The NNT increased to 3.2 (95% CI 2.3–4.8) when just TCAs were evaluated. Four trials used imipramine and when combined the NNT was 3.7 (95% CI 2.3–9.5), two trials used desipramine and when combined the NNT was 3.2 (1.9–9.7).

In patients with postherpetic neuropathy, two of the three studies had significant benefit seen in the odds ratio. The combined odds ratio was 6.8 (95% CI 3.4–14.3) and the NNT was 2.3 (95% CI 1.7–2.3). Both studies in atypical facial pain had a significant odds ratio that combined was 4.1 (95% CI 2.3–7.5) with an NNT of 2.8 (95% CI 2–4.7). For all pain indications, the TCAs have an NNT of 2.9 (95% CI 2.4–3.7). The authors also

evaluated the overall incidence of minor adverse effects with a calculated NNT of 3.7 (95% CI 2.9–5.2) and for major adverse effects an NNT of 22 (95% CI 13.5–58). A simpler way to view this data is that if 100 patients with neuropathic pain are treated with antidepressants, 30 patients will experience greater than 50% relief of their pain, 30 patients will have minor adverse effects, and 4 patients will have to discontinue treatment secondary to a major adverse effect.

In 1999, Sindrup and Jensen[19] published a meta-analysis evaluating all pharmacologic treatments for neuropathic pain also using the NNT. The NNT did not change for either postherpetic neuropathy or diabetic peripheral neuropathy from the previous McQuay analysis.[18] When TCAs were separated from other antidepressants for treatment of diabetic peripheral neuropathy the NNT was 2.5 (95% CI 2.0–3.0). The authors also separated the TCAs by receptor inhibition group imipramine, amitriptyline, and clomipramine as "balanced" reuptake inhibitors of both serotonin and norepinephrine and desipramine and maprotiline as selective norepinephrine reuptake inhibitors. The NNT in patients with diabetic peripheral neuropathy for balanced reuptake inhibitors was 2 (95% CI 1.7–2.5) and 3.4 (95% CI 2.3–6.6) for the selective norepinephrine reuptake inhibitors.

In 2000, Collins and colleagues[20] reported an updated meta-analysis for both antidepressants and anticonvulsants in patients with peripheral diabetic neuropathy and postherpetic neuralgia. The authors calculated the NNT for each pain indication and the number-needed-to-harm (NNH). Twelve studies were included in patients with diabetic peripheral neuropathy and the overall NNT was 3.4 (95% CI 2.6–4.7). When agents other than the TCAs were excluded from the analysis the relative benefit was 1.9 (95% CI 1.5–2.3) and the NNT was 3.5 (95% CI 2.5–5.6). The data in postherpetic neuropathy was pulled from three trials and the overall NNT was 2.1 (95% CI 1.7–3) for all antidepressants. The NNH for minor adverse effects of antidepressants compared with placebo was 2.7 (95% CI 2.1–3.9). The NNH for major adverse effects of antidepressants compared with placebo was 17 (95% CI 11–43).

The authors concluded that for every three people treated with TCAs for either pain condition, one patient would have greater than 50% pain relief, and one would have a minor adverse effect. A major adverse effect would occur in 1 person out of every 17 treated with an antidepressant resulting in withdrawal from therapy.

Topical Application of TCAs (Amitriptyline and Doxepin)

In 1999, Scott and colleagues reported a single patient's experience with topical amitriptyline to treat pain and depression.[21] The patient was unable to take medication orally secondary to severe inflammatory bowel disease. In the past the patient had responded to amitriptyline, but failed sertraline therapy for depression. For 19 days the patient received amitriptyline 80 mg per day administered intramuscularly and achieved a serum plasma concentration of 201 ng/mL. These injections were discontinued because of pain and the patient was switched to a transdermal amitriptyline gel at a dose of 150 mg. This formulation was specially compounded using a lecithin organogel base, as topical amitriptyline is not commercially available. Serum concentrations were monitored 7 days after the change in therapy and were in the therapeutic range (50 to 250 ng/mL). This patient's abdominal pain did not respond to either dosage form of amitriptyline. Even though the patient reported mood improvement, his psychiatrist determined the patient's depression did not respond to the transdermal formulation.

In 2000, McCleane[22] reported a randomized, double-blind, placebo-controlled study of the topical application of doxepin, capsaicin, and a combination of the two. A total of 200 patients with chronic neuropathic pain were enrolled in the trial with 151 patients able to be evaluated. Patients were randomized to placebo consisting of an aqueous cream (group A, 41 patients), 3.3% doxepin cream (group B, 41 patients), 0.025% capsaicin (group C, 33 patients), or 3.3% doxepin plus 0.025% capsaicin (group D, 36 patients). Commercially available doxepin and capsaicin were compounded with the placebo cream to yield the lower concentration and in the combination arm all three creams were mixed together. Patients were instructed to apply the cream three times daily in size equal to a grain of rice. They were to record study measurements using a visual analog score daily for the entire 4-week study period.

Baseline scores were similar between all four groups. The overall pain rating remained consistent in patients on placebo and decreased by 0.9 (95% CI 0.34–1.46) in the doxepin group ($P < 0001$), 1.12 (95% CI 0.44–1.8) in capsaicin group ($P < 0.001$), and 1.07 (95% CI 0.39–1.75) in the combination group ($P < 0.001$). All active treatment groups achieved a statistically significant difference versus placebo after 2 weeks of treatment. The rating for burning pain also remained at baseline for placebo group but increased in the doxepin, capsaicin, and combination group during the first week and then achieved a statistically significant decrease in all 3 active treatment groups in subsequent weeks. Sensitivity ratings and shooting pain were unchanged for patients receiving placebo and doxepin, but were decreased in the capsaicin group and the combination group.

Overall, side effects were minor and included drowsiness (doxepin groups), skin rash (doxepin), itching (doxepin), and headache (combination group). Eighty-one percent of patients receiving the capsaicin, 61 percent of patients on combination therapy, and 17 percent of patients on doxepin reported burning discomfort on application. The combination product had a quicker onset of pain score reduction during the first week of application.

An abstract was published in 2002[23] for a pilot study in oncology patients with chemotherapy-induced painful polyneuropathy. A total of eight patients were randomized to placebo or commercially available doxepin 5% cream applied three times a day. Patients were followed for 4 weeks, and pain was assessed using neuropathic pain scales at baseline and weekly. A reduction in thermal dysesthesia was demonstrated in the doxepin treatment ($P < 0.05$) and a trend toward reduction in pain intensity was observed ($P = 0.06$). There were no significant side effects reported.

Cancer Pain

There are very few trials that have been conducted with TCAs for the management of pain in oncology patients. Breitbart[9] lists 16 trials (both controlled and uncontrolled) with TCAs in oncology patients, starting in 1969 and ending in 1998. Over half of these trials are published in languages other than English and are not discussed in this chapter.

Ehrnrooth and colleagues[24] recently reported a randomized trial of opioids versus TCAs for radiation-induced mucositis pain in patients with head and neck cancer. Patients describe mucositis pain as burning and stinging, which mimics the pain seen with herpes zoster. This led the authors to try TCAs in some of their patients. On the basis of this success, they conducted a randomized trial to determine the overall efficacy of these agents. A total of 43 patients participated in the trial over a 4-year period. Patients were included if they had radiation-induced pain not sufficiently managed with "weak" analgesics (acetaminophen) and a biopsy-verified diagnosis of head and neck cancer. Patients were excluded if they had cancer-related pain before initiation of radiotherapy or were on opioids, TCAs, or nonsteroidal anti-inflammatory agents.

Patients were randomized to morphine 5 mg every 4 hours and as needed or nortriptyline 50 mg daily. Both agents were titrated to adequate pain relief and tolerability with a maximum dose of 150 mg/day for the nortriptyline arm. Patients over the age of 60 years received 25 mg of nortriptyline and all patients in this arm could receive acetaminophen for breakthrough pain. Patients with insufficient pain relief were allowed to have the opposite agent added to their regimen. Assessment of pain occurred at baseline; weekly during radiation; and at 2, 4, and 8 weeks after completion of radiation therapy. Pain was assessed using a 100-mm visual analog scale and a 5-point Likert scale. Patients also completed the Danish version of the McGill Pain Questionnaire, and depression was rated using Beck's Depression Inventory (BDI).

Twenty-two patients received morphine and twenty-one patients received nortriptyline. The groups were unbalanced in the size of elective field, dose, and time to onset of pain after radiation therapy began ($P < 0.05$). Two patients in each arm were not included in the analysis, one patient on the nortriptyline group had dry mouth and discontinued the trial and the remaining 3 patients did not complete the questionnaires. Patients receiving opioid therapy had lower VAS scores at week one and two compared with patients receiving nortriptyline ($P = 0.007$ and 0.04, respectively). Eleven of the patients on the nortriptyline arm had to receive morphine for pain relief, with eight patients being managed alone with nortriptyline. Patients on the nortriptyline arm had higher baseline BDI scores at baseline versus those receiving morphine and these scores decreased during treatment. Adverse effects did not differ significantly between treatment groups.

Given the small patient numbers and the differences between groups at baseline, it is difficult to draw any firm conclusions from this trial. However, patients receiving radiation who develop mucositis may benefit from the combination of opioids plus TCA.

Minotti et al.[25] evaluated the use of diclofenac, diclofenac plus codeine, and diclofenac plus imipramine in oncology patients with chronic pain. Patients were randomized to imipramine 10 mg three times a day (age > 65) or 25 mg three times a day (age < 65) plus diclofenac 50 mg four times a day; codeine 40 mg plus diclofenac 50 mg both agents dosed four times a day; or placebo plus diclofenac 50 mg four times a day. The dose of imipramine was titrated, but to maintain blinding a double-dummy technique was used. Pain ratings were measured using a 100-mm visual analog scale at baseline and after 3 days of therapy (day 4). Patients who had a decrease in pain intensity of at least 50% or below 40 mm were continued on the study for 1 week. Nonresponders were removed and placed on more appropriate analgesic therapy.

The study was appropriately powered to determine if imipramine plus diclofenac and codeine plus diclofenac were different than placebo plus diclofenac. A total of 184 patients were enrolled into the study. Four patients were not evaluated, one patient refused treatment, and three patients received concomitant steroid therapy. Baseline characteristics were similar between the three groups, with more than 50% of patients having bone metastases. Nociceptive pain was the primary complaint in 75.5% of patients enrolled in the study, and 24.5% of patients had neuropathic pain. Thirty patients received subcutaneous morphine during the first 3 days, and results were reported for all patients and for the

150 patients who did not receive morphine. However, the mean VAS scores were similar among all three groups at each visit and no significant difference was found at the end of study between the three groups. The majority of patients withdrew from the study due to inefficacy, with more patients in the codeine plus diclofenac group withdrawing for adverse effects.

The authors concluded that the addition of imipramine or codeine to diclofenac added no additional pain relief compared with diclofenac alone. The results are not surprising given the large number of patients with bone metastases (50%), which tend to respond better to a nonsteroidal anti-inflammatory drug, and the low numbers of patients with a neuropathic pain component (24.5%).

Ventafridda et al.[26] conducted a study on the effect of antidepressant drugs on the antinociceptive action of morphine in both humans and rats. Twenty-four patients who were on a consistent dose of morphine had plasma concentrations for morphine measured alone and after administration of chlorimipramine, amitriptyline, nortriptyline, or trazodone. Patients received the antidepressants for 3 days before plasma measurements. Both chlorimipramine and amitriptyline consistently increased the plasma concentration of morphine, whereas neither trazodone or nortriptyline had any effect on morphine concentrations. Both chlorimipramine and amitriptyline affect serotonin to a greater degree than trazodone or nortriptyline, and the activity of morphine has been tied to serotonin availability.

Magni and colleagues[27] published a survey regarding the use of antidepressants in cancer pain. The survey consisted of 13 questions and was sent to 79 Italian oncology centers. A total of 35 centers responded, and 22 of these used antidepressants for the management of cancer pain. The agents used varied from center to center and included amitriptyline (19 centers); clomipramine (9 centers); imipramine (7 centers); trazodone (5 centers); amineptine and mianserin (2 centers each); and doxepin, nomifensine, nortriptyline and viloxazine in 1 center each. A wide variety of doses were used in each center for the previously listed agents and the various centers reported widely varying incidences of adverse effects. The survey illustrates that TCAs are being used in cancer pain management as adjuvant analgesics, regardless of whether patients have underlying depression.

Breivik and Rennemo[28] performed a retrospective chart review of 111 patients receiving methadone for cancer pain over a 2.5-year period. Half of these patients were treated by the papers' authors and received other psychotropic medications as indicated for hallucination, confusion, nausea, overwhelming pain, depression and anxiety, or insomnia. The other half was treated with methadone during the same time period without adjuvant medications. Only 5 patients out of 56 (8.6%) received amitriptyline 25 to 100 mg for depression or insomnia, or both, (3 patients) or who were having overwhelming pain (2 patients). Overall, patients on combination therapy achieved good pain relief 80% of the time versus 67% in those not receiving adjuvant medications. In the 5 patients on amitriptyline, 3 reported good pain relief, 1 reported moderate, and 1 reported questionable pain relief.

Bourhis et al.[29] performed a trial in French oncology patients to assess overall pain infirmity and the use of psychotropic medications. One hundred patients were observed for 1 week without changes to their analgesic medications. Patients were rated based on level of confinement and pain invasion. Patients were then divided into 3 categories: (1) major syndrome (confinement indoors with total or partial invasion); (2) partial syndrome (confinement indoors without invasion); and (3) minor syndrome (neither confinement nor invasion). Only 19 of the 100 patients were receiving opioid therapy, and the other 81 were receiving "large doses of a minor analgesic." Once the initial evaluation was complete, these therapies were discontinued and the patients were started on psychotropic treatment with levomepromazine and trimipramine. Eight patients had previously received these medications unsuccessfully and were allowed to receive perimetazine, amitriptyline, or sulpiride.

Medication selection was based on patient symptoms, so patients who were depressed or quiet received trimipramine, agitated patients received levomepromazine, and patients with pain plus insomnia received trimipramine during the day and levomepromazine at night. A total of 78 out of 92 patients received trimipramine (48 as a single agent and 31 in combination with levomepromazine). Patients with major syndromes benefited greatest from therapy, followed by partial syndromes, and then minor syndromes. Interestingly, only half of the patients receiving opioid therapy had responses, whereas 43 of 53 patients who were opioid-naive responded to treatment. This led the authors to conclude that previous opioid exposure leads to resistance to psychotropic agents.

Other Studies

In 1999, Grond et al.[30] reported a prospective longitudinal survey of the assessment and treatment of neuropathic cancer pain following the World Health Organization (WHO) guidelines. Over 2 year period all oncology patients referred to an anesthesiology-based pain service were followed prospectively. All patients were treated according to the 1996 WHO guidelines for cancer pain relief (i.e., three-step process). At any point in treatment anticonvulsants, corticosteroids, or antidepressants could be added to treatment. Antidepressant agents were recommended for patients with burning neuropathic pain, with amitriptyline being the drug of choice. Anticonvulsant agents were recommended for patients with stabbing neuropathic

pain, with clonazepam being preferred and carbamazepine being an alternative. Corticosteroids were used in patients with neuropathic pain secondary to nerve compression, with dexamethasone being the preferred agent.

A total of 593 patients were referred over the 2 years with 380 having nociceptive pain, 32 having neuropathic pain, and 181 with a combination of nociceptive and neuropathic pain.

Overall, analgesics were prescribed to 99% of patients with nociceptive pain, 88% of patients with neuropathic pain, and 96% of patients with mixed pain syndromes. Adjuvant analgesics were prescribed in 35% of patients with nociceptive pain, 53% of patients with neuropathic pain, and 59% of patients with mixed pain syndromes. Antidepressants were the adjuvants prescribed in 8% of patients with nociceptive pain, 19% of patients with neuropathic pain, and 25% of patients with mixed pain. The average daily dose of amitriptyline was calculated to be 37 ± 23 mg. Pain intensity scores were significantly decreased from admission to last follow-up in all patient subtypes.

ADVERSE EFFECTS

The adverse effects of TCAs are directly related to their effect on muscarinic, histaminic, and alpha-1 receptors, with increasing incidence directly linked to the binding affinity to these receptors. Table 22–5 shows the relative frequency of the adverse effects discussed next for each agent.

Anticholinergic Effects

Anticholinergic effects appear to be responsible for the cognitive effects seen with TCAs. For older agents in this class, the cognitive effects are dose-related, with subtle cognitive impairment increasing to not-so-subtle impairment as dosages are increased. The elderly are more susceptible to the cognitive impairment associated with TCAs.[31]

Cardiac Side Effects

The TCAs do have cardiac side effects, including orthostatic hypotension, conduction abnormalities, and tachycardia. These agents have not been associated with hypertension or bradycardia. Research has shown that their cardiovascular effects are limited to orthostatic hypotension in patients who have no history of cardiac disease, with an overall incidence of 2% to 3%.[32] Elderly patients have a higher incidence of orthostatic hypotension and are at greater risk from fall injuries.

A recent article reviewed the safety of antidepressant drugs in cardiac patients.[33] TCAs affect cardiac tissue in a similar manner to other class I antiarrhythmics,

TABLE 22–5 Adverse Effects of Tricyclic Antidepressants[14,31,33,38–42,44]

Generic Name	Anticholinergic Effects	Conduction Abnormalities	Orthostatic Hypotension	Tachycardia	Sedation	Seizures	Sexual	Weight Gain
Amitriptyline	4+	3+	3+	3+	4+	3+	2+	4+
amoxapine	3+	2+	2+	2+	2+	3+	0	2+
Clomipramine	3–4+	3+	2+	2+	3–4+	4+	4+	4+
Desipramine	1+	2+	2+	1+	1–2+	2+	1+	1+
Doxepin	2–3+	2+	2+	2+	3–4+	3+	2+	4+
Imipramine	2–3+	3+	4+	2+	2–3+	3+	2+	4+
Nortriptyline	2+	2+	1+	1+	2+	2+	1+	1+
Protriptyline	2–3+	3+	2+	1+	1+	2+	1+	0
Trimipramine	2–4+	3+	3+	2+	3–4+	3+	2+	4+

- Use these agents with caution in patients with a seizure history—may lower seizure threshold.
- Do not administer any TCA within 14 days of a monoamine oxidase inhibitor (MAOI).
- Use with caution in hyperthyroid patients or those receiving thyroid supplementation.
- All TCAs may cause SIADH and alterations in glucose control.
- Amoxapine may cause extrapyramidal side effects.
- Symbols: 4+ = high, 3+ = moderate, 2+ = low, 1+ = very low, 0 = none, - = unknown.

SIADH, syndrome of inappropriate antidiuretic hormone; TCA, tricyclic antidepressant.

including prolongation of intraventricular conduction. Other concerning cardiac effects include postural hypotension, which is seen in up to 20% of cardiac patients receiving TCAs. Patients at an increased risk of experiencing postural hypotension have pretreatment orthostatic drops in systolic blood pressure greater than 10 mm Hg.

The authors concluded that imipramine or doxepin are acceptable agents to use in patients without left ventricular dysfunction or significant coronary artery disease. Imipramine and nortriptyline do not seem to alter left ventricular function in patients who have significant left ventricular dysfunction, defined as an ejection fraction of less than 40%. However, there is a high frequency of orthostatic hypotension in patients receiving imipramine; therefore, nortriptyline may be the preferred agent for this patient population. Nortriptyline seems to have the least effect on blood pressure of the TCAs studied to date.[33]

Due to the TCAs effects on cardiac function in patients with a cardiac history, these agents should not be used as the first line in this patient population for the management of pain.

Seizures

The TCA clomipramine has been linked to seizures, which appear to be dose-related.[31] Other tricyclic antidepressants may increase the risk of seizures, but the risk is usually due to dose and overaggressive use of these agents. One study found a 0.4% incidence of seizures in hospitalized patients who were receiving TCA for affective or panic disorder.

Sexual Dysfunction

The reported incidence of sexual dysfunction associated with TCAs ranges from 25% to 95% of all patients.[34,35] If a patient develops sexual dysfunction there are several published strategies for managing this adverse effect. The first step is to observe the patient for a period of time to ensure that the sexual dysfunction is not a temporary problem. In addition, the patient's medications should be reviewed for other agents that can also cause sexual dysfunction. If the patient continues to experience sexual dysfunction, the dose of the TCA should be lowered if possible. If this is not an option or it does not correct the problem, the TCA should be stopped and a different agent tried.

Syndrome of Inappropriate Antidiuretic Hormone (SIADH)

This adverse effect has been reported infrequently with TCAs. The mechanism behind this adverse effect is unknown; however, animal studies have shown that norepinephrine and serotonin increase antidiuretic hormone section by stimulation of alpha-1 adrenergic receptors and serotonin 5-HT_{1C} and 5-HT_2 receptors, respectively.[36] One study with clomipramine reported a 16.7% incidence of SIADH versus 1.1% with controls. The risk of developing SIADH with antidepressant medications appears to increase in patients who are greater than 65 years of age, smokers, or receiving concomitant diuretics.[31]

Spigset and Hedenmalm[36] published a survey of the World Health Organization Data Base for Spontaneous Reporting of Adverse Drug Reactions for hyponatremia secondary to antidepressants. Reports of hyponatremia existed for amitriptyline, clomipramine, desipramine, doxepin, imipramine, nortriptyline, and protriptyline. The majority of all cases of hyponatremia with antidepressant agents occurred within 1 month of starting treatment (74.9%) and more than half occurred within 2 weeks of starting treatment. A higher incidence of this adverse effect was reported in women and patients older than 70 years.

Therefore, TCAs may not be appropriate adjunct agents for pain management in patients with underlying malignancies that also cause SIADH, such as lung cancer.

Weight Gain

In patients with nononcologic chronic pain, weight gain does occur with TCAs usually secondary to decreased activity. Amitriptyline has been associated with increasing appetite in some patients.

CONCLUSION

The TCAs have been shown to be effective in the management of continuous dysesthetic pain and lancinating neuropathic pain. Studies have been conducted in postherpetic neuralgia, diabetic neuropathy, and central pain states in nononcology patients. These studies have shown pain relieving benefits after about 2 weeks, which seem to peak over a 2- to 4-week period.[5] There are limited clinical trials published using these agents in the oncology population. However, the existing data in oncology patients support the use of these agents as adjuvants for the relief of pain. The choice of a tricyclic agent should be based on the patient's overall symptoms, their risk of adverse effects with the specific agent, and the potential for drug interactions. The tables included in this chapter should aid in guiding your selection of a specific TCA for a patient.

Patients who are experiencing agitation, anxiety, and insomnia may benefit from the more sedating TCAs, including doxepin and amitriptyline.[5,13] Patients suffering from a loss of energy or psychomotor retardation may do better on nortriptyline.[5] Patients who have adequately treated congestive heart failure without symptomatic orthostatic hypotension or markedly impaired cardiac ejection fractions can receive nortriptyline or imipramine. Nortriptyline also seems to cause less orthostatic hypotension when compared with imipramine or amitriptyline.[37] Patients with a focused point of neuropathic pain may respond to the use of topical doxepin.

If a patient is currently receiving codeine, hydrocodone, or oxycodone for pain and has a decreased effect once a TCA is added, the patient may be a poor metabolizer via the CYP2D6 pathway and be unable to convert these drugs to morphine. Changing the patient to another opioid agent, such as morphine or fentanyl, may be appropriate. All of the available TCAs act as a substrate or inhibitor of CYP2D6 and should be used cautiously with paroxetine and fluoxetine both of which inhibit CYP2D6. This interaction could lead to significantly elevated levels of the TCA and toxicities. If a patient is already on a stable dose of paroxetine or fluoxetine, a TCA should be added at a low dose and slowly titrated.

REFERENCES

1. Foley KM: The treatment of cancer pain. N Engl J Med 313:84-95, 1985.
2. Stahl SM: Psychopharmacology of antidepressants. London, Martin Dunitz Ltd, 1997.
3. Stahl S: Basic psychopharmacology of antidepressants, Part 2: Estrogen as an adjunct to antidepressant treatment. J Clin Psychiatry 59(suppl 4):15-24, 1998.
4. Stahl SM: Selecting an antidepressant by using mechanism of action to enhance efficacy and avoid side effects. J Clin Psychiatry 59(suppl 18):23-29, 1998.
5. Teasell R, Merskey H: Antidepressants in rehabilitation. Phys Med Rehabil Clin N Am 10:237-253, 1999.
6. Sawynok J, Esser MJ, Reid AR: Antidepressants as analgesics: An overview of central and peripheral mechanisms of action. J Psychiatry Neurosci 26:21-29, 2001.
7. Berney A, Stiefel F, Mazzocato C, et al: Psychopharmacology in supportive care of cancer: A review for the clinician III. Antidepressants. Support Care Cancer 8(4):278-286, 2000.
8. Baumann TJ: Pain management. In: DiPiro JT, Talbert RL, Yee GC, Matzke GR, Wells BG, Posey LM (eds): Pharmacotherapy: A Pathophysiological Approach, 4th ed. Stamford, Conn, Appleton & Lange, 1999, pp 1014-1026.
9. Breitbart W: Psychotropic adjuvant analgesics for pain in cancer and aids. Psychooncology 7:33-45, 1998.
10. Frackiewicz EJ, Sramek JJ, Cutler NR: Gender differences in depression and antidepressant pharmacokinetics and adverse effects. Ann Pharmacother 34:80-88, 2000.
11. Sindrup SH, Gram LF, Skjold T, et al: Concentration-response relationship in imipramine treatment of diabetic neuropathy symptoms. Clin Pharmacol Ther 47:509-515, 1990.
12. McQuay HJ, Carroll D, Glynn CJ: Dose-response for analgesic effect of amitriptyline in chronic pain. Anaesthesia 48:281-285, 1993.
13. Portenoy RK: Adjuvant analgesic agents. Hematol Oncol Clin North Am 10:103-119, 1996.
14. Lexi-Comp: Lexi-comp clinical reference library online. November 15, 2003.
15. Flockhart DA: Cytochrome p-450 drug interaction table. http://medicine.iupui.edu/flockhart/. November 15, 2003.
16. Kalash GR: Psychotropic drug metabolism in the cancer patient: Clinical aspects of management of potential drug

interactions. Psychooncology 7:307–320, 1998.

17. Lynch ME: Antidepressants as analgesics: A review of randomized controlled trials. J Psychiatry Neurosci 26:30–36, 2001.

18. McQuay H, Tramer M, Nye B, et al: A systematic review of antidepressants in neuropathic pain [see comments]. Pain 68:217–227, 1996.

19. Sindrup S, Jensen TS: Efficacy of pharmacological treatments of neuropathic pain: An update and effect related to mechanism of drug action. Pain 83:389–400, 1999.

20. Collins SL, Moore RA, McQuay HJ, et al: Antidepressants and anticonvulsants for diabetic neuropathy and postherpetic neuralgia: A quantitative systemic review. J Pain Symptom Manage 20:449–458, 2000.

21. Scott MA, Letrent K, Hager KL, et al: Use of transdermal amitriptyline gel in a patient with chronic pain and depression. Pharmacotherapy 19:236–239, 1999.

22. McCleane G: Topical application of doxepin hydrochloride, capsaicin and a combination of both produces analgesia in chronic human neuropathic pain: A randomized, double-blind, placebo-controlled study. Br J Pharmacol 49:547–579, 2000.

23. Brice BL, Clark-Vetri RJ: Topical doxepin 5% cream for chemotherapy-induced painful polyneuropathy. Pharmacotherapy 22:1355, 2002.

24. Ehrnrooth E, Grau C, Zachariae R, et al: Randomized trial of opioid versus tricyclic antidepressants for radiation-induced mucositis pain in head and neck cancer. Acta Oncol 40:745–750, 2001.

25. Minotti V, Betti M, Ciccarese G, et al: A double-blind study comparing two single-dose regimens of ketorolac with diclofenac in pain due to cancer. Pharmacotherapy 18:504–508, 1998.

26. Ventafridda V, Bianchi M, Ripamonti C, et al: Studies on the effects of antidepressant drugs on the antinociceptive action of morphine and on plasma morphine in rat and man. Pain 43:155–162, 1990.

27. Magni G, Arsie D, De Leo D: Antidepressants in the treatment of cancer pain: A survey in Italy. Pain 29:347–353, 1987.

28. Breivik H, Rennemo F: Clinical evaluation of combined treatment with methadone and psychotropic drugs in cancer patients. Acta Anaesthesiol Scand 74(suppl): 135–140, 1982.

29. Bourhis A, Boudouresque G, Pellet W, et al: Pain infirmity and psychotropic drugs in oncology. Pain 5:263–274, 1978.

30. Grond S, Radbruch L, Meuser T, et al: Assessment and treatment of neuropathic cancer pain following WHO guidelines. Pain 79:15–20, 1999.

31. Settle EC, Jr. Antidepressant drugs: Disturbing and potentially dangerous adverse effects. J Clin Psychiatry 59(suppl 16):25–30, 1998.

32. Glassman AH: Cardiovascular effects of antidepressant drugs: Updated. J Clin Psychiatry 59(suppl 15):13–18, 1998.

33. Alvarez W, Jr, Pickworth KK: Safety of antidepressant drugs in the patient with cardiac disease: A review of the literature. Pharmacotherapy 23:754–771, 2003.

34. Hirschfeld RM: Management of sexual side effects of antidepressant therapy. J Clin Psychiatry 60(suppl 17):31–35, 1999.

35. Hirschfeld RM: Care of the sexually active depressed patient. J Clin Psychiatry 60(suppl 17):32–35, 1999.

36. Spigset O, Hedenmalm K: Hyponatremia in relation to treatment with antidepressants: A survey of reports in the world health organization data base for spontaneous reporting of adverse drug reactions. Pharmacotherapy 17:348–352, 1997.

37. Brown TM, Stoudemire A, Fogel BS, et al: Psychopharmacology in the medical patient. In: Stoudemire A, Fogel BS, Greenberg DB (eds): Psychiatric care of the medical patient. vol 2. New York, Oxford University Press, 2000 pp 329–372.

38. Westenberg HG: Pharmacology of antidepressants: Selectivity of multiplicity. J Clin Psychiatry 60(suppl 17):4–8, 1999.

39. Feighner JP: Mechanism of action of antidepressant medications. J Clin Psychiatry 60(suppl 4):4–11, 1999.

40. DeVane CL: Differential pharmacology of newer antidepressants. J Clin Psychiatry 59(suppl 20):85–93, 1998.

41. Kando JC, Wells BG, Hayes PE: Depressive disorders. In: DiPiro JT, Talbert RL, Yee GC, Matzke GR, Wells BG, Posey LM (eds): Pharmacotherapy: A Pathophysiologic Approach, 4th ed. Stamford, Conn, Appleton & Lange, 1999, pp 1141–1160.

42. Lipman AG: Analgesic drugs form neuropathic and sympathetically maintained pain. Clin Geriatr Med 12:501–515, 1996.

43. Greenblatt DJ, von Moltke LL, Harmatz JS, et al: Drug interactions with newer antidepressants: Role of human cytochromes p450. J Clin Psychiatry 59(suppl. 15): 19–27, 1998.

44. Roose SP: Tolerability and patient compliance. J Clin Psychiatry 60(suppl 17):14–17, 1999.

CHAPTER 23

Anticonvulsants

Brian E. McGeeney, MD, MPH

Since 1993 there have been eight novel anticonvulsants (antiepileptic drugs [AEDs]) approved by the U.S. Food and Drug Administration (FDA) and two new intravenous preparations of anticonvulsant (valproic acid and fosphenytoin) drugs.[1] These exciting additions have some advantages over the older agents phenytoin, carbamazepine, valproate, primidone, and ethosuximide. Both newer and older AEDs have great usefulness in a range of disorders beyond their anticonvulsant efficacy. The newer agents have advantages of better side effect profile, fewer drug interactions, fewer enzyme inductions, new mechanisms of action, and broad spectrum of activity. Blood levels of AEDs, a guide to treatment are less commonly employed with the newer agents. Guidelines for the use of the newer drugs and the management of epilepsy have been developed in the United States and the United Kingdom.[2-5] Although having a lot of similarities, there are also differences in the suggested treatment regimens. The UK guidelines are more conservative, recommending the use of the new medications as a first choice only in specific clinical conditions, such as contraindications to or lack of efficacy of older drugs. The long-term outcome and cost-effectiveness of the newer agents compared with the old is being conducted in a randomized controlled trial.[4] About 150,000 people in the United States are diagnosed with epilepsy every year and most are well controlled on a single agent. Of those, as many as 35% of individuals have continued seizures, and the newer agents allow greater options for monotherapy or adjunctive treatment. Although intended as anticonvulsants, these agents have frequent use in neuropathic pain, migraine prophylaxis, and bipolar disorder, among other conditions. The field of pain management in particular has seen large increases in the use of AEDs as adjuvant analgesics, particularly for neuropathic pain.[6] In the United States, five AEDs have FDA approval for pain syndromes: carbamazepine for trigeminal neuralgia, gabapentin and pregabalin for postherpetic neuralgia, pregabalin for painful diabetic peripheral neuropathy,

and divalproex and topiramate for migraine prophylaxis. There have been great advances in the understanding of these agents in recent years but much has yet to be learned. All AEDs modify the excitability of neurons and act on diverse molecular targets, known and unknown. Once a membrane target is identified, its contribution to the effect of interest has to be elucidated.

The main actions of AEDs can be summarized as modulation of voltage-gated sodium channels, modulation of voltage-gated calcium channels, or enhancing the gamma-aminobutyric acid (GABA) inhibitory system. Anticonvulsants still have a burden of side effects, such as rash, occurring in up to 10% of those taking phenytoin, carbamazepine, and lamotrigine. Most AEDs, such as valproate and carbamazepine, are known for their propensity to increase weight. Generally, lamotrigine, levetiracetam, and phenytoin are weight neutral, and topiramate and felbamate are associated with weight loss. Anticonvulsants are variably used in seizure prophylaxis in those with a brain lesion, such as a brain tumor, and no history of seizures. A recent meta-analysis was published of randomized controlled trials evaluating the efficacy of AED treatment compared with no AED treatment for seizure prophylaxis in patients with brain tumors.[7] The clinical trials included patients with primary brain tumors and metastases, all without a seizure history. Phenobarbital, phenytoin, and valproic acid were studied, and four of the five trials analyzed showed no statistical benefit of seizure prophylaxis. It was concluded that there was no benefit from prophylactic use of phenobarbital, phenytoin, or valproic acid to prevent seizures in those with brain tumors and no seizure history. Even with this study, an argument can be made that those tumors with a greater propensity to bleed, such as melanoma or choriocarcinoma may still benefit. There may be important drugs interactions with AEDs in the cancer patient. Enzyme-inducing anticonvulsant drugs may hasten the metabolism of steroids in the treatment of the cancer patient, and also reduce the effects of vinca alkaloids, methotrexate, and other chemotherapeutic agents.[8] Cisplatin and carmustine (BCNU) chemotherapy can reduce blood levels of AEDs.

MECHANISMS OF ACTION

The main actions of AEDs can be summarized as modulation of voltage-gated sodium channels, modulation of voltage-gated calcium channels, or enhancing the GABA inhibitory system.

Voltage-Gated Calcium Channels

Modulation of voltage-gated calcium channels is a major mechanism of action of some AEDs.[9] The intracellular free Ca^{2+} concentration is only 1/10,000 that of the extracellular environment and influx of calcium from calcium channels has important effects on the neuron. Voltage-gated calcium channels can be divided into high-voltage activated (HVA) and low-voltage activated (T-type). Hagiwara and colleagues[10] first suggested that different calcium channels existed, each with different kinetics for opening and closing. Electrophysiologic characteristics allowed a division into HVA and T-type channels, depending on the threshold of activation. The HVA group is further divided into L-type, P/Q type, N-type, and R-type.[11] They require a large membrane depolarization and are largely responsible for calcium entry and neurotransmitter release from presynaptic nerve terminals. Low-voltage channels regulate firing by participating in bursting and intrinsic oscillations. The spike and wave discharges from the thalamus in absence seizures are dependent on T-type calcium channels, and these discharges are inhibited by valproic acid or ethosuxamide. The N-type HVA calcium channels are thought to be largely responsible for neurotransmitter release at synaptic junctions and inactivate particularly quickly. The P/Q type calcium channel is so named because it was first described in the Purkinje cells of the cerebellum in 1989. The T-type channel (named after the transient currents elicited) starts to open with weak depolarization, near resting potential. The L-type channels are found in high concentration in skeletal muscle, and many other tissues such as neuronal and smooth muscle, where it has been most studied. The voltage-gated calcium channel is composed of five polypeptide subunits and is the target of many drugs. Calcium channels consist of an alpha protein along with several auxiliary subunits. The alpha protein forms the channel pore.

Pregabalin and gabapentin are amino acid derivatives of GABA and have been demonstrated to have antiseizure activity and analgesic activity in neuropathic pain. Both agents reduce nociceptive behavior in animal models of neuropathic pain or inflammation, in addition to the antiseizure effect. They bind to the alpha-2-delta subunit of voltage-gated calcium channels with high affinity.[9] The binding of gabapentin or pregabalin to the alpha-2-delta subunit results in inhibition of calcium influx at presynaptic voltage-gated calcium channels. The binding affinity correlates with their antinociceptive and anticonvulsant potencies. Animal models have demonstrated increased expression of the alpha-2 delta subunit of the calcium channel in the dorsal root ganglion secondary to peripheral nerve injury.[12] This subunit is not upregulated in all models of hyperalgesia. The increased expression may explain the relative selectivity of these agents for neuropathic or inflammatory pain. In addition to the actions listed previously, gabapentin has also been demonstrated to elevate GABA levels in the brain.[13] A number of other anticonvulsants can act on HVA calcium channels, including phenobarbital, lamotrigine, and possibly levetiracetam, although they are likely to have more important effects on other systems.

The T-type low voltage–activated calcium channels are also involved in the transmission of neuropathic pain from the periphery and in the spinal cord. Both ethosuxamide and zonisamide inhibit these channels. However, this channel is involved in thalamocortical bursting, and recent evidence suggests this has an inhibitory role on the transmission of pain centrally, hence the use of these medications may be of limited value as antinociceptive agents.

Voltage-Gated Sodium Channels

When neurons are depolarized and approaching an action potential, the voltage-gated sodium channels quickly change conformation in response and permit flow of sodium ions. As described by Hodgkin and Huxley, activation of sodium channels (and other voltage-gated ion channels) derives from outward movement of charged residues as a result of an altered electrical field across the membrane.[76] Sodium channels play an essential role in the action potential of neurons, as well as other electrically excitable cells such as myocytes. The flow of sodium ions is terminated by channel inactivation in a few milliseconds (fast inactivation). Sodium channels can cycle open and close rapidly, which may result in seizures, neuropathic pain, or paresthesias. The structure of the channel is essentially a rectangular tube whose four walls are formed from four subunits—four domains of a single polypeptide. A region near the N-terminus protrudes into the cytosol and forms an inactivating particle. It has recently been demonstrated that a short loop of amino acid residues acting as a flap or hinge blocks the inner mouth of the sodium channel resulting in fast inactivation.[14] The highly conserved intracellular loop is the inactivating gate that binds to the intracellular pore and inactivates it within milliseconds. Site-directed antibody studies against this intracellular loop have prevented this fast inactivation. Phenytoin does not appear to act directly on this mechanism. Phenytoin stabilizes sodium channels in a nonconducting state, separate to fast inactivation. Unlike local anesthetics the binding of phenytoin is slow and the unbinding is slow also.[15]

The voltage-gated sodium channel can be divided into an alpha subunit and one or more auxiliary beta subunits. At least nine alpha subunits have been functionally characterized, termed Nav 1.1 through Nav 1.9.[16] The sodium channels 1.8 and 1.9 are preferentially expressed on peripheral sensory neurons, where they are very important in nociception and may be a future target for channel-specific analgesics.[17] Seven of the nine sodium channel subtypes have been identified in sensory ganglia such as the dorsal root ganglia and trigeminal ganglia. The sodium channel 1.7 is also present in large amounts in the peripheral nervous system. Sodium channel 1.2 is expressed in unmyelinated neurons and Nav 1.4 and Nav 1.5 are muscle sodium channels. Sodium channel mutations have been described, resulting in well-recognized syndromes. A mutation of sodium channel 1.4 is responsible for hyperkalemic periodic paralysis and an inherited long QT syndrome can be caused by mutation of Nav 1.5. A mutation of Nav 1.1 has been shown to be responsible for a syndrome of generalized epilepsy.[18,19]

Increased expression of sodium channels have been demonstrated in peripheral and central sensory neurons in neuropathic pain and is one mechanism for hyperexcitability of pain pathways.[20] Anticonvulsants modulating the gating of sodium channels are phenytoin, lamotrigine, carbamazepine, oxcarbazepine, and zonisamide, with some evidence for topiramate and valproic acid. It is important to note that at clinical concentrations the sodium channel is only weakly blocked when hyperpolarized. When the neuronal membrane is depolarized there is a much greater inhibition in the channel.[9] Binding of the channel by anticonvulsants is slow compared with local anesthetics. The slow binding of AEDs ensures that the kinetic properties of the normal action potentials are not altered. Generally, AEDs have no role in the treatment of acute pain, although they have demonstrated efficacy for chronic pain conditions. Interestingly, the local application of phenytoin and carbamazepine has antinociceptive effect that is more potent than lidocaine.[21] It has been demonstrated that phenytoin, carbamazepine, and lamotrigine bind to a common recognition site on sodium channels, which is likely because of their two phenol groups that act as binding elements.[22] At normal resting potentials, AEDs have little effect on action potentials. In addition to the fast current of the open channel, there is also a persistent sodium current. This current, carried by persistent openings, is a small fraction of the fast current but may have an important role in regulating excitability. There is evidence that a number of AEDs also act by blocking the persistent sodium current, which is separate from the fast sodium current and includes phenytoin, valproate, and topiramate.

Gamma-Aminobutyric Acid Modulation

Gamma-aminobutyric acid (GABA) is the main inhibitory neurotransmitter in the CNS and acts through ligand-gated ion channels. The potentiation of GABA inhibitory transmission is an important mechanism of action of AEDs.[9] There is also evidence that GABA acts as a trophic factor during brain development.[23] GABA is synthesized from glutamate by two glutamic acid decarboxylase enzymes (GAD). GABA activity is rapidly terminated at the synapse by reuptake into nerve terminals and metabolized by a reaction catalyzed by GABA transaminase (GABA-T). Tiagabine is an AED that acts by inhibiting the GABA transporters, which remove GABA from the synaptic cleft. In this way, the effect of GABA is prolonged. The AED vigabatrin is a GABA analog that acts as an irreversible inhibitor of GABA-T, resulting in markedly elevated brain GABA levels. GABA acts through fast chloride permeable ionotropic (intrinsic channel pore) GABA-A receptors and also through slower metabotropic (G protein coupled) GABA-B receptors. Bicuculine is an antagonist of GABA-A but not GABA-B. An ionotropic GABA-C receptor has been recently described, also with an intrinsic chloride-sensitive channel but insensitive to the antagonist bicuculline.

A number of AEDs act on GABA system, either by direct action (benzodiazepines) on the GABA-A receptor or by indirect pathways like valproate and gabapentin, which increase GABA synthesis and turnover. Both topiramate and felbamate also modulate the GABA-A receptor. Mice lacking functional GABA-B receptors have been shown to exhibit seizures and hyperalgesia.[24]

Mutation of GABA receptor genes can cause epilepsy, such as a mutation of the alpha subunit (GABRA1) of the GABA-A receptor described in a French Canadian family with juvenile myoclonic epilepsy.[25] Bromides, first introduced by English physician Charles Locock in the 1850s, are now thought to act by enhancing the GABA-A receptor affinity for GABA and increasing the ion current. Drugs that enhance GABA activity generally have a broad spectrum of activity against seizure disorders, although they are not as effective against absence seizures. Generally GABA-A receptors are composed of alpha, beta, and delta subunits, with each containing a large N-terminal portion, four transmembrane regions, and a short C-terminal extracellular portion. Phenobarbital and other barbiturates act on sodium, calcium, and GABA-linked ion channels, but their most important action is on the GABA-A receptor, with a different action than the benzodiazepine family has on the GABA-A receptor. Barbiturates prolong openings of the channel leading to more passage of ions. Both topiramate and felbamate appear to also act in part through action at the GABA-A receptor. Benzodiazepines bind to the GABA-A receptor where the delta-2 subunit is necessary for their action. The action of benzodiazepines is conferred by the gamma-2 subunit and adjacent alpha1, alpha2, alpha3, or alpha5 subunits.

Glutamate Modulation

Glutamate is the main excitatory neurotransmitter in the CNS, and most of its actions are mediated through ionotropic (ligand-gated) receptors. There are also metabotropic (G-protein coupled) receptors. The ionotropic glutamate receptors are the N-methyl-D-aspartate (NMDA), alpha-amino-3-hydroxy-5-methyl-4-isoxazole-propionic acid (AMPA), and kainate receptor subtypes, which have numerous differences. The AMPA receptors show fast gating and desensitize strongly, whereas NMDA receptors gate more slowly, only weakly desensitize, and are blocked by magnesium in a strongly voltage-dependent manner. Efficient agonist action at NMDA receptors also requires the co-agonist glycine. The glutamate receptor ion channel has similarities with the K^+ channel. Ketamine is an NMDA antagonist, which is used in particular to treat refractory status epilepticus. In analgesic clinical trials, antagonists of glutamate have been disappointing. Felbamate is also an NMDA antagonist. The compound MK-801 has the highest affinity for the NMDA receptor. Lower affinity antagonists of NMDA include the medications memantine and ketamine. Among its many actions, topiramate selectively inhibits kainate receptors and to a lesser extent AMPA receptors. AMPA receptors are the primary mediators of fast excitatory transmission under basal signaling conditions.

SPECIFIC ANTICONVULSANT DRUGS

The remainder of this chapter discusses different anticonvulsant drugs and their specific properties. Starting and maintenance dosing regimens are shown in Table 23–1.

TABLE 23–1 Starting and Maintenance Dosing Regimens for Anticonvulsants	
Phenytoin	Loading 20 mg/kg. Maintain at 5–8 mg/kg, often 300 mg daily. BID or daily regimen orally. IV formulation infusion max 50 mg/kg.
Fosphenytoin	Loading 20 mg/kg. Up to 150 mg/min IV. Full loading by intramuscular route possible. Large volume IM tolerated well.
Carbamazepine	200 mg daily. Maintain 600–1200 mg daily, lower in elderly. TID regimen. Slow release forms (Tegretol XR, Carbatrol) given BID.
Oxcarbazepine	300 mg BID. Maintain 1200 mg/day. Max 2400 mg/daily. BID regimen.
Gabapentin	300 mg daily. Maintain 900–3600 mg daily.
Pregabalin	150 mg daily. Maintain 300–600 mg daily. TID or BID regimen.
Phenobarbital	Loading 20 mg/kg divided in two. Start orally at 60–90 mg daily. Maintain 90–120 mg daily.
Levetiracetam	500 mg BID. Maintain 1000–3000 mg.
Topiramate	25 mg daily. Maintain 200–400 mg/day BID regimen. For migraine 50–100 mg typically.
Valproic acid	250 mg daily. Depakene TID. Depakote BID. Depacon is IV formulation at 100 mg/mL, requires dilution, slow infusion a couple of times/day.
Zonisamide	100 mg once daily then BID with higher doses. Increase by 100 mg/wk. Maximum 400 mg daily.
Lamotrigine	50 mg daily (25 mg if taking valproic acid) increasing slowly over 4–6 wk to maintenance of 300–500 mg/day in a BID regimen.
Clonazepam	0.5 mg TID. Maintain 2–6 mg daily.

BID, twice daily; *IM*, intramuscular; *IV*, intravenous *TID*, three times a day.

Phenytoin and Fosphenytoin

Merrit and Punam[26] first described the utility of phenytoin in treating seizures when they described its ability to suppress electric shock–induced seizures in animals. Phenytoin was able to control seizures without producing sedation. In more recent times, Mattson and colleagues[27] performed a large blinded study of phenytoin, phenobarbital, primidone, and carbamazepine in 622 patients with new onset, partial, and secondarily generalized tonic-clonic seizures. Phenytoin and carbamazepine were the most efficacious and least toxic. Intravenous phenytoin is often used to treat status epilepticus where it acts quickly and is suitable for a loading dose. In addition to widespread use for seizures, with a 1942 report on its use in trigeminal neuralgia, phenytoin became the first AED to be used for neuropathic pain. Subsequent controlled trials investigating its analgesic potential have been unimpressive. Phenytoin is known for nonlinear metabolism, which is manifest as marked increases in plasma level with small dose increases after saturation of metabolism. Approximately 95% of a phenytoin dose is excreted as metabolites from the cytochrome P450 system. The half-life varies by dose and is between 12 and 36 hours, allowing for once daily administration. More frequent administration can reduce peak dose symptoms and a steady state concentration is not met for a couple of days given the long half-life. Phenytoin is still extensively used in the United States for the management of partial and generalized seizures, but it has a number of drawbacks.[28] It is highly protein bound, known for multiple drug interactions, and the intravenous formulation has drawbacks. Parenteral phenytoin is dissolved in 40% propylene glycol and 10% ethanol with a pH of 12, and intravenous administration can easily cause hypotension. The drug is administered at up to 50 mg per minute. Extravasation may cause a severe tissue reaction. The parenteral form cannot be given by the intramuscular route, unlike fosphenytoin, which is discussed later. Dilution should be with saline and not dextrose. Parenteral phenytoin crystallizes into insoluble phenytoin when admixed with solutions of 5% dextrose in water. Elimination follows first-order kinetics at low doses, after which degradation is saturated and zero-order kinetics characterizes the elimination. The therapeutic range is 10 to 20 µg/mL with a free level of 1 to 2 µg/mL. Only the free drug concentration is biologically active. Side effects include rash in 5% to 10% of patients. Phenytoin may cause a hypersensitivity syndrome manifesting in fever, rash, and lymphadenopathy. An association between erythema multiforme in patients on phenytoin undergoing whole brain radiation has been described and it would be prudent to avoid phenytoin in such circumstances.[29] Nystagmus occurs early in toxicity followed by ataxia progressing to encephalopathy. Phenytoin toxicity is reported to cause an exacerbation in seizures on rare occasions. The drug may result in birth defects called the fetal hydantoin syndrome. Phenytoin use is a risk factor for osteoporosis because of the multiple effects on calcium metabolism and supplemental vitamin D, and calcium is often recommended.[30] One study looked at the use of phenytoin, buprenorphine, or both together, for the relief of cancer pain. Seventy five cancer patients with various pain syndromes were studied, and there was a mild effect in favor of phenytoin.[31]

Fosphenytoin is a phosphate ester pro-drug and is entirely metabolized to phenytoin with a bioavailability of phenytoin at around 100%.[32] Fosphenytoin has certain advantages over phenytoin; namely, the ability to infuse intravenously in a rapid manner and availability for intramuscular injection. Disadvantages include cost when compared with generic phenytoin.

Carbamazepine

Carbamazepine has been used in the United States for a couple of decades to treat partial and generalized tonic-clonic seizures. The drug has an initial and adjunctive indication for seizure disorder. Besides an anticonvulsant indication, it also has FDA approval for trigeminal neuralgia and is used frequently for bipolar disorder. The drug was one of the first AEDs studied in neuropathic pain. The analgesic properties of carbamazepine were first reported in 1962.[33] It is chemically related to the tricyclic antidepressants and has been studied in postherpetic neuralgia, painful diabetic neuropathy, poststroke pain, and pain in Guillain–Barré syndrome, among other syndromes. Newer generation AEDs are often compared with carbamazepine for efficacy and side effects. A major clinical trial compared carbamazepine, phenytoin, phenobarbital, and primidone against each other for the treatment of partial and secondarily generalized tonic-clonic seizures.[27] Treatment success was greatest with carbamazepine and phenytoin. Results were intermediate with phenobarbital and worst with primidone. Carbamazepine exhibits nonlinear, time-dependent kinetics due to autoinduction. Metabolism involves oxidation to a 10-11 epoxide, which is further hydrolyzed. Both steps become more efficient with time, and the patient often needs an increase in dose after a few weeks of treatment. The half-life can shorten considerably. The autoinduction of enzymes is quickly reversed with discontinuation, so caution is advised in restarting after a few days of absence.[34] Generally, the dose does not correlate well with blood levels and the elderly require a smaller dose for adequate levels. The "therapeutic range" is 4 to 12 mg/dL, and the elimination half-life varies from 38 hours after a single dose to 12 hours after chronic monotherapy. The starting dose of carbamazepine is 100 mg or 200 mg a day, and it is available in an oral suspension, as well as tablet formulation. Carbamazepine is typically given twice daily. Enzyme-inducing drugs shorten the half-life of carbamazepine. The drug does not have the cosmetic side effects of phenytoin. Slow release formulations are available, reducing the serum fluctuations, which may reduce peak dose side effects. The development of rash, generally within the first few weeks, occurs in up to 10% of patients. It is suggested that a slow introduction reduces the chance of this side effect, which warrants discontinuation. Neurotoxicity generally occurs at levels greater than 12 mg/dL and often includes diplopia. The carbamazepine-10-11-epoxide is the major metabolite of carbamazepine and is responsible for a lot of the side effects. Hyponatremia is not uncommon with carbamazepine, although only a minority of patients will be symptomatic. The exact mechanism for hyponatremia is not clear, but it appears to be an effect on the renal tubules and not attributable to syndrome of inappropriate diuretic hormone (SIADH).

Oxcarbazepine

Oxcarbazepine is an AED with a chemical structure similar to carbamazepine but with a different metabolism.[35] Oxcarbazepine was developed as a structural variation of carbamazepine to avoid the production of the epoxide metabolite, implicated in a lot of the side effects. Oxcarbazepine does have other differences that separate it from carbamazepine. Clinical trials for the antiseizure effect have used doses from 600 to 2400 mg/day.[36] Rash occurs in about 3% of patients talking oxcarbazepine and cross reactions with carbamazepine have been reported. Hyponatremia also occurs with oxcarbazepine, more so in older patients, and it may be more frequent in patients taking oxcarbazepine than carbamazepine. In a postmarketing survey of 947 patients, 23% had a serum sodium level of lower than 135 mEq/L, and 1% required discontinuation of the medication.[37] Compared with carbamazepine, fewer patients will develop rash or hypersensitivity to oxcarbazepine. Oxcarbazepine is not associated with idiosyncratic hepatic or hematologic effects. Low serum thyroid hormone concentrations have been reported in patients on long-term treatment of oxcarbazepine for epilepsy. The mechanism of action of oxcarbazepine mainly involves blockade of sodium currents but differs from carbamazepine by modulating different types of calcium channels. Both oxcarbazepine and carbamazepine block sodium currents as described earlier, but oxcarbazepine does this at lower concentrations. Oxcarbazepine is metabolized by reduction and glucuronidation, resulting in a monohydroxy derivative (MHD). Oxcarbazepine metabolism is not induced or inhibited by the cytochrome P450 system, and its metabolites are passed in the urine. High-dose oxcarbazepine can cause some inhibition of CYP450 enzymes. When switching subjects from carbamazepine to oxcarbazepine, the practitioner should be aware of the effect of loss of enzyme induction on the metabolism of concurrent medications. Involvement of the hepatic cytochrome P450-dependent enzymes in the metabolism of the drug is minimal. This allows for better combining of oxcarbazepine with other AEDs such as valproate.[35] The bioavailability of the oral form is high (>95%).

Oxcarbazepine has limited but increasing data on the experimental use for pain. A recent study reported the antinociceptive effects of carbamazepine and oxcarbazepine in an inflammatory paw pressure test in rats.[75] The study demonstrated significant dose and time-dependent reduction in nociception with both agents individually. Furthermore, the challenge of caffeine (or a selective adenosine A1 receptor antagonist) to the model significantly reduced the antinociceptive effect of carbamazepine and oxcarbazepine. This is further evidence for the important role adenosine receptors (caffeine is a competitive antagonist at both adenosine A1 and A2 receptors) in the actions of carbamazepine and oxcarbazepine.

Phenobarbital

Phenobarbital has an FDA indication for monotherapy and adjunctive indication for partial and generalized tonic-clonic seizures. A parenteral form is available and it is often used to control status epilepticus. It is one of the oldest AEDs, and currently it is not used as much for monotherapy because it has been replaced by newer agents. The drug still retains an important place in the management of neonatal seizures because of its predictable pharmacokinetics and efficacy. It induces hepatic enzymes and is approximately 50% protein bound. The drug has a half-life of 4 days, and the blood level may be increased with the addition of valproate or tricyclic antidepressants. A concern in the use of phenobarbital is its effect on cognition and behavior. The drug has been associated with hyperactivity in children.

Pregabalin

Pregabalin has been demonstrated to have anticonvulsant, analgesic, and anxiolytic activity in animal models and in clinical trials.[38-45] As addressed earlier, the presumed mechanism of action is similar to gabapentin, binding to the alpha-2-delta subunit of voltage-gated calcium channels, resulting in inhibition of calcium influx. The pharmacokinetics are predictable, in contrast to those of gabapentin. The drug has high bioavailability and an elimination half-life of 6.3 hours. It does not bind to plasma proteins and does not undergo hepatic metabolism or have any effect on the cytochrome P450 system. The antiseizure activity of pregabalin has been studied at doses from 300 to 600 mg daily.[42-44] Three randomized double-blind trials of 5 to 8 weeks duration have been conducted using pregabalin for painful diabetic neuropathy.[38,39] Dosages ranged from 300 to 600 mg daily, administered in divided doses three times a day. There were significant improvements in pain and sleep score from one week on. Pregabalin was studied in four randomized double-blind placebo-controlled trials as adjunctive treatment with partial seizures.[42-44] Doses ranged from 50 mg to 600 mg daily and statistically significant reductions in seizure frequency were noted with pregabalin.

Gabapentin

Gabapentin is used as an adjunctive medication for partial seizures and generalized tonic-clonic seizures; however, most of its use in the United States is for neuropathic pain. Besides the binding to calcium channels, other effects have been described such as reducing the release of monoamines and possible sodium channel modulation on action potentials.[48,49] The drug is available in oral formulations and is absorbed by both diffusion and facilitated transport via an amino acid transport mechanism. The facilitated transport is saturable, leading to nonlinear kinetics and bioavailability somewhat related to dose. The drug is not metabolized and is eliminated unchanged in the kidneys. The half-life is roughly 6 hours. Those with renal impairment may need a smaller dose and patients on dialysis need a maintenance dose after dialysis as gabapentin is removed during dialysis. Gabapentin does not induce enzymes and is known for its lack of drug interactions and low protein binding. The most common side effects are somnolence, dizziness, fatigue, and weight gain. It is thought to be relatively safe even in overdose. It is generally given three times a day to control seizures and can be started at 300 mg nightly and increased briskly.[46] A liquid formulation at 50 mg/mL is available. Gabapentin has been studied in a wide range of pain syndromes, including multiple sclerosis–related central pains and spasms, complex regional pain, migraine, trigeminal neuralgia, HIV-related neuropathy, spinal cord injury pain, cluster headache, diabetic painful peripheral neuropathy, and postherpetic neuralgia where it has an FDA indication.[47]

Topiramate

Topiramate is a sulfamate-substituted derivative of D-fructose.[50] It has multiple mechanisms of action and has broad use in seizure disorders. Topiramate blocks voltage-sensitive sodium channels and limits sustained repetitive firing and binds to GABA-A receptors to enhance GABA activity through nonbenzodiazepine and nonbarbiturate mechanisms. The drug increases the opening frequency of chloride ion channels in GABA-A receptors and can block AMPA/Kainate glutamate receptors, acting as a negative modulator of glutamate at this receptor. Topiramate reduces the activity of L-type calcium channels and is a carbonic anhydrase inhibitor. Topiramate exhibits linear pharmacokinetics its dose range is exceeded and has a half-life of 19 to 25 hours. The oral bioavailability is about 85%, and topiramate is not affected by food. The drug is a mild enzyme inducer and increases the clearance of ethinylestradiol at doses greater than 200 mg a day. Enzyme-inducing drugs may reduce the serum level of topiramate. Common side effects include paresthesias (caused by inhibition of carbonic anhydrase), drowsiness, fatigue, and cognitive complaints. It also commonly causes dysgusia. The incidence of nephrolithiasis was 1.5% in clinical trials and mild weight loss is often noted. The propensity to reduce weight in some patients has led to investigations on its potential as a weight-reducing agent.[55] Two large trials on migraine prophylaxis with topiramate were published in 2004 and topiramate received FDA approval for this indication.[51,52] The particular mechanisms of action responsible for topiramate's efficacy in migraine are unknown. A recent study by Storer and colleagues demonstrates the inhibition of trigeminocervical neurons by topiramate consistent with its clinical effect. Anesthetized cats were studied with a microelectrode in the trigeminal nucleus and trigeminal activation by electrical stimulation of the superior sagittal sinus.[53] Three recent placebo-controlled studies on the use of topiramate for painful diabetic neuropathy did not demonstrate a significant pain-relieving effect.[54]

Levetiracetam

Levetiracetam is a newer AED, approved in 1999 as adjunctive therapy for partial seizures in adults. The drug has a number of favorable characteristics and is being investigated for adjuvant use in areas such as pain.[58] The drug has linear kinetics, is not significantly bound to plasma proteins (10%), has no important drug interactions, is of high oral bioavailability, and is eliminated partly unchanged by the kidneys. Hence, its pharmacokinetic characteristics are very favorable. It appears that inhibition of voltage-gated sodium channels or T-type calcium channels is not involved in the anticonvulsant effect of levetiracetam, which does not appear to have direct GABA-A receptor effects. Hence, the mechanism of action of levetiracetam does not involve modulation of the three main systems. Recent evidence suggests that levetiracetam reduces the inhibitory action of zinc and other negative allosteric modulators (beta-carbolines) on GABA and glycine-gated currents.[56] It has recently been shown that levetiracetam binds to SV2A, a synaptic vesicle protein, and this is thought to be involved in its anticonvulsant action. The protein SV2A interacts with the presynaptic protein synaptotagmin, considered the primary calcium sensor for regulating calcium-dependent exocytosis of synaptic vesicles.[57]

The most common side effects include somnolence, headache, and anxiety. Levetiracetam is not metabolized by the liver. There is no significant interaction with other AEDs or oral contraceptives.

Valproate

First synthesized in 1882, valproate became available in the 1960s as an antiepileptic agent and received FDA approval in 1978 as an immediate-release formulation.[59] The drug has a broad spectrum of use in seizure disorders, including absence seizures, and is now used extensively by psychiatrists for mood disorders. An enteric-coated formulation of divalproex sodium became available in 1983, which is a 1:1 ratio of sodium valproate and valproic acid. Valproic acid, but not divalproex, is available in generic form. Divalproex has FDA approval for monotherapy and adjunctive therapy for partial seizures, manic episodes associated with bipolar disorder, and migraine prophylaxis. Evidence for its use as an acute treatment for migraine is lacking but some experts will attest to its benefits (at a dose of 1000 mg IV), and it is used off-label for a range of other psychiatric problems. The exact molecular mechanisms responsible for its clinical effects are unknown. The catabolism of GABA is inhibited and the synaptic release of GABA is increased. Valproate is highly bound to plasma proteins although somewhat less in the elderly and those with liver or kidney disease. Valproate is extensively metabolized, the most significant pathway being conjugation with glucuronic acid, and this pathway can be saturated within the therapeutic range. The general "therapeutic range" is 50 to 100 μg/mL. Valproate has complex interactions with other anticonvulsants, but it should not alter the metabolism of steroid contraceptives because it does not induce enzymes. Levels above 125 μg/mL often cause toxic symptoms on the CNS including drowsiness and tremor. Valproate may alter the pharmacokinetics of other drugs. Both carbamazepine and phenobarbital can reduce the level of valproate by 30% to 40%. Valproate can displace phenytoin from its protein-binding sites, increasing the free fraction of phenytoin. The most frequent side effects include nausea, vomiting, tremor, and weight gain. Most of the gastrointestinal disturbances go away quickly. Valproate is known for idiosyncratic reactions unlike most other AEDs. Both hepatotoxicity and pancreatitis may occur, the hepatic effects more so in those less than 2 years of age.[60] Ammonia levels may increase, which, if severe, can cause encephalopathy. Valproate is a known tetratogen, increasing the risk of spina bifida in particular to 2% of infants born to mothers taking valproic acid.

Lamotrigine

Lamotrigine received FDA approval in 1994 and is used as an adjunctive agent for partial seizures and as monotherapy for partial and generalized seizures.[61,62] Compared with phenytoin and carbamazepine patients treated with lamotrigine were less likely to experience adverse events such as dizziness, somnolence, and cognitive impairment.[61] There is little dose-dependent toxicity, so monitoring of laboratory values is not necessary. The most concerning side effect is rash, known to occur more often with rapid titration and can present as Stevens-Johnson syndrome.[63] The risk of rash is similar to that found in phenytoin or carbamazepine at up to 5% to 10%. The risk of Stevens-Johnson syndrome is increased in those taking valproate. The enzyme-inducing drugs reduce the serum level of lamotrigine. Lamotrigine has no effect on liver enzymes, is metabolized via glucuronidation, and is 55% protein bound with a half-life of 30 hours. The drug does need a slow titration, requiring at least 4 to 6 weeks. The co-administration of valproate leads to higher levels of lamotrigine. Lamotrigine has been reported as useful for the neuropathic pain of sciatica.[64] Controlled trials have been conducted on the analgesic effects of lamotrigine on HIV-associated painful neuropathy, spinal cord injury pain, and central poststroke pain.[65-67] Lamotrigine 200 mg daily was moderately effective for poststroke pain and was not clearly effective for HIV-related neuropathy or spinal cord injury pain.

Tiagabine

Tiagabine became available in the United States in 1997 for partial seizures in those older than 12 years.[68] The drug blocks the uptake of GABA, prolonging its effect. It does not affect liver enzymes and is metabolized by the cytochrome P450 system. The half-life of about 8 hours is reduced considerably in the presence of enzyme-inducing medications. It has not been studied much in pain. In the animal tail flick model, it does have an antinociceptive effect, and it has been reported useful in a pilot study to treat tonic spasms in multiple sclerosis.[69,70]

Zonisamide

Zonisamide is indicated for adjunctive therapy in the treatment of partial seizures in adults and became available on the market in the United States in 2000.[71] It blocks repetitive firing of voltage-sensitive sodium channels and reduces voltage sensitive T-type calcium currents. It has a long half-life of approximately 65 hours and is completely absorbed. It may be administered once or twice daily. Zonisamide is metabolized by the cytochrome P450 system but does not induce enzymes. The most common side effects in trials were dizziness, ataxia, and anorexia. Zonisamide is contraindicated in those with sulfonamide allergy because it is a sulfonamide derivative, and the drug is approximately 40% bound to plasma proteins. Uncommon side effects include hyperthermia and oligohidrosis. There are case reports on usefulness in poststroke pain and headache.

Benzodiazepines

As described earlier, benzodiazepines facilitate the actions of GABA in the CNS as a result of their binding to the GABA-A receptor. Clonazepam and clobazam (clobazam is not available in the United States) are useful as adjunct treatment in refractory epilepsies.[74] Clonazepam is 47% protein bound and is extensively metabolized. Diazepam and lorazepam have extensive use in the emergency management of seizures and status epilepticus. The side effects of drowsiness, ataxia, and the development of tolerance to the antiseizure effect limit the usefulness of clonazepam and other benzodiazepines from chronic use. Diazepam is available as a rectal gel for quick onset in the acute management of seizures. Clonazepam is also used for chronic facial pain, and it has had some success in small clinical trials.[72] The only randomized double-blind trial of a benzodiazepine for pain was lorazepam when it was compared with amitriptyline in postherpetic neuralgia. Lorazepam was found to be less effective.[73]

Vigabatrin

Vigabatrin is an irreversible inhibitor of gamma-aminobutyric acid transaminase and is used as adjunctive therapy in those with partial seizures. It is not available in the United States. It is also useful in infantile spasms and is the drug of choice in children with infantile spasms secondary to tuberous sclerosis. It is more effective in partial seizures than generalized seizures. Headache and drowsiness are the most prevalent side effects. Visual field defects and psychiatric reactions have been reported. The drug is rapidly and completely absorbed after oral administration and does not exhibit significant protein binding. The drug is eliminated unchanged in the urine with minimal metabolism. The elimination half-life is 5 to 7 hours, but the pharmacodynamic half-life is considerably longer, enabling a once or twice daily dosing schedule. The role of vigabatrin in pain management is unknown.

REFERENCES

1. LaRoche SM, Helmers S: The new antiepileptic drugs. JAMA 291:605–614, 2004.
2. French JA, Kanner AM, Bautista J, et al: Efficacy and tolerability of the new antiepileptic drugs I: Treatment of new onset epilepsy. Neurology 62:1252-1260, 2004.
3. French JA, Kanner AM, Bautista J, et al: Efficacy and tolerability of the new antiepileptic drugs II: Treatment of refractory epilepsy. Neurology 62:1261-1273, 2004.
4. National Institute for Clinical Excellence. Newer drugs for epilepsy in adults. www.nice.org.uk/Docref.asp?d=110081. Accessed Jan 17 2005.
5. National Institute for Clinical Excellence. Newer drugs for epilepsy in children. www.nice.org.uk/Docref.asp?d=113359. Accessed Jan 17 2005.
6. Tremont-Lukats IW, Megeff C, Backonja MM: Anticonvulsants for neuropathic pain syndromes: Mechanisms of action and place in therapy. Drugs 60:1029-1052, 2000.
7. Sirven JI, Wingerchuk DM, Drazkowski JF, et al: Seizure prophylaxis in patients with brain tumors: A meta-analysis. Mayo Clin Proc 79:1489-1494, 2004.
8. Vecht CJ, Wagner GL, Wilms EB: Interactions between antiepileptic and chemotherapeutic drugs. Lancet Neurol 2:404-409, 2003.
9. Rogawski M, Loscher W: The neurobiology of antiepileptic drugs. Nat Rev Neurosci 10:685-692 2004. Review.
10. Hagiwara S, Ozawa S, S and O: Voltage clamp analysis of two inward current mechanisms in the egg cell membrane of a starfish. J Gen Physiol 65:617-644, 1975.
11. Yamakage M, Namiki A: Calcium channels – basic aspects of their structure, function, and gene encoding; anesthetic action on the channels—a review. Can J Anesth 49:151-164, 2002.
12. Luo ZD, Chaplan SR, Higuera ES, et al: Upregulation of dorsal root ganglion (alpha)2(delta) calcium channel subunit and its correlation with allodynia in spinal nerve-injured rats. J Neurosci 15;21:1868-1875, 2001.
13. Errante LD, Williamson A, Spencer D, et al. Gabapentin and vigabatrin increase GABA in the human neocortical slice. Epilepsy Res 49:203-210, 2002.
14. Golden AL: Mechanisms of sodium channel inactivation. Curr Opin Neurobiol 13:284-290, 2003.
15. Kuo CC, Bean BP: Slow binding of phenytoin to inactivated sodium channels in rat hippocampal neurons. Mol Pharmacol 46:716-725, 1994.
16. Yu F, Catterall W: Overview of the voltage-gated sodium channel family. Genome Biol 4:207, 2003. Review.
17. Priestley T: Voltage-gated sodium channels and pain. Curr Drug Targets CNS Neurol Disord 3:441-456, 2004.
18. Lossin C, Wang DW, Rhodes TH, et al: Molecular basis of an inherited epilepsy. Neuron 34:877-884, 2002.
19. Spampanato J, Kearney JA, de Haan G, et al: A novel epilepsy mutation in the sodium channel SCN1A identifies a cytoplasmic domain for beta subunit interaction. J Neurosci 24:10022-10044, 2004.
20. Gold MS, et al: Redistribution of Na v 1.8 in uninjured axons enables neuropathic pain. J Neurosci 23:158-166, 2003.
21. Todorovic SM, Rastogi AJ, Jevtovic-Todorvic V: Potent analgesic effects of anticonvulsants on peripheral thermal nociception in rats. Br J Pharmacol 140:255-260, 2003.
22. Kuo C: A common anticonvulsant binding site for phenytoin, carbamazepine, and lamotrigine in neuronal Na+ channels. Mol Pharmacol 54:712-721, 1998.
23. Owens DF, Kriegstein AR: Is there more to GABA than synaptic inhibition? Nat Rev Neurosci 3:715-727, 2002.
24. Schuler V, et al: Epilepsy, hyperalgesia, impaired memory, and loss of pre- and postsynaptic GABA(B) responses in mice lacking GABA(B(1)). Neuron 31:47-58, 2001.
25. Cossette P, Lortie A, Vanasse M, et al: Autosomal dominant juvenile myoclonic epilepsy and GABRA1 [review]. Adv Neurol 95:255-263, 2005.

26. Merrit HH, Putnam TJ: A new series of anti-convulsant drugs tested by experiments on animals. Arch Neurol Psychiatry 39:1003–1015, 1938.

27. Mattson RH, Cramer JA, Collins JF, et al: Comparison of carbamazepine, phenobarbital, phenytoin, and primidone in partial and secondarily generalized tonic-clonic seizures. N Engl J Med 18:313:145–151, 1985.

28. Antiepileptic drugs. In Browne TR, Holmes GL, ed. Handbook of Epilepsy. 3rd ed. Philadelphia, Lippincott Williams & Wilkins, 2004.

29. Ahmed I, Reichenberg J, Lucas A, Shehan JM: Erythema multiforme associated with phenytoin and cranial radiation therapy: A report of three patients and review of the literature. Int J Dermatol 43:67–73, 2004.

30. Orwoll ES, Klein RF: Osteoporosis in men. Endocr Rev 16:87–116, 1995.

31. Yajnik S, Singh GP, Singh G, Kumar M: Phenytoin as a coanalgesic in cancer pain. J Pain Symptom Manage 7:209–213, 1992.

32. Fischer JH, Patel TV, Fischer PA: Fosphenytoin: Clinical pharmacokinetics and comparative advantages in the acute treatment of seizures. Clin Pharmacokinet 42:33–58, 2003.

33. Blom S: Trigeminal neuralgia: Its treatment with a new anticonvulsant drug. Lancet 1:839–840, 1962.

34. Schaffler L, Bourgeois BF, Lunders HO: Rapid reversibility of autoinduction of carbamazepine metabolism after temporary discontinuation. Epilepsia 35:195–198, 1994.

35. Kalis MM, Huff NA: Oxcarbazepine, an antiepileptic agent. Clin Ther 23:680–700, 2001.

36. Barcs G, Walker EB, Elger CE, et al: Oxcarbazepine placebo-controlled, dose-ranging trial in refractory partial epilepsy. Epilepsia 41:1597–1607, 2000.

37. Friis ML, Kristensen O, Boas J, et al: Therapeutic experiences with 947 epileptic out-patients in oxcarbazepine treatment. Acta Neurol Scand 87:224–227, 1993.

38. Lesser H, Sharma U, LaMoreaux L, Poole RM: Pregabalin relieves symptoms of painful diabetic neuropathy: A randomized controlled trial. Neurology 63:2104–2110, 2004.

39. Rosenstock J, Tuchman M, LaMoreaux L, Sharma U: Pregabalin for the treatment of painful diabetic peripheral neuropathy: A double-blind, placebo-controlled trial. Pain 110:628–638, 2004.

40. Sabatowski R, Galvez R, Cherry DA, et al: Pregabalin reduces pain and improves sleep and mood disturbances in patients with post-herpetic neuralgia: Results of a randomized, placebo-controlled trial. Pain 109:26–35, 2004.

41. Pary R: High dose pregabalin is effective for the treatment of generalized anxiety disorder. Evid Based Ment Health 7:17, 2004.

42. Arroyo S, Anhut H, Kugler AR, et al: Pregabalin add-on treatment: A randomized, double blind, placebo-controlled, dose-response study in adults with partial seizures. Epilepsia 45:20–27, 2004.

43. Beydoun AA, Uthman BM, Ramsay RE, et al: Pregabalin add-on trial: Double-blind multi-center study in patients with partial epilepsy [abstract]. Epilepsia 41(suppl 7):253–254, 2000.

44. French JA, Kugler AR, Robbins JL, et al: Dose-response trial of pregabalin adjunctive therapy in patients with partial seizures. Neurology 60:1631–1637, 2003.

45. Dworkin RH, Corbin AE, Young Jr JP, et al: Pregabalin for the treatment of postherpetic neuralgia a randomized, placebo-controlled trial. Neurology 60:1274–1283, 2003.

46. Chadwick DW, Anhut H, Greiner MJ, et al: A double-blind trial of gabapentin monotherapy for newly diagnosed partial seizures. International Gabapentin Monotherapy Study Group 945-77. Neurology 51:1282–1288, 1998.

47. Rowbotham M, Harden N, Stacey B, et al: Gabapentin for the treatment of postherpetic neuralgia: A randomized controlled trial. JAMA 280:1837–1842, 1998.

48. Schlicker E, Reimann W, Gothert M: Gabapentin decreases monoamine release without affecting acetylcholine release in the brain. Arzneimittel-Forschung 35:1347, 1985.

49. Wail AW, McLean MJ: Limitation by gabapentin of high frequency action potential firing by mouse central neurons in cell culture. Epilepsy Res 17:1–11, 1994.

50. Glauser T: Topiramate. Epilepsia 40 (suppl 5):S71–S80, 1999.

51. Silberstein SD, Neto W, Schmitt J, Jacobs D: MIGR-001 Study Group. Topiramate in migraine prevention: Results of a large controlled trial. Arch Neurol 61:490–495, 2004.

52. Brandes JL, Saper JR, Diamond M, et al: Topiramate for migraine prevention: A randomized controlled trial. JAMA 291:965–973, 2004.

53. Storer RJ, Goadsby PJ: Topiramate inhibits trigeminovascular neurons in the cat. Cephalalgia 24:1049–1056, 2004.

54. Thienel U, Neto W, Schwabe SK, Vijapurkar U: Topiramate Diabetic Neuropathic Pain Study Group. Topiramate in painful diabetic polyneuropathy: Findings from three double-blind placebo-controlled trials. Acta Neurol Scand 110:221–231, 2004.

55. Astrup A, Caterson I, Zelissen P: Topiramate: Long term maintenance of weight loss by a low-calorie diet in obese subjects. Obese Res 12:1658–1669, 2004.

56. Rigo JM, Hans G, Nguyen L, et al: The anti-epileptic drug levetiracetam reverses the inhibition by negative allosteric modulators of neuronal GABA- and glycine-gated currents. Br J Pharmacol 136:659–672, 2002.

57. Lynch BA, Lambeng N, Nocka K, et al: The synaptic vesicle protein SV2A is the binding site for the antiepileptic drug levetiracetam. Proc Natl Acad Sci USA 101:9861–9866, 2004.

58. Price MJ: Levetiracetam in the treatment of neuropathic pain: Three case studies. Clin J Pain 20:33–36, 2004.

59. DeVane LC: Pharmacokinetics, drug interactions, and tolerability of valproate. Psychopharmacology Bulletin Summer 37(suppl 2):25–42, 2003.

60. Eadie MJ, Hooper WD, Dickinson RG: Valproate-associated hepatotoxicity and its biochemical mechanisms. Med Toxicol 3:85–106, 1988.

61. Brodie MJ, Richens A, Yuen AWC, et al: Double-blind comparison of lamotrigine and carbamazepine in newly diagnosed epilepsy. Lancet 345:476–479, 1995.

62. Steiner TJ, Dellaportas CI, Findley LJ: Lamotrigine monotherapy in newly diagnosed untreated epilepsy: A double blind comparison with phenytoin. Epilepsia 40:601–607, 1999.

63. Roujeau JC, Stern RS: Severe adverse cutaneous reactions to drugs. N Engl J Med 331:1272–1285, 1994.

64. Eisenberg E, Damunni G, Hoffer E, et al: Lamotrigine for intractactable sciatica: Correlation between dose, plasma concentration and analgesia. Eur J Pain 7:485–491, 2003.

65. Simpson DM, McArthur JC, Olney R, et al: Lamotrigine for HIV-associated painful sensory neuropathies: A placebo-controlled trial. Neurology 60:1508–1514, 2003.

66. Finnerup NB, Sindrup SH, Bach FW, et al: Lamotrigine in spinal cord injury pain: A randomized controlled trial. Pain 96:375–383, 2002.

67. Vestergaard K, Anderson G, Gottrup H, et al: Lamotrigine for central poststroke pain: A randomized controlled trial. Neurology 56:184–190, 2001.

68. Leach JP, Brodie MJ: Tiagabine. Lancet 351:203–207, 1998.

69. Giardina WJ, Decker MW, Porsolt, et al: An evaluation of the GABA uptake blocker tiagabine in animal models of neuropathic and nociceptive pain. Drug Dev Res 44:106–113, 1998.

70. Solaro C, Tanganelli P: Tiagabine for treating painful tonic spasms in multiple sclerosis: A pilot study. J Neurol Neurosurg Psychiatry 75:341, 2004.

71. Sackellares JC, Ramsey RE, Wilder BJ, et al: Randomized, controlled clinical trial of zonisamide as adjunctive treatment for refractory partial seizures. Epilepsia 45:610–617, 2004.

72. Smirne S, Scarlato G: Clonazepam in cranial neuralgias. Med J Aust 1:93–94, 1977.

73. Max MB, Schafer SC, Culnane M, et al: Amitriptyline, but not lorazepam relieves postherpetic neuralgia. Neurology 38:1427–1432, 1988.

74. Levy RH, Mattson RH, Meldrum BS, et al: Antiepileptic Drugs, 5th ed. Philadelphia, Lippincott Williams & Wilkins, 2002.

75. Tomic MA, Vuckovic SM, Stepanovic-Petrovic RM, et al: The anti-hyperalgesic effects of carbamazepine and oxcarbazepine are attenuated by the treatment with adenosine receptor antagonists. Pain 111:253–260, 2004.

76. Hodgkin AL, Huxley AF. A quantitative description of membrane current and its application to conduction and excitation in nerve. J Physiol 117:500–544, 1952.

CHAPTER 24

Topical and Oral Anesthetics

MARK S. WALLACE, MD, BRADLEY S. GALER, MD, AND ARNOLD R. GAMMAITONI, PharmD

The clinical use of the sodium channel blockers (SCBs) dates back to the 1940s, when reports emerged describing the analgesic effects of the systemically administered SCBs in acute pain.[1-3] Soon after it was recognized that SCBs were also effective in treating chronic painful conditions.[3-5] These initial reports led to an abundance of preclinical and clinical studies supporting the use of topical and systemic SCBs for the treatment of chronic pain.

Peripheral nerve injury and inflammation lead to a spontaneous and evoked pain that is thought to be in part mediated by voltage-sensitive sodium channels. The spontaneous pain occurs at the level of the injured axons and in the dorsal root ganglion cells. Preclinical studies have demonstrated that this spontaneous and evoked pain can be decreased with the delivery of SCBs. In addition, clinical studies are supporting the topical application of SCBs for the treatment of several pain syndromes.

This chapter discusses the use of the topical and systemically delivered SCBs for the treatment of cancer pain. The first part of the chapter reviews the neurophysiology of the sodium channel as it relates to pain transmission. The second part of the chapter reviews clinical literature on the use and efficacy of topical and systemically delivered SCBs in the treatment of cancer pain.

SODIUM CHANNEL BLOCKERS AND NOCICEPTION

Evidence suggests that both the spontaneous and evoked pain after nervous system injury is mediated in part by an increase in the density of voltage-sensitive sodium channels in the injured areas of the axon and dorsal root ganglion of the injured axon.[6-8] In animal models of neuropathic pain, it has been demonstrated that spontaneous and evoked pain is significantly diminished after delivery of sodium channel antagonists.[9-12]

Importantly, these effects occur at plasma concentrations that do not produce an afferent conduction block.[13]

The development of the spontaneous and evoked pain after nervous system injury is thought to be due to not only a change in number of sodium channels but also a change in the distribution and type of sodium channels. These changes occur at the area of injury, demyelination, and dorsal root ganglion. These sodium channels display marked pharmacologic differences from the uninjured state. For example, it is speculated that in the presence of injury, sodium channels on C fibers display a significant increase in affinity and an exaggerated response to sodium channel blockade as opposed to the uninjured state.[14] Therefore, it has been suggested that neuropathic pain is more responsive to SCBs than nociceptive pain. Indeed it has been demonstrated that the SCBs have no effect on acute nociceptive processing, whereas there is a significant effect on pain after tissue injury and nerve injury. At plasma lidocaine concentrations of up to 3 μg/mL, there are no prominent effects on acute heat, cold, or mechanical thresholds.[15,16] A similar lack of effect on acute nociceptive processing has been demonstrated with mexiletine, an oral bioavailable analog of lidocaine, at plasma concentrations of up to 0.5 μg/mL.[17] Two other studies have demonstrated a significant effect of intravenous (IV) lidocaine on acute ischemic pain (a model of acute nociceptive processing).[18,19] However, the plasma concentrations were above the 3 μg/mL plasma level, which typically exceeds the maximal tolerable dose. In contrast, IV lidocaine has been demonstrated to significantly reduce postoperative pain with achieved plasma levels of 1 to 2 μg/mL.[20,21] In addition, there are numerous reports on the efficacy of the SCBs in neuropathic pain disorders (discussed in the following section).

Sodium channels are present throughout the body including in the nerves, muscle, and heart. At least seven different sodium channels have been isolated, all with important biophysical and pharmacologic differences resulting in differing sensitivities to SCBs.

327

Sodium channels are classified by their sensitivity to tetrodotoxin (TTX), a potent SCB. TTX-sensitive (TTXs) sodium channels are blocked by small concentrations of TTX, whereas TTX-resistant (TTXr) sodium channels are not blocked even when exposed to high concentrations of TTX. The role of TTXs and TTXr sodium channels in nociception is controversial; however, as described previously it is clear that after nerve injury and during inflammation, there are dynamic and expression changes that occur in both TTXs and TTXr sodium channels.[22]

Proponents for the TTXr sodium channel as being important in nociception argue that because of their different voltage sensitivities of activation and inactivation, TTXr channels are still capable of generating impulses at depolarized potentials (which characterize the chronically damaged nerve fibers), whereas TTXs channels are inactivated and cannot contribute to excitability. For example, PN3 is a subclass of the TTXr sodium channel that is located only in the peripheral nervous system on small neurons in the dorsal root ganglion and is thought to be specific to pain transmission.[23] Animal models of experimental nerve damage have demonstrated changes in expression and distribution of the PN3 sodium channel; therefore, SCBs specific to the PN3 sodium channel could have important clinical implications.[24,25]

It has been demonstrated in animal models of spinal nerve ligation that application of TTX of approximately two orders of magnitude lower than those needed to block TTXr sodium channels resulted in a significant reduction of ectopic discharges in the dorsal root ganglion cells. This suggests that the TTXs subtype of sodium channels may be important in generating neuropathic pain.[26,27] Therefore, it is unclear as to what type, if any, of the sodium channels are important to the development of nociceptive pain.

Inflammation is also thought to lead to changes in sodium channel expression. In the presence of inflammation, sodium channel plasticity is thought to result from an increase in nerve growth factor (NGF). Whereas axotomy reduces the amount of NGF in the dorsal root ganglion (DRG), inflammation increases the amount of NGF in the DRG.[28] Patterns of sodium channel expression can be quite different between inflammation and nervous system injury; however, both tend to increase DRG excitability through these changes. In inflammatory conditions, such as osteoarthritis, animal studies have reported clinically active abnormal sodium channels, which when antagonized reduce spontaneous nociceptive activity and alleviate pain behaviors of the rodent.[10,11] Lidocaine, a topically and systemically administered SCB, has also been shown to inhibit the expression of nitric oxide and subsequent release of proinflammatory cytokines from T-cells and thus provides another potential analgesic mechanism for the lidocaine patch in the treatment of inflammatory pain conditions.[12]

CLINICAL USE OF SODIUM CHANNEL BLOCKERS IN PAIN

Topical Agents

Peripheral mechanisms of pain are inherent in most pain states including acute and chronic pain and neuropathic, inflammatory, and cancer pain. These peripheral mechanisms are believed to be clinically relevant sources of pain and thus appropriate targets for drug therapy.[29] Topical treatment by definition provides clinically meaningful levels of drug delivered directly to the peripheral tissues, including nerve and soft tissue, via a patch or poultice, without any relevant systemic activity.

Although there are many treatment options and combinations for pain, including cancer pain, the choice of treatment relies on three important criteria: (1) efficacy demonstrated in controlled clinical trials; (2) safety demonstrated in controlled clinical trials and subsequent clinical experience; and (3) favorable tolerability profiles (i.e., side effects, drug/drug interactions). The efficacy of treatment does not necessarily match its invasiveness and with increased invasiveness comes increased risks and costs. Due to the low risk and side effects associated with topical treatment, this mode of treatment is very attractive and should be considered early on in the pain treatment continuum when indicated. For some patients, topical medication can be at least as effective as systemic and more invasive therapies.[30,31] Two topical SCBs are currently available in the United States—the lidocaine patch 5% (Lidoderm®, Endo Pharmaceuticals Inc., Chadds Ford, Pa), and eutectic mixture of lidocaine 2.5% and prilocaine 2.5% (EMLA®, AstraZeneca Pharmaceuticals LP, Wilmington, Del). Analgesic effects of topical lidocaine patch and EMLA cream are summarized in Table 24–1.

Lidocaine Patch

The lidocaine patch is a 10-cm × 14-cm topical patch comprising an adhesive material containing 5% lidocaine (700 mg) in an aqueous base, which is applied to a nonwoven polyester felt backing and covered with a polyethylene terephthalate film-release liner. The release liner is removed prior to application. In addition to its sodium-channel–blocking activity, it has been suggested that the lidocaine patch acts as a protective

Pain Syndrome	Treatment	Design	NNT	Result	Reference
PHN	Lidocaine patch	RCDBX	35	↓ Pain at 4, 6, 9, 12 hr	Rowbotham, 1996
PHN	Lidocaine patch	RCDBX	32	↓ Pain, median time to exit >14 days vs 3.8 days with vehicle	Galer, 1999
PHN	Lidocaine patch	RCDBX	96	↓ All common neuropathic pain qualities	Galer, 2002
PHN	Lidocaine patch	Open label	332	↓ Pain and interference with quality of life	Katz, 2003
Neuropathic pain	Lidocaine patch	Open label	16	Moderate or better pain relief in 87%	Devers, 2000
Neuropathic pain	Lidocaine patch	RCDBX	40	↓ Pain over a period of 7 days (NNT = 4.4)	Meier, 2003
PHN	EMLA cream	Open label	12	↓ Pain after 6 hr	Stow, 1989
PHN	EMLA cream	Open label	11	↓ Paroxysmal pain and mechanical hyperalgesia with repeated application. No effect on ongoing pain	Attal, 1999
Postoperative pain	EMLA cream	RCDB	45	Time to 1st analgesic request ↑ and analgesic consumption on d 2-5 ↓. At 3 mo, pain ↓	Fassoulaki, 2000

TABLE 24–1 Analgesic Effects of Topical Lidocaine Patch and EMLA Cream

C, controlled; DB, double-blind; EMLA, eutectic mixture of local anesthetics; NNT, number needed to treat; PHN, postherpetic neuralgia; R, randomized; X, crossover.

barrier against cutaneous stimuli for patients with allodynia.[29,32] The lidocaine patch delivers lidocaine directly to the painful area to produce an analgesic effect without loss of sensation.[30] In addition, only a small amount (i.e., 3% ± 2%) of lidocaine has been found to be absorbed in healthy subjects treated with the lidocaine patch; therefore, it is unlikely that the pain relief from the lidocaine patch results from systemic absorption.[30,31,33] This is a major advantage over systemically administered SCBs, where efficacy is often limited by side effects. The most common adverse reactions are local, in the skin region directly underlying the patch, and generally tend to be mild, resolving without the need for intervention.[30,31] There have not been any serious systemic adverse events related to treatment with the lidocaine patch in six recent clinical trials.[30,31] Of the 450 patients studied in these trials, the most frequently reported systemic adverse event was mild-to-moderate headache (1.8%). Other, less common systemic adverse events included dizziness and somnolence (<1%).

The lidocaine patch is approved by the Food and Drug Administration (FDA) for the treatment of postherpetic neuralgia (PHN). The current FDA-approved labeling recommends that patients apply up to 3 lidocaine patches to the most painful areas of intact skin and wear them for no more than 12 hours in a 24-hour period. Increasing the dose to 4 lidocaine patches applied either once daily for 24 hours or twice daily every 12 hours for 3 consecutive days was shown to be safe and well tolerated in a pharmacokinetic study of 20 normal subjects. In this study, plasma lidocaine levels were 14.3% of those associated with cardiac activity and 4% of those typically associated with toxicity.[30] A regimen of four lidocaine patches worn for 18 hours/day for 3 consecutive days also was shown to be well tolerated in 20 normal subjects.[31] The lidocaine patch 5% should be used with caution in patients with severe hepatic disease and in those receiving antiarrhythmic or local anesthetic drugs. One to two weeks of therapy with the lidocaine patch may be required to determine whether a patient will experience satisfactory relief. However, one study reported that a very small subgroup of patients with PHN required up to 4 weeks of treatment with the lidocaine patch to obtain maximal benefit.[34] No dose escalation is necessary, and tolerance does not develop with the lidocaine patch.[35,36]

Although there are no specific studies on the efficacy of lidoderm patch in the treatment of cancer pain, there are numerous studies supporting the efficacy of the lidocaine patch in the treatment of numerous painful conditions, both nociceptive and neuropathic. Many of these studies include pain that can occur indirectly from cancer and cancer treatment (e.g., postherpetic neuralgia, peripheral neuropathy, low back pain, and osteoarthritis). In one study of refractory PHN, 24 of 35 patients reported slight or better pain relief (averaging scores at 4 and 6 hours), and 10 patients reported moderate or better relief.[32] An enriched enrollment study of 32 patients with PHN, who were known responders to the lidocaine patch, showed that the lidocaine patch provided significantly more pain relief than a vehicle patch, using "time to exit" as the primary endpoint.[35] In a prospective, randomized, controlled trial of 96 patients with PHN, the lidocaine patch was superior to a vehicle patch in reducing all common pain qualities associated with neuropathic pain (e.g., "burning," "dull," "deep," "superficial," and "sharp" pains).[37] Statistically significant reductions in pain interference with quality of life were noted with the lidocaine patch in a large (N = 332), open-label, effectiveness study.[34]

In addition to studies in PHN, there is one study supporting the use of the lidocaine patch in the treatment of a variety of other peripheral neuropathic pain conditions. In a randomized placebo-controlled crossover study in 40 patients with peripheral neuropathic pain, it was demonstrated that lidocaine patch significantly reduced pain over the 7-day treatment period. Number needed to treat was 4.4, which is comparable with other studies (NNT = 3.2–5.0).[38] In an open-label trial, the lidocaine patch improved pain in patients with a variety of refractory neuropathic conditions with allodynia, including post-thoracotomy pain, stump neuroma pain, intercostal neuralgia, painful diabetic polyneuropathy, meralgia paresthetica, complex regional pain syndrome, radiculopathy, and postmastectomy pain: 13 of 16 patients reported moderate or better pain relief with the lidocaine patch.[39]

A unique feature of the lidocaine patch 5% is that it provides analgesia without anesthesia. Even with dosing every 24 hours, both light touch and pinprick sensation have been shown to be preserved.[30]

Eutectic Mixture of Local Anesthetics

Eutectic mixture of local anesthetics (EMLA) cream is a mixture of lidocaine 2.5% and prilocaine 2.5%, which is available as an oil-based cream. It is generally applied to intact skin under an occlusive dressing. EMLA cream is approved by the FDA as a topical agent for use on normal, intact skin for local analgesia, on genital mucous membranes for superficial minor surgery, and as pretreatment for infiltration anesthesia.

Like the lidocaine patch, EMLA cream delivers the local anesthetic directly to the site of application. However, unlike the lidocaine patch 5%, EMLA cream causes a time-dependent sensory loss in the skin area (anesthesia) to which it is applied through sodium-channel–blocking activity. The onset of skin anesthesia depends primarily on the amount of cream applied. Skin anesthesia peaks 2 to 3 hours after application with an occlusive dressing and persists for 1 to 2 hours after removal. Disadvantages of EMLA cream as compared with lidocaine patch include poor patient compliance due to the inconvenience of using a cream and production of a sensory loss that can be annoying. Like the lidocaine patch, there is limited absorption of the local anesthetics found in EMLA cream. The peak blood levels of lidocaine and prilocaine absorbed with the application of EMLA cream 60 g to 400 cm^2 are well below systemic toxicity levels. Thus, minimal systemic side effects or drug/drug interactions have been noted with EMLA cream. Like the lidoderm patch the most common side effect is a local reaction at the site of application in up to 56% of patients. These reactions are usually mild and transient, resolving spontaneously within 1 to 2 hours.

Although there are numerous studies supporting the use of EMLA cream for the approved indication of skin anesthesia prior to blood draws and surgical incisions, there are few studies evaluating the efficacy in the treatment of acute and chronic pain conditions. In one small study in PHN (N = 12), EMLA cream 5% applied for 24-hour periods significantly improved mean pain intensity 6 hours after application as measured by a visual analog scale.[40] In another small study in PHN (N = 11), 5% EMLA cream applied daily under an adhesive occlusive dressing for 5 hours/day for 6 days had no significant effect on mean ongoing pain intensity as measured by a visual analog scale.[41] However, eight patients reported that the number of painful attacks decreased by 50%. EMLA cream had significant benefit in a subset of eight patients with tactile allodynia. In one double-blind, randomized study of women undergoing breast surgery for cancer (N = 45), EMLA cream 5% or placebo was applied 5 minutes prior to surgery and daily for 4 days during the postsurgical period. Acute pain at rest and with movement did not differ between the EMLA cream and control groups, and the analgesics consumed during the first 24 hours were the same. However, time to the first analgesia requirement was longer, and analgesic consumption during the second to fifth days was less in the EMLA cream group. Three months postoperatively, pain in the chest wall and axilla and total incidence and intensity of chronic pain were significantly less in the EMLA cream versus the control group. The use of analgesics at home and the feeling of abnormal sensations did not differ between the two groups.[42]

Thus, while both lidocaine patch 5% and EMLA cream have local anesthetics as their active ingredients, they differ dramatically in their clinical use profile, most likely due to their very different formulations and penetrating-enhancing chemicals.

Systemic Sodium Channel Blockers

Analgesic effects of systemic SCBs are summarized in Table 24–2.

Lidocaine

Lidocaine has been the most widely studied drug in the treatment of pain states.[43] When examined in patients reporting significant pain secondary to pain states, subanesthetic doses of systemic lidocaine produce clinically relevant relief in diabetes,[16,44] nerve injury pain states,[45-47] postherpetic neuralgia,[48] central pain,[49,50] fibromyalgia,[51] and migraine.[52,53] The efficacy of IV lidocaine on postoperative pain, which represents a nociceptive pain mechanism, yields conflicting results. Two randomized placebo-controlled trials using similar doses and achieving similar plasma lidocaine concentrations (1 to 2 µg/mL) showed conflicting results.[20,54] One large, open-label study in 302 subjects suggested an analgesic effect of lidocaine in postoperative pain.[21] These studies suggest a differential effect of lidocaine on neuropathic pain versus nociceptive pain. After nerve injury, sodium channels seem to play a substantive role in pain processing. However, the role of the sodium channels in pain processing after inflammation is unclear (see previous discussion). Although controversial, it is suggested that sodium channel blockade is less effective in nociceptive pain processing as opposed to neuropathic pain processing. Consistent with this theory, patients with peripheral nervous system injury report substantially more pain relief than those with pain of unknown etiology.[55] In addition, there appears to be a differential effect of IV lidocaine depending on the location of the nervous system injury. Galer et al. reported substantially better pain relief after peripheral nervous system injury as opposed to central nervous system injury.[55] It has also been suggested that IV lidocaine may lead to a reduction in sympathetic activity with resulting pain relief in sympathetically mediated pain. While some reduction in sympathetic activity has been demonstrated after systemic lidocaine,[56] this appears to be a minor consequence of lidocaine-evoked hypertension and tachycardia with reflex sympathetic attenuation.[14] Consistent with this, a recent study by Wallace et al. showed minimal effects of IV lidocaine on pain and allodynia of complex regional pain syndrome types I and II with plasma levels of up to 3 µg/mL plasma level.[57]

Lidocaine can also be delivered intranasally and has been studied with conflicting results. In acute migraine, intranasal lidocaine was shown to significantly decrease the pain and rescue medication.[58] However, a report in myofascial facial pain failed to show a significant difference among intranasal lidocaine, cocaine, and placebo.[59]

There are few studies on the effects of IV lidocaine on malignant pain. Three randomized, controlled trials failed to show an effect of IV lidocaine on cancer bone pain,[60] neuropathy secondary to cancer treatment,[61] and malignant plexopathy.[62] Brose and Cousins reported on three cancer patients with cancer-related neuropathic pain who responded to a continuous subcutaneous infusion of lidocaine. Plasma lidocaine levels were in the range of 2 to 5 µg/mL.[63] Kronenberg et al. reported on 83 hospice patients who received IV lidocaine 2 mg/kg over 20 minutes followed by 1 to 3 mg/kg/hour infusion for opioid refractory cancer pain. Fifty-eight percent experienced a major response (complete or nearly complete relief of pain); twenty-four percent had partial relief; and eighteen percent experienced no benefit. Although systemic lidocaine clearly is advantageous in peripheral neuropathic pain, the role in central neuropathic pain, nociceptive pain, and cancer pain is unclear and further studies are needed.

Lidocaine can be administered intravenously or subcutaneously; it is available in concentrations ranging from 5 to 200 mg/mL. The high concentration should be reserved for subcutaneous administration. The standard loading dose for pain is 2 mg/kg over 20 to 30 minutes followed by a continuous infusion of 1 to 3 mg/kg/hour. If monitoring plasma levels, the targeted concentration is in the range of 1 to 3 µg/mL, which is well below the cardiac and nervous system toxicity level.

Procaine

Procaine was one of the first local anesthetics to be used systemically for the treatment of pain. An advantage of procaine is the extremely low toxicity when administered systemically. A disadvantage is the extremely short half-life due to ester hydrolysis by plasma pseudocholinesterases and red cell esterases.[64] The earliest use of procaine was to supplement general anesthesia and to treat chronic musculoskeletal disorders.[3,65] It has also been shown anecdotally to be effective in the treatment of postherpetic neuralgia.[4,5] There is one controlled study using procaine 4 to 6.5 mg/kg that shows efficacy in postoperative pain.[66] There are no studies using procaine for the treatment of cancer pain.

Mexiletine

Mexiletine is an oral sodium channel antagonist that is structurally similar to lidocaine. Mexiletine has been reported to be effective in a variety of neuropathic pain

TABLE 24–2 Analgesic Effects of Systemic Local Anesthetics

Pain Syndrome	Treatment	Design	NNT	Result	Reference
Diabetic neuropathy	IV lidocaine 5 mg/kg	RCDBX	3	↑ Nociceptive flexion reflex thresholds	Bach, 1990
Diabetic neuropathy	IV lidocaine 5 mg/kg	RCDBX	15	↓ Pain	Kastrup, 1987
PHN	IV lidocaine 5 mg/kg	RCDBX	19	↓ Pain	Rowbotham, 1991
Central pain	IV lidocaine 1 mg/kg	CB	8	↓ Pain	Backonja, 1992
Peripheral nerve injury	IV lidocaine 1–3 µg/mL plasma level	RCDBX	11	↓ Pain	Wallace, 1996
Peripheral nerve injury	IV lidocaine 2 mg/kg vs 5 mg/kg	RCDBX	23	↓ Pain with both doses + dose response	Galer, 1996
Neuropathy: cancer treatment related	IV lidocaine 5 mg/kg	RCDBX	10	NS	Ellemann, 1989
Cancer-related bone pain	IV lidocaine 5 mg/kg	RCDBX	10	NS	Sjogren, 1989
Cancer malignant plexopathy	IV lidocaine 5 mg/kg	RCDBX	10	NS	Bruera, 1992
Postoperative pain	IV lidocaine 2 mg/min	RCDB	20	↓ Pain and opioid consumption	Cassuto, 1985
Postoperative pain	IV lidocaine 2 mg/kg/hr	RCDB	18	NS	Birch, 1987
Postoperative pain	IV lidocaine 1 g	Open label	302	↓ Pain	Bartlett, 1961
Fibromyalgia	IV lidocaine 5 mg/kg	RCDBX	11	↓ Pain	Sorensen, 1995
Migraine	IV lidocaine max 2.7 mg/kg	RCDB	76	↓ Pain	Bell, 1990
Migraine	IV lidocaine 1 mg/kg	RCDB	25	↓ Pain 1st 20 min after treatment	Reutens, 1991
Migraine	IN lidocaine max 1.1 mg/kg	RCDB	81	↓ Pain and rescue medication	Maizels, 1996
Facial Pain	IN lidocaine 29 mg	RCDBX	28	NS	Marbach, 1988
Postoperative pain	IV procaine 4-6.5 mg/kg	Open label	40	↓ Pain	Keats, 1951
Migraine	IN lidocaine				
Diabetic peripheral neuropathy	Mexiletine 10 mg/kg/day	RCDBX	16	↓ Pain	Dejgard, 1988
Diabetic peripheral neuropathy	Mexiletine 225–675 mg/day	RCDB	95	NS	Stracke, 1992
Diabetic peripheral neuropathy	Mexiletine 600 mg/day	RCDB	29	NS	Wright, 1997
Alcoholic peripheral neuropathy	Mexiletine 300 mg/day	Open label	5	↓ Pain	Nishiyama, 1995
Peripheral nerve injury	Mexiletine 750 mg/day	RCDBX	11	↓ Pain	Chabal, 1992
Peripheral neuropathic pain	Mexiletine 900 mg/day	RCDBX	20	NS	Wallace, 2000
Thalamic pain	Mexiletine 10 mg/kg/day	Open label	9	↓ Pain in 8 of 9 patients	Awerbuch, 1990
Spinal cord injury pain	Mexiletine 450 mg/day	RCDBX	11	NS	Chiou-Tan, 1996

Continued

TABLE 24–2 Analgesic Effects of Systemic Local Anesthetics—cont'd

Pain Syndrome	Treatment	Design	NNT	Result	Reference
Cancer pain	Mexiletine	Open label		NS	Chong, 1997
Trigeminal neuralgia	Tocainide	RCDBX	12	Equivalent to carbamazepine	Lindstrom, 1987
PHN	Flecainde	Open label	20	↓ Pain in 15 out of 20	Ichimata, 2001
Cancer pain	Flecainide	Open label		NS	Chong, 1997

C, controlled; DB, double-blind; IV, intravenous; IN, intranasal; NNT, number needed to treat; NS, not significant; PHN, postherpetic neuralgia; R, randomized; X, crossover.

syndromes including diabetic neuropathy,[67,68] alcoholic neuropathy,[69,70] peripheral nerve injury,[71-73] and thalamic pain.[74] However, more recent reports question the efficacy of oral mexiletine in neuropathic pain.[75-77]

There are two double-blind, placebo-controlled studies on mexiletine in neuropathic pain that showed an effect on spontaneous pain scores in diabetic neuropathy and peripheral nerve injury.[68,72] However, there are four double-blind, placebo-controlled studies that show no significant effect of mexiletine on neuropathic pain scores in diabetic neuropathy, spinal cord dysesthetic pain, and neuropathic pain with allodynia.[67,76-78] In a double-blind, randomized, placebo-controlled trial in diabetic neuropathy, Stracke et al. showed a significant decrease in specific components of neuropathic pain; however, they did not show any significant effect on pain scores using mexiletine doses up to 675 mg/day.[67]

There are few studies in the literature correlating plasma levels of mexiletine with analgesia. Nishiyama and Sakuta concluded that the minimum effective plasma concentration for alcoholic neuropathy was 0.66 µg/mL.[69] Wallace et al. showed that a peak level of 0.54 µg/mL plasma level did not result in pain relief if the pain was neuropathic.[78] The only other study that measured plasma concentrations was published by Galer et al. The mean highest tolerated dosage was 878 mg (range 400–1200 mg), with a mean serum level of 0.76 µg/mL. They found no correlation between mexiletine dose, serum level, and pain relief scores.[45] It is difficult to make firm conclusions on the predictive value of IV lidocaine on oral mexiletine success as claimed in the study by Galer et al. because there are several reports in the literature on a prolonged pain relief from a single IV lidocaine infusion.[16,79,80] This may explain the lack of correlation between serum mexiletine level and pain relief in their study.

There are several reports in the literature on the dose-limiting side effects of oral mexiletine.[45,76] These dose-limiting side effects often preclude achieving adequate therapeutic blood levels for pain relief. A study by Ando et al. in healthy volunteers showed that the maximum tolerated plasma level was 0.5 µg/mL, which

is likely subtherapeutic.[17] Dose-limiting side effects may account for the poor outcomes with this drug.

From studies evaluating the effective plasma level of mexiletine for the treatment of pain, it appears that the recommended daily dosage is in the range of 1200 to 1500 mg. However, as discussed previously, this may be difficult to achieve due to dose-limiting side effects, namely nausea. There are anecdotal reports of coadministering carafate to minimize the nausea, thus allowing higher doses.

Tocainide

Tocainide is a derivative of lidocaine with antiarrhythmic action, which can be delivered orally. It has been demonstrated to have analgesic efficacy in a number of animal studies; however, there are few studies in humans.[12,81,82] In a double-blind crossover comparator study with carbamazepine in trigeminal neuralgia, tocainide was found to be equivalent to carbamazepine.[83] Carbamazepine is FDA approved for the treatment of trigeminal neuralgia.

Flecainide

The analgesic effects of flecainide were reported by Dunlop in 1988.[84] Systemic flecainide has been demonstrated to suppress ectopic nerve discharge in neuropathic rats.[85] In spite of these reports, the clinical use of flecainide has been mixed. In an open-label trial, Ichimata et al. delivered IV flecainide to 20 patients with postherpetic neuralgia in which 15 responded. The responders received oral flecainide with chronic relief of the pain.[86]

The use of flecainide in cancer pain has been ineffective. In a pilot study of 21 cancer patients with inadequately controlled pain with opioid analgesics, flecainide was of no benefit in 17 cases, two cases had clear-cut analgesic benefit, and two cases had mild-moderate analgesic relief.[75] Bennett et al. reported on a case of paranoid psychosis due to flecainide toxicity in malignant neuropathic pain and cautioned on use of flecainide in this vulnerable population.[87]

REFERENCES

1. Bigelow N, Harrison I: General analgesic effects of procaine. JPET 81:368–373, 1944.

2. Gordon RA: Intravenous novocaine for analgesia in burns. Can Med Assoc 49:478–481, 1943.

3. Morton R, Spitzer K, Steinbrocker O: Intravenous procaine as an analgesic and therapeutic procedure in painful, chronic neuromusculoskeletal disorders. Anesthesiology 10:629–633, 1949.

4. Collins EB: The use of intravenous procaine infusion in the treatment of postherpetic neuralgia. Med J Aust 2:27–28, 1969.

5. Shanbrom E: Treatment of herpetic pain and postherpetic neuralgia with intravenous procaine. JAMA 176:1041–1043, 1961.

6. Cummins TR, Waxman SG: Down regulation of tetrodotoxin-resistant sodium currents and up regulation of a rapidly repriming tetrodotoxin-sensitive sodium current in small spinal sensory neurons after nerve injury. Neuroscience 17:3503–3514, 1997.

7. England JD, Happel LT, Kline DG: Sodium channel accumulation in humans with painful neuromas. Neurology 47:272–276, 1996.

8. Devor M, Govrin-Lippmann R, Angelsides K: Na channel immunolocalization in peripheral mammalian axons and changes following nerve injury and neuroma formation. J Neurosci 13:1976–1792, 1993.

9. Jett M, et al: The effects of mexiletine, desipramine and fluoxetine in rat models involving central sensitization. Pain 69:161–169, 1997.

10. Kamei J, et al: Antinociceptive effect of mexiletine in diabetic mice. Res Comm Chem Path Pharm 77:245–248, 1992.

11. Xu XJ, et al: Systemic mexiletine relieves chronic allodynia-like symptoms in rats with ischemic spinal cord injury. Anesth Analg 74:649–652, 1992.

12. Chabal C, Russell DA, Buchiel KJ: The effect of intravenous lidocaine, tocainide, and mexiletine on spontaneous active fibers originating in rat sciatic neuromas. Pain 38:333–338, 1989.

13. Devor M, Wall D, Catalan N: Systemic lidocaine silences ectopic neuroma and DRG discharge without blocking nerve conduction. Pain 48:261–268, 1992.

14. Chaplan SR, Bach FW, Yaksh TL: Systemic use of local anesthetics in pain states. In Yaksh TL et al (ed.): Anesthesia: Biologic Foundations. Philadelphia, Lippincott-Raven, 1997, pp 977–986.

15. Wallace MS, et al: Concentration-effect relations for intravenous lidocaine infusions in human volunteers: Effect on acute sensory thresholds and capsaicin-evoked hyperpathia. Anesthesiology 86:1262–1272, 1997.

16. Bach FW, et al: The effect of intravenous lidocaine on nociceptive processing in diabetic neuropathy. Pain 40:29–34, 1990.

17. Ando K, et al: Neurosensory finding after oral mexiletine in healthy volunteers. Reg Anesth and Pain Med 25:468–474, 2000.

18. Boas RA, Covino BG, Shahnarian A: Analgesic responses to I.V. Lignocaine Br J Anaesth 54:501–505, 1982.

19. Rowlingson JC, et al: Lidocaine as an analgesic for experimental pain. Anesthesiology 52:20–22, 1980.

20. Cassuto J, et al: Inhibition of postoperative pain by continuous low-dose intravenous infusion of lidocaine. Anesth Analg 64:971–974, 1985.

21. Bartlett EE, Hutaserani O: Xylocaine for the relief of postoperative pain. Anesth Analg 40:296–304, 1961.

22. Tanaka M, et al: SNS sodium channel expression increases in dorsal root ganglion neurons in the carrageenan inflammatory pain model. Neuroreport 9:967–972, 1998.

23. Sangameswaran L, et al: Structure and function of a novel voltage-gated tetrodotoxin-resistant sodium channel specific to sensory neurons. J Bio Chem, 1996. 27:5953–5956.

24. Tzoumaka E, et al: PN3 sodium channel distribution in the dorsal root ganglia of normal and neuropathic rats. Proc West Pharmacol, 40:69–72, 1997.

25. Novakovic S, et al: Distribution of the tetrodotoxin-resistant sodium channel PN3 in rat sensory neurons in normal and neuropathic conditions. J Neurosci 18:2174–2187, 1998.

26. Liu X, et al: Ion channels associated with the ectopic discharges generated after segmental spinal nerve injury in the rat. Brain Res 900:119–127, 2001.

27. Chung JM, Dib-Hajj SD, Lawson SN: Sodium channel subtypes and neuropathic pain. Proceedings of the 10th World Congress on Pain, 2003, 24:99–113.

28. Lee SE, et al: Expression of nerve growth factor in the dorsal root ganglion after peripheral nerve injury. Bran Res 769: 99–106, 1998.

29. Galer BS: Topical drugs for the treatment of pain. In Loeser JD: Bonica's Management of Pain. Hagerstown, Md, Lippincott Williams & Wilkins, 2001, pp 1736–1742.

30. Gammaitoni AR, Alvarez NA, Galer BS: Safety and tolerability of the lidocaine patch 5%, a targeted peripheral analgesic: A review of the literature. J Clin Pharmacol 43:111–117, 2003.

31. Gammaitoni AR, Davis MW: Pharmacokinetics and tolerability of lidocaine patch 5% with extended dosing. Ann Pharmacother 36:236–240, 2002.

32. Rowbotham MC, et al: Lidocaine patch: Double-blind controlled study of a new treatment method for post-herpetic neuralgia. Pain 65:39–44, 1996.

33. Comer AM, Lamb HM: Lidocaine patch 5%. Drugs 59:245–249, 2000.

34. Katz NP, et al: Lidocaine patch 5% reduces pain intensity and interference with quality of life in patients with postherpetic neuralgia: An effectiveness trial. Pain Med 3:324–332, 2002.

35. Galer BS, et al: Topical lidocaine patch relieves postherpetic neuralgia more effectively than a vehicle topical patch: Results of an enriched enrollment study. Pain 80:533–538, 1999.

36. Kanzai GE, Johnson RW, Dworkin RH: Treatment of postherpetic neuralgia: An update. Drugs 59:1113–1126, 2000.

37. Galer BS, et al: The lidocaine patch 5% effectively treats all neuropathic pain qualities: Results of a randomized, double-blind, vehicle-controlled, 3-week efficacy study with use of the neuropathic pain scale. Clin J Pain 18:297–301, 2002.

38. Meier T, et al: Efficacy of lidocaine patch 5% in the treatment of focal peripheral neuropathic pain syndromes: A randomized, double-blind, placebo-controlled study. Pain, 106:151–158, 2003.

39. Devers A, Galer BS: Topical lidocaine patch relieves a variety of neuropathic pain conditions: An open-label study. Clin J Pain 16:205–208, 2000.

40. Stow PJ, Glynn CJ, Minor B: EMLA cream in the treatment of post-herpetic neuralgia. Efficacy and pharmacokinetic profile. Pain 39:301–305, 1989.

41. Attal N, et al: Effects of single and repeated applications of a eutectic mixture of local anesthetic (EMLA) cream on spontaneous and evoked pain in post-herpetic neuralgia. Pain 81:203–209, 1999.

42. Fassoulaki A, et al: EMLA reduces acute and chronic pain after breast surgery for cancer. Reg Anesth and Pain Med 25:350–355, 2000.

43. Kalso E, et al: Systemic local-anaesthetic-type drugs in chronic pain: A systematic review. Eur J Pain 2:3–14, 1998.

44. Kastrup J, et al: Intravenous lidocaine infusion: A new treatment of chronic painful diabetic neuropathy? Pain 28: 69–75, 1987.

45. Galer BS, Harle J, Rowbotham MC: Response to intravenous lidocaine infusion predicts subsequent response to oral mexiletine: A prospective study. J Pain Symptom Manage 12:161–167, 1996.

46. Wallace MS, et al: Computer-controlled lidocaine infusion for the evaluation of neuropathic pain after peripheral nerve injury. Pain 66:69–77, 1996.

47. Marchettini P, et al: Lidocaine test in neuralgia. Pain 48:S63–S66, 1992.

48. Rowbotham M, Reisner-Keller L, Fields H: Both intravenous lidocaine and morphine reduce the pain of postherpetic neuralgia. Neurology 41:1024–1028, 1991.

49. Attal N, et al: Intravenous lidocaine in central pain: A double-blind, placebo-controlled, psychophysical study. Neurology 54:564–574, 2000.

50. Backonja M, Gombar K: Response of central pain syndromes to intravenous lidocaine. J Pain Sympt Manage 7:172–178, 1992.

51. Sorensen J, et al: Pain analysis in patients with fibromyalgia. Scand J Rheumatol 24:360–365, 1995.

52. Bell R, et al: A comparative trial of three agents in the treatment of acute migraine headache. Ann Emerg Med 19:1079–1082, 1990.

53. Reutens DC, et al: Is intravenous lidocaine clinically effective in acute migraine? Cephalgia 11:245–247, 1991.

54. Birch K, et al: Effect of IV lignocaine on pain and the endocrine metabolic responses after surgery. Br J Anaesth 59:721–724, 1987.

55. Galer BS, Miller KV, Rowbotham MC: Response to intravenous lidocaine infusion differs based on clinical diagnosis and site of nervous system injury. Neurology 43:1233-1235, 1993.

56. Ebert TJ, Mohanty PK, Kampine JP: Lidocaine attenuates efferent sympathetic responses to stress in humans. J Cardiothorac Vasc Anesth 5:437-443, 1991.

57. Wallace MS, et al: Concentration-effect relationship of intravenous lidocaine on the allodynia of complex regional pain syndrome types I and II. Anesthesiology 92:75-83, 2000.

58. Maizels JJ, et al: Intranasal lidocaine for treatment of migraine. JAMA 276:319-321, 1996.

59. Marbach JJ, Wallenstein SL: Analgesic, mood, and hemodynamic effects of intranasal cocaine and lidocaine in chronic facial pain of deafferentation and myofascial origin. J Pain Sympt Manage 3:73-79, 1988.

60. Sjogren P, et al: [Intravenous lidocaine in the treatment of chronic pain caused by bone metastases]. Ugeskr Laeger 151:2144-2146, 1989.

61. Ellemann K, et al: Trial of intravenous lidocaine on painful neuropathy in cancer patients. Clin J Pain 5:291-294, 1989.

62. Bruera E, Ripamonti C, Brenneis C: A randomized double-blind cross-over trial of intravenous lidocaine in the treatment of neuropathic cancer pain. J Pain Sympt Manage 7:138-140, 1992.

63. Brose WG, Cousins MJ: Subcutaneous lidocaine for treatment of neuropathic cancer pain. Pain 45:145-148, 1991.

64. Tucker GT, Mather LE: Clinical pharmacokinetics of local anesthetics. Clin Pharmacokinet 4:241-278, 1979.

65. Edmonds GW, et al: Intravenous use of procaine in general anesthesia. JAMA 141:761-765, 1949.

66. Keats AS, D'Alessandro GL, Beecher HK: A controlled study of pain relief by intravenous procaine. JAMA 147:1761-1763, 1951.

67. Stracke H, Meyer UE: Mexiletine in the treatment of diabetic neuropathy. Diabetes Care 15:1550-1555, 1992.

68. Dejgard A, Petersen P, Kastrup J: Mexiletine for treatment of chronic painful diabetic neuropathy. Lancet 1:9-11, 1988.

69. Nishiyama K, Sakuta M: Mexiletine for painful alcoholic neuropathy. Intern Med 34:577-579, 1995.

70. Nishiyama K, et al: Remarkable effect of a class Ib Na^+ channel blocker on painful alcoholic neuropathy. Clin Neurol 30:1140-1142, 1990.

71. Davis RW: Successful treatment for phantom pain. Orthopedics 16:691-695, 1993.

72. Chabal C, Jacobson L, Mariano A: The use of oral mexiletine for the treatment of pain after peripheral nerve injury. Anesthesiology 76:513-517, 1992.

73. Tanelian DL, Brose WG: Neuropathic pain can be relieved by drugs that are use-dependent sodium channel blockers: lidocaine, carbamazepine, and mexiletine. Anesthesiology 74:949-951, 1991.

74. Awerbuch G, Sandyk R: Mexiletine for thalamic pain syndrome. Internat J Neurosc 55:129-133, 1990.

75. Chong SF, Bretscher ME, Maillard JA: Pilot study evaluating local anesthetics administered systemically for treatment of pain in patients with advanced cancer. J Pain Sympt Manage 13:112-117, 1997.

76. Wright JM, Oki JC, Graves L: Mexiletine in the symptomatic treatment of diabetic peripheral neuropathy. Ann Pharmacother 31:29-34, 1997.

77. Chiou-Tan F, Tuel S, Johnson J: Effect of mexiletine on spinal cord injury dysesthetic pain. Amer J Phys Med Rehab 75:84-87, 1996.

78. Wallace MS, Magnuson S, Ridgeway B: Oral mexiletine in the treatment of neuropathic pain. Reg Anesth and Pain Med 25:459-467, 2000.

79. Arner S, Lindblom U, Meyerson B: Prolonged relief of neuralgia after regional anesthetic block. Pain 43:287-297, 1990.

80. Peterson P, et al: Chronic pain treatment with intravenous lidocaine. Neurol Res 8:189-190, 1986.

81. Erichsen HK, et al: A comparison of the antinociceptive effects of voltage-activated Na^+ channel blockers in two rat models of neuropathic pain. Eur J Pharmacol 458:275-282, 2003.

82. Franchini C, et al: Stereoselectivity in central analgesic action of tocainide and its analogs. Chirality 5:135-142, 1993.

83. Lindstrom P, Lindblom U: The analgesic effect of tocainide in trigeminal neuralgia. Pain 28:45-50, 1987.

84. Dunlop R, et al: Analgesic effects of oral flecainide. Lancet 1:420-421, 1988.

85. Ichimata M, et al: Flecainide reverses neuropathic pain and suppresses ectopic nerve discharge in rats. Neuroreport 12:1869-1873, 2001.

86. Ichimata M, et al: Analgesic effects of flecainide on postherpetic neuralgia. Int J Clin Pharmacol Res 21:15-19, 2001.

87. Bennett MI: Paranoid psychosis due to flecainide toxicity in malignant neuropathic pain. Pain 70:93-94, 1997.

CHAPTER 25

Bisphosphonates

ELENA CATALÀ, MD, PHD, AND Mª JOSÉ MARTINEZ, MD

Bone metastasis is common in primary cancers. Consequently, patients with advanced cancer can develop 30% to 90% of skeletal metastasis. Among primary tumors those that often metastasize are the following: breast cancer (47% to 85%), prostate cancer (33% to 85%), and lung cancer (32% to 60%).[1] Metastases mainly occur on the spine, ribs, and pelvis and at a lower rate on long bones such as the humerus or femur.

In breast cancer, the most common site of metastasis is the bone. However, patients who only present bone metastasis have a relatively long survival after diagnosis compared with patients who have visceral metastases. Mean survival is longer than 20 months, and about 10% of patients live 5 to 10 years longer after the diagnosis of the first bone metastasis.[2]

According to the type of primary tumor, bone metastases may be osteolytic (increase in bone resorption), osteoblastic (sclerotic events), or mixed.

In breast cancer the most common metastasis is osteolytic, but in prostate cancer it is osteoblastic.[3] Multiple osteolytic skeletal lesions characterize myeloma. Related morbidity and the resulting negative impact on patients' quality of life are significant. Pain is the most frequent symptom, accounting for 45% to 75% of cases and leading to performance disability.[4] When bones are involved, pathologic fractures might occur (10% to 20%); another frequent complication is hypercalcemia (10% to 15%).[1] Thus, more than 75% of patients with multiple myeloma suffer from pain, and half of them have vertebral fractures at the time of the diagnosis.

The source of pain might be the bone (direct bone involvement by the tumor with associated microfractures, increased endosteal pressure, or periosteal derangement), because of nerve structure compression (most frequently vertebral bone lesions) or soft tissue lesion on the area surrounding the involved bone.[5] Only the periosteum and blood vessels have nerve endings, so pain is elicited when bony structures are involved. Pain is also associated with the release of chemical mediators such as peptides, amines, prostaglandins, fatty acids, or potassium as a result of nociceptive fiber stimulation eliciting not only pain but also swelling and edema.[6,7]

Osteoclast activation is the main pathophysiologic action of bone metastasis even though the stimulation of osteoblastic activity and simultaneous bone formation are also detected.[8] More than direct bone destruction, malignant cells release different substances (paracrine, growth factors, proteolytic enzymes, prostaglandins) able to stimulate osteoclast activity in bone resorption and nociceptive receptors, thereby reducing the surrounding pH.[9] Macrophages present in the tumor mass may in turn become osteoclasts or produce substances that stimulate osteoclastic activity.[10,11]

In short, bone metastases might lead to a imbalance between bone formation and bone resorption. Metastatic cancer cells release substances that induce direct osteoclast proliferation and activity via the osteoblasts. Bone loss sometimes occurs in those sites with increased activity. By and large, osteolytic lesions associated with a net bone loss are more common and cause more morbidity including hypercalcemia, fractures, and pain.[6]

When most of these tumors metastasize, cure is no longer possible. Consequently, the treatment objective is to reduce patients' symptoms and improve quality of life. In the case of bone metastases, the most important pathogenic mechanism responsible for metastasis development and progression is bone resorption. Therefore, bisphosphonates are a very attractive treatment option because their main mechanism of action is to inhibit osteoclastic activity, responsible for bone resorption. However, there are other strategies focused on prevention and treatment, the most important being corticosteroids, nonsteroidal anti-inflammatory drugs or opioids, radiation therapy (external radiation or radiation therapy with radiopharmaceutical agents), surgery, chemotherapy, and hormone therapy, all of which can be associated with the concomitant use of bisphosphonates.

BISPHOSPHONATES

Background

Biological characteristics of bisphosphonates were discovered about 35 years ago.[12] The concept arises from prior studies with inorganic pyrophosphate shown to inhibit calcium phosphate precipitation and consequently ectopic calcification. Due to its lack of effectiveness when given orally and as a result of its fast hydrolysis, analogs with a similar physical and chemical activity but with the characteristic of being able to resist enzymatic hydrolysis and consequently being unable to be metabolically inactivated were sought. Meeting these requirements, bisphosphonates started to be developed as drugs.[13]

Chemical Structure

They are compounds chemically characterized by two C-P bonds. If these two bonds are located on the same carbon atom originating a P-C-P structure, compounds are then called germ bisphosphonates. Thus, these compounds are pyrophosphate analogs that contain a carbon atom instead of an oxygen atom (Figure 25-1). In the literature, however, they are often exclusively called bisphosphonates.

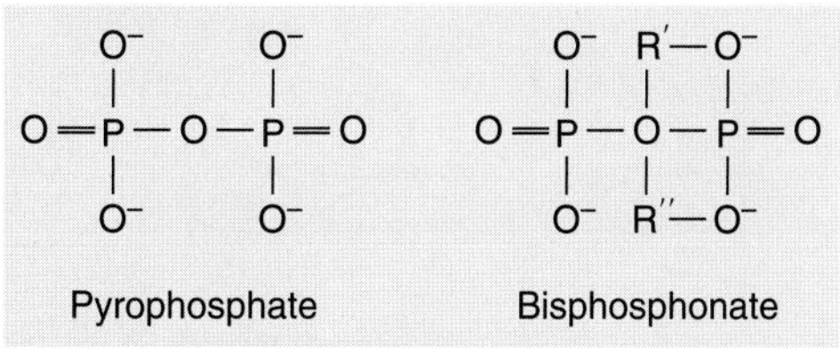

The P-C-P structure allows for a large number of likely variations to be made by changing two side chains of the carbon atom via the esterification of a phosphate resulting in first, second, and third generation bisphosphonates. The greatest difference concerning its chemical structure is the inclusion of amino radicals (aminobisphosphonates), thus varying its physical and

FIGURE 25–1 Chemical structure of pyrophosphate and bisphosphonate.

chemical features and consequently its own activity profile (Figure 25-2). The introduction of one or more nitrogen atoms in the chemical structure of bisphosphonates will determine its power, so that there is a difference between bisphosphonates that have an amino group (more powerful) and those that do not. In the past few years, new, more powerful molecules have been developed such as pamidronate, ibandronate, and zoledronate (Table 25-1).

In Vivo Activity

Bisphosphonates are strongly bound to calcium phosphate crystals, inhibiting their growth, aggregation, and dissolution. This significant effect is the basis for the use of these drugs as skeletal markers in nuclear medicine and the basis of their action on bone resorption when used as drugs.[13]

The main effect of pharmacologically active bisphosphonates is bone resorption inhibition, although its mechanism of action has not yet been totally elucidated. However, there is a general consensus on the role of bisphosphonates as inhibitors of osteoclastic activity.

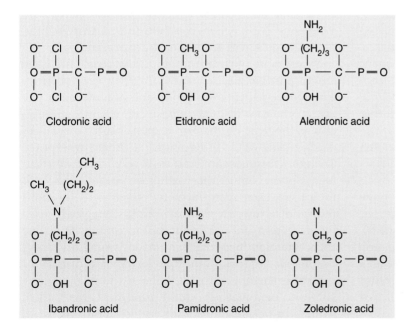

FIGURE 25–2 Chemical structure of various bisphosphonate drugs.

TABLE 25-1 Potency of the Bisphosphonates

Generic Name	Relative Potency	Route of Administration
Etidronic acid	1	PO, IV
Clodronic acid	10	PO, IV
Pamidronic acid	100	IV
Alendronic acid	1000	PO, IV
Ibandronic acid	10,000	PO, IV
Zoledronic acid	100,000	IV

IV, intravenously; *PO*, per os.

In fact, bisphosphonates alter osteoclast morphology, both in vitro and in vivo. The assumption proposed some time ago is interesting; bisphosphonates are deposited in the bone given their high affinity for minerals while osteoclasts are inhibited when incorporating bone that has bisphosphonates.[14-16] This assumption would therefore account for the fact that a single dose of bisphosphonates might remain active for a long time after discontinuation of the drug.

Pharmacokinetics

Given the small number of available studies, little is known on the pharmacokinetics of these drugs; however, we do know that they are not biodegradable, at least in relation with their P-C-P bond, and that their oral bioavailability is low (1% to 10%). The highest absorption occurs in the small intestine via passive diffusion, being diminished when given with food, mainly if food contains calcium or iron. Its plasma half-life is very short because it is soon deposited in the bone, in areas of bone formation and destruction.[17,18] The quantity of drug deposited in the bone will depend on the type of bisphosphonate delivered (lower in the clodronic acid and higher in alendronic, pamidronic, or zoledronic acids). When administered at clinically effective doses there is no apparent saturation in the fixation to the skeleton in human beings, at least for years or even decades. It might remain in the skeleton for many years, possibly for a lifetime as a result of the slowing of bone resorption in the area in which they are deposited. However, it has not been shown that the bisphosphonate deposited in the bones has any pharmacologic activity.

Bisphosphonate is not metabolized in the liver, the kidney being its only pathway of clearance.[13] Its renal clearance is high, suggesting the presence of a renal tubular secretory pathway.

Adverse Events

Bisphosphonate toxicity at the clinical dosage employed is not significant even though it is not free from mild adverse events. The most frequently described adverse events are the following[19]:

1. Transient hyperthermia within the first 24 to 48 hours since the administration that reverts with the use of acetaminophen
2. Thrombophlebitis in the infusion site
3. Increase of pain intensity after the first infusion
4. Gastrointestinal disorders such as nausea or vomiting more frequently present when the drug is used orally
5. Transient hypophosphoremia or hypocalcemia in patients with significant bone metastasis spreading. If hypocalcemia persists, secondary hyperparathyroidism might develop.
6. Pancytopenia, fatigue, and arthralgia
7. Renal function impairment, mainly if the drug is given intravenously and at a faster rate than scheduled. Consequently, renal function should be monitored (plasma creatinine levels and albuminuria) every 3 to 6 months in patients undergoing intravenous bisphosphonate treatment.[20] The simultaneous use of nephrotoxic drugs should be avoided.

USE OF BISPHOSPHONATES IN BONE TUMORS

Tumor osteolytic disease is a condition in which tumors of different sources induce bone destruction either by local or distant involvement[6] via the release to systemic circulation of products that stimulate bone resorption resulting in malignant humoral hypercalcemia. The causes of hypercalcemia are an increase in osteolysis, an increase in calcium renal resorption, or a likely dehydration.[21]

The most common clinical symptoms will be pain, fractures, and a hypercalcemic syndrome with multiple metabolic consequences.[22] Occasionally, patients might develop a hypercalcemic crisis, which represents a life-threatening emergency.

Some of the most important bone resorption markers are *N*-telopeptide, pyridinoline, deoxypyridinoline, hydroxyproline, calcium, and *N*-telopeptide–creatine ratio. However, their use is restricted to research trials.[23] The most important biochemical tests for bone metastasis will be calcemia, serum alkaline phosphatase, calciuria, hydroxyprolinuria, and urine pyridinoline. Nevertheless, the main parameters frequently used to follow up bone metastases are calcemia, calciuria, pain, fractures, and osteolytic foci.

Thus in the clinical setting of patients with bone metastases, bisphosphonates are the treatment of choice for the previously mentioned conditions, mainly because of their inhibitory activity on osteoclasts (main bone resorption mediators). Bisphosphonates are mainly indicated for the following:

1. Bone tumors with osteolytic lesions (breast, myeloma) and tumors with osteoblastic lesions as recently shown (prostate and third-generation bisphosphonates—zoledronate)[24]
2. Malignant humoral hypercalcemia[25]

Currently, however, and with the use of more powerful bisphosphonates in vitro evidence is coming up regarding the more direct effects on the bone tumor per se. It is being shown that third-generation bisphosphonates such as ibandronic acid or zoledronic acid are able to also inhibit the occurrence and progression of bone lesions and reduce the tumor burden.[26] This indirect effect is based on the inhibition that these drugs produce on bone resorption and osteoclastogenesis, which deprives tumor cells of essential growth factors.[27,28] This likely action is also related to their effect on the prevention of bone metastases. Although there is also in vitro and in vivo preclinical evidence it is too early to favor this indication.[29]

The most recent action described about these drugs is their likely beneficial effect on nociception (analgesic effect) that might not be related with its traditional mechanism on bone resorption.[30,31]

MAIN BISPHOSPHONATES CLINICALLY USED IN ONCOLOGY

Several generations of bisphosphonates have been developed since the early 1970s. In each of the following generations their chemical structure has been modified, resulting in more powerful compounds. If classified from the least to the most powerful agents, the following drugs are available (Table 25–1).

Etidronate (Etidronic Acid)

This is the least powerful of the clinically evaluated bisphosphonates so far and because there is no clear evidence in terms of its use in patients with metastatic bone pain, it is not used for that specific aim.[32] A further disadvantage is a likely inhibition of bone mineralization, which can lead to osteomalacia.

Clodronate (Clodronic Acid)

It belongs to the second generation of bisphosphonates with an intermediate power between etidronate and pamidronate. Like other bisphosphonates, it does not have negative effects on bone mineralization and can be administered orally or intravenously. Several studies have shown a moderate analgesic effect and a slowing effect on bone metastasis.[33,34] Recommended doses are 1600 mg/day orally and 600 mg every 3 weeks intravenously.[35] The approaches can be combined occasionally.

Pamidronate (Pamidronic Acid)

This is a second-generation aminobisphosphonate widely studied in the palliative treatment of patients with bone metastases, the most powerful agent known until not long ago.[36] Given its sound safety profile, even in patients with altered kidney function,[37] its higher effectiveness and its long-lasting action in comparison with the previously mentioned bisphosphonates it has recently become the drug of choice for the treatment of tumor hypercalcemia or as adjuvant treatment in patients with bone involvement.[38,39] The intravenous route is used because oral administration is associated with more gastrointestinal adverse events and lower clinical effectiveness.[5] Recommended doses range from 60 to 90 mg intravenously for 2 hours once a month.[35,40]

Alendronate (Alendronic Acid)

It also belongs to the aminobisphosphonate class. Even though its power is greater than that of pamidronate, its effectiveness and length of action is shorter; therefore, it has not been studied in tumor bone disease.

Ibandronate (Ibandronic Acid)

Ibandronate is a third-generation bisphosphonate, about 100 times more powerful than pamidronate.[41] There are few studies available that address it as bone tumor coadjuvant treatment. Doses used are 4 to 6 mg per month during a 2-hour infusion period.[35]

Zolendronate (Zoledronic Acid)

With the most recent appearance in clinical practice and the widest use in health institutions, the American Society of Clinical Oncology (ASCO) has recommended zolendronate in its clinical practice guide as the bisphosphonate of choice in patients with tumor bone disease.[20] A powerful third-generation bisphosphonate (100 times as powerful as pamidronate and 10,000 times as powerful as etidronate), it presents a second nitrogen atom in its molecule.[42] As an aminophosphonate, it inhibits osteoclastic activity (and possibly that of tumor cells) by preventing phenylization of proteins inhibiting the pharnesyl-diphosphate-synthetase (enzyme of the mevalonate pathway), leading to a loss of metabolites essential for the function of osteoclasts inducing apoptosis and cell death.[43,44] It is to be noted that its possible action is against bone tumors of osteoblastic nature like bone metastases in prostate cancer[24,45] or in solid tumors[46] (lung cancer) because a decrease in biochemical markers associated with bone resorption in osteoblastic bone metastasis is seen in patients treated with 4 mg of zoledronic acid in comparison with placebo.[42] Recommended doses are 4 mg intravenously infused for 15 minutes once a month.[42] When compared with pamidronate, zoledronic acid presents at least similar or greater effectiveness, fewer side effects, greater length of action and, above all, shorter delivery time.[47-49] On the other hand, its price is higher. Consequently, all these factors should be balanced when it comes to decide between these two medications.

SCIENTIFIC EVIDENCE

Several studies of the efficacy of bisphosphonates for treating pain and complications resulting from bone metastasis have been conducted to date and not all are summarized here. Four systematic reviews have been identified (Djulbegovic,[50] Pavlakis,[51] Ross,[52] and Wong[53]) that evaluated the efficacy of bisphosphonates on bone metastases, either regarding pain or complications (bone fractures, spinal compression, etc.), and in which data could be combined and meta-analyses performed.

Djulbegovic's systematic review[50] included 11 clinical trials[33,38,54-67] of bisphosphonates compared with placebo or with a group with no treatment. The trials were performed in patients with myeloma. It assessed the efficacy of bisphosphonates for treating bone pain and its complications.

Pavlakis's review[51] included 19 clinical trials[68-95] of bisphosphonates compared with standard treatment or other bisphosphonates in patients with breast cancer–related bone metastasis. It not only analyzed the bisphosphonates' efficacy in breast cancer–related bone complications but also their efficacy for the prevention of skeletal events in patients with early breast cancer.

Ross's systematic review[52] included 30 clinical trials[A] on bisphosphonates. They were randomized and compared with placebo, standard treatment, or with other bisphosphonates. These trials involved patients with myeloma and breast cancer. This review addressed complications associated with these bone tumors (fractures, spinal compression, and need for surgery or radiation therapy).

Wong's systematic review[53] included 30 clinical trials[B] on bisphosphonates, randomized, open or blind; compared with placebo, standard treatment, or with other bisphosphonates. It assessed the efficacy of bisphosphonates

on bone metastases–related pain regardless of the primary tumor.

In addition to the information from these reviews, another unpublished systematic review is added, performed by Roqué et al.[133] and sponsored in 2000 by the Instituto Carlos III that depends on the Spanish Health Department. That review evaluated 12 double-blind placebo-controlled clinical trials.[C] Bisphosphonates were used for the treatment of bone metastases–related pain and complications, regardless of the primary tumor.

Nevertheless, the search for clinical trials of these reviews was performed until 2001; therefore, data will be supported with the brief description of new randomized controlled clinical trials not included in those reviews published in 2003.

Evaluation of Bone Pain Related to Metastatic Lesions

As for the evaluation of bisphosphonates for treating bone metastasis–related pain, the Cochrane Library (Djulbegovic,[50] Pavlakis,[51] Wong[53]) published three systematic reviews, although only two included a meta-analysis (Djulbegovic[50] and Wong[53]).

Djulbegovic's review[50] evaluated the efficacy of bisphosphonates on bone complications related to multiple myeloma. Pain relief was considered as a secondary variable. Results of analysis for pain, though favoring bisphosphonates, showed heterogeneity and should therefore be interpreted with caution. Additionally, a further factor that contributed to questions about the results was that accepted clinical trials did not mask treatments so the effect of placebo of each intervention, especially on subjective variables as pain, could not be controlled.

Wong's review[53] studied the efficacy of bisphosphonates on bone metastasis–related pain. Studies in which pain was self-assessed by patients were included. However, inclusion criteria were wide because open clinical trials were accepted. The effect of placebo was not controlled either. Overall results of the meta-analysis of the variable pain relief were homogeneous and favored bisphosphonates: odds ratio (OR) 2.56 (95% confidence interval [CI] 1.57-4.18).

When performing the sensitivity analysis comparing the double or single-blinded clinical trials with open trials, results were more modest in the first group than in the second (OR 1.92 [95% CI 1.26-2.92] versus OR 5.29 [95% CI 2.13-13.15], respectively), thereby confirming the significance of masking all treatments to obtain a more reliable outcome.

[A]See references 33, 46, 48, 58, 59, 62, 63, 65, 68, 69, 72, 74, 77–79, 82, 84, 93, 96–115.

[B]See references 34, 54, 55, 57–59, 62, 65, 68, 70, 80, 84, 92, 116–132.

[C]See references 39, 55, 59, 68, 70, 80, 86, 124, 126, 127, 130–132.

Results of the meta-analysis of the number of patients with a reduction of analgesics were homogeneous and favored bisphosphonates, both in week 4 (OR 2.81 [95% CI 1.24-6.38]) and week 12 (OR 2.37 [95% CI 1.1-5.12]).

Finally, the review by Roqué et al[133] also followed the Cochrane guidelines and assessed double-blind clinical trials of bisphosphonates for treating pain related to bone metastasis and its complications. Inclusion criteria for the clinical trials were highly strict, considering that the main variable presents great subjectivity. Results, though favorable, were more modest than those observed in Wong's review.[53] Results of the analysis of the variable pain relief at week 4 were homogeneous and not significant (OR 1.80 [95% CI 0.93-3.46]), while at week 12 they were homogeneous and significantly favored bisphosphonates (OR 1.29 [95% CI 1.05-1.59]). Results of the analysis of the variable rate of patients with reduction or maintenance of analgesics were homogeneous and favored bisphosphonates (OR 1.26 [95% CI 1.08-1.46]).

Evaluation of Complications

Pathologic Fractures

Djulbegovic's systematic review[50] showed a beneficial effect of bisphosphonates on the prevention of pathologic fractures (OR = 0.59 [95% CI 0.45-0.78]; NNT 10 [95% CI 7-20]). Results obtained were similar to those in Ross's[52] systematic review (OR = 0.65 [IC 95% 0.55-0.78]) and Pavlakis's[51] (RR = 0.88 [95% CI 0.81-0.96]). However, Roqué's review[133] was unable to show differences with the placebo, possibly because the inclusion criteria were stricter and because recently published studies were not analyzed.

Hypercalcemia

Djulbegovic's review[50] showed no differences in the efficacy of bisphosphonates compared with the control group as to hypercalcemia. On the other hand, Ross's[52] and Roqué's[133] obtained homogeneous and favorable results for bisphosphonates (OR = 0.54 [0.36-0.81] and RR = 0.52 [0.39-0.71], respectively).

Need for Orthopedic Surgery

Only Ross's review[52] studied this variable and found no difference with the control group.

Need for Radiation Therapy

Both Ross's and Roqué's reviews[52,133] showed a decrease in the need for radiation therapy when bisphosphonates were administered (OR = 0.67 [0.57-0.79] and RR = 0.80 [0.66-0.98], respectively).

Spinal Compression

Both Ross's and Roqué's studies[52,133] agreed that there are no differences on the effect of bisphosphonates compared with the control group.

Survival

Djulbegovic's,[50] Pavlakis's,[51] Roqué's,[133] and Ross's[52] meta-analyses agreed that there are no differences in the survival of patients receiving bisphosphonates compared with the control group.

Evaluation by Active Drug, Route of Administration, Dosage, and Length of Treatment

There are different bisphosphonates evaluated in patients with bone metastasis. Ordered from the least to the most powerful they are as follows: etidronate, clodronate, pamidronate, ibandronate, and zoledronic acid (Table 25-1).

The largest number of randomized clinical trials to date comprises clodronate and pamidronate. Wong's[53] review evaluated pain relief in patients with bone metastases. An analysis by type of bisphosphonate was performed. Five clinical trials[62,116,120,124,129] used clodronate, which proved to be significantly favorable; whereas two clinical trials[119,132] used pamidronate and the result was not significant with respect to the control group (OR = 3.26 [95% CI 1.8-5.89] and OR = 2.35 [95% CI 0.77-7.15], respectively). It is likely that in the light of new data obtained from the recently published clinical trials, the results of Wong's review might be modified, especially in the evaluation of skeletal events. Two new clinical trials[134,135] performed with clodronate in prostate cancer, one used as an oral agent and the other as an intravenous agent, have shown no differences with respect to placebo. Pamidronate has been used as the benchmark in comparative studies carried out with zoledronate[47,48,88,98,113] and ibandronate.[136] A placebo-controlled clinical trial[137] with pamidronate in the early stages of myeloma favored pamidronic acid concerning the development of skeletal events. However, the result was not the same regarding patients' survival or disease progression. On the other hand, there are almost no comparative studies of clodronate and pamidronate. A clinical trial[138] that included 51 patients compared 1600 mg intravenous clodronate with 1600 mg oral clodronate and 60 mg intravenous pamidronate in advanced metastatic disease, showing a better effect of pamidronate. However, the number of patients included was too small to consider these results as reliable.

So far there have been too few studies on etidronic acid, and the sample size is small.[50] Ibandronate has been evaluated in two placebo-controlled clinical trials[139,140] and in one with pamidronate.[136] Results of one of the clinical trials[139] show that it has favorable effects on breast cancer when compared with placebo and that it is as effective as pamidronate for treating tumor hypercalcemia. The result of another clinical trial[140] on myeloma shows no difference with respect to placebo.

Although the clinical trials that evaluated the efficacy of zoledronic acid are recent, their acceptable design, the large number of patients included, results obtained, and the short delivery time turn this medication into the bisphosphonate of choice when compared with all other bisphosphonates. Zoledronic acid has been evaluated in placebo-controlled clinical trials in bone metastasis related to prostate,[24] lung,[46,111] and kidney[141] cancer with favorable results as far as the prevention of skeletal events and on the time elapsed until the first skeletal event occurs. It has also been compared with pamidronate,[47,48,98,113] showing similar efficacy, although in a recent study[48] in a subgroup of patients (breast cancer) results of zoledronic acid are better than those of pamidronate.

Pavlakis's review[51] evaluated efficacy of bisphosphonate by route of administration (intravenous or oral). The result of the analysis of three studies[68,80,73,74] of intravenous pamidronate was not conclusive because it was heterogeneous. On the other hand, a pooled analysis of three studies[82,85,86,90] of clodronic acid and one study[92] of pamidronate, both used orally, was carried out, showing homogeneity in the analysis and favorable results on efficacy (RR = 0.83 [0.73; 0.94]). However, these results are not consistent with the general overview that intravenous administration is more effective than oral administration, due to the poor intestinal absorption of bisphosphonates and based on the experience from several clinical trials recently developed that prove the efficacy of the intravenous approach. Therefore, the most recent review by Ross,[52] including new clinical trials, shows that both the oral and the intravenous approach are effective on reducing vertebral and nonvertebral fractures.

None of the systematic reviews included a subgroup analysis by dosage of bisphosphonate despite the existing recommended guideline for each one.

ASCO has recently published a guideline for the use of bisphosphonates in multiple myeloma.[20] The three bisphosphonates that have shown beneficial effects when compared with placebo are oral clodronate, intravenous pamidronate, and zoledronic acid. Later, however, the guideline only recommends pamidronate and zoledronic acid because clodronate is not marketed in

the United States and the time elapsed until the first skeletal event occurs is shorter in patients who receive clodronate than in those given the other two medications, although they have not undergone a head-to-head comparison.

We believe that clodronate should continue as a drug for reference in those countries in which its use is approved. It is one of the medications most widely used, and clinical trials show that there is a benefit in comparison with placebo in the treatment of pain and hypercalcemia resulting from bone metastasis. The clinician should weigh risks and benefits of each active drug.

The route of administration recommended by ASCO[20] is the intravenous route, and doses advised are 90 mg of pamidronic acid in a 2-hour infusion or 4 mg of zoledronic acid in an infusion of 15 minutes every 3 to 4 weeks. The most effective doses of clodronate are 1600 to 2400 mg/day orally.

As to the length of treatment, ASCO[20] recommends treating the patient until the patient's general performance status remarkably improves.

Evaluation by Type of Tumor

The effect of bisphosphonates has been extensively studied in primary tumors such as myeloma and breast cancer,[50-52] in which they have proved to be effective for the management of bone pain and the prevention of skeletal events.

Prostate cancer–related bone metastatic lesions, although predominantly osteoblastic, are also sensitive to the effects of bisphosphonates due to the coexistence of osteolytic components.[142] Clinical trials have also been carried out with different results according to the type of bisphosphonate: Two clinical trials[134,135] on clodronate have been negative (see references), and one clinical trial[24] on zoledronic acid compared with placebo has shown its effectiveness in the prevention of skeletal events.

Clinical trials[46,59,126-128,132] have also been developed in patients with bone metastasis regardless of their primary tumor and quite likely will be an area for further research.

Future Implications

Pavlakis's review[51] that evaluated the effects of bisphosphonates on preventing metastasis in patients with early breast cancer was not conclusive when a meta-analysis was performed on two clinical trials. However, there are ongoing Phase III clinical trials[143] of zoledronic acid for preventing breast and prostate cancer related bone metastases. Two clinical trials[144,145] on clodronate for preventing breast cancer–related bone metastasis have been published recently. Results are controversial because one clinical trial[144] shows negative results (see reference) whereas the other[145] shows positive results (see reference) with a significant reduction of mortality in patients at 2-year follow-up and a decrease in bone metastasis rate during treatment, though not during the follow-up period.

Likewise, the antitumor action of bisphosphonates is an area suitable for future research. On the basis of the results of most clinical trials carried out to the present day, we can say that their effects on patients' survival are null.

Similarly, we need a more homogeneous and standardized evaluation, which will allow setting up comparisons among the studies so as to have deeper knowledge on their effects on patients' quality of life.

CONCLUSION

Based on the findings discussed earlier, the following conclusions can be drawn:

1. Bisphosphonates are one of the main treatments in patients with tumor bone disease, either metastatic (breast, lung, colon) or primary (myeloma).
2. Bisphosphonates are the drugs of choice for cases of malignant humoral hypercalcemia.
3. The route of administration should be intravenous rather than oral because of its faster onset of action and effectiveness.[49]
4. Zoledronic acid is currently the treatment of choice given its quick onset of action and shorter infusion time. However, as pointed out, each health care institution should weigh the cost against the benefit because there are no great differences with pamidronate.
5. The use of oral clodronate is still justified in those countries where it is available because there are few comparative studies with pamidronate or zoledronic acid to disregard its use and there is evidence that seems to favor its effectiveness.
6. There is still lack of consensus regarding when to start treatment (in bone metastases) and how long treatment with bisphosphonates should last. Nevertheless, it seems reasonable to start treatment soon after a malignant bone tumor is detected. The length of treatment is also hard to define, but it is recommended not to discontinue treatment in spite of disease progression due to the palliative effects of bisphosphonates on bone complications.
7. Finally, due to the lack of evidence of a greater survival in patients treated with these medications and to their moderate analgesic action, we cannot set aside other treatments such as chemotherapy, radiation therapy, or concomitant analgesic therapy.

REFERENCES

1. Body JJ: Metastases bone disease: Clinical and therapeutic aspects. Bone 13(suppl 1): S57–S62, 1992.
2. Coleman RE, Rubens RD: The clinical course of bone metastases from breast cancer. Br J Cancer 55:61–66, 1997.
3. Keller ET: The role of osteoclastic activity in prostate cancer skeletal metastases. Drugs Today (Barce) 38:91–102, 2002.
4. Kanis JA, O'Rourke N, McCloskey EV: Consequences of neoplasia-induced bone resorption and the use of Clodronate. Int J Oncol 5:713–731, 1994.
5. Ripamonti C, Fulfaro F: Malignant bone pain: Pathophysiology and treatments. Curr Rev Pain 4:187–196, 2000.
6. Mercadante S: Malignant bone pain: Pathophysiology and treatment. Pain 69:1–18, 1997.
7. Bennet A: Role of biochemical mediators in peripheral nociception and bone pain. Cancer Surv 7:55–67, 1988.
8. Mundy GR: Bone resorption and turnover in health and disease. Bone 12(suppl 1): S9–S16, 1991.
9. Dodwell DJ: Malignant bone resorption: Cellular and biochemical mechanisms. Ann Oncol 3:257–267, 1992.
10. Mundy GR: Mechanisms of osteolytic bone destruction. Bone 12(suppl 1) S1–S6, 1991.
11. Sabatini M, Chavez J, Mundy GR, et al: Stimulation of tumor necrosis factor release from monocytic cells by the A375 human

melanoma via granulocyte-macrophage colony-stimulating factor. Cancer Res 5:2673–2678, 1990.
12. Fleisch H: Development of bisphosphonates. Breast Cancer Res 4:30–34, 2002.
13. Fleisch H: Bisphosphonates. Pharmacology and use in the treatment of tumor-induced hypercalcemic and metastatic bone disease. Drugs 42:919–944, 1991.
14. Flanagan AM, Chambers TJ: Inhibition of bone resorption by bisphosphonates: Interactions between bisphosphonates, osteoclasts, and bone. Calcif Tissue Int 49:407–415, 1991.
15. Berenson JR, Lipton A: Pharmacology and clinical efficacy of bisphosphonates. Curr Opin Oncol 10:566–571, 1998.
16. Rogers MJ, Gordon S, Benford HL, et al: Cellular and molecular mechanisms of action of bisphosphonates. Cancer 88:2961–2978, 2000.
17. Russell R, Rogers MJ, Frith JC, et al: The pharmacology of bisphosphonates and new insights into their mechanisms of action. J Bone Min Res 14:53–65, 1999.
18. Cheung WK, Brunner L, Schoenfeld S, et al: Pharmaco kinetics of pamidronate disodium in cancer patients after a single intravenous infusion of 30-60-90 mg dose over 4 or 24 hours. Am J Therap 1:228–235, 1994.
19. Vinholes J, Guo CY, Purohit OP, et al: Metabolic effects of pamidronate in patients with metastatic bone disease. Br J Cancer 73:1089–1095, 1996.

20. Berenson JR, Hillner BE, Kyle RA, et al: American society of clinical oncology clinical practice guidelines: The role of bisphosphonates in multiple myeloma. J Clin Oncol 20:3719–3736, 2002.
21. Bajorunas DR: Clinical manifestations of cancer-related hypercalcemia. Sem Oncol 17:16–25, 1990.
22. Vassilopoulou-Sellin R, Newman BM, Taylor SH, et al: Incidence of hypercalcemia in patients with malignancy referred to a comprehensive cancer center. Cancer 71:1309–1312, 1993.
23. Berenson JR, Vescio R, Henick K, et al: A phase I, open label, dose ranging trial of intravenous bolus zoledronic acid, a novel bisphosphonate, in cancer patients with metastatic bone disease. Cancer 91:144–154, 2001.
24. Saad F: Treatment of bone complications in advanced prostate cancer: Rationales for bisphosphonate use and results of a phase III trial with zoledronic acid. Semin Oncol 29(suppl 21):19–27, 2002.
25. Berenson JR: Treatment of hypercalcemia of malignancy with bisphosphonates. Sem Oncol 29(suppl 21): 12–18, 2002.
26. Clézardin P: The antitumor potential of bisphosphonates. Sem Oncol 29(suppl 21): 33–42, 2002.
27. Hiraga T, Williams PJ, Mundy GR, et al: The bisphosphonate ibandronate promotes apoptosis in MDA-MB-321 human breast cancer cells in bone metastases. Cancer Res 61:4418–4424, 2001.

28. Van Beek ER, Lowik CW, Papapoulus SE: Bisphosphonates suppress bone resorption by a direct effect on early osteoclast precursors without affecting the osteoclastogenic capacity of osteogenic cells: The role of protein geranylgeranylation in the action of nitrogen-containing bisphosphonates on osteoclast precursors. Bone 30:64–70, 2002.

29. Coleman R: Bisphosphonates for the prevention of bone metastases. Semin Oncol 29(suppl 21):43–49, 2002.

30. Bonabello A, Galmozzi MR, Bruzzese T, et al: Analgesic effect of bisphosphonates in mice. Pain 92:269–275, 2001.

31. Walker K, Medhurst SJ, Kidd BL, et al: Disease modifying and anti-nociceptive effects of bisphosphonate zoledronic acid in a model of bone cancer pain. Pain 100:219–229, 2002.

32. Belch AR, Bergsagel DE, Wilson K, et al: Effect of daily etidronate on the osteolysis of multiple myeloma. J Clin Oncol 9:1397–1402, 1991.

33. McCloskey EV, MacLennan IC, Drayson MT, et al: A randomized trial of the effect of clodronate on skeletal morbidity in multiple myeloma. MRC working party on leukemia in adults. Br J Haematol 100:317–325, 1998.

34. Ernst DS, Brasher P, Hagen N, et al: A randomized, controlled trial of intravenous clodronate in patients with metastatic bone disease and pain. J Pain Symptom Manage 13:319–326, 1997.

35. Fulfaro F, Casuccio A, Ticozzi C, et al: The role of bisphosphonates in the treatment of painful metastatic bone disease: A review of phase III trials. Pain 78:157–169, 1998.

36. Kellihan MJ, Mangino PD: Pamidronate. Ann Pharmacother 26:1262–1269, 1992.

37. Gucalp R, Theriault R, Gill I, et al: Treatment of cancer-associated hypercalcemia. Double-blind comparison of rapid and slow intravenous infusion regimens of pamidronate disodium and saline alone. Arch Intern Med 154:1935–1944, 1994.

38. Berenson JR, Lichtenstein A, Porter L, et al: Long-term pamidronate treatment of advanced multiple myeloma patients reduces skeletal events. J Clin Oncol 16:593–602, 1998.

39. Hortobagyi GN, Theriault RL, Lipton A, et al: Long-term prevention of skeletal complications of metastatic breast cancer with pamidronate. J Clin Oncol 16: 2038–2044, 1998.

40. Thurlimann B, Morant R, Jungi WF, et al: Pamidronate for pain control in patients with malignant osteolytic bone disease: A prospective dose-effect study. Support Care Cancer 2:61–65, 1994.

41. Muhlbauer RC, Bauss F, Schenk R, et al: BM 210955, a potent new bisphosphonate to inhibit bone resorption. J Bone Mineral Res 6:1003–1011, 1991.

42. Wellington K, Goa KL: Zoledronic acid: A review of its use in the management of bone metastases and hypercalcaemia of malignancy. Drugs 63:417–437, 2003.

43. Dunford JE, Thompson K, Coxon FP, et al: Structure-activity relationship for inhibition of farnesyl diphosphate synthase in vitro and inhibition of bone resorption in vivo by nitrogen-containing bisphosphonates. J Pharmacol Exp Ther 296:235–242, 2001.

44. Coxon FP, Helfrich MH, Van't Hof RJ, et al: Protein geranylgeranylation is required for osteoclast formation, function, and survival: Inhibition by bisphosphonates and GGTI-298. J Bone Miner Res 15: 1467–1476, 2000.

45. Corey E, Brown LG, Quinn JE, et al: Zoledronic acid exhibits inhibitory effects on osteoblastic and osteolytic metastases of prostate cancer. Clin Cancer Res 9:295–306, 2003.

46. Rosen LS, Gordon D, Tchekmedyian S, et al: Zoledronic acid versus placebo in the treatment of skeletal metastases in patients with lung cancer and other solid tumors: A phase III, double-blind, randomized trial – the zoledronic acid lung cancer and other solid tumors study group. J Clin Oncol 21:3150–3157, 2003.

47. Major P, Lortholary A, Hon J, et al: Zoledronic acid is superior to pamidronate in the treatment of hypercalcemia of malignancy: A pooled analysis of two randomized, controlled clinical trials. J Clin Oncol 19:558–567, 2001.

48. Rosen LS, Gordon D, Kaminski M, et al: Long-term efficacy and safety of zoledronic acid compared with pamidronate disodium in the treatment of skeletal complications in patients with advanced multiple myeloma or breast carcinoma: A randomized, double-blind, multicenter, comparative trial. Cancer 98:1735–1744, 2003.

49. Major PP, Lipton A, Berenson J, et al: Oral bisphosphonates: A review of clinical use in patients with bone metastases. Cancer 88:6–14, 2000.

50. Djulbegovic B, Wheatley K, Ross J, et al: Bisphosphonates in multiple myeloma (Cochrane Review). In: The Cochrane Library. Chichester, United Kingdom, Wiley, Ltd. Issue 4, 2003.

51. Pavlakis N, Stockler M: Bisphosphonates for breast cancer (Cochrane Review). In: The Cochrane Library. Chichester, United Kingdom, Wiley, Ltd. Issue 4, 2003.

52. Ross JR, Saunders Y, Edmonds PM, et al: Systematic review of role of bisphosphonates on skeletal morbidity in metastatic cancer. BMJ 327:469–472, 2003.

53. Wong R, Wiffen PJ. Bisphosphonates for the relief of pain secondary to bone metastases (Cochrane Review). In: The Cochrane Library. Chichester, United Kingdom, Wiley, Ltd. Issue 4, 2003.

54. Belch AR, Bergsagel DE, Wilson K: Effect of daily etidronate on the osteolysis of multiple myeloma. J Clin Oncol 9: 1397–1402, 14, 1991.

55. Berenson JR, Lichtenstein A, Porter L, et al: Efficacy of pamidronate in reducing skeletal events in patients with advanced multiple myeloma. Myeloma Aredia Study Group. N Engl J Med 334:488–493, 1996.

56. Abildgaard N, Rungby J, Glerup H, et al: Long-term oral pamidronate treatment inhibits osteoclastic bone resorption and bone turnover without affecting osteoblastic function in multiple myeloma. Eur J Haematol 61:128–134, 1998.

57. Brincker JW, Abildgaard N: Failure of oral pamidronate to reduce skeletal morbidity in multiple myeloma: A double-blind placebo-controlled trial. Br J Haematol 101:280–286, 1998.

58. Daragon A, Humez C, Michot CXLL: Treatment of multiple myeloma with etidronate results of a multicentre double-blind study. Eur J Med 2:449–452,1993.

59. Delmas PD, Charhon S, Chapuy MC, et al: Long-term effects of dichloromethylene diphosphonate (Cl2MDP) on skeletal lesions in multiple myeloma. Metab Bone Dis Rel Res 1:163–168, 1982.

60. Fontana A, Herrmann Z. Menssen HD, et al: Effects of intravenous ibandronate therapy on skeletal related events (SRE) and survival in patients with advanced multiple myeloma. Blood 92: (Supp 1):106, 1998.

61. Clemens MR, Fessele K, Heim ME: Multiple myeloma: Effect of daily dichloromethylene bisphosphonate on skeletal multiple myeloma: Effect of daily dichloromethylene bisphosphonate on skeletal complications. Ann Hematol 66:141–146, 1993.

62. Heim ME, Clemens MR, Queiber W, et al: Prospective randomized trial of dichloromethilene bisphosphonate (clodronate) in patients with multiple myeloma. Onkologie 18: 439–448, 1995.

63. Kraj M, Poglód R, Pawlikowsky J, Maj S: The effect of long-term pamidronate treatment on skeletal morbidity in advanced multiple myeloma. Acta Haematol Pol 31:379–389, 2000.

64. Kraj M, Póglod R, Pawlikowski J, et al: Effect of pamidronate on skeletal morbidity in myelomatosis. I. The results of the 12 months of pamidronate therapy. Acta Pol Pharm 57(suppl 1):113–116, 2000.

65. Lahtinen R, Laakso M, Palva I: Randomized, placebo-controlled multicentre trial of clodronate in multiple myeloma. Lancet 340:1049–1052, 1992.

66. McCloskey EV, Dunn JA, Kanis JA, et al: Long-term follow-up of a prospective, double-blind, placebo-controlled randomised trial of clodronate in multiple myeloma. Br J Haematol 113:1035–1043, 2001.

67. Terpos E, Palermos J, Tsionos K, et al: Effect of pamidronate administration on markers of bone turnover and disease activity in multiple myeloma. Eur J Haematol 65:331–336, 2000.

68. Hortobagyi GN, Theriault RL, Porter L, et al: Efficacy of pamidronate in reducing skeletal complications in patients with breast cancer and lytic bone metastases [Efficacy of pamidronate in reducing skeletal complications in patients with breast cancer and lytic bone metastases]. N Engl J Med 335:1785–1791, 1996.

69. Lipton A, Theriault RL, Hortobagyi GN, et al: Pamidronate prevents skeletal complications and is effective palliative treatment in women with breast carcinoma and osteolytic bone metastases. Cancer 88:1082–1090, 2000.

70. Theriault RL, Lipton A, Hortobagyi GN, et al: Pamidronate reduces skeletal morbidity in women with advanced breast cancer and lytic bone lesions: A randomized, placebo-controlled trial [Pamidronate reduces skeletal morbidity in women with advanced breast cancer and lytic bone lesions: A randomized, placebo-controlled trial]. J Clin Oncol 17:846–854, 1999.

71. Body JJ, Lichinitser MR, Diehl I, et al: Double-blind placebo-controlled trial of intravenous ibandronate in breast cancer

metastatic to bone. Proc Annu Meet Am Soc Clin Oncol. Abstract 2222, 1999.

72. Diel IJ, Lichinitser MR, Body JJ, et al: Improvement of bone pain, quality of life and survival time of breast cancer patients with metastatic bone disease treated with intravenous ibandronate. Proc Eur Com Clin Onc, Abstract 269, 1999.

73. Conte PF, Giannessi PG, Latreille J, et al: Delayed progression of bone metastases with pamidronate therapy in breast cancer patients: A randomized, multicenter phase III trial. Ann Oncol 5(suppl 7): S41–S44, 1994.

74. Conte PF, Latrielle J, Mauriac L, et al: Delay in progression of bone metastases in breast cancer patients treated with intravenous pamidronate: Results from a multinational randomized controlled trial. J Clin Oncol 14:2552–2559, 1996.

75. Diel IJ, Solomayer E-F, Costa SD, et al: Reduction in new metastases in breast cancer with adjuvant clodronate treatment. N Engl J Med 339:357–363, 1998.

76. Diel IJ, Marschner N, Kindler M, et al: Continual oral versus intravenous interval therapy with bisphosphonates in patients with breast cancer and bone metastases. Proc Annu Meet Am Soc Clin Oncol, Abstract 488, 1999.

77. Elomaa I, Blomqvist C, Grohn P, et al: Long-term controlled trial with diphosphonate in patients with osteolytic bone metastases. Lancet 1:146–149, 1983.

78. Elomaa I, Blomqvist C, Porkka, et al: Clodronate for osteolytic metastases due to breast cancer. Biomed Parmacother 42:111–116, 1988.

79. Elomma I, Blomqvist L, Porkka L, et al: Treatment of skeletal disease in breast cancer: A controlled clodronate trial. Bone 8(Supp 1):S53–S56, 1987.

80. Hultborn R, Gundersen S, Ryden S, et al: Efficacy of pamidronate in breast cancer with bone metastases: A randomized, double-blind placebo-controlled multi-center study. Anticancer Res 19:3383–3392, 1999.

81. Kanis JA, Powles T, Paterson S, et al: Clodronate decreases the frequency of skeletal metastases in women with breast cancer. Bone 19:663–667, 1996.

82. Kristensen B, Ejlertsen B, Groenvold M, et al: Oral clodronate in breast cancer patients with bone metastases: A random-ized study. J Intern Med 246:67–74, 1999.

83. Mardiak J, Bohunicky L, Chovanec J, et al: Adjuvant clodronate therapy in patients with locally advanced breast cancer: Long term results of a double blind randomized trial. Neoplasma 47:177–180, 2000.

84. Martoni A, Guaraldi M, Camera P, et al: Controlled clinical study on the use of dichloromethylene diphosphonate in patients with breast carcinoma metastasiz-ing to the skeleton. Oncology 48:97–101, 1991.

85. Powles T, Paterson S, Kanis JA, et al: Randomised placebo-controlled trial of clodronate in patients with primary operable breast cancer. J Clin Oncol 20:3219–3224, 2002.

86. Paterson S, Powles TJ, Kanis JA, et al: Double-blind controlled trial of oral clodro-nate in patients with bone metastases from breast cancer. J Clin Oncol 11:59–65, 1993.

87. Powles TJ, Paterson S, Nevantaus A, et al: Adjuvant clodronate reduces the incidence of bone metastases in patients with primary operable breast cancer. Proc Annu Meet Am Soc Clin Oncol. Abstract 468, 1998.

88. Rosen LS, Gordon D, Kaminski M, et al: Zoledronic acid versus pamidronate in the treatment of skeletal metastases in patients with breast cancer or proteolytic lesions of multiple myeloma: A Phase III, double-blind, comparative trial. Cancer J 7:377–387, 2001.

89. Saarto T, Blomqvist C, Virkkunen P, Elomaa I. Adjuvant clodronate treatment does not reduce the frequency of skeletal metastases in node-positive breast cancer patients: 5 year results of a randomized controlled study. J Clin Oncol 19:10–17, 2001.

90. Tubiana-Hulin M, Beuzeboc P, Mauriac L, et al: Double-blinded controlled study comparing clodronate versus placebo in patients with breast cancer bone metastases. Bull Cancer 88:701–707, 2001.

91. Cleton FJ, van Holten-Verzantvoort AT, Bijvoet OLM: Recent results in cancer research. Vol. 116, Berlin-Heidelberg, Springer-Verlag, 73–78, 1989.

92. Van Holten-Vaerzantvoort AT, Kroon HM, Bijvoet OLM, et al: Palliative pamidronate treatment in patients with bone metas-tases from breast cancer. J Clin Oncol 11:491–498, 1993.

93. Van Holten-Verzantvoort AT, Bijvoet OLM, Cleton FJ, et al: Reduced morbidity from skeletal metastases in breast cancer patients during long-term bisphosphonate (APD) treatment. Lancet 31:983–985, 1987.

94. Van Holten-Verzantvoort AT, Zwinderman AH, et al: The effect of supportive pami-dronate treatment on aspects of quality of life of patients with advanced breast cancer. Eur J Cancer 27:544–549, 1991.

95. Van Holten-Verzantvoort, Hermans J, Beex LVAM, et al: Does supportive pami-dronate treatment prevent or delay the first manifestations of bone metastases in breast cancer patients? Eur J Cancer 32:450–454, 1996.

96. Ausili-Cefaro G, Capirci C, Crivellari D, et al: Radiation therapy vs radiation therapy + pamidronate (Aredia) in elderly patients with breast cancer and lytic bone metastases: A GROG-GIOGER random-ized clinical trial. Rays 24(suppl 2):49–52, 1999.

97. Berenson JR: The efficacy of pamidronate disodium in the treatment of osteo-lytic lesions and bone pain in multiple myeloma. Rev Contemp Pharmacother 9:195–203, 1998.

98. Berenson JR, Rosen LS, Howell A, et al: Zoledronic acid reduces skeletal-related events in patients with osteolytic metasta-ses. Cancer 91:1191–1200, 2001.

99. Berenson JR: Zoledronic acid in cancer patients with bone metastases: Results of phase I and II trials. Semin Oncol 28 (suppl 6):25–34, 2001.

100. Brincker H, Westin J, Abildgaard N, et al: Failure of oral pamidronate to reduce skeletal morbidity in multiple myeloma: A double-blind placebo-controlled trial. Danish-Swedish

co-operative study group. Br J Haematol 101:280–286, 1998.

101. Ford JF: Pamidronate in the treatment of bone metastases: The European experi-ence. Br J Clin Pract Suppl 87:3–4, 1996.

102. Glover D, Lipton A, Keller A, et al: Intravenous pamidronate disodium treat-ment of bone metastases in patients with breast cancer. Cancer 74:2949–2955, 1994.

103. Gomez-Pastrana E, Velasco JG, Requena A, et al: Clinical and biochemical valuation of clodronate in tumoral osteolysis by bone metastases of breast cancer. Progresos de Obstetricia y Ginecologia 39:357–364, 1996.

104. Harris AL, Millward M, Tomkin K, et al: Randomised trial of aminoglutethamide and hydrocortisone with and without diso-dium pamidronate (APD) in patients with advanced postmenopausal breast cancer and bone metastases. In: Bijvoet OL, Lipton A (eds): Osteoclast inhibition in the management of malignancy-related bone disorders. Seattle, Hogrefe and Huber, A73, 1993.

105. Hultborn R, Gundersen S, Ryden S, et al: Efficacy of pamidronate in breast cancer with bone metastases: A randomized double-blind placebo controlled multicenter study. Acta Oncol 35 (suppl 5):73–74, 1996.

106. Laakso M, Lahtinen R, Virkkunen P, Elomaa I: Subgroup and cost-benefit analysis of the Finnish multicentre trial of clodronate in multiple myeloma. Br J Haematol 87:725–729, 1994.

107. Theriault R: Pamidronate in the treatment of osteolytic bone metastases in breast cancer patients. Br J Clin Pract Suppl 87:8–12, 1996.

108. Paterson AH, Powles TJ, Kanis JA, et al: Double-blind controlled trial of oral clo-dronate in patients with bone metastases from breast cancer. J Clin Oncol 11:59–65, 1993.

109. Hulin MT, Beuzeboc P, Mauriac L, et al: Double blind placebo controlled trial of oral clodronate in patients with bone metastases from breast cancer. Ann Oncol 5(suppl 8):198, 1994.

110. Unpublished data A. From R Murphy, Novartis pharmaceuticals to JR Ross and Y Saunders, 2001.

111. Rosen LS: Efficacy and safety of zoledronic acid in the treatment of bone metastases associated with lung cancer and other solid tumours. Semin Oncol 29 (suppl 21):28–32, 2002.

112. Unpublished data B. From R Murphy, Novartis pharmaceuticals to JR Ross and Y Saunders, 2001.

113. Rosen LS, Gordon D, Kaminski M, et al: Zoledronic acid versus pamidronate in the treatment of skeletal metastases in patients with breast cancer or osteolytic lesions of multiple myeloma: A phase III, double-blind, comparative trial. Cancer 7:377–387, 2001.

114. Unpublished data C. From R Murphy, Novartis pharmaceuticals to JR Ross and Y Saunders, 2001.

115. Saad F, Gleason DM, Murray R, et al: A randomized placebo controlled trial of zoledronic acid in patients with hormone refractory metastatic prostate cancer. J Natl Cancer Inst 94:1458–1468, 2002.

116. Arican A, Icli F, Akbulut H, et al: The effect of two different doses of oral clodronate on pain in patients with bone metastases. Med Oncol 16:204–210, 1999.

117. Cascinu S, Graziano F, Alessandroni P, et al: Different doses of pamidronate in patients with painful osteolytic bone metastases. Support Care Cancer 6:139–143, 1998.

118. Coleman RE, Houston S, Purohit OP, et al: A randomised phase II study of oral pamidronate for the treatment of bone metastases from breast cancer. Eur J Cancer 34:820–824, 1998.

119. Conte PF, Giannessi PG, Latreille J, et al: Delayed progression of bone metastases with pamidronate therapy in breast cancer patients: A randomized, multicenter phase III trial. Ann Oncol 5(suppl 7):S41–44, 1994.

120. Elomaa I, Kylmala T, Tammela T, et al: Effect of oral clodronate on bone pain. A controlled study in patients with metastatic prostatic cancer. Int Urol Nephrol 24:159–166, 1992.

121. Ernst DS, MacDonald RN, Paterson AH, et al: A double-blind, crossover trial of intravenous clodronate in metastatic bone pain. J Pain Symptom Manage 7:4–11, 1992.

122. Glover D, Lipton A, Keller A, et al: Intravenous pamidronate disodium treatment of bone metastases in patients with breast cancer: A dose-seeking study. Cancer 74:2949–2955, 1994.

123. Koeberle D, Bacchus L, Thuerlimann B, Senn HJ: Pamidronate treatment in patients with malignant osteolytic bone disease and pain: A prospective randomized double-blind trial. Supp Care Cancer 7:21–27, 1999.

124. Kylmala T, Taube T, Tammela TLJ, et al: Concomitant IV and oral clodronate in the relief of bone pain: A double blind placebo-controlled study in patients with prostate cancer. Br J Cancer 76:939–942, 1997.

125. Moiseyenko YM, Blinov NN, Semiglasov VU, Konsta MM: Randomized trial of two intravenous schedules of bonephos (clodronate) in patients with painful bone metastases. Voprosy Onkologii (Matters of Oncology) 44:725–728, 1998.

126. O'Rourke N, McCloskey E, Houghton F, et al: Double-blind, placebo-controlled, dose-response trial of oral clodronate in patients with bone metastases. J Cl Oncol 13:929–934, 1995.

127. Piga A, Bracci R, Ferretti B, et al: A double blind randomized study of oral clodronate in the treatment of bone metastases from tumors poorly responsive to chemotherapy. J Exp Clin Cancer Res 17:213–217, 1998.

128. Robertson AG, Reed NS, Ralston SH: Effect of oral clodronate on metastatic bone pain: A double-blind, placebo-controlled study. J Clin Oncol 13: 2427–2430, 1995.

129. Siris E, Hymann G, Canfield R: Effects of dichloromethylene diphosphonate in women with breast carcinoma metastatic to the skeleton. Am J Med 74:401–406, 1983.

130. Smith JA Jr: Palliation of painful bone metastases from prostate cancer using sodium etidronate: Results of a randomized, prospective, double-blind, placebo-controlled study. J Urol 141: 85–87, 1989.

131. Strang P, Nilsson S, Brandstedt S, et al: The analgesic efficacy of clodronate compared with placebo in patients with painful bony metastases from prostatic cancer. Anticancer Res 17:4717–4722, 1997.

132. Vinholes JJ, Purohit OP, Abbey ME, et al: Relationships between biochemical and symptomatic response in a double-blind randomised trial of pamidronate for metastatic bone disease. Ann Oncol 8:1243–1250, 1997.

133. Roqué M, Martínez MJ, Catalá E, et al: Control del dolor óseo por metástasis: revisión sistemática del tratamiento farmacológico con bifosfonatos, calcitonina y radiofármacos. Grant 00/10011, of the Instituto de Salud Carlos III, Subdirección General de Investigación Sanitaria, 2000.

134. Dearnaley DP, Sydes MR, Mason MD, et al: A double-blind, placebo-controlled, randomized trial of oral sodium clodronate for metastatic prostate cancer (MRC PR05 Trial). J Natl Cancer Inst 95:1300–1311, 2003.

135. Ernst DS, Tannnock IF, Winquist EW, et al: Randomized, double-blind, controlled trial of mitoxantrone/prednisone and clodronate versus mitoxantrone/prednisone and placebo in patients with hormone-refractory prostate cancer and pain. J Clin Oncol 21:3335–3342, 2003.

136. Pecherstorfer M, Steinhauer EU, Rizzoli R, et al: Efficacy and safety of ibandronate in the treatment of hypercalcemia of malignancy: A randomized multicentric comparison to pamidronate. Supp Care Cancer 11:539–547, 2003.

137. Musto P, Falcone A, Sanpaolo G, et al: Pamidronate reduces skeletal events but does not improve progression-free survival in early stage untreated myeloma: Results of a randomized trial. Leukemia and Lymphoma 44:1545–1548, 2003.

138. Jagdev SP, Purohit P, Heatley S, et al: Comparison of the effects of intravenous pamidronate and oral clodronate on symptoms and bone resorption in patients with metastatic bone diseases. Ann Oncol 12:1433–14388, 2001.

139. Body JJ, Diel JJ, Lichinitser MR, et al: Intravenous ibandronate reduces the incidence of skeletal complications in patients with breast cancer and bone metastases. Ann Oncol 14:1399–1405, 2003.

140. Messen HD, Sakalovà A, Fontana A, et al: Effects of long-term intravenous ibandronate therapy on skeletal-related events, survival, and bone resorption markers in patients with advanced multiple myeloma. J Clin Oncol 20:2353–2359, 2002.

141. Lipton A, Zheng M, Seaman J: Zoledronic acid delays the onset of skeletal-related events and progression of skeletal disease in patients with advanced renal cell carcinoma. Cancer 98:962–969, 2003.

142. Yoneda T: Cellular and molecular mechanisms of breast and prostate cancer metastasis to bone. Eur J Cancer 34:240–245, 1998.

143. Hotte SJ, Webert KE, Major PP: Zoledronic acid: An overview of its current and potential benefits in patients with malignancy. Today's Therapeutics Trends 20:197–219, 2002.

144. Saarto T, Blomqvist C, Virkkunen P, Elomaa I: Adjuvant clodronate treatment does nor reduce the frequency of skeletal metastases in node-positive breast cancer patients: 5-year results of a randomized controlled trial. J Clin Oncol 19:10–17, 2001.

145. Powles T, Paterson S, Kanis JA, et al: Randomized, placebo-controlled trial of clodronate in patients with primary operable breast cancer. J Clin Oncol 20:3219–3224, 2002.

CHAPTER 26

Cancer Pain Management in the Home Setting

NESSA COYLE, PhD, FAAN

Chronic pain associated with cancer is an extremely stressful situation for both patient and family. Surveys indicate that pain is experienced by 30% to 60% of cancer patients during active therapy and in more than two-thirds of those with advanced disease.[1-7] In addition, symptom clusters and multiple symptoms tend to be the norm not the exception in advanced cancer patients with pain.[8-10] These patients spend minimal time in the hospital and most of the time in their homes. The experience of chronic pain, therefore, is mainly a home experience, one that involves not only pain but also multiple other symptoms, and one that involves not only the patient but also their family and friends.[11-13] Unrelieved pain is incapacitating and undermines quality of life; it interferes with physical functioning and social interaction and is strongly associated with heightened psychological distress.[14-18] Uncontrolled severe pain, or episodes of excruciating pain in this setting, can lead to a desire for hastened death.[18]

The literature is replete with discussions about the prevalence of pain, its undertreatment, and barriers to adequate pain management.[19-24] Until recently, however, little attention had been given to factors affecting pain management in the home. A growing literature explores issues particular to the management of pain in the home. These include knowledge and attitudes about cancer pain and its management among patient and family members,[22,25,26] stress in family caregivers and community nurses,[26-31] the increasing use of technology in the home,[31,32] and communication.[33] Recognition of the "responsibility without adequate training or power" phenomenon that nurses commonly experience in the home care setting has been an impetus for the development of training programs for home care nurses in pain management. This same phenomenon is experienced by many families. Family caregivers are expected to play a primary role in cancer pain relief across all stages of the disease and yet they are frequently given little or no training on how

to do so.[29-31,34-37] Yet structured pain education programs for patients and family caregivers have been shown to result in positive outcomes for patients and their family caregivers.[38-40]

Understanding the factors that influence adequacy of pain management in the home has become increasingly important in the face of the current trend toward shorter inpatients hospital stays, earlier hospital discharges, and the expectation that extremely sick patients will be managed at home.[41-43] Family members, with community nursing support, are in the frontline of home pain management. Barriers have been described that hinder pain management in the home including patient and family fears of addiction, failure to report pain, and limited access to care.[27,35,36,38,39] The intense demands on family caregiving at home especially in the provision of 24-hour physical caregiving is well described.[41-43,46] Less attention has been placed on the emotional burden to the family of assuming responsibility for the patient's well-being in the home.[47,48] In addition, little has been written about the care of cancer patients with pain who are discharged home to a high-risk drug abuse environment. Encompassing a relatively small group of individuals, their needs can be great. However, with careful planning and close monitoring, safe pain management at home can be achieved for many.[49]

Most home environments offer substantial benefits to the individual with cancer and pain, but home care can also result in intense burdens for family caregivers, resulting in compromised care.[35,50] Home care is best viewed as a family experience, with the recognition that every aspect of care provided to the patient will affect that family system.[50]

An early, small, descriptive study (triad of 10) investigated the experience of managing pain at home from the perspectives of the patient, the primary family caregiver, and the home-care nurse encapsulates many of the important areas that affect pain management in the home.[26]

Areas of decision making and conflict mainly centered on the use of medications. Patients were preoccupied with decisions about which pain medication to take and how much of it to take. Negative side effects and meaning with regard to these medications contributed to conflicts in the patient's mind about whether they were doing the "right thing" in taking the pain medication.

Nearly all the patients assumed that their pain would increase with impending death. Patient's decisions about how to live with and cope with the pain included considerations of how what they did and said affected their health care professionals and family members. Sometimes these factors led the patient to deny the pain. Similarly, the decisions and conflicts that arose most often for family caregivers also related to pain medication and having to make decisions about which pill to give and when to give it. Compounding these decisions were concerns related to overdosing, adverse side effects, and addiction. Sometimes the family member admitted to withholding information from the patient or nurse in an attempt to benefit the patient in some way. So, for example, depending on the decision-making process of the family member, more or less medication might be given. Other studies conducted on knowledge and beliefs about pain management in cancer patients and their families found that although patients and families share similar beliefs about pain, family members tend to have a higher degree of emotional distress associated with observing pain in their loved ones.[51]

Effective pain management is dependent on an accurate assessment. When the patient is being cared for at home, the physician frequently relies on second- or third-hand information supplied by the family or home care nurse; on the severity of the pain; adequacy of relief; and presence of side effects. Correct interpretation of the patient and family's report of pain is essential. According to Elliot and colleagues[52] and suggested by the studies discussed earlier, three dimensions compose a patient's pain experience: cognitive factors (including attitude, belief, knowledge), sensory or physical input, and affective or emotional experience. Elliot and colleagues found that although patients and families reported parallel perceptions of the patient's cancer pain, family members consistently assessed the patient's level of pain somewhat higher than the patient did. This suggested to them the effect of observing rather than experiencing the pain. In addition, Ward and colleagues[34] reported that patient with increased concerns were less likely to use analgesics adequately. These studies, as well as others, document that family caregivers are often as affected by pain as the patient, and sometimes more so. There are important implications here for evaluating the efficacy of a pain management strategy, if the assessment is largely

TABLE 26–1 Difficulties Patients and Caregivers Encounter in Setting Up a Pain Management Regimen at Home
Obtaining the prescribed medication(s)
Accessing information
Tailoring prescribed regimens to meet individual needs
Managing side effects
Cognitively processing information
Managing new or unusual pain
Managing multiple symptoms simultaneously

From Schumacher KL, Koresawa S, West C, et al: Putting pain management regimens into practice in the home. J Pain Symptom Manage 23:369-382, 2002.

dependent on a family member's report.[27,31,35,46] The report of poorly controlled pain may be indicative of the family member's distress, as well as that of the patient. Areas of family distress include fatigue, lack of knowledge of pain management, concern about addiction, concern about harming the patient, and an overwhelming feeling of responsibility.[25,26,34] Family distress, as well as patient distress, must be addressed if pain is to be adequately managed. There is a close relationship between the two. The difficulties that patient and family caregivers commonly encounter when trying to put a pain management regimen into place at home are summarized in Table 26-1. They illustrate that patients and family caregivers need ongoing support and help with problem solving in order to optimize their pain management regimen.[53]

NONPHARMACOLOGIC PAIN MANAGEMENT IN THE HOME

In addition to the numerous and sometimes overwhelming responsibilities related to the pharmacologic management of pain in the home, patients and family caregivers use many nondrug strategies for pain relief. Although some of these techniques are taught in the hospital setting, they are seldom reinforced by the medical team once the patient is discharged home. Nondrug interventions include both physical and cognitive approaches. Physical approaches include interventions such as heat, cold, and massage. Cognitive strategies include relaxation, imagery, a variety of relaxation techniques, meditation, and prayer.[37,54-57] These nondrug strategies, especially those that are a "fit" with the patient values and belief system, can be enormously helpful in not only enhancing pain relief but also in giving the individual back a sense of control.

PLANNING FOR HOME PAIN MANAGEMENT: TRANSITION FROM HOSPITAL TO HOME

To facilitate discharge planning for patients with cancer-related pain and to ease the transition from hospital to home, it is useful to classify the patients into five groups. This classification helps individualize and organize care to meet the specific needs of a patient and family.[49] This is important as there are discharge-planning needs and home care needs specific to each group.

- Group I consists of patients with stable pain.
- Group II consists of patients requiring a parenteral route of opioid administration.
- Group III consists of patients who are imminently dying.
- Group IV consists of patients living in a setting where drug diversion is considered likely.
- Group V consists of patients who are to be discharged to an extended-care facility that becomes their home.

Common to all groups are the following needs: basic education on cancer pain management with the individualized home pain management regimen clearly written out in a language that the patient and family can understand; the pain management plan is financially feasible for the patient; the prescribed analgesics are available in the community; the patient and family feel secure with the discharge plan and follow-up; and the patient not be discharged if at all possible within 24 hours of a change in opioid drug or route of administration (Table 26–2).[49]

Group I consists of patients who have stable pain, and are, for example, using an oral, transmucosal, rectal, or transdermal route of opioid administration. These patients may or may not be pursuing a course of curative or life-prolonging therapy. The patient is usually followed on an outpatient basis with ongoing prescriptions written by his or her primary physician or nurse practitioner. The patient is instructed to contact the primary physician or nurse practitioner for any change in the quality, severity, or site of the pain and the occurrence of adverse side effects. Before the patient's discharge home, it is important that the community pharmacy is contacted to make sure that it has the necessary opioid in stock or are willing to obtain it if it does not.[49,58,59] It is good practice for the physician or pain management nurse to initiate contact with the patient within the first week of discharge to confirm that the pain is adequately controlled and that the patient and his or her family feel confident with his or her pain management approach. This initial telephone contact also confirms to the patient that his or her pain management is important and that he or she will continue to be monitored closely and have resources available to him or her even though the care is now on an ambulatory basis. Cost of medication on an outpatient basis can be a significant barrier for patients without a prescription plan.[60-62] The ability of a patient to both pay for and obtain their outpatient analgesic prescription must be established before discharge home. Often this information is not volunteered by the patient unless specifically asked. The social worker can be very helpful in this area. Table 26–3 gives a comparison of average opioid wholesale prices in the United States in 2001. For those patients without a prescription plan, the cost of opioid

---

TABLE 26–2 Factors That Facilitate Continued Pain Control During the Transition Period from Hospital to Home

Do **not** discharge a patient:
1. Within 24 hours of a change in route of opioid administration
2. Within 24 hours of a change in opioid drug
3. Without written instructions regarding their analgesic regimen
4. Without a 24-hr resource telephone number for pain management issues
5. Without a bowel regimen

If a patient is being discharged on other than the parenteral route of drug administration **make sure:**
1. That the prescribed drugs are available in the patient's community pharmacy
2. That the patient has an outpatient prescription plan or can afford to pay for the pain medication out of pocket
3. That the patient is given sufficient medication at time of discharge to continue the pain management regimen until they can get a prescription filled at a local pharmacy.

If a patient is being discharged on a parenteral infusion:
1. **Avoid** sending the patient home over the weekend if possible.
2. **Give** the patient a 48-hour supply of oral or injectable opioids to take home in case there is mechanical problem with the pump.

TABLE 26–3 Acquisition Costs of Long-Term Opioid Therapy: Comparison of Average Wholesale Prices in the United States in 2001[a]

Drug	Dose[b]	Schedule	AWP per dose ($US)	AWP per day ($US)
Mild-to-moderate pain				
Short-acting oral preparations				
Codeine	60 mg	q4h	0.80	4.80
Dextropropoxyphene	100 mg	q4h	0.33	1.98
Hydrocodone (+ paracetamol, acetaminophen)	10 mg	q4h	0.53	3.18
Oxycodone (+ acetaminophen)	10 mg	q4h	0.52	3.12
Moderate to severe pain				
Short-acting oral preparations				
Oxycodone, immediate release	20 mg	q4h	0.32	1.86
Morphine, immediate release	30 mg	q4h	0.31	1.86
Hydromorphone	8 mg	q4h	1.22	7.32
Levorphanol	4 mg	q4h	0.87	3.48
Transmucosal preparation				
Oral transmucosal fentanyl citrate	200 μg	q6h	6.95	27.80
	400 μg	q6h	8.93	35.72
	600 μg	q6h	10.91	43.64
	800 μg	q6h	12.90	51.60
	1200 μg	q6h	16.87	67.48
	1600 μg	q6h	20.83	83.32
Long-acting oral preparations				
Oxycodone, controlled release	60 mg	q12h	6.60	13.20
Morphine, controlled release (MS Contin)	90 mg	q12h	5.58	11.16
Morphine, controlled release (Kadian)	150 mg	q24h	9.63	9.63
Methadone	5 mg	q8h	0.09	0.27
Transdermal preparations				
Transdermal fentanyl	25 μg	q72h	12.33	4.11
	50 μg	q72h	20.37	6.79
	75 μg	q72h	32.63	10.88
	100 μg	q72h	40.65	13.55

AWP, average wholesale price; qxh, every x hours.

[a]AWP were averaged for all suppliers using the 2001 edition of RedBook™ for Windows version 4.0 (Medical Economic Data, Montvale, NJ, USA). Costs to patients are variable and approximately 10%–20% above AWPs for outpatients and 50%–200% above AWPs for inpatients. Costs to pharmacies are based on product volume discounts and can be considerably less than AWP.

[b]Doses are not intended to be equianalgesic.

[c]Mean AWP for available products multiplied by the number of doses required in a 24-hr period.

From Kornick CA: Benefit-risk assessment of transdermal fentanyl for the treatment for cancer pain. Drug Safety 26:969, 2003.

medications can be prohibitive. Several pharmaceutical companies have specific patient "hardship" programs. A social worker can again be very helpful in evaluating a patient's eligibility for these programs and accessing such resources.

If a patient's pain escalates once home, it is crucial to explore with the patient and family caregiver whether the pain medication is being taken as prescribed. It is not unusual that a pain management regimen is not adhered to once an individual goes home, for the variety of reasons described earlier.[63] The reasons for nonadherence need to be discussed in an open and frank manner. Tailoring a pain management regimen that fits in with the patient and family caregiver's values, goals, and capabilities is essential if symptom control is to be maintained at home.

Group II consists of patients who require a parenteral route of drug administration to control their pain. Although the majority of patients do well on the oral or transdermal route of opioid administration, some will require ongoing administration through a parenteral route.[64-66] The most common indications for a parenteral infusion in the cancer population are bowel obstruction or malabsorption, severe stomatitis, intractable nausea and vomiting, and dysphagia.[64-66] A parenteral opioid infusion is also considered for patients with rapidly escalating and unstable pain or those with frequent and severe episodes of breakthrough pain. In these situations, the use of patient-controlled analgesia in combination with the continuous parenteral infusion helps ensure more effective pain relief.[66] Finally, an opioid parenteral infusion may be considered if the oral route produces severe gastrointestinal side effects. Similar to Group I, these patients may or may not be pursuing a course of curative or life-prolonging therapy. They are not imminently dying and do not meet hospice criteria for long-term follow up. Discharge planning is more complex than for those in Group I and requires a team approach, with good communication between hospital and community. In some institutions a specific discharge planner, usually a nurse, plays an important role in organizing the home care plan once the needs have been identified by the team. The discharge planner facilitates referral to home care agencies (e.g., a home infusion company) and is able to identify insurance constraints or availability of drug constraints, so that alternative avenues may be sought to provide the patient and family with the care that they need.

It is rarely feasible to maintain peripheral IV access for continuous infusion in the home. Continuous infusions are usually only considered in patients who have an indwelling central venous port or other long-term central venous device. Placement of one of these devices is occasionally necessary before the patient's discharge home to accommodate a large volume of fluid (e.g., in the case of a fentanyl infusion). In most cases, however, a continuous subcutaneous infusion can accomplish the goals of therapy without the need for IV access.

The degree of support that is needed to maintain a parenteral infusion at home varies widely, depending on the patient and family characteristics. Specific educational issues need to be addressed with all patients. These include knowledge of drug effects and side effects; the use of rescue doses; operation of the infusion device, specifically turning the pump on and off and changing the battery; and changing the cassette or infusion bag. A minority of patients and their families never achieve a comfort level in changing the infusion cassette or bag. In those instances, the infusion home care nurse will usually make the necessary changes. It is mandatory that all patients and their families who are receiving a parenteral infusion at home have a 24-hour resource person available to them to troubleshoot the system (Table 26–4). The most common error encountered in a continuous infusion at home using a computerized pump is incorrect programming (e.g., failure to reprogram the pump when the concentration of the opioid in the cassette or bag is changed).[66] This leads to an inadvertent overdosing or underdosing of the patient. Such errors can be largely circumvented through the use of a flow chart kept in the patient's home. Errors will be picked up

TABLE 26–4	Parenteral Opioid Infusion at Home: Troubleshooting the System
Complaints of increased pain:	
Evaluate in context of the disease and psychological state Check needle site, pump setting, cassette content, and concentration Evaluate use and amount of "rescue" doses	
Complaints of increased side effects (e.g., sedation):	
Evaluate in context of disease and psychological state Check cassette for drug and concentration Check pump setting, correlate with cassette Evaluate use and amount of "rescue" doses Evaluate other drugs being used	

quite rapidly if the patient is being adequately monitored. The first sign of an incorrectly programmed pump might be increasing pain or the occurrence of side effects such as increasing sedation or nausea and vomiting.

The cost of a parenteral opioid home infusion may be high. It includes rental of the pump, involvement of a home infusion agency including pharmacy overheads, delivery of the premixed medication to the home, and availability of home infusion nurses on a 24-hour basis. However, the cost of poorly controlled pain is even higher in both human terms and from the need to re-hospitalize the patient for uncontrolled pain.[67-69] Medicare, Medicaid, and most private insurance cover the cost of home infusion pain management, as long as there is a clearly documented indication for such an approach. For Medicare and Medicaid patients, if an opioid other than morphine is being used, a letter is usually needed to explain why the alternative opioid has been chosen. The specific insurance requirements are drug specificity must be clarified before the patient's discharge.

Group III consists of patients who are imminently dying and want to go home. Patients in this group may or may not require a parenteral route of drug administration to control their pain. Systems are in place, however, to manage even the most complex patients at home if the family is strongly committed to this end. There are a variety of models in place to facilitate good pain control. Regardless of which model is selected as the optimal mechanism for the delivery of home pain management at end-of-life, the common theme for all models is one of an interdisciplinary team approach to care, with the patient and family at the center of such care.

Hospice care, the most widely available model of home care for the dying, focuses on optimizing quality of life in those not seeking, and unlikely to benefit from, life-sustaining treatment.[70] Hospice programs are run by both profit and not-for-profit organizations and have become part of the standard of care offered to patients nearing the end of life. Eligibility requirement for a hospice program is a life expectancy of 6 months or less. A major advantage for patients and families followed in a hospice home care program is regular home visits by the hospice nurse and a 24-hour emergency support from skilled hospice nurses with backup from the hospice medical staff. In addition, all medication related to the terminal illness are free. Because of the variety of hospice models, levels of sophistication, and depth of services offered, the needs of the patient and the services offered through the program should be evaluated before referral of a patient. For example, although most hospice programs have changed their policy toward the use of technology in end-of-life care, in contrast to an earlier "no high-tech" approach, severe restrictions on the financial reimbursement for programs may limit their ability to deliver care to patients requiring the parenteral route of opioid infusion to manage their pain. The physician who refers the dying patient to hospice care can remain as actively involved in the patient's ongoing pain management as he or she chooses to be. In some instances the referring physician remains the patient's primary physician and works with the hospice team in titrating the opioids to ensure comfort. In other instances, the referring physicians ask the hospice physician to assume that role.

Group IV consists of patients with chronic cancer-related pain, who are going home to an environment where it is suspected that drug diversion may occur. The patients themselves may or may not have a history of illicit drug use. In general, patients with a history of drug abuse are at risk for having their pain undertreated.[71,72] Three subgroups of patients can be identified: (1) patients who are actively using street drugs, (2) patients who are in methadone maintenance programs, and (3) patients who have not used illicit drugs for many years.[73]

Patients in the first subgroup strain the resources of the most sophisticated home management pain team and require tight control during opioid therapy. It must be recognized that these patients, like any other patient, may experience severe pain associated with their cancer but will probably require larger doses of opioids to control their pain because of the development of tolerance. One physician or nurse practitioner should be identified as the person to adjust analgesics and write all prescriptions, and one nurse identified as the person to organize and coordinate the patient's plan of care.[72] If the patient is on an oral drug regimen, it may be necessary to give only a 1-week supply of the opioid at a time. Giving a larger amount at one time invariably results in the patient "running out of the drug" regardless of the amount given. Psychiatric symptoms and comorbidities such as anxiety, depression, and bipolar disorders are frequently seen in this population

and need to be addressed.[71-73] A team approach is essential in the care of these patients. If the patient is in a methadone maintenance program it is important that the program be contacted for assistance in planning the patients' overall care.

For some patients being discharged home into a drug-abuse or chaotic environment, the use of an oral route of opioid administration is not feasible because of constant drug loss. Occasionally, these patients are placed on a parenteral route of opioid administration to ensure adequate pain control and safety, maintain tighter control on the amount of drug used, and to minimize the risk of drug diversion. In these situations, extra opioid cassettes are not left in the home and neither the patient nor the family is taught how to change the infusion cassette. Cassette changes are done by the home infusion nurse. In addition, cassettes and not bags are used for the infusion as there is less risk of "siphoning off" the medication. Personal experience using this approach with several patients has been extraordinarily successful. The patients' pain has been controlled and unaccounted for drug usage kept to a minimum. Patients also appear to appreciate the considerable amount of attention they receive. It is, however, time intensive and requires close coordination and communication between the prescribing physician or nurse practitioner, the home infusion pharmacist, and the home infusion nurse.

Group V consists of patients with cancer and pain who are unable to be cared for at home and are to be discharged to an extended-care facility. Such facilities are rarely able to accommodate a patient whose pain requires a parenteral route of opioid administration. These patients are frequently elderly, debilitated, and receiving polypharmacy for chronic medical conditions. They are at high risk for having their pain inadequately assessed and consequently to be undermedicated for pain.[74,75] In addition, the elderly and debilitated patient's therapeutic margin may be narrow, and the individual is at increased risk for developing troublesome side effects including sedation and confusion. Close monitoring is required, with careful dose titration and adjustment based on ongoing assessment. This requires training, skill, and an institutional system in place that screens for the presence of pain and adequacy of relief on a regularly scheduled basis. Until recently, the staff in long-term-care facilities had little training in pain management and end-of-life care. Such training is still limited, although the new Joint Commission on Accreditation of Healthcare Organizations (JCAHO) standards has made such training mandatory.[76]

In the current situation it is essential that verbal communication be established between the physician, nurse practitioner, or pain management advanced practice nurse from the discharging institution, and the physician and nursing supervisor from the extended-care facility.

This communication should take place before the patient's discharge to the facility. The two teams can then work together to ensure adequate pain relief for the patient. In the last 5 to 10 years some long-term care facilities have established contracts with community hospice programs and have developed palliative care approaches to the care of their residents. But because this is not the norm, the selection of a long-term care facility for someone with cancer and pain must be done with great care.

ADDITIONAL ASPECTS OF THE TRANSITION FROM HOSPITAL TO HOME

In preparing the patient with chronic pain and his or her family to go home, the focus is on security, clarification of the pain management plan, and communication.[49] A family meeting is often a useful method of consolidating this information.

Family Support

The central role of the family is acknowledged in the management of pain in the home. It is emphasized that the family will be given ongoing support and backup for their day-to-day pain management decisions, for example, when and how a rescue dose should be used, and the management of opioid side effects should they occur. Of note, the needs of the family when the patient is initially discharged home and his or her needs later on are different. When the patient is first discharged home the family is still learning the basic principles and skills required for pain management. Once these skills have been learned and a routine established, the need is for continuing support and validation.

Clarification and Written Instructions on the Pain Management Approach

It is essential that the patient and family are given specific, detailed, written instructions, in layman's terms, of the pain management approach, both pharmacologic and nonpharmacologic, to be used. The principle underpinning the pain management approach: that analgesics should be used to prevent pain rather than having to be "earned" through experiencing severe pain, is underscored. This principle encompasses addressing the concerns surrounding the prevalence of addiction when opioids are used to manage pain, and the clinical significance of tolerance (e.g., the patient or family's concerns that the opioids may no longer be effective if they are used early on in a disease process). In addition, safety issues surrounding opioids in the home need to be

reviewed. These include that the opioids be kept in a safe place out of reach of children; that unused opioids be flushed down the toilet or returned to the prescribing institution for disposal; that if parenteral opioids are used, a syringe and needle disposal kit be obtained; and that needles and syringes, however well wrapped, should not be disposed of in household garbage containers.[49]

Communication of Pain Severity, Pain Relief, and Pain Treatment Side Effects

The patient and family should have no ambiguity as to whom to call on a 24-hour basis if pain is not well controlled or if the patient experiences troublesome side effects. Tools of communication are reinforced. Such tools include keeping a daily diary to record pain level (e.g., using a numerical estimate such as a 0 to 10 scale or categorical scale such as none, slight, moderate, severe), medication taken, other pain relieving strategies used, extent and duration of pain relief, activity level, and interference with quality of life. Keeping a pain diary has been found to heighten the patient and caregiver's awareness of the pattern of pain, guide pain management behaviors, enhance a sense of control, and facilitate communication.[77]

Communicating with the Community: Facilitating Ongoing Pain Management at Home

To ensure that the pain management plan instituted in the hospital can be maintained at home, a series of steps can be taken. First, if home care nursing has been instituted, the home care nurse should be contacted to discuss the pain management plan. Second, the community pharmacy should be contacted to ensure that they have the prescribed opioids in stock or, if not, are willing to obtain the medication. In addition, it should be established specifically when the drugs are available in the community pharmacy, so that the patient is not left uncovered. In the event that the local pharmacy neither has nor can obtain the prescribed opioid, an alternative source for the patient must be located before discharge from the hospital. Third, the physician or nurse practitioner responsible for writing the opioid prescriptions and titrating the drug must be clearly identified. Fourth, the family should be instructed to establish a routine by which the amount of medication they have left is checked on a scheduled basis so that the medication does not "run out" (the Friday night and holiday syndrome). Some families find it helpful to keep a 1-week supply of the medication to the side, and when they need to go into that medication it reminds them to call their prescribing clinician for a new prescription.

These simple steps can help ease the transition from hospital to home for the patient with chronic pain and his or her family.[49]

Continuity of Care and Community Support for Complex Pain Management at Home

Continuity of care for cancer patients with pain is particularly important. Frequently patients receive their care in a variety of medical settings.[78,79] Numerous physicians, nurses, and other health care professionals are involved. Pain management may or may not have been considered a priority. Effective management approaches may be changed because of unfamiliarity with a specific technology (such as a continuous subcutaneous infusion) or with the community resources (such as a "high-tech" agency's ability to initiate or maintain an infusion in the home) or concern over the amount of opioid a patient is receiving. The hospice movement has addressed the need for continuity of care of the dying patient.[69] A similar need of the cancer patient with chronic pain who is not imminently dying and the importance of bridging the gap between hospital and community, has been recognized.[79] A palliative care approach, using hospital-based continuity of care or supportive care programs, which bring the expertise of a cancer center to the community, is seen as a valuable component to patient care and addresses the needs of the cancer patient with chronic pain earlier on in the disease process. Such a model of care is also important for dying patients who, either do not have access to a hospice program or who, for a variety of reasons, choose not to be followed by the hospice system of care.

An example of a long-running program that provides intensive palliative care to a small number of patients is the Supportive Care Program (SCP), a part of the Pain and Palliative Care Service at Memorial Sloan-Kettering Cancer Center in New York City.[79] This program utilizes institutional and community resources to optimize care for patients who are in need of palliative care but may have goals that still focus on prolongation of life. The program is a patient- and family-centered, nurse-coordinated program that provides 24-hour access to palliative care nurse practitioners; daily telephone contact (or more often if indicated); ongoing monitoring and treatment of symptoms; psychological support; and liaison and coordination among the physicians, nurses, and social workers involved in the care of the patient at home. Because this system of care is very time intensive, it is directed toward patients who have been identified as at high risk for poorly managed pain once discharged home (Table 26–5).

Communication, Monitoring, and Support

The use of the telephone is an important aspect of monitoring and managing pain on an outpatient basis.[79,81] In addition, it makes expert resources available to communities where this might not otherwise be the case. Continuity of care can also be fostered through 24-hour telephone availability of a pain management expert (usually an advanced practice nurse) to the patients, their families, and community professionals. In the Sloan-Kettering model, two advanced practice nurses working with an average of 85 complex cancer pain patients during a 1-year period, make or receive approximately 3200 telephone calls to these patients, their families, and community practitioners and nurses. The calls are related to pain management, symptom control, patient and family education and support, and professional education about and support of the management of pain at all stages of the disease.[79,82]

TABLE 26–5   Risk Factors for Poor Cancer Pain Control in the Home Setting

Complex pain syndromes
Advanced disease, rapidly escalating opioid requirements, and need for a parenteral or "unfamiliar" route of administration
Advanced disease and want to die at home but have poor community or social supports, or both
High levels of physiologic, psychological, and social fatigue, or an overwhelmed family
Memory or cognitive impairment
Discharge to an extended-care facility that does not have a pain management program
No outpatient prescription plan and financial burden
History of drug abuse or discharge to a "high risk" home environment

Telemonitoring has been widely used in a variety of chronic diseases. For the cancer patient with chronic pain, the use of a telemonitoring system may be a useful tool to reinforce patient and family teaching of medication use and nonpharmacologic approaches to pain control. The system is reasonably inexpensive and can be used through a TV or computer screen. As computers are becoming more commonplace in the home, use of web sites, e-mail and computer programs to reinforce patient and family teaching, and to document changes in the management approach are becoming more commonplace.

CONCLUSION

Although the basic principles of pain management are the same whether the patient is being cared for in an acute care setting, his or her home, or a long-term care facility, there is a major shift in responsibility for day-to-day pain management when the patient is to be cared for at home. What was primarily the responsibility of the nurse and physician team in the inpatient setting becomes the responsibility of the patient and family once the patient is home. Pain management in the home becomes a family experience, every aspect of care provided to the patient affecting the family system as a whole.

Successful pain management at home depends on an informed and confident patient and family with collaboration and effective communication between the physician or nurse practitioner, home care nurse and patient and family. Most importantly, a system of ongoing monitoring and support for the patient and family must be in place to ensure effectiveness of pain relief measures and early identification of undue stress on the part of the family. Careful discharge planning will help to facilitate appropriate pain management and support for the patient at home and for their family.

REFERENCES

1. Bonica JJ, Ventafridda V, Twycross RG: Cancer pain. In Bonica JJ (ed): The Management of Pain, 2nd ed. Philadelphia, Lea & Febiger, 1990, pp 400–460.
2. Vuorinen E: Pain as an early symptom in cancer. Clin J Pain 9:272–278, 1993.
3. Portenoy RK, Kornblith AB, Wong G, et al: Pain in ovarian cancer patients: Prevalence, characteristics, and associated symptoms. Cancer 74:907–915, 1994.
4. Portenoy RK, Miransky J, Thaler HT, et al: Pain in ambulatory patients with lung or colon cancer: Prevalence, characteristics and effect. Cancer 70:1616–1624, 1992.
5. Brescia FJ, Portenoy RK, Ryan M, et al: Pain, opioid use and survival in hospitalized patients with advanced cancer. J Clin Oncol 10:149–155, 1992.
6. Donnelly S, Walsh D: The symptoms of advanced cancer. Semin Oncol 22(suppl 3):67–72, 1995.
7. Caraceni A, Portenoy RK: An international survey of cancer pain characteristics and syndromes: IASP Task Force on Cancer Pain. International Association for the Study of Pain: Pain 82:263–274, 1999.
8. Gift AG, Stommel M, Jablonski A, Given W: A cluster of symptoms over time in patients with lung cancer. Nurs Res 52:393–400, 2003.
9. Walsh D, Donnelly S, Rybicki L: The symptoms of advanced cancer: Relationship to age, gender, and performance status in 1,000 patients. Supportive Care Cancer 8:175–179, 2000.
10. Miakowski C, Dodd M, Lee K: Symptom clusters: The new frontier in symptom management research. J Natl Cancer Inst Monogr 32:17–21, 2004.
11. McNally JC: Home care for oncology patients. Semin Oncol Nurs 12:177–178, 1996.
12. Seeber S, Baird SB: The impact of health care changes in home health. Semin Oncol Nurs 12:179–187, 1996.
13. Juarez E, Ferrell BR: Family and caregivers involvement in pain management. Clin Geriatr Med 12:531–547, 1996.
14. Ferrell BR, Dean G: The meaning of cancer pain. Semin Oncol Nurs 11:17–22, 1995.
15. Ferrell BR: The impact of pain on quality of life: A decade of research. Nurs Clin North Am 30:609–624, 1995.
16. Strang P: Existential consequences of unrelieved pain. Palliat Med 11:299–305, 1997.
17. Massie MJ, Holland JC: The cancer patient with pain: Psychiatric complications and their management. J Pain Symptom Manage 7:99–109, 1992.
18. Coyle N, Sculco L: Expressed desire for hastened death in 7 patients living with advanced cancer. Oncol Nurs Forum 31:699–709, 2004.
19. Cherny NI, Catane R: Professional negligence in the management of cancer pain: A case for urgent reforms (editorial; comment). Cancer 76:2181–2185, 1995.
20. Stjernsward J, Colleau SM, Ventafridda V: The World Health Organization Cancer Pain and Palliative Care Program: Past, present and future. J Pain Symptom Manage 12:65–72, 1996.
21. Von Roenn JH, Cleeland CS, Gonin R, et al: Physicians attitudes and practice in cancer pain management: A survey from the Eastern Cooperative Oncology Group. Ann Intern Med 119:121–126, 1993.
22. Grossman SA, Sheidler VR, Swedeen K, et al: Correlations of patient and caregiver ratings of cancer pain. J Pain Symptom Manage 6:53–57, 1991.
23. Cleeland CS, Gonin R, Hatfield AK, et al: Pain and its treatment in outpatients with metastatic cancer. N Engl J Med 330:592–596, 1994.
24. Cherny NI, Ho MN, Bookbinder M, et al: Cancer pain: Knowledge and attitudes of physicians at a cancer center. Proc Annu Meet Am Soc Clin Oncol 13, 1994.
25. Ward SE, Goldberg N, Miller-McCauley V, et al: Patient related barriers to management of cancer pain. Pain 52:319–324, 1993.
26. Taylor EJ, Ferrell BR, Grant M, et al: Managing cancer pain at home: The decisions and ethical conflicts of patients, family caregivers, and home care nurses. Oncol Nurs Forum 20:919–927, 1993.
27. Miaskowski C, Zimmer EF, Barrett KM, et al: Differences in patients' and family caregivers perceptions of the pain experience influence patient and family caregiver outcomes. Pain 72:217–226, 1997.
28. Yaeger KA, Miaskowski C, Dibble SL, et al: Differences in pain knowledge and perception of the pain experience between outpatients with cancer and their family caregivers. Oncol Nurs Forum 22:1235–1241, 1995.
29. Ferrell BR: The family. In Doyle D, Hanks GWC, MacDonald N (eds): Oxford Textbook of Palliative Medicine, 2nd ed. New York, Oxford University Press, 1998, pp 909–917.
30. Magrum LC, Bentzen C, Landmark S: Pain management in home care. Semin Oncol Nurs 15:202–218, 1996.
31. Coyle, N: Focus on the nurse: Ethical dilemmas with highly symptomatic patients dying at home. Hospice J 12:33–41, 1997.
32. Storey P, Hill HH Jr, St Louis RH, et al: Subcutaneous infusions for the control of cancer symptoms. J Pain Symptom Manage 5:33–41, 1990.
33. Wilkinson S, Bailey K, Aldridge J, et al: A longitudinal evaluation of a communication skills program. Palliat Med 13:341–348, 1999.
34. Ward SE, Berry PE, Misiewicz H: Concerns about analgesics among patients and family caregivers. Res Nurs Health 19:205–211, 1996.

35. Ferrell BR, Ferrell BA, Rhiner M, et al: Family factors influencing cancer pain management. Post Grad Med J 67(suppl 2): S64–S69, 1991.

36. Hileman JW, Lackley NR, Hassanein RS: Identifying the needs of home caregivers in patients with cancer. Oncol Nurs Forum 19:771–777, 1992.

37. Warner JE: Involvement of families in pain control of terminally ill patients. Hosp J 8:155–170, 1992.

38. Ferrell BR, Grant M, Chan J, et al: The impact of cancer pain education on family caregivers of elderly patients. Oncol Nurs Forum 22:1211–1218, 1995.

39. Ferrell BR, Grant M, Borneman T, et al: Family caregiving in cancer pain management. J Palliat Med 2:185–195, 1999.

40. West CM, Dodd MJ, Paul SM, et al: The PRO-SELF(c): Pain control program: An effective approach for cancer pain management. Oncol Nurs Forum 30:65–73, 2003.

41. Arras JD, Dubler NN: Bringing the hospital home. Hastings Center Report Sept. Oct., S19–S28, 1994.

42. Leonard KM, Enzle SS, McTavish J, et al: Prolonged cancer death: A family affair. Cancer Nurs 18:222–227, 1995.

43. Siegel KS, Ravei VH, Houts P, Mor V: Caregiver burden and unmet patient needs. Cancer 68:1131–1140, 1991.

44. Levine C (ed.): Always on call: When illness turns families into caregivers. New York: United Hospital Fund of New York, 2000.

45. Ferrell BR: The impact of pain on quality of life: A decade of research. Nursing Clin North Am 30:609–624, 1995.

46. Ferrell BR, Johnston-Taylor E, Grant M, et al: Pain management in the home: Struggle comfort and mission. Cancer Nurs 16:169–178, 1993.

47. Coyle N: Facilitating cancer pain control in the home: Opioid related issues. Curr Pain Headache Reports 5:217–226, 2001.

48. Ferrell BR, Hastie, BA: Home Care. In Berger AM, Portenoy RK, Weissman DE (eds): Principles and Practice of Palliative Care and Supportive Oncology, 2nd ed. Philadelphia, Lippincott Williams & Wilkins, 2002, pp 775–788.

49. Lobchuk MM, Kristjanson L, Degner L, et al: Perceptions of symptom distress in lung cancer patients: Congruence between patients and primary family caregivers. J Pain Symptom Manage 14:136–146, 1997.

50. Elliot BA, Elliot TE, Murray DM, et al: Patient and family members: The role of knowledge and attitudes in cancer pain. J Pain Symptom Manage 12:209–220, 1996.

51. Schumacher KL, Koresawa S, West C, et al: Putting pain management regimens into practice in the home. J Pain Symptom Manage 23:369–382, 2002.

52. Rhiner M, Ferrell BR: A structured non-drug intervention program for cancer pain. Cancer Pract 1:137–143, 1993.

53. Ferrell BR, Ferrell BA, Ahn C, et al: Pain management for elderly patients with cancer at home. Cancer 74:2139–2146, 1994.

54. Montbriand MJ: An overview of alternate therapies chosen by patients with cancer. Oncol Nurs Forum 21:1541–1554, 1994.

55. Pan CX, Morrison RS, Ness J, et al: Complementary and alternative medicine in the management of pain, dyspnea, and nausea and vomiting near the end-of-life: A systematic review. J Pain Symptom Manage 20:374–385, 2000.

56. Kanner RM, Portenoy RK: Unavailability of narcotic analgesics for ambulatory patients in New York City. J Pain Symptom Manage 1:87–89, 1986.

57. Morrison RS, Wallenstein S, Natale DK, et al: "We don't carry that": Failure of pharmacies in predominantly nonwhite neighborhoods to stock opioid analgesics. N Engl J Med 342:1203–1206, 2000.

58. Kornick CA, Santiago-Palma J, Moryl N, et al: Benefit-risk assessment of transdermal fentanyl for the treatment for cancer pain [review]. Drug Safety 26:969, 2003.

59. Ferrell BR, Griffith H: Cost issues related to pain management: report from the Cancer Pain Panel of the Agency for Health Care Policy and Research. J Pain Symptom Manage 9:221–234, 1994.

60. Ferrell BR: Pain: How patients and families pay the price. In Cohen MJM, Campbell JN (eds): Pain Treatment in the Crossroads, Vol 7. Seattle, International Association for the Study of Pain (IASP), 1996.

61. Miaskowski C, Dodd MJ, West C, et al: Lack of adherence with the analgesic regimen: A significant barrier to effective cancer pain management. J Clin Oncol 19:4275–4279.

62. Coyle N, Adelhardt J, Foley KM, et al: Character of terminal illness: Pain and other symptoms during the last four weeks of life. J Pain Symptom Manage 5:83–89, 1990.

63. Bruera E, MacMillan K, Paredes R, et al: Subcutaneous administration of narcotics for cancer pain: Results from 400 patients [meeting abstract]. Pain 43(suppl 5):497, 1990.

64. Coyle N, Cherney N, Portenoy RK: Subcutaneous opioid infusions at home. Oncology 8:21–27, 1994.

65. Grant M, Ferrell BR, Rivera LM, Lee J: Unscheduled hospital re-admissions for uncontrolled symptoms. Nurs Clin North Am 30:673–682, 1995.

66. Ferrell BR, Schaffner M: Pharmacoeconomics and medical outcomes in pain management. Semin Anesth 16:152–159, 1997.

67. Jacox A, Carr DB, Mahrenholz DM, et al: Cost considerations in patient-controlled analgesia. Pharmacoeconomics 12 (2 PT 1):109–120, 1997.

68. Egan KA, Labyak MJ: Hospice care: A model for quality end-of-life care. In Ferrell BR, Coyle N (eds): Textbook of Palliative Nursing. Oxford, Oxford University Press, 2001, pp 7–26.

69. Compton P: Substance abuse. In McCaffery M, Passero C (eds): Pain: Clinical Manual, 2nd ed. St Louis. Mosby, 1999, pp 428–466.

70. Passik SD, Portenoy RK: Substance abuse issues in palliative care. In Berger A, Portenoy RK (eds): Principles and Practice of Palliative Care and Supportive Oncology. Philadelphia, Lippincott Williams & Wilkins, 1998, pp 513–529.

71. Fulz JM, Sonay EC: Guidelines for the management of hospitalized narcotic addicts. Ann Intern Med 82:815–818, 1975.

72. Ferrell BA, Ferrell BR: Pain in the nursing home. J Am Geriatr Soc 38:409–414, 1990.

73. Ferrell BA, Ferrell BR, Rivera LM: Pain in the cognitively impaired nursing home patient. J Pain Symptom Manage 10: 591–598, 1995.

74. Joint Commission on Accreditation of Hospitals Organization (JCAHO) (2000). Available: http://www.jcaho.org.

75. Schumacher KL, Koresawa S, West C, et al: The usefulness of a daily pain management diary for outpatients with cancer-related pain. Oncol Nurs Forum 29:1304–1313.

76. Ventafridda V: Continuing care: A major issue for in cancer pain management. Pain 36:137–143, 1989.

77. Coyle N: Continuity of care for the cancer patient with chronic pain. Cancer (suppl 63): 2289–2293, 1989.

78. Nauright LP, Moneyham L, Williamson J: Telephone triage and consultation: An emerging role for nurses. Nurs Outlook 47:219–226, 1999.

79. Coyle N, Khojainova N, Francavilla JM, Gonzales GR: Audio-visual communication and its use in palliative care. J Pain Symptom Manage 23:171–175, 2002.

Nonpharmacologic Management
of Cancer Pain

CHAPTER 27

Psychological Interventions

ALLEN LEBOVITS, PhD

The multiplicity of pain etiologies, as well as pain syndromes, that cancer patients present with mandates the need for the multidisciplinary treatment of the patient with cancer pain.[1] Advances in chemotherapeutic and radiologic treatments, as well as earlier detection and diagnosis trends, have resulted in an increasing number of cancer patients who are surviving or living longer, thus creating the need for improved pain management and quality of life.[2] Nevertheless, significant barriers to effective pain control in patients who have cancer still remain despite the advances in pain management techniques.[3,4]

Cancer patients with pain also experience emotional distress, particularly depression[5] and anxiety,[6] which in turn can potentiate pain and suffering. Cancer patients who have pain are more depressed and report a poorer quality of life.[7-9] Because anxiety exacerbates pain,[6] it becomes especially important to address the emotional distress of cancer patients. Efforts to control pain and emotional distress using conventional means, such as analgesics, antidepressants, and anxiolytics, may lead to other side effects, such as somnolence, confusion, nausea, and constipation, all having an effect on quality of life. Cancer patients, particularly those in advanced stages of illness, such as patients in the palliative care setting, often cannot tolerate medications. The exploration of non-pharmacologic modalities to alleviate pain would therefore seem particularly worthwhile in this population.

Despite the often clear medical etiology in cancer pain, which distinguishes it from chronic noncancer pain, where the medical etiology often does not correlate with the reported level of pain intensity, psychological interventions nevertheless can play a significant role in cancer pain. Pain for the cancer patient has a different meaning than for the noncancer patient, often signifying progression of deteriorating health, which in turn can lead to a deteriorating psychological state.[10] Additionally, the traumatic effect of receiving a cancer diagnosis, as well as attendant emotional distress commonly associated with cancer treatment,[11] all necessitate a comprehensive psychological approach to the patient. Cancer pain, therefore, is similar to noncancer chronic pain in that it is not merely the product of physiological nociception but rather is a complex emotional experience as well.[10,12]

Evidence for the effectiveness of psychological approaches to cancer pain, based on meta-analyses, demonstrates their effectiveness in reducing cancer pain, particularly procedural and treatment-related pain.[13-15] When psychological strategies are used as adjuncts to medical treatments, more than 75% of patients were able to reduce their cancer pain compared with patients not receiving psychological interventions.[15,16]

EDUCATION

The initial step is educating the patient about pain, the mind–body relationship, attitudinal issues, and the expectations and goals of treatment. Clinical practice guidelines and research recommend that patient education about cancer pain be an integral component of treatment.[17-19] Cancer patients need to be informed that pain management is an important part of their care and to tell doctors about unrelieved pain. Additionally, cancer patients and their caregivers should be reassured that cancer pain can be effectively relieved. Educating patients about what to expect regarding pain after procedures or surgery has been demonstrated to significantly improve satisfaction with pain control.[20] Uncertainty about what will happen increases emotional distress. This is particularly true for cancer patients who may undergo many painful procedures for diagnosis and treatment, such as lumbar puncture and bone marrow aspiration. Painful procedures are often considered to be the most difficult part of the cancer experience, particularly for children. Information about the expected quality and duration of the procedure can decrease distress and improve coping.

A pain education program for cancer pain patients produced an increase in pain knowledge and a decrease in pain intensity.[21] Patients need to receive a rationale to understand why they are having pain, the benefits of a comprehensive approach to pain management, and the specific role of nonpharmacologic approaches, such as psychological intervention in the management of their pain. The effectiveness of this step depends on the patient's defensiveness, level of knowledge about the mechanism of pain, and attitudes about the mind–body relationship. The patient needs to be educated about the mind–body relationship according to the patient's ability to understand. Patient education materials such as instruction sheets, audiotapes, and particularly pain diaries[18] can supplement the clinician's efforts. Clinical practice guidelines on cancer pain recommend that all patients should receive a detailed written plan regarding the plan for pain management.[22]

Patient belief systems can interfere with attempts to deliver good pain management to the cancer patient.[10] In a study of public attitudes toward cancer pain, half of the respondents were concerned about the use of opioids for cancer pain, as well as the side effects associated with such therapy.[23] This same study also found a significant fear of cancer pain, which respondents felt would delay their seeking medical care. Patients need to be educated about cancer pain and opioid therapy.[24] Specific maladaptive attitudinal issues need to be addressed, such as the fear of addiction and nonadherence to medication protocols. The unwarranted fear of addiction in patients with cancer pain prevents patients from taking analgesics and adjuvants that might have a significant beneficial impact on pain, functional level, and quality of life.[25] Seventy-nine percent of cancer patients reported believing that a person could become addicted to pain medications.[26] Addiction is not a problem associated with good cancer pain management.[22] The misunderstanding of these issues, however, leads to undertreatment. Additionally, patients may refuse to take specific medications that have "addict" connotations to them, such as methadone and Oxycontin. Cancer patients often worry that their doctors and nurses may not see them as good patients if they complain about their pain.[26-28] As a result, many cancer pain patients take their opioids only when their pain is severe rather than following the recommended fixed schedule.[27] Patients need to be educated on effective communication skills about unrelieved pain with their health care providers.[18]

Additionally, nonadherence to medication protocols is a major problem that needs to be addressed as part of the psychoeducational intervention. Cancer patients take only about half of their prescribed analgesics.[29,30] Poor management of side effects, inadequate knowledge about analgesic titration, and fears about addiction have been noted as accounting for lack of adherence.[25,31] That patients should not give up on protocols too soon needs to be reinforced, to allow for example, the longer-acting tricyclic antidepressants to take effect. Effective educational methods can improve adherence with medications in cancer patients[18,32] and can lower pain intensity.[33] In addition, patients and their home care workers need to be educated about as-needed analgesics that often supplement and optimize the effectiveness of their fixed regimen.

COGNITIVE-BEHAVIORAL APPROACH

The most commonly used psychological approach in treating the patient with chronic pain is the cognitive-behavioral approach. The goal of cognitive-behavioral treatments is to enable the patient to reframe the belief that pain is uncontrollable to a belief that pain can be under his/her control.[34,35] It is based on the theory that thoughts, emotions, and behavior can influence the pain experience. Although the pain is not "cured," the patient may be better able to cope with it. Cognitive-behavioral therapies are recommended for cancer pain[36,37] and for the side effects commonly encountered with chemotherapy, such as nausea and vomiting,[38] as part of a multidisciplinary approach.[22] Meta-analyses have concluded that cognitive-behavioral methods for cancer pain are more effective than no treatment or attention placebo, and do have additive effects over that found with hypnosis or imagery alone.[39,40] Patients benefit from these nonpharmacologic approaches when delivered by trained professionals rather than patient untrained use.[41] Cognitive-behavioral approaches include hypnosis, relaxation (including guided imagery, progressive muscular relaxation, and meditation), biofeedback, coping skills training, cognitive restructuring, music therapy, supportive and group therapy, and stress management techniques.

Hypnosis

Hypnosis is a particularly effective therapeutic technique with pain patients that, of all the psychological techniques, has the strongest empirical support in the treatment of cancer pain.[10,13-16,42] It has been used and studied largely in cancer pain related to procedures, surgery, and chemotherapy. Up to 90% of patients benefit from the use of hypnosis.[42,43]

Hypnosis not only induces relaxation and a passive disregard of intrusive thoughts but can also introduce specific goals through suggestions. These suggestions enable patients to experience analgesia or reinterpretation of their pain. Posthypnotic suggestions allow the patient continued use of the new behavior and assistance in re-creating the relaxed state when needed after termination of hypnosis. In fact, suggestion appears to be the most important element in reducing pain.[44] It is unclear what the exact mechanism is to explain the efficacy of hypnosis,[42] with theories ranging from reductions in peak somatosensory event–related potentials[45] to decreased cortical arousal with increased occipital regional blood flow in areas involved with mental absorption and attention.[44,46] Length of treatment with hypnosis does not add to its effectiveness,[14,42] and individuals vary widely in their hypnotic susceptibility for reasons that are largely unknown.

In a famous study by Spiegel and Bloom,[47] women with metastatic breast carcinoma pain undergoing weekly group therapy with self-hypnosis had significantly lower pain ratings over 1 year than a control group. In another study, patients undergoing hypnosis reported a significant reduction in oral mucositis pain associated with bone marrow transplantation.[48] An NIH consensus conference on symptom management in cancer noted that hypnosis is particularly helpful with procedural pain and mouth sores.[3] A recent review of outcome studies utilizing hypnosis with chronic pain patients concluded that hypnosis is "consistently superior" to no treatment but only equally as effective as other treatments.[49] There is conflicting evidence about the use of the term "hypnosis" with patients, with a meta-analysis showing that it increases efficacy beyond relaxation and imagery,[43] but another study indicated the opposite.[50]

Relaxation

The primary component of the cognitive-behavioral approach is relaxation therapy, which is a systematic method of gaining awareness of physiologic processes and attaining both a cognitive and physiologic sense of tranquility.[51] Relaxation training is currently one of the most widely used cognitive psychological techniques in the management of chronic pain and is used extensively with individuals suffering from cancer pain. Relaxation training acts on pain by lowering anxiety,[52] altering sympathetic activity,[53] reducing generalized arousal and muscle tension,[54] as well as by its cognitive effects of distraction.[54,55] Studies report the effectiveness of relaxation in reducing pain,[56] with one study reporting pain reduction in 38% of advanced cancer patients in a hospice.[57] A comprehensive review of the literature on relaxation training and pain support the effectiveness of this approach with patients in pain.[58] A National Institutes of Health (NIH) technology panel, conducting an extensive scientific review of the literature, concluded that the evidence is "strong" (its highest rating) for the effectiveness of relaxation in reducing chronic pain.[55]

Although relaxation/imagery has been noted to significantly affect pain in a palliative care setting,[59]

research reviews have found that relaxation training is more effective than no treatment with chronic pain but only equally as effective as other self-regulation techniques.[49] Often the initial step of relaxation training is learning controlled diaphragmatic breathing that diverts the patient's attention and can induce the relaxation effect by itself. However, one needs to be vigilant with cancer patients, because deep inspirations can produce or exacerbate pain, particularly postoperatively or in those in advanced stages.

Live relaxation as well as audiotaped relaxation produced significant positive changes in pain sensation, intensity, and severity in cancer pain patients.[60] The live method was the most effective. A meta-analysis of 15 studies (totaling 742 cancer patients) evaluating the effects of relaxation on treatment side effects noted a statistically significant reduction in pain.[14] Specific relaxation strategies that have been shown to reduce pain levels in cancer patients include guided imagery, progressive muscle relaxation, and meditation.[61]

Guided Imagery

Relaxation methods may be most effective with pain when used with imagery.[48] Imagery-based relaxation methods may reduce pain through more of a structured focus than non–imagery-based relaxation methods. Imagery is emerging as a particularly effective tool for managing cancer pain.[61] A recent review of the literature on behavioral interventions for cancer treatment side effects concludes that methods involving relaxation and imagery hold the greatest promise for benefit to the patient with cancer.[62]

Guided imagery has the patient focus on a multisensory imaginary scene. Focusing on the different sensory modalities of the scene can make the image more engaging. Typically, the image is elicited from the patient, and the patient is guided through the image, substituting sensations such as warmth or numbness for pain. Patients need to set aside time to practice in a comfortable position without any interruptions. Imagery can work as an effective distraction technique. An alternative use of imagery is to have the patient focus on the pain rather than distract from it. In this technique, the patient might visualize the pain as a color, for example, red, and makes it less bright until it turns light pink corresponding to lower pain intensity. Relaxation and imagery have been shown to be effective in reducing pain levels in bone marrow transplant patients.[63]

Progressive Muscular Relaxation

In progressive muscular relaxation, patients are taught to alternately tense and relax major muscle groups throughout the body. Progressive muscle relaxation techniques may not be appropriate or well tolerated by patients with advanced cancer or physical limitations. Only nonpainful muscle groups and body locations are used. Patients learn to recognize and differentiate feelings of tension from relaxation and then apply these skills in situations that are painful. Sixteen muscle groups can be initially tensed and relaxed. The number of muscle groups is reduced as the patient becomes more proficient. The patient is instructed to focus on the pleasantness of the relaxation phase. Progressive muscle relaxation is recommended if a muscle tension is thought to be a major contributing factor to the patient's cancer pain.[22]

Meditation

Meditation is defined as "the intentional self-regulation of attention from moment to moment."[64] Concentration meditation, involving the focused attention on a point or object, such as a mantra, differs from mindfulness meditation, which emphasizes detached observation from one moment to the next of a changing field of objects. The primary advantage of mindfulness meditation is the ability to adapt a detached view of the pain sensation, which can lead to an "uncoupling" of the affective from sensory interpretation of pain. As a result, patients have lower levels of reactivity to pain. A study of 51 refractory chronic noncancer pain patients going through a mindfulness meditation program showed that 65% experienced a reduction of more than 33% in their pain ratings.[64]

Biofeedback

Biofeedback can be a particularly effective modality for teaching relaxation to chronic pain patients, as well as self-regulation of physiologic processes. Patients learn to modify specific physiologic processes based on auditory or visual feedback, or both. It is based on the educational paradigm that learning occurs with feedback, which then enables a desired response. Ongoing physiologic processes (such as muscle tension or surface electromyography (EMG), temperature, heart rate, sweat gland activity or basal skin response, and breath rate) can be monitored, and visual (through graphs, images, or games) and auditory (through tones or music) feedbacks are provided. The latest application of biofeedback is neurofeedback, which teaches patients to regulate electroencephelograph (EEG) activity or brain waves. Two studies, however, evaluating the effects of combined EMG and EEG protocols as well as combined EMG-electrodermal biofeedback training on cancer pain found that patients had difficulty transferring their acquired skills to the home.[65,66] Although some patients were able to reduce their levels of pain during the biofeedback sessions, most patients, particularly those with advanced disease, had difficulty reducing their pain levels.

Coping Skills Training

Revised guidelines for the management of cancer pain recommend that patients and their caregivers participate actively in their pain management.[22] Patients can learn to adopt more effective, active coping styles rather than the passive, ineffective coping styles such as catastrophizing, avoidance, and denial. Coping skills can be effective methods in reducing cancer pain,[13,16] particularly those who don't respond to hypnosis or imagery alone.[63]

Activity pacing, which involves the scheduling of rest periods so that patients do not overdo it and sabotage their progress, can be very beneficial for many pain patients. Overexertion, which often results in increased pain and prolonged rest, often has negative sequelae such as increased muscle tension and increased use of medications. Teaching patients to schedule their daily activities into periods of moderate activity followed by limited rest can increase their self-confidence.[67] Overly inactive patients are taught to initiate activities in a very limited fashion and gradually increase activities followed by rest. Patients are also taught to schedule pleasant and enjoyable activities during the day. Additionally, the use of pain diaries to help identify stressful situations or times of day that exacerbate pain can help patients regulate their behaviors and emotions to facilitate more adaptive pain coping skills.

Nearly a quarter of cancer patients undergoing radiotherapy report using alternative methods and an additional 31% are interested in such methods.[68] Of interest is their finding that the use of complementary methods by cancer patients is associated with active coping behavior rather than distress or poor compliance with medical treatment. Patients consider these techniques as supplementary to standard medical methods and as a means of avoiding passivity. It is also a method of coping with hopelessness. Thus, using complementary methods can be a positive adaptation on the part of cancer patients.

Cognitive Restructuring

Cognitive restructuring, or reframing, has been used effectively in cancer pain[69] and as part of an overall cognitive-behavioral treatment.[63,70] It is based on the theory that cognitions determine behavior, affect, and physiology (such as increased muscle tension). Patients learn to identify, challenge, and eventually change self-defeating thoughts (e.g., "I am worthless"). With this technique, pain patients are taught to identify maladaptive negative thoughts, which are often overgeneral or catastrophic statements about oneself or one's illness (e.g., "pain means I need more surgery" or "no one can help me") that pervade their thinking, and to replace them with more constructive and adaptive positive thoughts (e.g., "I can still do many important things"). Patients are taught to use their adaptive thoughts when confronted with pain or situations that lead to pain. Unless patients practice, they may relapse in face of stressful or difficult situations that can lead to increased depression and helplessness. Family and significant other support can be very influential in ensuring the promotion of the generalization and maintenance of the newly acquired cognitive skills.

Music Therapy

Pain has been found to be the most common reason for referral for music therapy in a palliative care setting.[71] Music therapy has been defined as the use of specifically prescribed music under the supervision of a music therapist to aid in the physiologic, psychological, and emotional integration of an individual.[72]

Music therapy can have a beneficial effect on mood and cancer pain when given a choice of music[73] as a method of relaxation and distraction.[74] Diversional and associative qualities of music may distract a patient's attention from the adverse nature of a stimulus. Music may also have a powerful effect on reducing the emotional components of pain, such as fear and anxiety, thus mediating the very perception of pain. Individual music preferences are an important factor to consider.[75]

A recent review of the literature on the effectiveness of music in alleviating pain in the palliative care setting is positive.[76] Music therapy can be an effective independent intervention for providing pain relief in cancer patients.[73] A randomized placebo-controlled crossover trial, however, did not find any effect of music on pain in nine terminally ill cancer patients.[77] The inability of this study, however, to detect the effects of music therapy on pain is attributed to the very small sample size.[59] Although music therapy can be an effective intervention in the relief of pain,[78,79] the literature in this area is scant, anecdotal, and lacking studies with good research design.[59] Studies have been plagued by lack of random assignment, small samples, and lack of control groups.[53]

Music may stimulate the release of endogenous opiates in the central nervous system, which can modulate the perception of the sensory and affective components of pain.[76] Other potential mediating mechanisms that have been postulated include an increased sense of control, reduction in anxiety, regulation of muscle tension, and distraction.[80,81] Music therapy may enable patients to control their pain by distracting their attention from the pain and by changing their emotional experiences.[72,82] Music may also distract by inhibiting pain through selective attention that is mediated by the thalamus, which alerts the prefrontal cortex to the sound rather than to the painful stimulus.[83]

Supportive and Group Therapy

Evidence for the effectiveness of supportive therapy in reducing cancer pain has been studied.[13,47,48] Support and reassurance with the opportunity to vent can be a useful adjunctive method in cancer pain treatment.[47,63] Additionally, support from professionals with expertise in cancer pain management is recommended as well.[22] Social support can be influential in reducing psychological disability.

Group therapy has become a popular form of psychological intervention for the chronic pain patient.[84] A recent meta-analysis of randomized controlled trials of cognitive-behavioral therapy for chronic pain found that most treatments were delivered in groups.[85] The advantages of group therapy are that pain patients learn they are not alone in their suffering, the group can be an effective support system, and patients can learn from other patients' pain coping skills. Patients will often accept challenges from other patients to improve functionality more readily than from an individual therapist whom patients may feel does not understand or appreciate their pain. The major goals of group therapy often are to promote behavior change, educate patients, and provide social support.[84]

Stress Management

Many cancer patients feel high levels of stress because of a cancer diagnosis and have difficulty coping with their illness. Often stress management interventions can be very helpful. Many patients readily acknowledge that stressors, such as return to work issues and conflicts with family and friends, can exacerbate pain. Reducing perceived stress can be very helpful in reducing levels of pain. The initial step in stress management programs is to identify one's stressors in daily life. This is frequently followed by cognitive-behavioral methods as outlined earlier, such as relaxation training and cognitive restructuring. Other important stress management interventions that can be particularly helpful to cancer pain patients include:

1. Sharing feelings and problems with others, such as significant others, patients, or professionals, can be an effective method of relieving stress. Patients with cancer often have great difficulty coping with the cancer diagnosis, decisions about treatment, and the ensuing medical and psychological sequelae. Internalizing emotions or keeping them pent up is generally considered to be unhealthy and has been correlated with a variety of medical conditions including chronic pain. Patients with strong support systems have been shown to cope more effectively with stress.

2. The use of humor can be an effective stress reducer. Laughing at one's problems and taking a humorous

perspective on difficult situations can facilitate stress reduction. Similarly, making time for fun and involvment in recreational activities can be a good distraction and breaks up the chronicity of stress.

3. If medically feasible, physical exercise on a regular basis, usually recommended to be done three times a week for 20–30 minutes can be a particularly effective stress reducer. Patients who have been physically inactive need to be cautioned to avoid injury by starting out slowly. Cancer pain patients should never initiate a physical exercise program without the guidance of a physiatrist or physical therapist. Swimming is considered to be one of the best cardiovascular exercises, particularly for chronic pain patients because there is limited stress placed on the joints.

4. Time management is an important intervention, particularly for "workaholics" or very disorganized patients. Time management consists of instructing patients to make daily lists of tasks to be done, prioritizing them with regard to their importance, estimating the amount of time each task takes, and possibly delegating the ones that others can do. If done properly, time management methods can relieve a significant amount of stress for pain patients who often feel overwhelmed trying to cope with their illness, their pain, and trying to reintegrate back into their work and social lives.

PSYCHOLOGICAL INTERVENTIONS WITH CHILDREN AND ADOLESCENTS

Research on the use of psychological interventions with children and adolescents in pain is less extensive than with adults. Much of the relevant literature has focused on procedure-related pain, in which distraction techniques are recommended,[22] particularly with children.[86,87] It is increasingly recognized that psychological interventions suitable for adults may not be appropriate in the pediatric setting. There may be specific psychological interventions for children and adolescents that are particularly efficacious with cancer pain. Because children often have active imaginations, they are receptive to imagery and relaxation methods. Although cognitive-behavioral methods have been consistently demonstrated to be effective in relieving headaches in children, the evidence for other types of chronic pain, particularly cancer pain, has not been as conclusively demonstrated.[88] There are only anecdotal descriptions and case studies reporting on the usefulness of cognitive-behavioral therapy in cancer pain patients.[88]

BARRIERS TO INTEGRATION OF PSYCHOLOGICAL THERAPIES

The integration of psychological interventions with conventional medical methods in the treatment of cancer pain is essential. This is highlighted by reports of increased mortality, including reduced cancer survival, as a result of unresolved pain.[89,90] In addition, the success of medical interventions, such as surgery and spinal cord implantation, in reducing pain has been shown to be largely dependent on psychosocial factors.[91] A review of 33 studies evaluating psychosocial interventions for cancer patients for all needs did not demonstrate the superiority of one method over another.[92] The authors of the review recommend that practitioners practice flexibility and use more than one method, a practice that appears prevalent in attempting to treat pain.

Despite the generally accepted efficacy of these methods with pain patients, their relative ease of implementation, and their very low side effect profile, barriers nevertheless still exist with the integration of psychological therapies into standard medical care.[55] Those are summarized in Table 27–1.

TABLE 27–1   Barriers to Integration of Psychological Therapies in Cancer Pain Management
Continued overemphasis on the biomedical model, both in clinical care and in medical education
Lack of standardization of psychological techniques
Lack of patient compliance in practicing these methods
Physician reluctance to prescribing psychological methods because of lack of awareness of the benefits of these techniques
Concerns regarding patient perception that referral reflects mental illness
Inconsistent and poor reimbursement by third party payers that hinder the delivery of services
Poorly defined credentialing criteria for providers of such services, which create an unreliability in the delivery of these methods
Psychosocial interventions are time-intensive and often necessitate many visits, which can impede physician and patient acceptance

These barriers to the integration and implementation of psychological therapies in the management of pain in cancer patients can hopefully be overcome with physician and patient education, as well as additional research.[55]

With cancer pain, often the emphasis is on the medical intervention, considering the psychological intervention only when medical management has failed. However, this may not be in the patient's best interest, considering clinical experience shows that psychological techniques, such as hypnosis, are less effective in later stages when pain may be more severe[93] or when the patient may be suffering from drug-induced adverse effects[10] such as compromised cognitive function from high doses of opioids. This would indicate a need for an earlier consideration of psychological techniques when pain levels are less severe or the patient is less medicated. This approach might also be beneficial for treatment side effects and might reduce medication requirements as well.

REFERENCES

1. Cleeland CS, Rotondi A, Brechner T, et al: A model for the treatment of cancer pain. J Pain Symptom Manage 1:209–215, 1986.
2. Portenoy RK: Pain and quality of life: Clinical issues and implications for research. Oncology 4:172–178, 1990.
3. NIH Consensus Conference. State of the Science Conference Statement on Symptom Management in Cancer: Pain, Depression, and Fatigue. National Institutes of Health, 2002, Bethesda, MD.
4. Cleeland CS: Documenting barriers to cancer pain management. In Chapman CR, Foley KM (eds): Current and Emerging Issues in Cancer Pain: Research and Practice. New York, Raven, 1993, pp 321–330.
5. Spiegel D, Giese-Davis J: Depression and cancer: Mechanisms and disease progression. Biol Psychiatry 54:269–282, 2003.
6. Breitbart, W: Psychiatric management of cancer pain. Cancer 63:2236–2342, 1989.
7. Burrows M, Dibble SL, Miaskowski C: Differences in outcomes among patients experiencing different types of cancer-related pain. Oncol Nurs Forum 25:735–741, 1998.
8. Heim H, Oei TPS: Comparison of prostate cancer patients with and without pain. Pain 53:159–162, 1993.
9. Serlin RC, Mendoza TR, Nakamura Y, et al: When is cancer pain mild, moderate or severe? Grading pain severity by its interference with function. Pain 61:277–284, 1995.
10. Roth RS, deRosayro AM: Cancer pain. In Block AR, Kremer EF, Fernandez E (eds): Handbook of Pain Syndromes: Biopsychosocial Perspectives. Mahwah, NJ, Lawrence Erlbaum Associates, 1999, pp 499–527.
11. Holland JC, Rowland J, Lebovits, AH, Rusalem R: Reactions to cancer treatment-assessment of emotional response to adjuvant radiotherapy as a guide to planned intervention. Symp Liaison Psychoth 2:347–358, 1979.
12. Turk DC, Fernandez E: On the putative uniqueness of cancer pain: Do psycho-logical principles apply? Behav Res Ther 28:1–13, 1990.
13. Devine EC: Meta-analysis of the effect of psychoeducational interventions on pain in adults with cancer. Oncol Nurs Forum 30:75–89, 2003.

14. Luebbert K, Dahme B, Hasenbring M: The effectiveness of relaxation training in reducing treatment-related symptoms and improving emotional adjustment in acute non-surgical cancer treatment: A meta-analytical review. Psycho-Oncology 210:490–502, 2001.
15. Montgomery GH, DuHamel KN, Redd WH: A meta-analysis of hypnotically induced analgesia: How effective is hypnosis? Int J Clin Exp Hypn 48:138–153, 2000.
16. Fernandez E, Turk DC: The utility of cognitive coping strategies for altering pain perception: a meta-analysis. Pain 38:123–135, 1989.
17. Agency for Health Care Policy and Research Management of Cancer Pain Rockville, MD, US Department of Health and Human Services, 1994.
18. West CM, Dodd MJ, Paul SM, et al: The PRO-SELF©: Pain Control Program—an effective approach for cancer pain management. Oncol Nurs Forum 30:65–73, 2003.
19. Ferrell BR, Rivera LM: Cancer pain education for patients. Semin Oncol Nurs 13:42–48, 1997.
20. Lebovits AH, Zenetos P, O'Neill DK, et al: Satisfaction with epidural and intravenous patient controlled analgesia. Pain Med 2:280–286, 2001.
21. de Wit R, van Dam F, Zandbelt L, et al: A pain education program for chronic cancer pain patients: Followup results from a randomized controlled trial. Pain 73:55–69, 1997.
22. American Pain Society: Guideline for the Management of Cancer Pain in Adults and Children Glenview, Illinois: American Pain Society, 2005.
23. Levin DN, Cleeland CS, Dar R: Public attitudes toward cancer pain. Cancer 56:2337–2339, 1985.
24. Elliott BA, Elliott TE, Murray DM, Braun BL, Johnson KM: Patients and family members: The role of knowledge and attitudes in cancer pain. J Pain Symptom Manage 12:209–220, 1996.
25. Schumacher KL, West C, Dodd M, et al: Pain management autobiographies and reluctance to use opioids for cancer pain management. Cancer Nurs 25:125–133, 2002.
26. Ward SE, Goldberg N, Miller-McCauley V, et al: Patient-related barriers to management of cancer pain. Pain 52:319–324, 1993.

27. Dar R, Beach CM, Barden PC, Cleeland CS: Cancer pain in the marital system. J Pain Symptom Manage 7:87–93, 1992.
28. Cleeland CS: The impact of pain on patients with cancer. Cancer 54:263–267, 1984.
29. DuPen SL, DuPen AR, Polissar N, et al: Implementing guidelines for cancer pain management: Results of a randomized controlled clinical trial. J Clin Oncol 17:361–370, 1999.
30. Miaskowski C, Dodd MJ, West C, et al: Lack of adherence with the analgesic regimen: A significant barrier to effective cancer pain management. J Clin Oncol 19:4273–4274, 2001.
31. Ersek M, Kraybill BM, Pen AD: Factors hindering patients' use of medications for cancer pain. Cancer Practice 7:226–232, 1999.
32. Oliver JW, Kravitz RL, Kaplan SH, Meyers FJ: Individualized patient education and coaching to improve pain control among cancer outpatients. J Clin Oncol 19:2206–2212, 2001.
33. Allard P, Maunsell E, Labbe J, Dorval M: Educational interventions to improve cancer pain control: A systematic review. J Palliat Med 4:191–203, 2001.
34. Bradley LA: Cognitive-behavioral therapy for chronic pain. In Gatchel RJ, Turk DC (eds): Psychological Approaches to Pain Management. New York, Guilford Press, 1996, pp 131–147.
35. Bradley LA, McKendree-Smith NL, Cianfrini LR: Cognitive-behavioral therapy interventions for pain associated with chronic illness: Evidence for their effectiveness. Semin Pain Med 1:44–54, 2003.
36. Cleeland CS: Nonpharmacologic management of cancer pain. J Pain Symptom Manage 2:523–528, 1987.
37. Fishman B, Loscalzo M: Cognitive-behavioral interventions in the management of cancer pain: Principles and applications. Med Clin North Am 71:217–286, 1987.
38. Burish TG, Tope DM: Psychological techniques for controlling the adverse side effects of cancer chemotherapy: Findings from a decade of research. J Pain Symptom Manage 7:287–301, 1992.
39. Sellick SM, Zara C: Critical review of 5 nonpharmacologic strategies for managing cancer pain. Cancer Prev Control 2:7–14, 1998.

40. Thomas EM, Weiss SM: Nonpharmacological interventions with chronic cancer pain in adults. Cancer Control 7:157–164, 2000.

41. Kwekkeboom KL: Pain management strategies used by patients with breast and gynecologic cancer with postoperative pain. Cancer Nurs 24:378–386, 2001.

42. Montgomery GH, Weltz CR, Seltz M, Bovbjerg DH: Brief presurgery hypnosis reduces distress and pain in excisional breast biopsy patients. Int J Clin Exp Hypn 50:17–32, 2002.

43. Kirsch I, Montgomery G, Sapirstein G: Hypnosis as an adjunct to cognitive-behavioral psychotherapy: A meta-analysis. J Consult Clin Psychol 63:214–220, 1995.

44. Rainville P, Duncan GH, Price DD, Carrier B, Bushnell MC: Pain affect encoded in human anterior cingulated but not somatosensory cortex. Science 277:968–971, 1997.

45. DePascalis V, Magurano MR, Bellusci A, Chen AC: Somatosensory event-related potential and autonomic activity to varying pain reduction cognitive strategies in hypnosis. Clin Neurophysiol 112: 1475–1485, 2001.

46. Rainville P, Hofbauer RK, Bushnell MC, Duncan GH, Price DD: Hypnosis modulates activity in brain structures involved in the regulation of consciousness. J Cogn Neurosci 14:887–901, 2002.

47. Spiegel D, Bloom J: Group therapy and hypnosis reduce metastatic breast carcinoma pain. Psychosom Med 45:333–339, 1983.

48. Syrjala KL, Cummings C, Donaldson G: Hypnosis or cognitive-behavioral training for the reduction of pain and nausea during cancer treatment: A controlled clinical trial. Pain 48:137–146, 1992.

49. Kessler R, Patterson DR, Dane J: Hypnosis and relaxation with pain patients: Evidence for effectiveness. Semin Pain Med 1:67–78, 2003.

50. Hendler CS, Redd WH: Fear of hypnosis: the role of labeling in patients' acceptance of behavioral interventions. Behav Ther 17:2–13, 1986.

51. Arena JG, Blanchard EB: Biofeedback and relaxation therapy for chronic pain disorders. In Gatchel RJ, Turk DC (eds): Psychological Approaches to Pain Management. New York, Guilford Press, 1996, pp 179–230.

52. Borkovec TD, Sides JK: Critical procedural variables related to the psychological effects of progressive relaxation: A review. Behav Res 17:119–125, 1979.

53. Good M, Stanton-Hicks M, Grass JM, et al: Relief of postoperative pain with jaw relaxation, music, and their combination. Pain 81:163–172, 1999.

54. Good M: A comparison of the effects of jaw relaxation and music on postoperative pain. Nurs Res 44:52–57, 1995.

55. NIH Technology Assessment Panel on Integration of Behavioral and Relaxation Approaches into the Treatment of Chronic Pain and Insomnia: Integration of behavioral and relaxation approaches into the treatment of chronic pain and insomnia. JAMA 276:313–318, 1996.

56. Syrjala KL, Chapko ME: Evidence for a biopsychosocial model of cancer treatment-related pain. Pain 61:69–79, 1995.

57. Fleming U: Relaxation therapy for far-advanced cancer. Practitioner 229: 471–475, 1985.

58. Turner JA, Chapman CR: Psychological interventions for chronic pain: A critical review. I. Relaxation training and biofeedback. Pain 12:1–21, 1982.

59. Pan CX, Morrison S, Ness J, Fugh-Berman A, Leipzig RM: Complementary and alternative medicine in the management of pain, dyspnea, and nausea and vomiting near the end of life: A systematic review. J Pain Symptom Manage 20:374–387, 2000.

60. Sloman R: Relaxation and the relief of cancer pain. Nurs Clin North Am 30: 697–708, 1995.

61. Graffam S, Johnson A: A comparison of two relaxation strategies for the relief of pain and its distress. J Pain Symptom Manage 2:229–231, 1987.

62. Redd WH, Montgomery GH, DuHamel KN: Behavioral interventions for cancer treatment side effects. J Natl Cancer Inst 93:810–823, 2001.

63. Syrjala KL, Donaldson GW, Davis MW, Kippes M, Carr JE: Relaxation and imagery or cognitive-behavioral training reduce pain during bone marrow transplantation: A controlled clinical trial. Pain 48:137–146, 1995.

64. Kabat-Zinn J: An outpatient program in behavioral medicine for chronic pain patients based on the practice of mindfulness meditation: Theoretical considerations and preliminary results. Gen Hosp Psychiatry 4:33–47, 1982.

65. Fotopolous SS, Cook MR, Graham C, et al: Cancer pain: Evaluation of electromyographic and electrodermal feedback. Prog Clin Biol Res 132D:33–53, 1983.

66. Fotopolous SS, Graham C, Cook MR: Psychophysiologic control of cancer pain. In Bonica JJ, Ventafridda (eds): Advances in Pain Research and Therapy, Vol 2. New York, Raven Press, 1979, pp 231–244.

67. Hirano PC, Laurent DD, Lorig K: Arthritis patient education studies, 1987–1991: A review of the literature. Patient Educ Couns 24:9–54, 1994.

68. Sollner W, Maislinger S, DeVries A, et al: Use of complementary and alternative medicine by cancer patients is not associated with perceived distress or poor compliance with standard treatment but with active coping behavior. Cancer 89:873–880, 2000.

69. Chen E, Zeltzer LK, Craske MG, Katz ER: Alteration of memory in the reduction of children's distress during repeated aversive medical procedures. J Consult Clin Psychol 67:481–490, 1999.

70. Liossi C, Hatira P: Clinical hypnosis versus cognitive-behavioral training for pain management with pediatric cancer patients undergoing bone marrow aspirations. Int J Clin Exp Hypn 47:104–116, 1999.

71. Gallagher LM, Huston MJ, Nelson KA, Walsh D, Steele AL: Music therapy in palliative medicine. Support Care Cancer 9:156–161, 2001.

72. Munro S, Mount B: Music therapy in palliative care. Can Med Assoc J 119: 1029–1034, 1978.

73. Beck SL: The therapeutic use of music for cancer-related pain. Oncol Nurs Forum 18:1327–1337, 1991.

74. Good M, Stanton-Hicks M, Grass JA, et al: Relaxation and music to reduce postsurgical pain. J Adv Nurs 33:208–215, 2001.

75. Good M, Picot BL, Salem SG, et al: Cultural differences in music chosen for pain relief. J Holist Nurs 18:245–260, 2000.

76. O'Callaghan CC: Pain, music creativity and music therapy in palliative care. Am J Hosp Palliat Care 13:43–49, 1996.

77. Curtis S: The effect of music on pain relief and relaxation of the terminally ill. J Music Ther 23:10–14, 1986.

78. Foley KM: The treatment of pain in the patient with cancer. CA Cancer J Clin 36:194–215, 1986.

79. Kerkvliet GJ: Music therapy may help control cancer pain. J Natl Cancer Inst 82:350–352, 1990.

80. Magill-Levreault L: Music therapy in pain and symptom management. J Palliat Care 9:42–48, 1993.

81. Hirsch S, Meckes D: Treatment of the whole person: Incorporating emergent perspectives in collaborative medicine, empowerment, and music therapy. J Psychosoc Oncol 18:65–77, 2000.

82. Brown CJ, Chen A, Dworkin SF: Music in the control of human pain. Music Ther 8:47–60, 1989.

83. Hardy SGP: Analgesia elicited by prefrontal stimulation. Brain Res 339:281–284, 1985.

84. Keefe FJ, Beaupre PM, Gil KM: Group therapy for patients with chronic pain. In Gatchel RJ, Turk DC (eds): Psychological Approaches to Pain Management. New York: Guilford Press, 259–282, 1996.

85. Morley S, Eccleston C, Williams A: Systematic review and meta-analysis of randomized control trials of cognitive behavioral therapy and behavior therapy for chronic pain in adults, excluding headache. Pain 80:1–13, 1999.

86. Broome ME, Lillis PP, McGahee TW, Bates T: The use of distraction and imagery with children during painful procedures. Oncol Nurs Forum 19:499–502, 1992.

87. Broome ME, Rehwaldt M, Fogg L: Relationships between cognitive-behavioral techniques, temperament, observed distress, and pain reports in children and adolescents during lumbar puncture. J Pediatr Nurs 13:48–54, 1998.

88. McGrath PA, Holohan AL: Psychological interventions with children and adolescents: Evidence for their effectiveness in treating chronic pain. Semin Pain Med 1:99–109, 2003.

89. McBeth J, Silman AJ, Macfarlane GJ: Association of widespread body pain with an increased risk of cancer and reduced cancer survival. Arthritis Rheum 48: 1686–1692, 2003.

90. Liebeskind JC: Pain can kill. Pain 44:3–4, 1991.

91. Nelson DV, Kennington M, Novy DM: Psychological selection criteria for implantable spinal cord stimulators. Pain Forum 5:93–103, 1996.

92. Iacovino V, Reesor K: Literature on interventions to address cancer patients' psychosocial needs: What does it tell us? J Psychosoc Oncol 15:47–71, 1997.

93. Hilgard ER, Hilgard JR: Hypnosis in the Relief of Pain. Los Altos: California, 1983.

CHAPTER 28

Physical Therapy

ANNALISE BIONDOLILLO, PT

Sources of pain in cancer patients can be direct (i.e., consequence of disease) and indirect (i.e., prolonged bed rest and inactivity). Physical therapists need to be aware of this in treating the patient with a cancer diagnosis. This chapter begins by briefly reviewing cancer pain syndromes from a perspective relevant to physical therapy (PT). The remainder of the chapter focuses on the procedures, treatment modalities, and techniques that will enable the physical therapist to effectively treat a patient with cancer-related pain.

Cancer pain syndromes can be broadly grouped into three categories:

1. Pain related to cancer and its spread.
2. Pain related to cancer therapy.
3. Pain unrelated to cancer or cancer therapy.[1]

PAIN RELATED TO CANCER AND ITS SPREAD

Cancer pain can develop when the tumor invades nerves and their related structures, bone, and the viscera. Tumor invasion can occur in contiguous structures or metastasize via blood or lymph systems. Additional complaints may accompany the cancer-related pain and may include loss of appetite, nausea, constipation, and shortness of breath. These can compound patient's pain, as well as contribute to anxiety and general decline in health.

Clinically, a variety of pain syndromes may present when a tumor invades nerves. These may include brachial, cervical, and lumbar plexopathies; peripheral and intercostal neuropathies; nerve root or cord compression; and trigeminal neuralgia. Pain can be well localized and confined to the area of involvement or radicular pain syndromes can develop. Transcutaneous electrical nerve stimulation (TENS) may be effective in treating nerve pain.

When tumor invades bone it can be the primary source of cancer (i.e., osteosarcoma) or the result of metastasis.

Bone pain is usually described as severe in nature and may require advanced understanding of pain management to effectively reduce the pain intensity. Bone pain can be a result of involvement of the bone itself, pathologic fractures, secondary to reflex muscle spasms, from connective tissue, or bone marrow replaced by tumor. Many cancers are known for their frequent metastasis to bone (i.e., lung cancer, breast cancer, prostate cancer, thyroid cancer, renal cancer, and multiple myeloma which by its nature produces lytic lesions in bones throughout the body). Usual sites of metastasis include the skull, ribs, spine, and pelvis. The location of tumor will affect activity level, weight-bearing status, and functional mobility in the patient.

Tumor can also invade the viscera. It may involve the organs themselves (which may not in themselves be sensitive to pain) or the pleural membranes. Organs most commonly affected include the lungs, pancreas, gastrointestinal tract, and the uterus. In addition to the local and referred pain, other symptoms might arise, including bleeding, constipation or change in bowel or bladder function, weight loss, and abdominal distension. Again, functional status of the patient will be affected.

PAIN RELATED TO CANCER THERAPY

Pain can be a result of the therapy used to actually reduce or eliminate the cancer. Patients have the potential to develop pain as a side effect of specific surgical procedures, chemotherapeutic agents, and radiation therapy.

Postsurgical pain syndromes can be differentially diagnosed from postoperative pain in that postsurgical pain syndromes develop almost immediately after the surgery or shortly thereafter and gradually increase in intensity. Acute postsurgical pain is initially intense and gradually lessens over time as healing occurs. Dramatic increase in postoperative pain may also be the result of infection or tumor recurrence.

Pain after radical neck dissection is caused by injury to the cervical plexus, cranial nerves, and cervical sympathetics at the time of surgery. Patients may describe pain as a tight, burning pain in the area of sensory loss, and a shock-like pain may also present. In addition to the pain, patients may express concern over cosmetic changes and functional loss of movement and strength in the jaw, neck, and shoulder. Physical therapists need to be aware of the nerves and muscles damaged, sacrificed, or preserved to best address muscle imbalances in the upper quarter caused by the surgery and radiation therapy. PT does not immediately address these deficits until the surgical area is well healed. Initially in the postoperative phase, the goal of therapy is regaining functional abilities in ambulation and transfers and normal mobility in the unaffected upper extremity.

Postmastectomy pain syndrome may occur in 10% of those women undergoing a simple or radical mastectomy.[2] It is caused by trauma to the intercostobrachial nerves. Pain can present as tight, constricting, or burning pain in the anterior chest wall, axilla, and upper arm. Pain will also be exacerbated by range of motion of the shoulder. A frozen shoulder may develop secondary to prolonged guarding posture in the involved upper extremity. Exquisite pain may be reproduced on palpation of axilla with trigger points identified. There is evidence to suggest that the incidence of postmastectomy pain syndrome increases in patients who develop complications such as delayed wound healing, infection, and hematoma in the region of the scar.[3] The role of physical therapy is to prevent disuse atrophy on the involved side and to educate patients in awareness and prevention of lymphedema and to promote joint and soft tissue mobility.

Postthoracotomy pain is caused by a disruption or irritation of the intercostal nerves. A thoracotomy is done to resect lung cancer. During the procedure, ribs may be fractured or intercostal tissues may be overstretched, which could lead to intercostal nerve damage. The patient may describe an aching sensation or "hot knife-like" pain in the distribution of the incision associated with sensory loss. There can also be exquisite pain on palpation of trigger points. TENS can be beneficial in treating this nerve pain. Myofascial release can reduce the connective tissue tightness and minimize trigger points.

Limb sparing procedures have reduced the need for amputation; however, salvage procedures have not eliminated the need for amputations altogether. Phantom limb pain occurs after an amputation, and is reportedly identical in nature and location as in the limb before surgery. The severity of the phantom limb pain that develops appears to be related to the duration of the preamputation pain and the presence of pain on the day of the surgery.[4] Pain usually lessens within 2 months of the surgery. Recurrent pain may indicate recurrent disease.

Stump pain differs from phantom limb pain in that it develops at the site of the surgical scar, not in the missing limb. Stump pain is believed to be caused by the development of a neuroma at the site of the nerve transection. Pain increases with activity and decreases with rest. It can be characterized by sharp, shooting sensations. Neuromas also can be responsible for phantom limb sensation that is described as an itching or burning feeling in the amputated extremity. Stump pain is localized on palpation and can be "shock-like" in nature. TENS can be beneficial in this patient population.

Radiation therapy techniques are used more frequently and selectively in the treatment of cancer. Pain caused by radiation therapy, however, is less common than with chemotherapy. Collateral damage from radiation techniques can occur to tissues adjacent to tumors. Nerve tissues are most susceptible to injury associated with fibrosis of the surrounding connective tissue, and secondary injury to the nerve. Brachial plexopathy (more commonly seen) and lumbar plexopathy may present with mixed motor and sensory deficits in the affected limb. Radiation myelopathy occurs when the spinal cord is included in the radiation field. Transient myelopathy is frequently seen approximately 4 months after radiation therapy in an area where the cervical spinal cord is exposed to treatment. Clinically, the patient would complain of "shock-like" sensations that are exacerbated by cervical flexion and exercise. Symptoms usually disappear in 2 to 36 months. Chronic progressive myelopathy occurs with prolonged exposure of the spinal cord to radiation. Incidence of myelopathy increases with greater exposure leading to increased pain at the spinal level involved with dysesthesias below the level of injury.[5] Physical therapy can be useful in maximizing functional mobility and trial of TENS for pain management.

Postchemotherapy pain is caused by the use of chemical agents that are toxic to peripheral nerves. This pain is seen with increasing frequency as patients survive longer and more effective chemotherapeutic agents are developed. The side effects from chemotherapy that are frequently presented to the physical therapist are: musculoskeletal pain, postherpetic neuralgia, headache, peripheral neuropathy, and steroid-induced pain syndromes. TENS can be effective in managing the "nerve" pain. Osteonecrosis and avascular necrosis associated with prolonged steroid use require weight-bearing modifications and adaptive equipment. For those withdrawing from steroids, myalgias, myopathies, and arthralgias may develop and can be treated symptomatically and with exercise.

Patients in the process of diagnosis and treatment of cancer undergo a variety of procedures that induce pain and may limit a patient's willingness to participate in a physical therapy program at any given time. Bone marrow biopsies are performed at the iliac rest with patient positioned prone. Local analgesics are given before the procedure, but may not fully mask the pain. Some patients opt for conscious sedation for the biopsy, which may leave the patient drowsy for a period of time and not the best PT candidate. Lumbar punctures are used for diagnostic, as well as therapeutic, reasons. Local anesthetics are used before the procedure. Excess leakage of cerebrospinal fluid may lead to a headache. Patients are usually confined to flat bed rest for a period of time after the puncture. Many patients continue to experience pain from frequent blood draws, but some patients have a mediport inserted, which eliminates this source of irritation.

PAIN UNRELATED TO CANCER OR CANCER THERAPY

Regardless of cancer pain, 10% of cancer patients may have pain from a nonmalignant source.[6] Degenerative joint disease in the cervical or lumbar spine, diabetic neuropathy, myofascial pain syndrome, postherpetic neuralgia, and chronic headaches may be causes of the patients' complaints. It may be difficult for the clinician to differentiate cause of the pain from a cancer or noncancer source. Cancer patients may also contribute to their pain by maintaining the same position for prolonged periods. This inactivity can lead to muscle weakness, joint and nerve compression, and prolonged elongation of soft tissues, all which contribute to the overall discomfort of the patient.

Lymphedema

Lymphedema is best defined as tissue swelling caused by a failure of lymph drainage.[7] It may be primary in type because of a genetic problem of lymph drainage, or secondary as a result of disruption or destruction of lymph channels from surgery, radiation, disease, or infection. Pain occurs in approximately 50% of patients with cancer-related lymphedema.[8] Onset of lymphedema is unpredictable and is differentiated from postoperative edema. Pain related to lymphedema has specific characteristics:

1. Use of the affected limb exacerbates pain, resting relieves it.
2. Patients complain of the limb feeling heavy and uncomfortable, with aching and tightness.
3. Both the pain and the swelling become worse throughout the day and are often worse during warm weather.
4. Analgesics are often ineffective and resting the arm in a supported position provides the only relief.

Patients may have difficulty sleeping if a comfortable position is not found and maintained.[9]

Treatment of lymphedema incorporates a specialized program of manual lymphatic drainage and compression bandaging or sleeves. Patient education on prevention and self-care is paramount as lymphedema is a lifelong problem.

PHYSICAL THERAPY TREATMENT OF CANCER PAIN

Significant numbers of cancer patients have physical limitations as a result of cancer or its treatment. Most commonly, this impairment results from prolonged bed rest and deconditioning syndrome or neurologic loss coupled with deconditioning.[10] In addition, patients may experience loss of appetite, sleep disturbances, impaired social roles with family and friends, and depression. Throwing pain syndromes into the mix further hampers patients' rehabilitation and affects quality of life.

Evaluation

To effectively treat the cancer patient who is in pain, a thorough evaluation of the patient is the first step. In an inpatient environment, the patient chart is more readily available than in an outpatient department. If available, review the entire patient medical history looking for cancer and noncancer sources for patient complaints of pain. In the outpatient setting, one has to rely on the patient or family member to provide an accurate history. Clinicians can also consult with the patient's physician for clarification. Interviewing the patient can uncover the onset, duration, intensity, site, quality, and frequency of the pain, which are important to establish a plan of care. One must not overlook the effect of the patient's condition on his or her quality of life.

Assessing the pediatric or mentally impaired patient presents different challenges. This patient might have more difficulty describing the quality or nature of the pain. The visual analog scale can be used in older children, but in younger children behavioral changes may be observed, (crying, facial grimacing, sweating, activity avoidance). They may be less likely to report pain if they think it will result in a painful procedure (needle stick). On the other hand, they may exaggerate their complaints to avoid a portion of treatment. Pain behaviors can be positively reinforced by sympathy or concern from others. Pain behaviors can also be reinforced by special attention, which can lead to lower performance expectations and avoiding difficult tasks or people.

This patient population may get reinforced pain behavior when pain medication is taken with the painful activity as opposed to on a regular fixed schedule. Pain triggers can develop when a child associates a time, place, or person with a painful event.[11]

Clinicians have to also consider the special needs of those patients at a palliative care level; patients who are not responsive to or not desiring curative treatment. Disability in patients at this level of care often comes from prolonged bed rest, deconditioning, and neurologic and musculoskeletal complications of cancer or its treatment. The physical therapist's role in this setting is to elevate the patient's level of function and comfort. Meaningful physical activity affects the patient's quality of life by maintaining a certain level of independence and by lessening the burden on the caregiver. Recommendations for adaptive equipment and environmental modifications help to elevate safety and independence. It is also important for patients to maintain social interaction at this time. Physical therapists who address the social, as well as physical, needs of the patient are contributing to an enhanced quality of life for the individual.

The next step is establishing goals for the patient. There is a lot to consider. The patient should be viewed as a whole and not just by an identified diagnosis. In establishing goals, one must consider the stage of the disease, comorbidities, type of pain, and psychological and sociocultural characteristics of the patient. Goals should be realistic and measurable. The patient's goals should also be incorporated and addressed. Understand that patients' need to have some control over their condition and therefore they need to play an active role in their treatment. Patients' perceptions of having control over their pain improves their satisfaction with the pain management techniques being used.[12] Ultimately, the goals of physical therapy are to restore function, reduce pain, and promote independence. In most cases, patients and their families view rehabilitation favorably.

Treatment Goals

Treatment should be done in a manner that leaves the patient with the highest functional status, fewest side effects, and best quality of life.

Multidisciplinary Plan

In the inpatient setting, coordination of care with physical therapy, occupational therapy, social work, nursing, dietary, pastoral care, psychology, case management, pharmacy, and physicians can be obtained more easily because all are under one roof. Studies conclude that significant functional gains are observed in hospitalized cancer patients who received interdisciplinary rehabilitation services.[13] Facilities often have rounds or multidisciplinary care meetings where all aspects of patient care can be discussed and plans for coordination of services to maximize patient outcomes can be determined. Multimodal management strategies offer patients the greatest improvement potential for chronic pain syndromes.[14] Combination of therapies provides patients with the skills and knowledge needed to increase their sense of control over pain.

Positioning and Handling

Careful attention to the patient reinforces a good relationship. Patients need to feel that they matter. Handling of patients must be secure enough to prevent sudden movement, but also gentle enough as to not aggravate symptoms. Informing the patient about what to expect may also reduce patient anxiety. Positioning and handling a sensory impaired individual requires extra attention to avoid soft tissue damage. Also note clothing, bedding, and lines, which may become irritants to the skin.

Position changes reduce pain and incidence of frozen joints, ulcers, and contractures. Cancer patients may lose the spontaneous pain-relieving movements that healthy people have; therefore, positioning has to be done for them and may require the use of pillows, splints, and other supports to maintain the correct posture. Custom-made or prefabricated wedges, supports, slings, and other equipment may be used. Sometimes inexpensive and readily available materials are put to use. The physical therapist may be involved in ordering the appropriate item needed, including hospital beds and wheelchairs.

In patients who are otherwise active and somewhat independent, instruction in correct postures and positioning through various activities of daily living (ADLs) can reduce the incidence and aggravation of pain. Incorporation of neutral spinal postures in sitting, standing, and sleep should be reviewed in an effort to reduce the spinal load.

Sitting

Hips should be flexed to 90 degrees and thighs should be parallel to the floor. Not all chairs and work situations accommodate for this, so use of a stool under the feet may allow for correct posture (Figure 28-1). The lumbar lordosis should be supported with a back support, small pillow, towel roll, or seat back. Shoulders should be centered over hips and head upright. Forward head posture is to be discouraged. A simple way of checking correct posture is to align ears, shoulders, and hips in a straight line in the saggital plane. Arms can be supported on pillows on the lap or resting at 90 degrees flexion at a workstation. Recliners are often used for

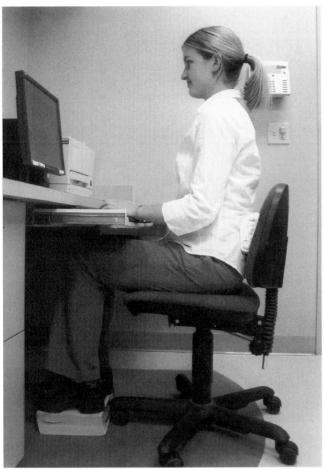

FIGURE 28-1   Neutral spinal posture—sitting.

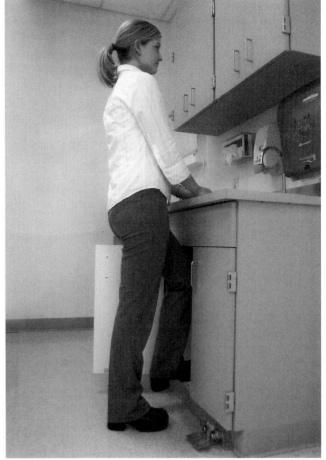

FIGURE 28-2   Neutral spinal posture—standing.

comfort care and occasionally as a substitute sleep surface. Many recliners encourage poor back posture in that rounding of the lumbar lordosis is noted in sitting and reclined positions. Support of the low back with whatever tools are available is important for comfort and spinal health.

Standing

The forward head posture is to be eliminated. Ears, shoulders, and hips should be aligned in the saggital plane (Figure 28-2). Back fatigue can settle in during prolonged standing. Alternately resting one foot on a 4- to 6-inch stool can be helpful in reducing low back strain, as long as shoulder and head posture remain erect.

Sleeping

It is often difficult to discourage a patient from lying prone, but considering the cervical strain from the prolonged rotational component, it is worth the effort. Lying supine with one pillow under the head and one or two pillows under the knees can be very comfortable (Figure 28-3). Very soft mattresses may allow for

flattening of the lumbar lordosis. Use of a small pillow or towel roll at the small of the back can correct this problem. Many patients prefer side lying. In this position, encourage a pillow between the knees to prevent lower trunk rotation, "hug" a pillow at chest level to prevent thoracic rotation, (Figure 28-4) and use one or two pillows to support the head and neck in a neutral

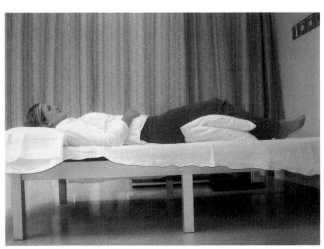

FIGURE 28-3   Neutral spinal posture—lying supine.

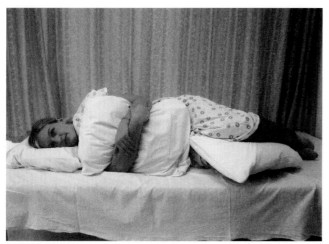

FIGURE 28–4   "Hugging" a pillow at chest level prevents thoracic rotation.

posture. Patients may not be able to maintain the correct position for the entire night, but at least they can get some benefit for a period of time and hopefully progress in their endurance of the correct posture. Individual variances may be needed given the patient's specific physical abilities, disease, surgical site, and endurance.

Heat and Cold

Heat increases blood flow to the skin and superficial tissues, which in turn reduces the blood flow to the deeper tissues. It induces vasodilation, which increases oxygen and nutrient delivery to damaged tissues. Heat increases the elastic properties of muscle which reduces joint stiffness. The gate control theory of pain also implies that pain can be reduced with heat.[15]

Heat can be administered in many forms in the cancer patient: hot packs, hot water bottles, hot/moist compresses, electric heating pads, gel packs, and hot tubs. The use of deep heat by means of diathermy or ultrasound can be used cautiously in the cancer patient, but never over a cancer site.[16]

Heat is contraindicated in an area of inflammation as it may accelerate the inflammatory process. Similarly, bleeding disorders can be aggravated by increased blood flow from heat. Caution should be used heating an area of reduced or diminished sensation as resultant tissue damage can occur. Appropriate insulation of the heat source and limited exposure time is warranted. Avoid using heat in an area of poor circulation as tissue necrosis can occur from the increased metabolic demands in the heated area. Some patients use topical pain creams that can burn when combined with heat. Cleaning the skin before treatment will eliminate that risk. Some recommend that heat not be applied to tissue that has been exposed to radiation therapy.[17]

Cold reduces blood flow initially upon application, which decreases inflammation and edema after injury. It decreases pain from muscle spasm by interrupting the cycle of nerve ischemia caused by muscle spasms. Cold decreases nerve conduction in peripheral nerves. Application of cold decreases local hyperesthesia. The gate control theory of pain also applies to ice therapy.[15]

Cold can be applied in the form of ice packs, gel packs, cold water bottle, ice massage with an ice cube, or coolant spray. At home, a bag of frozen vegetables is often available to use. Ice should not be applied directly to the skin, except for ice massage. Wrapping ice in an insulating layer of towels will reduce the risk of damage to the soft tissue and is more comfortable to the patient. It is also recommended that the ice application conform to the body part treated to evenly distribute the cold treatment.

The use of ice is contraindicated in patients with sensory or circulatory impairment (i.e., Raynaud's). Prolonged exposure to ice can cause burns. The U.S. Department of Health recommends ice and heat not be used on tissue damaged by radiation therapy.

Functional Mobility

Improved or maintained ambulation ability is important in reducing pain from prolonged inactivity and pressure. The benefits of ambulation include improved oxygen uptake, muscle elasticity, and range of motion, while also fighting fatigue.

Safety in ambulation is paramount. The patient needs to be evaluated for the type of device that best suits the patients' ability. Canes, walkers, and crutches are the most frequently used aids. The device then needs to be adjusted to fit the patient. Patients need to be properly instructed in the use of the device and clearly understand if they are safe to ambulate independently or require assistance. Some individuals may need instruction in the parallel bars before progressing to the device. Caregivers and staff also need to be informed of patients' ambulation ability and weight-bearing status so they can provide the necessary supervision or assistance. This is particularly important for those patients with bony metastases, who are prone to painful pathologic fractures.

For those who cannot ambulate, there are physical, as well as psychological, benefits to being out of bed and in a chair. Physically, there are increased demands on the circulatory system in sitting. Gravitational pressures on the body are distributed differently. Some chairs have wheels that allow patient to be mobile. Sitting upright leads to improved social interaction and the patient may feel less debilitated.

Providing patients with adaptive equipment such as raised toilet seats, shower benches, and handrails can affect patients' function, as well as preserve independence in ADLs. The use of slings, braces, or casts can provide temporary pain relief and support that can increase functional mobility.

Exercise

A persistent pain cycle is established when illness strikes. Serious illness leads to prolonged bed rest, which in turn encourages a loss in functional mobility. With this diminished capacity for movement, joint stiffness, shortened soft tissues, and weak muscles develop, all leading to increased pain. Therapeutic exercise is one tool used by physical therapists to break this pain cycle and enhance the patient's overall well-being. The numerous benefits of exercise are listed in Table 28–1.

There are additional positive outcomes from an exercise program: decreased stress and fatigue and improved relaxation. Moderate exercise may also improve immune function.[18] More importantly, exercise may assist the patient in obtaining some sense of control over their body, thus boosting their optimism.

The patient's overall condition must be considered when establishing an appropriate exercise program. Those confined to bed may only be able to tolerate passive range of motion (PROM) exercises. PROM addresses joint stiffness and muscle elasticity and is a prelude to active exercises. PROM should be done with proper handling of the patient. Grip should be firm, but comfortable. Movement through the limb's normal anatomic range should be slow and gentle initially, then gradually increase to patients' tolerance or soft tissue resistance. If the patient is nonverbal, watch for signs of distress such as facial grimacing or resistance to stretch.

Active range of motion is the next progression in therapeutic exercise, which increases muscle activity, strength, and coordination. The patient moves his or her joints through the available range of motion in gravity neutral or resisted planes. Range of motion is limited by joint mobility, pain, or limited endurance. Eventually, manual resistance or weights may be added to enhance muscle strengthening, and weight-bearing activities should be incorporated. A therapy ball is a cost-effective exercise tool that can be used for both strengthening and aerobic activities, with low impact on the joints. Some patients enjoy the balance and coordination challenges presented in therapy ball use, along with an interesting change of pace.

Aerobic exercise, such as walking, stationary bicycling, or swimming, are three of the best cardiovascular exercises one can do. Aerobic exercise is known to increase endurance, raise metabolism, and strengthen bones. Oxygenated blood is distributed to the muscles and all tissues, which assist in the healing process. Most rehabilitation centers have stationary bikes, treadmills, stair steppers, and the like, to work with patients. Some inpatients may be confined to their room or floor, which limits their use of physical therapy equipment. Using a stool for step up activities or simply walking in the halls may serve as a substitute. Therapy band–resistive exercises can also present an aerobic challenge.

The importance of diaphragmatic breathing exercise should not be overlooked when working with all patient populations. Although not as efficient as aerobic exercise, improving the level of oxygen in the blood aids in reducing muscle spasm and pain.

Soft Tissue Techniques

Some patients with cancer-related pain would like nothing more than a back rub as their treatment when physical therapy has so much more to offer. Despite the frequent misunderstanding of the concept of physical therapy, there are definite benefits to a therapeutic massage. Massage increases venous and lymphatic circulation, decreases muscle spasm, and aids relaxation. Massage may also stimulate the release of endogenous endorphins, which naturally reduce pain. However, it cannot strengthen muscle and is therefore not a substitute for exercise. There is something to be said for the "laying on of hands" (Figure 28–5). There is a soothing effect in massage that is interpreted as natural empathy and concern for the patient. There is increased confidence in physical therapists who use their hands to find the pain and apply treatment directly to the painful area, especially when physicians look at pain from a distance. Techniques in therapeutic massage are varied and apply to specific symptoms. Massage is contraindicated over areas of infection or underlying pathology.

Effleurage is a light stroking technique in which there is constant contact with the skin at all times. Effleurage is used generally for relaxation and reducing anxiety. Superficial blood flow is stimulated. The amount of pressure used determines the depth of soft tissue affected.

TABLE 28–1 Benefits of Exercise
Increased cardiovascular conditioning
Decreased joint stiffness
Increased range of motion
Decreased pain
Increased joint stability
Improved posture
Improved functional mobility
Increased bone density

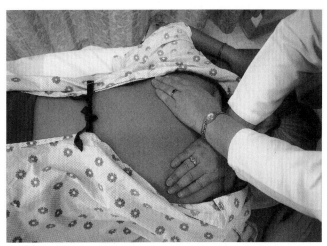

FIGURE 28–5 Therapeutic massage increases venous and lymphatic circulation, decreases muscle spasm, and aids relaxation. It has a soothing effect that is interpreted as natural empathy and concern for the patient.

This technique is usually gentle and nonpainful. Deeper stroking in the direction of venous flow can help reduce edema.

Petrissage is deeper and may be somewhat uncomfortable. Skin and deeper soft tissues are gripped, rolled, and maneuvered between the therapist's hands. It can be effective in reducing muscle spasm.

Deep friction massage is a more localized treatment for the release of adhesions or scar tissue. Techniques can be performed by the therapist or taught to the patient and performed independently depending on the area being treated. This is a painful technique that can be better tolerated by the applying of an ice massage locally over the treated area for up to 3 minutes before the massage. The strokes can be done in a circular or cross-friction manner, but one has to be careful to apply as much pressure as needed to effectively treat the underlying tissue. Too light pressure may cause blistering of the skin.

Manual lymphatic drainage (MLD) is a gentle massage technique used to mobilize lymph fluid from a congested area to areas of the body where fluid can drain normally.[19] When done correctly, the massage techniques should not induce pain from deep pressure. The amount of pressure used for MLD should only be enough to move the skin and tissues beneath. It is a specialized method of massage that requires detailed understanding of the lymph system and lymphedema to effectively treat this patient population.

Myofascial release (MFR) is a specialized technique used by physical therapists to treat soft tissue problems. Fascia is a thin connective tissue that surrounds and permeates every muscle, nerve, bone, organ, and vessel. Injury, disease, excessive strain, inflammation, and surgery can cause changes in the fascia that stimulate pain. Fascia is a three-dimensional network that connects the entire body. When fascia tightens, pain can be felt locally, regionally, or remotely from the injured area. The goal of MFR is to restore the elasticity of the fascia, so that restrictions in movement and function are eliminated.

Physical therapists can locate areas of fascial restrictions through palpation and range of motion. Myofascial trigger points are locally sensitive spots that can reduce in size and sensitivity with MFR. Gentle stretching techniques are applied to an area of fascial tightness and held until the therapist notes a "release" of the tissue. The therapist relies on feedback from the patient to determine the direction and flow of treatment. Myofascial release works with the patient, not on the patient. The patient is instructed in appropriate stretches and exercises to perform at home. This maximizes the benefit of treatment.

Transcutaneous Electrical Nerve Stimulation

There are several theories as to how TENS works:

1. Cutaneous electrodes deliver low-voltage electrical stimulation through peripheral nerve fibers for the purpose of diminishing the transmission of the pain signal to the brain, thus relieving pain (gate control theory of pain).
2. Endorphin levels are known to be elevated after treatment of TENS in those with chronic pain.[20] Endorphins are endogenous polypeptides with morphine-like properties that transmit, modify, and inhibit noxious stimuli.[21]
3. There is also the theory that positive results are just a placebo effect, and within a short period of time of TENS use, the benefits are drastically reduced. It is speculated that this occurs because of increased tolerance to the stimulation. Modulation settings in the unit may reduce this effect.
4. TENS application is taught to patients to be used independently (Figure 28–6). This gives them a sense of control over their symptoms and may be another reason for successful pain relief with TENS use.

There are a few contraindications for TENS. TENS should never be used over the carotid sinus, eyes, metal implants, or gravid uterus. It cannot be used in the patient with a cardiac pacemaker. Electrode placement over unhealthy skin from infection or inflammation is to be avoided. Lymphedema has been reported to worsen with TENS use. Patients with limited understanding caused by brain dysfunction should not use TENS.

Serious side effects from TENS use are rare. Most common is skin irritation from electrodes. Trying different electrodes or cleansing the skin before application may eliminate this problem.

There are many indications for TENS use in the patient with cancer pain. Postsurgical pain syndromes, phantom limb and stump pain, postradiation and

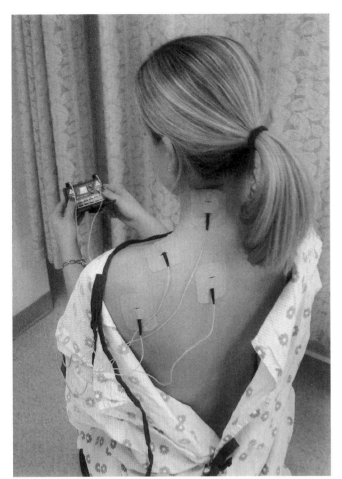

FIGURE 28–6 Patients are taught to use transcutaneous electrical nerve stimulation (TENS) independently, which gives them a sense of control over their symptoms.

postchemotherapy pain may all respond favorably to TENS treatment. Use of TENS to treat extremity and trunk pain appear to be most rewarding for pain relief, whereas perineal and pelvic pain are most difficult to control.[22]

Placement of electrodes for optimal pain relief may require some trial and error. There are some general principles in determining electrode placement. Initial application might be directly over the painful site as long as there is no active disease present. If relief is not sufficient, placement of electrodes proximal to the painful site in the same dermatome, adjacent dermatome, or over a larger nerve branch innervating the pain site may bring positive results. In areas of nerve compression or injury, stimulation should be proximal to the level of injury, where sensation is intact. In the case of neuropathic pain, TENS may be delivered to the contralateral side of the body in the same dermatome level as the injury if stimulation to the involved side is not tolerated.

When treating with TENS, electrodes should be of sufficient size and number to treat the involved area. Electrodes are available through a variety of distributors in many configurations and materials. Trial and error may also determine the placement of the electrodes on the patient that provides optimal patient comfort and pain relief. Electrodes may be set up in a medial–lateral line connecting to each channel, or a proximal distal line. Some feel a crossed pattern of the electrodes provides greatest benefit. The clinician has to also determine if the patient can duplicate the treatment independently. If assistance is required, does the patient have someone available? When wearing the TENS unit, patients need to have lead wires under clothing to avoid catching the wires on handles and knobs.

Depending on the model of TENS unit, various stimulation parameters may be offered. The simplest and easiest for patients to use is conventional TENS in which a constant impulse is delivered. It is also the easiest to accommodate to and may not provide long-term benefit. Many units offer modulated outputs in which frequency or amplitude vary, thus reducing the accommodation effect on patients. In both types of stimulation, a sensation of pins and needles is delivered through the electrodes, but the sensation can be soothing, some with gradual increased intensity, but usually without discomfort. Other modes of treatment include acupuncture-like TENS and Burst. These deliver a stronger sensation of pins and needles that some patients find noxious.

The clinician must also determine the frequency of TENS use, which maximizes treatment outcomes. TENS units can be worn 24 hours daily if desired. Initial treatment may start with limited time, and then gradually increase duration to reach the pain relief goal. Some patients find it difficult or disruptive to attempt to sleep with the unit on, therefore may use the stimulator up until bedtime. Others are successfully able to sleep with the unit on. Careful monitoring of patient participation and compliance with TENS unit use is required for successful pain management.

Patient Education

Pain education based on the evolving science of pain relief should be a part of the standard of physical therapy practice in pain management. Education provides important support for the patient with cancer and their caregivers. Pain-management education when done in a tailored fashion to individual needs that includes written materials, verbal instruction, or audio/video supplements, with follow up, significantly increases patient knowledge, and decreases pain intensity reported by patients. The patient then can be proactive in managing their pain, which will increase their sense of control over their pain.

ACKNOWLEDGMENT

The author would like to thank Laura Coons, DPT and Adam Cleaver, DPT for their research assistance during the preparation of this manuscript.

REFERENCES

1. Winston PCV, Henry FW, Ronald M: Cancer Pain Management: Principles and Practice. Boston, Butterworth-Heinemann, 1996, pp 279-292.
2. Granek I, Ashikari R, Foley KM: Postmastectomy pain syndrome: Clinical and anatomical correlates. Proc ASCO 3:122, 1983.
3. Winston PCV: Cancer Pain Management: Principles and Practice. Boston, Butterworth-Heinemann, 1996, p 285.
4. Bach S, Noreng MF, Tjellden NU: Phantom limb pain in amputees during the first 12 months following limb amputation, after preoperative lumbar epidural blockade. Pain 33:297, 1988.
5. Foley KM, Woodruff JM, Ellis FT: Radiation-induced malignant and atypical peripheral nerve sheath tumors. Arch Neurol 7:311, 1980.
6. Wall PD, Melzack R: Textbook of Pain, 3rd ed. Edinburgh, Churchill Livingstone, 1994, p 787.
7. Mortimer PS: Investigation and management of lymphoedema. Vasc Med Rev 1:1-20, 1990.
8. Alliot F, Miserey G, Cluzan R: The secondary upper limb lymphoedema can be painful and disturb the quality of life. World Lymphology Conference, Tokyo, 1990.
9. Carroll D, Rose K: Treatment leads to significant improvement: Effects of treatment on pain in lymphoedema. Professional Nurse 8:32-36, 1992.
10. Sliwa JA, Marciniak C: Physical rehabilitation of the cancer patient. Cancer Treat Res 100:75-89, 1999.
11. McGrath PA: Pain in Children. New York, Guilford Press, 1990.
12. Pellino TA, Ward SE: Perceived control mediates the relationship between pain severity and patient satisfaction. J Pain Symptom Manage 15:110-116, 1998.
13. Sabers SR, Kokal JE, Girardi JC, et al: Evaluation of consultation-based rehabilitation for hospitalized cancer patients with functional impairment. Mayo Clin Proc 74:855-861, 1999.
14. Barkin RL, Lubenow TR, Bruehl S, et al: Management of chronic pain. Part I. Disease -A-Month 42:389-454, 1996.
15. Melzack D, Wall PD: Pain mechanisms: A new theory. Science 15:971-978, 1965.
16. Lehmann JF, deLateur BJ: Therapeutic heat. In: Lehmann JF (ed): Therapeutic Heat and Cold, 4th ed. Baltimore, Williams & Wilkins, 1990, p 417-581.
17. Santiago-Palma J, Payne R: Palliative care and rehabilitation. Cancer 92:1049-1052, 1999.
18. Cannon JG: Exercise and resistance to infection. J Appl Physiol 74:973-981, 1993.
19. Mortimer PS, Badger C, Hall JG: Lymphoedema. In Doyle D, Hanks GWC, MacDonald N (eds): Oxford Textbook of Palliative Medicine, 2nd ed. New York, Oxford University Press, 1998, pp 657-665.
20. West AB: Understanding endorphins: Our natural pain relief system. Nursing 11:50-53, 1981.
21. Wilson RW: Endorphins. Am J Nurs 81:722-725, 1985.
22. Avellanosa AM, West CR: Experience with transcutaneous electrical nerve stimulation for relief of intractable pain in cancer patients. J Med 13:203-213, 1982.

CHAPTER 29

Occupational Therapy

SANDRA MEYERS, MS, OTR/L

This chapter describes occupational therapy intervention and palliative approaches for the cancer patient with pain that are used by the occupational therapists at Roswell Park Cancer Institute in Buffalo, New York. The occupational therapists at Roswell Park work with many cancer patients who receive palliative care, and a hospice room is available at the institute.

When the author joined Roswell Park in 1995, one responsibility was to become a member of the Cancer Pain Management Service to offer occupational therapy assessments, intervention, and education for cancer pain outpatients and inpatients of the institute. Other members of the Pain Management Service included anesthesiologists, a dentist/psychologist/specialist for head and neck pain, a pharmacist, a nurse practitioner, and a registered nurse for pain management. The team also included a research nurse, a pain psychologist, a physical therapist, a nutritionist, and interns. A patient's pain was measured on the Pain Intensity Scale with no pain (0), mild pain (1 to 4), moderate pain (5 to 7), and severe pain (9 to 10).[1] The comprehensive pain assessment questionnaire (CPAQ) and a Barriers Questionnaire were developed by some of the Pain Management Service members.[2] Occupational therapy referrals were received from weekly pain clinic patient rounds and by contacting the occupational therapists by pager.

The Pain Initiative Task Force was formed in 2001 to meet the Pain Management Quality Improvement required by the Joint Commission on Accreditation of Healthcare Organizations (JCAHO).[3] Roswell Park occupational therapists were members of the task force. Among the goals that the Pain Initiative Task Force met were ensuring staff competency with pain assessments for measuring pain as the fifth vital sign, developing policies and procedures that supported the appropriate prescription ordering for effective pain management, and addressing patient needs for symptom management in the discharge planning process.[3]

Pain is common in cancer. Three types of pain are somatic, which is felt with bone fractures or bone metastases; visceral, which is felt by the stretching and invasion of linings as in colon or stomach cancer; and neuropathic pain, which occurs from cancer spreading to the nervous system. Pain can also be caused from cancer chemotherapy, radiation, and surgery.[4,5] Pain is described as anything from dull aches to a burning sensation; it can worsen from physical activity. Sleep and appetite disturbances, a decrease in activity, and irritability can be caused by pain.[4]

Cancer pain is often managed by drugs. Nonsteroidal anti-inflammatory drugs (NSAIDs) are used for mild pain, weak opiates with simple analgesics are used for moderate pain, and strong opiates are used for severe pain. Alternative opiates (co-analgesics) and radio therapy neural blockade surgery can also relieve pain.[5] Intraspinal administration and patient-controlled analgesia (PCA) are also methods of pain control.[6] Patients' feelings of relief from trigger point injections have been observed.[2] Pain medication side effects can include nausea, vomiting, constipation, drowsiness, and urinary retention. Pain tolerance can also be different with individuals. Breakthrough pain can occur before the next dose of analgesia is due, and additional medication is given for it. Tolerance and dependence may occur, but physical dependence is not an addiction.[5] Pharmacologic pain control takes place at nerve endings, peripheral nerves, the dorsal horn, the spinothalamic tract, the midbrain, and the cortex. Cancer pain medication has to be supervised by palliative care specialists to achieve optimal pain control or relief for palliative patients.[7]

Medication may affect patient performance during occupational therapy evaluation and treatment sessions. Therapy may be better tolerated after receiving pain medication; otherwise, pain medication can make patients lethargic and sick, resulting in ineffective occupational therapy treatment.[4] For example, a patient recovering from surgery for a desmoid tumor was coming every day to the occupational therapy clinic for therapeutic activities to relieve depression. One day, she was unable to concentrate on her activity because her pain level was at a 7 out of 10, and she became tearful. Because of this, she asked to be returned to the nursing unit for her pain medication. The nursing unit was called before she arrived to be ready with her pain medicine. For the rest of her visits to occupational therapy clinic, the patient received her pain medication prior to the scheduled time for occupational therapy.

Roswell Park Cancer Institute provides acute care, bone marrow transplants, inpatient hospice care, and outpatient care. The Department of Occupational Therapy serves the entire population of patients. After a referral for occupational therapy has been received, an initial evaluation and goal-setting take place with the patient.

An occupational therapy evaluation at Roswell Park consists of several components. Included are a full assessment of the patient's activities of daily living status prior to admission, components of his or her usual lifestyle, individual priorities, personal goals, and desired outcomes for therapy.[4] A pain scale rating of the patient's pain is taken, and a fatigue rating on a scale of 0 to 10 is done for the patient. Active and passive range of motion are also measured. Manual muscle testing is measured if the patient's platelet count is higher than 50,000 per mm^3. Gross and fine motor coordination are tested along with sensation, light touch, proprioception, kinesthesia, sharp/dull discrimination, and temperature. Endurance is tested by measuring rest periods during the assessment.

Cognition, including orientation, judgment, memory, attention span and problem solving, and safety awareness are also evaluated. Psychosocial adjustment such as coping styles, emotional state, and support of family and friends are assessed. Overall vision, peripheral vision, depth perception, figure/ground perception, and use of corrective lenses are assessed. Static and dynamic balance in sitting and standing positions are evaluated. Activities of daily living performance are evaluated including feeding, grooming, bathing, dressing, and toileting. Leisure and work skills assessments, as well as kitchen assessments, are also provided depending on the roles and goals the patient chooses (Figure 29-1).[4]

After the occupational therapy assessment is completed and goals are set with the patient, a physician's order is needed to treat the patient. Occupational therapists at Roswell Park contribute to pain management in the following ways: physical management (orthotics, positioning, seating, and activities of daily living), patient teaching and education (work simplification, energy conservation, and fatigue management), and psychosocial support (distraction, or diversion, and communication).

Orthotics consist of fabrication and fitting of upper and lower extremity splints, slings, back supports, cervical collars, and specialized supports to help relieve pain (Figures 29-2 to 29-6). Back braces and neck braces are ordered from vendors to relieve pain and provide stability for patients with cancer that affects the spine (Figures 29-7 to 29-11).

In cases of prolonged bed rest in which neuropathy or severe weakness develops, wrist supports maybe needed if medial nerve involvement or if carpel tunnel symptoms are present (Figure 29-12).[8] Positioning and seating help prevent painful pressure ulcers and joint contractures when patients and families are taught the importance of frequent and correct positioning. Chair cushions and back supports increase the patient's comfort and time out of bed.[4] Multiboots or resting foot splints are designed to elevate patients' heels, to prevent skin breakdown and foot drop, to position patients' feet in a neutral position, and to help reduce painful edema (Figure 29-13). At Roswell Park, abduction pillows are cut in half lengthwise with an electric knife to be used to elevate patients' arms (Figure 29-14).

With activities of daily living, occupational therapy helps patients maintain or regain as much independence as possible with self-care. Pain patients are taught to use adaptive equipment when needed to perform activities in spite of pain or disability. Education in proper body mechanics may help reduce pain.[4] At Roswell Park, long-handled sponges and reachers are used to avoid excessive bending and straining. These sponges also have been used to apply topical pain medication (Figure 29-15).

Peripheral neuropathy and myelopathy are conditions that can result from chemotherapy, radiation treatment, tumor metastasis, and nerve resection surgery. They can cause a lack of pain sensation in touch, temperature, and position. The safety of the patient can be at risk when he or she is performing activities involving hot surfaces, such as accidentally touching a stove burner or a pot of boiling water.[4]

Shoulder dysfunction and impairment of activities of daily living can be caused by muscle atrophy, nerve damage, or arm swelling that may occur with pain, weakness, tingling, or numbness after breast surgery.[4] Patients who undergo axillary node dissection are at risk for developing sensory and motor deficits secondary to nerve trauma. Complaints of pain throughout the shoulder region are prevalent. The long thoracic nerve and the serratus anterior muscle are at risk. Movements of upward rotation, protraction, and elevation of the scapula are needed for performing routine activities of daily living such as brushing hair, putting on a shirt, or washing the back. Occupational therapy can be required for remedial or adaptive care.[4] In one study, occupational therapy was successful for the improvement of shoulder function except for active abduction. Independence in daily living and household activities was gained after accessory nerve palsy occurred following radical neck dissections; however, occupational therapy alone was not adequately effective for resting pain and motion pain.[9]

ROSWELL PARK CANCER INSTITUTE
Elm and Carlton Streets, Buffalo, New York 14263

Occupational Therapy Department

Patient Name:			Patient Number		Age	Sex	Pain
Evaluation Date		☐ Inpatient ☐ Outpatient					Score
☐ Initial Assessment	☐ Re-assessment	**Reason(s) for Referral**					0 – 10
Primary Diagnosis:		ADL's	Orthotics	ROM/Strengthening			
Onset Date:		Fine Motor	Cognition	Sensory			
		Fatigue	Endurance	Pain Management			

Precautions:	None	Falls	Seizures	Cardiac	Location of Pain
	Thrombocytopenia	Neutropenia	Isolation	Anemia	Description of Pain

Medical/Surgical History	
Living Situation	☐ House (# of Floors) # Steps to Enter ☐ Railing ☐ Apartment on Floor # ☐ Assisted Living ☐ Other
Comments:	
Bathroom	☐ Tub/Shower (curtain/door) ☐ Stall Shower (curtain/door) ☐ Tub ☐ Grab Bar ☐ Tub Seat ☐ Hand Shower
Persons in Household	☐ Lives Alone ☐ Spouse ☐ Significant Other ☐ Children ☐ Dep ☐ NonDep ☐ Caretaker
Comments	

Hearing Deficits	☐ None	☐ Mild	☐ Severe	☐ Hearing Aids
Visual Deficits	☐ None	☐ Mild	☐ Severe	☐ Glasses/Contacts
Speech Deficits	☐ None	☐ Mild	☐ Severe	

Comments	
Leisure, Recreational and Hobby Interests	
Vocational Status	**Occupation**

Cognitive Status	Intact	Impaired	**Comments**
Orientation			
Attention Span			
Direction Following			
Safety Awareness			
Problem Solving/Reasoning			
Judgment Skills/Memory			
Motivational Level			

Emotional Status	☐ Depressed ☐ Agitated ☐ Calm ☐ Anxious
	Comments
Pre-Admission ADL Status	
Adaptive Equip. Previously Used	
Fatigue Score 1 -10	
Endurance - No. of Rest Periods	

Functional Status as Measured by the FIM								
Level of Assistance	Indep. 7	Mod Indep 6	Sup Setup 5	Min. A 4	Mod A 3	Max A 2	Dependent 1	**Comments**
Grooming								
Feeding								
Dressing – UE								
Dressing – LE								
Bathing – UE								
Bathing – LE								
Toileting								
Transfers								
Kitchen Mgt								
Household tasks								
Shopping								
Laundry								
Cleaning								

FIGURE 29–1 An occupational therapy evaluation form and treatment plan from Roswell Park Cancer Institute. Pain assessment is included.

Continued

ROSWELL PARK CANCER INSTITUTE
Elm and Carlton Streets, Buffalo, New York 14263

Left						Right			Muscle Tone	
PROM	AROM	Strength				PROM	AROM	Strength	Right	Left
			SHOULDER	Abduction					☐ Normal	☐ Normal
				Adduction					☐ Hypertonic	☐ Hypertonic
				Flexion					☐ Hypotonic	☐ Hypotonic
				Extension					☐ Rigidity	☐ Rigidity
				Int. rotation					**Balance**	
				Ext. Rotation					Intact	Impaired
				Protraction					☐ Static Sitting	☐
				Retraction					☐ Dynamic Sitting	☐
				Elevation					☐ Static Standing	☐
				Depression					☐ Dynamic Standing	☐
			ELBOW	Flexion					Ambulatory Status:	
				Extension						
			FOREARM	Pronation					Devices for Ambulation:	
				Supination						
			WRIST	Flexion						
				Extension						
			FINGERS	Flexion						
				Extension						
			THUMB	Opposition						

Coordination	Intact	Impaired	Comments	Hand Function		
Gross Motor				Dominant	R	L
Fine Motor				Gross	R#	L#
Sensory Processing				Grasp		
Tactile				Tip Pinch		
Proprioceptive				Lateral Pinch		
Visual				3 Jaw Chuck		
Auditory				**Foot Splint Assessment**		
Gustatory				Prolonged	Y	N
Olfactory				Bed Rest		
Perceptual Skills				Edema	Y	N
Stereogonsis				Foot Drop	Y	N
Depth Perception				Skin Integrity	Int	Imp
Right/Left Discrim.				Comments		
Body Scheme						
Figure – Ground						

Assessment	
Patient's Goals	
Short Term Goals	Est. Time:
	Est. Time:
	Est. Time:
Long Term Goals	Est. Time:
Patient/Family/SO Participation in Goals	
Plan	
Discharge Planning	☐ Rehab ☐ Home Care ☐ Home ☐ Family
Signature	Date
Physician Signature	Date

FIGURE 29–1 cont'd

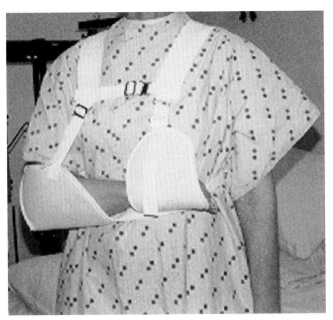

FIGURE 29–2   A sling used for breast cancer patients for painful arms from lymphedema.

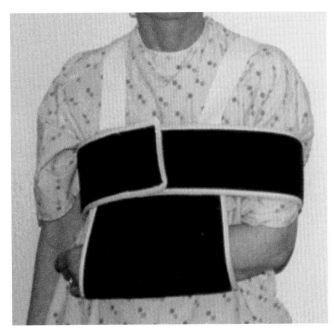

FIGURE 29–3   A shoulder immobilizer used for painful pathologic fractures of the humerus.

Patient teaching or education for pain management patients is addressed at Roswell Park by the Department of Occupational Therapy with instruction of work simplification, energy conservation, and fatigue management. Patients are helped to select the tasks most important to them and to set priorities within their limitations. Alternative methods and delegation of tasks are also considered. Energy conservation involves patients learning how to pace tasks and to schedule regular rest periods. The Fatigue Management Program from the Department of Occupational Therapy has been made possible by Quality of Life Grants from the Roswell Park Alliance Foundation. Factors such as decreased energy

level and increased pain are complaints a patient might have. Both can severely limit patients from engaging in purposeful activities such as going for walks, preparing meals, and socializing with friends. Chronic fatigue can be seen in patients with cancers affecting blood cell production and lymphatic system function such as leukemia, Hodgkin's disease, and multiple myeloma. Chemotherapy and radiation treatment can decrease red blood cell production, resulting in anemia. Surgery and cancer pain can greatly affect a patient's activity level and can result in long periods of bed rest and overall deconditioning.[4] Chronic disuse can lead to multiple

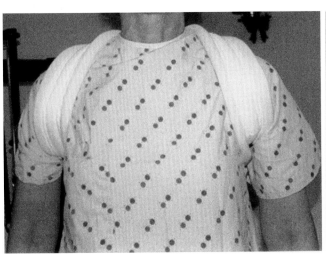

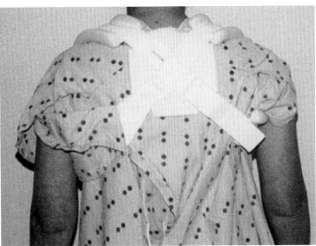

A   B

FIGURE 29–4   A clavicle strap used for painful pathologic fractures of the clavicle.

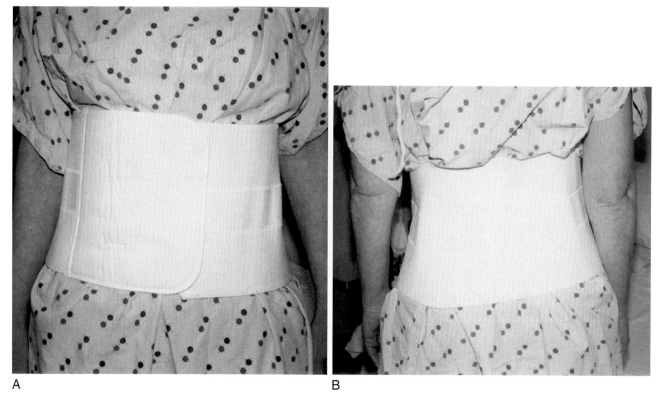

A

B

FIGURE 29–5   A low back support used for muscular pain.

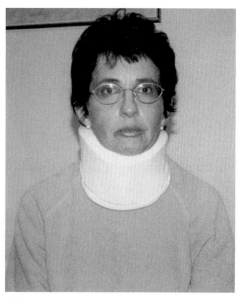

FIGURE 29–6   A cervical collar used for muscular pain.

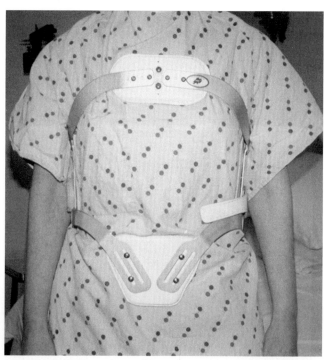

FIGURE 29–7   A thoracic lumbar hyperextension brace used for stability and relief of pain of thoracic lumbar sacral spine fractures and prevention of spinal-cord compression.

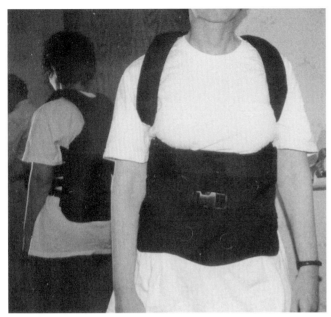

FIGURE 29–8 A thoracic lumbar sacral orthosis used for stability, prevention of spinal cord compression, and pain relief of thoracic, lumbar, and sacral spine.

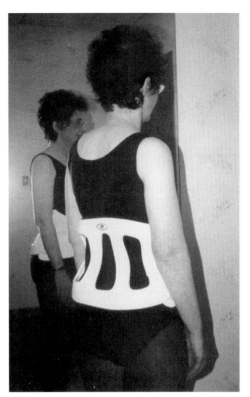

FIGURE 29–9 A Buffalo Brace for low back pain.

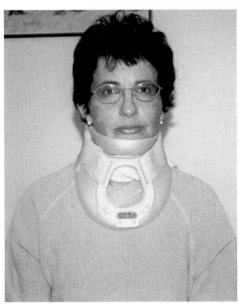

FIGURE 29–10 A Philadelphia Collar.

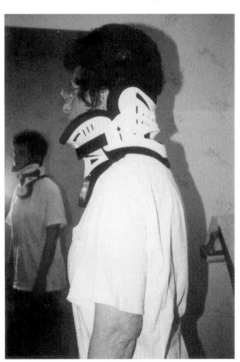

FIGURE 29–11 A Miami-Jay neck brace for cervical spine stability.

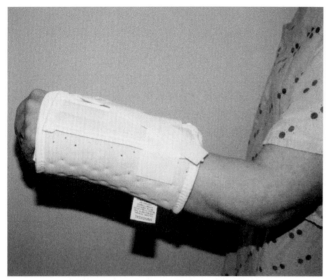

FIGURE 29–12 A wrist support used for carpel tunnel syndrome.

complications that affect the body's systems. The Fatigue Management Program addresses the measured level of fatigue from 0 to 10, a patient's sleep pattern, exercise, rest, pain, nutrition, leisure, and household tasks.

Additional methods of patient education about treatment of pain with occupational therapy include participation in a series of videotaped pain management lectures, an occupational therapy and pain kiosk that is available in the Pain Management Center, and participation in the Pain Management Support Group that was facilitated by the Division of Psychology and the Department of Physical Therapy.[3]

Psychosocial support including distraction, diversion, and communication are also ways that occupational therapy can intervene with pain patients. For more than

25 years, the Department of Occupational Therapy at Roswell Park has had a Diversional/Psychosocial Program for cancer patients.[10] Distraction, or diversion, is any activity that helps a patient focus his or her attention on something other than pain (Figure 29-16). Rhythmic breathing, speech, listening to music, walking, craft activities, and progressive muscular relaxation are all used to decrease awareness of pain. The occupational therapist helps each patient determine what works best. Relaxation can help one regain a sense of control over his or her psychological and emotional reactions as well as improve personal productivity on a daily basis. Certain types of muscle relaxation techniques significantly reduce overall muscle tension, which can result in a reduced level of pain.

Cognitive distraction during relaxation therapy can also account for decreasing pain because the person's mind is focusing on thoughts other than the discomfort, thereby inhibiting the awareness of pain.[4] Deep breathing is used as an effective form of relaxation when one is in a lot of pain and feels stressed or nervous. When one is anxious, he or she tends to take short and shallow breaths from the upper chest. Deep breathing exercises encourage the expansion of the abdomen, and breath becomes lower and longer.[4] If pain is felt all over, relaxation and imagery techniques can be incorporated into treatment sessions.[5] Positive or guided imagery is another relaxation technique devised to assist people in dealing with pain or reduced stress. An example would be imagining a setting that is calming, such as a beach.[5] At Roswell Park, the occupational therapists use relaxation, imagery tapes, and soft music with patients with pain (Figure 29-17).

Communication helps patients with pain. Through regular supportive visits from the occupational therapists, patients are given an opportunity to express their feelings and concerns. Patients are encouraged to identify meaningful goals and then plan how to reach them. Establishing areas of patient control helps to alleviate depression.[11]

Beyond physical disfigurement and emotional ravages of advanced malignancy, it is the pain of cancer that is the most dreaded. Physicians have the expertise to control the pain of these cancer patients who experience it. Other forms of pain that can be equally devastating are the pain of isolation, pain of abandonment, and pain of the loss of role. Occupational therapy treatment strategies can improve the quality of life and perception of pain for the hospice patient. Occupational therapists play an important part in giving patients an opportunity to live out their lives in a dignified and purposeful manner as their disease permits.[8] Occupational therapy has a unique contribution to make to the terminally ill person because of its focus on the use of time and the significance of time to the person who has little left.[8]

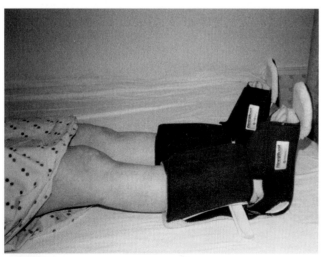

FIGURE 29–13 Multiboots used for prevention of foot drop as well as for pain from breakdown of skin in both heel and toe.

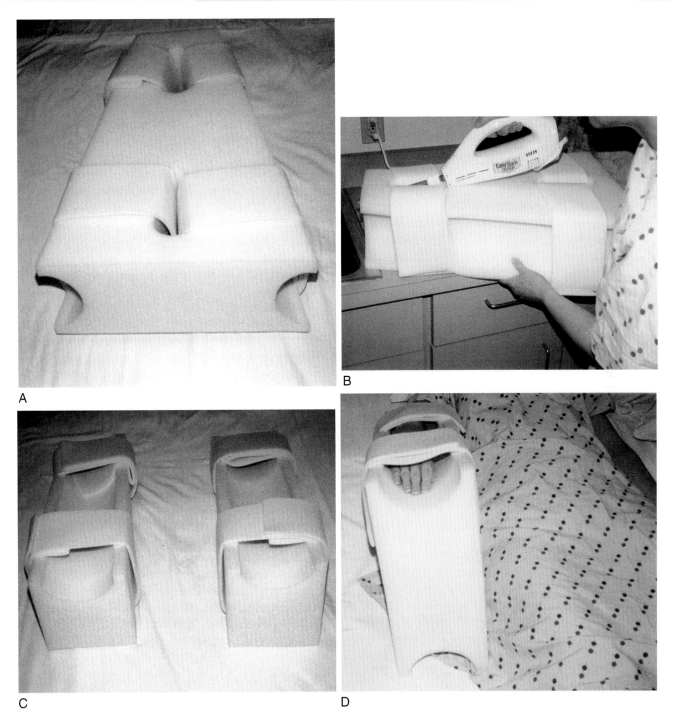

A

B

C

D

FIGURE 29–14   An abduction pillow used to elevate a patient's arm to reduce edema.

The occupational therapist who reestablishes a sense of worth in the terminally ill cancer patient by maximizing his or her occupational roles makes a significant contribution to the reduction of the cancer patient's pain.[8] Provision of a pleasant environment with familiar possessions, quality time, the gift of touch, the provision of friends, tapes or CDs, books or television programs, assistance with attaining a degree of independence, and granting choices will decrease feelings of isolation and help minimize pain.[8]

Occupational therapists have worked with hospice patients who had become dependent on the caregiver for feeding, bathing, and dressing and enabled them to achieve a degree of independence in every area. It is possible for cancer patients to make significant gains in self-care and resume work roles in the last few months of their lives.

Arts and crafts activities can reassure a patient of his or her ability to function on some level, and handmade gifts enable a role reversal when the patient

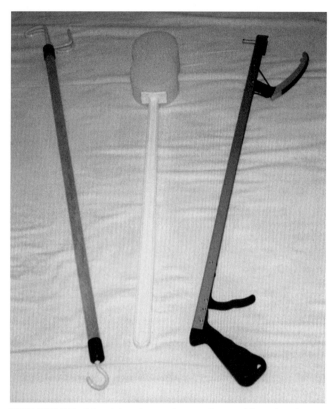

FIGURE 29–15 Adaptive equipment for reaching, dressing, hygiene, and application of topical medicine to control pain.

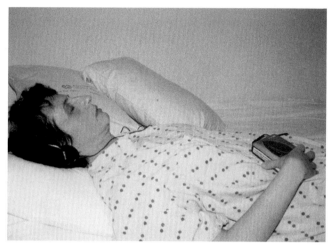

FIGURE 29–17 A relaxation tape to help reduce awareness of pain.

becomes the giver. Keeping a journal, writing a family history or autobiography, and reminiscing are more than diversional activities. Poetry is also a modality. The more a patient can do for himself or herself and the more interest he or she has up until the last moments of life, the better quality of that life and death. Occupational therapy emphasizes the quality of life, the dignity and comfort of the individual, and the need for making choices for hospice patients.[8]

The author, who has also worked in home hospice care, thinks of occupational therapy as the granting of last wishes for home hospice patients. For example, one patient's goal was to travel to New England one last time before she died. She was a paraplegic cancer patient living on the second floor of her home. With the help of the family, an outdoor elevator was installed outside her room so she would be able to access her station wagon for the trip.

CONCLUSION

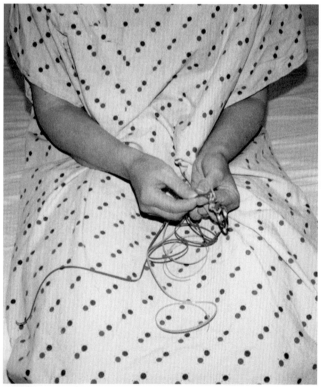

FIGURE 29–16 A patient focuses on diversional activity to help reduce awareness of pain.

Occupational therapy concentrates on the physical and psychological approaches to pain.[11] Pain is a multidimensional experience with sensory as well as cognitive and affective components that are affected by environmental contingencies.[5] Pain is likely to cause distress, and psychological distress can increase a patient's perception of pain.[8] Occupational therapy plays an important role in pain management of the cancer patient, both as part of the pain team and in hospice care. Occupational therapy has helped many cancer patients live each day more comfortably and meaningfully.

REFERENCES

1. Jacox A, Carr DB, Payne R, et al: Management of Cancer Pain. Clinical Practice Guideline No. 9 Alt CPR Publication No. 94-0592. Rockville, MD, Agency for Health Care Policy and Research, U.S. Department of Health and Human Services, Public Health Service, March 1994, p 26.
2. Sist T: A Multidisciplinary Team Approach to Assessment and Management of Pain and Other Symptoms in Head and Neck Cancer Patients. Unpublished, 2000.
3. Sist T: Pain Management Quality Improvement Initiatives. Unpublished, September 2001.
4. Kumiega K: Windows to Cancer Rehabilitation: An Occupational Therapy Treatment Guide. Bisbee, AZ, Imaginart International, 1997, pp 25-27, 37, 38, 40, 41, 61, 65, 78, 84, 85.
5. Cooper J: Celphane Hume: Occupational Therapy in Oncology and Palliative Care. San Diego, CA, Singular Publishing Group, 1997, pp 61-65.
6. American Pain Society: Principles of Analgesic Use in the Treatment of Acute Pain and Cancer Pain, 4th ed. Glenview, IL, 1999, pp 39-43.
7. Kaye P: A-Z of Hospice and Palliative Medicine. Northampton, EPL Publications, 1994.
8. Cromwell FS: Occupational Therapy and the Patient with Pain. New York, Haworth Press, 1984, pp 62-67, 126, 128.
9. Chida S, Shimada Y, Matsunaga T, et al: Occupational Therapy for Accessory Nerve Palsy after Radical Neck Dissection. Tohoku J Exp Med 196:157, 2002.
10. Mehls J: Diversional Occupational Therapy for Cancer Survivors. Regional Cancer Report, March 1983, pp 3, 11.
11. Turk DC, Fernandez E: Pain: A cognitive-behavioral perspective. In Watson M (ed): Cancer Patient Care: Psychosocial Treatment Methods. Leicester, BPS, 1983.

CHAPTER 30

Acupuncture Therapy

M. KAY GARCIA, DrPH, MSN, RN, LAc, AND JOSEPH S. CHIANG, MD

Public interest in complementary and alternative therapies, both for the maintenance of wellness and the treatment of disease, has grown rapidly in the United States in recent years.[1-4] Integrating complementary and alternative therapies proven to be effective into the current mainstream health care system in a well-regulated environment is an important step toward achieving goals set forth by the Department of Health and Human Services in *Healthy People 2010*.[6] Unfortunately, the mechanistic parameters of many such therapies remain unclear, and the need for quality research evaluating integrative clinical practice remains. This chapter discusses complementary, alternative, and integrative medicine with a focus on Traditional Chinese Medicine (TCM) and, more specifically, acupuncture for pain control in cancer patients.

HEALTH CARE POLICY ON COMPLEMENTARY AND ALTERNATIVE MEDICINE

With the arrival of the 21st century, a multibillion-dollar industry in complementary and alternative medicine (CAM) has emerged.[7] Overall estimates of CAM use in the United States range from 28.9% to 42%.[1-5] To maximize the benefit to public health and ensure the quality of care, in 1998, Congress established the National Center for Complementary and Alternative Medicine (NCCAM) at the National Institutes of Health (NIH). The purpose of the NCCAM is to stimulate, develop, and support CAM-related research.[8] Also in 1998, the Office of Cancer Complementary and Alternative Medicine (OCCAM) was established to coordinate and enhance the activities in this arena of the National Cancer Institute (NCI).[9] Finally, in response to public demand for more information and direction, the White House Commission on Complementary and Alternative Medicine Policy was created in March 2000. Among the recommendations made by the commission were: (1) Federal

agencies should receive increased funding for clinical, basic science, and health services research of CAM therapies; (2) The federal government should consider enacting legislative and administrative incentives to stimulate private sector investment in CAM research of products that may not be patentable; (3) Federal, private, and nonprofit sectors should support research of CAM modalities and approaches designed to improve self-care and promote wellness, and; (4) These sectors should support innovative CAM research of core questions posed by new areas of scientific study that might expand understanding of health and disease.[10]

The World Health Organization (WHO) subsequently established specific objectives regarding CAM use that address policy; safety, efficacy and quality; access, and rational use.[11] The challenges of meeting these objectives are many, but considering the global economic and public health impact of CAM, they are challenges that must be addressed. Efforts by the WHO and the U.S. government to establish meaningful health care policies regarding CAM are extremely important for ensuring the safe and appropriate use of these therapies.

Guidelines for Use of Complementary and Alternative Medicine

The American Cancer Society (ACS) has published guidelines to assist patients and physicians in making decisions about CAM use.[12] According to the guidelines, patients should be encouraged to gather as much information about CAM therapies as possible from reputable sources and share that information with their doctor. Patients also should be instructed to bring a list of questions and a complete list of all dietary supplements, including dosage, to follow-up visits, and to promptly report any changes to the list. It is particularly important for physicians to inform patients of the risks involved in delaying or forgoing conventional treatment. Asking informed and appropriate questions can help patients to recognize fraudulent claims and avoid

TABLE 30–1   Questions to Ask About Complementary and Alternative Methods
When evaluating a complementary or alternative treatment, consider the following questions:
What claims are made for the treatment? Does it claim to cure cancer? Does it claim to enable the conventional treatment to work better? Does it claim to relieve symptoms or side effects? What are the credentials of the people or organizations supporting the treatment? Are they recognized experts in cancer treatment? Have their findings been published in trustworthy medical journals? Be skeptical of treatments promoted by people or organizations giving vague credentials such as "expert."
How is the method promoted? Is it promoted only in the mass media (e.g., books, magazines, TV, radio)? Is it mentioned in scientific journals?
What are the costs of the therapy?
Is the method widely available for use within the health care community, or is it controlled with limited access to its use?
Does the method require that you forgo conventional therapy? If so, will doing so affect any chances for cure? Is the cancer stage likely to advance during the delay?
From the American Cancer Society, http://www.cancer.org, with permission.

potential illness or injury. Tables 30-1 and 30-2 provide patients and physicians with a list of questions to ask to ensure that CAM treatments are being provided by a reputable practitioner or group.

In cancer treatment, it is important to distinguish complementary, alternative, and integrative medicine. Many complementary therapies may be used safely as adjuncts to conventional standards of practice. Alternative treatments, on the other hand, imply therapies that are used in place of current accepted medical care.[11] Patients should be warned that alternative approaches in the absence of conventional treatment delay accurate diagnosis and treatment and may be life-threatening. Patients are often reluctant to discuss their use of adjunctive treatments with their physician, yet such a conversation initiated by the physician in an open-minded, non-judgmental way that allows for an exploration of the associated risks and benefits is extremely important to the overall outcome of cancer treatment.[12] As we learn more about nonconventional therapies through research, we may discover that an integrative approach to medicine (i.e., a method that combines conventional diagnostic and treatment methods with nonconventional therapies empirically proven to be effective) enhances patient outcome and improves health care delivery overall.

HISTORY OF ACUPUNCTURE

TCM is a complete system of health care that has been practiced in China for thousands of years. According to the WHO, TCM is used to treat at least 200 million people annually and accounts for nearly 40% of all health care provided in China. The primary disciplines within TCM include acupuncture; herbology; food therapy; Tui na, or Chinese bodywork; Tai chi (therapeutic exercise); and Qi gong (meditative/energy therapy). Acupuncture is among the most popular of these

TABLE 30–2   Spotting Fraudulent or Questionable Therapies
In addition to the questions in Table 30-1, use the following checklist to avoid falling prey to fraudulent or questionable treatment methods. If the safety and validity of the treatment are questionable, discuss it with a doctor or health care provider before trying it.
Is the treatment based on an unproven theory?
Does the treatment promise a cure for all cancers?
Do the promoters say not to use conventional medical treatment?
Is the treatment or drug a secret that only certain people can give?
Is the treatment or drug offered by only one individual?
Does the treatment require travel to another country?
Do the promoters attack the medical or scientific establishment?
From the American Cancer Society, http://www.cancer.org, with permission.

therapies and is used in at least 78 countries worldwide.[11]

In the West, acupuncture therapy has grown substantially more common over the past few decades. In 1971, James Reston, a journalist for the *New York Times*, wrote a front-page article describing how his postoperative pain from an emergency appendectomy was relieved by acupuncture while traveling in Beijing.[13] Three months later, a group of U.S. physicians visiting hospitals in China observed acupuncture for surgical analgesia and reported their observations in the *Journal of the American Medical Association*.[14] Growing public interest ensued, and in 1972, President Richard Nixon, accompanied by his personal physician, witnessed several surgeries using acupuncture-assisted anesthesia.[15] The NIH subsequently sponsored a team of physicians to study the health care system in China, and as a result, several studies attempting to elucidate the underlying mechanisms of action for acupuncture were initiated, textbooks of TCM were translated into English, and training programs were established.[16]

Prior to Nixon's visit to China, little information about acupuncture was available in the United States. There is documented evidence, however, of acupuncture being used in clinical practice as early as 1826, when Franklin Bache, a Philadelphia physician and grandson to Benjamin Franklin, concluded in a published report that he had found acupuncture to be an effective treatment for pain due to rheumatism and neuralgia among prisoners at the Pennsylvania state penitentiary.[17] Sir William Osler also endorsed acupuncture as an effective treatment for lumbago and sciatica in *The Principles and Practice of Medicine*,[18] and interestingly, brief passages on acupuncture appeared in a Civil War surgeon's manual and in two medical treatises written in 1876 and 1880.[19]

In the late 1970s and early 1980s, researchers demonstrated that acupuncture analgesia was associated with the stimulation of endogenous opioid peptides and biogenic amines through the central nervous system,[20-25] and although later work revealed this as an isolated mechanism of action, these findings helped give acupuncture scientific credibility in the minds of medical professionals.[26] As a result, clinical training programs in acupuncture techniques and guidelines for education, practice, and regulation have been developed, and programs in integrative medicine are beginning to appear in medical schools, nursing schools, and hospitals throughout the United States.

THEORY OF ACUPUNCTURE: EAST MEETS WEST

Acupuncturists use many different models and approaches to understand and apply treatment. These models range from a metaphysical paradigm used by those traditionally trained to a strictly neurophysiologic approach incorporated by physicians who use acupuncture exclusively for pain control. Although the former may seem untenable to the Western scientific community, it is useful in treating problems that are not well described by the latter. Acupuncture sometimes has effects on the body that are difficult to explain in purely scientific terms, and a symptom complex that does not easily fit a given set of diagnostic criteria may elucidate a meaningful clinical pattern when analyzed using a different model. In TCM, emphasis is placed on function, not structure. As a result, certain aspects of human physiologic functional relationships are emphasized that are not directly addressed by Western biomedicine. In TCM, it is more important to understand the relationships between variables and the functional "whole" of the patient than it is to identify the specifics of a single pathology. Diagnoses in TCM are made according to manifestations of the root cause, as opposed to the sequelae of illness, as in Western biomedical practice.[27] This contrasts sharply with the Western allopathic medical approach of focusing on an isolatable illness or injury and attempting to change or remove a precise underlying cause.

Eastern Perspective of Traditional Chinese Medicine

Although there are many theoretical foundations underlying the practice of TCM and acupuncture, basic to all approaches is yin-yang theory (Figure 30–1). The constructs within this framework are relatively simple, but yin-yang thinking is substantially different from the classical Aristotelian dogma underlying Western medicine.

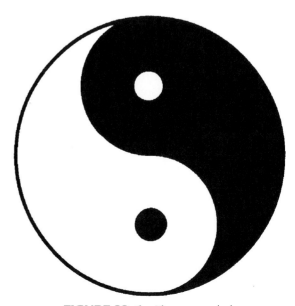

FIGURE 30–1 Yin-yang symbol.

Within yin-yang conceptualization, qualities may be simultaneously opposite and complementary. Yin always possesses characteristics of yang and vice versa. So while being opposites, yin and yang are also interdependent, can transform into each other, and can consume each other. Physiology and pathology represent variations along a continuum of health and illness. Thus, a state of good health is determined by the dynamic balance between opposing yin-yang forces.[28]

In TCM, acupuncture is based on the premise that there are well-defined patterns of Qi (pronounced *chee*) flow throughout the body. The concept of Qi has been discussed by Chinese philosophers throughout time, and the symbol representing Qi in the Chinese language indicates something that is simultaneously material and immaterial. Some authors define Qi as matter + energy or "mattery," thus expressing the same continuum of matter and energy explained by modern particle physics.[28]

In ancient Chinese thought, Qi was believed to be a fundamental and vital substance of the universe, with all phenomena being produced by its changes. There are many types of Qi classified according to source, function, and distribution. It is considered one of the human body's fundamental substances, helping to maintain normal activities, permeating all parts of the body, and flowing along organized pathways known as acupuncture channels, or meridians. TCM practitioners believe that a balanced flow of Qi throughout the system is required for good health, and imbalances can be corrected by acupuncture stimulation.[27,28]

It is also important to recognize that the Blood of Chinese medicine has broader characteristics and functions than blood in Western medicine. In TCM, Blood is a yin substance and is a dense and material form of Qi. It circulates continuously throughout meridian pathways as well as through blood vessels, although the former carries relatively more Qi while the latter carries relatively more Blood. The primary functions of Blood are to nourish, maintain, and moisten various parts of the body and to provide the material foundation for mental, emotional, and spiritual activities. Qi and Blood are inseparable, and without Qi, Blood would be an inert fluid.[27,28]

Western Perspective on Mechanisms of Action

Since the late 1950s, numerous studies have been published in China hypothesizing the underlying mechanisms of action for acupuncture, and by the mid-1990s, compelling evidence describing a neurohumoral model for acupuncture analgesia could be found in the English literature. More recently, basic scientific research has revealed that bioelectromagnetic, as well as neurohumoral, mechanisms are responsible for the effects of acupuncture on various types of health problems. The stimulation of acupuncture points is believed to cause biochemical changes that affect the body's natural healing abilities. The primary mechanisms of these changes include enhanced conduction of bioelectromagnetic signals, activation of opioid systems, and activation of the autonomic and central nervous systems causing the release of various neurotransmitters and neurohormones.[26]

ACUPUNCTURE POINTS

Many studies have described acupuncture point morphology,[29-44] relating the so-called "acupoints" to areas on the skin surface with decreased electrical resistance and increased conductance. Most acupoints are palpable as a surface depression located along the cleavage between muscles. They generally correspond to peripheral, cranial, and spinal nerve endings and are often hypersensitive. According to Bossy, they have a surface area of 1 to 5 mm^2.[30]

In 1979, Senelar used statistical evaluation of a large number of histologic sections from rabbits, cats, mice, and human cadavers to describe acupoint morphology as a lymphatic trunk coupled to a large arteriole accompanied by a satellite vein. This lymph–arteriole–venous system creates a passageway between the skin and deeper tissue and is located in a vertical column of loose connective tissue surrounded by the thick, dense connective tissue of skin.[31] This sleeve of connective tissue, through which neurovascular, lymphatic, and tendinomuscular structures pass enhances the conduction of bioelectric energy.[32] Approximately 80% of traditional acupuncture points have this morphologic organization,[33] which may partially explain the effects of acupuncture in soft tissue disease.

In the 1980s, observations from both conventional light microscopy and electron microscopy confirmed a high concentration of microvesicles and perineural cells situated at the contact zones of sympathetic nerve terminations at the walls of large vessels.[33] Other studies in the 1980s described these thin-walled vascular structures as sinuous, organized in a series of closed loops, and surrounded by a web of unmyelinated cholinergic nerve fibers from the autonomic nervous system. Nerves are located proximal to the vasculature, with additional myelinated nerves woven among the blood and lymph vessels leading to superficial levels of the dermis. The epidermis thins at the acupuncture point and has a corresponding modification of collagen fibers.[34]

Acupuncture points can be categorized in various ways.[32,35] One approach separates points according to their relationship with known neural and tendinomuscular structures. For example, Type I acupoints correspond to motor points located where a nerve enters muscle.

Maximal muscle contraction with minimal electrical stimulation is achieved at these points. Type II points are located on superficial nerves in the sagittal plane at dorsal and ventral midlines. Type III points are located in areas with a high density of superficial nerves and nerve plexi, and Type IV points are found where tendons join muscles.

Several studies have investigated the correlation between acupuncture points, motor points, and trigger points. In 1977, one group of researchers reported a 71% correlation between trigger points and acupuncture points.[45] Trigger points are hypersensitive regions in muscle tissue that can be palpated as taut bands. They are similar to acupuncture points in that they may lie within areas where referred pain is experienced or be located some distance away. The increased sensitivity of acupuncture points is not fully understood; however, hyperalgesia may arise spontaneously from local irritation or from excitation of somatic or visceral structures distant from the painful point. Stimulation of trigger points can provide long-lasting analgesia similar to that achieved through acupuncture. The high correlation between acupuncture points used to treat pain and myofascial trigger points suggests similar underlying mechanisms for analgesia.[32]

With greater pain intensity, both the number of sensitive acupuncture points and the diameter of the sensitive area increase. Points become tender in a predictably progressive order, and the tenderness disappears in reverse order as healing occurs.[46] Mann describes the general mechanism by which diseased organs are able to refer pain, sensitivity, or muscle contraction to acupuncture or trigger points as a viscerocutaneous reflex and states the pathways of referred pain appear to follow autonomic and sensorimotor, myotomal, and dermatomal distributions for each spinal segment. Acupuncture may cause excitation of a cutaneovisceral reflex, allowing stimulation of a point on the skin to influence the neurologic excitation of corresponding organs.[47] The characteristics of acupuncture point morphology and related tissues allow for the transmission and integration of bioelectromagnetic and neurohumoral information between systems.[32]

CHANNELS AND COLLATERALS

According to TCM theory, specific pathways known as meridians or channels carry Qi and Blood throughout the body. These pathways differ from neurovascular systems as defined by modern anatomy and physiology and comprise an infinite network linking all fundamental substances and organs. There are 12 regular channels and 8 extra channels, each with divergent branches and numerous divisions known as collaterals.

Channel/meridian theory assumes that blockage or disorder within the system can be identified using a systematic method of differential diagnosis and that treatment strategies can be developed based on restoring orderly flow.[27]

Several attempts have been made to explain acupuncture channels in modern scientific terms, and most, but not all, channels follow the pathways of major nerves, vessels, and fascial cleavage planes.[26] During acupuncture treatment, patients frequently describe a sensation of numbness, aching, heaviness, or warmth along the channel pathway.[48] Many TCM clinicians consider this phenomenon, sometimes called De Qi sensation, to be essential for effective therapy and suggest it carries the therapeutic signal to the target area.[26,27,49] After needling a point on the stomach channel in one study, fluoroscopic imaging revealed peristalsis was different among patients who experienced De Qi compared with those who did not. Furthermore, gastrographs registered decreased frequency and increased amplitude in gastric contractions when the sensation was felt in the abdominal area.[50] Some studies have shown surgical analgesia is also more effective when De Qi is felt.[51]

De Qi sensation has been shown to travel along channel pathways at 1 to 10 cm/s. This rate varies depending on the subject and the type of needle stimulation but is considerably slower than visceral or somatic nerve conduction.[52,53] De Qi appears to be primarily a peripheral phenomenon, as it can be blocked by chilling, local anesthetic, and mechanical pressure.[54,55] Some investigators, however, have stated that it can travel to phantom limbs, implying participation by the central nervous system.[56]

Darras and colleagues attempted to identify the network of acupuncture channels and collaterals by comparing the trajectory of a radioactive tracer, technetium-99, injected into real acupuncture points with the trajectory of the tracer injected into sham points. The tracer was observed with a scintillation camera and revealed that diffusion patterns from the real acupuncture points corresponded to classically described channels, whereas a centrifugal diffusion pattern without linearity was observed at the sham points. Furthermore, radioisotope diffusion moved beyond a tourniquet that blocked surface peripheral blood circulation. Tracer injected into lymphatic vessels showed they also were distinct from acupuncture channels. Because the migration rate of the tracer did not correspond to vascular or lymphatic circulation rates, the authors concluded that diffusion did not appear to be via either the vascular or lymphatic system.[57]

Mussat evaluated the electrical propagation along traditionally defined acupuncture pathways. He concluded acupuncture channels carry a measurable charge, due to lower resistance and increased conductance, that is relatively independent from surrounding tissue and propagation of an electrical current between acupuncture points follows the organization of classical channel theory. He demonstrated that: (1) placing a barrier needle between needles placed at two points along the same channel can increase the resistance of the channel; (2) electrical current introduced into a channel on the upper extremity can be captured in its corresponding channel on the lower extremity; and (3) current introduced into one channel can be captured in the internally–externally related channel, according to TCM theory, of the same extremity after a 5-minute latent period.[58]

BIOELECTROMAGNETIC PROPERTIES OF POINTS AND CHANNELS

Ancient Chinese scholars were unable to identify electro-ionic migration patterns or discuss electron flow between needles. They were, however, able to recognize patterns and qualities of response and subjectively quantify the distribution and actions of a phenomenon they referred to as Qi. Although no single discipline can definably illustrate the presence or absence of acupuncture channels and collaterals according to classical theory, combined evidence from many different approaches can provide a basic scientific explanation for ancient Chinese conceptualizations.

In brief, the mechanical act of needling an acupuncture point stimulates a bioelectric response initiating polarization and ionizing tissues along preferential pathways, in part because of the piezoelectrical characteristics of collagen (i.e., the property of a material that results in polarization when subjected to mechanical strain and a change in conformation when subjected to an electric field).[59] Adding an electrical stimulus (i.e., electroacupuncture) causes further morphologic changes and alterations in the alignment of collagen fibers.[32] Increased conductance along the meridian system is further supported by a high density of gap junctions at the epithelia of acupuncture points. Gap junctions facilitate intercellular communication and increase electric conductivity through hexagonal protein complexes that form channels between adjacent cells. In both cell culture and animal tests, gap junction genes have been shown to behave as classical tumor suppressor genes that help restore growth regulatory properties to metastatic cancer cells.[60-62]

The exploration of bioelectromagnetic phenomena in living systems is an emerging area of study, and speculative theories have been proposed regarding the manipulation of the body's endogenous electromagnetic fields through acupuncture. As research in this area continues, a more comprehensive and dynamic explanation of the effects of acupuncture on physiologic functional relationships will become apparent.

NEUROHUMORAL MECHANISMS OF ACUPUNCTURE

Awareness that acupuncture analgesia was at least partially mediated through endogenous opioids was first demonstrated in 1976. Shortly after opiate receptors were discovered in the periaqueductal gray, the limbic system, and the periventricular gray matter of the central nervous system (CNS), it was discovered that acupuncture analgesia could be reversed by naloxone, a pure antagonist at all known opioid receptors.[63] Acupuncture can change concentrations of serotonin and biogenic amines, including opioid peptides, met-enkephalin, leu-enkephalin, β-endorphin, and dynorphin. These are involved in the activation of descending tracts that inhibit transmission of nociceptive information in the spinal cord and also inhibit ascending tracts transmitting nociceptive information. When large, unmyelinated A-d fibers that sense touch and pressure are stimulated with an acupuncture needle, impulses from small, unmyelinated C-fibers transmitting ascending nociceptive information are blocked by a gate of inhibitory interneurons in the substantia gelatinosa of the spinal cord, releasing neurotransmitters such as γ-aminobutyric acid and enkephalins and resulting in the inhibition of transmission of pain impulses to the brain. There is also a regional effect, because A-d fibers transmit cranially and caudally in the dorsolateral funiculus before entering the substantia gelatinosa to stimulate inhibitory interneurons.[32,64,65]

Functional magnetic resonance imaging (fMRI) studies suggest stimulation of acupuncture points can initiate multiple endogenous pathways of analgesia by the neuromodulation and integration of neurotransmitter and pain control systems at various levels. The release of serotonin, endogenous opioids, and other neurotransmitters leads to an alteration of nociceptive processing and perception, and quantifiable changes in specific areas of the human brain have been observed with fMRI following acupuncture. In patients who experienced De Qi sensation, unilateral needling has been shown to activate structures of the descending antinociceptive pathways and cause deactivation of multiple limbic areas subserving pain perception (i.e., activation of the hypothalamus and nucleus accumbens and deactivation of the rostral part of the anterior cingulated cortex, amygdala formation, and hippocampal complex). Superficial tactile stimulation caused a signal increase in the somatosensory cortex but did not cause signal decreases in deeper structures as was observed with true acupuncture. When combined with fMRI studies in which brain function is localized, observations suggest that stimulation of specific points can initiate multiple endogenous pathways of analgesia through neuromodulation and integration of neurotransmitter and pain control systems at various levels of the CNS.[32,66]

Acupuncture points have also been found to have a higher temperature and a higher metabolic rate, and to release more carbon dioxide than surrounding tissues.[67,68] Needle stimulation at an acupuncture point causes erythema and heat to develop, and patients often report a feeling of warmth at the site. Furthermore, unilateral stimulation can cause cutaneous skin temperatures to rise bilaterally. Local vasodilation, decreased sympathetic tone, and increased cholinergic efferent impulses may all contribute to this effect and may play an important role in relieving chronic pain.[69] Vasodilation is also mediated by the physical irritation of the needle and stimulates the release of histamine and other vasodilators.

Although acupuncture has been most widely recognized for pain control, stimulation of certain points can also affect the viscera and immune system, partially through the multifaceted role of opioids. Acupuncture promotes neuroendocrine modulation of the hypothalamus–pituitary axis, which interacts with the immune system to modulate cellular function.[32,70-74] Because opioid receptors are found on neurons and lymphocytes, they provide communication between the CNS and the immune system.

Morphogenetic Singularity Theory

A speculative but compelling theory regarding acupuncture involves developmental biology and suggests the meridian system is related to the bioelectric field in morphogenesis and growth control. According to the Morphogenetic Singularity Theory, acupoints originate from organizing centers in morphogenesis, and channel distribution is not solely determined by nerves, muscles, or blood vessels but is the result of the morphogenesis of both internal and external structures. Although compatible with neurohumoral constructs, this theory explains several long-standing puzzles that the neurohumoral model cannot. For example, the theory helps explain indications for specific acupoints and meridians, such as the Du channel (also called governing vessel), whose distributions do not follow any major nerve, lymphatic, or blood vessels.[75]

ACUPUNCTURE RESEARCH IN CANCER CARE

Since use of CAM therapies has skyrocketed in the United States in recent years, research designed to explore the integration of conventional health care with these therapies is greatly needed. The strongest evidence thus far for the efficacy of acupuncture has been demonstrated in the areas of nausea, vomiting, and pain control.

A review of the literature reveals acupuncture is superior to placebo and various other controls for nausea associated with pregnancy, surgery, and chemotherapy. Meta-analysis has further revealed acupuncture's efficacy is similar to that of antiemetic drugs in preventing early postoperative nausea and vomiting.[76,77]

A randomized, blinded, controlled trial conducted in France investigated the use of auricular acupuncture for cancer pain. Ninety patients were randomly divided into three groups: one group received two courses of auricular acupuncture; one received acupuncture at placebo auricular points; and one group received auricular seeds at placebo points. Efficacy was based on a decrease in pain intensity 2 months after randomization using a visual analog scale (VAS). At 2 months, pain intensity decreased by 36% from baseline among the treatment group versus 2% among patients in the two placebo groups ($P < 0.0001$).[78] A nonrandomized preliminary study of 20 subjects conducted by the same authors had also revealed a significant decrease in pain intensity after receiving auricular acupuncture. All patients had a chronic pain syndrome related to their cancer diagnosis. The authors further reported that improvement was not limited to a reduction in pain. Some patients stated that they felt better in general and wanted to interrupt analgesic treatment.[79]

In 1999, a German study reported positive findings for the use of acupuncture to treat pain in breast cancer patients. Forty-eight patients (group I) who received acupuncture after ablation and axillary lymphadenectomy were compared with 32 patients (group II) who had the same surgical procedure but no acupuncture. Group I showed greater improvement in terms of the maximum abduction angle reached without pain and the maximum tolerable pain barrier after the first treatment, on postoperative days 5 and 7, and at the time of discharge ($P < 0.001$ in each situation). Pain in the operative field at rest was significantly lower in the treatment group on day 5 ($P < 0.01$) but not on day 7 or at discharge ($P > 0.05$). Pain during arm movements was significantly less in the treatment group on days 5 and 7 ($P < 0.01$) and at discharge ($P < 0.001$). The authors concluded that acupuncture was effective in this study population for reducing pain and improving arm mobility.[80]

Another randomized clinical trial conducted in China studied pain control in patients with stomach cancer. The results showed similar outcomes in the acupuncture and Western medicine groups at 2 months. According to the authors, long-term outcome measures were superior for the acupuncture group.[81]

A pilot study from Sweden investigated the use of acupuncture for treating vasomotor symptoms in seven men with prostate cancer. Treatment was provided twice weekly for 2 weeks and then once a week for 10 weeks.

Of the six subjects who completed the full course of therapy, all had a substantial decrease (70%) in the number of hot flushes. At 3 months after treatment, the number of hot flushes was still 50% lower than before therapy. Although this was a nonrandomized pilot study, the results merit further evaluation.[82]

Another pilot study of 20 subjects evaluated acupuncture for the relief of cancer-related breathlessness. Outcome measures included pulse rate, respiratory rate, oxygen saturation level, and patient-rated VAS scores for breathlessness, pain, anxiety, and relaxation. Seventy percent of patients reported a substantial benefit from acupuncture treatment. VAS scores for breathlessness, relaxation, and anxiety were significantly improved up to 6 hours after acupuncture treatment ($P < 0.005$, $P < 0.001$, respectively). There was also a significant reduction in respiratory rate ($P < 0.02$), which was sustained for 90 minutes after acupuncture. Again, these results warrant further investigation of acupuncture for the management of breathlessness.[83]

Several studies have explored placebo effects related to acupuncture therapy, and researchers have questioned why the public has turned to therapies that have been less rigorously tested than conventional treatments. Psychosocial issues may be a major reason.[84] One study designed to determine whether acupuncture treatment outcomes are associated with a patient's degree of general hopefulness, expectations regarding treatment, attributions of health status, and beliefs about mind-body dualism and patient–provider relationship factors revealed the following: (1) most patients achieved their goals with acupuncture treatment; (2) higher patient expectations led to less favorable outcomes; (3) outcome was not due to the placebo effect; (4) patients who received a greater number of different types of CAM therapies had better outcomes, and (5) patients who assigned more control to the health care provider had less favorable outcomes. The negative correlation between positive expectations from acupuncture and goal attainment led the author to conclude that perceived positive outcomes were not due to the placebo effect because if they were, the more patients expected from acupuncture, the more, not less, positive their outcomes would have been.[85]

Although acupuncture has been used to treat a wide range of problems from fatigue to specific diseases, in cancer treatment, its use is often limited to palliative care and the relief of symptoms such as nausea, vomiting, insomnia, fatigue, anxiety/depression, pain, and various gastrointestinal or genitourinary complaints.[12] Although most studies investigating the use of acupuncture in cancer patients have been conducted outside the United States, one descriptive study regarding the integration of acupuncture services into an oncology clinic in San Diego reported a 30% improvement among 60% of the patients referred (89 patients with 444 total visits) over a 4-month period. No untoward effects were recorded. The most common reasons for referral included pain (53%), xerostomia (32%), hot flashes (6%), and nausea/loss of appetite (6%). In a follow-up survey, irrespective of response to therapy, 86% of respondents considered it "very important" to continue providing acupuncture services.[86] Additional cancer-related projects are under way or are being developed to evaluate the use of acupuncture for the prevention of postoperative paralytic ileus, the treatment of radiation-induced xerostomia, chemotherapy-induced hot flashes, peripheral neuropathies, impotence, urinary incontinence, and wound healing.[87]

Issues in Acupuncture Research

Identifying research methodologies that are scientifically sound yet sensitive to the TCM paradigm is difficult. Often, we find ourselves guilty of comparing the proverbial apples with oranges, and in many instances, it may be inappropriate to apply an Eastern treatment to a Western diagnosis without first understanding the relationships between Eastern and Western diagnoses. The subset of signs and symptoms deemed clinically relevant often differs between Eastern and Western perspectives even though the patient may have a single chief complaint. For example, in TCM, the prescribed treatment for someone with a migraine headache varies from one patient to another. Thus, a research protocol designed to study migraine headaches must give consideration to the process of TCM differential diagnosis and cannot be based simply on the Western diagnosis of "migraine headache." While the scientific community is unwilling to accept the outcome of studies that are not well designed, TCM practitioners are just as unwilling to accept the outcome of studies that ignore current standards of clinical practice.[88] Although the fact that TCM has been used as a primary source of health care by millions of people for thousands of years provides some degree of pragmatic validity, if it is to be integrated into a Western model of health care, the two systems must merge so that the strengths of one overcome the weaknesses of the other.

Designing and conducting valid and reliable acupuncture research presents many challenges. Because standard TCM clinical practice calls for individualized treatment, studies from which meaningful results can be drawn have been relatively few. Misleading conclusions, either false negative or false positive, occur for a variety of reasons including inadequate treatment regimens as well as inappropriate controls. Determining an adequate study design and optimal treatment plan is extremely complex, and a number of factors must be considered beyond symptomatology and patient characteristics.

For example, the specific points selected and number of points used, type of needle, depth of needle insertion, method of stimulation, duration of treatment, and number and frequency of sessions may all affect outcome. Seemingly, the art and science of practice are both important aspects of care, but this poses many problems from a researcher's perspective. Although the specific question under study determines the choice of controls, the use of sham points or the use of penetrating sham procedures and nonpenetrating methods such as mock transcutaneous electrical nerve stimulation (TENS) or inactivated laser to either real or sham point locations and blinding of patients, assessors, investigators, analysts, acupuncturists, and other participants are all important considerations for ensuring the accuracy of findings. Recommendations for optimizing treatment and controls have been developed,[89] but debate in this area continues.

TYPES OF TREATMENT

Electroacupuncture and Acupuncture Analgesia

The most common technique for acupoint stimulation involves the penetration of the skin by thin, solid, metallic needles stimulated either manually or electrically. In the United States, the manufacture and use of acupuncture needles is regulated by the Food and Drug Administration (FDA), and compliance with Good Manufacturing Practices and single-use standards of sterility are required. Guidelines and standards for the clean and safe clinical practice of acupuncture have been established by the National Acupuncture Foundation. This nationally accepted protocol reflects Occupational Safety and Health Administration (OSHA) requirements, and successful completion of a certification examination in clean-needle technique is required by most states before licensure to practice is granted.[90]

Electroacupuncture involves the passage of electrical energy through acupuncture points by attaching battery-operated electronic devices to the needles. This technique allows for more accurate and uniformly regulated stimulation than can be achieved using manual stimulation of the needles alone.[91] According to Han, specific frequencies of electrical stimulation induce the gene expression of specific neuropeptides in the central nervous system. A frequency of 2 Hz induces the gene expression of endorphins in the diencephalons, which act on anxiolytic mu receptors. A frequency of 2 to 15 Hz causes the release of β-endorphin and met-enkephalin in the brain and dynorphin in the spinal cord and is more effective in relieving deep and chronic pain than is higher-frequency stimulation (100 Hz), which causes the release

of dynorphin alone. In the periaqueductal gray matter, the effects of acupuncture may be predominantly mediated by the enkephalins and β-endorphin. In the spinal cord, effects are predominantly due to enkephalins and dynorphin.[92-95] A synergistic effect from these three types of opioids is likely to occur in response to simultaneous stimulation from acupuncture as they bind to their respective receptors.[32] Although some authors state the frequency of stimulation may be of greater importance than classical rules for needle placement,[95] pain relief achieved through acupuncture treatment cannot be explained by this mechanism alone because the analgesic effect is much longer than the half-life of endorphins.

Auricular Acupuncture

Auricular acupuncture is a commonly practiced technique involving the stimulation of specific points on the ear. Although it has long been used in China for a variety of conditions, auricular diagnosis and treatment has become a unique branch of TCM throughout other parts of the world since the late 1980s. When internal disorders occur, changes such as tenderness, decreased cutaneous electrical resistance, morphologic changes, or discoloration may appear at specific ear points.[96]

In classical TCM literature, there are many references to stimulating specific points on the ear with needles, moxibustion, and massage to both prevent and treat disease. Ancient Chinese clinicians classified and recorded information about the ear on silk scrolls discovered in the excavation of the No. 3 Han Tomb at Mawangdui, Changsha City in 1973. Two of these scrolls, titled *Moxibustion Classic with Eleven Yin-Yang Channels*, discuss the "ear meridian." Other descriptions of auricular acupuncture appear in the earliest existing classic of TCM, the *Huang Di Nei Jing*.[97] Citations of treatments using points on the ear are also found in Egyptian tomb paintings and in ancient Persian medical references.[98]

In France in the early 1950s, Paul Nogier systematically mapped the auricular/body correspondences. His teachings spread from France to Germany, Japan, and finally to China, where his charts were screened, verified, and refined in clinical practice.[99-101] In 1960, Xu Zuolin, a physician at the Beijing Pingan hospital, published a paper summarizing the application of auricular therapy for 255 cases, and in 1970, the *Hanging Wall Chart of Acupoints*, published by the Peoples' Liberation Army (PLA) hospital in Gang Zhou, illustrated 107 auricular acupoints. Since that time, the number used in clinical practice has expanded to include points on both anterior and posterior portions of the ear.[97]

More recently, authors have discussed auriculotherapy as a reflex somatotropic microsystem.[102] Many such systems have been described in the human body and range from the very simple to quite complex. In TCM, three primary somatotropic microsystems involve the tongue, radial pulse, and ear. The first two are used for diagnostic purposes only. Theorists have speculated that reflex somatotropic systems behave as bioholographic phenomena, with each cell containing information about the whole organism. This view reflects ancient Chinese beliefs that man is a microcosm expressing harmony of a natural order within the overall universe.[27]

In his text, *Acupuncture Energetics: A Clinical Approach for Physicians*, Helms states afferent excitation arriving at a modulating center in the brain may trigger efferent impulses that change the sensitivity of the skin on surface reflex zones. This may involve the reticular formation in the brainstem, which functions as a modulating intersection activating and inhibiting cranial, spinal, somatic, visceral, and autonomic neurologic impulses. This reticular unit may respond to input by patterning topographic regions of the body and subsequently activating the thalamic reticular formation involved in pain modulation, influencing somatic motor and sensory functions, and regulating viscera through the autonomic nervous system.[26]

Scalp Acupuncture

Although ancient Chinese clinicians needled acupuncture points on the scalp, Jiao Shunfa first described treatment of various diseases using a systematic approach to scalp acupuncture in the early 1970s.[103] Like auriculotherapy, scalp acupuncture is considered to be a microreflex system that involves needling areas directly above corresponding nerve centers.[26] It has been used to treat problems such as chronic headaches, facial paralysis, cerebrovascular disease, enuresis, vertigo, cerebral palsy, and epilepsy.[103] To date, few controlled studies evaluating the use of scalp acupuncture have been conducted in the United States.

CONCOMITANT THERAPIES

In China and many parts of the world, other therapies are used as adjuncts to acupuncture. These include moxibustion; cupping; gua sha, or scraping; Tui na; Qi gong; Tai chi; and herbal and food therapy. The same diagnostic paradigm and treatment strategies used for acupuncture are used to develop a treatment plan utilizing these techniques.

Moxibustion

Moxibustion (moxa) is an ancient technique that uses heat from burning preparations of the herb *Artemisia vulgaris* (mugwort) to stimulate the circulation of Qi and Blood. Ancient clinicians believed moxa was effective in treating a variety of disorders and regular use could prevent illness. Today, many TCM practitioners use moxa in an effort to strengthen the immune system.[96]

Moxa can be applied using a variety of direct and indirect methods. Direct moxa was used in ancient times and is still used in some cultures today. It involves placing a moxa cone directly on the skin at specified acupuncture points and allowing it to burn to completion. Blistering and scarring occur at the site. A nonscarring method is also used in which the moxa cone is removed and replaced with a new one before burning to completion. With indirect moxa, the cone is insulated from the skin with slices of ginger, garlic, or salt. The type of insulating material chosen depends on the specific indication. With indirect moxa, the cones may also be placed directly on the acupuncture needles. Finally, the indirect method may be applied using a cigar-like stick of tightly rolled moxa held near the skin at acupuncture sites. The patient is instructed to indicate when he or she feels warmth, and individual acupoints may be heated or groups of points warmed in succession along the channel being treated to stimulate Qi and Blood flow.[96] Indirect moxa is most often used to treat chronic conditions. Although a few recent studies from China and Japan have evaluated the effects of moxa on the immune system, with one reporting moxa smoke induces cytotoxicity by its pro-oxidant action,[104-107] its use for cancer pain has not been systematically evaluated. Furthermore, fire safety concerns and the potential for allergic reactions limit its usefulness as an adjunctive treatment modality.

Cupping and Scraping (Gua Sha)

Another treatment often combined with acupuncture therapy is cupping. In this technique, the inside of a small jar or cup is heated to create negative pressure. The cup is then attached to the surface of the skin using the vacuum created by the heat. In ancient times, bamboo jars were used; today, glass or plastic cups are most common. The cups may be left in place for 5 to 10 minutes or may be continuously applied and removed along the meridian pathway. Experienced clinicians may also be able to carefully slide the cup along the chosen meridian. The cups are removed by placing a finger at its edge on the skin to release the vacuum. After removal, the area is massaged lightly for patient comfort and to further stimulate Qi and Blood flow. The suction from the cups may leave a painless mark on the skin,[96] and informed consent should be obtained prior to using this adjunctive therapy. Although it has not been evaluated specifically for cancer pain, cupping is frequently combined with acupuncture to treat various pain syndromes, including myofascial pain and fibromyalgia.[26,96]

Another therapeutic approach used by TCM clinicians is scraping or gua sha. In gua sha, some form of oil or lubricant is placed on the skin followed by scraping with a smooth-edged instrument such as a coin or porcelain spoon. Again, this is done to stimulate circulation to specific areas and is used to treat chronic pain. The procedure is somewhat uncomfortable, and a mark or bruise is left on the skin surface for 3 to 5 days. There have been reports in the literature of marks left from this procedure being mistaken for abuse. Physicians should be aware that it is a common practice in Asian culture and can be recognized by the pattern of the mark. Although there are no published randomized trials evaluating the use of gua sha for pain, there is considerable anecdotal evidence that it mobilizes stagnant blood and body fluid thereby relieving pain.[26] This procedure has not been evaluated and may not be appropriate for cancer-related pain. It should not be used in areas where tissue is fragile or near skin lesions of any type.

Tui Na

Tui na (Chinese bodywork) is based on the theory of meridians and collaterals and is a special form of massage that uses techniques specific to Chinese medicine. It involves stimulation of areas along specific pathways and is considered a major area of specialty within TCM.[108] In the United States, examination and certification in Chinese bodywork are provided through the National Certification Commission for Acupuncture and Oriental Medicine. To be eligible for the national board examination, applicants must demonstrate the successful completion of an educational program or apprenticeship documenting at least 500 contact hours. A significant portion of those hours must be dedicated to direct patient care.[109]

Qi Gong and Tai Chi

Qi gong is a form of mental and physical exercise that has been practiced in China for thousands of years.[110] It is mentioned in ancient Chinese books such as the *I Ching* (Book of Changes) and the *Huang Di Nei Jing* (Yellow Emperor's Classic of Internal Medicine). The *I Ching* was written in 2852 BCE by Fu Xi. The *Huang Di Nei Jing* was written around 2697–2597 BCE. Its authorship is attributed to the great Huang Di (Yellow Emperor) who ruled during the middle of the third millennium BCE and who symbolizes the vital spirit of Chinese civilization.[111,112] The book provides the accumulated knowledge of many generations underlying the philosophy and foundation of acupuncture, Qi gong, and Tai chi and is used in colleges and universities of TCM even today.

Although there are different schools of Qi gong, in general, the practice involves meditation, special breathing techniques, and physical exercises that can be either static or dynamic. Buddhist and Taoist monks practice many ancient Qi gong techniques, and masters believe the practice enables them to accumulate, store, and consume energy in a controlled manner, strengthens their resistance to illness and injury, and can be used as an aid in healing others.[111,112] Studies have shown that breathing exercises, such as those used in Qi gong, may be effective for treating breathlessness in lung cancer patients.[113,114] Although the underlying mechanisms of Qi gong are not well understood, it partially blocks sympathetic activity, and in cancer patients, it may be effective in treating certain types of sympathetic-related chronic pain syndromes caused either by disease or cancer treatment.

Tai chi, a form of Qi gong, was originally developed by Chang San Feng in the 13th century. Involving slow, controlled movements coordinated with special breathing techniques, Tai chi is based on a defensive form of martial arts. The original form of Tai chi included 12 movement sequences known as the 12 Chi Disruption Forms. It later evolved into the Wu Dang Mountain Tai chi style. During the 19th century, it was further developed by Yang Lu Chan and became known as The Old Yang Style of Tai chi. Today, many forms of Tai chi are practiced in China,[112,115] and practitioners believe it is an effective form of exercise to promote Qi and Blood flow, maintain balance, and promote longevity.

Herbal and Food Therapy

TCM practitioners often combine acupuncture with the use of herbal or food therapy. It is not the purpose of this chapter to discuss the topic of herbs or therapeutic dietary guidelines, but the same diagnostic paradigm and treatment strategies used in acupuncture therapy are used to select herbal supplements and foods intended to correct imbalances that cause illness.

In TCM, single herbs are rarely given. Rather, formulas containing many plant, mineral, or animal substances are given in pill, tincture, powder, or loose herb form. Loose herbs are decocted into teas and taken in divided doses over a 24-hour period.[116] Because of the vast interest in and use of herbal supplements by the public and especially by cancer patients, it is important that research to explore herb–drug interactions be conducted and that physicians familiarize themselves with this growing area. Because patients are often reluctant to discuss the use of herbal supplements with their doctor, asking questions in an open-ended, nonjudgmental way during history taking is imperative.[12]

ADVERSE EFFECTS OF ACUPUNCTURE

Several publications have investigated the safety of acupuncture treatment.[117-121] One prospective survey following 34,000 consultations with professional acupuncturists (members of the British Acupuncture Council) reported no serious adverse events; serious adverse events were defined as requiring hospital admission, prolonging hospital stays, permanently disabling, or resulting in death (95% CI: 0 to 1.1 per 10,000 treatments). Only 43 significant minor adverse events were reported (1.3 per 1000 treatments; 95% CI: 0.9 to 1.7), including severe nausea, fainting, aggravation of symptoms, pain, bruising, and psychological and emotional reactions.[117]

Another large-scale project investigated all first-hand case reports of complications and adverse effects of acupuncture identified in the English language between 1965 and 1999. Over the 35-year period, only 202 incidents were identified in reports from 22 countries. Complications from acupuncture included infections (primarily hepatitis) and organ, tissue, and nerve injury. Other minor adverse effects included cutaneous disorders, hypotension, fainting, and vomiting. Fewer adverse events have been reported since 1988 because of improvements in clinical practice, standardization of clean-needle techniques, and better training of practitioners.[118] A multicenter survey conducted in Norway, reported that, like any treatment intervention, acupuncture has adverse effects but is safe when performed according to established guidelines.[119]

When compared with other treatments, acupuncture is considered to be relatively safe. Most serious adverse events occur as a result of improper needle placement secondary to inadequate training of personnel, not using single-use disposable needles, or poor technique when cleaning the area before needling. In other words, most adverse events from acupuncture are due to a lack of education or negligence on the part of the practitioner and are not due to the treatment itself. The side effects reported when acupuncture is performed correctly by properly trained personnel are relatively minor and most commonly include fainting, nausea, vomiting, bruising, and mild pain.[117-120]

Special precautions should be taken when performing acupuncture on cancer patients. First, care should be taken with immune-suppressed patients, and needles should not be placed in the vicinity of the tumor. Second, because acupuncture may mask the symptoms of tumor progression, full knowledge and understanding of the clinical stage of disease and treatment methods is necessary. According to Filshie, an unstable spine, severe clotting disorders, neutropenia, and lymphedema are contraindications for acupuncture. Additionally, semipermanent needles should not be used in patients with valvular heart disease or in vulnerable neutropenic patients.[121] Electroacupuncture should also not be used in patients with cardiac pacemakers.

CREDENTIALING OF ACUPUNCTURE PROVIDERS

Selecting a qualified practitioner is an important decision, and guidelines have been recommended by NIH/NCCAM.[122] Specific requirements for credentialing acupuncturists vary from state to state, but training programs in the United States have a standardized, clinically based curriculum and are formally accredited by the Accreditation Commission for Acupuncture and Oriental Medicine.[123] In addition, a nonprofit organization, the National Certification Commission for Acupuncture and Oriental Medicine (NCCAOM), was established in 1982 to promote nationally recognized standards of competence and safety. The primary mission of NCCAOM is to protect the public interest in quality care by examining and certifying competence in the practice of acupuncture, Chinese herbology, and Asian bodywork (tui na) through national board examinations. The first comprehensive written examination administered by NCCAOM for acupuncture was given in March 1985. In 2004, testing for competency in basic principles of biomedicine was added. Most states now require successful completion of the NCCAOM board examination for licensure to practice acupuncture.[109]

CONCLUSION

With an explosion of interest in CAM therapies in recent years,[1-4] several steps have been taken to ensure the quality of care and safety to public health. Health care policy has been developed in the United States, and the NCCAM was established at the NIH to stimulate, develop, and support CAM-related research.[8] The NCI also established the OCCAM to coordinate and enhance activities specific to CAM as it relates to the prevention, diagnosis, and treatment of cancer.[9] Specific objectives addressing policy; safety, efficacy and quality; access; and rational use have also been set forth in the *WHO Traditional Medicine Strategy 2002–2005*.[11]

The history of acupuncture spans thousands of years, but its popularity in the United States has grown substantially since the early 1970s, following a front-page article published in the *New York Times* by James Reston describing his personal experience with acupuncture during a visit to China.[13] Interest continued to grow after President Richard Nixon's visit in 1972, and since that time, programs in training and research have been developed.[15,16]

Acupuncture practitioners use many different approaches for diagnosing and treating patients, ranging from the purely metaphysical to the strictly neurophysiologic. Although integrating ancient concepts into a health care delivery system relying solely on modern scientific methods is difficult, it is an endeavor worthy of exploration as certain aspects of human physiologic functional relationships are emphasized in TCM that are not directly addressed by Western biomedicine. Thus, integrating therapies that have been demonstrated to be empirically effective, such as acupuncture, into mainstream health care in a well-regulated environment could lead to a dramatic medical paradigm shift, benefiting the general health of the public.[88]

When performing acupuncture on cancer patients, certain precautions should be observed. Care should be taken to avoid placing needles in the vicinity of the tumor, and understanding the clinical stage of disease and treatment regimen is necessary. According to Filshie, specific contraindications in this population include an unstable spine, severe clotting disorders, neutropenia, and lymphedema and semipermanent needles should not be used in vulnerable neutropenic patients or in patients with valvular heart disease.[121] Finally, electroacupuncture should be avoided in patients with a cardiac pacemaker.

Several promising studies are beginning to elucidate the mechanisms and efficacy of acupuncture in a variety of areas related to cancer. As our understanding improves of how this ancient tradition works, our ability to optimize treatment regimens will also improve. As we endeavor to learn more about therapies such as acupuncture, our focus should not be limited to clinical medicine. As a group, cancer patients are frequent users of CAM approaches,[12] and future research should also consider the social, cultural, political, and economic contexts of Traditional Chinese Medicine.

REFERENCES

1. Eisenberg DM, Kessler RC, Foster C, et al: Unconventional medicine in the United States: Prevalence, costs and patterns of use. N Engl J Med 328:246-252, 1993.
2. Eisenberg DM, Davis RB, Ettner SL, et al: Trends in alternative medicine use in the United States, 1990-1997: Results of a follow-up national survey. JAMA 280: 1569-1575, 1998.
3. Astin JA: Why patients use alternative medicine: Results of a national study. JAMA 279:1548-1553, 1998.
4. Ni H, Simile C, Hardy AM: Utilization of complementary and alternative medicine by United States adults: Results from the 1999 national health interview survey. Med Care 40:353-358, 2002.
5. Barnes PM, Powell-Griner E, McFann K, et al: Complementary and alternative medicine use among adults: United States, 2002. Advance Data from Vital and Health Statistics, CDC 343:1-20, 2004.
6. United States Department of Health and Human Services (DHHS): Healthy People 2010. McLean, VA: International Medical Pub, 2000.
7. Bodeker G, Kronenberg F: A public health agenda for traditional, complementary, and alternative medicine. Am J Public Health 92:1582-1591, 2002.
8. National Institutes of Health (NIH). National Center for Complementary and Alternative Medicine (NCCAM) [Online]. http://www.nccam.nih.gov.
9. National Cancer Institute (NCI). Office of Cancer Complementary & Alternative Medicine (OCCAM). [Online]. http://www3.cancer.gov/occam/.
10. White House Commission on Complementary and Alternative Medicine Policy: Final Report. Washington, DC: DHHS, 2002 [Online]. www.whccamp.hhs.gov.
11. World Health Organization: WHO Traditional Medicine Strategy 2002-2005. Geneva, World Health Organization, 2002.
12. American Cancer Society: American Cancer Society's Guide to Complementary and Alternative Cancer Methods. Atlanta, American Cancer Society, 2000.
13. Reston J: Now about my operation in Peking. New York Times, July 26, 1971: pp 1, 6.
14. Dimond EG: Acupuncture anesthesia: Western medicine and Chinese traditional medicine. JAMA 218:1558-1563, 1971.
15. Tkach W: I have seen acupuncture work. Today's Health 50:50-56, 1972. [cited in Helms JM: Acupuncture Energetics: A Clinical Approach for Physicians. Berkeley, CA, Medical Acupuncture Publishers, 1997, p 3].
16. Chen JYP: Medicine and Public Health in the People's Republic of China. J.R. Quinn (ed). U.S. Department of Health, Education and Welfare: National Institutes of Health, John S. Fogarty International Center, 65-90, 1972. [cited in Helms, p 3].
17. Bache F: Cases illustrative of the remedial effects of acupuncture. North American Medical and Surgical Journal 2:311-321, 1826. [cited in Helms, p 5].
18. Osler W: The Principles and Practices of Medicine, 1st ed. New York, Appleton, 1892, pp 282, 820. [cited in Helms, p 4].
19. Warren E: An Epitome of Practical Surgery. Richmond, VA, West and Johnston, 1863, p 228. [cited in Helms, p 4].
20. Mayer DJ, Price DD, Rafii A: Antagonism of acupuncture analgesia in man by the narcotic antagonist naloxone. Brain Res 121:368-372, 1977.
21. Pomeranz B, Cheng R: Suppression of noxious responses in single neurons of cat spinal cord by electroacupuncture and its reversal by the opiate antagonist naloxone. Exp Neurol 64:327-341, 1979.
22. Clement-Jones V, McLoughlin L, Tomlin S, et al: Increased beta-endorphin but not met-enkephalin levels in human cerebrospinal fluid after acupuncture for recurrent pain. Lancet 2: 946-949, 1980.
23. Pert A, Dionne R, Ng L, et al: Alterations in rat central nervous system endorphins following transauricular electroacupuncture. Brain Res 224:83-93, 1981.
24. Han JS, Terenius L: Neurochemical basis of acupuncture analgesia. Annu Rev Pharmacol Toxicol 22:193-220, 1982.
25. Han JS, Xie GX: Dynorphin: Important mediator for electroacupuncture analgesia in the spinal cord of the rabbit. Pain 18:367-376, 1984.
26. Helms JM: Acupuncture Energetics: A Clinical Approach for Physicians. Berkeley, CA, Medical Acupuncture Publishers, 1997.
27. Kaptchuk T: The Web That Has No Weaver: Understanding Chinese Medicine. Chicago, Congdon & Weed, 1983.
28. Maciocia G: The Foundations of Chinese Medicine: A Comprehensive Text for Acupuncturists and Herbalists. New York, Churchill Livingstone, 1998.
29. Huang YC: Anatomy and classification of acupoints. Probl Vet Med 4:12-15, 1992.
30. Bossy J, Sambuc P: Acupuncture et système nerveaux: Les acquis. Acupuncture et Médecine Traditionnelle Chinoise. Paris, Encyclopédie des Médecines Naturelles, IB-1, 1989. [cited in Helms, p 26].
31. Senelar R: Caractéristiques morphologiques des points chinois. In: Niboyet JEH (ed): Nouveau Traité d'Acupuncture. Moulins-lès-Metz: Maisonneuve, 1979, pp 247-277. [Cited in Helms, p 26.]

32. Mittleman E, Gaynor JS: A brief overview of the analgesic and immunologic effects of acupuncture in domestic animals. JAVMA 217:1201–1205, 2000.

33. Senelar R, Auziech O: Histophysiologie du point d'acupuncture. Acupuncture et Médecine Traditionnelle Chinoise. Paris, Encyclopédie des Médecines Naturelles, IB-2C, 1989. [Cited in Helms, p 27.]

34. Auziech O: Étude Histologique des Points Cutanés de Moindre Résistance Électrique et Analyse de Leurs Implications Possibles Dans la Mise en Jeu des Mécanismes Acupuncturaux. Montpellier, Thèse de Médecine, 1984. [Cited in Helms, p 27.]

35. Gunn CC: Type IV acupuncture points. Am J Acupunct 5:51–52, 1977.

36. Dung HC: Anatomical features contributing to the formation of acupuncture points. Am J Acupunct 12:139–143, 1984.

37. Kendall DE: A scientific model for acupuncture: Part I. Am J Acupunct 17:251–268, 1989.

38. Dolson AL: Acupuncture from a pathologist's perspective: Linking physical to energetic. Med Acupunct 10:25–31, 1998.

39. Becker RO, Reichmanis M: Electrophysiologic correlates of acupuncture points and meridians. Psychoenergetic Systems 1:195–212, 1976.

40. Reichmanis M, Marino AA, Becker RO: DC skin conductance variation at acupuncture loci. Am J Chin Med 4:69–72, 1976.

41. Still J: Relationship between electrically active skin points and acupuncture meridian points in the dog. Am J Acupunct 16:55–71, 1988.

42. Niboyet JEH, Mery A: Compte-rendu recherches expérimentales sur les méridiens; chez le vivant et chez le cadavre. Actes des IIIème Journées Internationales d'Acupuncture, 1957, pp 47–51. [Cited in Helms, p 20.]

43. Grall Y: Contribution à l'Étude de la Conductibilité Électrique de la Peau. Algiers: Thèse de Médecine, 1962. [Cited in Helms, p 21.]

44. Human Anatomy Department of Shanghai Medical University: A relationship between points of meridian and peripheral nerves. Acupuncture Anesthetic Theory Study. Shanghai: Shanghai Peoples Publishing House, 1973. [Cited in Helms, p 27.]

45. Melzack R, Stillwell DM, Fox EJ: Trigger points and acupuncture points for pain: Correlations and implications. Pain 3:3–23, 1977.

46. Dung HC: Three principles of acupuncture points. Am J Acupunct 12:263–266, 1984.

47. Mann F: Acupuncture: The Ancient Chinese Art of Healing and How It Works Scientifically. New York, Random House, 1971, pp 5–16.

48. Deng L, Gan Y, He S, et al: Acupuncture techniques. In Cheng Y (ed): Chinese Acupuncture and Moxibustion. Beijing, Foreign Languages Press, 1997, 325–326.

49. Cooperative Group of Investigation of PSAC: Advances in Acupuncture and Acupuncture Anesthesia. Beijing, The Peoples' Medical Publishing House, 1980.

50. Meng Z, et al: New development in the researches of meridian phenomena in China during the past five years. Zhen Ci Yan Jiu 9:207–222, 1984.

51. Cooperative Group in Research of PSC, Fujian Province: Studies of relation between propagated sensation along channels and effectiveness of clinical acupuncture analgesia. In Zhang XT (ed): Research on Acupuncture, Moxibustion, and Acupuncture Anesthesia. Beijing, Science Press, 1986.

52. Eckman P: Acupuncture and science. Int J Chin Med 1:3–8, 1984.

53. Xuetai W: Research on the origin and development of Chinese acupuncture and moxibustion. In Zhang XT (ed): Research on Acupuncture, Moxibustion, and Acupuncture Anesthesia. Beijing, Science Press, 1986, p 791.

54. Xiao YJ, Su DG: Effect of local refrigeration on ECG changes of EA in Neiguan acupoint. In Second National Symposium of Acupuncture and Moxibustion and Acupuncture Anesthesia. Beijing, 1984: Paper 291. [Cited in Helms, p 23.]

55. Research Group of Acupuncture Anesthesia, Fujian: Studies of phenomenon of blocking activities of channels and collaterals. In Zhang XT (ed): Research on Acupuncture, Moxibustion, and Acupuncture Anesthesia. Beijing, Science Press, 1986, pp 653–667.

56. Xue CC: The phenomenon of propagated sensation along channels (PSAC) and the cerebral cortex. In Zhang XT (ed): Research on Acupuncture, Moxibustion, and Acupuncture Anesthesia. Beijing, Science Press, 1986, pp 668–683.

57. Darras JC, et al: Visualisation isotopique des méridiens d'acupuncture. Cahiers de Biothérapie 95:13–22, 1987. [Cited in Helms, p 23.]

58. Mussat M: Les Réseaux d'Acupuncture: Étude Critique et Expérimentale. Paris, Librairie Le Francois, 1974, pp 255–300. [Cited in Helms, pp 24–25.]

59. Shamos MH, Lavine LS: Piezoelectricity as a fundamental property of biological tissues. Nature 213:267–269, 1967.

60. Fan JY: The role of gap junctions in determining skin conductance and their possible relationship to acupuncture points and meridians. Am J Acupunct 18:163–170, 1990.

61. Zheng JY, Fan JY, Zhang YJ, et al: Further evidence for the role of gap junctions in acupoint information transfer. Am J Acupunct 24:291–296, 1996.

62. Hirschi KK, Xu CE, Tsukamoto T, et al: Gap junction genes Cx26 and Cx43 individually suppress the cancer phenotype of human mammary carcinoma cells and restore differentiation potential. Cell Growth Differ 7:861–870, 1996.

63. Pomeranz B, Chiu D: Naloxone blockade of acupuncture analgesia: Endorphin implicated. Life Sciences 19:1757–1762, 1976.

64. Kendall DE: A scientific model for acupuncture: Part II. Am J Acupunct 17:343–360, 343–360, 1989.

65. Melzack R, Wall PD: Pain mechanisms: A new theory. Science 150:971–979, 1965.

66. Wu MT, Hsieh JC, Xiong J, et al: Central nervous system pathway for acupuncture stimulation: Localization of processing with functional MR imaging of the brain-preliminary experience. Radiology 212:133–141, 1999.

67. Zhang D, Fu W, Wang S, et al: Displaying of infrared thermogram of temperature character on meridians. Zhen Ci Yan Jiu 21:63–67, 1996.

68. Eory A: In-vivo skin respiration (CO_2) measurements in the acupuncture loci. Acupunct Electrother Res 9:217–223, 1984.

69. Lee MH, Ernst M: The sympatholytic effect of acupuncture as evidenced by thermography: A preliminary report. Orthop Rev 12:67–72, 1983.

70. Petti F, Bangrazi A, Liguori A, et al: Effects of acupuncture on immune response related to opioid-like peptides. J Tradit Chin Med 18:55–63, 1998.

71. Matthews PM, Froelich CJ, Sibbitt WL, et al: Enhancement of natural cytotoxicity by beta-endorphin. J Immunol 130:1658–1662, 1983.

72. Bianchi M, Jotti E, Sacerdote P, et al: Traditional acupuncture increases the content of beta-endorphin in immune cells and influences mitogen induced proliferation. Am J Chin Med 19:101–104, 1991.

73. Moss CS: Acupuncture stimulation of endogenous opioids and effects on the immune system. Clin Ecol 88:140–143, 1987.

74. Sin YJ, Sedgewick AR, Mackay MB, et al: Effect of electric acupuncture on acute inflammation. Am J Acupunct 11:359–362, 1983.

75. Shang C: Mechanism of acupuncture: Beyond neurohumoral theory. 2003. [Acupuncture.com]

76. Vickers AJ: Can acupuncture have specific effects on health? A systematic review of acupuncture antiemesis trials. J R Soc Med 89:303–311, 1996.

77. Lee A, Done ML: The use of nonpharmacologic techniques to prevent postoperative nausea and vomiting: A meta-analysis. Anesth Analg 88:1362–1369, 1999.

78. Alimi D, Rubino C, Pichard-Leandri E, et al: Analgesic effect of auricular acupuncture for cancer pain: A randomized, blinded, controlled trial. J Clin Oncol 21:4120–4126, 2003.

79. Alimi D, Rubino C, Leandri EP, et al: Analgesic effects of auricular acupuncture for cancer pain. J Pain Symptom Manage 19:81–82, 2000.

80. He JP, Friedrich M, Ertan AK, et al: Pain-relief and movement improvement by acupuncture after ablation and axillary lymphadenectomy in patients with mammary cancer. Clin Exp Obstet Gynecol 26:81–84, 1999.

81. Dang W, Yang J: Clinical study on acupuncture treatment of stomach carcinoma pain. J Tradit Chin Med 18:31–38, 1998.

82. Hammar M, Frisk J, Grimas O, et al: Acupuncture treatment of vasomotor symptoms in men with prostatic carcinoma: A pilot study. J Urol 161:853–856, 1999.

83. Filshie J, Penn K, Ashley S, et al: Acupuncture for the relief of cancer-related breathlessness. Palliat Med 10:145–150, 1996.

84. Cauffield J: The psychosocial aspects of complementary medicine. Pharmacotherapy 20:1289–1294, 2000.

85. So DW: Acupuncture outcomes, expectations, patient-provider relationship, and the placebo effect: Implications for health promotion. Am J Public Health 92:1662–1667, 2002.

86. Johnstone PA, Polston GR, Niemtzow RC, et al: Integration of acupuncture into the oncology clinic. Palliat Med 16:235–239, 2002.

87. Chiang JS: Unpublished data.
88. Giordano J, Garcia MK, Boatwright D, et al: Complementary and alternative medicine in mainstream public health: A role for research in fostering integration. J Altern Complement Med 9:441-445, 2003.
89. White AR, Filshie J, Cummings TM, et al: Clinical trials of acupuncture: Consensus recommendations for optimal treatment, sham controls and blinding. Complement Ther Med 9:237-245, 2001.
90. National Acupuncture Foundation: The theory and practice of clean needle technique. In Mitchell B, Davis E, McCormick J, et al (eds): Clean Needle Technique Manual for Acupuncturists: Guidelines and Standards for the Clean and Safe Clinical Practice of Acupuncture. Washington, DC, National Acupuncture Foundation, 1997, pp 10-22.
91. Altman S: Techniques and instrumentation: Electroacupuncture. In Schoen AM (ed): Veterinary Acupuncture: Ancient Art to Modern Medicine. St Louis, Mosby, 1994, pp 95-102.
92. Han JS: Physiologic and neurochemical basis of acupuncture analgesia. In Han JS (ed): The Neurochemical Basis of Pain Relief by Acupuncture. Beijing, Beijing Medical University, 1987, pp 589-597.
93. Pomeranz B: Electroacupuncture and transcutaneous electrical nerve stimulation. In Stux G, Pomeranz B (ed): Basics of Acupuncture, 2nd ed. Berlin, Springer-Verlag, 1991, pp 250-260.
94. Han JS: The Neuro-chemical Basis of Pain Control by Acupuncture. Beijing, Hu Bei Technical and Science Press, 1998.
95. Ulett G: Acupuncture: archaic or biologic? Am J Public Health 93:1037, 2003.
96. Deng L, Gan Y, He S, et al: Acupuncture Techniques. In Cheng Y (ed): Chinese Acupuncture and Moxibustion. Beijing, Foreign Languages Press, 1997, pp 491-512.
97. Huang LC: Auriculotherapy: Diagnosis and Treatment. Bellaire, TX, Longevity Press, 1996, p 3.
98. Nogier P: Treatise of Auriculotherapy. Moulins-lès-Metz: Maisonneuve, 1972. [Cited in Helms, p 135.]
99. Nogier P: Introduction Pratique Á L'Auriculothérape. Moulins-lès-Metz,

Maisonneuve, 1978. [Cited in Helms, p 135.]
100. Nogier P: From Auriculotherapy to Auriculomedicine. Moulins-lès-Metz, Maisonneuve, 1983. [Cited in Helms, p 135.]
101. Nogier P, Nogier R: The Man in the Ear. Moulins-lès-Metz: Maisonneuve, 1985. [Cited in Helms, p 135.]
102. Taillandier J: Réflexothérapies et micro-systèmes en acupuncture. Bases physiologiques et thérapeutiques. Acupuncture et Médecine Traditionnelle Chinoise. Paris, Encyclopédie des Médecines Naturelles, II-1, 1989. [Cited in Helms, p 132.]
103. Jiao S: Scalp Acupuncture and Clinical Cases. Beijing, Foreign Languages Press, 1997.
104. Chen Y, Zhao C, Chen H, et al: Effects of "moxibustion serum" on proliferation and phenotypes of tumor infiltrating lymphocytes. J Tradit Chin Med 23:225-229, 2003.
105. Liu J, Yu RC, Tang WJ: Influence of combined therapy of guben yiliu III, moxibustion and chemotherapy on immune function and blood coagulation mechanism in patients with mid-late stage malignant tumor. Zhongguo Zhong Xi Yi Jie He Za Zhi 22:104-106, 2002.
106. Liu J, Yu RC, Rao XQ: Study on effect of moxibustion and guben yiliu III combined with chemotherapy in treating middle-late stage malignant tumor. Zhongguo Zhong Xi Yi Jie He Za Zhi 21:262-264, 2001.
107. Hitosugi N, Ohno R, Hatsukari I, et al: Induction of cell death by pro-oxidant action of moxa smoke. Anticancer Res 22:159-163, 2002.
108. Wang G, Fan Y, Guan Z, et al: Chinese massage. In Zhang E (ed): A Practical English-Chinese Library of Traditional Chinese Medicine. Shanghai, Publishing House of Shanghai University of Traditional Chinese Medicine, 1988.
109. National Certification Commission for Acupuncture and Oriental Medicine: General Information Brochure. NCCAOM, 2003. [http://www.nccaom.org/om_first.htm]
110. Bi YS, Sun H, Guo Y, et al: Chinese Qigong. In Zhang E (ed): A Practical English-Chinese Library of Traditional Chinese Medicine. Shanghai, Publishing

House of Shanghai University of Traditional Chinese Medicine, 1988.
111. Ni M: The Yellow Emperor's Classic of Medicine: A New Translation of the Neijing Suwen with Commentary. Boston, Shambhala, 1995.
112. Brecher P: Secrets of Energy Work. London, Dorling Kindersley, 2001, pp 16-17.
113. Hately J, Laurence V, Scott A, et al: Breathlessness clinics within specialist palliative care settings can improve the quality of life and functional capacity of patients with lung cancer. Palliat Med 17:410-417, 2003.
114. Corner J, Plant H, A'Hern R: Non-pharmacological intervention for breathlessness in lung cancer. Palliat Med 10:299-305, 1996.
115. Yang JM: Advanced Yang Style Tai Chi Chuan Martial Applications. Jamaica Plain, MA, YMAA Publication Center, 1996.
116. Bensky D, Barolet R: Chinese Herbal Medicine: Formulas & Strategies. Seattle, Eastland Press, 1990.
117. MacPherson H, Thomas K, Walters S, et al: A prospective survey of adverse events and treatment reactions following 34,000 consultations with professional acupuncturists. Acupunct Med 19:93-102, 2001.
118. Lao L, Hamilton GR, Fu J, et al: Is acupuncture safe? A systematic review of case reports. Altern Ther Health Med 9:72-83, 2003.
119. Ernst G, Strzyz H, Hagmeister H: Incidence of adverse effects during acupuncture therapy: A multicentre survey. Complement Ther Med 11:93-97, 2003.
120. Chung A, Bui L, Mills E: Adverse effects of acupuncture. Which are clinically significant? Can Fam Physician 49:985-989, 2003.
121. Filshie J: Safety aspects of acupuncture in palliative care. Acupunct Med 19: 117-122, 2001.
122. National Center for Complementary and Alternative Medicine: Selecting a complementary and alternative medicine (CAM) practitioner. NIH/NCCAM, 2003. [http://nccam.nih.gov/health/practitioner/index.htm].
123. Accreditation Commission for Acupuncture and Oriental Medicine: Handbook. Greenbelt, MD: ACAOM, 2003. [http://acaom.org/handbook.htm].

Interventional Techniques for Cancer Pain Management

CHAPTER 31

Neurolytic Celiac Plexus Block

GILBERT Y. WONG, MD, AND PAUL E. CARNS, MD

Patients with pancreatic cancer often present with the symptoms of pain, nausea, lack of appetite, and weight loss. Unfortunately, pancreatic adenocarcinoma is surgically resectable in only 10% to 20% of patients[1] and the long-term benefits of chemotherapy and radiation therapy are limited.[2] The pain associated with pancreatic cancer is typically located in the upper abdomen, often radiating to the mid-back. The quality of the pain is frequently described as being constant, gnawing, and visceral. At the time of diagnosis of pancreatic cancer, 26% of patients had mild pain, 36% had moderate pain, 11% had severe pain, and only 27% had no discomfort.[3] Importantly, cancer pain has been shown to be associated with significant loss of quality of life (QOL).[4,5] To optimize the QOL of these patients, palliative care with adequate pain control is an essential priority.[6]

PAIN PATHWAYS

The nerves of the pancreas[7] can receive nociceptive stimulation[8] that is transmitted to the celiac plexus. The celiac plexus is a sympathetic nervous system structure that transmits both visceral afferent and efferent information for the majority of the upper abdominal viscera. The splanchnic nerves are composed of sympathetic nerve fibers that synapse at the celiac plexus and pass through the diaphragmatic crus to reach the spinal cord. The nociceptive information received is then transmitted by sensory and sympathetic nerves to the thalamus and cortex of the brain and perceived as pain. The ascending pain information may also be modulated by descending mechanisms.[9]

Pain Mechanisms in Pancreatic Cancer

There are a number of possible mechanisms that may be involved in the pain associated with pancreatic cancer.[10] Pancreatic cancer may directly infiltrate, stretch, or injure the nerves of the pancreas[7] causing neuritis and neuropathic pain. Additionally, it has been shown that ductal adenocarcinoma of the pancreas can express and secrete neurolytic enzymes permitting tumor spread along nerve sheaths[11] contributing to the neuritis. In addition, pancreatic cancer frequently metastasizes to the retroperitoneal lymph nodes including those in close proximity to the celiac axis and surrounding neural ganglia. These affected lymph nodes may potentially infiltrate or stretch the surrounding neural tissues also causing neural irritability.

Pancreatic cancer may also cause a form of localized pancreatitis, which may contribute to pain.[12] Nerves within the pancreas may then become sensitized to both chemical and mechanical stimuli[8] associated with the ongoing inflammatory processes. In chronic pancreatitis (without pancreatic cancer), increased numbers of eosinophils infiltrate perineural areas.[13] Due to localized inflammation, injury to the perineural sheath can result in the development of hypersensitivity to a variety of noxious chemical stimuli including prostaglandins, bradykinins, acidosis, histamine, and others.[14] Also, the increased presence of neurotransmitters in afferent pancreatic nerves in patients with pancreatitis may support this theory.[15]

The presence of increased ductal and interstitial pancreatic pressures may contribute to the pain associated with pancreatitis, which may also potentially occur in pancreatic cancer.[12,15,16] Intraductal pancreatic pressure has been found to be abnormally high in chronic pancreatitis.[17-20] Visceral afferent nerves already sensitized from noxious chemical stimuli found in both pancreatitis and pancreatic cancer can become hypersensitive to mechanical stimuli, which may occur with increased pancreatic pressure.[8] Surgical drainage to relieve increased pancreatic pressure improves pain in 70% to 80% of patients.[21,22] Increased pancreatic parenchymal pressure may also contribute to the pain. The increased pressure of the parenchyma within a finite space, limited by a fibrotic pancreatic capsule, may result in increased vascular resistance with reduced pancreatic blood flow, resulting in further neural irritability and pain from ischemia.[15,16]

Repeated visceral afferent stimulation from the previously described pain mechanisms associated with pancreatic cancer may result in a centrally sensitized pain state. Tissue injury or visceral inflammation may increase afferent input to the spinal cord by activation of previously silent nociceptors (pain receptors) in the viscera.[8] With repeated ongoing stimulation, these peripheral nerve endings may have increased sensitivity and their threshold to stimulation decreased, resulting in a prolonged and enhanced response to stimulation. Activation of these newly recruited peripheral nerve fibers can contribute to an afferent barrage of pain information to the spinal cord. A consequence of this increased activity at the spinal cord is the increased tonic release of neurotransmitters (glutamate, substance P, and others) that can alter the excitability of spinal neurons.[23,24] At this level of the central nervous system, these spinal neurons become more easily excitable, resulting in an expanded peripheral receptive field, which is the perceived area of pain.[24] After tissue damage or irritation, this central sensitization may result in the amplification of pain from peripheral input that was previously interpreted as being normal or physiologic. As a result, patients may have decreased thresholds to pain, enhanced responses to painful stimuli, and expanded areas of perceived pain.

Currently, an animal model of pancreatic cancer pain, simulating the human experience of pain in pancreatic cancer, is being characterized and developed (P. Mantyh, personal communication). The key goals of such an animal model of pancreatic cancer pain are to better understand the mechanisms of pain in such a visceral cancer state and then to identify effective mechanism-based analgesic therapies. Novel pain-relieving therapies identified in the model will then be translated to clinical trials in humans.

TREATMENT OF PANCREATIC CANCER PAIN

Systemic analgesic medications and neurolytic celiac plexus block are the two mainstay therapies used in treatment of pancreatic cancer pain. Rather than being mutually exclusive, these therapies used in combination may provide the most effective pain relief with pancreatic cancer.

Systemic Analgesic Therapy

The Agency for Health Care Policy and Research (AHCPR) recommends the World Health Organization (WHO) analgesic ladder as an effective and validated approach in the pharmacologic treatment of cancer pain,[25] including pancreatic cancer pain management.[26,27] This simple method uses a stepwise approach to individualize patient therapy, beginning with nonopioids, progressing to opioids for mild to moderate pain, and then to continue titration of opioids for moderate to severe pain.[25,28] These analgesics are prescribed on a scheduled basis with additional doses as needed for breakthrough pain.

Although pain management with opioid medications may be acceptable for many patients, there are certain disadvantages. A study evaluating the use of the WHO analgesic ladder in cancer patients found the most frequent side effects were dry mouth (39% of the days of follow-up), drowsiness (38%), constipation (35%), and nausea and vomiting (22%). A lack of any significant opioid-related side effects was noted in only 24% of the days of follow-up.[28]

Neurolytic Celiac Plexus Block

Neurolytic celiac plexus block (NCPB) is the most commonly used interventional procedure for the palliation of pain from pancreatic cancer[29] and other upper abdominal tumors.[30] In the past, the use of NCPB in the treatment of pancreatic cancer pain was often reserved for patients who were receiving inadequate analgesia or were intolerant of opioid medications. Although the AHCPR suggests reserving nerve blocks in the management of cancer pain until nearly all other pain relief modalities have failed,[25] there is evidence that NCPB may be a useful adjunct for the relief of pancreatic cancer pain.[26,31,32] Because earlier implementation of NCPB may provide more effective pain relief, a paradigm shift to its inclusion in therapy sooner rather than later should be considered.[27,33,34]

Outcome Studies for Neurolytic Celiac Plexus Block

The efficacy of NCPB for treatment of upper abdominal cancer pain has previously been evaluated by meta-analysis.[29] The authors identified 24 papers: two randomized controlled trials, one prospective case series, and 21 uncontrolled retrospective case series. Most of the published reports describing NCPB involved patients with upper abdominal pain due to pancreatic cancer. With available data, the authors concluded that NCPB has long-lasting benefit for 70% to 90% of patients with pancreatic and other intra-abdominal cancers.[29] A systematic review of the literature has also been conducted and reported in an evidence-based report sponsored by the Agency for Healthcare Research and Quality.[35]

Several smaller, randomized controlled trials comparing NCPB with pharmacologic therapy in the management of pancreatic cancer pain have been reported.[36-38] All of these studies included limited numbers of subjects (10 to 12 patients to each randomized treatment arm) and were not double-blinded. The findings of these smaller studies suggest that NCPB provides more effective analgesia during the first 4 weeks following the procedure compared with systemic analgesic medications.[37,38] Also, patients randomized to receive NCPB had significantly decreased opioid consumption along with fewer opioid-induced side effects lasting from 50 days following the procedure[36,37] up to the time of death.[38] Finally, patients randomized to NCPB have less deterioration in QOL estimates over time compared with patients receiving systemic analgesic medications only.[37]

In the first, larger, randomized controlled trial involving unresectable pancreatic cancer patients, those receiving intraoperative chemical splanchnicectomy (splanchnic neurolysis) at the time of exploratory laparotomy had improved pain control until their death compared with those receiving placebo control.[32] There was also a significant decrease in opioid requirements in the chemical splanchnicectomy group compared with the placebo group. Particular strengths of this investigation were the large total number of subjects ($n = 137$) and the use of double blinding. In a very small subgroup of patients with significant pain ($n = 34$), there was the observation of increased survival time in those receiving the chemical splanchnicectomy compared with controls.

Recently, the Mayo Clinic Pancreatic Cancer Pain Study Team conducted a randomized, double-blinded, sham-controlled trial to evaluate the effect of NCPB on pain relief, QOL, and survival in patients with unresectable pancreatic adenocarcinoma.[26] This clinical trial randomized eligible patients ($n = 100$) to receive either NCPB or systemic analgesic therapy (SAT) alone, along with a sham injection. All study patients could receive additional opioids managed by a physician blinded to the treatment assignment. Baseline pain was similar between NCPB and SAT groups (4.4 ± 1.7 and 4.1 ± 1.8, respectively). At the first week following randomization, pain intensity (2.1 ± 1.4 and 2.7 ± 2.1, respectively) and QOL were both significantly ($P < 0.001$) improved, with a larger decrease in pain for patients with NCPB compared with patients on SAT ($P = 0.005$). From repeated measure analysis, pain was also significantly ($P = 0.013$) lower for NCPB vs. SAT over time. However, opioid consumption ($P = 0.93$), frequency of opioid side effects (all $P > 0.10$), and QOL ($P = 0.46$) were not significantly different between groups. Fewer NCPB patients reported moderate or severe pain ($\geq 5/10$) compared with SAT patients in the first 6 weeks (14% vs. 40%, $P = 0.005$). One year following randomization, 16% of NCPB patients and 6% of SAT patients were alive. However, survival did not differ significantly between groups ($P = 0.26$, proportional hazards regression).

The results of this study suggest that NCPB improves pain relief in pancreatic cancer patients compared with optimized SAT alone, but does not affect QOL or survival.

The analgesic benefit derived from NCPB has been suggested to vary depending on the location of the intra-abdominal cancer and extent of metastases. In a study of 50 pancreatic cancer patients, the efficacy of NCPB was compared between patients with cancer of the head of the pancreas (36 patients) and patients with cancer of the body and tail of the pancreas (14 patients). Patients with cancer of the head of the pancreas had improved response to NCPB in regard to percent responding, relative decrease in pain scores, longer duration of pain relief, and survival time compared with patients with cancer of the pancreas body and tail. Patients with pancreatic cancer of the body and tail had extensive metastases (95% of patients in this group) involving the liver and mesenteric lymph nodes compared with more localized disease in patients with cancer of the head of the pancreas. The authors suggest that lymphatic metastases surrounding the celiac axis may limit the spread of the neurolytic agent resulting in less effective neurolysis. Another study suggests that NCPB can provide significant relief in either early or late disease, as defined by opioid requirements.[34] However, in a randomized clinical trial involving NCPB for unresectable pancreatic cancer, NCPB provided significant pain relief even though the majority of study patients (66 out of 100) had advanced stage IV (widely metastatic) disease.[26] With regard to timing, there are some data to suggest that earlier implementation of NCPB may provide better analgesia and that delay are not necessary, because the effectiveness of NCPB may continue with disease progression.

With regard to choice of percutaneous technique, a long-term prospective randomized trial evaluated three different posterior approaches to NCPB in pancreatic cancer patients: transaortic, classic retrocrural, and bilateral chemical splanchnicectomy.[27] No differences in analgesia were found among the three groups (each group with 20 to 21 patients). All patients were followed weekly until their death. Importantly, NCPB provided complete pain relief until death in 10% to 24% of patients when used alone, but 80% to 90% of patients also required systemic analgesic therapy. This finding may be related to the likelihood that pancreatic cancer pain is not limited to visceral celiac pain, but may also have neoplastic involvement of other somatic or nervous system structures in the advanced stages of disease.[36] These observations emphasize the role of NCPB as an important adjuvant analgesic technique, which is a part of a multimodal analgesic approach to the management of upper abdominal cancer pain. In a study involving pancreatic cancer of the body and tail ($n = 39$), patients were randomized to NCPB by transaortic technique and splanchnic nerve block.[39] Splanchnic nerve block patients had improved pain intensities and decreased opioid requirements compared with NCPB. Further study may assist clinicians in selection of the most effective approach to neurolytic block based on location of the pancreatic tumor.

The potential duration of a NCPB, estimated at 3 to 6 months or longer[26,27,32,40] may match or outlast the median survival time of 6 months following the diagnosis of pancreatic cancer.[41] However, some patients who benefit from an initial NCPB will subsequently experience return or worsening of their pain. If necessary, the NCPB may be repeated.

Relevant Neural Anatomy for Neurolytic Celiac Plexus Block and Splanchnicectomy

The celiac plexus is involved in nociceptive transmission from the upper abdominal viscera including the pancreas (Figures 31-1 and 31-2). Originating from higher levels (greater [T5-T10], lesser [T10-11], and least [T12]), splanchnic nerves comprise preganglionic efferent and visceral afferent nerve fibers. These splanchnic nerves traverse the posterior mediastinum and enter the abdomen through the diaphragmatic crus to synapse at the right and left celiac ganglia, forming the celiac plexus (see Figures 31-1 and 31-2). The celiac ganglia can range in diameter from 0.5 to 4.5 cm and vary in position from the T12-L1 disc space to the middle of the L2 vertebral body.[42] Typically, the celiac plexus is located anterolateral to the aorta, immediately caudal to the celiac artery's origin, at the cephalad border of the L1

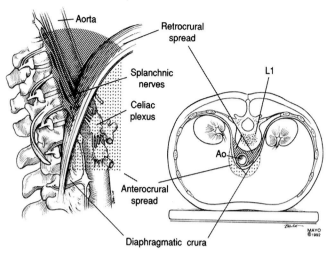

FIGURE 31-2   The lateral and cross-sectional views of the celiac plexus, splanchnic nerves, and anatomy relevant to celiac plexus block. The areas of retrocrural and anterocrural spread of injected solution, anatomically defined by the diaphragm, are shown.

vertebral body. From the celiac ganglia, the postganglionic efferent fibers then innervate their target visceral structures. There may also be some parasympathetic contributions, which originate from the cranial-sacral levels of the spinal cord, to the celiac plexus. The visceral afferent fibers that receive nociceptive information about pain from the pancreas travel with the autonomic efferent fibers to the celiac plexus. The visceral afferent fibers then pass without interruption to the dorsal root ganglia, where their cell bodies are located. They continue with the other afferent fibers in the dorsal root and terminate in the dorsal horn of the thoracic cord (T5-L2). At least one synapse occurs before the nociceptive information is relayed to higher brain centers.

Technique of Neurolytic Celiac Plexus Block

NCPB can be performed with a variety of techniques by either posterior or anterior approaches.[43,44] The posterior approach involves the percutaneous insertion of needles through the back directed to the targeted structures. The anterior approach can be performed by percutaneous, endoscopic, or surgical techniques.

Posterior Approaches

The most commonly used method for NCPB involves the posterior approach with percutaneous insertion of needles directed toward the celiac plexus or splanchnic nerves.[44] The patient is placed in a prone position and needles are inserted bilaterally slightly below the inferior ribs (T12) at points approximately 7 to 7.5 cm from the midline (Figure 31-3). Radiographic guidance is typically used to direct the needles toward the celiac plexus, which is located at the anterior-lateral aspect

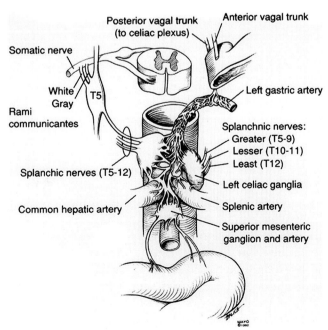

FIGURE 31-1   The celiac plexus conveys visceral afferent information from the upper abdominal viscera, including the pancreas, to the greater, lesser, and least splanchnic nerves.

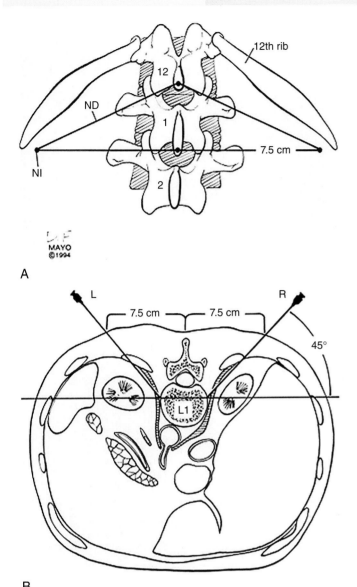

FIGURE 31–3 Percutaneous celiac plexus block from a bilateral posterior percutaneous approach. A, An isosceles triangle formed by the lower border of the 12th ribs (7–7.5 cm from the midline) to the T12-L1 vertebral interspace in retrocrural technique. B, Cross-sectional image of initial needle placement at the L1 vertebral body initially directed 45 degrees from the horizontal plane (or "table top").

of the first lumbar vertebral body. The celiac plexus consists of a network of neural ganglia surrounding the aorta. On the left side (aortic side), once the needle advances past the vertebral body, it should be inserted an additional 1 cm, or until the dense wall of the aorta is identified by pulsations transmitted through the length of the needle. On the right side, the needle can be inserted another 1 cm beyond the anterior plane of the vertebral body. A variation of this technique uses a single needle placed on the left side with the patient in a right lateral decubitus position.[45] Prior to the injection of any substance, the needle is carefully examined to rule out the presence of cerebrospinal fluid, blood,

or urine. The needle position is then confirmed with injection of several milliliters of an appropriate radiocontrast agent. It is important to ensure that there is no spread of radiocontrast to the epidural or intrathecal spaces, psoas muscle (encases the lumbar plexus), nerve roots, or vascular structures, especially the aortic wall. Then, 10 mL of 0.5% bupivacaine is injected on each side. If there are no neurologic deficits after 10 minutes, 10 mL of neurolytic agent (absolute alcohol) is injected on each side, which will spread to the celiac plexus or splanchnic nerves (see Figures 31-2 and 31-3) to interrupt nerve transmission for 3 to 6 months. Previously, it was common to perform a diagnostic celiac plexus block with local anesthetic only, a day or two prior to the NCPB.[33] However, clinical observation and evidence suggest that nearly all patients receiving diagnostic celiac block receive temporary benefit and subsequently proceed to the actual neurolytic procedure.[33] As a result, many clinicians now perform the NCPB without need for a diagnostic celiac plexus block, consideration being given to its relative safety and analgesic efficacy.[27,32]

The final needle tip position, relative to the diaphragmatic crura, defines the NCPB as being anterocrural or retrocrural (anterior or posterior to the diaphragm, respectively) based on the attachment of the diaphragmatic crura to the vertebral bodies and discs and longitudinal ligament[44,46] (see Figure 31-2). The placement of the needles at the level of L1 vertebral body will increase the probability of an anterocrural block, or a true celiac plexus block, which is the technique described previously.[44,46] The transaortic approach has also been advocated as another technique to accomplish anterocrural NCPB.[27,47] From the left side, a single needle is inserted through the aorta so that the final needle tip is anterior to the aorta at the lower portion of L1 vertebral body. Using a posterior approach but with a more superior placement of needles at T12 will likely result in a retrocrural block or a splanchnic nerve block. The accurate determination of a block as being anterocrural or retrocrural requires radiographic imaging. A previous study comparing anterocrural and retrocrural approaches with NCPB suggests that there is no significant difference in analgesia.[27]

Anterior Approaches

There are a variety of techniques that have been described for the anterior approach to NCPB. One technique involves the percutaneous placement of a single needle through the abdominal wall, and possibly the stomach, intestine, and pancreas, to the preaortic region of the celiac plexus.[48,49] This anterior percutaneous technique uses computed tomography (CT) imaging or ultrasound guidance to guide and confirm needle placement. The endoscopic ultrasound–guided NCPB is another anterior approach, in which an endoscope is placed through the upper gastrointestinal tract into the stomach. A needle for injection is then advanced through the posterior wall of the stomach into the preaortic region of the celiac plexus, using ultrasound imaging of the aorta and surrounding structures.[10,50] Another anterior technique is a chemical splanchnicectomy at the time of open abdominal surgery.[32,51-53] The stomach can be retracted to expose the celiac axis to inject neurolytic solution on either side of the aorta in the retroperitoneal compartment, immediately posterior to the lesser omentum.[10]

Radiographic Guidance

Currently, there seems to be consensus to use some form of radiographic guidance in performing NCPB, to both guide needle placement and confirm correct needle location for injection. Fluoroscopy has been commonly used in this procedure.[54] Some have advocated the use of CT imaging for greater accuracy, especially given the possibility of anatomic distortions with tumor spread.[54,55] A meta-analysis evaluating NCPB was unable to conclude that the success of the block or frequency of adverse effects were significantly improved with radiographic guidance, including CT imaging, compared to nonradiographic methods.[29]

Neurolytic Celiac Plexus Block Complications and Adverse Effects

NCPB is a relatively safe procedure. However, there are theoretical concerns and mild clinical side effects that may be associated with this procedure.[56] The potential risk and benefits of NCPB must be considered in the context of a suffering cancer patient with a typically poor prognosis.

Effective neurolysis of the celiac plexus and splanchnic nerves, which are primarily structures of the sympathetic nervous system, can result in relatively unopposed parasympathetic effect in the splanchnic region. As a result, vasodilation of the splanchnic vasculature may precipitate orthostatic hypotension in some individuals. Despite this, most patients compensate well with these fluid shifts.[30] Additionally, increased parasympathetic outflow to the viscera can cause bowel hypermotility, resulting in diarrhea that is typically transient.

Neurologic complications are the most worrisome concerns associated with NCPB. Although uncommon, potentially long-term neurologic deficits may include sensory and motor deficits of the trunk and lower extremities; loss of bladder or bowel control, or both; and impotence in males. In a case series of 2730 NCPBs, major complications were limited to 4 cases of neurologic deficit (frequency of <0.2%) ranging from loss of anal or bladder control to paraplegia.[57] The mechanisms of these complications may include spread of injected solution into the intrathecal or epidural space or to the

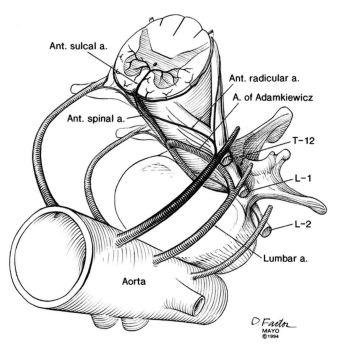

FIGURE 31–4 Arterial supply of the spinal cord at the level of low thoracic and high lumbar vertebrae. The most common major feeding artery, artery of Adamkiewicz, typically occurs at vertebral level T9-T11.

thoracic and lumbar nerve roots. Injury or spasm of the arteries supplying blood to the spinal cord may result in neural injury due to ischemia (Figure 31–4).[58]

CONCLUSION

Achieving the highest possible quality of life throughout the course of disease is the most important goal in the management of the patient with pancreatic cancer. However, optimal quality of life can only be achieved with effective palliation of pain. The two mainstay pain control therapies, systemic analgesic therapy and NCPB, should not be mutually exclusive alternatives in the effort to provide effective pain control in pancreatic cancer. Instead, the combination of these therapies may ultimately provide the most effective pain relief for these patients. Therefore, in the management of unresectable pancreatic cancer pain, implementation of earlier rather than later NCPB is an option that clinicians should strongly consider.

ACKNOWLEDGMENTS

Supported in part by the Cancer Treatment Research Foundation, Ehlers Family Program for Psychosocial Oncology and Spiritual Care at Mayo Clinic Cancer Center, and Mayo Clinic and Foundation. We also thank David Factor for essential illustrations and Linda Husser for secretarial support.

REFERENCES

1. Warshaw AL, Fernandez-del Castillo C: Pancreatic carcinoma. New Engl J Med 326:455–465, 1992.
2. Hawes RH, Xiong Q, Waxman I, et al: A multispecialty approach to the diagnosis and management of pancreatic cancer. Am J Gastroenterol 95:17–31, 2000.
3. Grahm AL, Andren-Sandberg A: Prospective evaluation of pain in exocrine pancreatic cancer. Digestion 58:542–549, 1997.
4. Owen JE, Klapow JC, Casebeer L: Evaluating the relationship between pain presentation and health-related quality of life in outpatients with metastatic or recurrent neoplastic disease. Qual Life Res 9:855–863, 2000.
5. Skevington SM: Investigating the relationship between pain and discomfort and quality of life, using the WHOQOL. Pain 76:395–406, 1998.
6. Foley KM, Gelband H: Improving Palliative Care for Cancer. Washington, DC, National Academy Press, 2001.
7. Nagakawa T, Mori K, Nakano T, et al: Perineural invasion of carcinoma of the pancreas and biliary tract. Br J Surg 80:619–621, 1993.
8. Gebhardt GF: Visceral pain mechanisms. In: Chapman CR, Foley KM (eds): Current and Emerging Issues in Cancer Pain. New York, Raven Press, 99–111, 1993.
9. Sorkin LS (ed): Basic Pharmacology and Physiology of Acute Pain Processing. Philadelphia, WB Saunders, 1997.
10. Wong GY, Wiersem MJ, Sarr MG: Palliation of pain in adenocarcinoma of the pancreas. In: Cameron JL (ed): American Cancer Society Atlas of Clinical Oncology: Pancreatic Cancer. Hamilton, Ontario, BC Decker Inc, 2001.
11. Kayahara M, Nagakawa T, Futagami F, et al: Lymphatic flow and neural plexus invasion associated with carcinoma of the body and tail of the pancreas. Cancer 78:2485-2891, 1996.
12. Reber HA: Pancreatic cancer: Presentation of the disease, diagnosis and surgical management. J Pain Symptom Manage 3:164–170, 1988.
13. Keith RG, Keshavjee SH, Kerenyi NR: Neuropathology of chronic pancreatitis in humans. Can J Surg 28:207–211, 1985.
14. Bockman DE, Buchler M, Malfertheiner P, Beger HG: Analysis of nerves in chronic pancreatitis. Gastroenterology 94:1459-1469, 1988.
15. Malfertheiner P, Dominguez-Munoz JE, Buchler MW: Chronic pancreatitis: Management of pain. Digestion 55(Suppl 1):29–34, 1994.
16. Karanjia ND, Reber HA: The cause and management of pain of chronic pancreatitis. Gastroenterol Clin North Am 19:895–904, 1990.
17. Bradley EL: Pancreatic duct pressure in chronic pancreatitis. Am J Surg 144:313–315, 1982.
18. Madsen P, Winkler K: The intraductal pancreatic pressure in chronic obstructive pancreatitis. Scand J Gastroenterol 17:553–554, 1982.
19. Okazaki K, Yamamoto Y, Ito K: Endoscopic measurement of papillary sphincter zone and pancreatic main ductal pressure in patients with chronic pancreatitis. Gastroenterology 91:409–418, 1985.
20. Okazaki K, Yamamoto Y, Kagiyama S, et al: Pressure of papillary sphincter zone and pancreatic main duct in patients with chronic pancreatitis in the early stage. Scand J Gastroenterol 23:501–507, 1988.
21. Holmberg JT, Isaksson G, Ihse I: Long-term results of pancreatico-jejunostomy in chronic pancreatitis. Surg Gynecol Obstet 160:339–346, 1985.
22. Prinz RA, Greenlee HB: Pancreatic duct drainage in 100 patients with chronic pancreatitis. Ann Surg 194:313–318, 1981.
23. Woolf CJ, Thompson SW: The induction and maintenance of central sensitization is dependent on N-methyl-D-aspartic acid receptor activation: Implications for the treatment of post-injury pain hypersensitivity states. Pain 44:293–299, 1991.
24. Dubner R: Neuronal plasticity in the spinal and medullary dorsal horns: A possible role in central pain mechanisms. In: Casey KL (ed): Pain and Central Nervous System Disease: The Central Pain Syndromes. New York, Raven Press; 1991, pp 143–155.
25. Jacox A, Carr DB, Payne R, et al. (eds): Management of Cancer Pain. Rockville, MD, Agency for Health Care Policy and Research, U.S. Department of Health and Human Services, Public Health Service, March, 1994.
26. Wong GY, Schroeder DR, Carns PE, et al: Effect of neurolytic celiac plexus block on pain relief, quality of life, and survival in patients with unresectable pancreatic cancer. JAMA 291:1092–1099, 2004.
27. Ischia S, Ischia A, Polati E, Finco G: Three posterior percutaneous celiac plexus block techniques: A prospective randomized study in 61 patients with pancreatic cancer pain. Anesthesiology 76:534–540.
28. Ventrafridda V, Tamburini M, Caraceni A, De Conno F, Naldi F: A validation study of the WHO method for cancer pain relief. Cancer 59:850–856, 1987.
29. Eisenberg E, Carr DB, Chalmers TC: Neurolytic celiac plexus block for treatment of cancer pain: A meta-analysis. Anesth Analg 80:290–295, 1995.
30. Brown DL, Bulley CK, Quiel EL: Neurolytic celiac plexus block for pancreatic cancer pain. Anesth Analg 66:869–873, 1987.
31. Lillemoe KD: Palliation of pain: Operation. J Gastrointest Surg 3:345–347, 1999.
32. Lillemoe KD, Cameron JL, Kaufman HS, et al: Chemical splanchicectomy in patients with unresectable pancreatic cancer: A prospective randomized trial. Ann Surg 217:447–457, 1993.
33. Rykowski JJ, Hilgier M: Efficacy of neurolytic celiac plexus block in varying locations of pancreatic cancer. Anesthesiology 92:347–354, 2000.
34. de Oliveira R, dos Reis MP, Prado WA: The effects of early or late neurolytic sympathetic plexus block on the management of abdominal or pelvic cancer pain. Pain 110:400–408, 2004.
35. Goudas L, Carr DB, Bloch R, et al: Management of Cancer Pain. Evidence Report/Technology Assessment No.35.
Rockville, MD, Agency for Healthcare Research and Quality: (Prepared by the New England Medical Center Evidence-based Practice Center under Contract No 290-97-0019). AHCPR Publication No. 02-E002; 2001 October, 2001.
36. Polati E, Finco G, Gottin L, et al: Prospective randomized double-blind trial of neurolytic coeliac plexus block in patients with pancreatic cancer. Br J Surg 85:199–201, 1998.
37. Kawamata M, Ishitani K, Ishikawa K, et al: Comparison between celiac plexus block and morphine treatment on quality of life in patients with pancreatic cancer pain. Pain 64:597–602, 1996.
38. Mercadante S: Celiac plexus block versus analgesics in pancreatic cancer pain. Pain 52:187–192, 1993.
39. Ozyalcin SN, Talu GK, Camlica H, Erdine S: Efficacy of coeliac plexus and splanchnic nerve blockades in body and tail located pancreatic cancer pain. Eur J Pain: EJP 8:539–545, 2004.
40. Moore DC: Intercostal nerve block combined with celiac plexus (splanchnic) block. In: Moore DC (ed): Regional Block, 4th ed. Springfield, IL, Charles C Thomas Publisher, 1981.
41. Saltzburg D, Foley KM: Management of pain in pancreatic cancer. Surg Clin North Am 69:629–649, 1989.
42. Ward EM, Rorie DK, Nauss LA, Bahn RC: The celiac ganglia in man: Normal anatomic variations. Anesth Analg 58:461–465, 1979.
43. Wong GY: Palliation of pain in unresectable pancreatic cancer. J Gastrointest Surg 3:348–350, 1999.
44. Wong GY, Brown DL: Celiac plexus block for cancer pain. In: Urmey W (ed): Techniques in Regional Anesthesia and Pain Management. Philadelphia, WB Saunders, 1997, pp 18–26.
45. Hilgier M, Rykowski JJ: One needle transcrural coeliac plexus block: Single shot or continuous technique, or both. Reg Anesth 19:277–283, 1994.
46. Boas RA: Sympathetic blocks in clinical practice. Intern Anesthesiol Clin 4:149–182, 1978.
47. Ischia S, Luzzani A, Ischia A, Faggion S: A new approach to the neurolytic block of the coeliac plexus: The transaortic technique. Pain 16:333–341, 1983.
48. Matamala AM, Lopez FV, Martinez LI: The percutaneous approach to the celiac plexus using CT guidance. Pain 34:285–288, 1988.
49. De Cicco M, Matovic M, Balestreri L, et al: Single-needle celiac plexus block. Anesthesiology 87:1301–1308, 1997.
50. Gunaratnam NT, Wong GY, Wiersema MJ: Endosonography-guided celiac plexus block for the management of pancreatic pain. Gastrointest Endosc 52(suppl):S28–S34, 2000.
51. Copping J, Willix R, Kraft R: Palliative chemical splanchnicectomy. Arch Surg 94:418–420, 1969.
52. Flanigan DP, Kraft RO: Continuing experience with palliative chemical splanchnicectomy. Arch Surg 113:509–511, 1978.

53. Gardner AM, Solomou G: Relief of pain of unresectable carcinoma of pancreas by chemical splanchnicectomy during laparotomy. Ann Roy Coll Surg Engl 66:409–411, 1984.

54. Ischia S, Polati E, Finco G, Gottin L, Benedini B: 1998 Labat Lecture: the role of the neurolytic celiac plexus block in pancreatic cancer pain management: Do we have the answers? Reg Anesth Pain Med 23:611–614, 1998.

55. Moore DC, Bush WH, Burnett LL: Celiac plexus block: A roentgenographic, anatomic study of technique and spread of solution in patients and corpses. Anesth Analg 60:369–379, 1981.

56. Wong GY, Brown DL: Celiac plexus block: side effects and complications. In: Atlee JL (ed): Complications in Anesthesia. Philadelphia, WB Saunders, 1999.

57. Davies DD: Incidence of major complications of neurolytic coeliac plexus block. J Royal Society of Medicine 86:264–266, 1993.

58. Wong GY, Brown DL: Transient paraplegia following alcohol celiac plexus block. Reg Anesth 20(4):352–355, 1995.

CHAPTER 32

Intraspinal Therapy

CHERYL WHITE, MD, AND ARUN RAJAGOPAL, MD

The prevalence of pain approaches 80% to 90% in patients with advanced cancer who are undergoing disease treatment.[1,2] This sobering statistic has been one of the driving factors in the development and implementation of rational guidelines for symptomatic management and palliative care by the World Health Organization.[3,4] Unfortunately, approximately 10% to 20% of patients may not achieve relief from the "three-step ladder" approach.[5]

Although the taxonomy of pain syndromes is discussed in Chapter 1, it is important for clinicians to understand various pain mechanisms and perform comprehensive pain assessments if they are to make rational treatment decisions relating to the care of the terminally ill. The International Association for the Study of Pain (IASP) Task Force surveyed pain characteristics in large patient populations in an effort to develop uniformity in characterization of cancer pain syndromes, a greater understanding of their pathophysiology, and information relating to opioid and adjuvant responsiveness.[6] Mercadante and Portenoy define opioid responsiveness as a degree of analgesia achieved as a dose is titrated to an endpoint defined as either the development of intolerable side effects or occurrence of acceptable analgesia.[7]

Although opioid management is usually the mainstay of treatment for nociceptive pain, specific strategies have been outlined for patients unable to achieve an appropriate balance between satisfactory pain management and unacceptable side effects, despite use of the WHO analgesic ladder and an exhaustive attempt at conservative measures. It is at this point that ablative and neurointerventional procedures, such as implantable neuraxial therapy, must be considered. Yaksh and Wang's early work with opiate receptors in spinal administration has led to widespread use of intraspinal opioids and to the development of other spinal adjuvant agents.[8,9] Patients fail to respond to analgesic regimens for any number of reasons, including pain mechanisms, disease progression, development of tolerance, pain related to therapeutic measures, and unacceptable side effects. Krames describes a continuum of approaches to pain syndromes in which nociceptive versus neuropathic elements predominate (Figure 32-1).[10] Generally, neuraxial opioid therapy is reserved for intractable somatic pain syndromes, whereas neuropathically mediated mechanisms more favorably respond to neuromodulative techniques. There are, unfortunately, syndromes with combined features that complicate effective treatment.

The decision to proceed with interventional pain control must be undertaken with the utmost care. Appropriate patient selection, life expectancy, and type of implantable device, as well as choice of infusion agent, its mode of administration, and potential complications are factors to be considered.

SPINAL PHARMACOLOGY

Selection of appropriate agents for spinal delivery requires a basic understanding of spinal pharmacology. The mechanisms of dorsal horn neurophysiology are extremely complicated, and a thorough discussion is beyond the scope of this chapter. In overview, neurotransmitters and peptide mediators are derived from three principal sources: primary afferent neurons, spinal relay neurons, and descending inhibitory pathways.

Peripheral injury resulting in afferent fiber stimulation causes increased spontaneous firing of excitatory synaptic transmission and release of neurotransmitters, such as glutamate, substance P, and calcitonin gene-related peptide, which are closely approximated to modulatory spinal interneurons. Phosphorylation of receptors such as N-methyl-D-aspartate (NMDA) and alpha methyl propionic acid (AMPA) increases membrane excitability and calcium conductance, effectively amplifying signal transmission to dorsal horn interneurons.[11,12] The term "spinal plasticity" refers to the ability of the central nervous system (CNS) to adapt pain processing in the face of repetitive signaling via conformational or phosphorylative changes in receptor and ion channels,[13] and it is instrumental in the perpetuation of chronic pain states.

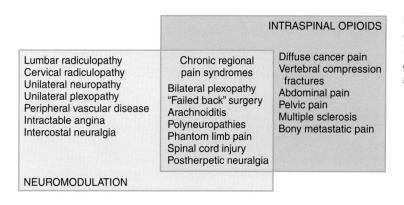

| Lumbar radiculopathy
Cervical radiculopathy
Unilateral neuropathy
Unilateral plexopathy
Peripheral vascular disease
Intractable angina
Intercostal neuralgia

NEUROMODULATION | Chronic regional
pain syndromes
Bilateral plexopathy
"Failed back" surgery
Arachnoiditis
Polyneuropathies
Phantom limb pain
Spinal cord injury
Postherpetic neuralgia | INTRASPINAL OPIOIDS

Diffuse cancer pain
Vertebral compression
fractures
Abdominal pain
Pelvic pain
Multiple sclerosis
Bony metastatic pain |

FIGURE 32–1 Response and overlap of various chronic pain syndromes to neuromodulation versus intraspinal opioids. *(Modified from Krames EI: Implantable devices for pain control: Spinal cord stimulation and intrathecal therapies. Best Pract Res Clin Anaesth 16:619–649, 2002.)*

Hammonds's review of GABA receptors describes three different types and their role in nociception.[14] The GABA-A receptor is a dual binding site with an ion-gated channel whose activation results in a chloride influx and neuronal hyperpolarization. Histologic studies reveal as many as 12 to 15 different subtypes of GABA-A scattered throughout the CNS. Methods now exist to genetically target these subtypes,[14] which have allowed further preclinical study in rodent models. There are several subunits within the binding sites at which other substances, such as barbiturates, steroids, and inhalational anesthetic gases, are thought to bind, modulating expression of the receptor complex. This has been useful in the investigation of the various roles of GABA-mediated pharmacology on anxiety, memory, seizure disorders, and the actions of various pharmacologic agents, as well as the significance of the B receptor subunit and its role in allodynia and hyperalgesia.

GABA-B receptors function via a G protein complex, promoting inhibition of cAMP, increase in potassium conductance, and hyperpolarization of afferent terminals. Hyperactive polysynaptic segmental reflexes or supraspinal descending facilitatory pathways respond to its GABA-B effects of inhibition of evoked release of excitatory neurotransmitters (e.g., glutamate) and substance P.[15]

GABAergic modulation in dorsal horn interneurons is most likely effected at the primary afferent fibers via presynaptic inhibition.[16] It is suggested that normal encoding of low to moderate intensity stimuli depends on the tonic and intrinsic functionality of GABAergic and glycinergic receptors and that spinal receptors and competitors such as A-1 receptor agonist adenosine, N-type calcium channel blockers, and NMDA antagonists are thought to downregulate release of excitatory peptides. There is also evidence for the role of muscarinic facilitation of spinal antinociception via dorsal horn GABAergic interneurons by cholinergic agents.[17-20]

GABA's close approximation to and interaction with NMDA receptors may play a pivotal role in the mechanism of central sensitization and "wind up." Afferent excitatory potentials relieve the normally quiescent NMDA ion channels of Mg^{2+} and facilitate Ca^{2+} influx, promoting long-term conformational changes, altered plasticity, and perhaps the development of tolerance to antinociceptive therapy.[21,22] Hyperpolarization and membrane stabilization of dorsal horn interneurons make NMDA activation more difficult.[23] Receptor-specific antagonism in a rodent model found that inhibitory modulation is minimized and NMDA receptor activity is readily recruited, even in the absence of noxious stimulation.[24-26]

Opioids and alpha-2 agonist agents act presynaptically to inhibit release of excitatory neurotransmitters and postsynaptically by hyperpolarization of cell membranes.[27,28] Although their actions are synergistic, they appear to act by different pathways and are not affected by cross-tolerance.[29] Alpha-adrenergic stimulation in the receptor-dense region of the dorsal horn and brainstem decreases sympathetic outflow and blocks nociceptive transmission at the level of the spinal cord.[30]

Cyclooxygenase (COX) isoenzymes are present in spinal sites and spinal prostaglandins have also been implicated in central sensitization. The intrathecal administration of NSAIDs attenuates excitatory neuropeptide release in the rodent model.[31] Although both COX1 and COX2 enzymes are implicated in the production of allodynia after peripheral nerve injury, COX1 may play a greater role.[32,33]

Opioids

Morphine is the only FDA-approved opioid for spinal use and remains the gold standard for neuraxial use. Other opioids, such as fentanyl, hydromorphone, sufentanil, and methadone, are often used and depending on lipid solubility, have various effects on spinal spread and subsequent supraspinal effects. Both epidural and intrathecal routes can be effective for intractable pain; however, the agent and dose chosen depend on individual properties of each. The general conversion for intraspinal use is 1/10th of parenteral dose for epidural use and 1/100th for intrathecal. Because of incomplete cross-tolerance among different opioid classes, methadone may be effective for its combination mu-agonist and NMDA-antagonist properties.

Midazolam

Analgesic synergism with local anesthetics has been demonstrated.[34,35] A pilot study in which humans received long-term polyanalgesia with a combination of opioids, clonidine, and midazolam noted a slower rate of opioid dose escalation with multimodal therapy, suggesting a favorable effect on opioid tolerance.[36] Although this is encouraging, there appear to be histologic changes and spinal cord toxicity associated with its use in animal studies.[37]

Neostigmine

There are reports documenting facilitation of analgesia by intraspinal neostigmine.[38-40] Side effects appear to be dose-related, and they include nausea, vomiting, somnolence, leg weakness, and hemodynamic changes.[41,42] In combination therapy with opioids, neostigmine appears to prolong analgesia.[43]

Clonidine

Clonidine is used most often in refractory neuropathically mediated pain. Its actions are thought to be synergistic with opioids and local anesthetics, which account for its analgesic efficacy by other routes of administration.[44] Because its site of action is distinct from that of opioids, it has a potential role in opioid-induced tolerance and treatment-limiting side effects.[45-47] Side effects include hemodynamic changes, including hypotension, sedation, and rebound hypertension. Newer agents, such as dexmedetomidine, may be clinically useful in the future, as they appear to have fewer adverse effects.[48]

Ketamine

Although its role in the setting of acute pain is limited, the use of ketamine in chronic neuropathic pain is expanding. The addition of spinal ketamine significantly enhances antinociceptive effects of mu opioid agonists in preclinical investigations,[49-51] and its NMDA-antagonist activity may be useful in chronic neuropathic pain. It may serve to reduce the development of opioid tolerance, especially when administered via the intrathecal route.[52,53] Clinical usefulness of intrathecal ketamine is limited by its dysphoric side effects; however, it may have a synergistic role in smaller doses when administered in conjunction with opioids or local anesthetics.[54] Long-term safety has not been established, and there are a few reports of histopathologic changes associated with intrathecal use. In preclinical studies, dextromethorphan, also a potent NMDA antagonist, does not appear to possess the dysphoric properties of ketamine; however, no intrathecal formulation currently exists for clinical use.[55-57]

Ketorolac

Ketorolac has been shown to be effective in preclinical studies, both alone and in combination with clonidine.[58,59] A phase 1 assessment of intrathecal ketorolac by Eisenach and colleagues showed no serious side effects,[60] though clinical use in humans has yet to be established.

Adenosine

Adenosine has been shown to reduce areas of mechanical hypersensitivity and allodynia in neuropathic pain.[61] Animal studies have demonstrated a lack of significant intrathecal morphologic changes associated with chronic administration.[62] Phase 1 safety profiles look promising for use with newer formulations in humans.[63]

Amitriptyline

Initial animal studies on amitriptyline in neuropathic pain models demonstrated its effect on thermal hyperalgesia, regardless of the route of administration, though interestingly, it did not affect allodynia.[64] Intrathecal administration was shown to favorably affect potentiation of systemic opioids,[65,66] which suggests that it may have a role in future clinical use.

Ziconotide

Ziconotide is a prototypical N-type calcium channel blocker, which, when administered intrathecally, has been shown to produce dose-dependent antinociception and reduction of allodynia. Side effect profiles also appear to be dose related[67] and include hemodynamic instability, as well as CNS symptoms of nystagmus, sedation, confusion, and ataxia. The proposed mechanism of action of N-type calcium blockers when administered in central sites is inhibition of calcium influx.

Baclofen

The clinical use of intrathecal baclofen was first proposed in 1984.[68,69] Its subsequent use has been well documented and is currently one of the only two agents approved by the FDA for intrathecal use. It is indicated for use in spasticity-related pain of cerebral palsy and damage of upper motor neuron origin with deafferentation pain such as stroke, encephalopathy, traumatic brain injury, multiple sclerosis, or spinal cord injury.[70-73]

Acute interruption of systemic baclofen administration produces a clinical withdrawal syndrome which may evolve as early as 1 to 3 days with manifestations of agitation, insomnia, confusion, delusions, muscular rigidity, hallucinations, seizures, psychosis, hemodynamic instability, disseminated intravascular coagulation, rhabdomyolysis, neuroleptic malignant syndrome, cardiac dysrhythmias and failure, dyskinesia, hyperthermia, and increased spasticity.[74,75] Long-term safety and effectiveness of infusion therapy is documented,[76-79] and it appears that there is evidence for the development of tolerance; presumably caused by decreased receptor affinity or down-regulation of GABA receptors during chronic treatment.[80]

Local Anesthetics

Local anesthetic agents, by virtue of their sodium channel antagonism, have been widely used in combination with opioids and other adjuvant agents for epidural or intraspinal use. Chronic neuraxial infusions alone or in combination with other agents have been shown to have additive effects and are more effective in neuropathic pain. Bupivacaine is the most widely used of this class. Cancer patients receiving long-term infusions have shown no significant adverse effects, especially at relevant clinical doses.[81,82] Mixtures for neuraxial infusion are reported to maintain their stability for as long as 3 months.[83] The use of lidocaine has decreased because of reports of neurotoxicity when used in high concentration.

IMPLANTABLE DRUG DELIVERY SYSTEMS

Penn first described an implantable programmable pump for morphine infusion in 1984 and DuPen described a permanent exteriorized silicone epidural catheter for self-administration of opioids in 1987.[84,85] Figure 32-2 shows the DuPen epidural catheter consisting of a two-piece catheter, tunneling rod, guide wire, 14-gauge Tuohy needle, and connectors. The epidural

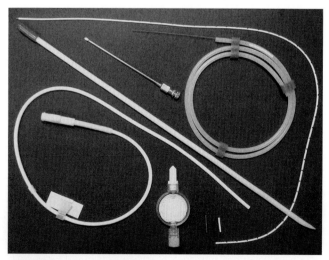

FIGURE 32–2 DuPen catheter, shown with two-piece epidural catheter, guide wire, tunneling rod, 14-gauge Tuohy needle, and connectors.

catheter is shown with distance markings, and the subcutaneous catheter is shown with bacterial-resistant cuff. Catheter types include polyethylene, polyamide, polyurethane, and silicone-rubber.[86] Early infusion systems consisted of percutaneous ports for intermittent epidural administration and implantable constant infusion systems,[87] which are still available for use. Because of the need for programmability, an implantable, programmable, battery-powered system was subsequently developed in the late 1980s. The various infusion systems are outlined in Table 32-1. Basic to all fully implanted systems is a drug reservoir, a chamber containing a propellant such as Freon, and a bellows assembly, which separates the two.

Filling the drug reservoir compresses the two-phase charging fluid, which expands with normal body temperature, forcing the infusate through a filter-impedance assembly before exiting the pump. The programmable pump contains an electronic programming module and a peristaltic motor, which determines rate of infusion via microprocessors. A telemetric receiver and transmitter are common between the pump and its programmer, enabling interrogation and transmission. Potential benefits of a totally implantable system include reduced infection risk because there are no external components, although percutaneous reservoir refilling does compromise the system to a limited degree.[88]

There are several decisions to consider when selecting the type of neuraxial infusion device: epidural versus intrathecal route; percutaneous versus implantable ports; and intermittent, constant, or programmable infusion mode.[89]

The choice of epidural versus intrathecal therapy depends on proposed duration of therapy, technical aspects such as epidural fibrosis and metastasis and factors such as lipophilicity of the opioid chosen for use. Lipophilic agents, when used in the epidural space, create a risk for systemic side effects due to absorption.[90] Table 32-2 outlines major differences between epidural and intrathecal infusion therapy.

The system most widely used at our institution is the Medtronic Synchromed infusion pump (Figure 32-3). The reservoir volume is either 10 or 18 cc, and the choice is generally determined by patient size. Either a one- or two-piece catheter system can be used, although the one-piece system is usually easier. Alternatively, a tunneled intrathecal or epidural catheter may be used for a shorter expected duration of therapy.

Patient Selection

Appropriate patient selection is crucial before implantation, and the type of pain syndrome may profoundly influence the success of treatment. In general, somatic nociceptive pain, which is present in multiple sites,

TABLE 32–1 Comparison of Neuraxial Delivery Systems

Type	Description	Risk and Associated Considerations	Infusion Type	Use Duration
Percutaneous catheter	Intrathecal or epidural insertion	Infection. Epidural fibrosis, encapsulation	Bolus	Acute postoperative pain, drug trials, inability to undergo invasive procedures
Tunneled catheter	Intrathecal or epidural	Less infection risk	Bolus or continuous	Anticipated use for weeks to months
Implanted reservoir	Surgical implantation, percutaneous filling. Costly	Less infection or catheter failure risk than percutaneous or tunneled catheters	Bolus or continuous	Anticipated use for months to years
Implanted mechanical delivery system	Surgical implantation, percutaneous access. Patient-activated dose titration	Not FDA approved	Bolus	Anticipated use for months to years
Implanted drug delivery pump	Continuous delivery; periodic pump refills	Dose change requires pump refill with different concentrations	Continuous	Anticipated use for months to years
Programmable implanted delivery pump	Allows dose programming without solution exchange	Most costly	Continuous with bolus capability	Anticipated use for months or years

such as in metastatic cancer or some nonmalignant pain syndromes, responds more favorably to intrathecal therapy. A single or unilateral pain site with radicular, lancinating, burning, or shooting pain often typifies a neuropathic etiology, usually indicating neurostimulation may be better suited to successful therapy. Krames and others outline appropriate criteria helpful for patient selection[91] (Table 32–3).

Traditionally, life expectancy of over 3 months duration has been the point at which it is more economically feasible to consider an implantable intrathecal pump versus a tunneled epidural catheter with external delivery system.[92,93] The patient's current functional levels and realistic expectations of pain relief may also affect success of intraspinal therapy, and it is important to portray achievable goals rather than emphasizing

TABLE 32–2 Epidural versus Intrathecal Routes of Administration

Factors	Intrathecal	Epidural
Suitability	Long term	Short term
Catheter tip occlusion	Granuloma	Fibrosis
Side effects	Less frequent	More frequent
Pump refill	Less frequent	More frequent
Dosing	Lower amount	Higher amount
Implantation complications	Greater	Less
Long-term complications	Fewer	Greater
Infection rate	Equivocal	Equivocal

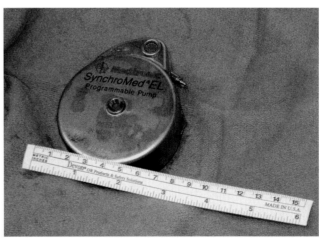

FIGURE 32–3 The Medtronic Synchromed programmable pump.

TABLE 32–3   Criteria for Patient Selection for Implantable Therapies
Identified pathology consistent with pain
Failure of all conservative therapies
Intolerable side effects, despite use of adjuvants
No further identifiable surgical or medical correction is indicated
Psychological assessment and clearance has been obtained
Opioid-responsive pain syndrome
Successful preimplantation trial of neuraxial therapy
Absence of contraindications to proposed procedure

complete pain relief and resumption of functionality. A thorough psychological evaluation is critical preoperatively to evaluate affective or sensory components or maladaptive coping skills, which may be addressed before consideration for therapy. Olson has outlined several risk factors in chronic pain that are predictive of poor outcome.[94] These include major psychopathology, mood disorder, addictive issues, potential for self-harm, anxiety, catastrophization, and a high degree of distress. In general, when psychological and social issues overshadow medical and nociceptive factors, the outcome is less likely to be successful. The patient's social, economic, and emotional support systems are also critical in their long-term care. A general outline of absolute and relative contraindications is shown in Table 32–4. The reader is also referred to select readings on patient selection for long-term intrathecal therapy.[95,96]

Trial of Intraspinal Opioid Therapy

The intraspinal trial itself functions as a screening tool in evaluating drug efficacy versus toxicity. It is presumed that patients who present for evaluation have demonstrated prior opioid responsiveness for a period. Issues to be resolved with screening trial include efficacy, tolerance, improvement in level of functioning, and effect on quality of life as endpoints. Options for trial include single shot opioids, percutaneous epidural or intrathecal catheters, and implanted temporary catheters. There is ongoing debate about which trial method is superior.

"Single shot" or bolus dose of morphine is usually 0.2 to 1.0 mg (intrathecal) or 3.5 to 7.5 mg per day (epidural) or more, depending on the patient's MEDD. Bolus dose proponents argue that the incidence of drug-related side effects is best evaluated with this method, whereas proponents of a continuous trial maintain that it best simulates the postimplantation state.[97] Continuous infusion also permits change of dose or drug and may be optimal for accurate assessment of side effects. Adequate trial length also continues to be debated, with longer periods necessarily culling potential placebo-responders. Criteria that portend an effective trial include overall reduction in pain scores by 50%, improvement in function, reduction of side effects, and reduction of oral or systemic analgesic agents.[98] The management of systemic opioid medications during intraspinal trial depends on the trial method selected and on practitioner preference. Many convert 50% of baseline opioid therapy into intraspinal route when using a continuous infusion trial in an effort to minimize withdrawal symptoms and provide adequate "breakthrough" dosing.

TABLE 32–4 Absolute and Relative Contraindications to Intraspinal Infusion Analgesic Therapy	
Absolute Contraindications	**Relative Contraindications**
Systemic infection	Poor healing capacity
Known allergies to metals and/or plastic materials used	Limited patient support system
Known allergies to proposed medications for infusion	Body habitus not compatible with pump placement
Aplastic anemia	
Uncorrectable coagulopathy	
Intravenous drug abuse history	
Nonopioid responsive pain or failed trial	
Poor patient compliance and cooperation	
Untreated psychopathology	

Other Preimplantation Considerations

Before surgery, the clinician should determine optimal placement of the battery-operated pump. The pump should not be positioned in the way of restrictive clothing such as belt lines or bra straps, nor should it be placed near or on ribs, lower abdominal quadrants, in the vicinity of a radiation port, or prior surgical scar. Postoperative arrangements should be solidified regarding follow-up care, transportation to the clinic, refill schedules, safety precautions, scheduling of appointments, and self-care responsibilities such as routine infection survey.

Implantation Procedure

The implantation procedure is conducted under strict aseptic technique with appropriate preoperative antibiotic administration. An overview of the technique is shown in Figure 32–4. Adequate time spent with the patient before surgery to determine location of pump placement greatly assists outcome. General anesthesia is almost always indicated for patient comfort, and the patient is positioned in the lateral decubitus position with the proposed pump implantation side in the nondependent position. Meticulous attention should be paid to proper padding of extremities and spinal alignment.

1. Survey via fluoroscopy, appropriate intraspinous level for insertion. The patient must be positioned for an anterior–posterior projection image.
2. A Tuohy needle is then placed via a paramedian approach, either percutaneously or through a 4-cm to 7-cm paramedian skin incision. This approach minimizes potential catheter occlusion and facilitates tunneling later in the procedure. Confirm free flow of cerebrospinal fluid (CSF).
3. An intrathecal catheter is then threaded through the spinal needle. Never withdraw the catheter through the needle because it is extremely fragile and is easily sheared.
4. Document free CSF flow and clamp the catheter to the sterile drapes to prevent dislodgment.
5. The abdominal incision is now made with a 10-cm lower quadrant to Scarpa's fascia. Using blunt dissection and undermining, a pocket is made to accommodate the pump, taking care to allow enough room for closure without undue tension on suture lines. Meticulous hemostasis must be ensured to minimize the occurrence of a pump pocket hematoma.
6. Create a tunnel for the intrathecal catheter from the pump pocket toward the spinal incision, using the supplied malleable tunneling tool.
7. Anchor the spinal catheter securely to the fascia with nonabsorbable suture, and ensure freedom from kinking before passing the spinal catheter toward the pump pocket. This step is crucial in preventing catheter dislodgment or kinking. CSF free flow must again be confirmed after this step.
8. Position the pump in the subcutaneous pocket after appropriately warming, de-airing, and filling. A Dacron pouch may be used if desired, or anchoring sutures may be placed. It is important to ensure adequate fixation of the pump to discourage movement or flipping.
9. Carefully close all incisions with interrupted absorbable sutures for fascia and either nonabsorbable suture or staples for the skin.

Complications

1. Infection: wound infection, meningitis, or epidural abscess.
2. Hematoma: pocket hematoma, seroma, hygroma, epidural hematoma, or intrathecal hemorrhage.
3. Neurologic events: nerve injury, arachnoiditis, cauda equina injury, CSF leak, and hygroma.
4. Catheter-related complications: catheter breakage, kinking or dislodgment, tip obstruction or allergic reaction to catheter materials.
5. Pump-related complications: pump dislodgment or torsion, programming or telemetric failures, battery failures, rotor failures, or allergic reaction to pump material.
6. Infusate-related complications: medication side effects; contamination of infused agents; allergies to infusates; errors in mixing, reconstituting, or refilling infusates.
7. Hypogonadism: reported in long-term intrathecal opioid therapy, as well as systemic therapy,[99,100] and continuing investigation is ongoing.

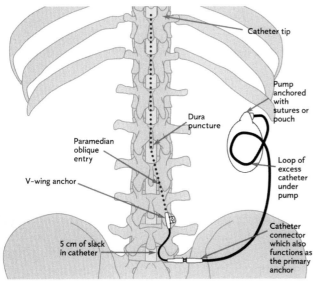

FIGURE 32–4 Overview of implantation technique for intrathecal catheter and pump. Note the position of anchoring and connecting devices. *(Reprinted with permission of Medtronic, Inc.)*

8. There are also reports of abuse of intrathecal medications by "pump-raiding".[101]

Programming Considerations

Various infusion modes are currently available with most models of programmable pumps, enabling customization of drug delivery. They either operate via single- or continuous-cycle infusion or can be programmed to deliver single or periodic bolus doses of medication as desired. Upon initial insertion and programming of an implanted system in the operating room, care must be taken to warm and purge the pump of air and prime it with the appropriate dose of agent to be infused. Refilling and reprogramming the pump with a different concentration of drug entails the programming of a "bridge bolus" of medication to facilitate delivery of the new concentration agent in a timely manner to the intrathecal space. At our institution the following formula is used for such a calculation:

Bridge bolus dose (mg)
= (volume of implanted catheter length in mL)
× (concentration of new drug in mg/mL)

(Note: Implanted catheter length is usually approximately 0.4 mL)

0.4 mL × (former concentration of drug in mg/mL)

Time for bridge bolus delivery (hours)
= hourly rate of new drug dose (mg/hour)

It is important that the patients carry with them written information pertaining to their pump, model, manufacturer, appropriate pain clinic and manufacturer contact information, as well as future appointment and refill dates.

Complications of Long-Term Indwelling Catheters

Indwelling epidural catheters, by virtue of their presence as a foreign body, incite an inflammatory reaction in epidural tissue, with the attraction of fibroblasts and development of a well-organized sheath around the epidural catheter. The abundance of epidural venous plexus and lack of a blood–brain barrier afford the organization of several populations of inflammatory cells in the epidural space.

Long-term infusion of substances in the intrathecal space is more problematic and less understood. Catheter tip inflammatory masses are a rare but significant occurrence that can result in progressive loss of pain control, withdrawal symptoms, or even neurologic events such as spinal cord compression. New neurologic events, such as dose escalation, change in quality of pain, sensory changes, hyperalgesia, myelopathy, incontinence, gait disturbance, or paraparesis, must raise a high index of suspicion for mass–effect and emergent magnetic resonance imaging (MRI) is indicated.

Inflammatory catheter tip masses were first reported in the early 1990s. These growths appeared to differ from the fibrotic masses seen with chronically implanted epidural catheters and did not appear to emanate from an infectious etiology. Although the true incidence of this phenomenon is probably underreported, the circumstances appear to be different from chronic fibrotic masses previously reported in chronic epidural implantation, largely because of the privileged blood–brain barrier. The location of granulomas outside the arachnoid membrane speaks to an extra-neuraxial origin.

A review of the clinical case data by Coffey and Burchiel in 2000 hypothesized mechanisms of mass formation to be affected by both chemical characteristics of infused opioids and their concentration and placement within the neuroaxis.[102] Hassenbusch and Yaksh identified 92 cases since 1992 and evaluated clinical and demographic factors borne out in the review of the literature: duration of intrathecal therapy (mean 25 to 29 months), drug administered (usually morphine), placement of the intrathecal catheter (usually thoracic) in areas of potentially low CSF flow, daily dose of opioid (greater than 10 mg/day), concentration of opioid (greater than 25 mg/mL, which probably represented pharmacy compounding) and type of chronic pain (cancer vs. noncancer).[103] There have been no reported cases of intrathecal catheter tip masses with long-term baclofen infusion.

Proposed factors, which were initially thought to be contributory to the formation of catheter tip masses, have been investigated and subsequently dismissed. These include infectious causes, allergic or inflammatory reaction to silicone or catheter materials, contamination of the infusate, pyrogens or endotoxins, catheter tip design faults, surgical trauma, and predisposing patient conditions such as arachnoiditis.

The most accepted explanations for clinical data implicate properties of intrathecal drugs themselves, especially morphine, in combination with CSF flow properties and catheter placement along the spinal cord. Thoracic catheter levels are most frequently used, and ventral placement related to insertion technique is common. In an effort to maximize time between pump refills, a highly concentrated agent and slower infusion rates are utilized, making the catheter tip the nidus of potential mass formation. The current hypotheses include mass effect upon medullary structures and localized disruption of spinal CSF flow and drug distribution patterns.

Routine follow-up and refill visits should be used to thoroughly assess and document changes in the

TABLE 32–5   Diagnosis and Treatment of Catheter Tip Masses

Diagnostic Clues	Treatment Options
Diminishing analgesia or rapid dose escalation not commensurate with disease process Sensory changes including paresthesias or new-onset radicular pain Loss of bowel or bladder function Motor weakness or gait difficulties Proprioceptive changes Reflex hypoactivity or hyperactivity Pain upon injection of catheter tip	Surgical removal of the catheter and mass Withdrawal of the spinal catheter to a lower level, if force is not required Discontinue opioid infusion and infuse preservative-free saline through the catheter, if no symptoms The clinician may or may not elect to replace an intrathecal catheter at a lower lumbar level Eventual substitution of another opioid

neurologic examination that arouse an index of suspicion for catheter tip masses (Table 32-5).[104] Neurodiagnostic imaging should be sought with any suspicion for catheter tip masses and some advocate routine imaging for screening purposes. An MRI with and without gadolinium or computed tomography (CT) myelography best serves to detect enhancing lesions. If the catheter's access port is to be injected with contrast material, close attention should be paid to the avoidance of overdose, injection of intrathecal air, or the possibility of injecting directly into the mass. It is suggested that flow through the CSF catheter should be documented before study. Treatment of catheter tip masses has been outlined by a consensus panel (see Table 32-5).[105]

CONCLUSION

A review of the literature conducted, including randomized controlled trials and systematic reviews, revealed favorable outcomes for intrathecal therapy, including overall efficacy and cost effectiveness when used long term as opposed to medical management.[106] Visual analog scales, composite toxicity score, and estimated survival were favorably affected as compared with medical

therapy alone.[107] In other surveys, analgesia was rated as excellent or good in over 95% of more than 429 patients with improvements in daily functioning and quality of life.[108] Smith and others have compared implantable therapy with conservative medical management in refractory cancer pain.[109] Decreased toxicity and overall improvement in side effect–related symptoms were documented in implanted patients and visual analog pain score were somewhat favorably affected. There may be a favorable effect on survival versus medical management alone.

In summary, intraspinal analgesic therapy, when administered to appropriately selected patient populations, is a valuable tool in improving chronic, intractable cancer pain when other conservative measures have failed or when intolerable side effects predominate over acceptable analgesia. Alternative opioids, as well as several newer, nonopioid agents are also undergoing investigation and are gaining greater acceptance for clinical use. Successful intraspinal analgesic management requires an understanding of amenable pain syndromes, adequate management resources, and a low threshold for potential complications. Commitment on the part of the patient, as well as the care team, must include frequent, regular communication and long-term follow-up.

REFERENCES

1. Brescia FJ, Adler D, Gray G, et al: Hospitalized advanced cancer patients: a profile. J Pain Symptom Manage 5:221–227, 1990.
2. Portenoy RK: Management of cancer pain. Lancet North Am Educ 353:1695–1700, 1999.
3. Ventafridda V, Tamburinit M, Caracent A, et al: A validation study of the WHO method for cancer pain relief. Cancer 59:850–856, 1987.
4. Zech D, Grond S, Lynch J, et al: Validation of World Health Organization Guidelines for

cancer pain relief: A 10 year prospective study. Pain 63:65–76, 1995.
5. Lesage P, Portenoy RK: Trends in cancer pain management. Cancer Control 6:136–145, 1999.
6. Portenoy RK: Report from the International Association for the Study of Pain Task Force on cancer pain. J Pain Symptom Manage 12:93–96, 1996.
7. Mercadante S, Portenoy RK: Opioid poorly responsive cancer pain. Part 1: Clinical considerations. J Pain Symptom Manage 21:144–150, 2001.

8. Yaksh TL, Rudy TA: Analgesia mediated by a direct spinal action of narcotics. Science 192:1357–1358, 1976.
9. Wang JK, Nauss LA, Thomas JE: Pain relief by intrathecally applied morphine in man. Anesthesiology 50:149–151, 1979.
10. Krames EI: Implantable devices for pain control: Spinal cord stimulation and intrathecal therapies. Best Pract Res Clin Anaesth 16:619–649, 2002.
11. Woof CJ, Bennett GJ, Doherty M, et al: Towards a mechanism based classification of pain? Pain 77:227–229, 1998.

12. Woof CJ, Decostered I: Implications for recent advances in the understanding of pain physiology for the assessment of pain in patients. Pain 6:S141–S147, 1999.

13. Woolf CJ, Salter MW: Neuronal plasticity: Increasing the gain in pain. Science 288:1765–1769, 2000.

14. Hammond DL: Role of spinal GABA in acute and persistent nociception: JJ Bonica Lecture 2001. Reg Anesth Pain Med 26:551–557, 2001.

15. Davidoff RA: Antispasticity drugs: Mechanism of action. Ann Neurol 17:107–116, 1985.

16. Walker SM, Goudas LC, Cousins MJ, et al: Combination spinal analgesic chemotherapy: A systematic review. Anesth Analg 95:674–715, 2002.

17. Chen SR, Pan HL: Spinal GABAb receptors mediate antinociceptive actions of cholinergic agents in normal and diabetic rate. Brain Res 965:67–74, 2003.

18. Baba H, Kohno T, Okamoto M, et.al: Muscarinic facilitation of GABA release in substantia gelatinosa of the rat spinal dorsal horn. J Physiol 508(Pt1):83–93, 1998.

19. Hwang JH, Hwang KS, Kim JU, et al: The interaction between intrathecal neostigmine and GABA receptor agonists in rats with nerve ligation injury. Anes Analg 93:1297–1303, 2001.

20. Hwang JH, Hwang KS, Leem JK, et al: The antiallodynic effects of intrathecal cholinesterase inhibitors in a rat model of neuropathic pain. Anesthesiology 90:492–499, 1999.

21. Coderre TJ, Fundytus ME, McKenna JE, et al: The formalin test: A validation of the weighted scores method of behavioural pain rating. Pain 54:43–50, 1993.

22. Coderre TJ: The role of excitatory amino acid receptors and intracellular messengers in persistent nociception after tissue injury in rats. Mol Neurobiol 7:229–246, 1994.

23. Portenoy RK: Evolving role of NMDA-receptor antagonists in analgesia. J Pain Symptom Manage 19:1–64, 2000.

24. Dickenson AH, Chapman V, Green GM: The pharmacology of excitatory and inhibitory amino-acid mediated events in the transmission and modulation of pain in the spinal cord. Gen Pharmacol 28:633–638, 1997.

25. Kaneko M, Hammond DL: Role of spinal gamma-aminobutyric acid: A receptor in formalin-induced nociception in the rat. J Pharmacol Exp Ther 282:928–938, 1997.

26. Dickenson AH, Sullivan AF: Differential effects of excitatory amino acid antagonists on dorsal horn nociceptive neurons in the rat. Brain Res 506:31–39, 1990.

27. Mercadante S, Portenoy RK: Opioid poorly-responsive cancer pain. Part 3: Clinical strategies to improve opioid responsiveness. J Pain Symptom Manage 21:338–354, 2001.

28. Bennett G, Deer T, Du Pen S, et al: Future directions in the management of pain by intraspinal drug delivery. J Pain Symptom Manage 20:S44–S50, 2000.

29. Luo L, Puke MJC, Wiensenfeld-Hallin Z: The effects of intrathecal morphine and clonidine on the prevention and reversal of spinal cord hyperexcitability following sciatic nerve section in the rat. Pain 58:245–252, 1994.

30. Yaksh TL: Pharmacology of spinal adrenergic systems which modulate spinal nociceptive processing. Pharmacol Biochem Behav 22:845–858, 1985.

31. Southall MD, Michail RL, Vasko MR: Intrathecal NSAIDS attenuated inflammation-induced neuropeptide release from rat spinal cord slices. Pain. 78:39–48, 1998.

32. Ma W, Du W, Eisenach JC: Role for both spinal cord COX-1 and COX-2 in maintenance of mechanical hypersensitivity following peripheral nerve injury. Brain Res 937:94–99, 2002.

33. Zhu X, Conklin D, Eisenach JC: Cyclooxygenase-1 in the spinal cord plays an important role in postoperative pain. Pain 104:15–23, 2003.

34. Serrao JM, Marks RL, Morley SJ, et al: Intrathecal midazolam for the treatment of chronic mechanical low back pain: A controlled comparison with epidural steroid in a pilot study. Pain 48:5–12, 1992.

35. Nishiyama T: The post-operative analgesic action of midazolam following epidural administration. Eur J Anaesthesiol 12:369–374, 1995.

36. Rainov NG, Volkmar H, Burkert W: Long-term intrathecal infusion of drug combinations for chronic back and leg pain. J Pain Symptom Manage 22:862–871, 2001.

37. Bennett G, Serafini M, Burchiel K, et al: Evidence-based review of the literature on intrathecal delivery of pain medication. J Pain Symptom Manage 20:S12–S36, 2000.

38. Almeida RA, Lauretti GR, Mattos AL: Antinociceptive effect of low-dose intrathecal neostigmine combined with intrathecal morphine following gynecologic surgery. Anesthesiology 98:495–498, 2003.

39. Grant GJ, Piskoun B, Bansinath M: Intrathecal administration of liposomal neostigmine prolongs analgesia in mice. Acta Anaesthesiol Scand 46:90–94, 2002.

40. Naguib M, Yaksh TL: Antinociceptive effects of spinal cholinesterase inhibition and isobolographic analysis of the interaction with mu and alpha 2 receptor systems. Anesthesiology 80:1338–1348, 1994.

41. Hood, DD, Eisenach JC Tuttle, R: Phase 1 safety assessment of intrathecal neostigmine methylsulfate in humans. Anesthesiology 82:331–343, 1995.

42. Klalmt JG, Garcia LV, Prado WA: Analgesic and adverse effects of a low dose of intrathecally administered hyperbaric neostigmine alone or combined with morphine in patients submitted to spinal anaesthesia: Pilot studies. Anaesthesia 54:27–31, 1999.

43. Omais M, Lauretti GR, Paccola CA: Epidural morphine and neostigmine for postoperative analgesia after orthopedic surgery. Anesth Analg 95:1698–1701, 2002.

44. Eisenach JC, Hood DD, Curry R: Intrathecal, but not intravenous, clonidine reduces experimental thermal or capsaicin-induced pain and hyperalgesia in normal volunteers. Anesth Analg 87:591–596, 1998.

45. Mercadante S, Portenoy RK: Opioid poorly-responsive cancer pain, Part 3: Clinical strategies to improve opioid responsiveness. J Pain Symptom Manage 21:338–354, 2001.

46. Walker SM, Goudas LC, Cousins MJ, et al: Combination spinal analgesic chemotherapy: a systematic review. Anes Analg 95:674–715, 2002.

47. Dunbar SA: Alpha-2-adrenergic agonists in the management of chronic pain. Bailliere's Clin Anaesthesiol 14:471–481, 2000.

48. Kawamata T, Omote K, Yamamoto H, et al: Antihyperalgesic and side effects of intrathecal clonidine and tizanadine in a rat model of neuropathic pain. Anesthesiology 98:1480–1483, 2003.

49. Havarth G, Joo G, Dobos I, et al: The synergistic antinociceptive interactions of endomorphine with dexmedetomidine and/or S (+)-ketamine in rats. Anesth Analg 93:1018–1024, 2001.

50. Felsby S, Nielson J, Arendy-Nielson L, et al: NMDA receptor blockade in chronic neuropathic pain: A comparison of ketamine and magnesium chloride. Pain 64:238–291, 1996.

51. Yang CY, Wong CS, Chang JY, et al: Intrathecal ketamine reduces morphine requirements in patients with terminal cancer pain. Can J Anaesth 43:79–83, 1996.

52. Miyamoto H, Saito Y, Kirihara Y, et al: Spinal coadministration of ketamine reduces the development of tolerance to visceral as well as somatic antinociception during spinal morphine infusion. Anesth Analg 90:136–141, 2000.

53. Burton AW, Lee DH, Saab C, et al: Preemptive intrathecal ketamine injection produces a long lasting decrease in neuropathic pain behaviors in a rat model. Reg Anesth Pain Med 24:208–213, 1999.

54. Kathirvel S, Sadhasivam S, Saxena A, et al: Effects of intrathecal ketamine added to bupivacaine for spinal anaesthesia. Anaesthesia 55:899–904, 2000.

55. Karpinski N, Dunn J, HansenL, et al: Subpial vacuolar myelopathy after intrathecal ketamine: Report of a case. Pain 73:103–105, 1997.

56. Stotz M, Oehen HP, Gerber H: Histological findings after long-term infusion of intrathecal ketamine for chronic pain: A case report. J Pain Symptom Manage 18:223–228, 1999.

57. Beltrutti DP, Trompeo AC, Di Santo S: The epidural and intrathecal administration of ketamine. Curr Rev Pain 3:458–472, 1999.

58. Malmberg AB, Yaksh TL: Antinociceptive actions of spinal nonsteroidal anti-inflammatory agents on the formalin testing the rat. J Pharmacol Exp Ther 263:136–146, 1992.

59. Conklin DR, Eisenach JC: Intrathecal ketorolac enhances antinociception from clonidine. Anesth Analg 96:191–194, 2003.

60. Eisenach JC, Curry R, Hood DD, Yaksh TL: Phase 1 safety assessment of intrathecal ketorolac. Pain 99:599–604, 2002.

61. Eisenach JC, Curry R, Hood DD: Dose response of intrathecal adenosine in experimental pain and allodynia. Anesthesiology 97:938–942, 2002.

62. Rane K, Karlsten R, Sollevi A, et al: Spinal cord morphology after chronic intrathecal administration of adenosine in the rat. Acta Anaesth Scand 43:1035–1040, 1999.

63. Eisenach JC, Hood DD, Curry R: Phase 1 safety assessment of intrathecal injection of an American formulation of adenosine in humans. Anesthesiology 96:24–28, 2002.

64. Esser MJ, Sawynok J: Acute amitriptyline in a rat model of neuropathic pain: Differential symptom and route effects. Pain 80:643–653, 1999.

65. Eisenach JC, Gabhart GF: Intrathecal amitriptyline: Antinociceptive interactions with intravenous morphine and intrathecal clonidine, neostigmine and carbamylcholine in rats. Anesthesiology 83:1036–1045, 1995.

66. Cerda SE, Tong C, Deal DD, et al: A physiologic assessment of intrathecal amitriptyline in sheep. Anesthesiology 86:1094–1103, 1997.

67. Penn RD, Paice JA: Adverse effects associated with the intrathecal administration of ziconotide. Pain 85:291–296, 2000.

68. Penn RD, Savoy SM, Corcos D, et al: Intrathecal baclofen for severe spinal spasticity. N Engl J Med 320:1517–1521, 1989.

69. Penn RD, Kroin JS: Intrathecal baclofen alleviates spinal cord spasticity [letter]. Lancet 1:1078, 1984.

70. Stempien L, Tsai T: Intrathecal baclofen pump use for spasticity: A clinical survey. Am J Phys Med Rehabil 79:536–541, 2000.

71. Loubser PG, Akman NM: Effects of intrathecal baclofen on chronic spinal cord injury pain. J Pain Symptom Manage 12:241–247, 1996.

72. Herman RM, D'Luzansky SC, Ippolito R: Intrathecal baclofen suppresses central pain in patients with spinal lesions: A pilot study. Clin J Pain 8:338–345, 1992.

73. Taira T, Kawamura H, Tanikawa T, et al: A new approach to control central deafferentation pain: Spinal intrathecal baclofen. Stereotact Funct Neurosurg 65:101–105, 1995.

74. Alden TD, Lytle RA, Park TS, et al: Intrathecal baclofen withdrawal: A case report and review of the literature. Child's Nerv Syst 18:522–525, 2002.

75. Coffey RJ, Edgar TS, Francisco GE, et al: Abrupt withdrawal from intrathecal baclofen: Recognition and management of a potentially life-threatening syndrome. Arch Phys Med Rehabil 83:735–741, 2002.

76. Albright AL, Gilmartin R, Swift D, et al: Long-term intrathecal baclofen therapy for severe spasticity of cerebral origin. J Neurosurg 98:291–295, 2003.

77. Campbell WM, Ferrel A, McLaughlin JF, et al: Long-term safety and efficacy of continuous intrathecal baclofen. Dev Med Child Neurol 44:660–665, 2002.

78. Korenkov AI, Niendorf WR, Darwish N, et al: Continuous intrathecal infusion of baclofen in patients with spasticity caused by spinal cord injuries. Neurosurg Rev 25:228–230, 2002.

79. Sampson FC, Hayward A, Evans G, et al: Functional benefits and cost/benefit analysis of continuous intrathecal baclofen infusion for the management of severe spasticity. J Neurosurg 96:1052–1057, 2002.

80. Nielson JF, Hansen HJ, Sunde N, et al: Evidence of tolerance to baclofen in treatment of severe spasticity with intrathecal baclofen. Clin Neurol Neurosurg 104:142–145, 2002.

81. Sjoberg M, Karlsson PA, Nordborg C, et al: Neuropathological findings after continuous intrathecal administration of morphine and bupivacaine for pain treatment in cancer patients. Anesthesiology 76:173–186, 1992.

82. Kedlaya D, Reynolds L, Waldman S: Epidural and intrathecal analgesia for cancer pain. Best Pract Res Clin Anaesth 16:651–665, 2002.

83. Hildbrand KR, Elsberry DD, Deer TR: Stability, compatibility and safety of intrathecal bupivacaine administered chronically via an implantable delivery system. Clin J Pain 17:239–244, 2001.

84. Penn RD, Paice JA, Gottschalk W et al: Cancer pain relief using chronic morphine infusion: Early experience with a programmable implanted drug pump. J Neurosurg 61:302–306, 1984.

85. DuPen SL, Peterson DG, Bogosian AC, et al: A new permanent exteriorized epidural catheter for narcotic self-administration to control cancer pain. Cancer 59:986–993, 1987.

86. Buchheit T, Rauck R: Subarachnoid techniques for cancer pain therapy: When, why and how? Curr Rev Pain 3:198–205, 1999.

87. Coombs DW, Saunders RL, Baylor MS, et al: Relief of continuous chronic pain by intraspinal narcotics infusion via an implanted reservoir. JAMA 250:2236–2239, 1983.

88. Levy R: Implanted drug delivery systems for control of chronic pain. In North RB, Levy R (eds): Neurosurgical Management of Pain. New York, Springer-Verlag, 1997, pp 302–324.

89. Waldman SD, Coombs DW: Selection of implantable narcotic delivery systems. Anesth Analg 68:377–384, 1989.

90. Kedlaya D, Reynolds L, Waldman S: Epidural and intrathecal analgesia for cancer pain. Best Pract Res Clin Anaesth 16:651–665, 2002.

91. Prager J, Jacobs M: Evaluation of patients for implantable pain modalities: medical and behavioral assessment. Clin J Pain 17:206–214, 2001.

92. Hassenbusch SJ: Cost modeling for alternate routes of administration of opioids for cancer pain. Oncology 13(Suppl 2):63–67, 1999.

93. Krames ES: Practical issues when using neuraxial infusion. Oncology 13(Suppl 2):37–44, 1999.

94. Olson K: The physician and psychological services: Treating chronic pain. Minneapolis: NCS Assessments, 1992.

95. Krames ES, Olson K: Clinical realities and economic considerations: Patient selection in intrathecal therapy. J Pain Symptom Manage 14:S3–S12, 1997.

96. Prager J, Jacobs M: Evaluation of patients for implantable pain modalities: Medical and behavioral assessment. Clin J Pain 17:206–214, 2001.

97. Oakley J, Staats PS: The use of implanted drug delivery systems. In Raj RP (eds): Practical Management of Pain, 3rd ed. St. Louis, Mosby, 2000, pp 768–778.

98. Krames ES: Implantable devices for pain control: spinal cord stimulation and intrathecal therapies. Best Pract Res Clin Anaesth 16:619–649, 2002.

99. Rajagopal A, Vassilopoulou-Sellin R, Palmer L, et al: Hypogonadism and sexual dysfunction in male cancer survivors receiving chronic opioid therapy. J Pain Symptom Manage 26:1055–1061, 2003.

100. Abs R, Verhelst J, Maeyaert J, et al: Endocrine consequences of long term intrathecal administration of opioids. J Clin Endocrinol Metab 85:2215–2222, 2000.

101. Burton AW, Conroy B, Garcia E, et al: Illicit substance abuse via an implanted intrathecal pump. Anesthesiology 89:1264–1267, 1989.

102. Coffey RJ, Burchiel K: Inflammatory mass lesions associated with intrathecal drug infusion catheters: Report and observations on 41 patients. Neurosurgery 50:78–87, 2002.

103. Yaksh TL, Hassenbusch S, Burchiel K, et al: Inflammatory masses associated with intrathecal drug infusion: A review of preclinical evidence and human data. Pain Med 3:300–312, 2002.

104. Information about inflammatory masses: Intrathecal drug infusion. Medtronic Educational Brief. Minneapolis, Medtronic Incorporated, 2003.

105. Hassenbusch S, Burchiel K, Coffey RJ, et al: Management of intrathecal catheter-tip inflammatory masses: a consensus statement. Pain Med 3:313–323, 2002.

106. Implantable spinal infusion devices for chronic pain and spasticity. In New and Emerging Techniques-Surgical: Rapid Review. In Australian Safety and Efficacy Register of New Interventional Procedures. Melbourne, Royal Australian College of Surgeons, 2003.

107. Bennett G, Serafini M, Burchiel K, et al: Evidence-based review of the literature on intrathecal delivery of pain medication. J Pain Symptom Manage 20:S12–S36, 2000.

108. Paice JA, Winkelmuller W, Burchiel D, et al: Clinical realities and economic considerations: efficacy of intrathecal pain therapy. J Pain Symptom Manage 14(Suppl):S14–S26, 1997.

109. Smith TJ, Staats PS, Deer T, et al: Randomized clinical trial of an implantable drug delivery system compared with comprehensive medical management for refractory cancer pain: Impact on pain, drug-related toxicty and survival. J Clin Oncol 20:4040–4049, 2002.

CHAPTER 33

Spinal Cord Stimulation

ALLEN W. BURTON, MD, AND SAMUEL J. HASSENBUSCH, III, MD, PHD

Neurostimulation describes the use of pulsed electrical energy near the spinal cord (or other neural structures) to control pain.[1,2] This technique was first applied in the intrathecal space and finally in the epidural space as described by Shealy in 1967.[2] Today, neurostimulation most commonly involves the implantation of leads in the epidural space to transmit this pulsed energy across the spinal cord or near the desired nerve roots. Most of this chapter concentrates on spinal cord stimulation (SCS), sometimes called dorsal column stimulation. This technique has notable analgesic properties for neuropathic pain states, anginal pain, and peripheral ischemic pain. The same technology can be applied in deep brain stimulation, cortical brain stimulation, and peripheral nerve stimulation (PNS).[3-6] These techniques are mainly in the realm of the neurosurgeon but are described in this chapter for completeness. The role of these techniques in cancer pain syndromes is described in the last section of the chapter.

SPINAL CORD STIMULATION

Mechanism of Action

Neurostimulation began shortly after Wall and Melzack proposed the gate control theory in 1965.[7] This theory proposed that painful peripheral stimuli carried by C-fibers and lightly myelinated A-delta fibers terminated at the substantia gelatinosa of the dorsal horn (the gate). Large myelinated A-beta fibers responsible for touch and vibratory sensation also terminated at "the gate" in the dorsal horn. It was hypothesized that their input could be manipulated to "close the gate" to the transmission of painful stimuli. As an application of the gate control theory, Shealy implanted the first spinal cord stimulator device for the treatment of chronic pain.[2] This technique was noted to control pain and has undergone numerous technical and clinical refinements in the ensuing years. Although the gate theory was initially proposed as the mechanism of action, the underlying neurophysiologic mechanisms are not clearly understood.

The neurophysiologic mechanisms of action of SCS are not completely understood; however, recent research has given us insight into effects occurring at the local and supraspinal levels, and through dorsal horn interneuron and neurochemical mechanisms.[8,9] Linderoth and others have noted that the mechanism of analgesia when SCS is applied in neuropathic pain states may be very different from those involved in analgesia caused by limb ischemia or angina. Experimental evidence points to SCS having a beneficial effect at the dorsal horn level by favorably altering the local neurochemistry in that zone, thereby suppressing the hyperexcitability of the wide dynamic range interneurons. Specifically, there is some evidence for increased levels of GABA release, serotonin, and perhaps suppression of levels of some excitatory amino acids including glutamate and aspartate. In the case of ischemic pain, analgesia seems to be obtained through restoration of a favorable oxygen supply and demand balance—perhaps through a favorable alteration of sympathetic tone.

Technical Considerations

Spinal cord stimulation is a technically challenging interventional/surgical pain management technique. It involves the careful placement of an electrode array (leads) in the epidural space, a trial period, anchoring the lead(s), positioning and implantation of the pulse generator or radio frequency (RF) receiver, and the tunneling and connection of the connecting wires. This author advocates a collaborative effort between neurosurgeon and anesthesiologist for optimal success with neurostimulation.

Electrodes are of two types: catheter or percutaneous versus paddle or surgical (Figure 33–1). These electrodes are connected to an implanted pulse generator (IPG) or an RF unit (Figure 33–2). Currently, three companies, Medtronic Inc., American Neuromodulation Systems Inc.,

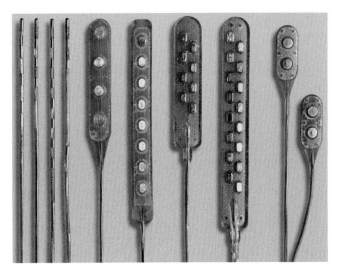

FIGURE 33–1 Neurostimulator leads (left to right): percutaneous type to paddle type (*Courtesy of ANS, Inc.*).

and Advanced Bionics, manufacture neurostimulation equipment (Appendix 1). Interested readers are directed to these companies for further specific information on the equipment.

A stimulator trial may be accomplished in two ways: "straight percutaneous" or "implanted lead." In both the trial methods, under fluoroscopy and sterile conditions, a lead is introduced into the epidural space with the standard epidural needle placement. The lead is steered under fluoroscopic imaging into the posterior paramedian epidural space up to the desired anatomic location. Trial stimulation is undertaken to attempt to "cover" the painful area with an electrically induced paresthesia. After the painful area is "captured" either with one or two leads, the two techniques diverge.

In the straight percutaneous trial, the needle is withdrawn, an anchoring suture placed into the skin, and a sterile dressing is applied. When the patient

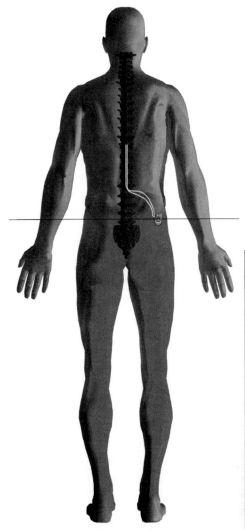

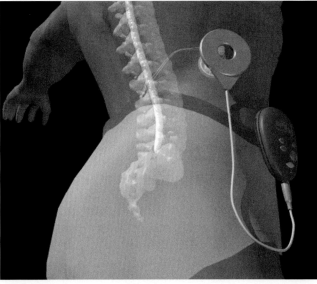

A   B

FIGURE 33–2 *A*, Schematic view of an implanted pulse generator (IPG) system implanted. *B*, Schematic view of an implanted radiofrequency spinal cord stimulation system (*A courtesy of Medtronic, Inc. B courtesy of ANS, Inc.*).

returns after a trial of several days, the dressing is removed, suture clipped, and the lead removed and discarded, regardless of the success of the trial. When the patient returns for implant, a new lead is placed in the location of the trial lead and connected to an implanted IPG.

In the "implanted lead" trial after successful positioning of the trial lead(s), local anesthetic is infiltrated around the needle(s) and an incision is made, cutting down to the supraspinous fascia to anchor the leads securely using nonabsorbable suture. Then a temporary extension piece is tunneled away from the back incision and out through the skin. This exiting piece is secured to the skin using a suture, antibiotic ointment, and a sterile dressing. If the trial is successful, at the time of implant the back incision is opened up, the percutaneous lead is cut, pulled out through the skin site, and discarded. The permanent lead(s) that were used for the trial are hooked to new extension(s) and tunneled to an implanted IPG.

The "implanted lead" method has the advantages of saving the cost of new electrodes at implant and ensuring that the implanted lead position matches the trial lead position. Advantages of the "percutaneous lead" approach include avoiding the cost of two trips to the operating room (even for an unsuccessful trial to remove the anchored trial lead); avoiding an incision and postoperative pain during the trial, which may confuse trial interpretation by the patient; and the percutaneous temporary extension has a risk for infection. The percutaneous extension must be anchored and meticulously dressed or the risk of infection may be higher than with the straight percutaneous technique.[10] Most consider 50% or greater pain relief to be indicative of a successful trial; although the ultimate decision also should include other factors such as activity level and medication intake. To paraphrase, some combination of pain relief, increased activity level, and decreased medication intake is indicative of a favorable trial.

A trial with paddle-type electrodes requires the "implanted lead" approach, with the significant addition of a laminotomy to slip the flat plate electrode into the epidural space. Some physicians trial the patient with the "straight percutaneous" approach and, if successful, will send the patient to a neurosurgeon for a paddle-type implant. The author's preference is to do a "straight percutaneous" trial, with an implant using nonpaddle-type electrodes.

The IPG/RF unit is generally implanted in the lower abdominal area or in the posterior superior gluteal area. It should be in a location the patient can access with their dominant hand for adjustment of their settings with the patient-held remote control unit. The decision to use a fully implantable IPG or an RF unit depends on several considerations. If the patient's pain pattern

requires the use of many anode/cathode settings with high power settings during the trial, consideration of an RF unit should be given. The IPG battery life will largely depend on the power settings utilized, but the newer IPG units (Synergy or Genesis XP) will generally last several years at average power settings.

Patient Selection

Appropriate patients for neurostimulation implant must meet the following criterion: the patient has a diagnosis amenable to this therapy (i.e., neuropathic pain syndromes) and has failed conservative therapy, significant psychological issues have been ruled out, and a trial has demonstrated pain relief.[11] However, pure neuropathic pain syndromes are relatively less common than the mixed nociceptive/neuropathic disorders, including failed back surgery syndrome (FBSS). Also, many patients with chronic pain will have some depressive symptomatology, but psychological screening can be extremely helpful to avoid implanting patients with major psychological disorders. An interesting study by Olson and colleagues revealed a high correlation between many items on a complex psychological testing battery and favorable response to trial stimulation.[12] This is to say that overall mood state is an important predictor of outcomes.

A careful trial period is advocated to avoid the failed implant. Trials of different lengths have been advocated; the risks of a longer trial are mainly infection, whereas the risks of too short of a trial are misreading success. We use a 5 to 7 day trial with the use of oral antibiotics. We encourage the patient to be as active as possible in their usual environment, with the exception of limiting bending/twisting movements. Despite advances in the understanding of diagnosis which respond to neurostimulation, increased understanding of and improved psychological screening, improved multilead systems, clinical failures of implanted neurostimulator devices remain too common and pain practitioners must critically evaluate their own outcomes and adhere to strict selection criterion outlined earlier.

Complications

Complications with SCS range from simple, easily correctable problems, such as lack of appropriate paresthesia coverage, to devastating complications such as paralysis, nerve injury, and death. Before the implantation of the trial lead, an educational session should occur with the patient and significant family members. This meeting should include a discussion of possible risks and complications. In the postoperative period, the caregiver should be involved in identifying problems and alerting the health care team.

North and colleagues reported their experience in 320 consecutive patients treated with SCS between 1972 and 1990.[13] A 5% rate of subcutaneous infection was seen and is consistent with the literature. The predominant complication consisted of lead migration or breakage. This remains the "Achilles' heel" of neurostimulation. In an earlier series, bipolar leads required electrode revision in 23% of patients. The revision rate for patients with multichannel devices was 16%. Failure of the electrode lead was observed in 13% of patients and steadily declined over the course of the study. When analyzed by implant type (single-channel percutaneous, single-channel laminectomy, and multichannel), the lead migration rate for multichannel devices was approximately 7%. Analysis of hardware reliability for 298 permanent implants showed that technical failures (particularly electrode migration and malposition) and clinical failures had become significantly less common as implants evolved into programmable, "multichannel" devices.

Studies by Barolat and May reported lead revision rates caused by lead migration of 4.5% and 13.6% and breakage of 0% and 13.6%, respectively.[14,15] Infections occurred in 7% and 2.5% of cases, respectively. No serious complications were seen in either study. These studies are representative of the complication rate of neurostimulation therapy.

Infections range from simple infections at the surface of the wound to epidural abscess. The patient should be instructed on wound care and recognition of signs and symptoms indicative of infection. Many superficial infections can be treated with oral antibiotics or simple surgical exploration and irrigation. At the authors' center, the standard includes prophylactic intraoperative antibiotics and oral coverage postoperatively for 10 days.

If infection reaches the tissues involving the devices, in most cases the implant should be removed. In such cases, one should have a high index of suspicion for an epidural abscess. Abscess of the epidural space can lead to paralysis and death if not identified quickly and treated aggressively. In the case of temporary epidural catheters (somewhat analogous to a percutaneous stimulator trial), Sarubbi and Vasquez discovered only 20 well-described cases.[16] The mean age of these 22 patients was 49.9 years, the median duration of epidural catheter use was 3 days, and the median time to onset of clinical symptoms after catheter placement was 5 days. The majority of patients (63.6%) had major neurologic deficits, and 22.7% also had concomitant meningitis. *Staphylococcus aureus* was the predominant pathogen. Despite antibiotic therapy and drainage procedures, 38% of the patients continued to have neurologic deficits. These unusual but serious complications of temporary epidural catheter use require efficient and accurate diagnostic evaluation and treatment because the consequences of delayed therapy can be substantial. Schuchard reported an infection with *Pasteurella* during an "implanted lead"

trial, which required explanting the system.[17] The author (AB) has experienced one similar case with *S. aureus* requiring explant of the entire system (unpublished data).

Programming

There are four basic parameters in neurostimulation, which may be adjusted to create stimulation paresthesias in the painful areas, thereby mitigating the patient's pain. They are amplitude, pulse width, rate, and electrode selection.[18]

Amplitude is the intensity or strength of the stimulation measured in volts (V). The voltage may be set from 0 to 10 V, with lower settings typically used over peripheral nerves and with paddle-type electrodes. Pulse width is a measure in microseconds (μsec) of the duration of a pulse. Pulse width is usually set between 100 and 400 μsec. A larger pulse width will typically give the patient a broader coverage. Rate is measured in hertz (Hz) or cycles per second, between 20 and 120 Hz. At lower rates, the patient feels more of a thumping, whereas at higher rates, the feeling is more of a buzzing. Electrode selection is a complex topic that has been the subject of some research by Barolat and colleagues, who provided mapping data of coverage patterns based on lead location in 106 patients.[19] The primary target is the cathode ("−"), with electrons flowing from the cathode(s) "−" to the anode(s) "+." Most patients' stimulators are programmed with electrode selection changed until the patient obtains anatomic coverage, then the pulse width and rate are adjusted for maximal comfort. The patient is left with full control of turning the stimulation off and on, and the voltage up and down to comfort.

We use an analogy of a stereo to discuss programming with patients. Amplitude is the "volume control," the pulse width is "how many speakers are on (mono vs. surround sound)," and the rate is the "bass or treble control." The lowest acceptable settings on all parameters are generally used to conserve battery life. Other programming modes that save battery life include a cycling mode during which the stimulator cycles full on/off at patient-determined intervals (minutes, seconds, or hours). The patient's programming may change over time and reprogramming needs are common. Both neurostimulator manufacturing companies are very helpful to clinicians with patient reprogramming assistance. Many busy pain practices designate a stimulator nurse to handle patient reprogramming needs.

OUTCOMES

The most common use for SCS in the United States is FBSS, whereas in Europe, peripheral ischemia is the predominate indication. With respect to clinical outcomes, it makes sense to subdivide the outcomes based on diagnosis. In a review of the available SCS literature, most evidence falls within the level IV (limited) or level V (indeterminate) categories due to the invasiveness of the modality and inability to provide blinded treatment. Because of rapidly evolving SCS technology, recognition must also be given to the time frame within which a study was performed. Basic science knowledge, implantation techniques, lead placement locations, contact array designs, and programming capabilities have changed dramatically from the time of the first implants. These improvements have lead to decreased morbidity and much greater probability of obtaining adequate paresthesia coverage and subsequent improved outcomes.[20] Thus, even a level II review study, such as the one by Turner with FBSS patients from 1966 to 1994, reported less positive outcomes than Barolat's level IV FBSS study in 2001.[21,22] The author believes this represents the effect of improving technology.

Failed Back Surgery Syndrome

There has been one recent prospective, randomized study on FBSS. North and colleagues[23] selected 50 patients as candidates for repeat laminectomy. All the patients had undergone previous surgery and were excluded from randomization if they presented with severe spinal canal stenosis, extremely large disc fragments, a major neurologic deficit such as foot drop, or radiographic evidence of gross instability. In addition, patients were excluded for untreated dependency on narcotic analgesics or benzodiazepines, major psychiatric comorbidity, the presence of any significant or disabling chronic pain problem, or a chief complaint of low back pain exceeding lower extremity pain. Crossover between groups was permitted after the 6-month follow-up. Of the 26 patients who had undergone reoperation, 54% (14 patients) crossed over to SCS. Of the 24 who had undergone SCS, 21% (5 patients) opted for crossover to reoperation. For 90% of the patients, long-term (3-year follow-up) evaluation has shown that SCS continues to be more effective than re-operation, with significantly better outcomes by standard measures and significantly lower rates of crossover to the alternative procedure. Additionally, patients randomized to reoperation used significantly more opioids than those randomized to SCS. Other measures assessing activities of daily living and work status did not differ significantly.

Two prospective case series have been done. The first, by Barolat examined the outcomes of patients with intractable low-back pain treated with epidural SCS utilizing paddle electrodes and an RF stimulator.[24] In four centers, 44 patients were implanted and followed with the visual analog scale (VAS), the Oswestry Disability Questionnaire, the Sickness Impact Profile (SIP), and a patient satisfaction rating scale. All patients

had back and leg pain and all had at least one previous back surgery, with most (83%) having two or more back surgeries, and 51% having had a spinal fusion. Data were collected at baseline, 6 months, 12 months, and 2 years.

All patients showed a reported mean decrease in their 10-point VAS scores compared with baseline. The majority of patients reported fair to excellent pain relief in both the low back and legs. At 6 months 91.6% of the patients reported fair to excellent relief in the legs and 82.7% of the patients reported fair to excellent relief in the low back. At one year 88.2% of the patients reported fair to excellent relief in the legs and 68.8% of the patients reported fair to excellent relief in the low back. Significant improvement in function and quality of life was found at both the 6-month and 1-year follow-ups using the Oswestry and SIP, respectively. The majority of patients reported that the procedure was worthwhile (92% at 6 months, 88% at 1 year). The authors concluded that SCS proved beneficial at 1 year for the treatment of patients with chronic low back and leg pain.

The second multicenter prospective case series was published by Burchiel in 1996.[25] The study included 182 patients with a permanent system after a percutaneous trial. Patient evaluation of pain and functional levels was performed before and 3, 6, and 12 months after implantation. Complications, medication usage, and work status also were monitored. A 1-year follow-up evaluation was available for 70 patients. All pain and quality-of-life measures showed statistically significant improvement, whereas medication usage and work status did not significantly improve during the treatment year. Complications requiring surgical interventions were experienced by 17% (12 of 70) of the patients.

There have been two systematic review articles on neurostimulation. Turner completed a meta-analysis from the articles related to the treatment of FBSS by SCS from 1966 to 1994.[26] They reviewed 39 studies that met the inclusion criteria. The mean follow-up period was 16 months with range of 1 to 45 months. Pain relief exceeding 50% was experienced by 59% of patients with a range of 15% to 100%. Complications occurred in 42% of patients, with 30% of patients experiencing one or more stimulator-related complications. However, all the studies were case control investigations. Based on this review, the authors concluded that there was insufficient evidence from the literature for drawing conclusions about the effectiveness of SCS relative to no treatment or other treatments, or about the effects of SCS on patient work status, functional disability, and medication use.

The second systematic review article on neurostimulation was written by North and Wetzel[27] and consisted of a review of case control studies and two prospective control studies. They concluded that if a patient reports a reduction in pain of at least 50% during a trial, as determined by standard rating methods, and demonstrates improved or stable analgesic requirements and activity levels, significant benefit may be realized from a permanent implant. The authors conclude that the bulk of the literature appears to support a role for SCS (in neuropathic pain syndromes) but caution that the quality of the existing literature is marginal because they are largely case series.

Complex Regional Pain Syndrome

Research of high quality regarding SCS and complex regional pain syndrome (CRPS) is limited, but existing data are overwhelmingly positive in terms of pain reduction, quality of life, analgesic usage, and function.

Kemler and colleagues published a prospective, randomized, comparative trial to compare SCS versus conservative therapy for CRPS.[28] Patients with a 6-month history of CRPS of the upper extremities were randomized to undergo trial SCS (and implant if successful) and physiotherapy versus physiotherapy alone. In this study, 36 patients were assigned to receive a standardized physical therapy program together with SCS, whereas 18 patients were assigned to receive therapy alone. In 24 of the 36 patients, randomized to SCS, along with physical therapy, the trial was successful, and permanent implantation was performed. At a 6-month follow-up assessment, the patients in the SCS group had a significantly greater reduction in pain, and a significantly higher percentage were graded as much improved for the global perceived effect. However, there were no clinically significant improvements in functional status. The authors concluded that in short term, SCS reduces pain and improves the quality of life for patients with CRPS involving the upper extremities.

Several important case series have been published on the use of neurostimulation in the treatment of CRPS. Calvillo reported a series of 36 patients with advanced stages of CRPS (at least 2 years duration) who had undergone successful SCS trial (>50% reduction of pain).[29] They were treated with either SCS, or PNS, and in some cases with both modalities. Thirty-six months after implantation, the reported pain measured on VAS was an average of 53% better, and this change was statistically significant. Analgesic consumption decreased in the majority of patients. Forty-one percent of patients had returned to work with modified duties. The authors concluded that in late stages of CRPS, neurostimulation (with SCS or PNS) is a reasonable option when alternative therapies have failed.

Another case series reported by Oakley is remarkable in that it used a sophisticated battery of outcomes tools to evaluate treatment response in CRPS using SCS.[30] The study followed 19 patients and analyzed the results from the McGill Pain Rating Index, the SIP, Oswestry Disability Profile, Beck Depression Inventory, and VAS. Nineteen patients were reported as a subgroup enrolled at two centers participating in a multicenter study of efficacy/outcomes of SCS. Specific preimplant and postimplant tests to measure outcome were administered. Statistically significant improvement in the SIP-physical and psychosocial subscales was documented. The McGill Pain Rating Index words chosen and sensory subscale also improved significantly, as did VAS scores. The Beck Depression Inventory trended toward significant improvement. All patients received at least partial relief and benefit from their device, with 30% receiving full relief. Eighty percent of the patients obtained at least 50% pain relief through the use of their stimulators. The average percent of pain relief was 61%. The authors concluded that patients with CRPS benefit significantly from the use of SCS, based on average follow-up of 7.9 months.

A literature review by Stanton-Hicks of SCS for CRPS consisted of seven case-series. These studies ranged in size from 6 to 24 patients. Results were noted as "good to excellent" in greater than 72% of patients over a time period of 8 to 40 months. The review concluded that SCS has proven to be a powerful tool in the management of patients with CRPS.[31]

A retrospective, 3-year, multicenter study of 101 patients by Bennett evaluated the effectiveness of SCS applied to complex regional pain syndrome I (CRPS I) and compared the effectiveness of octapolar versus quadrapolar systems, as well as high-frequency and multiprogram parameters.[32] VAS was significantly decreased in the group using the dual-octapolar system, with reductions in overall VAS approaching 70%. Of the dual-octapolar group, 74.8% used multiple arrays to maximize paresthesia coverage. VAS reduction in the group using quadrapolar systems approached 50%. Quadrapolar systems (86.3%) and dual-octapolar systems (97.2%) continued to be used. Overall satisfaction with stimulation was 91% in the dual-octapolar group and 70% in the quadrapolar group ($P < 0.05$). The authors concluded that SCS is effective in the management of chronic pain associated with CRPS I and that the use of dual-octapolar systems with multiple-array programming capabilities appeared to increase the paresthesia coverage and thus further reduce pain. High-frequency stimulation (>250 Hz) was found to be essential in obtaining adequate analgesia in 15% of the patients using dual-octapolar systems. (This frequency level was not available to those with quadrapolar systems.)

Peripheral Ischemia and Angina

Cook reported in 1976 that SCS effectively relieved pain associated with peripheral ischemia.[33] This result has been repeated and noted to have particular efficacy in conditions associated with vasospasm such as Raynaud's disease.[34] Many studies have shown impressive efficacy of SCS to treat intractable angina.[35] Reported success rates are consistently greater than 80%, and these indications already widely used outside of the United States, are certain to expand within the United States.

COST EFFECTIVENESS

Cost effectiveness of SCS (in the treatment of chronic back pain) was evaluated by Kumar and colleagues in 2002.[36] They prospectively followed 104 patients with FBSS. Of the 104 patients, 60 were implanted with an SCS using a standard selection criterion. Both groups were monitored over a period of 5 years. The stimulation group annual cost was $29,000 versus $38,000 in the control group. The authors found 15% return to work in the stimulation group versus 0% in the control group. The higher costs in the nonstimulator group were in the categories of medications, emergency center visits, x-rays, and ongoing physician visits.

Bell performed an analysis of the medical costs of SCS therapy in the treatment of patients with FBSS.[37] The medical costs of SCS therapy were compared with an alternative regimen of surgeries and other interventions. Externally powered (external) and fully internalized (internal) SCS systems were considered separately. No value was placed on pain relief or improvements in the quality of life that successful SCS therapy can generate. The authors concluded that by reducing the demand for medical care by FBSS patients, SCS therapy can lower medical costs and found that, on average, SCS therapy pays for itself within 5.5 years. For those patients for whom SCS therapy is clinically efficacious, the therapy pays for itself within 2.1 years.

Kemler performed a similar study that looked at "chronic reflex sympathetic dystrophy (RSD)" using outcomes and costs of care before and after the start of treatment.[38] This essentially is an economic analysis of the Kemler RSD outcomes paper. Fifty-four patients with chronic RSD were randomized to receive either SCS together with physical therapy (SCS + PT; $n = 36$) or physical therapy alone (PT; $n = 18$). Twenty-four SCS + PT patients responded positively to trial stimulation and underwent SCS implantation. During 12 months of follow-up, costs (routine RSD costs, SCS costs, out-of-pocket costs) and effects (pain relief by VAS, health-related quality of life [HRQL] improvement by EQ-5D) were assessed in both groups. Analyses were carried out up to 1 year and up to the expected time of death. SCS was both more effective and less costly than the

standard treatment protocol. Because of the high initial costs of SCS in the first year, the treatment per patient is $4,000 more than control therapy. However, in the lifetime analysis, SCS per patient is $60,000 cheaper than control therapy. In addition, at 12 months, SCS resulted in pain relief (SCS + PT [–2.7] versus PT [0.4] [$P < 0.001$]) and improved HRQL (SCS + PT [0.22] versus PT [0.03] [$P = 0.004$]). The authors found SCS to be both more effective and less expensive as compared with the standard treatment protocol for chronic RSD.

PERIPHERAL, CORTICAL, AND DEEP BRAIN STIMULATION

Besides stimulation of the spinal cord, neurostimulation can successfully be used at other locations in the peripheral and central nervous systems to provide analgesia.

Peripheral nerve stimulation was introduced by Wall and Sweet in the mid-1960s.[39] This technique has shown efficacy for peripheral nerve injury pain syndromes, as well as CRPS, with the use of a carefully implanted paddle lead using a fascial graft to help anchor the lead without traumatizing the nerve.[40]

Motor cortex and deep brain stimulation are techniques that have been explored to treat highly refractory neuropathic pain syndromes, including central pain, deafferentation syndromes, trigeminal neuralgia, and others.[41] Deep brain stimulation has become a widely used technique for movement disorders, but much less so for painful indications, although there have been many case reports of usefulness in treating highly refractory central pain syndromes.[42]

Applications of Neurostimulation in Cancer Pain

As has been described earlier, neurostimulation is most efficacious in neuropathic pain states. In active cancer pain, pure neuropathic pain states are unusual. Applications exist in this patient population, including (but not limited to) chemotherapy-induced painful peripheral neuropathy, postherpetic neuralgia, phantom limb pain, and postradiation plexopathies.[43,44] In treating patients who are cancer "survivors" some treatment principles must be kept in mind. When a patient who has had cancer develops a severe pain syndrome, a meticulous workup must be undertaken to rule out recurrent cancer. Also, at this time, magnetic resonance imaging (MRI) is contraindicated with an implanted SCS. Many cancer patients have surveillance MRIs periodically and advance communication with a patient's oncologist or primary physician is essential before implantation of an SCS system.

CONCLUSION

Spinal cord stimulation is an invasive, interventional surgical procedure. The difficulty of randomized clinical trials in such situations is well recognized. Based on the present evidence with two randomized, one prospective trial, and multiple retrospective trials, the evidence for SCS in properly selected populations with neuropathic pain states is moderate. Clearly, this technique should be reserved for patients who have failed more conservative therapies. With appropriate selection and careful attention to technical issues, the clinical results are overwhelmingly positive.

Linderoth has written some principles of neurostimulation which have been slightly modified here[45]:

- SCS mechanism of action is not completely understood but influences multiple components and levels within the CNS with both interneuron and neurochemical mechanisms.
- SCS therapy is effective for many neuropathic pain conditions. Stimulation-evoked paresthesia must be experienced in the entire painful area. No consistent evidence exists for the efficacy of neurostimulation in primary nociceptive pain conditions.
- Stimulation should be applied with low intensity, just suprathreshold for the activation of the low-threshold, large-diameter fibers, and should be of nonpainful intensity. To be effective, SCS must be applied continuously (or in cycles) for at least 20 minutes before the onset of analgesia. This analgesia develops slowly and typically lasts several hours after cessation of the stimulation.
- SCS has demonstrated clinical and cost effectiveness in FBSS and CRPS. Clinical effectiveness has also been shown in peripheral ischemia and angina.
- Multicontact, multiprogram systems improve outcomes and reduce the incidence of surgical revisions. Insulated paddle-type electrodes probably decrease the incidence of lead breakage, prolong battery life, and show early superiority in quality of paresthesia coverage and analgesia in FBSS as compared with permanent percutaneous electrodes.
- Serious complications are exceedingly rare but can be devastating. Meticulous care must be taken during implantation to minimize procedural complications. The most frequent complications are wound infections (approximately 5%) and lead breakage or migration (approximately 13% each for permanent percutaneous leads and 3% to 6% each for paddle leads).

Appendix: Manufacturers of Neurostimulation Equipment

- Medtronic Inc, 710 Medtronic Parkway, Minneapolis, MN, 55432, USA. 763-514-5604. www.medtronic.com
- American Neuromodulation Systems, Inc, 6501 Windcrest Drive, Suite 100, Plano, TX, 75024, USA. 800-727-7846. www.ans-medical.com.
- Advanced Bionics, 25129 Rye Canyon Loop, Valencia, CA 91355, USA. 800-678-2575. www.advancedbionics.com.

REFERENCES

1. Kumar K, Nath R, Wyant GM: Treatment of chronic pain by epidural spinal cord stimulation: A 10-year experience. J Neurosurg 5:402–407, 1991.
2. Shealy CN, Mortimer JT, Resnick J: Electrical inhibition of pain by stimulation of the dorsal columns: Preliminary reports. J Int Anesth Res Soc 46:489–491, 1967.
3. Kumar K, Toth C, Nath RK: Deep brain stimulation for intractable pain: A 15 year experience. Neurosurgery 40:736–746, 1997.
4. Nguyen JP, Lefaucher JP, Le Guerinel C, et al: Motor cortex stimulation in the treatment of central and neuropathic pain. Arch Med Res 31:263–265, 2000.
5. Campbell JN, Long DM: Stimulation of the peripheral nervous system for pain control. J Neurosurg 45:692–699, 1976.
6. Melzack R, Wall PD: Pain mechanisms: A new theory. Science 150:971–979, 1965.
7. Shealy CN, Mortimer JT, Resnick J: Electrical inhibition of pain by stimulation of the dorsal columns: Preliminary reports. J Int Anesth Res Soc 46:489–491, 1967.
8. Oakley J, Prager J: Spinal cord stimulation: Mechanism of action. Spine 27: 2574–2583, 2002.

9. Linderoth B, Foreman R: Physiology of spinal cord stimulation: Review and update. Neuromodulation 2:150–164, 1999.
10. May MS, Banks C, Thomson SJ: A retrospective, long-term, third-party follow-up of patients considered for spinal cord stimulation. Neuromodulation 5:137–144, 2002.
11. Burchiel KJ, Anderson VC, Wilson BJ, et al: Prognostic factors of spinal cord stimulation for chronic back and leg pain. Neurosurgery 36:1101–1111, 1995.
12. Olson KA, Bedder MD, Anderson VC, Burchiel KJ, Villenueva MR: Psychological variables associated with outcome of spinal cord stimulation trials. Neuromodulation 1:6–13, 1998.
13. North RB, Kidd DH, Zahurak M, James CS, Long DM: Spinal cord stimulation for chronic, intractable pain: Two decades' experience. Neurosurgery 32:384–395, 1993.
14. Barolat G, Oakley J, Law J, North R: Epidural spinal cord stimulation with a multiple electrode paddle lead is effective in treating low back pain. Neuromodulation 4:59–66, 2001.
15. May MS, Banks C, Thomson SJ: A retrospective, long-term, third-party follow-up of patients considered for spinal cord stimulation. Neuromodulation 5: 137–144, 2002.
16. Sarubbi F, Vasquez J: Spinal epidural abscess associated with the use of temporary epidural catheters: Report of two cases and review. Clin Infect Dis 25:1155–1158, 1997.
17. Schuchard M, Clauson W: An interesting and heretofore unreported infection of a spinal cord stimulator: Smitten by a kitten revisited. Neuromodulation 4:67–71, 2001.
18. Alfano S, Darwin J, Picullel B: Programming Principles in Spinal Cord Stimulation: Patient Management Guidelines for Clinicians, Medtronic, Inc, Minneapolis, 2001, pp 27–33.
19. Barolat G, Massaro F, He J, Zeme S, Ketcik B: Mapping of sensory responses to epidural stimulation of the intraspinal neural structures in man. J Neurosurg 78:233–239, 1993.
20. North RB, Kidd DH, Zahurak M, James CS, Long DM: Spinal cord stimulation for chronic, intractable pain: Experience over two decades. Neurosurgery 32:384–394, 1993.

21. Turner JA, Loeser JD, Bell KG: Spinal cord stimulation for chronic low back pain: A systematic literature synthesis. Neurosurgery 37:1088–1095; discussion 1095–1096, 1995.

22. Barolat G, Oakley J, Law J, North RB: Epidural spinal cord stimulation with a multiple electrode paddle lead is effective in treating low back pain. Neuromodulation 4:59–66, 2001.

23. North RB, Kidd DH, Farrokhi F, Piantadosi SA: Spinal cord stimulation versus repeated lumbosacral spine surgery for chronic pain: A randomized, controlled trial. Neurosurgery 56:98–106; discussion 106–107, 2005.

24. Barolat G, Oakley J, Law J, North R: Epidural spinal cord stimulation with a multiple electrode paddle lead is effective in treating low back pain. Neuromodulation 4:59–66, 2001.

25. Burchiel KJ, Anderson VC, Brown FD, et al: Prospective, multicenter study of spinal cord stimulation for the relief of chronic back and extremity pain. Spine 21: 2786–2794, 1996.

26. Turner JA, Loeser JD, Bell KG: Spinal cord stimulation for chronic low back pain: A systematic literature synthesis. Neurosurgery 37:1088–1095, 1995.

27. North R, Wetzel T: Spinal cord stimulation for chronic pain of spinal origin. Spine 27:2584–2591, 2002.

28. Kemler MA, Barendse GA, van Kleef M, et al: Spinal cord stimulation in patients with chronic reflex sympathetic dystrophy. N Engl J Med 343:618–624, 2000.

29. Calvillo O, Racz G, Didie J, Smith K: Neuroaugmentation in the treatment of complex regional pain syndrome of the upper extremity. Acta Orthopeadica Belgica 64:57–63, 1998.

30. Oakley J, Weiner R: Spinal cord stimulation for complex regional pain syndrome: A prospective study of 19 patients at two centers. Neuromodulation 2:47–50, 1999.

31. Stanton-Hicks M: Spinal cord stimulation for the management of complex regional pain syndromes. Neuromodulation 2:193–201, 1999.

32. Bennett D, Alo K, Oakley J, Feler C: Spinal cord stimulation for complex regional pain syndrome I (RSD): A retrospective multicenter experience from 1995-1998 of 101 patients. Neuromodulation 2:202–210, 1999.

33. Cook AW, Oygar A, Baggenstos P, Pacheco S, Kleriga E: Vascular disease of extremities: Electrical stimulation of spinal cord and posterior roots. NY State J Med 76:366–368, 1976.

34. Broseta J, Barbera J, De Vera JA: Spinal cord stimulation in peripheral arterial disease. J Neurosurg 64:71–80, 1986.

35. Eliasson T, Augustinsson LE, Mannheimer C: Spinal cord stimulation in severe angina pectoris-presentation of current studies, indications, and clinical experience. Pain 65:169–179, 1996.

36. Kumar K, Malik S, Demeria D: Treatment of chronic pain with spinal cord stimulation versus alternative therapies: Cost-effectiveness analysis. Neurosurgery 51:106–115, 2002.

37. Bell G, North R: Cost-effectiveness analysis of spinal cord stimulation in treatment of failed back surgery syndrome. J Pain Symptom Manage 13:285–296, 1997.

38. Kemler M, Furnee C: Economic evaluation of spinal cord stimulation for chronic reflex sympathetic dystrophy. Neurology 59:1203–1209, 2002.

39. Wall PD, Sweet WH: Temporary abolition of pain in man. Science 155:108–109, 1967.

40. Hassenbusch SJ, Stanton-Hicks M, Shoppa D: Long-term results of peripheral nerve stimulation for reflex sympathetic dystrophy. J Neurosurg 84:415–423, 1996.

41. Tsubokawa T, Katayama Y, Yamamoto T, et al: Chronic motor cortex stimulation in patients with thalamic pain. J Neurosurg 78:393–401, 1993.

42. Limousin P, Krack P, Pollack P, et al: Electrical stimulation of the subthalamic nucleus in advanced Parkinson's disease. NEJM 339:1105–1111, 1998.

43. Cata J, Cordiella J, Burton AW, Dougherty P, Hassenbusch SJ: Spinal cord stimulation effectively treats chemotherapy related painful peripheral neuropathy. J Pain Symptom Manage 27:72–78, 2004.

44. Harke H, Gretenkort P, Ladleif HU, Koestr P, Rahman S: Spinal cord stimulation in postherpetic neuralgia and in acute herpes zoster pain. Anesth Analg 94: 694–700, 2002.

45. Linderoth B, Meyerson BA: Spinal cord stimulation: Mechanisms of action in surgical management of pain. Burchiel K (ed): Thieme Medical Pub, Inc, New York, 2002, pp 505–526.

CHAPTER 34

Vertebroplasty and Kyphoplasty

Ronald A. Alberico, MD, Ahmed Abdel-Halim, MD, and Syed Hamed S. Husain, DO

It is well documented that malignant disease frequently metastasizes to bones. The length of time a patient suffers with metastatic disease increases the likelihood of bony involvement. As we become better at treating patients with malignancy, bony involvement will become more prevalent. Between 30% and 70% of bone metastases involve the vertebrae.[1] The result is chronic back pain caused by bone involvement in the majority of patients with metastatic disease and in those with marrow infiltrating diseases such as multiple myeloma and leukemia. Most bony metastases compromise the strength of the involved bone. In the vertebral bodies this decreased bone strength leads to pathologic compression fractures in 8% to 30% of patients, frequently without trauma.[2,3] It would appear that the physiologic load to the spine acting in isolation is sufficient to fracture the pathologically involved vertebral body. Other causes of vertebral compression fractures in patients with malignant disease include secondary osteoporosis from malnutrition, radiation treatments, or chronic steroid administration.

The consequences of pathologic compression fractures of the vertebral bodies are well documented in the osteoporotic population.[4] These complications include an acceleration of bone mineral loss caused by inactivity, perpetuating the likelihood of additional fractures. Inactivity also brings the risk of embolic and thrombotic complications in the lungs, as well as the lower extremities. The biomechanical effects of kyphosis secondary to vertebral body fractures include an increased risk of falling, a shift of biomechanical forces anteriorly thereby increasing risk of additional fractures, and physiologic decreases in lung capacity and appetite.[5,6] These processes describe a downward spiral that is known to significantly decrease the lifespan of patients after their first compression fracture. One study correlated a person's first vertebral compression fracture with significant increases in 1-year mortality.[7] This study revealed that the 1-year mortality of osteoporotic patients suffering one compression fracture is 23% higher than

age-matched controls! This number increases to greater than 30% for patients with multiple fractures.

Historically, medicine has had little to offer cancer patients with painful vertebral compression fractures that did not respond well to analgesic therapy. The surgical options frequently are not possible in this population because of the overall suboptimal health of the patients and the relatively long recovery time. Surgeons also avoid patients with multilevel disease.[8] As a result, surgery is reserved for those with anatomic compression of the spinal canal contents by retropulsion of bone. Therapeutic and palliative radiation therapy is an alternative to surgery for malignant bone pain and spinal canal compromise caused by epidural extension of tumor. Palliative radiation can be ineffective in up to 30% of patients, however, and cannot be given if maximal doses to the spine were already delivered for tumor treatment of the spine or adjacent structures. Radiation may also contribute to secondary osteoporosis, thereby increasing the risk of compression fracture, particularly after therapeutic doses. In recent years, the intravenous administration of bisphosphonates has shown some efficacy for those with chronic bone pain and may help prevent pathologic fractures, but its efficacy in pain relief for patients who have already suffered fractures is not established.[9] With the exception of surgery, none of the treatments listed addresses the issue of altered biomechanical forces in the spine and the other consequences of kyphosis.

In recent years interventional techniques have significantly improved our ability to perform minimally invasive procedures. The advantage of these procedures is that they frequently can be performed on patients who are otherwise too sick to endure more extensive techniques, while providing a significant improvement in response to that of medical therapy alone. The remainder of this chapter will describe the two minimally invasive procedures that are designed to address vertebral compression fractures and the associated chronic back pain. Both procedures have advantages and disadvantages, which will be discussed, as well as indications, contraindications, and risks. This chapter will not act as a tutorial for performing the techniques because that would require formal training in an established course with the guidance of experienced instructors.

VERTEBROPLASTY

Percutaneous vertebroplasty was first described by Galibert and Deramond in France in 1987.[10] The initial procedure was designed for treatment of a painful vertebral body hemangioma. The procedure itself can be summarized as a percutaneous fixation of pathologic vertebral compression fractures by injection of poly-methyl-methacrylate (PMMA) through a needle inserted into the vertebral body. Most procedures use a transpediculate approach for needle insertion to avoid segmental arteries that extend along the side of the vertebral body. Vertebroplasty is usually performed with the patient in the prone position, using strict sterile technique, conscious sedation, local anesthesia, and fluoroscopic guidance. Approaches have been described using one or two pediculate needles with similar results.[11,12] The fluoroscopic target is well defined anatomically, and success at accessing the pedicle with proper fluoroscopic technique and knowledge of the patient anatomy is dependent upon adequate visualization of the target during the procedure (Figure 34–1).

Indications and Contraindications

There are two main groups of patients that may benefit from vertebroplasty: those with pathologic fractures and associated pain and those with progressive vertebral compression from pathologic fractures. All patients must have a vertebral compression fracture that is related to a pathologic process to qualify for treatment at this time. Trauma-associated fracture without pathologic bone is not treated because of more definitive surgical options that are available. It is also felt that the small amount of space available in the trabecular network of normal bone increases the likelihood of cement extravasation during the injection process. For those patients with painful compression fractures, the pain should be directly related to the vertebral fracture on clinical examination, limit patient mobility or quality of life, and require chronic medication for control. Some patients that are more difficult to assess in terms of pain localization can benefit from imaging with magnetic resonance imaging (MRI) or bone scan.[13] Those patients with increased uptake on bone scan or demonstrable edema within the bone on MRI are more likely to obtain pain relief than those without imaging abnormality beyond simple compression. For patients with progressive vertebral compression deformity over time demonstrated on x-ray, MRI, or computed tomography (CT), vertebroplasty is indicated to arrest the progress of the deformity. The contraindications to

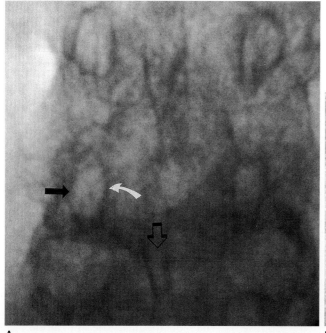
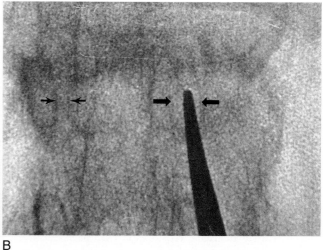

A   B

FIGURE 34–1   *A,* An anterior-posterior (AP) view of the spine shows the lateral wall (black arrow) and medial wall (curved white arrow) of the pedicle. Note the spinous process projects in the midline (open arrow). *B,* This oblique view of the spine shows a clamp projected over the midline of the pedicle. The large arrows point to the lateral and medial wall of the pedicle. The small arrows demonstrate the proximity of the lateral wall of the spinous process and the medial wall of the other pedicle when the obliquity is optimized for a two-needle approach (small arrows). A single needle approach would project the spinous process on top of the pedicle.

vertebroplasty include active osteomyelitis, all contraindications to conscious sedation, severe (> 30%) preexisting stenosis of the spinal canal, existing coagulopathy or thrombocytopenia (platelet count < 80,000), pregnancy, and hypersensitivity to PMMA or other implanted devices. Coagulopathy and thrombocytopenia can, of course, be corrected before the procedure. Epidural or intradural neoplastic disease compressing or encasing the thecal sack or nerve roots is also a contraindication to treatment. Relative contraindications include a dehiscent posterior cortical wall in the effected vertebral body, an inability of the patient to attain the prone position, and difficulty visualizing the vertebral structures at fluoroscopy. Ongoing or future radiation therapy is not a contraindication for vertebroplasty. PMMA has been shown to be unaffected by radiation at therapeutic doses in vitro.[14]

Efficacy

The literature on vertebroplasty is extensive and has evaluated both osteoporotic fractures and fractures secondary to solid and marrow-based malignancy.[15-18] Rates of pain relief after treatment vary somewhat among the reports. Pain relief is generally realized within 5 days of treatment and is maximal within 2 weeks. Pain relief is generally assessed with visual analog scale (VAS) and reported as complete, improved, unchanged, or worse. Reported relief is less frequent for cancer patients than for those with osteoporosis but still significant at 50% to 80% in most series. Lack of equivalent efficacy in the cancer patients is undoubtedly caused by multifactorial sources of pain in that population. Durability of pain relief in vertebroplasty is also demonstrated in some studies with follow-up assessment extending to 2 to 5 years. Despite the success with vertebroplasty, the procedure does not attempt to correct kyphotic deformity or to reestablish normal vertebral body height.

The exact mechanism of pain relief in vertebroplasty and kyphoplasty is not yet established. Potential sources of pain relief include fixation of chronically mobile bone fragments. Other possibilities include thermal neurolysis. PMMA polymerization is an exothermic process that can produce temperatures close to 70° C. It is theorized that this may damage nerve endings in the affected bone, thereby decreasing the pain response.

Procedure

In our institution, vertebroplasty is performed by neuroradiology and is almost exclusively done as an outpatient procedure. Patients are initially evaluated as to the source of pain and appropriate level or levels to treat by the neuroradiologist through a clinic appointment and are scheduled for an ambulatory surgery appointment on the day of treatment. The patients are instructed to take nothing orally after midnight the day of treatment and are confirmed to have a normal coagulation profile and platelet count before proceeding. Almost all vertebroplasties are performed successfully with conscious sedation administered by the operating physician in cooperation with a nurse. The nurse performs appropriate monitoring and documentation during the procedure. The majority of cases require 2 to 4 mg of intravenous Versed and 150 to 250 µg of fentanyl for patient comfort over the course of 1 to 2 hours. Lidocaine, 1%, is used over each access point for anesthesia and care is taken to infiltrate the region directly over the entry site into the bone. All patients receive a dose of antibiotics and 100 mg of Solu-Cortef intravenously during the procedure. Some centers also mix tobramycin powder with the PMMA before injection for prophylaxis. No more than three levels are treated at one setting primarily because of the negative effects of prolonged prone positioning, but also to avoid high volumes of PMMA injection and associated potential toxicity of unpolymerized monomer. Vertebroplasty can usually be performed with one needle for each treated level (Figure 34–2). The large majority of patients are discharged the afternoon of the procedure. Instructions given to the patient include restrictions on heavy lifting (> 5 pounds) for 1 week, restrictions on submerging the wounds for 1 week (showers are allowed), and instructions regarding signs and symptoms of infection. Patients are told to expect discomfort from the needle tracts for 5 to 7 days and that their existing pain medicine can be taken as directed for this pain. The patient is contacted by telephone 2 days after the procedure either by the operating physician or by a nurse. Follow-up visits are arranged at 2 weeks and 3 months after the procedure in the vertebroplasty clinic.

Although minimally invasive, vertebroplasty is not without risk. Complications have been shown to include fracture (of the vertebral body being treated and of ribs related to prone positioning), infection, major vessel or nerve injury, epidural hematoma, cerebral spinal fluid leak, and cement extravasation. Cement extravasation is the most frequent and occasionally the most serious complication potentially resulting in cord compression (<0.5%), nerve root compression (1% to 2%) and pulmonary emboli (<1%). The complication rate has been demonstrated to be directly related to the volume of injected PMMA.[15-19] Fortunately, pain relief is not related to volume of injection and seems to occur with relatively small amounts of injected PMMA (2 to 4 mL).[20,21] Proper technique is critical in avoiding complications. To successfully perform vertebroplasty procedures, optimal visualization of the PMMA during the injection process is required. This is best done with a fully functional angiography suite with biplane or single plane high-quality fluoroscopy. Alternatively, similar safety can be achieved

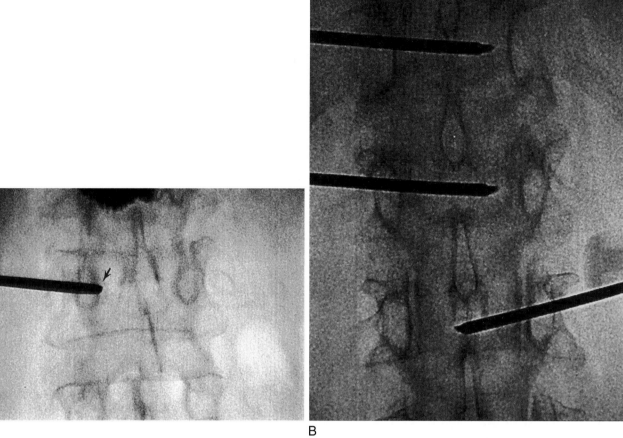

FIGURE 34–2   The images show stages of a vertebroplasty from start to finish. *A,* The pedicle needle in the anterior-posterior (AP) projection appears to extend beyond the medial wall of the pedicle, but this is an artifact of projection. The true needle position can only be seen with a combination of two orthogonal views or with a view down the needle barrel. *B,* The needle is advanced until the tip crosses the midline in the AP projection as seen here in these three levels.

with high-quality portable fluoroscopy in an operating room setting, but poor quality portable fluoroscopy opens the door for major undetected extravasation of PMMA. We should note that the great majority of cement extravasations are asymptomatic (Figure 34–3).

KYPHOPLASTY

Although it has been shown to be effective for painful vertebral compression fractures, several concerns about vertebroplasty exist in the medical community. The fact that kyphotic deformity has been shown in the literature to significantly affect the biomechanics of the spine has lead some physicians to question the wisdom of stabilizing a compressed vertebral body without reduction of the deformity. Other concerns about the use of vertebroplasty center on the injection process itself. Vertebroplasty uses an injection of relatively low viscosity PMMA into a

collapsed vertebral body. The result is a stabilization of the bone fragments without reduction of the deformity and a relatively high rate of cement extravasation (30% to 60%).[19-21] Although extravasation in most cases is asymptomatic, there is a definite risk of neurologic compression and associated severe deficits. Because vertebroplasty does not address the issue of deformity, techniques were advanced to correct that deficiency, and kyphoplasty was conceived. Kyphoplasty was first performed in 1998.[22] After initial success, more structured evaluation of the technique was undertaken as part of the FDA approval process for the inflatable bone tamp (IBT). The IBT is a balloon similar to an angioplasty balloon that is inserted into the compressed bone and inflated in order to reduce the fracture and create a cavity for the delivery of the PMMA (see Figure 34–3). In 2001, Belkoff and colleagues investigated the use of the IBT for reduction of vertebral compression fractures in vitro.[23] Liebermann and colleagues, also in 2001,

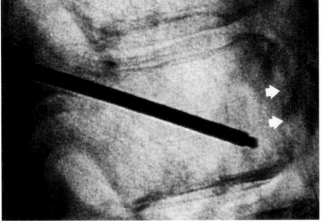

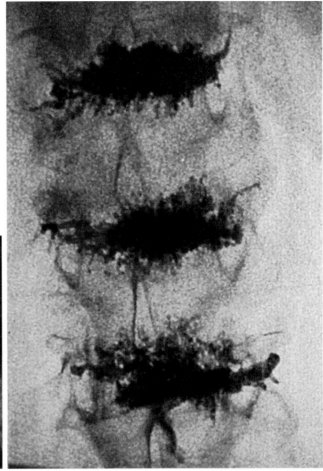

C   D

FIGURE 34-2   cont'd C, The lateral projection shows the optimal position of the needle tip relative to the anterior vertebral body wall (arrows). D, The AP view after completion reveals excellent bilateral filling of all three levels.

established the efficacy of percutaneous fixation and reduction of vertebral fractures using the IBT as a phase I evaluation in a series of patients with osteoporotic compression fractures.[24] In their study of 70 kyphoplasty procedures in 30 patients, a significant increase in vertebral body height was seen in 70% of cases with an average of 47% recovery of lost vertebral height. Thirty percent of treated levels had no increase in vertebral body height. There was statistically significant improvement in bodily pain, physical and social function, and mental health after the procedure. Extravasation of cement was seen in only 8.6% of levels treated and was asymptomatic in all cases. The findings of these studies support the use of kyphoplasty as an alternative to vertebroplasty in the osteoporotic population.

Although the kyphoplasty technique presented an attractive alternative to vertebroplasty in the osteoporotic population, its use in malignancy has not been established. Concerns about kyphoplasty, in particular the inflation of the IBT in bones that are infiltrated with solid tumor, are centered on the potential asymmetric

strength of these pathologic bones. If sclerotic bone was present anteriorly in the vertebral body with osteolytic foci posteriorly, it is conceivable that the IBT would cause a retropulsion of the posterior vertebral wall and subsequent neuronal compression. Liquid or marrow-based malignancy such as multiple myeloma was considered similar to osteoporotic bone in that the weakness of the bone was more likely diffuse; however, this also had not been established experimentally.

In 2002, a report on 55 kyphoplasty procedures performed in patients with multiple myeloma established the technique as safe and effective in this population.[25] The series demonstrated restoration of 34% of lost vertebral height in approximately 70% of treated levels. Cement extravasation occurred in 4% based on review of postprocedure radiographs. Pain relief was significant in all patients treated based on short form 36 health survey (SF36) data completed before and after treatment. In 2003, a report of vertebroplasty and kyphoplasty for malignant compression fractures included kyphoplasty performed at nine levels involved with solid

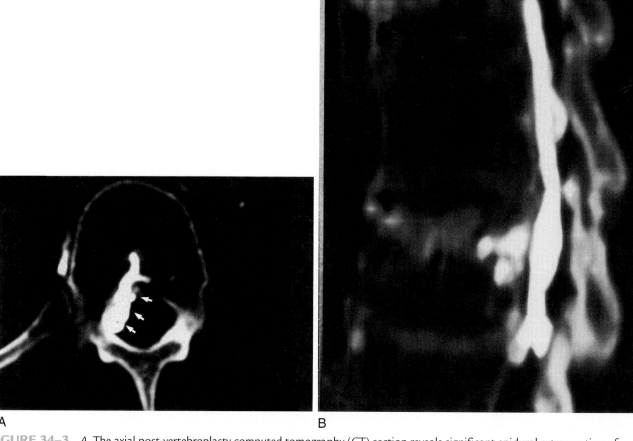

A   B

FIGURE 34–3   *A,* The axial post-vertebroplasty computed tomography (CT) section reveals significant epidural extravasation of polymethylmethacrylate (arrows). *B,* The sagittal reformatted image from the CT image reveals the cement extravasation extended for three levels. This patient was asymptomatic from the extravasation but complained of persistent unchanged pain after the procedure.

tumor processes. No complications occurred in this study and pain relief was achieved in 84% of procedures. Cement extravasation did not occur in the kyphoplasty group.[26] Although more work needs to be done with regard to kyphoplasty in solid tumor metastases, initial results are promising.

The durability of pain relief and vertebral height restoration after kyphoplasty has recently been evaluated.[26] In a study of 96 patients with 133 fractures, pain relief and vertebral height restoration were similar to that reported by other groups. Cement extravasation during kyphoplasty remained lower than that reported for vertebroplasty at 8% in this group. Furthermore, at 1 year the 26 patients available for follow-up had no decrease in height of the treated levels and maintained levels of pain relief. An impressive component of this study is that 10 out of 12 patients who were wheelchair-bound preoperatively were fully ambulatory at follow-up.

Why should we continue to consider patients for vertebroplasty if kyphoplasty is shown to have less frequent cement extravasation, efficacy with regard to fracture reduction, and better efficacy for pain relief? The answers lie in the mechanics of the techniques. Vertebroplasty is almost always done with conscious sedation as an outpatient procedure. Frequently, a single needle approach is possible, and a smaller (13 gauge) access system can be used. Kyphoplasty requires a dual needle approach with a 4.5-mm access diameter to accommodate the IBT insertion. Additional needle exchange and IBT inflation steps increase the complexity and duration of kyphoplasty compared with vertebroplasty (Figure 34–4). General anesthesia or heavy sedation is required, and many sites admit patients for overnight recovery. Kyphoplasty requires a higher degree of skill during insertion of the access system because of its large size, although those with vertebroplasty experience rarely have difficulty. The large access system also limits the ability to treat severely compressed vertebrae. Finally, kyphoplasty is considerably more expensive than vertebroplasty. A vertebroplasty at a single level can be

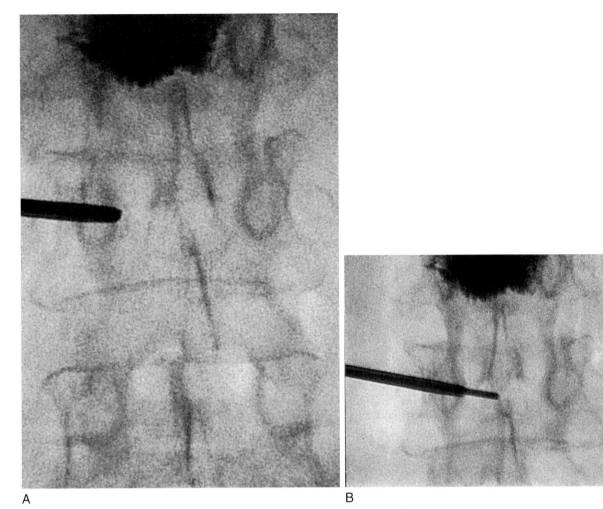

A

B

FIGURE 34–4   Images *A–I* demonstrate the steps involved in kyphoplasty. *A*, The guide needle is typically 11 gauge, and here it is positioned before advance along the pedicle. *B*, After the needle is positioned, a guide pin is advanced through the needle to maintain an access corridor for advancing the larger working needle.

Continued

performed with approximately $200 worth of equipment plus the use of the room, whereas kyphoplasty requires disposable IBT devices that cost more than $3000 per level in addition to anesthesiology, increased time in the room, and potential overnight admission.

The preoperative evaluation and clinic appointments for kyphoplasty and vertebroplasty are identical. The interventionalist should decide, based on the patient's health, severity, and location of compressed levels, which procedure or combination of procedures is most appropriate for each patient. The selection process itself is evolving as the technology and indications continue to expand.

CONCLUSION

As with all invasive techniques, maximal safety for vertebroplasty and kyphoplasty is achieved with maximal information. Efficacy is dependent on meticulous technique and appropriate patient selection. This is optimally achieved with a multidisciplinary approach with cooperation among the interventionalist, the neurosurgeon, or orthopedic surgeon, the radiation oncologist/oncologist, and the pain management team. The preoperative evaluation must include a complete physical examination, including detailed neurologic assessment, appropriate imaging, and blood work including platelet count and coagulation profile. The interventionalist should have adequate support in the event of a complication in the form of available surgical options and medical management in the treatment center. Anyone performing these techniques should undergo dedicated training under direct supervision of an experienced instructor. High-quality fluoroscopic equipment is required, as is knowledge of fluoroscopic landmarks and operative techniques. Attempting to perform these procedures without any one of these components will potentially lead to serious complications such as paralysis or death.

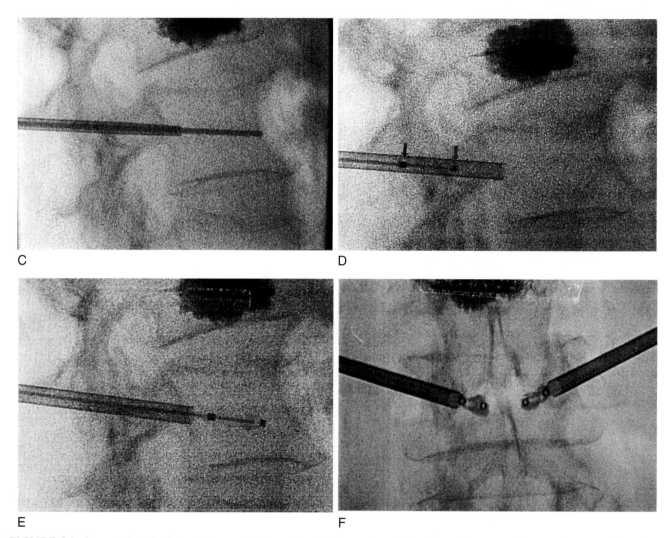

FIGURE 34–4 cont'd *C*, The lateral view reveals the guide pin is inserted to within a few millimeters of the anterior cortex. Note the needle remains only a few millimeters deep to the pedicle. *D*, The lateral view reveals the position of the working cannula after exchange over the guide pin. The distal markers of the inflatable balloon tamp (IBT) are visible in the cannula lumen (arrows). *E*, The IBT has been advanced into the vertebral body after a hand drill was used to clear away a cavity for it. *F*, After placement of the second working cannula and IBT, this anterior-posterior (AP) view shows good central position of the IBTs within the bone.

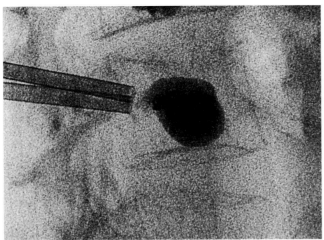

G

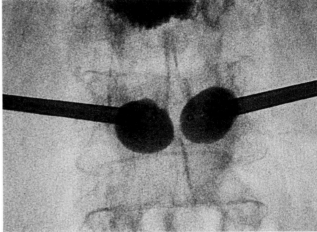

H

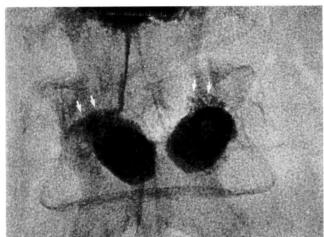

I

FIGURE 34–4 cont'd *G*, The lateral view shows the IBTs after inflation to create the cavity that will accept the polymethylmethacrylate. The IBTs are seen in the AP projection in image *H*. *I*, The final image with needles and IBTs removed. Polymethylmethacrylate fills the cavities created by the IBTs and extends minimally into the adjacent trabecular bone (arrows).

REFERENCES

1. Janjan N: Bone metastases: Approaches to management. Semin Oncol 28, suppl 11:28–34, 2001.
2. Patel B, DeGroot H: Evaluation of the risk of pathologic fractures secondary to metastatic bone disease. Othopedics 24:612–617, 2001.
3. Bunting R, Lamont-Havers W, Schweon D, et al: Pathological fracture risk in rehabilitation of patients with bony metastases. Clin Orthop 249:256–264, 1985.
4. Riggs LR, Melton LJ: The worldwide problem of osteoporosis: Lessons from epidemiology. Bone 17:505s–511s, 1995.
5. Schlaich C, Minne HW, Bruckner T, et al: Reduced pulmonary function in patients with spinal osteoporotic fractures. Osteoporos Int 8:261–267, 1998.
6. Silverman S: The clinical consequences of vertebral compression fracture. Bone 13:27–32, 1992.
7. Kado DM, Browner WS, Palermo L, et al: Vertebral fractures and mortality in older women: A prospective study. Study of osteoporotic fractures research group. Arch Intern Med 159:1215–1220, 1999.

8. Greenberg MS: Handbook of Neurosurgery. 5th ed. New York, Theime Medical Publishers, 2001.
9. Body JJ: Effectiveness and cost of bisphosphonates therapy in tumor bone disease. Cancer 97 supp:859–865, 2003.
10. Galibert P, Deramond H, Rosat P, et al: Note preliminaire sur le traitment des angiomes vertebraux par vertebroplastie acrylique percutanee. Neurochirurgie 33:166–168, 1987.
11. Evans AJ, Jensen ME, Kip KE, et al: Vertebral compression fractures: Pain reduction and improvement in functional mobility after percutaneous polymethylmethacrylate vertebroplasty-retrospective report of 245 cases. Radiology 226:366–372, 2003.
12. Deramond H, Depriester C, Galibert P, et al: Percutaneous vertebroplasty with polymethylmethacrylate: Techniques, indications, and results. Radiol Clin North Am 36:533–546, 1998.
13. Baur A, Stabler A, Arbogast S, et al: Acute osteoporotic and neoplastic vertebral compression fractures: Fluid sign at MR imaging. Radiology 225:730–735, 2002.

14. Murray JA, Bruels MC, Lindberg RD: Irradiation of polymethylmethacrylate: In vitro gamma radiation effect. J Bone Joint Surg 56A:311–312, 1974.
15. Garfin SR, Yuan HA, Reiley MA: Kyphoplasty and vertebroplasty for the treatment of painful osteoporotic compression fractures. Spine 26: 1511–1515, 2001.
16. Lane JM, Johnson CE, Khan SN, et al: Minimally invasive options for the treatment
17. Lin JT, Lane JM: Nonmedical management of osteoporosis. Curr Opin Rheumatol 14:441–446, 2002.
18. Fourney DR, Schomer DF, Nader R, et al: Percutaneous vertebroplasty and kyphoplasty for painful vertebral compression fractures in cancer patients. J Neurosurg 98(spine 1):21–30, 2003.
19. Moreland DB, Landi MK, Grand W: Vertebroplasty: Techniques to avoid complications. Spine J 1:66–71, 2001.
20. Cotton A, Dewatre F, Cortet B, et al: Percutaneous vertebroplasty for osteolytic metastases and myeloma: Effects of the

percentage of lesion filling and the leakage of methyl methacrylate at clinical follow-up. Radiology 200:525–530, 1996.

21. Tomeh AG, Mathis JM, Fenton DC, et al: Biomechanical efficacy of unipeducular versus bipedicular vertebroplasty for the management of osteoporotic compression fractures. Spine 24:1772–1776, 1999.

22. Wong W, Reilly MA, Garfin S: Vertebroplasty/kyphoplasty. Journal of Women's Imaging 2:117–124, 2000.

23. Belkoff SM, Mathis JM, Fenton DC, et al: An ex vivo biomechanical evaluation of an inflatable bone tamp used in the treatment of compression fracture. Spine 26:151–156, 2001.

24. Lieberman IH, Dudeney S, Reinhardt MK, et al: Initial outcome of "kyphoplasty" in the treatment of painful osteoporotic vertebral compression fractures. Spine 26:1631–1637, 2001.

25. Dudeney S, Lieberman IH, Reinhardt MK, et al: Kyphoplasty in the treatment of osteolytic vertebral compression fractures from multiple myeloma. J Clin Oncol 20:2382–2387, 2002.

26. Ledlie JT, Renfro M: Balloon kyphoplasty: one-year outcomes in vertebral body height restoration, chronic pain, and activity levels. J Neurosurg 98(spine 1):36–42, 2003.

CHAPTER 35

Neurosurgical Procedures for Cancer Pain Management

ROBERT A. FENSTERMAKER, MD

In recent years, the role of the neurosurgeon with regard to cancer pain management has evolved significantly as more effective medical pain management strategies have been devised. In particular, a shift in emphasis to surgical methods for the treatment of patients with pain caused by spinal metastatic disease has occurred. These procedures are designed to decompress neural elements and to reconstruct and stabilize the spine, which is a frequent source of pain caused by malignancy. Surgical techniques to decompress neural structures and create spinal stability provide excellent pain relief and help to prevent or even reverse serious coexisting neurologic deficits. Consequently, these methods have become the principle focus of neurosurgical cancer pain management in recent years. However, for cancers affecting the head and neck, chest wall, extremities, and visceral organs of the abdomen and pelvis, other traditional stereotactic and functional neurosurgical techniques may still find application in selected cases. These techniques are employed to produce specific lesions in neuroanatomic pathways that mediate nociception. Although improvements in pharmacologic therapy have led to a significant reduction in the use of these particular neurosurgical methods, there continues to be a limited role for cordotomy and other ablative procedures in the management of patients with unremitting cancer pain.

METASTATIC DISEASE OF THE SPINE

Metastatic disease of the spinal column continues to be a major source of pain and neurologic disability in cancer patients. Magnetic resonance imaging (MRI) has greatly improved our understanding of the pathologic anatomy of spinal metastases and their effect on the structural integrity of the spine. Newer surgical techniques permit greater access to the affected spinal segments for tumor removal, as well as better methods to reconstruct and stabilize the spine. Consequently, the approach to such tumors and the pain that they produce has changed substantially. Improved diagnostic and treatment methods now permit the use of surgical strategies at an earlier stage of the disease, with excellent results for both pain control and preservation of neurologic function over the patient's remaining life span. Hence, in addition to the prevention or alleviation of neurologic deficit, pain control is becoming an important primary indication for surgical intervention in an increasing number of cases.

Over 90% of patients with spinal metastases have pain at the time of their initial presentation.[1-3] One key to early diagnosis of spinal metastases is the recognition that back pain in the setting of malignancy often precedes evidence of objective neurologic dysfunction. Ordinarily, pain precedes the onset of neurologic deficit by weeks to months. However, both may occur abruptly after minor trauma, such as a fall, leading to pathologic spinal fracture. Pain arises from periosteal or ligamentous involvement by tumor, irritation of the spinal dura, nerve root (radicular) compromise, pathologic fracture, or vertebral collapse with creation of an abnormal motion segment. In each of these instances, pain is frequently exacerbated by motion of the spine, indicating its mechanical origin. Patients without bony destruction by tumor, but who have epidural metastatic disease, frequently do not have mechanical back pain, making the early diagnosis of spinal involvement more difficult in such cases.

In contrast with pain, weakness is uncommon at the onset of disease. However, by the time of diagnosis, 75% of patients have a demonstrable motor deficit and 60% have either bowel or bladder dysfunction.[1-3] Progressive compression of the spinal cord or cauda equina leads to paraparesis or quadriparesis, impaired sensation, and autonomic dysfunction. Early in the course of disease, loss of pinprick and light-touch sensation may be patchy.

Later, a distinct loss of sensation below the affected spinal level often develops, indicating significant spinal cord compromise. With cervical and thoracic lesions, deep tendon reflexes are often brisk and extensor plantar responses (Babinski signs) and ankle clonus are observed. The speed of neurologic progression can be quite variable depending upon the degree and rate of bone destruction and spinal cord compression, with acute or subacute development of paraparesis and rapid progression to paraplegia and incontinence. In addition to pain, associated neurologic deficits have a marked impact on the patient's quality of life. Therefore, controlling both pain and neurologic deficit are critical goals of medical, surgical, and radiation oncologic management of metastatic spinal tumors.

SURGICAL INDICATIONS

Bony destruction by metastatic tumor often produces structural spinal instability leading to back pain and radicular symptoms (pain, numbness, and paresthesias), as well as progressive neurologic deficits. One factor underlying this phenomenon is the development of an abnormal motion segment in the spine caused by vertebral destruction and collapse. Kyphotic spinal deformity may develop with retropulsion of tumor or bone fragments into the spinal canal. In contrast with the symptoms produced by tumor tissue within the spinal canal, the pain and neurologic deficit produced by displacement of bone either into the canal or against exiting spinal nerve roots frequently does not respond consistently to radiation therapy. Similarly, the pain produced by mechanical instability and abnormal motion may not respond to radiation therapy. Thus, in certain cases surgery to decompress the neural elements and to reestablish the structural integrity of the spine may be required for truly effective pain management.

For patients with lumbar or thoracic spinal tumor involvement, bed rest and elimination of a weight-bearing posture often provide significant short-term pain relief. These measures may also prevent neurologic progression temporarily but will do little to reverse it once it is present. When attempting to mobilize such a patient, pain often recurs unless effective bracing with a thoracolumbar orthosis is used. Similarly, for cervical pain and instability, the use of a firm cervical collar may be of substantial temporary benefit. Such measures are frequently overlooked in favor of pharmacologic interventions, which may be less effective and may produce sedation, confusion, and autonomic side effects. It has long been recognized that high-potency glucocorticoids such as dexamethasone and methylprednisolone are often of great benefit in relieving neurologic deficit and pain. Consequently, these should be employed early and throughout the course of radiation therapy. Ultimately, however, immobilization and corticosteroids alone are only of short-term benefit.

In the presence of a tumor of known histology that is likely to be radiosensitive, the patient with stable neurologic function and no spinal instability is usually treated primarily with high-potency corticosteroids, orthotic bracing, and radiation therapy. This approach will frequently lead to a significant improvement in pain and, to a lesser extent, ambulatory status.[1-3] In patients with advanced disease and short life expectancy, these measures may be all that are necessary to provide satisfactory management. With extended survival, however, preservation of neurologic function and maintenance of pain relief for longer periods of time may become problematic.

In addition to pain, other potential indications for surgical intervention include: (1) the need for a histologic diagnosis, (2) the presence of a radioresistant tumor, (3) neurologic deterioration during or after radiotherapy, (4) the presence of bone within the spinal canal, and (5) the existence of spinal instability or progressive spinal deformity. In each case, a recommendation regarding surgery must be predicated upon a number of factors. Such things as tumor histology, extent of systemic disease, life expectancy, and relevant comorbidities must be weighed carefully, along with the anticipated technical feasibility of surgery for a given tumor. Generally, patients with extensive systemic disease who have less than 3 to 4 months to live are considered poor candidates for the kind of surgical procedures described here.

Surgical decompression and stabilization are performed to alleviate back and radicular pain and prevent further neurologic compromise. Surgery can even reverse some existing neurologic deficits, provided that they are not too severe or long-standing. Moreover, in some patients who have not yet developed neurologic dysfunction, pain alone may be a sufficient indication for surgical intervention. Because the best neurologic results are obtained in patients with the least preoperative neurologic deficit, an emphasis on early surgery in appropriately selected patients has led to high rates of pain control, neurologic preservation, and fewer systemic complications. Thus, pain need not be refractory to medical management before considering surgical intervention.

Neurologic deterioration during ongoing radiotherapy may be caused by tumor swelling or radioresistance, untreated spinal instability, or retropulsion of bone into the spinal canal. In such cases, urgent operative intervention by one of the methods described below may become necessary. Also, some patients will eventually develop recurrent spinal cord compression at a previously irradiated site caused by progression of tumor. In such instances, surgery is usually the only remaining alternative since further radiotherapy is likely to exceed the tolerance of the spinal cord without much chance of providing further local tumor control.

SURGICAL DECOMPRESSION

Before the availability of (1) high-potency corticosteroid therapy, (2) high field-strength MRI, (3) anterior surgical approaches to the spine, and (4) effective methods and technology for spinal stabilization, laminectomy and radiotherapy were the principle means of treating metastatic spinal tumors. In a few cases, laminectomy alone may be sufficient to provide decompression, improve neurologic function, and relieve pain. However, the routine use of laminectomy, without regard to the specific anatomic pathology, will fail at an unacceptably high rate. There are several reasons why laminectomy fails to control pain and prevent progressive neurologic deficit. First, tumors that compress the spinal cord usually originate from bony vertebral metastases, most of which are located anterior to the spinal cord within the vertebral body. For this reason, laminectomy may not provide direct access to the site of pathology for adequate decompression. In contrast, an anterior surgical exposure permits direct decompression of the spinal canal contents and pain-sensitive structures. Second, when the anterior spinal elements are weakened by metastatic disease, overall spinal stability may be further compromised by surgical removal of the posterior supporting elements (i.e., lamina, spinous processes, facet joints, and ligaments). Thus, in the setting of advanced vertebral body destruction, laminectomy without concomitant internal fixation risks promoting further vertebral body collapse and kyphotic angulation, potentially leading to increased spinal cord and nerve root compression.

As a result of the poor results obtained with laminectomy, attention initially turned to anterior approaches to the spine to treat metastatic disease.[4-6] Harrington reported 52 patients with metastatic spinal tumors treated with anterior vertebral body resection and postoperative radiation therapy with excellent neurologic results.[4] Sundaresan and colleagues described their results of anterior vertebral body resection and fusion with bone cement (methyl methacrylate) for metastatic disease.[5] Overall, 70% of those who were nonambulatory preoperatively became ambulatory after surgery. These figures are similar to those reported by Siegal and Siegal, 80% of whose patients were ambulatory following vertebral body resection compared to 28% preoperatively.[6] Subsequently, a number of other clinical series, which have included use of the anterior approach, have reported excellent results in terms of pain control and preservation of ambulation and neurologic function.[7-18]

For tumors involving the thoracic spine, the anterolateral transthoracic and the posterolateral extracavitary approaches are generally preferred. In the lumbar spine, the anterolateral retroperitoneal and lateral extracavitary approaches both provide excellent exposure and similar overall results as well.[5,6,17,18] To obtain immediate spinal stability, surgical decompression is usually combined with the application of some type of instrumentation. As a group, these approaches produce the least iatrogenic instability while permitting extensive tumor resection and providing secure, immediate, spinal stabilization. Although not directly comparable, most studies indicate that the rate of neurologic improvement in nonambulatory patients is considerably higher in those treated by anterior surgery than those treated with either radiotherapy alone or with simple laminectomy.[1-7,13]

In recent years, the wider availability and expertise in the use of spinal instrumentation and improvements in the various systems have led to a return of interest in posterior surgical approaches to treat metastatic disease using these devices to secure immediate postoperative stability (Figure 35–1).[11,19-22] The ability to provide immediate stabilization has encouraged efforts at more complete tumor resection via posterior approaches,

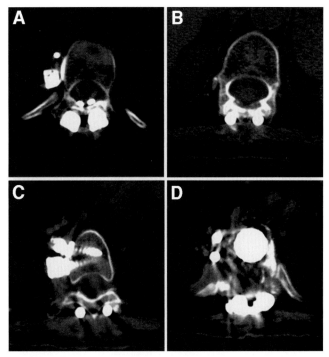

FIGURE 35–1 Postoperative computed tomography (CT) scan of a 44-year-old woman with severe back and T10 radicular pain caused by a destructive tumor of the T10 vertebral body with involvement of both anterior and posterior spinal elements. Instrumentation consists of pedicle screws and laminar hooks (*A*) and rods (*B*) for posterior stabilization. Vertebral body screws (*C*), together with cylindrical titanium cages filled with methyl methacrylate (*D*) are used for anterior spinal fixation and vertebral body reconstruction respectively.

which had previously been considered quite limiting.[21] Although these approaches do not completely solve the problem of access to tumor in the vertebral body located anterior to neural structures, they are quite effective at preventing or delaying neurologic progression and relieving mechanical and radicular pain.[19-22] Both anterior and the newer extended posterior surgical approaches provide excellent exposure for resection of tumor at thoracic and lumbar levels. Consequently, rather than relying solely on either an anterior or posterior approach, most spine surgeons now tailor their surgical attack to the specific anatomic pathology as defined by preoperative imaging studies.[9-13]

As with lumbar and thoracic surgical methods, several approaches are also possible at cervical levels (Figure 35–2).[23-25] Anterior corpectomy and fusion with instrumentation may be used either alone or in combination with posterior decompression and fixation, as dictated by the pathologic anatomy. Modifications of these well-established strategies are often required to gain exposure for adequate decompression and tumor resection at the cervico-thoracic junction and for disease of the T1 through T3 vertebral bodies.[26] Specifically, resection of the manubrium or median sternotomy may be required here. In addition, a combined thoraco-abdominal exposure with splitting of the diaphragm may be required for disease involving T11 through L2. Consequently, surgical procedures to address the pathology and re-create spinal stability can be devised for virtually all spinal levels. Given the challenge in predicting survival, the larger issue is frequently that of appropriate patient selection for these complex and invasive procedures.

Advanced, multilevel, spinal metastatic disease may preclude effective stabilization because vertebrae above or below the site of major pathology are also involved by tumor and cannot provide a secure interface for spinal instrumentation. In addition, patients with complete paraplegia are unlikely to obtain significant functional benefit, such as regaining ambulation or protective sensation. Thus, surgery may be considered futile in such patients. Even in these individuals, however, pain caused by progressive spinal deformity may be an overriding factor. Therefore, surgery may still be indicated in some patients with paraplegia to permit them to assume a sitting posture without pain or progression of their spinal deformity.

Although the surgical approaches described here are generally well tolerated and frequently lead to an improvement in quality of life, reported surgical mortality ranges from 0% to 10%. Thus, comorbidities and the extent of the primary disease must be considered carefully in the selection of patients for major spinal operations.[5,6,10,13,14,17,18] Similar rules apply to patients in whom extended posterior approaches are being contemplated. Although minimally invasive endoscopic surgical techniques for anterior tumor resection have been described by a few surgeons, these methods have not yet achieved widespread use.[27,28]

SPINAL STABILIZATION

After surgical decompression, immediate stabilization with spinal instrumentation may be required to prevent further compromise of the spinal cord and nerve roots by unchecked motion of the adjacent intact vertebrae.

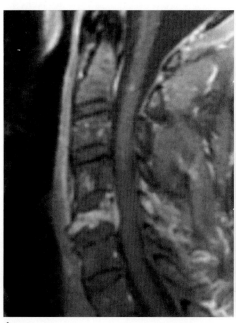
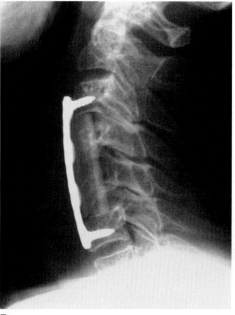

A   B

FIGURE 35–2 Imaging studies of a 62-year-old man with severe neck pain and bilateral C5 radiculopathies caused by metastatic carcinoma of the esophagus. Magnetic resonance imaging (MRI) scan of vertebral body metastases at C4 and C5 with epidural disease and partial C5 collapse (*A*) and postoperative plain lateral cervical spine film (*B*) after tumor resection and fusion with fibular strut graft and an anterior cervical plating device.

This type of rigid fixation is quite effective at preventing the development of an abnormal motion segment with persistence of pain. Early in the development of anterior spinal tumor surgery, stability was often achieved with bone cement (methyl methacrylate) held in place by metal pins inserted into the vertebrae above and below the resected vertebral body tumor.[4] Although this remains an effective approach that is simple and inexpensive, a number of different devices have been created in an effort to improve on this early method. One type of device consists of a cylindrical cage, which provides a metallic scaffold to replace the support previously provided by the diseased vertebral body. The cage is filled with bone cement to provide additional support or bone graft to promote bony fusion. In addition, a number of plating and rod systems have been devised to create additional immediate support for rigid anterior spinal fixation at the site of vertebral body resection. A host of spinal instrumentation systems is available for posterior stabilization as well. These devices provide a diversity of ways to obtain rigid fixation of the affected spinal segments once the neural elements have been adequately decompressed.

The traditional surgical approach to metastatic spinal disease was laminectomy, a technique that now plays a limited role in overall management. Laminectomy remains useful as a primary surgical approach for tumors that arise posterior to the dural sac, but do not threaten to destabilize the spine. In such cases, decompression via laminectomy can be performed by itself with removal of epidural tumor posterior and lateral to the spinal cord. In such cases, additional efforts to provide immediate fixation are not necessary. If additional spinal structures like pedicles and facet joints are involved by tumor and are not intact, or must be removed, stabilization using rods, hooks, or pedicle screws is usually advisable. More extensive tumors that involve both anterior and posterior elements of the spine may require combined anterior and posterior approaches to obtain adequate tumor resection, and in some cases, complete vertebrectomy may even be indicated.[21,22] In modern clinical series of spinal surgery for metastatic tumor, the most consistent finding is that surgery provides excellent pain control. However, in addition to tumor removal and neural decompression, spinal stabilization may be required to obtain optimum pain relief and preserve neurologic function.

SURGERY VERSUS PERCUTANEOUS VERTEBROPLASTY

The technique of injecting methyl methacrylate into diseased vertebral bodies under fluoroscopic control (vertebroplasty) can be very effective at relieving back pain caused by osteoporotic spinal fractures. Vertebroplasty can also be used to provide support against further subsidence of bone following destruction by some metastatic processes.[29,30] In such cases, pain relief may be rapid and sustained. As a minimally invasive approach, vertebroplasty can be particularly useful in older patients, or in those whose comorbidities preclude the type of direct surgical interventions described earlier. It is also particularly useful when there is significant pain caused by vertebral collapse and instability but little or no spinal cord or cauda equina compression or retropulsion of bone into the spinal canal. This technique is most useful in tumors that produce diffuse infiltration and weakening of the cancellous part of the vertebral body (e.g., multiple myeloma), rather than extensive destruction of cortical bone. Moreover, when a number of contiguous levels are involved, extensive weakening of bone or the advanced state of systemic disease in general may preclude a direct surgical approach. Hence, vertebroplasty may be better suited for such individuals. Effective tumor treatment by radiotherapy may actually be associated with an acceleration of vertebral weakening and collapse. Thus, vertebroplasty may be quite useful under these particular circumstances.

If a patient has a significant neurologic deficit, direct surgical intervention is usually the most effective way to arrest its progression. In addition, most solid or highly vascular tumors such as renal cell carcinoma are probably best treated with a direct surgical approach. Vertebroplasty should probably be reserved for patients with tumors that do not have a prominent epidural component or retropulsion of bone into the spinal canal. Similarly, the technique may not be feasible when tumor has destroyed the posterior cortex of the vertebral body. Incompetence of the posterior vertebral cortex could lead to extrusion of acrylic material into the spinal canal with further neurologic compromise. Under such circumstances, surgical decompression and stabilization are preferred. Clearly, however, percutaneous vertebroplasty will play an important and increasing role in the management of back pain caused by metastatic disease, particularly in patients without neurologic deficit.

ABLATIVE NEUROSURGICAL TECHNIQUES

Historically, ablative neurosurgical procedures played an important role in the management of cancer pain. However, the effectiveness of modern pharmacologic methods of pain control has greatly reduced dependence on these techniques. Nevertheless, functional neurosurgical methods continue to represent an effective option for cancer pain management and should be given serious consideration under appropriate circumstances.

For example, percutaneous radiofrequency cordotomy is of great potential benefit in properly selected patients whose pain cannot be controlled adequately by other means. With appropriate patient selection and careful technical application, patients may still benefit greatly from this and other well-established ablative procedures.

Cordotomy

Percutaneous high cervical cordotomy was used frequently before the introduction of intraspinal opiate therapy, more effective systemic medication regimens, and a multidisciplinary approach to cancer pain management. Cordotomy has proven to be highly effective and remains useful in properly selected patients in whom other methods have failed. The procedure has been used most effectively for the treatment of lateralized nonvisceral pain caused by cancer. Earlier methods of open surgical cordotomy have been largely supplanted by percutaneous radiofrequency lesion generation, although open cordotomy remains an option.[31] The earliest attempts to perform percutaneous cordotomy employed needles with radioactive tips and direct electrical coagulation to create lesions in the spinothalamic tract of the spinal cord.[32] The unpredictable size of such lesions led to the development of better approaches. Radiofrequency thermocoagulation with image guidance has since proved to be the most reliable means of controlling lesion size and location.[32-41]

Percutaneous cordotomy involves insertion of an electrode with an uninsulated tip into the substance of the spinal cord along its anterolateral surface via the spinal neural foramen located between the first and second cervical vertebrae. Under fluoroscopic control, the electrode is introduced through the ventral portion of the neural foramen.[33-37,39] The needle is repositioned in response to measurements of impedance and clinical responses to electrophysiologic stimulation.[35] When the electrode has been correctly positioned, electrical stimulation will produce stereotypical sensations in the contralateral half of the body on the side of the patient's pain. A short-acting anesthetic agent is administered while a radiofrequency current is passed through the needle. In this manner, a relatively symmetric tissue volume surrounding the uninsulated tip of the electrode is heated while the electrode temperature is maintained at a constant level for a specified time. Upon rapid awakening, the patient is tested for diminished pinprick sensation over the affected side of the body. Repeated lesioning and pinprick testing are employed to assist in enlarging the lesion to obtain sufficient dermatomal coverage.

The principle advantage of cordotomy is the rapid and frequently excellent degree of pain relief that can be achieved. Pain caused by unilateral involvement of the lateral chest or abdominal wall, lumbosacral plexus, pelvis, or lower extremity may be particularly well-suited for treatment by cordotomy. Brachial pain may also be treated, although with somewhat greater difficulty and higher chance of early failure. Pain syndromes involving the visceral organs, the spine, and those that cross the midline or are clearly bilateral are generally not responsive to unilateral cordotomy.

Because pain relief may decline over a period of months to years after the procedure, the use of cordotomy should be reserved for patients with pain caused by malignancy. Pain that is bilateral or of visceral origin responds poorly to unilateral cordotomy, with the best results being obtained in patients who have pain from a well-localized source below the cervical dermatomes. It has been especially useful for treating chest wall pain caused by mesothelioma.[41-43] As with all ablative lesions placed in the central nervous system, great care must be exercised in the performance of cordotomy to ensure that the lesion is confined to the target site. It must not be allowed to spread to motor pathways via improper electrode positioning or use of excessive temperatures or time of tissue heating. Also, treated patients have markedly reduced sensitivity to noxious stimuli and must be cautioned to avoid injury to areas of the body rendered hypoesthetic by the procedure.

Since the introduction of percutaneous high cervical (C1-C2) cordotomy, complications such as incontinence, hemiparesis, and sleep apnea (Ondine's curse) have been noted in a relatively small percentage of patients.[35,38,39,44] In an effort to reduce such adverse events, some neurosurgeons have advocated an anterior lower cervical approach, rather than the lateral upper cervical method.[38] The anterior lower cervical approach appears to reduce the risk of sleep apnea, making bilateral lesions safer when at least one is performed at the lower level. Incontinence and motor deficits have also been reported to be less frequent with the low-anterior approach, and the possibility of selective segmental lesion production has been cited as a benefit of this method as well.[38] Thus, lesions can be produced in thoracic and lumbar distributions with preservation of sacral fibers to reduce the incidence of urinary incontinence. Clearly, the anterior cervical method is unsuitable for pain of brachial origin.

After percutaneous cordotomy, approximately 90% of patients obtain initial pain relief that is sufficient to allow discontinuation or marked reduction of narcotic analgesics.[39-41] By 1 year after treatment, 40% of patients have significant recurrence of pain. Hence, cordotomy is most effective for those with short life expectancy with a fairly high rate of relapse being expected in patients who survive longer than a year.

Patients with unilateral pain syndromes respond much better to cordotomy than do those with bilateral pain. Consequently, patients must be screened carefully in this regard. For those with bilateral or axial pain, unilateral cordotomy may relieve symptoms on the opposite side, only to see the development of more severe pain on the previously less-affected side.[45] In such cases, bilateral cordotomy may be considered.[40,46] As indicated earlier, the second lesion should be placed via the lower anterior cervical route to minimize the chance of producing incontinence and sleep apnea.

Although serious complications may occur with cordotomy, the rate of significant neurologic problems is relatively low. These have been minimized by a combination of techniques including graded lesioning, careful electrophysiologic stimulation, and the use of newer imaging modalities during the procedure.[33-37,40] The principle limitation of cordotomy rests with the relatively short duration of pain control that is seen in some patients. However, given the effectiveness and relative safety of the technique, hesitancy regarding its invasive nature should not preclude its use when pharmacologic means fail.

As noted earlier, even high cervical cordotomy may not relieve pain caused by disease affecting the cervical dermatomes, as with radiation-induced brachial plexopathy. For this condition in particular, the use of dorsal root entry zone (DREZ) lesions has been reported to be efficacious, even with respect to "burning" pain sensations.[47] The DREZ technique provides sustained pain relief, but requires a multilevel cervical laminectomy or laminoplasty. As with the other ablative spinal cord procedures, it is not widely used at this time.

Midline Thoracic Myelotomy

An improved understanding of the neuroanatomic substrate underlying the effectiveness of open midline myelotomy has prompted a reexamination of this technique in recent years. The history of midline myelotomy, which was originally used over 30 years ago for the relief of visceral pain, has been reviewed by Gildenberg.[48] Willis and colleagues defined a possible anatomic basis for the effectiveness of this procedure when they identified nociceptive pathways in the posterior columns of the spinal cord.[49] Subsequently, Nauta reported on the use of this technique at low thoracic levels to control pelvic visceral pain in a small series of patients.[50] Others have reported good results with open punctate myelotomy at both upper thoracic levels to treat abdominal pain and at lower thoracic levels to treat pain caused by pelvic malignancy; however, these studies have included only small numbers of patients.[51-53] As with cordotomy, computed tomography (CT)-guidance can be used to perform midline myelotomy by percutaneous methods.[54] The safety of this method of lesion production has yet to be established in larger series.

STEREOTACTIC NEUROSURGERY

Pain of maxillofacial or upper brachial origin that is unresponsive to medical management may be addressed by the use of stereotactic ablative procedures or by electrical stimulation of the periaqueductal gray region. Ablative procedures include mesencephalic tractotomy, cingulotomy, and lesioning of a variety of medial thalamic targets, such as the nucleus medialis dorsalis. Mesencephalic tractotomy has been used for cephalic and brachial cancer pain with some success.[55,56] However, its use has never been widely adopted because of the potential for serious neurologic complications. As an alternative, medial thalamotomy is probably safer, but it tends to be less effective.[57] For cancer pain, cingulotomy has been used by a small number of surgeons. In addition to maxillofacial pain, cingulotomy is potentially useful for patients with pain caused by widespread metastatic disease or bilateral or midline pain that is poorly responsive to opioids.[58,59]

Neurophysiologic studies have implicated the cingulum in the affective response to pain perception, and cingulotomy has been used for some time to treat pain caused by malignancy. In particular, bilateral cingulotomy has been used to reduce the "suffering" occasioned by the extreme anxiety that is sometimes associated with severe, refractory pain caused by malignancy. Cingulotomy has been reported to be effective in approximately 50% of such patients, but seizures, transient confusion, and urinary incontinence are potential complications of this treatment.[58,59] In addition, cognitive deficits may occur.[60] As with cordotomy, intracranial stereotactic ablative procedures usually become less effective with time. Although the results of cingulotomy for treatment of cancer pain have not been studied in large numbers of patients and its use is considered controversial, the procedure is moderately effective. It may be useful for pain of the head, neck, or brachial region or for diffuse pain unrelieved by medical management.

In the past, radiofrequency lesions were created in the cingulate gyri following air-contrast cerebral ventriculography. More recently, MRI has supplanted ventriculography to assist in localization of the cingulum for lesioning.[58,59] Although modern imaging helps to ensure correct electrode placement, radiofrequency lesioning of the cingulum and other deep thalamic targets still requires introduction of an electrode into the brain with potentially serious attendant risks. Consequently, ablative stereotactic techniques of this type are best reserved for those few patients with truly intractable pain that does not respond to intensive efforts at medical management.

Stereotactic Radiosurgery

Traditionally, stereotactic neurosurgical ablative procedures like thalamotomy, cingulotomy, and retro-Gasserian rhizotomy have been performed using electrodes placed into deep intracranial targets with image guidance. Some have advocated performing these procedures using gamma knife stereotactic radiosurgery instead. The best example of the use of gamma knife for pain control is in the benign, but intensely painful condition known as trigeminal neuralgia (i.e., tic douloureux). Although conventional ablative procedures are still used for this condition, gamma knife stereotactic radiosurgery has been used in a growing number of patients for precise, high-dose irradiation of a very small volume of tissue in the retro-Gasserian segment of the affected trigeminal nerve. Accurate targeting of the nerve is accomplished using modern imaging techniques (MRI), a stereotactic neurosurgical head frame, and sophisticated computer planning software. In addition to idiopathic trigeminal neuralgia, facial pain caused by tumor involvement of the skull base may be helped by this technique. To date, however, success rates for relief of tumor-associated trigeminal pain have been somewhat lower than with true trigeminal neuralgia.[61]

The gamma knife contains multiple sources of Co^{60} from which beams of radiation are directed by precise collimation to a common target point. Using a stereotactic frame that is fixed rigidly to the patient's head, the target point is identified by MRI with respect to the external frame. In this manner, the point of intersection of the beams, or "isocenter," can be positioned precisely within the retro-Gasserian segment of the trigeminal nerve or other deep brain structure. A small, nearly spherical lesion can be created using a high dose of radiation administered in a single treatment session. The chief advantage of this technique is that no opening in the skull is required to create a lesion deep within the intracranial compartment. The minimally invasive nature and demonstrated safety of gamma knife stereotactic radiosurgery has led to increasing use in the treatment of certain benign and malignant brain tumors. These same characteristics have generated interest in using the gamma knife as a functional neurosurgical tool, for which it was originally developed.

Use of the gamma knife to perform thalamotomy and pallidotomy for Parkinson's disease is currently under investigation.[62] As with cordotomy, guidance of lesion placement with radiofrequency electrodes is assisted by intraoperative assessment of electrophysiologic correlates. Recently, it has been suggested that these types of functional neurosurgical lesions can be placed accurately using gamma knife radiosurgery without performing invasive electrophysiologic studies, although the safety and effectiveness of this method are still under investigation.[63] Radiosurgical thalamotomy has been reported to be of some benefit in the treatment of chronic intractable pain of benign origin.[64] However, its effectiveness for the treatment of cancer pain appears to be only fair.[65]

Another effective means to control pain caused by prostate and breast carcinoma in particular is by ablation of the pituitary gland (i.e., hypophysectomy). Conventionally, hypophysectomy for pain control has been performed by stereotactic injection of alcohol or liquid nitrogen into the gland.[66-68] In addition, direct surgical obliteration by an open transphenoidal route has been used successfully.[69] Gamma knife stereotactic radiosurgery also has been employed in a limited fashion for hypophysectomy with some reports of success.[70-72]

The safety and effectiveness of any functional neurosurgical ablation rests upon the surgeon's ability to target these critical structures with a high degree of precision. Therefore, the utility of radiosurgical lesioning will ultimately depend on being able to identify the correct brain target based solely on imaging information, without the aid of electrophysiologic monitoring. This is not a significant problem with pituitary ablation, but it is more problematic when targeting small thalamic nuclei or other deep brain structures that may vary in location and geometry from one patient to another. A second factor that might limit the effectiveness of gamma knife functional neurosurgery is the time interval between treatment and pain relief, although this has not been observed to be a problem in the cases reported to date.[64,73] Thus, the role of gamma knife radiosurgery in the treatment of cancer pain and its relationship to conventional functional neurosurgical procedures remains to be defined.

REFERENCES

1. Black P: Spinal metastasis: current status and recommended guidelines for management. Neurosurgery 5:726–746, 1979.
2. Gilbert RW, Kim JH, Posner JB: Epidural spinal cord compression from metastatic tumor: Diagnosis and treatment. Ann Neurol 3:40–51, 1978.
3. Zaidat OO, Ruff RL: Treatment of spinal epidural metastasis improves patient survival and functional state. Neurology 58:1360–1366, 2002.
4. Harrington KD: Anterior cord compression and spinal stabilization for patients with metastatic lesions of the spine. J Neurosurg 61:107–117, 1984.
5. Sundaresan N, Galicich JH, Lane JM, et al: Treatment of neoplastic epidural cord compression by vertebral body resection and stabilization. J Neurosurg 63:676–684, 1985.
6. Siegal T, Siegal T: Surgical decompression of anterior and posterior malignant epidural tumors compressing the spinal cord: A prospective study. Neurosurgery 17:424–432, 1985.
7. Sundaresan N, Scher H, DiGiacinto GV, et al: Surgical treatment of spinal cord compression in kidney cancer. J Clin Oncol 4:1851–1856, 1986.
8. McAfee PC, Zdeblick TA: Tumors of the thoracic and lumbar spine: Surgical treatment via the anterior approach. J Spinal Disord 2:145–154, 1989.
9. Onimus M, Papin P, Gangloff S: Results of surgical treatment of spinal thoracic and lumbar metastases. Eur Spine J 5:407–411, 1996.
10. Jackson RJ, Loh SC, Gokaslan ZL: Metastatic renal cell carcinoma of the spine: Surgical treatment and results. J Neurosurg 94(1 Suppl):18–24, 2001.
11. Klekamp J, Samii H: Surgical results for spinal metastases. Acta Neurochir (Wien) 140:957–967, 1998.
12. Buchelt M, Windhager R, Kiss H, et al: Surgical management of spinal metastases. Z Orthop Ihre Grenzgeb 134:263–268, 1996.
13. Sundaresan N, DiGiacinto GV, Hughes JE, et al: Treatment of neoplastic spinal cord compression: Results of a prospective study. Neurosurgery 29:645–650, 1991.
14. Walsh GL, Gokaslan ZL, McCutcheon IE, et al: Anterior approaches to the thoracic spine in patients with cancer: Indications and results. Ann Thorac Surg 64:1611–1618, 1997.
15. Goutallier D, Lewertowski JM: Treatment of metastases of thoracic and lumbar vertebrae with predominant corporeal involvement by osteotomy of the vertebral body and anterior approach with cement and screwed plate. Rev Chir Orthop Reparatrice Appar Mot 78:319–332, 1992.
16. Fenstermaker RA, Ratcheson RS: Malignant tumors of the thoracic spine. In Barrow DL (ed): Perspectives in Neurological Surgery. St. Louis, Quality Medical Publishing, Inc, 1991, pp 1–23.
17. Fourney DR, Abi-Said D, Rhines LD, et al: Simultaneous anterior-posterior approach to the thoracic and lumbar spine for the radical resection of tumors followed by reconstruction and stabilization. J Neurosurg 94(2 suppl):232–244, 2001.
18. Graham AW III, MacMillan M, Fessler RG: Lateral extracavitary approach to the thoracic and thoracolumbar spine. Orthopedics 20:605–610, 1997.
19. Bridwell KH, Jenny AB, Saul T, et al: Posterior segmental spinal instrumentation (PSSI) with posterolateral decompression and debulking for metastatic thoracic and lumbar spine disease: Limitations of the technique. Spine 13:1383–1394, 1988.
20. O'Neil J, Gardner V, Armstrong G: Treatment of tumors of the thoracic and lumbar spinal column. Clin Orthop 227:103–112, 1988.
21. Cahill DW, Kumar R: Palliative subtotal vertebrectomy with anterior and posterior reconstruction via a single posterior approach. J Neurosurg 90(1 suppl):42–47, 1999.
22. Akeyson EW, McCutcheon IE: Single-stage posterior vertebrectomy and replacement combined with posterior instrumentation for spinal metastasis. J Neurosurg 85:211–220, 1996.
23. Miller DJ, Lang FF, Walsh GL, et al: Coaxial double-lumen methylmethacrylate reconstruction in the anterior cervical and upper thoracic spine after tumor resection. Neurosurgery 92(2 suppl):181–190, 2000.
24. Caspar W, Pitzen T, Papavero L, et al: Anterior cervical plating for the treatment of neoplasms in the cervical vertebrae. J Neurosurg 90(1 suppl):27–34, 1999.
25. Jonsson B, Jonsson H, Karlstrom G, Sjostrom L: Surgery of cervical spine metastases: A retrospective study. Eur Spine J 3:76–83, 1994.
26. Seol HJ, Chung CK, Kim HJ: Surgical approach to anterior compression in the upper thoracic spine. J Neurosurg 97(3 suppl):337–342, 2002.
27. McAfee PC, Regan JR, Fedder IL, et al: Anterior thoracic corpectomy for spinal cord compression performed endoscopically. Surg Laparosc Endosc 5:339–348, 1995.
28. McLain RF: Spinal cord decompression: an endoscopically assisted approach for metastatic tumors. Spinal Cord 39:482–487, 2001.
29. Cotten A, Dewatre F, Cortet B, et al: Percutaneous vertebroplasty for osteolytic metastases and multiple myeloma: Effects of the percentage of lesion filling and the leakage of methyl methacrylate at clinical follow-up. Radiology 200:525–530, 1996.
30. Weill A, Chiras J, Simon JM, et al: Spinal metastases: Indications for and results of percutaneous injection of acrylic surgical cement. Radiology 199:241–247, 1996.
31. Jones B, Finlay I, Ray A, Simpson B: Is there still a role for open cordotomy in cancer pain management? J Pain Symptom Manage 25:179–184, 2003.
32. Mullan S, Harper PV, Hekmatpanah J, et al: Percutaneous interruption of spinal pain tracts by means of a strontium[90] needle. J Neurosurg 20:931–939, 1963.
33. Fenstermaker RA, Sternau L, Takaoka Y: CT-assisted percutaneous anterior cordotomy: Technical note. Surg Neurol 43:147–150, 1995.
34. Freidberg SR, Takaoka Y: Technique of high cervical percutaneous cordotomy. Symposium on surgical techniques. Surg Clin North Am 53:291–300, 1973.
35. Gildenberg PL, Zanes C, Flitter M, et al: Impedance measuring device for detection of penetration of the spinal cord in anterior percutaneous cervical cordotomy: Technical note. J Neurosurg 30:87–92, 1969.
36. Kanpolat Y, Akyar S, Caglar S, et al: CT-guided percutaneous selective cordotomy. Acta Neurochir (Wien) 123:92–96, 1993.
37. Krol G, Arbit E: Percutaneous lateral cervical cordotomy: Target localization with water-soluble contrast medium. J Neurosurg 79:390–392, 1993.
38. Lin PM, Gildenberg PL, Polakoff PP: An anterior approach to percutaneous lower cervical cordotomy. J Neurosurg 25:553–560, 1966.
39. Rosomoff HL, Brown CJ, Shestak P: Percutaneous radiofrequency cervical cordotomy: Technique. J Neurosurg 23:639–644, 1965.
40. Sander M, Zuurmond W: Safety of unilateral and bilateral percutaneous cervical cordotomy in 80 terminally ill cancer patients. J Clin Oncol 13:1509–1512, 1995.
41. Stuart G, Cramond T: Role of percutaneous cervical cordotomy for pain of malignant origin. Med J Aust 158:667–670, 1993.
42. Jackson MB, Pounder D, Price C, et al: Percutaneous cervical cordotomy for the control of pain in patients with pleural mesothelioma. Thorax 54:238–241, 1999.
43. Kanpolat Y, Savas A, Ucar T, Torum F: CT-guided percutaneous selective cordotomy for treatment of intractable pain in patients with malignant pleural mesothelioma. Acta Neurochir (Wien) 144:595–599, 2002.
44. Sanders M, Zuurmond W: Safety of unilateral and bilateral percutaneous cervical cordotomy in 80 terminally ill cancer patients. J Clin Oncol 13:1509–1512, 1995.
45. Nagaro T, Adachi N, Tabo E, et al: New pain following cordotomy: Clinical features, mechanisms, and clinical importance. J Neurosurg 95:425–431, 2001.
46. Amano K, Kawamura H, Tanikawa T, et al: Bilateral versus unilateral percutaneous high cervical cordotomy as a surgical method of pain relief. Acta Neurochir Suppl (Wien) 52:143–145, 1991.
47. Zeidman SM, Rossitch EJ, Nashold BS: Dorsal root entry zone lesions in the treatment of pain related to radiation-induced brachial plexopathy. J Spinal Disord 6:44–47, 1993.
48. Gildenberg PL: Myelotomy through the years. Stereotact Funct Neurosurg 77:169–171, 2001.
49. Willis WD, Al-Chaer ED, Quast MJ, Westlund KN: A visceral pain pathway in the dorsal column of the spinal cord. Proc Natl Acad Sci (USA) 96:7675–7679, 1999.
50. Nauta HJ, Soukup VM, Fabian RH, et al: Punctate midline myelotomy for the relief of visceral cancer pain. J Neurosurg 92(2 suppl):125–130, 2000.
51. Becker R, Gatscher S, Sure U, Bertalanffy H: The punctuate midline myelotomy concept for visceral cancer pain control-case report

and review of the literature. Acta Neurochir (suppl) 79:77–78, 2002.

52. Watling CJ, Payne R, Allen RR, Hassenbusch S: Commissural myelotomy for intractable cancer pain: Report of two cases. Clin J Pain 12:151–156, 1996.

53. Kim YS, Kwon SJ: High thoracic midline dorsal column myelotomy for severe visceral pain due to advanced stomach cancer. Neurosurgery 46:85–90, 2000.

54. Vilela Filho O, Araujo MR, Florencio RS, et al: CT-guided percutaneous punctate midline myelotomy for the treatment of intractable visceral pain: A technical note. Stereotact Funct Neurosurg 77:177–182, 2001.

55. Fabrizi F, Fabrizi AP, Gaist G: Stereotactic mesencephalic tractotomy in the treatment of chronic cancer pain. Acta Neurochir (Wien) 99:38–40, 1989.

56. Cohadon F, Laporte A: Value of stereotaxic mesencephalic tractotomy in neoplastic cervicofacial pain. Rev Laryngol Otol Rhinol (Bord) 106:9–10, 1985.

57. Tasker RR: Thalamotomy. Neurosurg Clin North Am 1:841–864, 1990.

58. Hassenbusch SJ, Pillay PK, Barnett GH: Radiofrequency cingulotomy for intractable cancer pain using stereotaxis guided by magnetic resonance imaging. Neurosurgery 27:220–223, 1990.

59. Wong ET, Gunes S, Gaughan E, et al: Palliation of intractable cancer pain by MRI-guided cingulotomy. Clin J Pain 13(3):260–263, 1997.

60. Cohen RA, Kaplan RF, Zuffante P, et al: Alteration of intention and self-initiated action associated with bilateral anterior cingulotomy. J Neuropsychiatry Clin Neurosci 11:444–453, 1999.

61. Pollack BE, Iuliano BA, Foote RL, Gorman DA: Stereotactic radiosurgery for tumor-related trigeminal neuralgia. Neurosurgery 46:576–582, 2000.

62. Lindquist C, Kihlstrom L, Hellstrand E: Functional neurosurgery: A future for the Gamma Knife? Stereotact Funct Neurosurg 57:72–81, 1991.

63. Young RF, Vermeulen SS, Grimm P, Posewitz A: Electrophysiological target localization is not required for the treatment of functional disorders. Stereotact Funct Neurosurg 66(suppl 1):309–319, 1996.

64. Young RF, Jacques DS, Rand RW, et al: Technique of stereotactic medial thalamotomy with the Leksell Gamma Knife for treatment of chronic pain. Neurol Res 17:59–65, 1995.

65. Steiner L, Forster D, Leksell L, et al: Gammathalamotomy in intractable pain. Acta Neurochir (Wien) 52:173–184, 1980.

66. Lloyd JW, Rawlinson WA, Evans PJ: Selective hypophysectomy for metastatic pain: A review of ethyl alcohol ablation of the anterior pituitary in a Regional Pain Relief Unit. Br J Anaesth 53:1129–1133, 1981.

67. Duthie AM, Ingham V, Dell AE, Dennett JE: Pituitary cryoablation: The results of treatment using a transphenoidal cryoprobe. Anaesthesia 38:448–451, 1983.

68. Yanagida H, Corssen G, Trouwborst A, Erdmann W: Relief of cancer pain in man: alcohol-induced neuroadenolysis versus electrical stimulation of the pituitary gland. Pain 19:133–141, 1984.

69. Smith JA, Eyre HJ, Roberts TS, Middleton RG: Transphenoidal hypophysectomy in the management of carcinoma of the prostate. Cancer 53:2385–2387, 1984.

70. Sloan PA, Hodes J, John W: Radiosurgical pituitary ablation for cancer pain. J Palliat Care 12:51–53, 1996.

71. Hayashi M, Taira T, Chernov M, et al: Gamma knife surgery for cancer pain-pituitary gland-stalk ablation: A multi-center prospective protocol since 2002. J Neurosurg 97(5 Suppl):433–437, 2002.

72. Liscak R, Vladyka V: Radiosurgical hypophysectomy in painful bone metastases of breast carcinoma. Cas Lek Cesk 137:154–157, 1998.

73. Friehs GM, Noren G, Ohye C, et al: Lesion size following gamma knife treatment for functional disorders. Stereotact Funct Neurosurg 66(suppl 1):320–328, 1996.

CHAPTER 36

Chemotherapy for Cancer Pain Management

MILIND JAVLE, MD, AND G VARMA, MD

A patient's first question after receiving the diagnosis of cancer is usually "Can it be cured?" The second question, which sometimes does not occur for several days, is often "Will I be in pain, and if the disease is not cured, will I die in pain?"[1] Unfortunately, even today most common cancers in the advanced stages are not curable and survival prolongation with modern therapies is usually measured in months. Although providers often tout modest survival improvements as significant therapeutic gains, patient and family perceptions of therapeutic benefit include an improvement in quality of life (QOL), alleviation of pain, and other distressing symptoms related to cancer.

More than 30% of cancer patients have pain at the time of diagnosis and 65% to 85% experience pain when the disease is advanced.[2] Pain management strategies have traditionally focused on analgesic therapy and the use of invasive procedures. However, an optimal integrated program should include anticancer therapy. Anticancer therapy, including chemotherapy, hormonal therapy, targeted agents, and biologic response modifiers, may provide palliation by decreasing tumor burden.[3] The perceived role of chemotherapy for advanced cancer has changed, and the concept of "palliative chemotherapy" has gained ground. Research studies from the 1970s and 1980s focused on tumor regression and response rates, often at the cost of substantial toxicity. Recent studies, however, often include QOL endpoints in clinical trial design. Indeed, it may be possible to ameliorate distressing symptoms such as pain for many patients with advanced cancer using appropriate systemic therapy.

Palliative chemotherapy is defined as treatment in circumstances in which its administration is unlikely to result in a major survival gain but is likely to lead to an improvement in tumor-related symptoms. The palliation/toxicity balance from such an intervention should clearly favor symptom relief. When choosing to treat with a palliative intent, the issues of patient selection, agent selection, assessment of response, and balancing toxicity with clinical benefit need to be addressed. A summary of current research in this area is presented in this chapter.

CHEMOTHERAPEUTIC AGENTS AND PALLIATION

Studies exploring the role of palliative chemotherapy have been conducted in advanced solid tumors, including cancers of the lung, pancreas, breast, and prostate. Selected studies are summarized in Table 36–1.

Advanced pancreatic cancer is associated with a high incidence of tumor-related symptoms such as pain, anorexia, and deterioration of performance status. The concept of clinical benefit response was introduced to assess the palliative efficacy of chemotherapy agents. In an important study by Burris and colleagues,[4] 126 patients with advanced symptomatic pancreatic cancer were randomized to receive either gemcitabine or 5-fluorouracil (5-FU). The primary efficacy measure was clinical benefit response, a composite measurement of pain (analgesic consumption and pain intensity), Karnofsky performance status (KPS), and weight. Clinical benefit required a sustained (≥ 4 weeks) improvement in at least one parameter without worsening in any others.

Twenty-three percent of the patients in the gemcitabine arm versus 4.8% in the 5-FU arm had a positive clinical benefit response on the basis of reduced pain intensity, decreased analgesic consumption, and improved performance status ($P = 0.0022$). The duration of clinical benefit was 18 weeks for gemcitabine and 13 weeks for 5-FU. The median survival was 5.65 months for the gemcitabine patients and 4.41 months for the 5-FU patients ($P = 0.0025$). Both drugs were well tolerated. World Health Organization (WHO) grade 4 neutropenia was reported in 6.9% of gemcitabine patients and 3.3%

TABLE 36–1 Select Trials of Palliative Chemotherapy

Disease	Agent	Palliative Response (%)	Disease Response (%)	Reference
Metastatic pancreatic cancer	gemcitabine	23	11	4
Metastatic colon cancer	irinotecan	42	11	8
Metastatic prostate cancer	mitoxantrone + prednisone	29	44% PSA response	10
Metastatic non–small cell lung cancer	Docetaxel	Decreased analgesic requirement noted	5.8	13
Metastatic breast cancer	doxorubicin + vinorelbine	60	38	17

PSA, prostate-specific antigen.

of 5-FU patients ($P = 0.18$). There were no serious infections in either group. The clinical benefit response of gemcitabine in pancreatic cancer patients was not negated by treatment-related toxicities. In this study, the radiologic response rate with gemcitabine was a meager 11%; yet, the agent was rapidly incorporated into treatment guidelines for pancreatic cancer because of its palliative role.

Studies in other advanced gastrointestinal malignancies such as gastric, biliary, and colorectal cancer reported similar palliative benefit with systemic chemotherapy.[5-7] A recent study investigated the palliative benefit of irinotecan in 5-FU refractory colorectal cancer patients.[8] This study was designed to prospectively determine the palliative benefit of irinotecan using improvement in disease-related symptoms (DRS) as the primary study endpoint. Patients had advanced colorectal cancer refractory to 5-FU with at least one DRS defined as (1) KPS 60% to 80%, (2) baseline analgesic use 10 mg morphine or equivalent per day or more, or (3) disease-related pain score greater than 1 cm on a 10-cm linear analog self-assessment (LASA) scale. Patients received irinotecan 125 mg/m² weekly for 4 weeks on a 6-week schedule. The primary endpoint was palliative response defined as at least 50% decrease in pain score or analgesic usage, or 10% increase in KPS, from baseline for 4 weeks. QOL was assessed by the European Organization for Research and Treatment of Cancer Quality-of-Life Questionnaire Core 30 (EORTC QLQ-C30) version 2 instrument. A total of 65 patients were entered into the study. A palliative response was achieved in 27 patients (42%), and improvement in pain score predominated. LASA and EORTC QLQ-C30 showed parallel changes in DRS. The radiologic response rate was 11% (complete responses and partial responses, $n = 46$); 23 patients achieved stable disease. The authors' conclusion was that irinotecan provides a rate of palliative benefit greater than the radiologic response rate.

Metastatic prostate cancer is yet another example in which systemic chemotherapy may have a palliative role. Although the initial response to hormonal therapy is very common, eventually the cancer becomes androgen independent, which leads to pain, weight loss, and other symptoms of advanced disease. As these patients are often elderly men with comorbid health problems, they have not been regarded as chemotherapy candidates. The response to commonly used chemotherapeutic agents, as measured by radiologic or prostate-specific antigen (PSA) criteria is suboptimal.[9] Tannock and colleagues[10] explored the palliative benefits of chemotherapy in 161 hormone-refractory prostate cancer patients. These patients were randomized to receive mitoxantrone plus prednisone or prednisone alone. The primary endpoint was palliative response defined as a 2-point decrease in pain as assessed by a 6-point scale completed by patients, without an increase in analgesic consumption. This response had to be maintained during 2 consecutive evaluations at least 3 weeks apart. QOL was evaluated with a series of LASA scales and the prostate cancer-specific QOL instrument (PROSQLI). Palliative response was observed in 23 of 80 (29%) patients who received mitoxantrone and prednisone and in 10 of 81 (12%) patients who received prednisone alone ($P = 0.01$). The duration of palliation was longer in patients who received chemotherapy, with a median of 43 weeks and 18 weeks for chemotherapy arm and prednisone alone arm, respectively ($P < 0.0001$). There was no difference in overall survival. Most responding patients had an improvement per QOL scales and a decrease in PSA. This study was unique in its design as unlike its historical counterparts, palliation was defined as its primary endpoint.

The survival benefit obtained with chemotherapy administration in advanced non–small cell lung cancer (NSCLC) patients has been demonstrated by numerous meta-analyses.[11,12] Recent trials in NSCLC have successfully incorporated QOL as an endpoint. These studies also favor chemotherapy with regard to QOL. A recent study examined the role of docetaxel in comparison with best supportive care (BSC) in 104 patients with NSCLC who had previously been treated with platinum-based chemotherapy.[13] Survival improvement was the primary endpoint of the study. Secondary endpoints included assessment of response (docetaxel-arm only), toxicity, and QOL. A modest survival improvement was noted in the docetaxel arm and the use of all tumor-related medications was less common in docetaxel-treated patients, compared with BSC patients ($P = 0.02$). Fewer docetaxel patients than BSC patients required morphine or morphine-equivalent medications for pain. Nonmorphine analgesic use was also less frequent in docetaxel patients (39% vs. 55%; $P = 0.03$). Fewer docetaxel patients required palliative radiotherapy. The palliative role of chemotherapy for NSCLC has been confirmed by several additional studies both in the first- and second-line settings, for the young and the elderly, for good and marginal performance status patients.[14-16]

Pain, lethargy, and anorexia are commonly reported in patients with metastatic breast cancer. In the study by Norris et al., 303 patients with metastatic breast cancer were randomized to receive doxorubicin or doxorubicin plus vinorelbine.[17] Major trial endpoints included overall survival, QOL, response rate, and time to disease progression. Changes from baseline were defined using patient responses to a QOL questionnaire (EORTC QLQ-C30) and graded toxicity data. The most common baseline symptom recorded was cancer pain (38%) and on the QOL questionnaire, it was tiredness (89%). As reported, of the 111 assessable patients with cancer pain at baseline, 67 (60.4%) improved and 31 (27.9%) remained stable. Analysis of change in cancer pain, using QOL data, demonstrated very similar results where 62.7% of patients had improvement and 24.5% remained stable. Patients with complete response (CR) and partial response (PR) were far more likely to have an improvement in pain (84.9%) than the patients with progressive disease. Objective tumor response was 38% for the doxorubicin and vinorelbine arm and 30.5% for the doxorubicin arm alone; this difference was not statistically significant. The authors concluded that symptom improvement is seen in some patients with metastatic breast cancer with systemic chemotherapy.[18]

These studies demonstrated a common pattern: although these cancers were not regarded as exceptionally chemosensitive, palliation of pain and other tumor-related symptoms could be achieved with systemic chemotherapy. Palliative responses were noted more often than "objective" responses.

SYSTEMIC THERAPIES FOR BONE METASTASES

Systemic therapy for cancer also includes hormonal agents (commonly for breast and prostate cancer) and specific agents for bony metastases, including bisphosphonates and radionuclides such as phosphorus-32 (32P) and strontium-89 (89Sr). These agents play an important role in palliation of pain. Bone metastases lead to skeletal morbidity, including bone pain, pathologic fractures, spinal cord compression, and hypercalcemia of malignancy. These complications are caused by soluble factors that stimulate osteoclasts to resorb bone. Bisphosphonates such as pamidronate inhibit osteoclastic activity, reduce bone resorption, and lower calcium levels in hypercalcemia of malignancy. They are used for the prevention or palliation of pain and skeletal events associated with bony metastases particularly from multiple myeloma and breast cancer.[19,20] Recent studies have investigated the palliative role of bisphosphonates in other solid tumors such as prostate and NSCLC. A large ($n = 429$), placebo-controlled study by Saad and colleagues,[21] in patients with metastatic prostate cancer indicated a reduction of skeletal events with zoledronic acid as compared with placebo. Small and colleagues[22] reported contradictory results (no decrease in skeletal-related events) in the same disease with pamidronate. In both studies there was little impact on analgesic scores and QOL indices. A recent placebo-controlled study of zoledronic acid in lung cancer and other solid tumors reported improvement in skeletal related events (SRE), defined as pathologic fracture, spinal cord compression, radiation therapy, and surgery to the bone. There was no significant improvement, however, in the mean composite pain score or QOL outcomes.

The reason for this disparity (improved SRE without a parallel benefit in analgesia) is unclear. An extremely large study may be needed to delineate a small effect from bisphosphonates and none of the studies mentioned earlier included pain relief as a primary endpoint. A Cochrane review of 30 randomized trials, with 3682 patients with bone metastases concluded that there is evidence to support the effectiveness of bisphosphonates in providing pain relief from bony metastases.[23] In conclusion, for diseases such as multiple myeloma and metastatic breast cancer, there are sufficient data to support routine use of these agents to reduce SRE. In other solid tumors with bony metastases, bisphosphonates should be considered when radiotherapy or analgesics, or both, are inadequate for the management of painful bony metastases.

Palliation of bone pain with narcotic analgesics often results in side effects such as lethargy and constipation, which may seriously impair QOL. Radiopharmaceuticals are efficacious in treating bone pain secondary to metastases. These include phosphorus-32, strontium-89, rhenium-186, samarium-153, and tin-117m. An ideal radiopharmaceutical agent would localize in osseous areas only and not lead to adverse effects on normal tissues, including bone marrow. The half-life of the

TABLE 36–2   Comparison of Three Approved Radiopharmaceuticals for Bone Pain Palliation[22–25]

Agent	Half-Life (d)	Mean Response	Pain Relief (wk)
^{32}P	14.26	74%	10
^{89}Sr	50.53	80%	10
^{153}Sm	1.95	77%	10

agent should be long enough for cytocidal doses to be administered; yet the dose should be low enough for outpatient dosing.[24] None of the previously listed agents meet all of these criteria. Phosphorus-32 can be safely administered orally as an outpatient; it is inexpensive but can lead to myelosuppression. Strontium-89 is the most widely used agent and leads to a 60% to 80% palliative response rate. Strontium-89 has been compared with radiotherapy, and no significant difference has been noted.[25] A small study ($n = 31$) compared phosphorus-32 with strontium-89, and no difference was noted between the two in the time to onset of response or time to maximum relief or duration of response.[26] Samarium-153 is associated with early marrow recovery, thereby allowing repeated dosing.[27] Rhenium-186 is an approved agent in Europe and results in a similar degree of myelosuppression as strontium. Tin (Sn)-117, unlike the previously listed agents, releases electrons and not beta particles. Thus tissue penetration and myelosuppression is lower than with other agents. Response rate with this compound is about 75%.[28] Select radiopharmaceuticals and their properties are listed in Table 36–2.

All of these radiopharmaceuticals share some common properties. These agents are effective in osteoblastic and not osteolytic lesions; therefore, painful areas have to be scintigraphically positive for therapy to be useful. Further, their administration may be associated with a flare phenomenon. Hence, they are contraindicated in the presence of impending cord or nerve root compression. Myelosuppression and disseminated intravascular coagulation are also known contraindications to their administration. At the present time, studies combining radiopharmaceuticals with bisphosphonates, chemotherapeutic agents, and each other are in progress.

ASSESSMENT OF PALLIATIVE RESPONSE

Efficacy of chemotherapy and systemic treatments (such as those discussed earlier) for the palliation of pain must be evaluated scientifically by randomized controlled trials using appropriate QOL instruments. In recent years, several QOL and symptom-based instruments have emerged that are useful in the evaluation of

palliative response. The simplest scales for the measurement of pain include numeric rating scale (NRS), visual analog scale (VAS), and a verbal descriptor scale (VDS).[29] These "quantify" pain numerically. Other, more sophisticated instruments measure multidimensional aspects, including the sensory and affective components of pain. These include the McGill Pain Questionnaire, Brief Pain Inventory, and the Memorial Pain Assessment Card,[30] which are often used in conjunction with other established QOL measures such as FACT-G (Functional Assessment of Cancer Therapy) and the EORTC QLQ-C30. These instruments are multidimensional constructs that measure symptoms (fatigue, pain, and nausea) and quantitate physical, social, and emotional aspects of functioning. Depending on the nature of the clinical trial, it may be necessary to supplement these QOL instruments with additional modules such as the FACT-L in lung cancer, FACT-O in ovarian cancer, and FACT-E in esophageal cancer. These provide additional information related to that specific cancer such as breathing difficulties or cough with lung cancer and dysphagia in esophageal cancer. There are several methodologic issues in the design of clinical trials with palliative endpoints. These include selection of an appropriate trial-specific instrument, definition of response, timing of assessments, and handling of missing data.[31]

BALANCING TOXICITY WITH CLINICAL BENEFIT

Clinical benefit from chemotherapy must exceed its toxicity for the treatment to be truly palliative in nature. Careful monitoring and treatment of toxicities such as nausea or emesis, asthenia, and mucositis can maintain this balance. Fortunately, the advent of 5-hydroxytryptamine receptor 3 (5-HT3) antagonists has made management of acute emesis easier. With modern antiemetics, acute emesis can be controlled in more than 70% of patients receiving highly emetogenic chemotherapy.[32] The control of delayed nausea and emesis is less satisfactory, with 50% complete responses noted with standard antiemetic regimens. The recent approval of neurokinin-1 antagonist, aprepitant, and 5-HT3 antagonist, palonosetron, which has a longer half-life of 40 hours, may significantly improve delayed nausea and emesis associated with highly and moderately emetogenic chemotherapy regimens.[33] Similarly, increasing usage of hemopoietic growth factors and drugs like methylphenidate may help alleviate asthenia, which remains a difficult problem with chemotherapy.[34]

The Oncology Drugs Advisory Committee (ODAC) has recommended that QOL improvement or survival, or both, should be the basis for approval of new drugs in cancer.[35] Newer targeted agents are likely to have an important role because they have a greater specificity and lower toxicity than cytotoxic agents. Recent experience with gefitinib (Iressa) may be a useful illustration of such a strategy.[36] Gefitinib is an orally active, selective epidermal growth factor receptor, tyrosine-kinase inhibitor that blocks signal transduction pathways implicated in proliferation. Gefitinib was investigated in two large phase II trials in advanced NSCLC.[37,38] These studies were conducted in pretreated patient population, and symptom relief was one of the primary endpoints. Symptom improvement was noted in more than 40% of treated patients; the median time to improvement was 8 and 10 days in the two studies. Patients with objective response were more likely to experience symptomatic improvement in both studies. This improvement was achieved with mild toxicity. The majority of adverse events noted were grade 1 or 2 (diarrhea and skin rash). Gefitinib represents a new class of targeted agents that may change the treatment paradigm for advanced cancer. Indeed, it is likely that targeted agents will also be used for disease palliation in the near future.

PHARMACOECONOMICS

The effect of the anticancer agents on overall health care costs is an important area of research because it may be possible to reduce the costs of expensive interventions such as radiotherapy and hospitalization with judicious use of anticancer agents in the setting of advanced cancer.

Economic considerations should not limit access to palliative chemotherapy; yet, in the present era of cost containment, cost-effectiveness has become important for all aspects of heath care, including palliative care. There are little prospective, randomized data regarding the cost-effectiveness of palliative chemotherapy. Most available data are from retrospective analyses of studies that compared chemotherapy with best supportive care.[39,40] There are no concrete examples as yet of chemotherapy reducing the cost of care. Yet, these studies conducted in NSCLC, prostate cancer, and gastrointestinal cancer suggest that palliative benefit can be obtained at seemingly acceptable cost-effectiveness ratios.

PATIENT PERCEPTION OF PALLIATIVE CHEMOTHERAPY

No real progress in this field can be made without an accurate assessment of patient expectations. Unfortunately, there are limited data on patient perceptions of the role of palliative chemotherapy. Available data regarding patient perceptions of palliative chemotherapy are conflicting. A study conducted in United Kingdom assessed treatment preferences of patients

with NSCLC.[41] Only 22% of patients said they would choose chemotherapy over best supportive care for a 3-month improvement in survival. A majority would choose chemotherapy for an improvement in symptoms, even if this were not associated with any survival improvement. In contrast, Slevin and colleagues[42] reported that the majority of patients offered chemotherapy will accept the same for only 1% chance of cure. Further, 40% would choose chemotherapy if it could prolong life by only 3 months; in contrast, their treating doctors were much less willing to accept chemotherapy as their own treatment if asked the same question. A study from Canada examined the palliative role and cost-effectiveness of chemotherapy for women with relapsed or recurrent ovarian cancer.[43] EORTC QLQ-C30 and FACT-O were used to assess QOL improvement, and the investigators developed their own questionnaire to assess patient expectations. All patients were informed of the palliative, noncurative intent of their chemotherapy and then required to fill out a questionnaire. Despite the clear and specified "palliative" intent of chemotherapy, the majority of patients expected to live longer, and 42% expected a moderately high or a high chance of cure. Clearly, patient and physician perceptions regarding the intent of chemotherapy for advanced cancers do not coincide.

CONCLUSION

"Best supportive care" without anticancer therapy does not represent the "best" palliative option for advanced cancer. In many patients, chemotherapy represents a useful strategy to improve QOL. It is clear in many trials that objective response results in symptom improvement. Therefore, there may not be a dichotomy between palliative chemotherapy and chemotherapy administered with the intent of achieving an objective response. Anticancer therapy may include chemotherapeutic agents, hormonal treatments, bisphosphonates, radiopharmaceuticals, and targeted agents. Judicious selection of the agent is required to achieve a favorable benefit/toxicity ratio. Targeted agents such as gefitinib, erlotinib, and bevacizumab may be particularly favorable in this setting. Supportive medications such as modern 5-HT3 receptor antagonists and hemopoietic growth factors will help alleviate common toxicities from chemotherapy such as nausea, emesis, and fatigue. Cost-effectiveness and patient expectations from these therapies are areas that need further research.

ACKNOWLEDGMENTS

The authors are grateful to Donald Trump, MD, and Nithya Ramnath, MD, for reviewing the manuscript.

REFERENCES

1. Roger C: The Cancer Pain Sourcebook. Lincolnwood, IL, McGraw-Hill/Contemporary, 2001.
2. Levy M: Pharmacologic treatment of cancer pain. New Engl J Med 335:1124–1132, 1996.
3. Kurman MR: Systemic therapy in the palliative treatment of cancer pain. In Patt RB (ed): Cancer Pain. Philadelphia, Lippincott, 1993, pp 251–274.
4. Burris HA 3rd, Moore MJ, Andersen J, et al: Improvements in survival and clinical benefit with gemcitabine as first-line therapy for patients with advanced pancreas cancer: a randomized trial. J Clin Oncol 15:2403–2413, 1997.
5. Nordin K, Steel J, Hoffman K, Glimelius B: Alternative methods of interpreting quality of life data in advanced gastrointestinal cancer patients. Br J Cancer 85:1265–1272, 2001.
6. Hoffman K, Glimelius B: Evaluation of clinical benefit of chemotherapy in patients with upper gastrointestinal cancer. Acta Oncol 37:651–659, 1998.
7. Glimelius B, Erkstrom K, Hoffman K, et al: Randomized comparison between chemotherapy plus best supportive care with best supportive care in advanced gastric cancer. Ann Oncol 8:163–168, 1997.
8. Michael M, Hedley D, Oza A, et al: The palliative benefit of irinotecan in 5-fluorouracil-refractory colorectal cancer: Its prospective evaluation by a Multicenter Canadian Trial. Clin Colorectal Cancer 2:93–101, 2002.
9. Raghavan D, Koczwara B, Javle M: Evolving strategies of cytotoxic chemotherapy for advanced prostate cancer. Eur J Cancer 33:566–574, 1997.
10. Tannock IF, Osoba D, Stockler MR, et al: Chemotherapy with mitoxantrone plus prednisone or prednisone alone for symptomatic hormone-resistant prostate cancer: A Canadian randomized trial with palliative end points. J Clin Oncol 14:1756–1764, 1996.
11. Souquet PJ, Chauvin F, Boissel JP, et al: Polychemotherapy in advanced non small cell lung cancer: A meta-analysis. Lancet 342:19–21, 1993.
12. Marino P, Pampallona S, Preatoni A, et al: Chemotherapy vs supportive care in advanced non-small-cell lung cancer. Results of a meta-analysis of the literature. Chest 106:861–865, 1994.
13. Shepherd FA, Dancey J, Ramlau R, et al: Prospective randomized trial of docetaxel versus best supportive care in patients with non-small-cell lung cancer previously treated with platinum-based chemotherapy. J Clin Oncol 18:2095–2103, 2000.
14. Hainsworth JD, Erland JB, Barton JH, et al: Minnie Pearl Cancer Research Network. Combination treatment with weekly docetaxel and gemcitabine for advanced non-small-cell lung cancer in elderly patients and patients with poor performance status: Results of a Minnie Pearl Cancer Research Network phase II trial. Clin Lung Cancer 5:33–38, 2003.
15. Jatoi A, Stella PJ, Hillman S, et al: Weekly carboplatin and paclitaxel in elderly non-small-cell lung cancer patients (>/=65 years of age): A phase II north central cancer treatment group study. Am J Clin Oncol 26:441–447, 2003.
16. Eckardt J: Single-agent chemotherapy for non-small cell lung cancer. Lung Cancer 41(Suppl 4):S17–S22, 2003.
17. Norris B, Pritchard KI, James K, et al: Phase III comparative study of vinorelbine combined with doxorubicin versus doxorubicin alone in disseminated metastatic-recurrent breast cancer: National Cancer Institute of Canada Clinical Trials Group Study MA8. J Clin Oncol 18:2385–2394, 2000.
18. Geels P, Eisenhauer E, Bezjak A, Zee B, Day A: Palliative effects of chemotherapy: Objective tumor response is associated with symptom improvement in patients with metastatic breast cancer. J Clin Oncol 18:2395–2405, 2000.
19. Hortobagyi G, Theriault R, Porter l, Blayney D, et al: Efficacy of pamidronate in reducing skeletal complications in patients with breast cancer and lytic bone metastases. Protocol 19 Aredia Breast Cancer Study Group. N Engl J Med 335:1785–1791, 1996.
20. Berenson J, Leichenstein A, Porter L, et al: Efficacy of pamidronate in reducing skeletal events in patients with advanced multiple myeloma. Myeloma Aredia Study Group. N Engl J Med 334:488–493, 1996.
21. Saad F, Gleason DM, Murray R, et al: Zoledronic Acid Prostate Cancer Study Group. A randomized, placebo-controlled trial of zoledronic acid in patients with hormone-refractory metastatic prostate carcinoma. J Natl Cancer Inst 94:1458–1468, 2002.
22. Small EJ, Smith MR, Seaman JJ, Petrone S, Kowalski MO: Combined analysis of two multicenter, randomized, placebo-controlled studies of pamidronate disodium for the palliation of bone pain in men with metastatic prostate cancer. J Clin Oncol 21:4277–4284, 2003.
23. Wong R, Wiffen PJ: Bisphosphonates for the relief of pain secondary to bone metastases. Cochrane Database Syst Rev 2:CD002068, 2002.
24. Silberstein EB, Eugene L, Saenger SR: Painful osteoblastic metastases: The role of nuclear medicine. Oncology 15:157–163, 2001.
25. Quilty PM, Kirk D, Bolger JJ, et al: A comparison of the palliative effects of strontium-89 and external beam radiotherapy in metastatic prostate cancer. Radiother Oncol 31:33–40, 1994.
26. Nair N: Relative efficacy of 32P and 89Sr in palliation of skeletal metastases. J Nucl Med 40:256–261, 1999.
27. Sandeman T, Budd R, Martin J: Samarium-153 labeled EDTMP for bone metastases from cancer of the prostate. Clin Oncol 4:160–164, 1992.
28. Srivastava SC, Atkins HL, Krishnamurthy GT, et al: Treatment of metastatic bone pain with tin-117m stannic diethylenetriamine-pentaacetic acid: A phase I/II clinical study. Clin Cancer Res 4:61–68, 1998.
29. Acute Pain Management Guidelines Panel. Acute Pain Management Operative or Medical Procedures and Trauma. Clinical Practice Guideline. AHCPR Publication No. 92-0032. Rockville, MD, Agency for Health Care Policy and Research, Public Health Service, US Department of Health and Human Services, 1992.
30. Paice J: Pain. In: Yarbro C, Frogge M, Goodman M (eds): Cancer Symptom Management (2nd ed). Sudbury, MA, Jones and Bartlett Publishers, 1999, pp 118–147.
31. Jacobsen PB, Weitzner MA: Evaluation of palliative endpoints in oncology clinical trials. Cancer Control 6:471–477, 1999.
32. Hesketh P, Harvey W, Harker W, et al: A randomized double blind comparison of intravenous ondansetron alone and in combination with intravenous dexamethasone in patients with high dose cisplatin induced emesis. J Clin Oncol 12:596–600, 1994.
33. Navari R: Pathogenesis based treatment and chemotherapy induced nausea and vomiting- two new agents. J Support Oncol 1:89–103, 2003.
34. Bruera E, Driver L, Barnes EA, et al: Patient-controlled methylphenidate for the management of fatigue in patients with advanced cancer: A preliminary report. J Clin Oncol 21:4439–4443, 2003.
35. Beitz J, Gnecco C, Justice R: Quality of life endpoints in cancer clinical trials: The US Food and Drug Administration perspective. J Natl Cancer Inst Monogr 20:7–9, 1996.
36. Natale R, Zaretsky S: ZD 1839 (Iressa): What's in it for the patient? The Oncologist 7(Suppl 4):25–30, 2002.
37. Fukouka M, Yano S, Giaccone G, et al: Final results from a phase II trial of ZD 1839 for patients with advanced non small cell lung cancer (IDEAL 1). Proc Am Soc Clin 21:299a (A1195), 2002.
38. Kris M, Natale R, Herbst R, et al: A phase II trial of ZD 1839 (Iressa) in advanced non small cell lung cancer patients who had failed platinum and docetaxel based regimens (IDEAL 2). Proc Am Soc Clin Oncol 21:292a (A1166), 2002.
39. Leighl NB, Shepherd FA, Kwong R, et al: Economic analysis of the TAX 317 trial: Docetaxel versus best supportive care as second-line therapy of advanced non-small-cell lung cancer. J Clin Oncol 20:1344–1352, 2002.
40. Bloomfield DJ, Krahn MD, Neogi T, et al: Economic evaluation of chemotherapy with mitoxantrone plus prednisone for symptomatic hormone-resistant prostate cancer: Based on a Canadian randomized trial with palliative end points. J Clin Oncol 16:2272–2279, 1998.
41. Silvestri G, Pritchard R, Welch HG: Preferences for chemotherapy in patients with advanced non-small cell lung cancer: descriptive study based on scripted interviews. BMJ 317:771–775, 1998.
42. Slevin ML, Stubbs L, Plant HJ, et al: Attitudes to chemotherapy: Comparing views of patients with cancer with those of doctors, nurses, and general public. BMJ 300:1458–1460, 1990.
43. Doyle C, Crump M, Pintilie M, Oza AM: Does palliative chemotherapy palliate? Evaluation of expectations, outcomes, and costs in women receiving chemotherapy for advanced ovarian cancer. J Clin Oncol 19:1266–1274, 2001.

CHAPTER 37

Radiation Therapy for Cancer Pain Management

PATRICK TRIPP, MD, AND MICHAEL KUETTEL, MD, MBA, PHD

Approximately 1.3 million new cases of cancer are diagnosed every year in the United States.[1] More than 70% of patients eventually develop symptoms from the primary disease or metastases, with pain described as the most frequent and incapacitating symptom. Often, the patient's ability to function is impaired.[2] Pain may be incapacitating and constant, or may be represented by "mechanical allodynia," some normally nonpainful activity perceived as painful, such as coughing or turning in bed.

Pain associated with direct tumor involvement is the most common type of cancer pain, with direct involvement of bone being the most common site.[3] Bone pain is a frequent symptom in advanced cancer. Estimates for cancer patients who report bone pain range from 28% to 70%.[4,5] Undoubtedly, these wide-ranging estimates depend on subjective factors such as patient reporting versus physician reporting.

Although cancer spread to bone typically does not involve vital organs, painful bone metastases affect patient quality of life and survival. Bone metastases can cause intractable pain, pathologic fracture, hypercalcemia, and neurologic deficits, including spinal cord compression and markedly reduced activity and comfort levels.

Radiation therapy remains a cornerstone of palliative management of bone pain. In cancer patients, pain relief is widely recognized as an important endpoint in itself.[6,7] Often radiation dose and fractionation schedule for palliation do not carry near the morbidity of the dose required for cure. Thus, palliative radiotherapy provides maximum relief with little risk to the suffering patient.

Pain relief involves response to the various components of pain, which can be broken down into sensory, reactive, and cognitive evaluative elements. Sensory elements are characteristic physical findings and symptoms including severity, location, quality, duration of pain, and relief from therapy. Reactive elements describe the social and psychological effects that often accompany pain, including anxiety, depression, suffering, what pain

means relative to disease progression, and perceived availability of relief.[8,9] Finally, pain can be described in cognitive evaluative terms, with the patient's attitudes and beliefs about pain playing a role in the patient's care.[10]

Radiation therapy plays an important part in pain relief, either alone or as part of overall management. The patient who requires radiation for relief from pain often has end-stage disease, but the spectrum of patients treated with palliative radiation also includes breast cancer patients who may live for many years after a course of radiation therapy or patients with indolent lymphoma who may require radiation to a specific painful site before going on with systemic therapy that may continue for many years. This chapter examines the role for radiation in pain relief, either alone, in combination with typical analgesics such as narcotics, and as part of newer approaches to management of pain, which may include hormonal or chemotherapy.

PALLIATION OF PAIN FROM BONE METASTASES

More than 100,000 patients in the United States are newly diagnosed with bone metastases each year.[11] Patterns of care studies show that sites treated with external beam irradiation include both weight-bearing and non–weight-bearing bones, with the goals of pain relief or return of function.[12] Multiple studies have demonstrated that patients treated with palliative radiation can anticipate a 70% to 90% response rate.[13–21] Recent large randomized trials confirm these response rates, with 72% to 78% of patients finding relief when single-fraction radiotherapy is used and 69% to 78% of patients responding when a more conventional protracted radiation course is used.[22,23]

Typically studies have examined outcome in terms of pain relief achieved, duration of response relative to remaining survival (or "net pain relief"), and need for re-irradiation. A review of 12 published fractionation trials found that pain relief was difficult to assess, with extent and duration of relief not always clear, and with confounding influence of simultaneous interventions, analgesics, hormones, chemotherapy, and bisphosphonates unclear.[24] However, in general, more than 40% of patients can expect at least 50% pain relief, and about 30% can expect complete pain relief at 1 month.[24] Given that analgesic drug regimens are often ineffective, radiotherapy has an important role in the management of bone pain.[25]

Median survival after diagnosis and treatment of bone metastases usually ranges from 5 to 12 months.[11] Higher median survivals have been reported in more recent series,[26] which may reflect growing recognition of the importance of palliative care. Alternately, reports of longer median survival may reflect the fact that many of the more recent trials examining the role of radiation in bone metastases excluded patients with more destructive metastases, such as patients with fracture or spinal cord compression.[16–21,26,27] Eligibility criteria for these more recent trials selected for patients who stood the best chance for long survival.

Five- to 12- month survival after diagnosis of bone metastases is reported in multiple trials describing various sites of disease and different primary tumors. However, drawing general conclusions from studies of cancer patients with bone metastases is difficult, as typically studies have included heterogeneous patient populations with an array of uncontrolled variables. Furthermore, many of these variables have been independent of the treatment regimen to which patients have been assigned.[11] A woman with good performance status and a diagnosis of breast cancer and solitary painful rib metastasis can anticipate a very different outcome from a patient with widely metastatic lung cancer who is urgently radiated to thoracic spine vertebral bodies and spinal cord to prevent spinal cord compression.

Bone metastases studies are unlike other studies for several reasons. Often, patients with many different primary tumor sites and histology are included. Next, patients with a range of disease extent and location are included, so that results from patients with solitary rib metastases are grouped with patients who have extensive widespread bone and systemic disease. Typically, outcome measures examined include requirements for further narcotic use and for re-irradiation. Various studies have relied on patients to report results using "pain scores" or some other measure to add objective quantification to a subjective endpoint.[11] For these reasons, despite multiple randomized trials carried out over the past 30 years, development of treatment guidelines based on the available data is difficult. As a result, the treatment approach in a given clinical scenario is left to the judgment of the treating physician.

Mechanism of Bone Metastases Pain and Pain Relief from Radiation

Bone pain from metastases is thought to arise from either a "mechanical" component such as gross tumor infiltration of bone, a "biologic" component that includes changes in the bone microenvironment, or some combination of these factors. "Mechanical" pathophysiology includes disease-induced bone loss and replacement of bone by metastatic tumor.[28] The mechanical pain model also includes physical stress to bone caused by impinging tumor or tumor infiltration of pain receptors.[11] Clinicians have long observed that asymptomatic metastases can transform into painful metastases in a short period of time. Such onset of pain may represent increased bone invasion and may represent an early marker of disease progression.[29]

Although these explanations may seem obvious or easily inferred, clinical observation suggests that the pathophysiology of bone pain may be more complex. The "biologic" model of bone pain has been developed from the observation that only a small proportion of bone metastases become painful. Moreover, the factors that convert painless metastases into painful ones are unknown.[30] Investigators have suggested that bone pain may be caused by tumor-stimulating chemical pain receptors.[11] Neuropathic pain characteristically responds to gabapentin-class drugs but not to morphine, whereas inflammatory pain characteristically responds to morphine but not to gabapentin. These responses are explained by the fact that the physiologic neurochemical markers that characterize chronic neuropathic pain are distinct from markers that characterize inflammatory pain. Mouse studies suggest that bone cancer pain may represent a third category, with distinct neurochemical features, such as increased neuronal expression of c-Fos for example.[31]

Evidence from a mouse model suggests that central nervous system (CNS) sensitization may also be a component of bone cancer pain. The sense of mechanical allodynia may derive from a "revving up" of the CNS, in effect lowering the patient's pain sensory threshold.[28]

The range of explanations for bone cancer pain from common-sense inferences to studies suggesting cellular changes in neurotransmitters underscores the lack of understanding of what causes bone cancer pain. The mechanism of pain relief provided by radiation is not well understood. Authors have suggested cell kill, biologic cascade, host response, or some combination of these factors accounts for pain relief.

Historically, radiation's role in providing relief from bone pain was thought to be from cell kill and tumor shrinkage, the same factors that clinicians use to assess radiation response in the curative setting. Using this model, shrinkage of disease would inevitably lead to less mechanical pressure and less infiltration of the bone and its pain receptors at the site of metastases.

Bone metastases from breast and prostate tumors tend to respond better to radiation than metastases from a lung cancer primary tumor.[11,14,23,27,32,33] Some authors have suggested that this observation of "site-specific" response indicates that cell kill is the mechanism by which radiation provides pain relief.[32] In this model, the suspected mechanism of radiation relieving bone pain is related to decreased tumor burden.[28]

But several observations do not support a cell kill model. First, a dose–response relationship, which would support tumor shrinkage or cell kill required for pain relief, has not been proven.[13–15,18,20,22] In this light, tumor shrinkage or cell kill alone to account for pain relief seems unlikely.[23]

Moreover, tumor shrinkage alone cannot account for the rapid relief of pain which sometimes follows radiation.[35] These observations have prompted investigators to examine the bone microenvironment to look for clues into radiation's mechanism of pain relief. Authors have speculated that radiation's potential role may include inhibiting cells that secrete prostaglandins, which are well-described mediators in the pain response.[35] By inference from known mechanisms of drug action and pain response in laboratory animals, prostaglandin E_2 has been suggested as one potential mediator.[36]

Cytokines such as TGF-β may also be involved in radiation's mechanism of pain relief. Low-dose radiation has been associated with activation and induction of TGF-β isoforms.[37,38] And TGF-β1 is known to be involved in bone development and remodeling.[39] Given these observations, authors have suggested that low-dose radiation may aid bone healing by induction of TGF-β.[23]

Finally, the patient's response to radiation has been suggested as playing a role in radiation's mechanism of pain relief. Radiation may induce some physiologic change in the patient, which contributes to relieving pain. For example, in breast cancer patients, recalcification of lytic metastases appears earlier after radiation compared with the rate of response after chemotherapy or hormones,[40,41] suggesting that radiation's mechanism of pain relief includes bone healing as well. The real answer to the pathophysiology of bone pain and pain relief likely includes all of these mechanisms.

Local External-Beam Radiation

Goals of local external-beam radiation include providing pain relief, maximizing convenience, and providing durable response. An area of ongoing controversy is the study of the optimal dose and fractionation regimen. The two basic approaches are conventional protracted moderate-dose regimen or relatively low-dose single-shot treatment regimen. The problem has long been an area

of research, and practice patterns are not always backed by data.

Building on results established in early trials, which showed high rates of pain relief regardless of dose-fractionation regimen,[42,43] investigators have attempted to show that a single-shot regimen is equivalent to a more protracted course. In support of this approach, a meta-analysis that included more than 3200 patients from 16 dose-fractionation trials showed no difference in complete response or overall response rates[44] (Table 37–1). And a methodologic review of the literature that included many of the same patients and trials found 43 different fractionation schedules examined in 12 trials, with no differences in pain relief obtained from single or multiple fraction schedules.[24]

Selecting the optimal regimen is not straightforward. Most important, the outcome measure "pain relief" does not adequately address all issues in palliative radiation for bone metastases. Thus, authors of a different review that included one more recent trial and 11 of the same 12 trials described in the methodologic review described earlier argued that higher dose-fractionated regimens produced better frequency, magnitude, and duration of response than single-shot regimens.[11]

DOES A DOSE–RESPONSE RELATIONSHIP EXIST?

Many investigators have looked for a dose–response relationship in palliative treatment of bone metastases. Studies show mixed results, but many appear to support a dose–response relationship. Radiation Therapy Oncology Group (RTOG) prospective trial 74-02 examined different radiation treatment schedules.[13] Enrollment was 1016 patients, 266 with solitary metastases and 750 with multiple sites of metastases. Patients were stratified by solitary site of metastases versus multiple sites of metastases, use of internal fixation, and participating institution. Patients with solitary metastases were randomized to either 40.5 Gy in 15 fractions at 2.7 Gy per fraction over 3 weeks or 20 Gy in 5 fractions at 4 Gy per fraction over 1 week. Fractionation schedules for patients with multiple sites of metastases were 30 Gy in 10 fractions over 2 weeks, 15 Gy in 5 fractions over 1 week, 20 Gy in 5 fractions over 1 week and 25 Gy in 5 fractions over 1 week.

Results for patients with solitary metastases showed that overall 91% of patients saw at least minimal relief, 83% had partial relief, and 57% of patients achieved complete relief. No differences in pain relief were reported between the two fractionation schedules, and recurrence of pain was at median 15 weeks for 57% of the patients in each of the two arms of the study.[13]

TABLE 37–1 Randomized Trials of Radiotherapy Fractionation for Painful Bone Metastases

Author/Country/Year Published	Treatment Arms	Number of Patients Randomized (Assessable)
Trials comparing single-fraction vs. multifraction radiotherapy		
Hartsell et al,[49] RTOG 97-14, US, 2003	8 Gy single 30 Gy/10 fractions	949 (897)
Kirkbride et al, Canada, 2000	8 Gy single 20 Gy/5 fractions	398 (278)
Bone Pain Trial Working Party,[23] UK/New Zealand, 1999	8 Gy single 20 Gy/5 fractions	761 (681)
Steenland et al,[22] Dutch Bone Metastases Trial, Holland 1999	8 Gy single 24 Gy/6 fractions	1171 (1073)
Koswig and Budach,[34] Germany, 1999	8 Gy single 30 Gy/10 fractions	107 (107)
Nielsen et al,[21] Denmark, 1998	8 Gy single 20 Gy/5 fractions	241 (207)
Gaze et al,[20] UK, 1989	10 Gy single 22.5 Gy/5 fractions	265 (240)
Cole,[16] UK, 1989	8 Gy single 24 Gy/6 fractions	29 (29)
Price et al,[14] UK, 1986	8 Gy single 30 Gy/10 fractions	288 (97)
Trials comparing different multifraction regimens		
Niewald et al,[18] Germany, 1996	20 Gy/5 fractions 30 Gy/15 fractions	100 (100)
Rasmusson et al,[26] Denmark, 1995	15 Gy/3 fractions 30 Gy/10 fractions	217 (127)
Hirokawa et al, Japan, 1988	25 Gy/5 fractions 30 Gy/10 fractions	128 (128)
Okawa et al,[15] Japan, 1988	20 Gy/10 fractions (bid) 30 Gy/15 fractions	80 (80)
Madsen, Denmark, 1983	20 Gy/2 fractions 24 Gy/6 fractions Solitary metastases	57 (57)
Tong et al,[13] RTOG 74-02, US, 1982	40 Gy/15 fractions 20 Gy/5 fractions Multiple metastases 15 Gy/5 fractions 20 Gy/5 fractions 25 Gy/5 fractions 30 Gy/10 fractions	266 (146) 750 (613)
Trials comparing single fractions at different doses		
Jeremic et al,[19] Yugoslavia, 1998	4 Gy vs 6 Gy vs 8 Gy	327 (327)
Hoskin et al, UK, 1992	4 Gy vs 8 Gy	270 (196)

Modified from Wu JS, Wong R, Johnston M, et al: Cancer Care Ontario Practice Guidelines Initiative Supportive Care Group: Meta-analysis of dose-fractionation radiotherapy trials for the palliation of painful bone metastases. Int J Radiat Oncol Biol Phys 55:594–605, 2003.

For patients with multiple bone metastases the numbers were similar, with 89% of patients experiencing minimal pain relief, 83% obtaining partial relief, and 53% achieving complete relief. Median duration of pain control was 12 weeks for each of the fractionation schedules, and 54% of the patients had recurrent pain.[13]

First results of RTOG 74-02 appeared to show that low-dose, short-course schedules were as effective as higher-dose, more protracted regimens. However, reanalysis of the RTOG data using logistic regression multivariate analysis, with solitary metastases and multiple metastases grouped together and endpoints pain relief, narcotic score, and requirement for re-treatment showed an apparent dose–response relationship.[45,46] The "pain relief" endpoint was defined as no continued use of narcotics. In the reanalysis, using the endpoint "combined complete response," pain relief was significantly related to the number of fractions and the total dose delivered, with improved response at higher doses.

Further evidence for a dose–response relationship has been found in trials comparing different single moderate-dose fractions. Improved pain relief has been documented at higher versus lower doses.[14,19] In addition, one trial found improved pain relief with doses greater than 40 Gy when compared with doses less than 40 Gy.[33] A trial comparing conventional fractionation 40 to 46 Gy, "short course" 30 to 36 Gy, and "fast course" 8 to 28 Gy found improved pain relief with higher total dose delivered using a multifraction regimen.[32]

"Net pain relief" is used by some authors to describe duration of pain relief compared with duration of survival. This is an important concept, as advocates who argue that single-shot radiotherapy for bone metastases provides equivalent results will point to patient convenience as a key quality of life issue. But even using this measure, one prospective randomized trial found improved "net pain relief" with 30 Gy in 15 fractions when compared with 20 Gy in 5 fractions.[18]

Perhaps confusing the picture of dose–response relationship, some investigators have found a primary site-specific response. Multiple trials have found favorable responses for bone metastases from primary prostate and breast cancers as compared with metastases from lung and other primary sites. Metastases from prostate and breast tumors have superior outcomes. such as rate of complete relief,[33] minimum duration of relief,[46] and time to progression after radiotherapy,[22] when compared with metastases from lung cancer. Reinforcing the particularly poor prognosis of bone metastases from lung cancer, other studies have found that lung cancer confers a worse outcome no matter what the dose fractionation schedule,[11,13,23,27] and that bone metastases from lung cancer are least responsive to radiation therapy.[32]

Using the measure "net pain relief" to compare duration of response of bone metastases from different primary sites, bone metastases from prostate and breast primary tumors were again found to respond better compared with bone metastases from lung primary sites.[32,33] Although these results may reflect the more aggressive natural history or more extensive tumor burden of lung cancer versus typically more indolent prostate and breast cancers, these studies do appear to support a more aggressive biology of bone metastases from lung cancer as well.

Understanding the radiobiology of fractionated radiation therapy allows a better perspective to understand external-beam radiation therapy for palliation of pain and radiation therapy to bone metastases in particular. Radiation therapy has two mechanisms of cell kill: at low doses, chromosome breaks are the consequence of a single electron set in motion by the absorption of x- or γ-rays, and the probability of an interaction is directly proportional to dose. A second mechanism at work at higher doses involves chromosome breaks from two separate electrons, and the probability of a lethal interaction is then proportional to the square of the dose. Thus, cell kill by radiation is proportional to dose and to the square of the dose. The "linear-quadratic model" expresses cell kill as a function of these two mechanisms, and the "α/β ratio" represents the dose at which linear and quadratic contributions to cell kill are equal. Finally, the "biologically effective dose" (BED) represents a means to compare total doses when dose per fraction and total dose are not equal.[47]

Thus, with 46 fractionation schedules identified in 17 dose-fractionation trials, BED can provide a means to compare various total doses and doses per fraction. One study pooled results from five dose-fractionation trials and calculated BED for each dose-fractionation schedule using the linear quadratic model.[48] Complete response of bone pain to radiotherapy intervention was chosen as an endpoint because it was seen as least susceptible to bias. Although acknowledging the limitations of a retrospective analysis, results showed a clear dose–response relationship for pain relief when the entire range of doses from five trials was examined, and on the basis of these findings the authors recommended further testing of high dose regimens.[48]

Although intriguing, lumping five studies together and fitting their methods to a mathematical formula does not carry the same weight as evidence from randomized controlled trials. In addition, these authors included only 1723 patients studied in five trials. At least 13 randomized trials were published before the study, and these trials, in addition to three large prospective randomized trials including an additional 2829 patients,[22,23,49] do not provide such a clear result.[24,44]

Recently reported results of RTOG 97-14 show no change in response to radiation at higher doses.[49] Eligibility for this trial was limited to patients with breast and prostate cancer primary tumors. Patients were randomized to 8 Gy in a single fraction versus 30 Gy in 10 fractions, and treatment could be delivered to a maximum of three sites. First reported results of the trial showed no differences in rates of partial response or complete response no matter the dose-fractionation scheme, with overall response rate of 66%. Pain response was similar whether the patient was on bisphosphonates, and at 3 months 33% of the patients no longer required narcotics. With eligibility restricted to patients with breast and prostate primary tumors, results of this trial were relatively "clean" compared with previous trials that included more heterogeneous populations. At least for patients with one to three bone metastases from breast and prostate cancer, evidence supports giving a single 8 Gy fraction.

The Dutch Bone Metastases Study provides further evidence for the efficacy of a single-fraction regimen.[22] This trial randomized 1171 patients with primary tumors from all sites except renal cell carcinoma and melanoma to single-fraction 8 Gy versus 24 Gy in 6 fractions. Overall, 71% of patients reported pain relief, and no differences between the groups were found with regard to response to radiation, requirement for pain medication, quality of life, and side effects. The single important difference found in the study was that re-treatment was required in 25% of patients in the single-fraction arm versus only 7% of patients in the multifraction arm.[22]

Finally, the Bone Pain Trial Working Party in the United Kingdom[23] reported results that reinforce findings of the RTOG and the Dutch Study. The trial randomized 765 patients to single-fraction 8 Gy versus multifraction regimens of either 20 Gy in 5 fractions or 30 Gy in 10 fractions. Patients with primary tumors from all sites were included. The trial showed no statistically significant differences between the groups in terms of first improvement in pain, time to complete pain relief, or time to first increase in pain, with 78% of patients reporting some pain relief. Similar to the findings in the Dutch Study, 23% of patients in the single-fraction 8 Gy group required re-treatment versus only 10% of patients in the multifraction higher dose groups. The study's authors concluded that 8 Gy in a single fraction is the treatment of choice for the majority of patients with bone metastases.

Perhaps the real answer for whether a dose–response relationship exists is buried somewhere in the data collected from multiple trials over 30 years. Undoubtedly, primary tumor site plays a role in response of bone metastases to radiotherapy, and undoubtedly patient characteristics such as performance status and extent of disease contribute to a good or poor outcome. Results of three large recent trials done by the RTOG, Dutch Bone Metastases Study, and Bone Pain Trial Working Party in the United Kingdom show that for the majority of patients, single-fraction 8 Gy provides equivalent pain relief to multifraction regimens.

Other Endpoints

Typically, bone metastases dose-fractionation trials have examined rates of partial or complete relief, duration of relief, and rates of re-irradiation required. Some trials have looked at survival relative to response as well, and some studies have reported a strong relationship between response of bone metastases and survival.[14,18] Other studies have found a relationship between primary site and survival regardless of the dose and fractionation schedule.[22,46] This supports the clinical observation that survival after radiotherapy for bone metastases is usually not related to the response of the metastases but to the progression of systemic disease elsewhere.

Other endpoints examined have included bone healing versus pain relief. A randomized prospective trial used computed tomography (CT) scan bone density measurements to determine recalcification rates of bone after radiotherapy at single-shot 8 Gy versus 30 Gy in 10 fractions. This trial reported a trend in improved recalcification for all primary sites and statistically significant improved bone healing for breast cancer, but the rate of recalcification was not related to pain relief, which showed no differences between the two fractionation schedules.[34]

Another significant outcome that trials have examined is the rate of re-treatment after radiotherapy to bone metastases. In general, re-treatment appears to be required more often in patients treated with single-fractions versus patients treated with multiple-fraction regimens.[10,13,21,26] Re-treatment has proven safe, effective, and well tolerated,[50,51] and even a second single-shot 4 Gy re-treatment has proved safe and effective, with no apparent difference between previous responders and previous nonresponders in terms of complete relief and overall response rate.[52]

Reasons for a higher rate of re-treatment among patients treated with single-shot regimen are unclear. A closer examination of re-treatment in the Dutch Bone Metastases Study is instructive. In this trial, which compared single-fraction 8 Gy against 24 Gy in 6 fractions, re-treatment was required in 25% of the single-fraction patients versus 7% of the multifraction patients. Mean time to re-treatment was 14 weeks in the single-fraction group versus 23 weeks in the multifraction group, but analysis seemed to show that the level of pain measured by patient-reported pain score was not the only reason to re-treat. In this study, regardless of pain score, patients in the single-fraction group were re-treated more often, showing an apparent greater readiness to re-treat in patients who received only one fraction. Moreover, the interval to re-treatment was shorter in the single-fraction group. Although the shorter interval may show shorter duration of response in the single-fraction group, the shorter interval may also represent only a greater willingness to re-treat.[22]

Typically, requirement for re-treatment has been seen as a drawback to a single-shot regimen. But re-treatment can also be seen as an advantage of the single-shot approach, with response rates of 75% in previous responders and 50% in previous nonresponders, with no increased toxicity.[50,51,53]

Tolerance and Toxicity

In general, trials examining radiotherapy for bone metastases report adverse events poorly. But from available reports, depending on location of bone metastases and field size, treatment toxicity for palliative radiotherapy to bone metastases ranges from mild to moderate. One trial that compared single-fraction 8 Gy versus 24 Gy in 6 fractions[16] reported lethargy related to field size rather than dose. In addition, nausea and vomiting were reported in 77% of the patients in the single-fraction group compared with 33% of the patients in the multifraction group.[16]

A common perception is that fractionated radiotherapy is more effective in preventing pathologic fracture and spinal cord compression.[54] But this perception is not supported by available evidence. RTOG 74-02[13] did not report nausea, vomiting, lethargy, or low blood counts but did report rates of pathologic fracture in the treatment field. Patients with solitary metastases who were treated to the higher dose had an 18% postradiation fracture rate versus a 4% rate at the lower dose. Half of the fractures reported in RTOG 74-02 occurred during the first 4 weeks after treatment, suggesting regression of tumor and subsequent instability of bone or possibly that an increase in patient activity precipitated the fracture.

Many trials excluded patients with impending pathologic fracture or spinal cord compression.[16-21,26,27] Nonetheless, reports of rates of pathologic fracture and spinal cord compression range from 3% to 9%.[19,21,23,55] Among trials that report complications, the methodologic review of 12 trials found no obvious differences between fractionation schedules in incidence of nausea and vomiting, diarrhea, or pathologic fracture.[24] Interestingly, trials do not report marrow toxicity, but concern about this adverse effect is often cited by referring physicians as a basis of nonreferral.[11]

Reimbursement Issues and Patterns of Care

The question of cost and the radiation oncology reimbursement system also influences treatment decisions. In a progressively cost-conscious health care setting,

a single-shot regimen seems obviously less costly.[26] However, clinical observations suggest the difference in costs between a single-shot regimen and a regimen of 5 or even 10 fractions is limited. Compared with curative dose-fractionation radiotherapy, even protracted course palliative radiation has relatively fewer fractions. A large proportion of costs is independent of the number of fractions and the total dose.[22] In addition, if higher rates of re-treatment required in patients treated with single-fraction regimen are taken into account, the apparent cost difference between regimens is reduced further still. Some authors argue that despite this negligible monetary difference, the economic savings of single-fraction regimens can be measured in saving radiotherapy capacity.[22]

An analysis of the Dutch Bone Metastases Trial compared quality-adjusted life expectancy and costs to society for patients receiving either single-fraction 8 Gy or multifraction 24 Gy in six fractions.[56] Using a patient-reported health classification system, subjective reporting of patient health problems was transformed into a score on a societal utility scale, with a number to represent the general public's attitude toward the particular patient's health condition, ranging from "optimal health" to "worse than death." Costs of radiotherapy, including medical costs such as the treatment itself and nonmedical costs such as transportation, were estimated using guidelines for cost effectiveness analyses. To estimate costs of different radiotherapy schedules, cost items were assigned to treatment costs independent of dose-fractionation schedule, such as physician services; cost items proportional to the number of fractions in a given schedule; and costs proportional to the radiation dose delivered. The analysis found that the multifraction schedule carried significantly higher medical costs than the single-fraction regimen, even when allowing for re-treatments. In addition, the analysis found that single-fraction radiotherapy provided equal quality of life and was thus more cost-effective than the multifraction schedule.[56]

The effect of the radiotherapy financing system on dose-fractionation treatment decisions was examined in an analysis of payment methods and radiotherapy practice at 170 European radiotherapy centers.[57] The study found two basic approaches to reimbursement: a case payment system more often used at university hospitals and a fee-for-service system more often used in private clinics. Results included significantly lower number of fractions and lower total dose, less use of shielding blocks, and less use of isodose calculations when a case payment system was used, with the type of center (private center versus university hospital) found to independently influence the fractionation regimen.[57]

These findings no doubt speak to the predominance of private clinics in the United States, and perhaps the consequent finding that radiation oncologists in the

United States tend to prescribe a more protracted dose-fractionation regimen. The Patterns of Care Study (PCS) survey of palliative care found the most commonly practiced schedule 30 Gy in 10 daily fractions.[12] Despite publication of trials that show equivalence of a single-shot regimen to a protracted conventional regimen in at least some primary sites, an updated PCS shows that long fractionation schemes continue to be used by 90% of practitioners in 96% of cases in the United States.[58]

The most recent American College of Radiology (ACR) bone metastases expert panel supports this treatment pattern, with a recommendation for 20 Gy in 5 fractions, 30 Gy in 10 fractions, or 35 Gy in 14 fractions in most situations. Recommendations updated as recently as June 2000 describe single-fraction 6 Gy dose appropriate only for rib metastases.[59,60]

Not surprisingly, until the RTOG 97-14 trial of 8 Gy single-fraction versus 30 Gy in 10 fractions in prostate and breast cancer bone metastases,[49] none of the trials to evaluate single-fraction radiotherapy for palliation of pain from bone metastases were carried out in the United States. The ACR attributes this pattern to lack of experience with daily doses more than 4 Gy and a perception that because single-fraction radiotherapy is less costly it must be inferior. This rationale does not appear to be based on evidence of multiple trials, which shows the safety and efficacy of single-shot regimens. Furthermore, although RTOG 97-14 is the first RTOG trial to study single-shot fractionation in localized external-beam treatment, the RTOG has a substantial track record in examining single-shot therapy in hemibody irradiation.[54]

But even outside the United States, extensive data to support a single-fraction regimen over an extended radiotherapy course has not been widely embraced. A questionnaire sent to 565 radiotherapy centers in 19 Western European countries found practice patterns are shaped largely by factors unrelated to patient or disease characteristics. The study reported that single-fraction regimens were more likely to be used in centers with larger patient loads and at university versus private centers.[61] The shift toward using single-fraction regimens at university centers relative to private clinics may reflect differences in reimbursement methods or may show greater acceptance of clinical trial results at university centers.[62]

The study of practice patterns in Western European countries found that the country in which the center was located independently predicted which schedule would be used, with centers in Germany, Austria, and Switzerland reporting more protracted fractionation regimens relative to Holland and England.[61] In Canada, a survey of 300 practicing radiation oncologists that described different palliative treatment scenarios found that most practitioners used the same regimen in each of the scenarios, and most frequently this regimen was 20 Gy in 5 fractions.[63]

Clinician judgment shaped by tradition and previous training appears to guide treatment policy more than multiple randomized studies that show single-shot fractionation radiotherapy, with at least equivalent results. A survey of radiation oncologists in Australia and New Zealand found that the reasons most commonly used to back a fractionated regimen were influence of training and goals to minimize recurrent pain, whereas reasons cited to support single-fraction regimen included results of randomized trials and patient convenience.[64]

Patient Understanding and Preferences

Some authors have suggested that treatment decisions should include patient expectations and preferences. A small study using a seven-question survey that collected information from patients about expectations before consultation at a radiation center in Canada yielded some curious findings. Most patients were not familiar with the concept of radiation treatment and were not given information from referring physicians about radiation treatment. One third of patients had concerns about treatment efficacy, and a small number of patients anticipated that palliative radiotherapy would cure their metastatic cancer and prolong their lives.[65] Certainly, clarification of such questions is required before any course of palliative radiotherapy.

When patients recognize what options are offered and what radiotherapy means in terms of pain relief and survival, they can be more involved in the decision-making process. A radiotherapy clinic in Singapore entered 62 patients into a study to determine what choices an informed patient would prefer. The dose-fractionation regimens offered were borrowed from the Dutch Bone Metastases Study, either 24 Gy in 6 fractions or 8 Gy in 1 fraction. Advantages and disadvantages of each approach were thoroughly explained to the patient. Most patients chose the multifraction regimen, and nearly all patients expressed positive opinions regarding participation in the decision.[66]

Local External-Beam Radiotherapy Conclusions and Recommendations

Some authors have suggested a staging system for bone metastases.[67] Results from bone metastases trials have identified prognostic markers a staging system would include, such as primary disease site, extent of bone metastases, previous failed therapies, patient performance status, and expected survival. Such a system might identify the subset of patients likely to benefit from a multifraction higher dose radiation course. Many trials have found patient characteristics such as initial pain score, response to therapy, and primary tumor site and histology to be more important than treatment dose in determining outcome,[13,14,16,18,27,46] with consistent findings that poor performance status in general and lung cancer in particular confer worse prognosis regardless of treatment regimen.[11,23]

Certainly, further trials examining multifraction higher dose radiation regimens versus a single-fraction regimen are not required. Recent results from trials carried out by the RTOG, Dutch Bone Metastases Study, and the Bone Pain Trial Working Party, as well as the meta-analysis including these studies and 14 previous trials, consistently show no difference between regimens in terms of pain relief.[22,23,43,49] Additionally, these studies show slightly higher rates of re-treatment among patients treated with a single-shot regimen but no significant differences in toxicity.[22,23,43] Using this evidence, we can safely recommend that pain from most bone metastases can be relieved with 8 Gy in 1 fraction, while bearing in mind that objectives other than pain relief may determine a clinician's choice of dose prescription.

Future trials examining appropriate radiotherapy for painful bone metastases might include typical patient and tumor factors, as well as less traditional measures such as patient perception and involvement. Rather than focus on what has been exhaustively studied over the last 30 years, endpoints of future trials should include parameters designed to promote consistency in data collection and reporting.[68] In addition, studies should include economic effect of treatment and quality of life evaluations such as examined by other trials.[22,49]

Hemi-Body (Wide-Field) Radiation Therapy for Palliation of Bone Metastases

Indications for hemi-body irradiation (HBI) include multiple painful sites of bone metastases. Developed in the 1970s,[69] HBI provides the fastest and most effective pain relief in cancer with widespread bone metastases.[70] Compared with radiation therapy to multiple local fields, single-dose HBI for multiple bone metastases has proven faster for achieving relief from bone pain.[70-72]

Effective and tolerable HBI dose was established by RTOG Trial 78-10, which examined increasing single-dose HBI for patients with multiple painful bone metastases. The toxicity and dose–response study enrolled 168 patients. Results showed that HBI provided pain relief in 73% of patients, with two thirds of patients seeing more than 50% relief. Of patients who responded to HBI, 50% responded within 2 days and 80% responded within 1 week. Pain control was found to be durable, without need for re-treatment. The safest and most effective doses tested were 6 Gy for upper body HBI and 8 Gy for lower- or middle-body HBI. Patients with tumors from all sites found relief, but response and

complete response rates were particularly good for patients with primary breast and prostate cancers.[71]

In patients with bone metastases, clinicians have long observed that patients previously irradiated for primary-site disease tended to have less frequent incidence of bone metastases at that site. In particular, patients with prostate cancer treated to the pelvis and para-aortic lymph node fields, including the lumbar spine, were observed to have fewer lumbar spine bone metastases compared with rib and lower extremity metastases.[73]

Building on this finding and the experience of RTOG 78-10, investigators examined the potential role for HBI in treating occult disease. Unlike many bone metastases trials with endpoints of pain relief, RTOG Trial 82-06 studied delay in disease progression after single-fraction HBI. The trial randomized 499 patients who had completed standard fractionation 30 Gy in 10 fractions to local known symptomatic sites to receive either single-fraction 8 Gy HBI or no further therapy. Time to disease progression was improved in patients who received HBI, with median time to new disease at 12.6 months after HBI versus new disease at median 6.3 months for patients not treated with HBI. Although bone marrow toxicity was higher in the patients who received HBI, the toxicity was transitory. Other life-threatening toxicities were not higher in the HBI arm, and in general, the additional radiation therapy was well tolerated.[74]

RTOG Trial 88-22 was designed to determine the maximum tolerated dose of HBI when used to treat occult bone metastases. The trial enrolled 144 patients with solitary painful site metastases from prostate or breast primary cancers. Initially, patients were treated to the painful site to 30 Gy in 10 fractions. This was followed by HBI to one of five dose levels between 10 and 20 Gy, delivered in 2.5 Gy fractions. The study found that 17.5 Gy was the maximum tolerated dose. Major dose-limiting toxicity was hematologic. When compared with single-fraction HBI, the fractionated regimen provided reduction in the rate of appearance of new disease, but a dose–response effect on appearance of new disease was not established.[75]

Results from a single institution study suggested that fractionated HBI required further investigation. In this retrospective review, 75 patients were treated using one of three different fractionation schemes: single dose with dose escalation from 4 to 10 Gy, split course HBI with two 4-Gy fractions separated by a 2-week rest period, and daily fractionation with total dose ranging from 9 to 15 Gy divided into fractions of 3 Gy each. Results showed that fractionation was effective for pain relief, with reported complete pain relief ranging from 13% in the split-course group to 49% in the daily fractionation group. Fractionation was found to eliminate the need for premedication and close patient monitoring required with single-dose high fraction HBI. In addition, fractionation allowed higher total dose, which the authors found produced better and more durable responses to pain, as well as improvement in overall quality of life.[76]

A study comparing single-shot HBI with fractionated HBI for prostate cancer patients with bone metastases reinforced these results. At a single institution, patients with hormone-refractory prostate cancer and widespread painful bone metastases were treated with HBI using either a single high-dose fraction or multiple fractions. Among the 14 patients treated using the single-shot regimen to 6 or 8 Gy depending on whether the upper or lower hemi-body was irradiated, 13 of the 14 patients achieved complete or partial relief. But in the same group, 10 of the patients (71%) eventually required re-treatment within the initial field because of recurrent bone pain or spinal cord compression.[77]

In the group treated with fractionated radiation, the most common dose schedule was 27 Gy delivered at 3 Gy per fraction in 9 fractions. Only two patients in this group (13%) required re-treatment. The two groups showed a significant difference in duration of response between the two groups but no difference in median survival. Toxicity, including bone marrow suppression and nausea, was similar in both groups.[77]

With fractionation of HBI established as the standard, a follow-up study was sponsored by the International Atomic Energy Agency (IAEA).[70] Given that approximately 50% of bone metastases occur in patients in developing countries, the study's endpoint was an economically sound way to deliver palliative radiation. The study randomized 156 patients, including 136 patients from developing countries. Patients were stratified by location of primary tumor and treated according to one of three HBI fractionation schedules: 15 Gy in 5 daily fractions, 8 Gy in two 4-Gy fractions delivered in the same day, or 12 Gy delivered in 2 daily doses of 3 Gy each on 2 consecutive days. Toxicity was worse for the patients in the arm that received two 4-Gy fractions in a single day, and these patients had worse results for pain relief and survival. The schedule that delivered 12 Gy in four fractions over 2 days had no worse toxicity than the previously standard fractionation HBI. Patients in this arm saw equal pain relief and survival as in the conventional fractionation arm, with the exception of patients with prostate primary cancers, who appeared to benefit from the more protracted course.[70]

Each of these studies has found that dose-limiting toxicities with HBI can include nausea, bone marrow suppression, and radiation pneumonitis. Nausea can be controlled by premedication, although fractionated regimens showed that premedication was not required. Up to a third of patients require packed red blood cell transfusions for anemia induced by the regimen.

This rate may reflect pretreatment performance status and clinical scenario as much as toxicity induced from HBI. Finally, for upper body HBI, partial lung shielding can minimize lung dose and thus reduce the risk of pneumonitis.[71,74,76,77]

Radiopharmaceuticals

Radiopharmaceuticals are indicated for multiple painful sites of bone metastases. The toxicity profile of radiopharmaceuticals is slightly different, with some authors recommending radiopharmaceuticals over HBI in certain clinical situations.[78] A review of seven trials of radiopharmaceuticals including 397 patients showed that compared with external-beam radiotherapy, radioisotopes alone provided a similar extent and duration of relief.[24]

The mechanism of action of radiopharmaceuticals is very different from the mechanism of external-beam radiation therapy. Also called "unsealed sources" by the nuclear regulatory commission, the radioisotope is usually attached to a chemical moiety with an affinity for hydroxyapatite in bone. This allows radiation to select for areas of osteoblastic metastases. Typical side effects from these internal emitters are minimal to moderate drop in platelet and white blood cell counts and occasionally a "flare" of pain at administration, a 2- to 3-day period in which pain at sites of bone metastases is temporarily worse. Pain relief is usually within 1 to 2 weeks, and time to relief may range from 5 days to 4 weeks.[79]

Indications for treatment with radiopharmaceuticals include widespread bone metastases, with unsealed source used as either single-agent therapy or in conjunction with localized external-beam radiation therapy. Radioisotopes are appropriate for metastases that show increased uptake (which represents increased osteoblast activity) on technetium 99m methylenediphosphonate (Tc-99m-MDP) bone scan. Importantly, metastases that appear osteolytic on plain film x-rays characteristically "light up" on bone scan because in the vast majority of bone metastases osteoblasts are stimulated no matter the net loss or gain of bone apparent on plain film x-rays. The ideal radiopharmaceutical has selective uptake in metastases relative to bone, rapid clearance from soft tissue and normal bone, and distribution predicted by Tc-99m-MDP bone scan and is simple to produce in a reactor for commercial use, with a short half-life with maximum beta energy between 0.8 and 2.0 MeV.[79]

In light of toxicity concerns, radiopharmaceutical use is not appropriate in patients with poor performance status, impending pathologic fracture, or low platelet or white blood cell counts. Use is not appropriate if myelosuppressive chemotherapy is planned. In addition, use is not indicated if bone scan at the site of pain does not show Tc-99m-MDP uptake.[80]

The radiopharmaceutical most commonly used to treat widespread painful bone metastases is strontium-89 (89Sr). The mechanism of 89Sr is to combine with calcium in hydroxyapatite in osteoblastic bone metastases.[81] 89Sr has been compared with external-beam radiation in randomized trials.[82,83] Compared with conventional external-beam radiation, 89Sr showed no significant difference in median survival, with similar efficacy and duration of pain relief. The trials found significantly fewer new pain sites in the patients treated with 89Sr compared with patients treated with local or hemi-body radiotherapy.[82,83]

A phase III trial conducted at eight Canadian Cancer Centers examined the role for systemic 89Sr in conjunction with localized external-beam radiation to treat widespread painful bone metastases from hormone-refractory prostate cancer. Fractionation schemes for localized radiation included 30 Gy in 10 fractions over 2 weeks or 20 Gy in 5 fractions in 1 week. 89Sr dose was 10.8 mCi, delivered intravenously within 1 week of completion of local radiation therapy. Results showed that patients given 89Sr reported significantly improved pain control, a reduced requirement for re-irradiation, and a reduced requirement for analgesic medication for 4 months as compared with those treated with localized radiation alone. Patients receiving 89Sr had no improvement in survival, but pain was improved and thus patient functional status was improved. Not surprisingly, patients in the 89Sr arm had more frequent incidence of hematologic toxicity, including decreased platelet and white blood cell counts.[84]

New approaches in using radiopharmaceuticals have included combinations with chemotherapy and hormonal therapy. Randomized trials with small numbers of patients have shown enhancement of patient response to pain without significant adverse effects using 89Sr in combination with cisplatinum and carboplatinum.[29,85] In addition, a survival advantage was found in patients with bone metastases from prostate cancer using consolidation 89Sr with weekly doxorubicin.[86,87] Not all combinations with chemotherapy provide improved response. A phase I study using gemcitabine as a radiosensitizer for 89Sr in patients with androgen independent prostate cancer was stopped when investigators determined that an overall response rate of more than 10% was unlikely in patients treated with this combination.[88]

89Sr has also been used in combination with hormonal therapy. A dose and toxicity study at a single institution examined vinblastine and estramustine as radiosensitizers in 44 patients with bone metastases from prostate cancer refractory to one or more alternative hormone therapies. Results showed 21 patients with at least a 50% decline in prostate specific antigen (PSA), with median duration of response 23 weeks and median

survival 13 months. The authors concluded that 89Sr can be delivered safely and repeatedly and may decrease the need for external-beam radiotherapy.[89]

Radiopharmaceutical agent selection considers ease of use, relative toxicity, effectiveness, and cost. An ACR survey showed that radiopharmaceutical use in the United States is mostly limited to 89Sr.[59] The radiopharmaceuticals approved by the Food and Drug Administration (FDA) for use in the United States are 89Sr, 32P, and 153Sm lexidronam. Although 89Sr is more widely used in the United States, 32P has been studied for safety and efficacy as well. A small trial comparing 32P with 89Sr found no differences in efficacy, with complete relief of pain in nearly half of patients in each arm of the trial. Patients treated with 32P had a higher rate of granulocytopenia, but none were neutropenic, and none required treatment for decreased blood counts.[90]

153Sm lexidronam has been found safe and effective in trials. In this second-generation radiopharmaceutical, lexidronam serves as a chelating agent for 153Sm and forms a metal complex that localizes preferentially to osteoblastic metastases, thus giving a higher target to nontarget ratio. 153Sm lexidronam gave pain relief to 72% of patients in a double-blind, placebo-controlled trial.[91] In a dose escalation study, very high doses were found safe and effective, with many patients able to discontinue opiate use.[92]

Despite the apparent support in the literature for use of radiopharmaceuticals, they are not widely embraced in the United States. ACR bone metastases expert panel members have been disappointed with results using this type of radiation, with one explanation for poor results being the low dose of 89Sr allowed by the FDA. The randomized trial in Canada used a dose of 10.8 mCi, whereas the maximum allowed dose in the United States is 4 mCi.[58,93] But radiopharmaceuticals seem safe and effective and may even have a cost advantage.[78] Their use deserves further investigation.

RADIATION THERAPY FOR PALLIATION OF PAIN AT OTHER SITES

Palliation of Neurologic Pain

Spinal cord compression can have catastrophic effects on neurologic motor function. In 90% of patients, the presenting symptom is progressively worsening pain.[94,95] Treatment for spinal cord compression includes high-dose steroids and either emergent radiation therapy or surgery to prevent permanent motor weakness or paraplegia.[95]

Widely accepted indications for surgical intervention are bone compression of the spinal cord, spinal instability, and progression of clinical signs despite radiation therapy.[95] One study randomized 101 patients with spinal cord compression to surgery followed by radiotherapy versus radiotherapy alone.[96] The study showed that patients first treated with surgical decompression retained the ability to walk, maintained continence, and maintained functional scores significantly longer than patients treated with radiation alone, although no difference in survival was found between the two groups.[96]

More frequently, the radiation oncologist is called to manage spinal cord compression using radiation alone, with the role for radiation therapy in spinal cord compression widely accepted. As with bone metastases treatment, radiation dose and fractionation scheme are not well established. An evidence-based guideline was developed from a review of 24 studies describing treatment of spinal cord compression.[95] Radiation therapy dose varied within and among centers and ranged from single-shot 8 Gy to 40 Gy in 20 fractions over 4 weeks. No single regimen was superior to others for any cohort of patients. Many centers commonly prescribe 30 Gy in 10 fractions, a regimen supported by consensus expert opinion.[95]

The spinal cord can be re-irradiated, which may be considered for recurrent, progressive painful disease. Because radiation myelopathy is one of the most devastating complications in radiation oncology, re-treatment of the spinal cord is considered only for patients who are not surgical candidates because of other medical problems, irreversible motor symptoms, or widespread extent of disease.[97] However, radiobiologically, the spinal cord is considered a late-reacting tissue. Given the usually short life expectancy of patients with spinal cord compression, radiation therapy for treating progressive pain is a reasonable option. Moreover, a review of human and animal data suggested little risk of radiation myelopathy for total doses less than the BED 128 Gy.[98] This review suggested that for patients who received 30 Gy in 10 fractions, re-treatment doses can range from 25 Gy in 10 fractions if delivered at least 6 months after first treatment to 30 Gy in 10 fractions if delivered more than 2 years after first treatment.[98] Results of studies describing re-irradiation of the spinal cord have been mixed. One series showed development of radiation myelopathy 4 to 25 months after re-treatment,[99] whereas another described little risk of radiation myelopathy during the lifetime of the patient.[100] One series showed that most patients who were re-irradiated to the spinal cord experienced some pain relief or complete pain relief.[101]

Neurologic pain from invasion of lumbar-sacral plexus can cause debilitating pelvic pain. Radiation therapy has a role for palliative control of pain, bleeding, and obstructive symptoms from uncontrolled gynecologic or gastrointestinal primary tumors or metastases. One study examined the role for chemoradiation in patients who presented with metastatic rectal cancer.[102] Patients were treated with 30 Gy in 6 fractions, 45 Gy in 25 fractions, or 35 Gy in 14 fractions. Pain, bleeding, and obstructive symptoms resolved in 94% of patients. A dose–response effect was found, with BED less than 35 Gy predicting a worse outcome. Only 4 of 80 patients suffered grade 3 acute gastrointestinal or skin complications.[102]

Pain from recurrent rectal cancer has also been treated with radiotherapy. As with re-irradiation of the spinal cord, re-treatment historically was considered inappropriate because of perceived increased risk for damage to small bowel, bladder, soft tissues, and bone. But patients who present with recurrent rectal cancer have few options for pain relief. A review of re-irradiation in 52 patients with recurrent rectal cancer after prior pelvic radiotherapy describes outcome for these patients.[103] Median initial radiation dose was 50.4 Gy. Median re-irradiation dose was 30.6 Gy, delivered either at conventional fractionation of 1.8 to 2.0 Gy per day or at 1.2 Gy twice per day (to reduce late side effects). Total cumulative dose ranged from 66.6 Gy to 104.9 Gy, with median cumulative dose 84.4 Gy, and 90% of the patients were treated with concurrent 5-fluorouracil (5-FU) chemotherapy. The review found that 65% of the patients experienced complete pain relief, with the response durable until death for most patients. Median overall survival after re-treatment was 12 months.[103]

Invasion of the celiac neurologic plexus from advanced pancreatic cancer can also cause debilitating pain. Reports have described various radiotherapeutic approaches including conventional external beam radiation therapy with chemotherapy,[104,105] use of neutrons,[106] intraoperative radiation therapy[107-109] and radioactive implants for recurrent pelvic wall tumors.[110] Rates of pain control range from 50% to 90% in studies that have addressed pain relief as an endpoint. None of these approaches appears superior to the others. Given the frequent clinical scenario of a patient with a poor performance status and limited life expectancy, conventional external-beam radiation with or without chemotherapy to 30 Gy in 10 fractions is a reasonable option.

Palliation of Lung and Chest Pain

Most lung cancer patients present with incurable disease. The Medical Research Council (MRC) in England conducted randomized trials to determine the optimal palliative radiation dose for patients presenting with incurable lung cancer. The first MRC trial in non–small cell lung cancer (NSCLC) studied patients with untreated inoperable NSCLC that was too advanced for long-term palliative radiotherapy. Effective palliation of symptoms, including pain, was achieved with equivalent results for 17 Gy in 2 fractions 1 week apart versus 30 Gy in 10 fractions daily, with 80% of patients reporting improvement in pain.[111]

The second MRC trial built on these results. The second trial included only patients with poor performance status, as investigators expected that patients with inoperable disease but good performance status would benefit from a multifraction higher dose regimen. Patients were randomized to either 17 Gy in 2 fractions or 10 Gy in 1 fraction. Results showed that of the 59% of patients who presented with pain as one of their symptoms, 72% in the single-fraction group and 59% in the 2-fraction group achieved at least some pain relief, with no reported *P*-value. Duration of pain control was similar in both arms.[112]

The National Cancer Institute of Canada (NCIC) recognized that despite these results, radiation oncologists were slow to adopt a single-fraction 10 Gy dose for poor performance NSCLC patients.[113] Potential explanations for not following the evidence established in the MRC trials included lack of experience with large single-fraction doses, concerns about acute toxicity, and uncertainty about which patient population stood to benefit. Against this background, the NCIC designed a trial to compare single-fraction 10 Gy with the Canadian standard of 20 Gy in 5 fractions, with the following endpoints: palliation of symptoms, toxicity, quality of life, and survival.[113] Eligibility requirements included stage IV disease or bulky, locally advanced, inoperable disease; inability to tolerate chemotherapy; greater than 10% body weight loss over 6 months; or poor performance status. Results showed that patients treated to 20 Gy in 5 fractions had better improvements in pain (*P* = 0.0008), better quality of life, and significantly longer median survival when compared with the single-fraction group, with no significant difference found in treatment-related toxicity.[113]

These findings were supported by a review of 8 trials of palliative thoracic radiotherapy. The effect of radiation treatment on survival of poor performance patients with inoperable NSCLC is not clear, as no study randomized patients to palliative radiotherapy versus supportive care alone. Nevertheless, the benefit of palliative radiation in this patient population seemed clear, as palliation of pain ranged from 60% to 80%.[114]

Further support for conventional protracted regimen versus a single-shot approach was provided by a quality of life study in the Netherlands in which eligible patients had inoperable disease and poor performance status.[115] Among the symptoms reported at entry, 62% of patients reported chest wall pain. Patients were treated four times per week to 30 Gy in 10 fractions, and patients completed a quality of life questionnaire. Findings included 60% of patients reporting pain relief. Patients also reported improvements in functioning and global quality of life,[115] suggesting that conventional protracted fractionation radiotherapy regimens are most appropriate for this subgroup of patients.

As with other sites, little information is available on re-irradiation of the lung for palliation of pain and other symptoms. Records of 1500 lung cancer patients over a 15-year period were reviewed at a single institution, and 23 patients who underwent re-irradiation for recurrent disease, metastases, or new primary were identified.[116] Median re-treatment dose was 30 Gy. Among the patients who reported thoracic pain before re-irradiation, most described an improvement in pain control after re-irradiation.[116]

CONCLUSION

Canadian primary care physicians were surveyed to determine their attitudes toward radiation therapy offered for the palliation of pain. The study found that primary care physicians perceived stumbling blocks in access to radiation oncology services, and the physicians acknowledged that they were not comfortable with their radiotherapy knowledge.[117] Certainly, many radiation oncologists can give anecdotal reports of referred patients who are over-drugged on narcotics and referred too late for palliative radiotherapy services. But many patients with cancer pain are ideal candidates for radiotherapy, which offers outpatient control of pain with low morbidity, thus enabling the patient to continue functioning.

A report counted the number of studies of palliative care or symptom control presented at the annual meeting of the American Society for Therapeutic Radiology and Oncology (ASTRO). Despite that 40% of radiation oncology services are delivered for palliation of pain or other symptoms, only 1.3% of 3511 abstracts submitted in an 8-year period studied palliative radiotherapy.[118] Research in radiotherapy for palliation of pain and other symptoms should be more actively supported, for the radiation oncologist's role in pain management is an important part of patient care.

Many unanswered questions open the door to continuing research in palliative radiation. Although recently published RTOG 97-14 trial results[49] support single-fraction palliative radiation in the population of breast and prostate cancer patients with bone metastases, radiation for pain control applies to many different clinical circumstances. And although the population of patients requiring radiation for pain control appears heterogeneous, RTOG 97-14 proves that well-designed trials with specific goals and limited eligibility criteria are possible in this setting. Trials can be designed to define subsets of patients who stand to benefit most from radiation versus some other palliative therapy, either alone or in combination with other therapies. In addition, once the efficacy of radiation for pain control is established, optimal dose and fractionation schemes can be designed and tested in trials, bearing in mind that for this group of patients in particular quality of life is of utmost importance.

REFERENCES

1. Jemal A, Murray T, Samuels A, et al: Cancer statistics, 2003. CA Cancer J Clin 53:5–26, 2003.

2. Cleeland CS, Gonin R, Hatfield AK, et al: Pain and its treatment in outpatients with metastatic cancer. N Engl J Med 330:592–596, 1994.

3. Foley K: Supportive care and quality of life. In DeVita S, Hellman S, Rosenberg S (eds): Cancer Principles and Practice of Oncology, 6th ed. Philadelphia, Lippincott Williams and Wilkins, 2001.

4. Anderson PR, Coia LR: Fractionation and outcomes with palliative radiation therapy. Semin Radiat Oncol 10:191–199, 2000.

5. Mercadante S: Malignant bone pain: Pathophysiology and treatment. Pain 69:1–18, 1997.

6. Cassel EJ: The nature of suffering and the goals of medicine. N Engl J Med 306:639–645, 1982.

7. American Society of Clinical Oncology. Outcomes of cancer treatment for technology assessment and cancer treatment guidelines. ASCO. J Clin Oncol 14:671–679, 1996.

8. Cleeland CS: Measurement and prevalence of pain in cancer. Semin Oncol Nurs 1:87–92, 1985.

9. Clark WC: Pain sensitivity and the report of pain. Anesthesiology 40:272–287, 1974.

10. Melzack R: The McGill Pain Questionnaire: Major properties and scoring methods. Pain 1:277–299, 1975.

11. Ratanatharathorn V, Powers WE, Moss WT, et al: Bone metastasis: Review and critical analysis of random allocation trials of local field treatment. Int J Radiat Oncol Biol Phys 44:1–18, 1999.

12. Coia LR, Hanks GE, Martz K, et al: Practice patterns of palliative radiotherapy for the United States 1984-1985. Int J Radiat Oncol Biol Phys 14:1261–1269, 1988.

13. Tong D, Gillick L, Hendrickson FR: The palliation of symptomatic osseous metastases: Final results of the Study by the Radiation Therapy Oncology Group. Cancer 50:893–899, 1982.

14. Price P, Hoskin PJ, Easton D, et al: Prospective randomized trial of single and multifraction radiotherapy schedules in the treatment of painful bony metastases. Radiother Oncol 6:247–255, 1986.

15. Okawa T, Kita M, Goto M, et al: Randomized prospective clinical study of small, large and twice-a-day fraction radiotherapy for painful bone metastases. Radiother Oncol 13:99–104, 1988.

16. Cole DJ: A randomized trial of a single treatment versus conventional fractionation in the palliative radiotherapy of painful bone metastases. Clin Oncol (R Coll Radiol) 1:59–62, 1989.

17. Kagei K, Suzuki K, Shirato H, et al: A randomized trial of single and multifraction radiation therapy for bone metastasis: A preliminary report. Gan No Rinsho 36: 2553–2558, 1990, Japanese, as translated and reported in Ratanatharathorn V, Powers WE, Moss WT, et al: Bone metastasis: Review and critical analysis of random allocation trials of local field treatment. Int J Radiat Oncol Biol Phys 44:1–18, 1999.

18. Niewald M, Tkocz HJ, Abel U, et al: Rapid course radiation therapy vs. more standard treatment: A randomized trial for bone metastases. Int J Radiat Oncol Biol Phys 36:1085–1089, 1996.

19. Jeremic B, Shibamoto Y, Acimovic L, et al: A randomized trial of three single-dose radiation therapy regimens in the treatment of metastatic bone pain. Int J Radiat Oncol Biol Phys 42:161–167, 1998.

20. Gaze MN, Kelly CG, Kerr GR, et al: Pain relief and quality of life following radiotherapy for bone metastases: A randomised trial of two fractionation schedules. Radiother Oncol 45:109–16, 1997.

21. Nielsen OS, Bentzen SM, Sandberg E, et al: Randomized trial of single dose versus fractionated palliative radiotherapy of bone metastases. Radiother Oncol 47: 233–240, 1998.

22. Steenland E, Leer JW, van Houwelingen H, et al: The effect of a single fraction compared to multiple fractions on painful bone metastases: A global analysis of the Dutch Bone Metastasis Study. Radiother Oncol 52:101–109, 1999. Erratum in: Radiother Oncol 53:167, 1999.

23. Bone Pain Trial Working Party. 8 Gy single fraction radiotherapy for the treatment of metastatic skeletal pain: Randomized comparison with a multifraction schedule over 12 months of patient follow-up. On behalf of the Bone Pain Trial Working Party. Radiother Oncol 52:111–121, 1999.

24. McQuay HJ, Collins SL, Carroll D, et al: Radiotherapy for the palliation of painful bone metastases. Cochrane Database Syst Rev 2000.

25. McQuay HJ, Jadad AR: Incident pain. Cancer Surv 21:17–24, 1994.

26. Rasmusson B, Vejborg I, Jensen AB, et al: Irradiation of bone metastases in breast cancer patients: A randomized study with 1 year follow-up. Radiother Oncol 34: 179–184, 1995.

27. Hoskin PJ, Price P, Easton D, et al: A prospective randomized trial of 4 Gy or 8 Gy single doses in the treatment of metastatic bone pain. Radiother Oncol 23:74–78, 1992.

28. Clohisy DR, Mantyh PW: Bone cancer pain. Cancer 97(3 Suppl):866–873, 2003.

29. Sciuto R, Festa A, Rea S, et al: Effects of low-dose cisplatin on 89Sr therapy for painful bone metastases from prostate cancer: A randomized clinical trial. J Nucl Med 43:79–86, 2002.

30. Portenoy RK, Lesage P: Management of cancer pain. Lancet. 353:1695–1700, 1999.

31. Honore P, Rogers SD, Schwei MJ, et al: Murine models of inflammatory, neuropathic and cancer pain each generates a unique set of neurochemical changes in the spinal cord and sensory neurons. Neuroscience 98:585–598, 2000.

32. Arcangeli G, Giovinazzo G, Saracino B, et al: Radiation therapy in the management of symptomatic bone metastases: The effect of total dose and histology on pain relief and response duration. Int J Radiat Oncol Biol Phys 42:1119–1126, 1998.

33. Arcangeli G, Micheli A, Arcangeli G, et al: The responsiveness of bone metastases to radiotherapy: The effect of site, histology and radiation dose on pain relief. Radiother Oncol 14:95–101, 1989.

34. Koswig S, Budach V: [Remineralization and pain relief in bone metastases after different radiotherapy fractions (10 times 3 Gy vs. 1 time 8 Gy). A prospective study] Strahlenther Onkol 175:500–508, 1999. German. (Findings are reported in abstract, available in English.)

35. Bates T, Yarnold JR, Blitzer P, et al: Bone metastasis consensus statement. Int J Radiat Oncol Biol Phys 23:215–216, 1992.

36. Bennett A: The role of biochemical mediators in peripheral nociception and bone pain. Cancer Surv 7:55–67, 1988.

37. Barcellos-Hoff MH, Derynck R, Tsang ML, et al: Transforming growth factor-beta activation in irradiated murine mammary gland. J Clin Invest 93:892–899, 1994.

38. Barcellos-Hoff MH, Dix TA: Redox-mediated activation of latent transforming growth factor-beta 1. Mol Endocrinol 10:1077–1083, 1996.

39. Mostov K, Werb Z: Journey across the osteoclast. Science 276:219–220, 1997.

40. Coombes RC, Dady P, Parsons C, et al: Assessment of response of bone metastases to systemic treatment in patients with breast cancer. Cancer 52:610–614, 1983.

41. Crone-Munzebrock W, Spielmann RP: Quantification of recalcification of irradiated vertebral body osteolyses by dual-energy computed tomography. Eur J Radiol 7:1–5, 1987.

42. Vargha ZO, Glicksman AS, Boland J: Single-dose radiation therapy in the palliation of metastatic disease. Radiology 93:1181–1184, 1969.

43. Allen KL, Johnson TW, Hibbs GG: Effective bone palliation as related to various treatment regimens. Cancer 37:984–987, 1976.

44. Wu JS, Wong R, Johnston M, et al: Cancer Care Ontario Practice Guidelines Initiative Supportive Care Group. Meta-analysis of dose-fractionation radiotherapy trials for the palliation of painful bone metastases. Int J Radiat Oncol Biol Phys 55:594–605, 2003.

45. Blitzer PH: Reanalysis of the RTOG study of the palliation of symptomatic osseous metastasis. Cancer 55:1468–1472, 1985.

46. Gillick LS, Goldberg S: Technical Report No. 185R, Final Analysis RTOG Protocol No. 74-02. Boston, Department of Biostatistics, Sidney Farber Cancer Institute, 1981.

47. Hall E: Radiobiology for the Radiobiologist, 5th ed. Philadelphia, Lippincott Williams and Wilkins, 2000.

48. Ben-Josef E, Shamsa F, Youssef E, et al: External beam radiotherapy for painful osseous metastases: Pooled data dose response analysis. Int J Radiat Oncol Biol Phys 45:715–719, 1999.

49. Hartsell WF, Scott C, Bruner DW, et al: Phase III randomized trial of 8 Gy in 1 fraction vs. 30 Gy in 10 fractions for palliation of painful bone metastases: Preliminary results of RTOG 97-14. Int J Radiat Oncol Biol Phys 57(S124), 2003.

50. Mithal NP, Needham PR, Hoskin PJ: Retreatment with radiotherapy for painful

bone metastases. Int J Radiat Oncol Biol Phys 29:1011–1014, 1994.

51. Jeremic B, Shibamoto Y, Igrutinovic I: Single 4 Gy re-irradiation for painful bone metastasis following single fraction radiotherapy. Radiother Oncol 52:123–127, 1999.

52. Jeremic B, Shibamoto Y, Igrutinovic I: Second single 4 Gy reirradiation for painful bone metastasis. J Pain Symptom Manage 23:26–30, 2002.

53. Jeremic B: Comment on: Single fraction RT for bone mets, are all questions answered? Radiother Oncol 54:185–186, 2000.

54. Chander SS, Sarin R: Single fraction radiotherapy for bone metastases: Are all questions answered? Radiother Oncol 52:191–193, 1999.

55. Uppelschoten JM, Wanders SL, de Jong JM: Single-dose radiotherapy (6 Gy): Palliation in painful bone metastases. Radiother Oncol 36:198–202, 1995.

56. van den Hout WB, van der Linden YM, Steenland E, et al: Single- versus multiple-fraction radiotherapy in patients with painful bone metastases: Cost-utility analysis based on a randomized trial. J Natl Cancer Inst 95:222–229, 2003.

57. Lievens Y, Van den Bogaert W, Rijnders A, et al: Palliative radiotherapy practice within Western European countries: Impact of the radiotherapy financing system? Radiother Oncol 56:289–295, 2000.

58. Ben-Josef E, Shamsa F, Williams AO, et al: Radiotherapeutic management of osseous metastases: A survey of current patterns of care. Int J Radiat Oncol Biol Phys 40:915–921, 1998.

59. Rose CM, Kagan AR: The final report of the expert panel for the radiation oncology bone metastasis work group of the American College of Radiology. Int J Radiat Oncol Biol Phys 40:1117–1124, 1998.

60. Kagan AR, Rose CM, Bedwinek JM, et al: Bone metastases. American College of Radiology. ACR Appropriateness Criteria. Radiology 215(Suppl):1077–1104, 2000.

61. Lievens Y, Kesteloot K, Rijnders A, et al: Differences in palliative radiotherapy for bone metastases within Western European countries. Radiother Oncol 56:297–303, 2000.

62. van der Linden YM, Leer JW: Impact of randomized trial-outcome in the treatment of painful bone metastases; patterns of practice among radiation oncologists. A matter of believers vs. non-believers? Radiother Oncol 56:279–281, 2000.

63. Chow E, Danjoux C, Wong R, et al: Palliation of bone metastases: A survey of patterns of practice among Canadian radiation oncologists. Radiother Oncol 56:305–314, 2000.

64. Roos DE: Continuing reluctance to use single fractions of radiotherapy for metastatic bone pain: An Australian and New Zealand practice survey and literature review. Radiother Oncol 56:315–322, 2000.

65. Chow E, Anderson L: Patients with advanced cancer: a survey of the understanding of their illness and expectations from palliative radiotherapy for symptomatic metastases. Clin Oncol (R Coll Radiol) 13:204–208, 2001.

66. Shakespeare TP, Lu JJ, Back MF, et al: Patient preference for radiotherapy fractionation schedule in the palliation of painful bone metastases. J Clin Oncol 21:2156–2162, 2003.

67. Janjan NA, Declos ME, Ballo MT, et al: Palliative Care. In Cox JD, Ang KK (eds): Radiation Oncology Rational Technique Results, 8th ed. St. Louis, Mosby, 2003.

68. Chow E, Wu JS, Hoskin P, et al: International consensus on palliative radiotherapy endpoints for future clinical trials in bone metastases. Radiother Oncol 64:275–280, 2002.

69. Fitzpatrick PJ, Rider WD: Half body radiotherapy. Int J Radiat Oncol Biol Phys 1:197–207, 1976.

70. Salazar OM, Sandhu T, da Motta NW, et al: Fractionated half-body irradiation (HBI) for the rapid palliation of widespread, symptomatic, metastatic bone disease: A randomized phase III trial of the International Atomic Energy Agency (IAEA). Int J Radiat Oncol Biol Phys 50:765–775, 2001.

71. Salazar OM, Rubin P, Hendrickson FR, et al: Single-dose half-body irradiation for palliation of multiple bone metastases from solid tumors. Final Radiation Therapy Oncology Group report. Cancer 58:29–36, 1986.

72. Salazar OM, Rubin P, Keller B, et al: Systemic (half-body) radiation therapy: Response and toxicity. Int J Radiat Oncol Biol Phys 4:937–950, 1978.

73. Kaplan ID, Valdagni R, Cox RS, et al: Reduction of spinal metastases after preemptive irradiation in prostatic cancer. Int J Radiat Oncol Biol Phys 18:1019–1025, 1990.

74. Poulter CA, Cosmatos D, Rubin P, et al: A report of RTOG 8206: A phase III study of whether the addition of single dose hemibody irradiation to standard fractionated local field irradiation is more effective than local field irradiation alone in the treatment of symptomatic osseous metastases. Int J Radiat Oncol Biol Phys 23:207–214, 1992.

75. Scarantino CW, Caplan R, Rotman M, et al: A phase I/II study to evaluate the effect of fractionated hemibody irradiation in the treatment of osseous metastases: RTOG 88-22. Int J Radiat Oncol Biol Phys 36:37–48, 1996.

76. Salazar OM, DaMotta NW, Bridgman SM, et al: Fractionated half-body irradiation for pain palliation in widely metastatic cancers: Comparison with single dose. Int J Radiat Oncol Biol Phys 36:49–60, 1996.

77. Zelefsky MJ, Scher HI, Forman JD, et al: Palliative hemiskeletal irradiation for widespread metastatic prostate cancer. Int J Radiat Oncol Biol Phys 17:1281–1285, 1989.

78. Malmberg I, Persson U, Ask A, et al: Painful bone metastases in hormone-refractory prostate cancer: Economic costs of strontium-89 and/or external radiotherapy. Urology 50:747–753, 1997.

79. Silberstein EB: Systemic radiopharmaceutical therapy of painful osteoblastic metastases. Semin Radiat Oncol 10:240–249, 2000.

80. McEwan AJ: Use of radionuclides for the palliation of bone metastases. Semin Radiat Oncol 10:103–114, 2000.

81. Janjan NA: Radiation for bone metastases: Conventional techniques and the role of systemic radiopharmaceuticals. Cancer 80(8 Suppl):1628–1645, 1997.

82. Quilty PM, Kirk D, Bolger JJ, et al: A comparison of the palliative effects of strontium-89 and external beam radiotherapy in metastatic prostate cancer. Radiother Oncol 31:33–40, 1994.

83. Bolger JJ, Dearnaley DP, Kirk D, et al: Strontium-89 (Metastron) versus external beam radiotherapy in patients with painful bone metastases secondary to prostatic cancer: Preliminary report of a multicenter trial. UK Metastron Investigators Group. Semin Oncol 20(3 Suppl 2):32–33, 1993.

84. Porter AT, McEwan AJ, Powe JE, et al: Results of a randomized phase-III trial to evaluate the efficacy of strontium-89 adjuvant to local field external beam irradiation in the management of endocrine resistant metastatic prostate cancer. Int J Radiat Oncol Biol Phys 25:805–813, 1993.

85. Sciuto R, Maini CL, Tofani A, et al: Radiosensitization with low-dose carboplatin enhances pain palliation in radioisotope therapy with strontium-89. Nucl Med Commun 17:799–804, 1996.

86. Logothetis C, Tu SM, Navone N: Targeting prostate cancer bone metastases. Cancer 97(3 Suppl):785–788, 2003.

87. Tu SM, Millikan RE, Mengistu B, et al: Bone-targeted therapy for advanced androgen-independent carcinoma of the prostate: A randomised phase II trial. Lancet 357:336–341, 2001. Erratum in: Lancet 357:1210, 2001.

88. Pagliaro LC, Delpassand ES, Williams D, et al: A Phase I/II study of strontium-89 combined with gemcitabine in the treatment of patients with androgen independent prostate carcinoma and bone metastases. Cancer 97:2988–2994, 2003.

89. Akerley W, Butera J, Wehbe T, et al: A multi-institutional, concurrent chemoradiation trial of strontium-89, estramustine, and vinblastine for hormone refractory prostate carcinoma involving bone. Cancer 94:1654–1660, 2002.

90. Nair N: Relative efficacy of 32P and 89Sr in palliation in skeletal metastases. J Nucl Med 40:256–261, 1999.

91. Serafini AN, Houston SJ, Resche I, et al: Palliation of pain associated with metastatic bone cancer using samarium-153 lexidronam: A double-blind placebo-controlled clinical trial. J Clin Oncol 16:1574–1581, 1998.

92. Anderson PM, Wiseman GA, Dispenzieri A, et al: High-dose samarium-153 ethylene diamine tetramethylene phosphonate: Low toxicity of skeletal irradiation in patients with osteosarcoma and bone metastases. J Clin Oncol 20:189–196, 2002.

93. Leibel SA: ACR appropriateness criteria. Expert Panel on Radiation Oncology. American College of Radiology. Int J Radiat Oncol Biol Phys 43:125–168, 1999.

94. Janjan N: Bone metastases: Approaches to management. Semin Oncol 28(4 Suppl 11):28–34, 2001.

95. Loblaw DA, Laperriere NJ: Emergency treatment of malignant extradural spinal cord compression: An evidence-based guideline. J Clin Oncol 16:1613–1624, 1998.

96. Patchell R, Tibbs PA, Regine WF, et al: A randomized trial of direct decompressive-surgical resection in the treatment of spinal cord compression caused by metastasis [abstract 2], ASCO 2003.

97. Morris DE: Clinical experience with retreatment for palliation. Semin Radiat Oncol 10:210–221, 2000.

98. Endicott TJ, Ford JM, Withers HR, et al: Re-irradiation of the spinal cord: Development of a dose fractionation schedule. Int J Radiat Oncol Biol Phys 45(Suppl 3):173–174, 1999.

99. Wong CS, Van Dyk J, Milosevic M, et al: Radiation myelopathy following single courses of radiotherapy and re-treatment. Int J Radiat Oncol Biol Phys 30:575–581, 1994.

100. Schiff D, Shaw EG, Cascino TL: Outcome after spinal re-irradiation for malignant epidural spinal cord. Ann Neurol 37: 583–589, 1995.

101. Grosu AL, Andratschke N, Nieder C, et al: Re-treatment of the spinal cord with palliative radiotherapy. Int J Radiat Oncol Biol Phys 52:1288–1292, 2002.

102. Crane CH, Janjan NA, Abbruzzese JL, et al: Effective pelvic symptom control using initial chemoradiation without colostomy in metastatic rectal cancer. Int J Radiat Oncol Biol Phys 49:107–116, 2001.

103. Lingareddy V, Ahmad NR, Mohiuddin M: Palliative re-irradiation for recurrent rectal cancer. Int J Radiat Oncol Biol Phys 38:785–790, 1997.

104. Gastrointestinal Tumor Study Group: Radiation therapy combined with Adriamycin or 5-fluorouracil for the treatment of locally unresectable pancreatic carcinoma. Cancer 56:2563, 1985.

105. Gastrointestinal Tumor Study Group: Treatment of locally unresectable carcinoma of the pancreas: Comparison of combined-modality therapy (chemotherapy plus radiotherapy) to chemotherapy alone. J Natl Cancer Inst 80:751, 1988.

106. Cohen L, Woodruff KH, Hendrickson FR, et al: Response of pancreatic cancer to local irradiation with high-energy neutrons. Cancer 56:1235–1241, 1985.

107. Zerbi A, Fossati V, Parolini D, et al: Intraoperative radiation therapy adjuvant to resection in the treatment of pancreatic cancer. Cancer 73:2930–2935, 1994.

108. Abe M, Shibamoto Y, Ono K, et al: Intraoperative radiation therapy for carcinoma of the stomach and pancreas. Front Radiat Ther Oncol 25:258–269; discussion 330–333, 1991.

109. Dobelbower RR Jr, Konski AA, Merrick HW 3rd, et al: Intraoperative electron beam radiation therapy (IOEBRT) for carcinoma of the exocrine pancreas. Int J Radiat Oncol Biol Phys 20: 113–119, 1991.

110. Syed AM, Puthawala AA, Neblett DL: Interstitial iodine-125 implant in the management of unresectable pancreatic carcinoma. Cancer 52:808–813, 1983.

111. Medical Research Council. Inoperable non-small-cell lung cancer (NSCLC): A Medical Research Council randomized trial of palliative radiotherapy with two fractions or ten fractions. Report to the Medical Research Council by its Lung Cancer Working Party. Br J Cancer 63:265–270, 1991.

112. Medical Research Council: A Medical Research Council (MRC) randomized trial of palliative radiotherapy with two fractions or a single fraction in patients with inoperable non-small-cell lung cancer (NSCLC) and poor performance status. Medical Research Council Lung Cancer Working Party. Br J Cancer 65:934–941, 1992.

113. Bezjak A, Dixon P, Brundage M, et al: Clinical Trials Group of the National Cancer Institute of Canada. Randomized phase III trial of single versus fractionated thoracic radiation in the palliation of patients with lung cancer (NCIC CTG SC.15). Int J Radiat Oncol Biol Phys 54:719–728, 2002.

114. Numico G, Russi E, Merlano M: Best supportive care in non-small cell lung cancer: Is there a role for radiotherapy and chemotherapy? Lung Cancer 32: 213–226, 2001.

115. Langendijk JA, ten Velde GP, Aaronson NK, et al: Quality of life after palliative radiotherapy in non-small cell lung cancer: A prospective study. Int J Radiat Oncol Biol Phys 47:149–155, 2000.

116. Gressen EL, Werner-Wasik M, Cohn J, et al: Thoracic re-irradiation for symptomatic relief after prior radiotherapeutic management for lung cancer. Am J Clin Oncol 23:160–163, 2000.

117. Barnes EA, Parliament M, Hanson J, et al: Palliative radiotherapy for patients with bone metastases: Survey of primary care physicians. Radiother Oncol 67:221–223, 2003.

118. Barnes EA, Palmer JL, Bruera E: Prevalence of symptom control and palliative care abstracts presented at the Annual Meeting of the American Society for Therapeutic Radiology and Oncology. Int J Radiat Oncol Biol Phys 54:211–214, 2002.

CHAPTER 38

Management of Visceral Pain Due to Cancer-Related Intestinal Obstruction

MELLAR P. DAVIS, MD, AND DANIEL HINSHAW, MD

There are several characteristics of visceral pain processing that facilitate our understanding of the clinical presentation of patients with primary abdominal cancers and bowel obstruction. Not every type of visceral injury evokes pain. Extensive visceral cutting or burning, for example, fails to elicit pain and, thus, viscera are exceptions to Sherrington's concept of pain.[1,2] First, a poor correlation exists between visceral pain and tissue injury. Second, patterns of referred pain are influenced by convergence of somatic and visceral afferents on the same dorsal horn neurons within the spinal cord.[3] Third, clinically visceral pain is poorly localized, midline, and perceived as deep in part because of poor representation within the primary somatosensory cortex.[4,5] Fourth, visceral pain, more common than somatic pain, is accompanied by autonomic responses.[3,6] As a fifth unique feature, only a minority of visceral afferents are sensory, most relate to motor or reflex responses and few have specialized sensory terminals.[7,8] And a sixth unique feature, pain severity is transmitted by the sum of activity from nonspecific sensory receptors within mucosa, smooth muscle, and serosa.[9] Neurotransmission from both high-threshold nociceptors and "silent" nociceptors is recruited for the pain experience.[1,10]

ANATOMIC INFLUENCES ON VISCERAL PAIN

The perception and psychological processing of visceral pain are distinctly different from somatic pain.[11] Such anatomic differences include: (1) a low number of visceral nociceptors compared with somatic nociceptors, (2) lack of specialization, (3) visceral polymodal nociceptors, (4) convergence with somatic afferents on dorsal horn laminae resulting in referred pain, (5) hypersensitivity that is both peripherally and centrally mediated but not by "wind up" characteristic of somatic pain, (6) unique ascending tracts through the dorsal column, (7) low and poor representation within primary somatosensory cortex, (8) rich input through the medial thalamus to the limbic cortex, amygdala, anterior cingulate, and insular cortex, and (9) close association with autonomic nerves.[2,6,11,12]

Visceral receptors are found in mucosa, muscle, and serosa of hollow organs and mesentery but not in parenchyma of solid organs.[10] Somatic tissues have highly specialized abundant receptors that discriminate between various types of stimuli, these are largely lacking in viscera. Only the mesentery contains Pacinian corpusles.[1,10] Hollow organs contain low- and high-threshold mechanoreceptors. Low-threshold receptors are regulatory, whereas high-threshold receptors depolarize only on noxious mechanical stimuli. Visceral pain is the summation of nociceptive input and recruitment of high-threshold and silent nociceptors rather than activation of specific nociceptors. These nonspecialized, high-threshold nociceptors fire at once to produce a central summation of sensory input interpreted as pain.[1] Inflammation lowers the threshold for nociceptor firing, resulting in sensitization of and pain experienced at lower distension pressures.[1] In addition, "silent" nociceptors are also recruited with inflammation into firing at lower thresholds or sensitized by hypoxemia and ischema.[1,3,11] Acute pain is the sum of high threshold nociceptors activated at high pressures where chronic noxious stimuli recruit previously unresponsive or silent nociceptors through hypoxemia or inflammation.[2,6,11] As pressure rises, there is afferent recruitment but also changes from phasic to monotonous or tonic afferent discharges. Pain sensations correlate with generated intracolonic or small bowel pressures and increased wall tension rather than intraluminal volume.[13] As a result, patients may have ileus without pain.[14] Mechanoreceptors in the muscular layer adapt slowly to pressures but in the serosa adapt rapidly.[15]

Mechanoreceptors are either poorly myelinated A-delta or unmyelinated C-fibers. There is a distinct lack of A-beta fibers within viscera. Large myelinated fibers characteristic of somatosensory afferents are only found within the pacinian corpuscles of the mesentery.[1,2,10] The vast majority of visceral afferents are arborizing small myelinated or unmyelinated fibers that terminate as free nerve endings. There are no distinctive anatomic characteristics that separate them from low-threshold, reflex generating afferents.[1] Organization of these mechanoreceptors remains diffuse as there is an absence of a separate peripheral sensory pathway. Visceral afferents travel with autonomic pathways in abdomen and pelvis. Stimulated nociceptors release both substance P and calcitonin gene-related protein (CGRP) within synapses of the dorsal horn. Tachykinin receptors, nerve growth factor receptors, and kappa opioid receptors are found on peripheral nociceptors and dorsal horn afferents transmitting visceral pain.[6,16-26]

Activation of visceral afferents results in up-regulation of nitric oxide synthase in the spinal cord dorsal horn and causes expression of the oncogene C-fos in laminae I, V, VII, X of the dorsal horn within the thoraco-lumbar spine.[20] In addition to C-fos in spinal cord, C-fos is also expressed in the limbic lobe, amygdala, and paraventricular hypothalamic nuclei when visceral nociceptors are stimulated.[2,11] Stimulation results in increased norepinephrine production within the locus coeruleus.[6] When kappa receptor agonists bind to peripheral visceral afferents, substance P release is prevented and expression of C-fos is reduced within the dorsal horn.[23-25]

Even though sensory afferents travel with autonomics, it is inappropriate to identify these nociceptors as sympathetic or parasympathetic sensory afferents. Sensory fibers do not belong to the autonomic system. Proper designation is either splanchnic or pelvic sensory afferents.[1,27] Splanchnic afferents have neuronal cell bodies originating in the lower thoracic and upper lumbar dorsal root ganglia, which innervate upper abdominal viscera, small bowel, and most of the colon to the transverse colon (Figure 38-1). Pelvic afferents terminate at S2-5 sacral cord and innervate a portion of the transverse, descending, and sigmoid colon and rectum.[1,2] This neuroanatomic distribution of afferents predicts that bilateral splanchnicectomy, celiac plexus block, and superior hypogastric plexus block will relieve visceral pain.[1]

Visceral afferents do have a large number of ventral root projections into the spinal cord and to the dorsal horn.[2] As a result, dorsal rhizotomy may fail to relieve visceral pain. Intraspinal distribution of afferent fiber terminals has a wider presentation than cutaneous nociceptors although both visceral and somatic afferents converge on the same laminae within the dorsal horn (Figure 38-2).[27] Such convergent projections lead to viscero-somatic referred hypersensitivity and viscero-visceral hyperalgesia.[15]

HYPERSENSITIVITY

Hypersensitivity is pain produced by innocuous stimuli (allodynia) or exaggerated response to pain (hyperalgesia). Primary visceral hypersensitivity as mentioned is caused by peripheral reduction in nociceptive thresholds. Secondary hypersensitivity is a central neuroplastic reaction to activated C-fibers and convergence. Central hypersensitivity is maintained by glutamate release that binds to N-methyl-D-aspartate (NMDA) receptors.[2,3,5] Activation of the NMDA receptor leads to nitric oxide synthase expression, nitric oxide production, and prostaglandin production.[28-38] Convergence leads to somatic hypersensitivity and referred pain, which can mislead physicians as to etiology and location of the source of pain. Central hypersensitivity reduces thresholds within somatic metameric (homologously innervated) sites producing muscle spasm and cutaneous hypersensitivity and well-localized somatic pain. The size of the area of somatic hypersensitivity and severity of referred pain directly reflects the degree of visceral afferent activation by noxious stimuli. In animal models, even muscle and subcutaneous tissue changes occur. Subcutaneous tissue hypertrophies and muscle atrophies at sites of pain referral.[5]

Viscero-visceral hypersensitivity is also caused by overlapping metameric convergence on the thoraco-lumbar dorsal horn. Clinically, this can be seen as overlapping pain patterns between esophageal and myocardial tissues with the development of "unstable angina" at the onset of gallbladder distension in someone with coronary disease. Somatic central sensitization characterized by "wind up" of intraneurons within the dorsal horn does not occur with visceral pain.[1] Hypersensitivity can be blocked by counter irritant or painless stimuli within somatic areas innervated by the same converging visceral afferent. Opioids hyperpolarize visceral afferents and prevent release of substance P and CGRP (Table 38-1). Intraspinal mu and delta opioid agonists will reduce visceral pain by binding to their receptors within the various laminae of the dorsal horn.[14,27,39,40] Ketamine, which blocks NMDA receptors, can influence visceral hypersensitivity.[30] Dexamethasone, which inhibits neuronal nitric oxide synthase gene expression, has been effective in treating visceral pain and bowel obstruction.[31-33] Nonsteroidal anti-inflammatory drugs reduce dorsal horn levels of prostaglandin stimulated by inflammatory cytokines and NMDA receptor activation and reduce visceral pain.[22,33,36,37] Gabapentin reduces glutamate levels and reduces hypersensitivity associated with celiac pain.[34] Finally, viscerosomatic referral may be related to impaired descending inhibitory signals through the periaqueductal gray, which is reversed by serotonin and norepinephrine receptor agonists.[36,39]

FIGURE 38–1 Visceral afferents to the spinal cord. CG, celiac ganglion; SMC, superior mesenteric ganglion; IMG, inferior mesenteric ganglion.

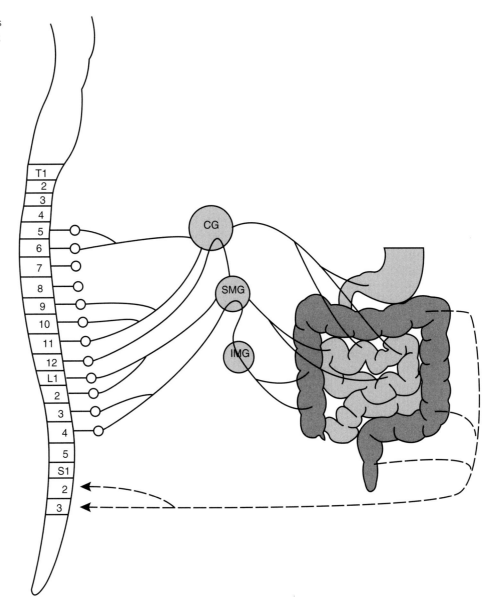

Ascending pathways are unique to visceral pain processing and include: (1) dorsal column ascending secondary sensory afferents, (2) spinal trigeminal to the parabrachioamygdaloid tract, and (3) the spinohypothalamic pathway.[1] Both ventrolateral and dorsal column postsynaptic neurons mediate nociception. The dorsal column is most important for visceral pain and is the reason why midline myelotomy uniquely reduces visceral pain (Figure 38–3).[6,41,42] Ascending tracts go through both the medial and lateral thalamus to the limbic lobe and somatosensory cortex respectively.[6] Somatic pain is dominantly displayed somatotopically as a homuncular representation within the primary somatosensory cortex. However, visceral pain is primarily represented in the secondary somatosensory cortex (S_2) and is only sparsely represented within the primary somatosensory cortex.[12] Visceral pain is well represented in the limbic lobe, including the anterior cingulate and insular cortex and amygdala, which accounts for the strong affective response to visceral pain.[5,12] The distinctly different activation pattern between primary somatosensory cortex on the one hand and the insular cortex and anterior cingulate cortex on the other hand may account for the ability to discriminate visceral pain from somatic pain.[4,30,43] The anatomic differences between visceral and somatic presentation within somatosensory cortex and the visceral nociceptor rich representation within limbic lobe accounts for differences in pain response. Somatic pain produces agitation, hyperactivity, and a "fight or flight" response associated with hypertension. Visceral pain produces behavioral

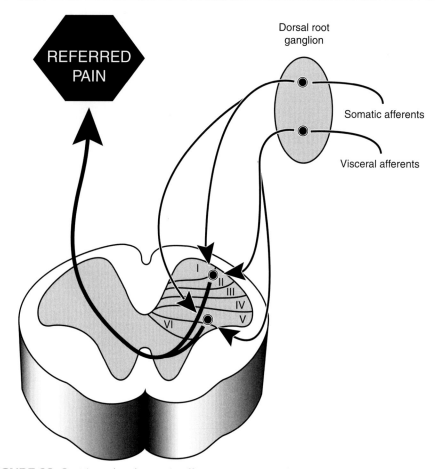

FIGURE 38–2 Visceral and somatic afferents converge on lamina 1 and 2 of the dorsal horn.

TABLE 38–1 Potentially Useful Agents in the Management of Visceral Pain

Kappa opioid agonist	Peripheral kappa receptor agonists on visceral afferents reduces substance P and calcitonin gene-related peptide
Mu and delta opioids	Central mu and delta receptors reduces primary nociceptors actually and central hypersensitivity through periaqueductal grey
Nonsteroidal anti-inflammatory drugs	Block spinal cord and peripheral prostaglandin and central hypersensitivity
Ketamine, methadone	Block dorsal horn NMDA receptors
Corticosteroids	Block expression of spinal cord nitric oxide synthase and reduces hypersensitivity
Gabapentin	Reduces central glutamate levels and NMDA binding for hypersensitivity
Alpha-2-adrenoreceptor agonists (clonidine)	Facilitate descending inhibitory tracts through periaqueductal grey
Tricyclic antidepressants	Facilitate descending tract inhibitory tracts in periaqueductal grey
Anticholinergics	Reduce colic and reduce intestinal secretion
Somatostatin	Inhibits vasointestinal peptide and decreases colic and intestinal secretion. Reduces central hypersensitivity.

NMDA, *N*-methyl-D-aspartate.

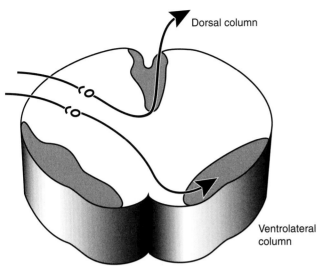

FIGURE 38–3 Visceral afferents ascend through the dorsal funiculus.

quiescence, decreased reactivity to the environment, and nausea associated with hypotension.[44] The reflex inhibition of gastrointestinal motility associated with visceral pain is through stimulation of dorsal motor neurons of the vagus within the medulla, clinically producing nausea and gastroparesis.[5,45]

SUMMARY OF VISCERAL PAIN

At early stages visceral pain is a misleading, vague sensation in the midline, causing deep discomfort, and is poorly localized by the patient and accompanied by both an emotional response and autonomic barrage. Late manifestations are somatic and referred pain hypersensitivity within the metameric spinal level of the visceral nociceptor terminus. This referred pain will be sharp, well localized, and associated with allodynia and muscle spasm. In addition, viscero-visceral hypersensitivity may affect another visceral organ innervated by the same spinal segment. Referred pain can result in a misdiagnosis of somatic pain or a delay in diagnosis.[5,12]

Bowel Obstruction As Initial Presentation

Cancer is the most common cause of bowel obstruction in patients without a prior history of hernia or laparotomy.[46] Acute intussusception in adults is commonly associated with a benign (67%) or malignant (33%) intestinal tumor. Small bowel intussusception is caused by metastases, whereas colonic intussusception is associated with a colon primary if associated with cancer.[47,48] Overall, small bowel obstruction is most commonly

caused by postoperative adhesions (70%), tumor (20%), bezoar, hernia, volvulus, and intussusception. Colonic obstructions are the result of tumor (8% to 29%), ulcerative colitis, diverticulitis or diverticular stricture, adhesions (rarely), fecal impaction, intra-abdominal abscess, and volvulus.[47] Patients who present with acute abdominal pain who are older than 50 years are three times more likely to have intestinal obstruction than those younger than 50. Incidence of cancer as a cause of abdominal pain, and obstruction is 24% for patients who are older than 50 years.[49]

BOWEL OBSTRUCTION IN PATIENTS WITH A HISTORY OF CANCER

Gastrointestinal and ovarian cancer are the most common intra-abdominal primaries to obstruct the bowel.[50] The incidence ranges from 5% to 51% and 10% to 28% with ovarian and gastrointestinal cancers respectively. Patients with gynecologic cancers are more likely to have small bowel (77%) than colonic (23%) obstructions. Postoperative adhesions account for 15% of bowel obstructions in patients with a history of gynecologic cancer.[51] More than two thirds of patients with a previous history of cancer who present with small bowel obstruction will have recurrent disease.[52] Most patients with a history of cancer who present with bowel obstruction will have small bowel obstruction (two thirds), colonic obstruction (one third), or both (one tenth).[53]

The median time from diagnosis of the primary to bowel obstruction caused by recurrent disease is 23 months compared with 56 months for the minority who develop bowel obstruction from primaries originating from extra-abdominal sites.[50] Common extra-abdominal cancers that obstruct the bowel are breast and lung cancer and melanoma.[54,55] In contrast, the mean latency between operation and bowel obstruction for patients with bowel obstruction caused by adhesions is 8 years.[56] Patients who develop bowel obstructions 5 years after the original operation for their intra-abdominal primary usually have adhesions.

Bowel obstruction is most commonly caused by external compression of the bowel lumen by the adjacent tumor or by omental or mesenteric masses or by abdominal or pelvic adhesions. Postradiation fibrosis may cause bowel obstructions in a minority.[57-60] Intraluminal obstruction is either from an intraluminal polypoid mass or annular constriction from circumferential growth of tumor in the bowel wall. Linitis plastica tumor infiltrates the bowel wall diffusely causing a desmoplastic, hard, rigid, nonfunctioning bowel segment and obstructive symptoms. Intestinal motility disorders mimic obstruction and include pseudo-obstruction from infiltration of mesenteric, myenteric, or splanchnic plexus, resulting in loss of motility.[61] Paraneoplastic autoimmune neuropathy or myopathy leads to destruction of gut neuronal networks or smooth muscle leading to obstructive symptoms. This is often associated with small cell lung cancer.[61,62]

Bowel obstruction is not infrequently caused by several factors. Inflammation, edema, constipating drugs (particularly clonidine, antimuscarinics, antihistaminics, and opioids), and fecal impaction may convert a low-grade partial obstruction into a symptomatic or complete bowel obstruction.[60,63]

Concerns for possible malignant obstruction are raised when a patient with advanced malignancy presents with nausea, vomiting, and failure to pass feces. Accurate characterization of associated pain or pains is critical to confirm the diagnosis. A detailed history of pain occurring in conjunction with associated episodes of obstructive symptoms will also clarify the nature and location of the underlying process and may suggest potential interventions for symptomatic relief.

The nature of the pain should be determined with the temporal pattern of pain and onset of nausea and vomiting and obstipation. Continuous visceral pain is usually deep, diffuse, and midline in location. Questions that help distinguish abdominal pain of musculoskeletal origin from visceral etiology are: (1) "Does taking a deep breath aggravate your pain?" (2) "Does twisting your back worsen your abdominal symptoms?" (3) "Has there been any change in bowel since the onset of your symptoms?" (4) "Does eating food aggravate your symptoms?" and (5) "Has there been any change in your weight since the onset of your symptoms?" The first two questions specify pain of musculoskeletal origin, if the answers are affirmative, and the last three questions center on visceral pain. The specificity of these questions is 96% and sensitivity 67%.[64] If abdominal pain is associated with a known history of intra-abdominal malignancy before the onset of obstructive symptoms, it is important to know if the pain characteristics have changed. A recent exacerbation of stable abdominal pain initially experienced at presentation may be a herald of progressive disease and pre-date obstructive symptoms. In contrast, in the absence of a prior known or symptomatic intra-abdominal malignancy, new onset of obstructive symptoms in a cancer patient with an extra-abdominal primary may not necessarily equate with cancer-related obstruction.[58] Many patients have early satiety, which is a common symptom in patients with an advanced cancer and not necessarily associated with bowel obstruction. Benign causes of bowel obstruction, such as adhesions from a prior unrelated laparotomy or an incarcerated hernia, may coincidentally occur in cancer patients.

The clinician needs to know whether the pain is well localized, or referred, vague, and diffuse. Somatic pain associated with cancer is fairly well localized, whereas colic on a backdrop of continuous pain is operationally a peristaltic wave impinging against an obstructed bowel segment. In addition with chronic obstruction, it produces visceral hypersensitivity from secondary bowel inflammation and ischemia and will refer pain to somatic sites such as the flank, abdomen, and chest.[2] Patients frequently have more than one distinctive pain. Patients may have colic, continuous pain, referred pain, and pain related to other metastatic sites. Continuous intraabdominal pain will occur in 90% of patients with a bowel obstruction and colic in 75%.[58] The pain pattern for the continuous pain may differ from that of the intermittent pain. The relationship of the pain to other symptoms, particularly nausea and vomiting, is key to the history of bowel obstruction. The temporal relationship between the onset of nausea, vomiting, and colicky pain will clarify this association. The pain and colic crescendo ends in vomiting followed by a short period of relief, only to recur again. The relationship of symptoms to the last bowel movement and flatus will also help clarify etiology. The gradual onset over several days of nausea and later vomiting, with mild colicky pain followed by obstipation is more typical of distal (colonic) obstruction, whereas the relatively sudden onset of nausea and vomiting, with severe colic and normal stools is characteristic of a more proximal obstruction. It is important to note exacerbating or relieving factors to pain. For instance, colic is relieved by vomiting and pain induced by retroperitoneal metastases may be partially relieved by assuming the fetal position or bending over. Cancer patients on opioids for obstructive symptoms may have temporary mitigation of the distress with the use of opioids because of the opioids' anticholinergic properties. Opioids, however, will also precipitate colic in the opioid bowel syndrome through disinhibited circular smooth muscle leading to segmental contraction. Opioids inhibit longitudinal muscle and propagation of peristalsis. Even worse, severe opioid-induced obstipation mimics obstruction. Physicians may inappropriately increase opioids in the opioid bowel syndrome where aggressive use of laxatives or nonabsorbable opioid antagonists such as naloxone methylnaltreone or alvimopan should be the treatment of choice.

Patients who have a prior bowel obstruction are at a higher risk for developing a recurrent obstruction. When this occurs, the current pain may be similar to the original obstructive symptoms and recognized by the patient. Emotional distress is an integral part of the patient's experience. Continuous nausea and intermittent vomiting with only temporary relief results in anxiety, reduced pain tolerance, and increased abdominal wall soreness from vomiting as a secondary pain. Thresholds for continuous pain are reduced by the psychic experience of unrelieved symptoms.

An important differential in malignant obstruction is obstructing adhesions from a prior operation, an incarcerated hernia, or recurrent tumor. Prior laparotomy is associated with a risk of adhesions. However, a recent history of a laparotomy that demonstrates asymptomatic intra-abdominal cancer should raise a significant concern about cancer-related bowel obstruction. A careful review of the patient's recent bowel habits should be made, including frequency and quality of bowel movements in relation to the degree of symptom relief with defecation. Patients on anticholinergics or other constipating medications and opioids are at an even greater risk for the opioid bowel syndrome, which needs to be kept in mind particularly if laxatives were not started with the initiation of opioid therapy. Autonomic dysfunction and gastroparesis are common in cancer patients, leading to early satiety, nausea, vomiting, and delayed gastrointestinal motility that mimics bowel obstruction. Patients with gastroparesis may respond well to prokinetic agents such as metoclopramide. In contrast, pain is worsened by metoclopramide in high-grade mechanical obstruction, and the onset of colic with metoclopramide therapy indicates that mechanical bowel obstruction is a likely cause.

The type of cancer, location, and usual pattern of metastases exert an important influence on the pattern of symptoms that evolve from cancer-related obstruction. Upper gastrointestinal malignancies produce proximal obstructive symptoms such as dysphagia, rapid onset of nausea and vomiting, and food intolerance, which is temporally and qualitatively different from distal obstructions, which are usually associated with colicky pain, slower onset to nausea, and limited oral intake. Cancers that are even more distal have less intense colic and more signs than symptoms. Distal obstructions are associated with more feculent vomitus. Metastatic disease extensively infiltrates the small bowel mesentery or producing ascites, interferes with peristaltic function sufficiently to minimize visceral colicky pain but not continuous pain, pressure, or vomiting. A matted bowel may prevent abdominal distension as a physical sign.

Physical findings yield important clues to the nature of the underlying intra-abdominal process accounting for the obstruction and provides potential avenues for treatment. The clinician needs to weigh the patient's fitness for undergoing invasive therapies. Patients with far advanced disease who are not surgical candidates should not be put through radiographic procedures for curiosity's sake. In this situation, the opioid bowel syndrome should be exempted from the differential by rectal examination and rectal laxatives followed by medical therapy. Careful prognostication of individual patients and projected survival immediately before the onset of obstructive symptoms is an essential element in the evaluation for surgery. Such prognostication is typically dependent on the patient's performance status (the ability to perform activities of daily living), the nature of the obstruction, current stage of the disease, and previous treatment. Marked cachexia in conjunction with a poor or declining performance status, previous chemotherapy, radiation and/or surgery precludes an aggressive approach to diagnosis because surgical benefits are small and directs the goals of care to medical management.

Abdominal distension, varying degrees of diffuse tenderness, and high-pitched bowel sounds with or without peristaltic rushes are typical features on abdominal examination. These features may or may not be prominent in any given patient with malignant bowel obstruction. Nothing in the physical examination will definitively differentiate between benign and malignant obstruction. However, the presence of palpable masses and ascites certainly favors cancer. Diagnostic imaging includes a radiographic plain abdominal film in the supine and upright positions, ultrasound, computerized tomography (CT), and magnetic resonance imaging (MRI). Sensitivity and specificity for plain x-rays are 69% to 50% and 75% to 57%, respectively.[65,66] Plain films of the abdomen are quite useful and may confirm the presence, the extent, and the level of obstruction because multiple air fluid levels may be found in the small bowel with or without air in the colon or rectum. Right-sided colonic distension and rapid taper and absence of air in the rectum suggests colonic or rectal obstruction. Contrast studies including upper gastrointestinal series, a dedicated small bowel series, or barium enema more precisely locate the point of obstruction. A major disadvantage to barium studies is the possible retention of contrast proximal to the obstruction, with aggravation of the obstruction by inspissated barium. Because of the risk of this complication, water-soluble contrast (i.e. gastrograffin) is preferable. Gastrograffin also has the potential advantage of relieving a partial small bowel obstruction from adhesions or a fecal impaction caused by opioids. CT of the abdomen and pelvis is increasingly recognized as the most useful procedure in diagnosing a bowel obstruction (Figure 38–4). The diagnostic accuracy is 92%, sensitivity 92%, and specificity 71%.[67-69] CT imaging offers an excellent perspective regarding the overall cancer through imaging extramural tumor volume. Tumor-related ascites or large masses at points of obstruction are well demonstrated by CT scans, and CT can assist with more accurately staging the extent of cancer within the abdomen.[66-69] Unfortunately, CT scans are not very effective in identifying multiple peritoneal implants as causes of cancer-related obstruction (Figure 38–5). CT scans will also detect rare complications such as strangulation or intussusception.[67] Finally, virtual colonoscopy has the potential to visualize the entire colon preoperatively, whereas standard colonoscopy is unable to do so.[70,71]

Ultrasound has a high degree of sensitivity (100%) and specificity (84%) in experienced hands. However, CT scans are clearly superior in clarifying etiology (87%) compared with ultrasound (23%).[65]

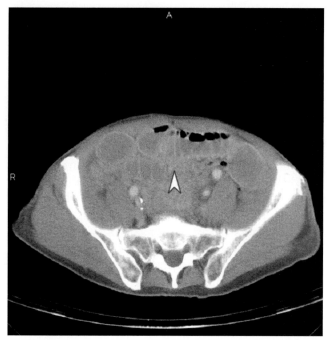

FIGURE 38–4   Computed tomography (CT) of complete small bowel obstruction near the terminal ileum in a patient with a history of gastric resection for adenocarcinoma 11 years earlier. Arrowhead identifies the point of transition from proximal dilated bowel to distal decompressed bowel. The obstruction was secondary to postoperative adhesions. *(Courtesy of Charles Marn, MD, Department of Radiology, VA Ann Arbor Healthcare System and University of Michigan, Ann Arbor, MI.)*

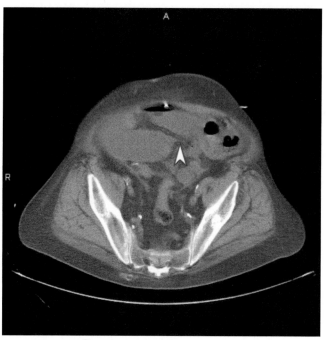

FIGURE 38–5   Computed tomography (CT) image of complete small bowel obstruction near the terminal ileum in a patient who was status postresection of a primary small bowel adenocarcinoma 10 months earlier. Arrowhead identifies the point of transition from proximal dilated to distal decompressed bowel. Laparotomy revealed multiple peritoneal implants not visualized on CT imaging in addition to the main recurrent tumor mass obstructing the bowel. *(Courtesy of Charles Marn, MD, Department of Radiology, VA Ann Arbor Healthcare System and University of Michigan, Ann Arbor, MI.)*

Endoscopic evaluation of the proximal and distal gastrointestinal tract serves as a useful adjunct to identifying and localizing a primary or recurrent obstructing cancer. Endoscopic access to an obstructing intraluminal lesion may allow for endoluminal stent placement or dilatation to restore a functional lumen. Radiographic studies with endoscopy, particularly conventional CT or virtual colonoscopy, will be critical to identifying secondary obstructing lesions inaccessible to endoscopy, which preclude the use of endoscopic stenting to palliate multiple sites of obstruction.

Although there is little debate that bowel obstruction is a surgical problem, bowel obstruction presenting in the context of advanced malignancy is not so clearly or uniformly amenable to surgical correction. A major principle to palliation is that whenever possible effective relief of distressing symptoms is best obtained by treating the underlying cause or causes of the symptoms (e.g., radiation therapy for painful osseous metastases). The rationale for an invasive and operative approach to palliating the pain, nausea, and vomiting of malignant bowel obstruction is based upon this principle. With this in mind, the challenge remains to determine which patients will actually benefit from an operative approach

to relieving their distress.[72-82] Retrospective reviews of multiple case series have identified a number of patient characteristics associated with poor outcomes after attempted surgical correction of malignant bowel obstruction. Major contraindications are: (1) extensive intra-abdominal carcinomatosis by imaging studies, (2) prior laparotomy, (3) extensive intra-abdominal disease with dysmotility seen on radiographic studies, (4) massive ascites, and (5) multiple palpable intra-abdominal masses on physical examination (Table 38–2).[58,75,80,82] Relative contraindications to surgical management are: (1) extensive and symptomatic tumor burden outside of the abdomen, (2) poor performance status, (3) cachexia, and (4) prior radiation to the abdomen or pelvis.[58] Successful surgical intervention is associated with: (1) a single site of obstruction, (2) absence of palpable abdominal masses, (3) ascites of less than 3 liters, and (4) preoperative weight loss of less than 9 kg. Patients who have nonmalignant adhesions as a cause for obstruction derive the greatest benefit from surgical management.[73] Successful outcomes have been defined in terms of survival, relief of symptoms for 60 days after operation, and ability to return home.[81] Cancer site correlates with the success or failure of operative intervention. Obstructions related to colorectal

TABLE 38–2 **Poor Prognostic Factors**
Widespread tumor
Extra-abdominal metastases
Massive ascites
Extensive radiation and chemotherapy
Cancer cachexia and poor performance score
Advanced age

cancer are likely to respond to operative treatment to a greater degree than obstruction secondary to advanced ovarian cancer.[58] Malignant bowel obstruction is rarely an emergency, and has a low risk of strangulation, unlike obstruction from benign causes.[82]

Due consideration should be taken to carefully assess patients for selection before embarking on an operative intervention because the procedure can be both complicated and disappointing to patient and surgeon. A critical and potentially neglected part of this assessment is the patient's understanding of treatment goals (as well as the surgeon's understanding of the patient's goals of care). Most surgically determined outcomes are retrospective and relatively poor in quality as evidence-based guidelines. Control of symptoms is poorly defined, but in the few studies available 42% to 80% have their symptoms improved depending on criteria.[77] Recurrent obstruction in 10% to 50% and 30 day mortality ranges from 5% to 32%.[77] Benefits from surgical therapy are also directly related to duration of disease-free interval. Adhesive bowel obstructions are most likely the cause of obstruction, if there is a long disease interval (5 years from initial resection).[75,77]

INFORMED CONSENT AND MANAGEMENT OF BOWEL OBSTRUCTION

Most reports of operative treatment for malignant bowel obstruction have concentrated on survival and technical success as outcomes.[47,58,82] The quality and durability of symptom relief after major surgery, particularly when the primary goal of surgery is palliative, have been neglected perhaps because of the subjective nature of such assessments and secondarily to the surgeons focus on technical success rather than patient-derived goals. No prospective effort to ascertain the specific and realistic goals in fully informed patients with malignant bowel obstruction before surgical treatment has been reported. A major barrier to a truly informed consent between

surgeons and cancer patients is the often poor level of understanding about prognosis that should inform the discussion. A full appreciation of the projected survival based on a careful assessment of reported and observed performance status before obstruction is usually absent from surgical evaluation. Clearly, a bowel obstruction complicating the course of an advanced malignancy only tends to shorten survival further and surgery will not prolong it. An experienced assessment of prognosis can be expressed in terms of months versus weeks or months versus days to weeks. Even such an imprecise estimate is extremely valuable for informing the discussion about procedures that result in a prolonged hospital course and consume a major portion of the remaining time of a patient's life. In the process of informed consent it may be difficult for surgeons and other providers to give due respect to priorities that the patient may have that are often foreign to health care providers whose primary focus is to treat a condition that usually results in the discharge of a healthy recovering patient. Such a process must be a dialog with much listening on the part of the provider with the expressed intent to hear and understand the specific short-term goals (for only short-term goals can be realistically considered). If an operative intervention is a reasonable fit within such a framework, with all the caveats of potential risks and complications, then it may represent a reasonable option for the patient. Surgical intervention should be seriously considered, after careful assessment of performance status, the nature of the neoplasm, and a favorable imaging study (e.g., suggesting a single point of obstruction without ascites or carcinomatosis). The patient may have months of life ahead after correction of the obstruction. An operation will not guarantee relief of pain. Indeed, at least in the short term it will add new incisional pain to the current misery with the hope of symptomatic relief in the first few days after the procedure with a reduction in obstructive symptoms. A realistic picture of the early postoperative outcome must be shared with the patient during informed consent. This must include morbidity and mortality, even though imprecisely known in retrospective studies.

Minimal invasive surgery with laparoscopy for the treatment of bowel obstruction is, in general, not clearly defined.[82] The presence of large distended loops of small bowel has typically made it very difficult to maneuver a laparoscope in a safe manner to treat a conventional obstruction secondary to adhesions. Laparoscopic bypass of a radiation-related bowel obstruction has been reported.[80] Such an approach may be limited by dense adhesions or carcinomatosis, or both, and require advanced laparoscopic skills. Although direct laparoscopic approaches to treating conventional bowel obstruction may have limitations, laparoscopic visualizations of the peritoneal cavity and malignant bowel obstruction may provide much needed staging information (e.g., confirming the presence of carcinomatosis not seen on CT scan or identifying multiple previously unsuspected sites of obstructions) that will guide an effective open surgical procedure or prevent an unnecessary laparotomy.

Interventions at the time of laparotomy for malignant bowel obstruction vary depending on operative findings.[82] If the actual point of obstruction is due to a benign cause (e.g., adhesion from before surgery), the problems may be easily corrected by lysis of adhesions with exploration made to determine the status of any gross tumor implants. Obstructions by single site recurrences (either intraluminal or extraluminal) may be amenable with fairly definitive chances for relief by resection of the involved bowel with primary anastomosis or surgical bypass of unresectable lesions. Multiple sites of obstruction associated with disease progression may be very difficult or impossible to resolve operatively. Less attractive but sometimes effective approaches include surgical bypass of multiple points of obstruction and proximal diverting ileostomy or colostomy for obstructions involving the distal small bowel, colon, or rectum, respectively. Finally, gastric intubation and percutaneous gastric tube placement should be considered even if only as a temporary measure. Tumor infiltration or compression of the mesentery may impair bowel motility, thus limiting the actual relief experienced after correction of the mechanical obstruction. Unfortunately, recurrent obstruction is not uncommon.[82]

For patients with obstructive lesions involving the proximal or distal portion of the gastrointestinal tract that can be reached by endoscopy, placement of an expandable stent may be a very effective option to relieve obstructive symptoms.[83-89] Stents have been used both for definitive palliation and as temporizing measures in preparation for surgical resection.[83-87] Stenting may be particularly useful when more invasive surgical procedures are not appropriate or feasible because of limited survival or prohibitive risk. Stents have been effective for obstructions of the esophagus, duodenum, sigmoid, colon, and rectum. Covered stents have been extremely useful in the control of fistulas complicating malignant obstructions.[88] An alternative approach has been to combine expandable wire mesh stents with periodic laser treatment to limit tumor ingress into the bowel lumen. Endocavitary I-192 radiation can also be used in conjunction with stents or laser, or both.[90] Stent migration potentially diminishes effectiveness as bridges through obstructed sites, particularly in places not amenable to being well anchored such as at the gastroesophageal junction. When feasible, stents are an attractive option from a palliative care standpoint because they can represent a durable therapy better than dilatation and laser alone and less invasive and morbid than an open procedure.

If successful, they will usually resolve the obstructive symptoms more quickly than an operation.

Another option that can be initiated at the time of laparotomy for malignant obstructions particularly if operative relief of the obstruction is not possible or questionable is the creation of a venting gastrostomy or jejunostomy, or both.[91-95] Recently, percutaneous endoscopy techniques have made it possible to place a percutaneous endoscopic gastrostomy (PEG), which is extended in some patients to the jejunum (PEJ) and permits venting of gastrointestinal secretions, using a minimally invasive approach without laparotomy.[96] Feeding and venting may be possible with PEJ.[96] Such an approach has made it possible for many patients to have limited oral intake and has facilitated home care. The best indication for the use of a PEG is a patient with a survival limited to days to weeks who still has intractable nausea and vomiting from obstruction despite aggressive medical management. Successful symptomatic relief is often predicted by response to the temporary use of nasogastric suctioning before placement of PEG or PEJ.

Quality of life has rarely been reported (e.g., successful discharge to home).[81] Actual measurement of specific symptom relief (i.e., relief of pain, nausea, and vomiting) has largely been lacking. Furthermore, it has been difficult to determine whether operative treatment has consistently or effectively prolonged the life of patients. Selection bias does play a role in most series. Ethically it would be problematic to randomize often desperate and vulnerable patients to a noninterventional limb of a study when they might otherwise have been reasonable surgical candidates based on the criteria mentioned earlier. Although randomization of therapies may be difficult to impossible to implement, careful assessment of patient perceptions regarding relief of specific symptoms, as well as a return to previous preoperative performance status, would be useful outcome measures for future prospective trials. The issue of prognostication is critical because the incidence of postoperative morbidity is high.[58,82] In these debilitated patients the cost of treatment (i.e., prolongation of hospitalization) needs to be balanced against the hope of quality time remaining.

Nasogastric intubation with continuous suctioning is an inadequate long-term palliation solution. Nasogastric suctioning is reasonable for: (1) preoperative management, and (2) as a prelude to medical management by PEG placement.[58,97,98]

Early administration of opioids during assessment of patients presenting with undifferentiated abdominal pain and possible obstruction is appropriate and not associated with undesirable detriments to diagnostic accuracy or physical examination.[99,100] If the findings on the initial evaluation are such that mechanical obstruction is unlikely, treatment should consist of removing potentially offending drugs that influence bowel motility such as anticholinergics, tricyclic antidepressants, and opioids (if possible). Substituting ketorolac for morphine or adding ketorolac and reducing morphine in patients who are on chronic opioids may allow normal peristalsis to return.[101] It is important to exclude sepsis, peritonitis, and recent spinal cord compression within the differential diagnosis of abdominal pain and potential bowel obstruction or ileus. If the rectum is full of feces and the patient is on opioids, rectal measures such as bisacodyl suppositories, phosphate soda enemas, or mineral oil enemas will relieve the obstipation, nausea, vomiting, and abdominal pain. Otherwise, oral naloxone 5 mg daily (which is not readily absorbed) or methylnaltrexone or alvimopan, which does not cross into the central nervous system, may produce laxation without reducing analgesia.[102-105]

If colic is absent and bowel obstruction only partial, a trial of metoclopramide 30 to 60 mg subcutaneous or intravenous over 24 hours dose and 10 mg every 4 hours as needed with escalation to 120 mg over 24 hours may reverse and relieve gastroparesis and partial blockage.[50,57,106] Metoclopramide should not be used if colic or complete obstipation is present or with anticholinergics that block its peristaltic action. Doses need to be halved in patients with hepatic or renal failure.

With extreme ileus (Ogilvie syndrome) neostigmine subcutaneous 1 to 2.5 mg every 6 hours may rapidly decompress the colon. The patient may require telemetry. Care must be taken in those with cardiac disease, asthma, hypotension, peptic ulcers, hypothyroidism, and renal disease.[107-110]

If bowel obstruction is complete or colic and nausea are worsened by metoclopramide or domperidone then haloperidol 5 mg subcutaneous or intravenous over 24 hours with 1 mg every 4 hours as needed may be used for nausea.[50,58] Doses can be increased to 10 mg (equivalent to 20 mg oral). Alternatively, where available, cyclizine 50 mg subcutaneous every 8 hours or 150 mg over 24 hours is used with some relief of nausea.[58,111,112] If nausea persists, several options are available: (1) add dexamethasone 8 mg parenteral in the morning and at noon, (2) methotrimeprazine 2.5 to 5 mg once to twice a day subcutaneous,[58,113-115] (3) Olanzapine 5 mg oral or as a zydius dissolvable disc. Other agents that can be added are hyoscine butylbromide subcutaneous for colic and nausea and octreotide infusions for refractory symptoms. Octreotide is given at 100 to 600 μg per 24 hours either intermittently or as a continuous infusion.[58,116-127] Ondansetron has been used clinically, although there is sparse data justifying use. Ondansetron 8 mg IV or subcutaneous every 8 hours are usual doses. As a warning, oral ondansetron has been associated with bowel obstruction by case report.[126]

Colic is relatively opioid resistant and best treated by antimuscarinics.[127] Hysocine butylbromide as mentioned earlier is helpful. Glycopyrrolate starting with 0.1 mg

subcutaneous or intravenous every 6 hours and increasing doses to 0.2 mg subcutaneous or intravenous is an alternative.[128] Both are quaternary amines and do not penetrate the blood–brain barrier and, thus, are a low risk for delirium.

Analgesics should be used per the World Health Organization stepladder. Acetaminophen 1 g every 6 hours or ketorolac 15 to 60 mg parenteral every 6 hours reduces pain. Ketorolac should not be given with corticosteroids or in renal failure. Both gastric ulcer prophylaxis and hydration are necessary with the use of ketorolac.

Opioids are important for continuous pain. Parenteral morphine 0.5 to 1 mg per hour continuous infusion in the opioid naive is a reasonable starting dose.[58,129,131,132] Provision for rescue doses hourly or every 2 hours should be made. If patients are able and willing, patient controlled analgesia (PCA) is a reasonable alternative means for opioid delivery. Other opioids are fentanyl and methadone, which may have a less detrimental effect on bowel motility.[130-132] If pain is not severe, tramadol, a weak opioid with monoamine reuptake inhibition and also less constipating than morphine, has been reported to be helpful. Starting doses are 50 mg parenteral where available or oral every 6 hours up to 400 mg per day except in the elderly, in whom the maximum dose is 300 mg.[133]

LAXATIVE USE IN BOWEL OBSTRUCTION

With complete bowel obstruction, all oral laxatives should be discontinued, although docusate, a wetting agent, may be continued. A special diet, low residue in nature, with frequent small feedings should be prescribed to those who are able to tolerate a diet. The overall goals of medical therapy are the control of pain, with nausea and vomiting limited to once daily.

If the obstruction is low (i.e., colonic or distal small bowel) attempts at oral medications can be made if symptoms are well controlled by parenteral infusion. Morphine, methadone, tramadol, glycopyrrolate, cyclizine, meclizine, hydroxyzine (as a cyclizine substitute), dexamethasone, haloperidol, nonsteroidal anti-inflammatory drugs (NSAIDs), and olanzapine can be taken by mouth and prescribed based on symptom cluster.

INTRAVENOUS HYDRATION AND NUTRITION

Hydration may be important. Hydration should not be overly exuberant but should replace vomitus and insensible loss. A positive fluid balance or volumes exceeding 2 L per day will lead to additional symptoms. Hydration status correlates poorly with either thirst or dry mouth.[58]

Those particular symptoms can usually be managed with local measures. Over rehydration can produce ascites, pleural effusions, and pulmonary edema associated with elevated renin levels.[134] Modest hydration, either intravenous or by hypodermoclysis, can be safely done either in the hospital or at home.[135,136] Hypodermoclysis with normal saline or two-thirds normal saline with 5% dextrose using 1 to 1.5 L overnight can be done at home.[58]

Total parenteral nutrition is generally more burdensome than helpful for patients with an expected short survival. Patients with slow growing tumors and good performance score may benefit from caloric replacement. Palliative response should be assessed, and if patients fail to respond or are losing strength despite parenteral nutrition, the nutrition should be discontinued. A short trial of therapy may be helpful to assess benefits. Most patients with cancer cachexia are not improved by parenteral nutrition.[58,137]

NEUROLYTIC BLOCKS AND VISCERAL PAIN

Celiac Plexus Block

The celiac plexus can be invaded by direct extension of tumor arising from pancreas or stomach or by nodal metastasis from upper abdominal primaries (Table 38–3). Celiac-related pain is characterized by epigastric midline pain that extends to the left or right upper quadrant or through to the back, or both. It is relieved by assuming a fetal position. It is often mistaken for musculoskeletal pain caused by referral to somatic structures. NSAIDs relieve the pain. Recently gabapentin has improved celiac pain by case report. Doses of gabapentin were 100 mg every 8 hours and titrated to comfort.[138] Celiac plexus block should be used early if possible when disease is limited. The success rate is greater in less advanced disease. Celiac plexus blocks should also be used when

TABLE 38–3	Surgical Invasive Therapies to Reduce Pain
Spinal opioids	
Celiac ganglion block	
Superior mesenteric ganglion block	
Inferior mesenteric ganglion block	
Hypogastric or splanchnic nerve block	
Midline myelotomy	

opioid toxicity, particularly constipation, is a major problem. Neurolysis will produce pain relief and laxation and, thus, relieve two symptoms with one procedure. Studies comparing celiac plexus block with morphine plus NSAIDs demonstrate improved pain control and marginal improvement in quality of life with neurolysis.[139,140] Celiac plexus blocks may only partially relieve pain and work temporarily requiring repeated procedures or the use of a celiac catheter with intermittent use of bupivacaine or splanchnic block.[141,142] Common complications of celiac plexus block are diarrhea and hypotension, both of which are usually temporary.[142-144]

Bilateral splanchnic neurolysis is accomplished by CT-guided needle placement in the retrocrural space. Substantial relief of upper abdominal pain caused by cancer has been reported in 20 of 21 patients.[145] Splanchnic neurolysis can be used in place of a celiac plexus block when such blocks fail to produce a response or are not feasible.

SUPERIOR HYPOGASTRIC PLEXUS BLOC

A relatively favorable risk-benefit ratio occurs with superior hypogastric plexus block and should be considered early with cancer pain in the lower abdomen or pelvis.[146] A coaxial imaging technique or CT may be used for guidance.[147,148] Neurolytic superior hypogastric plexus blocks reduce opioid use on average by 40% in the 75% who do respond.[149,150] Patients may require more than one procedure for response. A temporary bupivacaine block similar to celiac plexus block is used to determine benefit before permanent block.

CONCLUSION

Visceral pain has a distinctively different presentation compared with somatic pain, which is rationally understood by neuroanatomic differences between visceral and somatic pain processing. The symptom cluster of bowel obstruction is recognizable as nausea, vomiting, colic, and continuous pain that usually requires a triple drug combination of antiemetics, antimuscarinics, and opioids for relief. It is important to determine a patient's eligibility for corrective surgery based on prognostic criteria and obtain informed consent based on discussions centered on goals of care. Patients with intractable visceral pain benefit from neurolytic blocks of splanchnic nerves and celiac and superior hypogastric plexus depending on location of pain.

REFERENCES

1. Cervero F: Sensory innervation of the viscera: Peripheral basis of visceral pain. Phys Rev 7:95–138, 1994.
2. McMahon SB: Are there fundamental differences in the peripheral mechanisms of visceral and somatic pain? Behav Brain Sci 20:381–391, 1997.
3. Cervero F: Visceral pain: Central sensitisation. Gut 47(suppl IV):56–57, 2000.
4. Ladabaum U, Minoshima S, Owyang C: Pathobiology of visceral pain: Molecular mechanisms and therapeutic implications v. central nervous system processing of somatic and visceral sensory signals. Am J Physiol Gastrointest Liver Physiol 279:G1–G6, 2000.
5. Giamberardino MA: Recent and forgotten aspects of visceral pain. Eur J Pain 3:77–92, 1999.
6. Joshi SK, Gebhart GF: Visceral pain. Curr Rev Pain 4:499–506, 2000.
7. Gebhart GF: Pathobiology of visceral pain: Molecular mechanisms and therapeutic implications IV. Visceral afferent contributions to the pathobiology of visceral pain. Am J Physiol Gastrointest Liver Physiol 278: G834–G838, 2000.
8. Gebhart GF, Su X, Joshi S, et al: Peripheral opioid modulation of visceral pain. Ann N Y Acad Sci 909:41–50, 2000.
9. Gebhart GF: J.J. Bonica Lecture—2000: Physiology, pathophysiology, and pharmacology of visceral pain. Reg Anesth Pain Med 25:632–638, 2000.
10. Gebhart GF: Pathobiology of visceral pain: Molecular mechanisms and therapeutic implications v. central nervous system processing of somatic and visceral sensory signals. Am J Physiol Gastrointest Liver Physiol 278:G834–G38, 2000.
11. Cervero F: Visceral hyperalgesia revisited. Lancet 356:1127–1128, 2000.
12. Hobson AR, Aziz Q: Central nervous system processing of human visceral pain in health and disease. News Physiol Sci 18:109–114, 2003.
13. Petersen P, Gao C, Arendt-Nielsen K, et al: Pain intensity and biomechanical responses during ramp-controlled distension of the human rectum. Dig Dis Sci 48:1310–1316, 2003.
14. Janig W, Koltzenburg M: Receptive properties of sacral primary afferent neurons supplying the colon. Amer Physio Soc 65:1067–1077, 1991.
15. Garrison DW, Chandler MJ, Foreman RD: Viscerosomatic convergence onto feline spinal neurons from esophagus, heart and somatic fields: Effects of inflammation. Pain 49:373–382, 1992.
16. Kamp EH, Beck DR, Gebhart GF: Combinations of neurokinin receptor antagonists reduce visceral hyperalgesia. J Pharmacol Exp Ther 299:105–113.
17. Lamb K, Kang YM, Gebhart GF, et al: Nerve growth factor and gastric hyperalgesia in the rat. Neurogastroenterol Motil 15: 355–361, 2003.
18. Friedrich AE, Gebhart GF: Modulation of visceral hyperalgesia by morphine and cholecystokinin from the rat rostroventral medial medulla. Pain 104:93–101, 2003.
19. Black D, Trevethick M: The kappa opioid receptor is associated with the perception of visceral pain. Gut 43:312–313, 1998.
20. Bonaz B, Riviere PJ, Sinniger V, et al: Fedotozine, a kappa-opioid agonist, prevents spinal and supraspinal Fos expression induced by a noxious visceral stimulus in the rat. Neurogastroenterol Motil 12:135–147, 2000.
21. Friedrich AE, Gebhart GF: Effects of spinal cholecystokinin receptor antagonists on morphine antinociception in a model of visceral pain in the rat. J Pharmacol Exp Ther 292:538–544, 2000.
22. Friese N, Diop L, Chevalier E, et al: Involvement of prostaglandins and CGRP-dependent sensory afferents in peritoneal irritation-induced visceral pain. Regul Pept 70:1–7, 1997.
23. Sengupta JN, Snider A, Su X, Gebhart GF: Effects of kappa opioids in the inflamed rat colon. Pain 79:171–85, 1999.
24. Junien JL, Riviere P: Review article: The hypersensitive gut—peripheral kappa agonists as a new pharmacological approach. Aliment Pharmacol Ther 9:117–126, 1995.
25. Delgados-Aros S, Chial HJ, Camilleri M, et al: Effects of a k-opioid agonist, asimadoline, on satiation and GI motor and sensory functions in humans. Am J Physiol Gastrointest Liver Physiol 284: G558–G566, 2003.
26. Sengupta JN, Su X, Gebhart GF: Kappa, but not mu or delta, opioids attenuate responses to distention of afferent fibers innervating the rat colon. Gastroenterology 111:968–980, 1996.
27. Gebhart GF: Visceral nociception: Consequences, modulation and the future. Eur J Anaesth 10(suppl):24–27, 1995.
28. Kolhekar R, Gebhart GF: Modulation of spinal visceral nociceptive transmission by NMDA receptor activation in the rat. J Neurophysiol 75:2344–2353, 1996.
29. Sarkar S, Hobson AR, Furlong PL, et al: Central neural mechanisms mediating human visceral hypersensitivity. Am J Physiol Gastrointest 281:G1196–G1202, 2001.
30. Miyamoto H, Saito Y, Kirihara Y, et al: Spinal coadministration of ketamine reduces the development of tolerance to visceral as well as somatic antinociception during spinal morphine infusion. Anesth Anal 90:136–144, 2000.
31. Cavicchi M, Whittle BJ: Regulation of induction of nitric oxide synthase and the inhibitory actions of dexamethasone in the human intestinal epithelial cell line, Caco-2: Influence of cell differentiation. Br J Pharmacol 128:705–715, 1999.
32. Pfeilschifter J, Eberhardt W, Hummel R, et al: Therapeutic strategies for the inhibition of inducible nitric oxide synthase: Potential for a novel class of anti-inflammatory agents. Cell Bio Inter 20:51–58, 1996.
33. Schwarz PM, Gierten B, Boissel JP, et al: Expressional down-regulation of neuronal-type nitric oxide synthase I by glucocorticoids in N1E-115 neuroblastoma cells. Mol Pharmacol 54:258–263, 1998.
34. Feng Y, Cui M, Willis WD: Effect of anticonvulsant gabapentin on visceral nociception and its relationship with amino acid neurotransmitters released from spinal cord. Beijing Da Xue Bao 35:307–310, 2003.
35. Baker AK, Hoffman VLH, Meert TF: Interactions of NMDA antagonists and an a^2 agonist with μ, δ and χ opioids in an acute nociception assay. Acta Anaesth Delg 53:203–212, 2002.
36. Fioramonti J, Bueno L: Centrally acting agents and visceral sensitivity. Gut 51 (suppl I):i91–i95, 2002.
37. Maves TJ, Pechman PS, Mellar ST, Gebhart GF: Ketorolac potentiates morphine antinociception during visceral nociception in the rat. Anesthesiology 80:1094–1101.
38. Mercadante S, Casuccio A, Agnello A, et al: Analgesic effects of nonsteroidal anti-inflammatory drugs in cancer pain due to somatic or visceral mechanism. J Pain Symptom Manage 17:351–356, 1999.
39. Mertz H: Review article: Visceral hypersensitivity. Ali Pharm Ther 17:623–633, 2003.
40. Mertz H: Role of the brain and sensory pathways in gastrointestinal sensory disorders in human. Gut 51(suppl 1): i29–i33, 2002.
41. Palecek J, Paleckova V, Willis WD: Fos expression in spinothalamic and postsynaptic dorsal column neurons following noxious visceral and cutaneous stimuli. Pain 104:249–257, 2003.
42. Kim YS, Kwon SJ: High thoracic midline dorsal column myelotomy for severe visceral pain due to advanced stomach cancer. Neurosurgery 46:85–90, 2000.
43. Strigo IA, Duncan GH, Boivin M, et al: Differentiation of visceral and cutaneous pain in the human brain. Neurophysiol 89:3294–3303, 2003.
44. Nakagawa T, Katsuya A, Tanimoto S, et al: Differential patterns of c-fos mRNA expression in the amygdaloid nuclei induced by chemical somatic and visceral noxious stimuli in rats. Neuro Lett 344:197–200, 2003.
45. Zhang X, Jiang C, Tan Z, et al: Vagal motor neurons in rats respond to noxious and physiological gastrointestinal distention differentially. Eur J Neuro 16:2027–2038, 2002.
46. Leow CK: Re: The etiology of intestinal obstruction in patients without prior laparotomy or hernia. Am Surg 65: 390–391, 1999.
47. Dervenis C, Delis S, Filippou D, et al: Intestinal obstruction and perforation: The role of the surgeon. Dig Dis 21:68–76, 2003.
48. Omori H, Asahi H, Inoue Y, et al: Intussusception in adults: A 21-year

experience in the university-affiliated emergency center and indication for nonoperative reduction. Dig Surg 20: 433–439, 2003.

49. Telfer S, Fenyo G, Holt PR: Acute abdominal pain in patients over 50 years of age. Scand J of Gastro 144:47–50, 1988.

50. Davis MP, Nouneh C: Modern management of cancer-related intestinal obstruction. Curr Onc Rep 2:343–350, 2000.

51. Krebs HB, Goplerud DR: Mechanical intestinal obstruction in patients with gynecologic disease: A review of 368 patients. Am J Obstet Gyn 157:577–583, 1987.

52. Butler JA, Cameron BL, Morrow M: Small bowel obstruction in patients with a prior history of cancer. Am J Surg 162:624–628, 1991.

53. Tang E, Davis J, Silberman H: Bowel obstruction in cancer patients. Arch Surg 130:832–836, 1995.

54. Stenbygaard LE, Sorensen JB: Small bowel metastases in non-small cell lung cancer. Lung Ca 26:95–101, 1999.

55. Hao XS, Li Q, Chen H: Small bowel metastases of malignant melanoma: Palliative effect of surgical resection. Jpn J Clin Onc 29:442–444, 1999.

56. Sos EVJ, Yepes AV, Vizcaino SV: Adhesive small bowel obstruction: temporary evolution and derived practical consequences. Rev Esp Enferm Dig 95:328–332, 2003.

57. Ripamonti C, De Conno F, Ventafridda V, et al: Management of bowel obstruction in advanced and terminal cancer patients. Ann Onc 4:15–21, 1993.

58. Ripamonti C, Twycross R, Baines M: Clinical-practice recommendations for the management of bowel obstruction in patients with end-stage cancer. Support Care Cancer 9:223–233, 2001.

59. Ripamonti C, Bruera E: Palliative management of malignant bowel obstruction. Int J Gyn Ca 12:135–143, 2002.

60. Ripamonti C: Management of bowel obstruction in advanced cancer. Curr Opin Onc 6:351–357, 1994.

61. Chinn JS, Schuffler MD: Paraneoplastic visceral neuropathy as a cause of severe gastrointestinal motor dysfunction. Gastroenterology 95:1279–1286, 1988.

62. Schuffler MD, Baird HW, Fleming CR, et al: Intestinal pseudo-obstruction as the presenting manifestation of small-cell carcinoma of the lung: A paraneoplastic neuropathy of the gastrointestinal tract. Ann Int Med 98:129–134, 1983.

63. George CF: Drugs causing intestinal obstruction: A review. J Roy Soc Med 73:200–204, 1980.

64. Sparkes V, Prevost AT, Hunter JO: Derivation and identification of questions that act as predictors of abdominal pain of musculoskeletal origin. Eur J Gastroenterol Hepatol 15:1021–1027, 2003.

65. Suri S, Gupta S, Sudhakar PJ: Comparative evaluation of plain films, ultrasound and CT in the diagnosis of intestinal obstruction. Acta Radiol 40:422–428, 1999.

66. Maglinte DD, Reyes BL, Harmon BH, et al: Reliability and role of plain film radiology and CT in the diagnosis of small-bowel obstruction. Am J Roentgenol 167:1451–1455, 1996.

67. Donckier V, Closset J, Van Gansbeke D, et al: Contribution of computed tomography to decision making in the management of adhesive small bowel obstruction. Br J Surg 85:1071–1074, 1998.

68. Daneshmand S, Hedley CG, Stain SC: The utility and reliability of computed tomography scan in the diagnosis of small bowel obstruction. Am Surg 65:922–926, 1999.

69. Bogusevicius A, Pundzius J, Maleckas A, et al: Computer-aided diagnosis of the character of bowel obstruction. Int Surg 84:225–228, 1999.

70. Fenlon HM, McAneny DB, Nunes DP, et al: Occlusive colon carcinoma: Virtual colonoscopy in the preoperative evaluation of the proximal colon. Radiology 210:423–428, 1999.

71. Sosna J, Morrin MM, Copel L, et al: Computed tomography colonography (virtual colonscopy): Update on technique, applications, and future developments. Surg Tech Int 11:102–110, 2003.

72. Zoetmulder FAN, Helmerhorst JM, Coevorden PE, et al: Management of bowel obstruction in patients with advanced ovarian cancer. Eur J Cancer 30A:1625–1628, 1994.

73. Aabo K, Pedersen H, Bach F, et al: Surgical management of intestinal obstruction in the late course of malignant disease. Acta Chir Scand 150:173–176, 1984.

74. Dean A, Bridge D, Lickiss JN: The palliative effects of octreotide in malignant disease. Ann Acad Med 23:212–215, 1994.

75. Woolfson RG, Jennings K, Whalen GF: Management of bowel obstruction in patients with abdominal cancer. Arch Surg 132:1093–1097, 1997.

76. Feuer DJ, Broadley KE, Shepherd JH, et al: Systematic review of surgery in malignant bowel obstruction in advanced gynecological and gastrointestinal cancer. Gyn Onc 75:313–322, 1999.

77. Feuer DJ, Broadley KE, Shepherd JH, Barton DP: Surgery for the resolution of symptoms in malignant bowel obstruction in advanced gynaecological and gastrointestinal cancer. The Cochrane database of systematic reviews. Issue 4, CD002764, 2002.

78. Redman CW, Shafi MI, Ambrose S, et al: Survival following intestinal obstruction in ovarian cancer. Eur J Surg Onc 14:383–386, 1988.

79. Rubin SC, Hoskins WJ, Benjamin I, et al: Palliative surgery for intestinal obstruction in advanced ovarian cancer. Gyn Onc 34:16–19, 1989.

80. Krebs HB, Goplerud DR: Surgical management of bowel obstruction in advanced ovarian carcinoma. Obstet Gync 61:327–330, 1983.

81. DiSantis DJ, Ralls PW, Balfe DM, et al: The patient with suspected small bowel obstruction: imaging strategies. American College of Radiology. ACR appropriateness criteria. Radiology 215(suppl):121–124, 2000.

82. Krouse RS, McCahill LE, Easson AM, et al: When the sun can set on an unoperated bowel obstruction: Management of malignant bowel obstruction. J Am Coll Surg 195:117–128, 2002.

83. Boorman P, Soonawalla Z, Sathananthan N, et al: Endoluminal stenting of obstructed colorectal tumours. Ann R Coll Surg Engl 81:251–254, 1999.

84. Bethge N, Breitkreutz C, Vakil N: Metal stents for the palliation of inoperable upper gastrointestinal stenoses. Amer J Gastro 93:643–645, 1998.

85. Paul DL, Pinto PI, Fernandez LR, et al: Palliative treatment of malignant colorectal strictures with metallic stents. Cardio Int Radiol 22:29–36, 1999.

86. Mainar A, De Gregorio-Ariza MA, Tejero E, et al: Acute colorectal obstruction: Treatment with self-expandable metallic stents before scheduled surgery-results of a multicenter study. Radiology 210:65–69, 1999.

87. Tejero E, Fernandez-Lobato R, Mainar A, et al: Initial results of a new procedure for treatment of malignant obstruction of the left colon. Dis Colon Rectum 40:432–436, 1997.

88. Lapenta R, Assisi D, Grassi A, et al: Palliative treatment of esophageal tumors. J Exp Clin Cancer Res 21:503–507, 2002.

89. Nash CL, Gerdes H: Methods of palliation of espohageal and gastric cancer. Surg Onc Clin North Am 11:459–483, 2002.

90. Mischinger HJ, Hauser H, Cerwenka H, et al: Endocavitary Ir-192 radiation and laser treatment for palliation of obstructive rectal cancer. Eur J Surg Onc 23:428–431, 1997.

91. Malone JM, Koonce T, Larson DM, et al: Palliation of small bowel obstruction by percutaneous gastrostomy in patients with progressive ovarian carcinoma. Obstet Gyn 68:431–433, 1986.

92. Campagnutta E, Cannizzaro R, Gallo A, et al: Palliative treatment of upper intestinal obstruction by gynecological malignancy: The usefulness of percutaneous endoscopic gastrostomy. Gyn Onc 62:103–105, 1996.

93. Adelson MD, Kasowitz MH: Percutaneous endoscopic drainage gastrostomy in the treatment of gastrointestinal obstruction from intraperitoneal malignancy. Obstet Gyn 81:467–471, 1993.

94. Cunningham MJ, Bromberg C, Kredentser DC, et al: Percutaneous gastrostomy for decompression in patients with advanced gynecologic malignancies. Gyn Onc 59:273–276, 1995.

95. Brooksbank MA, Game PA, Ashby MA: Palliative venting gastrostomy in malignant intestinal obstruction. Pall Med 16:520–526, 2002.

96. Scheidbach H, Horbach T, Groitl H, et al: Percutaneous endoscopic gastrostomy/jejunostomy (PEG/PEJ) for decompression in the upper gastrointestinal tract: Initial experience with palliative treatment of gastrointestinal obstruction in terminally ill patients with advanced carcinomas. Surg Endosc 13:1103–1105, 1999.

97. Jong P, Sturgeon J, Jamieson CG: Benefit of palliative surgery for bowel obstruction in advanced ovarian cancer. Can J Surg 38:454–457, 1995.

98. Picus D, Marx MV, Weyman PJ: Chronic intestinal obstruction: Value of percutaneous gastrostomy tube placement. Am J Roentgenol 150:295–297, 1988.

99. Thomas SH, Silen W: Effect on diagnostic efficiency of analgesia for undifferentiated abdominal pain. Br J Surg 90:5–9, 2003.

100. Thomas SH, Silen W, Cheema F, et al: Effects of morphine analgesia on

diagnostic accuracy in emergency department patients with abdominal pain: A prospective, randomized trial. J Am Coll Surg 196:18–31, 2003.

101. Joishy SK, Walsh D: The opioid-sparing effects of intravenous ketorolac as an adjuvant analgesic in cancer pain: Application in bone metastases and the opioid bowel syndrome. J Pain Symptom Manage 16:334–339, 1998.

102. Kurz A, Sessler DI: Opioid-induced bowel dysfunction: Pathophysiology and potential new therapies. Drugs 63:649–671, 2003.

103. Choi YS, Billings JA: Opioid antagonists: A review of their role in palliative care, focusing on use in opioid-related constipation. J Pain Symptom Manage 24:71–90, 2002.

104. Yuan CS, Wei G, Foss JF, et al: Effects of subcutaneous methylnaltrexone on morphine-induced peripherally mediated side effects: A double-blind randomized placebo-controlled trial. J Pharm Exp Ther 300:118–123, 2002.

105. De Ponti F: Methylnaltrexone progenics. Curr Opin Invest Drugs 3:614–620, 2002.

106. Fainsinger RL, Spachynski K, Hanson J, et al: Symptom control in terminally ill patients with malignant bowel obstruction (MBO). J Pain Symptom Manage 9:12–18, 1994.

107. Quigley EM: Acute intestinal pseudo-obstruction. Curr Threat Options Gastro 3:273–286, 2000.

108. Davis MP, Walsh D: Gastrointestinal motility disorders chapter 7 in Gastrointestinal Symptoms. In Ripamonte C, Bruera E (eds): Advanced Cancer Patients. New York, Oxford University Press, 2002.

109. Ponec RJ, Saunders MD, Kimmey MB: Neostigmine for the treatment of acute colonic pseudo-obstruction. N Engl J Med 341:137–141, 1999.

110. De Giorgio R, Barbara G, Stanhellini V, et al: Review article: The pharmacological treatment of acute colonic pseudo-obstruction. Aliment Pharm Ther 15:1717–1727, 2001.

111. Baines MJ: ABC of palliative care: nausea, vomiting, and intestinal obstruction. Br J Surg 315:1148–1150, 1997.

112. Thorsen AB, Yung NS, Leung AC: Administration of drugs by infusion pumps in palliative medicine. Ann Acad Med Sing 23:209–211, 1994.

113. Philip J, Lickiss N, Grant PT, et al: Corticosteroids in the management of bowel obstruction on a gynecological oncology unit. Gyn Onc 74:68–73, 1999.

114. Feuer DJ, Broadley KE: Corticosteroids for the resolution of malignant bowel obstruction in advanced gynaecological and gastrointestinal cancer. Cochrane Database of Systematic Reviews 2: CD001219, 2000.

115. Feuer DJ, Broadley KE, Shepherd JH, et al: Systematic review and meta-analysis of corticosteroids for the resolution of malignant bowel obstruction in advanced gynaecological and gastrointestinal cancers. Gyn Onc 75:313–322, 1999.

116. Mangili G, Franchi M, Mariani A, et al: Octreotide in the management of bowel obstruction in terminal ovarian cancer. Neo Onc 61:345–348, 1996.

117. Mercadante S, Kargar J, Nicolosi G: Octreotide may prevent definitive intestinal obstruction. J Pain Symptom Manage 13:352–355, 1997.

118. Mystakidou K, Tsilika E, Kalaidopoulou O, et al: Comparison of octreotide administration vs conservative treatment in the management of inoperable bowel obstruction in patients with far advanced cancer: A randomized, double-blind, controlled clinical trial. Anticancer Res 22: 1187–1192, 2002.

119. Mercadante S, Ripamonti C, Casuccio A, et al: Comparison of octreotide and hyscine butylbromide in controlling gastrointestinal symptoms due to malignant inoperable bowel obstruction. Support Care Cancer 8:188–191, 2000.

120. Mercadante S, Maddaloni S: Octreotide in the management of inoperable gastrointestinal obstruction in terminal cancer patients. J Pain Symptom Manage 7:496–498, 1992.

121. Mercadante S, Spoldi E, Caraceni A, et al: Octreotide in relieving gastrointestinal symptoms due to bowel obstruction. Pall Med 7:295–299, 1993.

122. Mercadante S: Letter to the editor: Scopolamine butylbromide plus octreotide in unresponsive bowel obstruction. J Pain Symptom Manage 16:278–279, 1998.

123. Khoo D, Hall E, Motson R, et al: Palliation of malignant intestinal obstruction using octreotide. Eur J Cancer 30A:28–30, 1994.

124. Pandha HS, Waxman J: Octreotide in malignant intestinal obstruction. Anticancer Drugs 7(suppl 1):5–10, 1996.

125. Ripamonti C, Panzeri C, Groff L, et al: The role of somatostatin and octreotide in bowel obstruction: Pre-clinical and clinical results. Tumori 87:1–9, 2001.

126. Lebrun C, Chichmanian RM, Peyrade F, et al: Recurrent bowel occlusion with oral ondansetron with effects of the intravenous route: A previously unknown event. Ann Onc 8:919–920, 1997.

127. De Conno F, Caraceni A, Zecca E, et al: Continuous subcutaneous infusion of hyoscine butylbromide reduces secretions in patients with gastrointestinal obstruction. J Pain Symptom Manage 6: 484–486, 1991.

128. Davis MP, Furste A: Glycopyrrolate: A useful drug in the palliation of mechanical bowel obstruction. J Pain Symptom Manage 18:153–154, 1999.

129. Frank C: Medical management of intestinal obstruction in terminal care. Can Fam Phys 43:259–265, 1997.

130. Mercadante S, Sapio M, Serretta R: Treatment of pain in chronic bowel subobstruction with self-administration of methadone. Support Care Cancer 5:327–329, 1997.

131. Mercadante S, Caligara M, Sapio M, et al: Subcutaneous fentanyl infusion in a patient with bowel obstruction and renal failure. J Pain Symptom Manage 13:241–244, 1997.

132. Daeninck PJ, Bruera E: Reduction in constipation and laxative requirements following opioid rotation to methadone: A report of four cases. J Pain Symptom Manage 18:303–309, 1999.

133. Grond S, Radbruch L, Meuser T, et al: High-dose tramadol in comparison to low-dose morphine for cancer pain relief. J Pain Symptom Manage 18:174–179, 1999.

134. Morita T, Tei Y, Inoue S, et al: Fluid status of terminally ill cancer patients with intestinal obstruction: an exploratory observational study. Support Care Cancer 10:474–479, 2002.

135. Fainsinger RL, MacEachern T, Miller MJ, et al: The use of hypodermoclysis for rehydration in terminally ill cancer patients. J Pain Symptom Manage 9:298–302, 1994.

136. Steiner N, Bruera E: Methods of hydration in palliative care patients. J Pall Care 14:6–13, 1998.

137. Philip J, Depczynski B: The role of total parenteral nutrition for patients with irreversible bowel obstruction secondary to gynecological malignancy. J Pain Symptom Manage 13:104–111, 1997.

138. Pelham A, Lee MA, Regnard CB: Gabapentin for coeliac plexus pain. Pall Med 16:355–356, 2002.

139. Kawamata M, Ishitani K, Ishikawa K, et al: Comparison between celiac plexus block and morphine treatment on quality of life in patients with pancreatic cancer pain. Pain 64:597–602, 1996.

140. Mercadante S: Celiac plexus block versus analgesics in pancreatic cancer pain. Pain 52:187–192, 1993.

141. Vranken JH, Zuurmond WWA, de Lange JJ: Increasing the efficacy of a celiac plexus block in patients with severe pancreatic cancer pain. J Pain Symptom Manage 22:966–977, 2001.

142. Polati E, Finco G, Gottin L, et al: Prospective randomized double-blind trail of neurolytic coeliac plexus block in patients with pancreatic cancer. Br J Surg 85:199–201, 1998.

143. Okuyama M, Shibata T, Morita T, et al: A comparison of intraoperative celiac plexus block with pharmacological therapy as a treatment for pain of unresectable pancreatic cancer. J Hepa Panc Sur 9:372–375, 2002.

144. Yamamuro M, Kusaka K, Kato M, et al: Celiac plexus block in cancer pain management. Tohoku J Exp Med 192: 1–18, 2000.

145. Fujita Y: CT-guided neurolytic splanchic nerve block with alcohol. Pain 55: 363–366, 1993.

146. Patt RB, Reddy SK, Black RG: Neural blockade for abdominopelvic pain of oncologic origin. Int Anesth Clin 36: 87–104, 1998.

147. Stevens DS, Balatbat GR, Lee FM: Coaxial imaging technique for superior hypogastric plerus block. Reg Anesth Pain Med 25:643–647, 2000.

148. Cariati M, De Martini G, Pretolesi F, et al: CT-guided superior hypogastric plexus block. J Comput Assist Tomogr 26:428–431, 2002.

149. Plancarte R, de Leon-Casasola OA, El-Helaly M, et al: Neurolytic superior hypogastric plexus block for chronic pelvic pain associated with cancer. Reg Anesth 22:562–568, 1997.

150. De Leon-Casasola OA, Kent E, Lema MJ: Neurolytic superior hypogastric plexus block for chronic pelvic pain associated with cancer. Pain 54:145–151, 1993.

CHAPTER 39

Hypophysectomy

Luis Aliaga, MD, PhD, and Rubén Martinez-Castejon, MD

Pituitary ablation has been employed for several decades as an effective technique to reduce untreatable cancer pain, mainly in breast and prostate cancer.[1-4] It was first performed by an open surgery procedure (transcranial hypophysectomy) with the intention of producing regression of metastatic breast or prostatic carcinoma, but pain relief was a more consistent effect even in the absence of tumor regression. Because of limitations for major surgery in patients with advanced cancer, less aggressive techniques were developed. Forrest and Brown obtained neuroadenolysis by the insertion of radon via transsphenoidal spaces.[5] Others studied the effects by inserting radioisotopes or injecting alcohol.[6] Moricca in 1958 performed chemical neuroadenolysis by placing multiple needles into the adenohypophysis and injecting small amounts of absolute alcohol.[7] This technique has been modified by many authors by decreasing the number of needles used,[8] by using a stereotactic head frame[3] or by using a needle-through-a-needle technique (thus eliminating the need for the stereotactic frame).[9] Levin et al. described the injection of ethyl alpha-cyanomethacrylate resin through the needle to reduce the occasional occurrence of cerebrospinal fluid leakage.[3] Neuroadenolysis has also been performed by injecting phenol and by cryosurgery, radiosurgery, external radiotherapy, and radiofrequency.[10,11]

MECHANISMS OF PAIN RELIEF

The exact mechanism by which pituitary adenolysis produces analgesia remains unclear. It was expected that hormonal depletion could reduce tumor progression and pain. However, the correlation between analgesia and hormonal depletion has not been proved,[12] and neither has the correlation between analgesia and tumor regression.[13] Pain relief usually occurs within hours of the operation, preceding an objective tumor remission, and 40% to 60% of the patients that finally obtain pain relief do not show tumor regression.[14] Other mechanisms proposed are that an analgesic effect may be mediated by beta-endorphins[12] and that pain relief might be a result of a hypothalamic pain-suppressing capability triggered by hypophysectomy.[14]

INDICATIONS AND CONTRAINDICATIONS

Pituitary ablation is indicated for patients with advanced cancer, hormonally dependent or not, secondary to widespread metastases whose pain cannot be controlled by other methods and whose life expectancy is not longer than 3 to 6 months. At present, new hormonal treatments (aromatase inhibitors in breast cancer, LH-RH analogs, nonsteroidal antiandrogens, LH-RH antagonists, and Gn-RH agonists in prostate cancer),[15,16] new opioid presentations (transdermal) and wide experience with other techniques of neuroablation such as radiofrequency of sympathetic ganglia or neurostimulation of the spinal cord have limited the use of hypophysectomy for bilateral, diffuse cancer pain, bilateral facial or upper body cancer pain, intractable visceral pain, and in some occasions when all other appropriate pain-relieving measures have failed.[17]

Absolute contraindications for hypophysectomy are coagulopathy, local infection, empty sella syndrome, and a significant increase in intracranial pressure.

DESCRIPTION OF TECHNIQUE

Over the past 40 years pituitary destruction has been performed by different techniques: (a) transcranial hypophysectomy, (b) transsphenoidal hypophysectomy,[1,10] (c) radiation-induced hypophysectomy,[18] (d) radiofrequency thermal coagulation, (e) cryogenic hypophysectomy,[19,20] and (f) chemical hypophysectomy with alcohol.[3,8,9,21]

Both transcranial and transsphenoidal options are major surgical procedures and are now rarely indicated because less invasive options are available. Radiation-induced pituitary destruction has been performed by either transsphenoidal surgery or external radiation with little damage to surrounding structures. In a recent prospective multicenter protocol, nine patients underwent gamma knife radiosurgery targeted at the pituitary gland-stalk with sustained pain resolution that took effect after several days.[18] Pain relief with this technique does not always have the immediacy that is to be desired for a population with a short life expectancy and a high level of suffering.

One of the most useful techniques is probably transsphenoidal injection of absolute alcohol into the pituitary fossa[21] (Figure 39–1). Under low anesthesia or with local anesthesia, and with a C-arm fluoroscope, a special cannula is placed through the anterior wall of the sella turcica into the pituitary gland. Then after a confirmative contrast injection, absolute alcohol is injected gradually in amounts of 0.1 to 0.2 mL per minute to a total of 1 to 6 mL depending on the size of the sella. There are no adequate endocrinologic and anatomic data correlated with pain relief to serve as a guide in determining the amount of alcohol to inject. When using volumes of 1 or 2 mL, it is sometimes necessary to repeat alcohol injections because of inadequate pain relief.[22-24] For example, in Miles series, 122 patients with all forms of cancer (56% breast or prostate cancer) underwent chemical neuroadenolysis, with good results in 75% of the cases (sufficient pain relief to discontinue narcotic therapy). However, 30% of patients needed a second injection and 9% a third.[23] Pupillary size is carefully observed during injection because of the risk of optic pathway damage. Pupillary dilatation indicates that alcohol is outside the sella and is in contact with an oculomotor nerve. For this reason opioids are not recommended preoperatively and intraoperatively to avoid pupillary miosis. Alcohol infusion has to be discontinued and the needle withdrawn to a more anterior position.[17] When done at the first sign of ocular involvement, any disturbance in vision is transitory.[15] Bonica recommends infusing 200 to 500 mg of hydrocortisone intravenously immediately in these cases.[25] A cyanomethacrylate resin seal in the sella hole is placed to avoid cerebrospinal fluid leakage. The risk of hypopituitarism is unpredictable. For this reason all patients will receive pituitary hormone replacement therapy. Transient diabetes insipidus occurs in 40% of patients and is the leading cause of morbidity and mortality in these patients when untreated. Vasopressin therapy[17] should be given to patients unable to drink as much as they excrete or when urine output exceeds 2.5 L a day.

To reduce complications resulting from the spread of alcohol to neighboring structures, some authors have performed pituitary ablation with a cryoprobe, which can be passed up through the needle into the gland to produce a series of localized lesions. They reported pain relief as good, if not better, than that obtained with alcohol, with minimal vision and hormonal disturbances.[19]

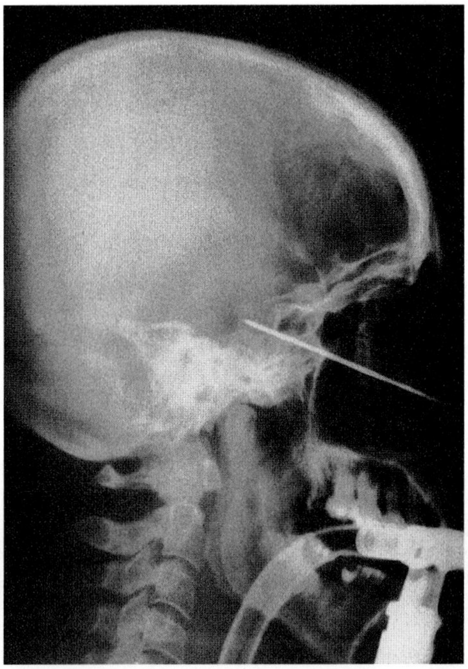

FIGURE 39–1   Lateral view radiograph showing the needle at the pituitary gland through the sella turcica space.

RESULTS

Most authors report pain relief in 70% to 90% of patients and complete pain relief in 60%. Most investigators report better results for breast and prostate cancer patients (hormone-dependent tumors) (41% to 95%) and worse results in hormonally independent tumors (69%).[26] Ramirez and Levin in a review of 13 series reported pain relief of 70% to 75% with little difference between surgical and chemical hypophysectomy in 867 patients, without distinguishing results in hormonal-dependent or independent tumors.[14] The duration of pain relief is variable. In the Bonica trial pain relief is observed almost immediately in some cases, but it takes several hours to even 2 days in others after neuroadenolysis with alcohol.[25] Two thirds will experience pain relief for 3 months or less.[27] However, pain-free periods of almost a year have been reported.[9] In the series reported by Levin, 82 patients had stereotactic chemical hypophysectomy (63% breast or prostate cancer) with good results in 84% of the patients. The duration of pain relief was limited by death due to malignant underlying disease rather than the recurrence of pain.[3]

COMPLICATIONS

Most patients complain of frontal bilateral headache, self-limited in about 48 hours, and in approximately 40% of patients diabetes insipidus can occur. Transient increases of body temperature are observed in 35% of patients (1–2°C) probably due to an alteration of the hypothalamus temperature-regulating mechanism.[17] An increase in pulmonary secretions similar to cardiac heart failure is seen in 20% of the patients. Transient disturbances in vision are reported in less than 10%, although with higher rates in one series,[27] and are permanent in 5% of patients. More severe complications such as cerebrospinal fluid leakage or pituitary hemorrhage or infection are rare (1%). The overall mortality reported is 2% to 6.5%.[28]

action is observed in some cases. Because of its facility it can be performed in patients in poor physical condition and repeated when pain recurs or when failing to achieve pain control the first time without impairing patient's mental faculties. Complete or partial pain relief is achieved in 70% to 85% of patients, beginning any time between minutes and 2 days and lasting around 3 to 5 months in most cases. When skilled personnel and usual radiologic equipment are available, it can be performed in any hospital, even in Third World countries. For these reasons neuroadenolysis is still a technique to keep in mind when confronted with bilateral, diffuse cancer pain, bilateral facial or upper body cancer pain, intractable visceral pain, and when all other appropriate pain-relieving measures have failed.

CONCLUSION

Neuroadenolysis is a useful tool to manage diffuse, advanced cancer pain not controlled with other neurolytic techniques or narcotics. A cancer-arresting

REFERENCES

1. Hardy J, Grisoli F, Leclercq TA, Somma M: Transsphenoidal hypophysectomy in metastasizing breast cancers. Experience from 160 cases. Nouv Presse Med 4:2387–2390, 1975.
2. Levin AB, Benson RC Jr, Katz J, Nilsson T: Chemical hypophysectomy for relief of bone pain in carcinoma of the prostate. J Urol 119:517–521, 1978.
3. Levin AB, Katz J, Benson RC, Jones AG: Treatment of pain of diffuse metastatic cancer by stereotactic chemical hypophysectomy: Long-term results and observations on mechanism of action. Neurosurgery 6:258–262, 1980.
4. Silverberg GD: Hypophysectomy in the treatment of disseminated prostate carcinoma. Cancer 39:1727–1731, 1977.
5. Forrest APM, Brown DA: Pituitary radon implant for breast cancer. Lancet 1:1054, 1955.
6. Lewis JL, Baxton L: Discussione dell' Adunanza Scientifica del 21 Diciembre 1957. Boll Mene Soc Tosco-umbra Chir 19:78, 1958.
7. Ventaffridda V, DeConno F: Moricca's operation at the National Cancer Institute of Milan. In Ischia S, Lipton S, Maffezzoli GF (eds): Pain Treatment. New York, Raven Press, 1993, pp 85–90.
8. Corssen G, Holcomb MC, Moustapha I, et al: Alcohol-induced adenolysis of the pituitary gland: A new approach to control of intractable cancer pain. Anesth Analg 56:414–421, 1977.
9. Waldman SD, Feldstein GS, Allen ML: Neuroadenolysis of the pituitary: Description of a modified technique. J Pain Symptom Manage 2:45–49, 1987.
10. Osenbach RK: Neurosurgical options for the management of intractable pain. In Tollison CD, Satterthwaite JR, Tollison JW (eds): Practical Pain Management, 3rd ed. Philadelphia, Lippincott, Williams and Wilkins, 2002, p 187.
11. Molet J, Parés P, Bartumeus F: Tratamiento neuroquirúrgico del dolor. In Aliaga L, Baños JE, Barutell C, et al (eds): Tratamiento del Dolor. Teoría y Práctica, 2nd ed. Barcelona, Publicaciones Permanyer, 2002, pp 559–572.
12. Sasaki K: The study of neuro-adrenolysis of pituitary gland on cancer pain and experimental approach to reveal its mechanism of pain relief. Hokkaido Igaku Zasshi 60:24–37, 1985.
13. Smith JA Jr, Eyre HJ, Roberts TS, Middleton RG: Transsphenoidal hypophysectomy in the management of carcinoma of the prostate. Cancer 53:2385–2387, 1984.
14. Ramirez LF, Levin AB: Pain relief after hypophysectomy. Neurosurgery 14:499–504, 1984.
15. Ruffion A, Fontaine E, Staerman F: Hormonal therapy in metastatic prostatic cancer. Prog Urol 13:334–341, 2003.
16. Persad R: Hosp Leuprorelin: A leading role in advanced prostate cancer therapy. Med 64:360–363, 2003.
17. Waldman SD: Neuroadenolysis of the pituitary: Indications and technique. In Waldman SD and Winnie AP (eds): Interventional Pain Management. Philadelphia, WB Saunders, 1996, pp 519–525.
18. Hayashi M, Taira T, Chernov M, et al: Gamma knife surgery for cancer pain-pituitary gland-stalk ablation: A multicenter prospective protocol since 2002. J Neurosurg 97(5 suppl):433–437, 2002.
19. Duthie AM, Ingham V, Dell AE, Dennett JE: Pituitary cryoablation: The results of treatment using a transsphenoidal cryoprobe. Anaesthesia 38:448–451, 1983.
20. Gonski A, Sackelariou R: Cryohypophysectomy for the relief of pain in malignant disease. Med J Aust 140:140–142, 1984.
21. Moricca G, Arcuri E, Moricca P: Neuroadenolysis of the pituitary. Acta Anaesthesiol Belg 32:87–99, 1981.
22. Madrid JL: Chemical hypophysectomy. Adv Pain Res Ther 2:373–380, 1979.
23. Miles J: Chemical hypophysectomy. Adv Pain Res Ther 2:381–391, 1979.
24. Moricca G: Neuroadenolysis for diffuse unbearable cancer pain. Adv Pain Res Ther 1:863–869, 1976.
25. Bonica JJ: Neurolytic blockade and hypophysectomy. In Bonica JJ, Loeser JD, Chapman CR, Fordyce WE (eds): The Management of Pain. Philadelphia, Lea and Febiger. 1990, pp 1980–2039.
26. Takeda F, Uki J, Fuse Y, Kitani Y, Fujita T: The pituitary as a target of antalgic treatment of chronic cancer pain: A possible mechanism of pain relief through pituitary neuroadenolysis. Neurol Res 8:194–200, 1986.
27. Cook PR, Campbell FN, Puddy BR: Pituitary alcohol injection for cancer pain: Use in a district general hospital. Anaesthesia 39:540–545, 1984.
28. Gybels JM, Tasker RR: Central neurosurgery. In Wall PD, Melzak R (eds): Textbook of Pain, 4th ed. New York, Churchill Livingstone, 1999, p 1330.

CHAPTER 40

Neurolytic Techniques for Cancer Pain Management

RICARDO PLANCARTE-SANCHEZ, MD, JORGE GUAJARDO-ROSAS, MD, AND MARIA DEL ROCIO GUILLÉN-NUÑEZ, MD

Nerve destruction using chemicals to promote analgesia had been extensively used in the early part of the 20th century for management of pain. With the advent of newer analgesics and the development of less invasive techniques for pain management, its use has markedly diminished. However, it still has its uses in specific patient populations, such as those who suffer from inadequate analgesia or opioid side effects or patients in underdeveloped countries who face economic limitations and thus cannot receive pharmacologic therapy. In appropriately selected patients, use of interventional techniques such as epidural and intrathecal neurolysis can achieve adequate pain relief with minimal or no side effects.

In 1863, Luton[1] was the first to publish a report of neurolysis over painful areas. He reported good results with subcutaneous injections of silver nitrate and hypertonic sodium chloride. In 1905, La Porte[2] reported using ethanol as a neurolytic agent, which he selected for being less caustic and less toxic. He started with a 45% concentration and increased it up to 80% over a period of 8 days. Afterward, he used another agent he referred to as guaiacol (2-methoxyphenol), which was later shown to be related to phenol.[3]

Fifty years later, in 1955, Maher described the administration of phenol through a subarachnoid route.[4] The required concentration was high (7.5%); thus he used glycerol as a solvent. This helped concentrate the phenol as it gradually liberated from glycerin.[5] Two years later, Maher reported an extradural injection, but this was not convenient for radiographic control and never became popular. In 1959 Kelley, Gautier-Smith, and Nathan restarted using intrathecal neurolysis with 10% phenol in various cases of painful spasticity of the central type.[5]

More recently, Racz, Heavener, and Haynsworth[6] reported the epidural administration of phenol as a safe technique providing a 24-hour pain relief. Another useful insight from this study was that this form of neurolysis namely affects sensory fibers. Thus, the risk of motor deficit is less than with a subarachnoid neurolysis. Thus, it is an inhibition of the preganglionic nociception that interferes with the somatic and sympathetic components.

NEUROLYTIC AGENTS

Neurolytic agents are chemical agents used since the beginning of the 20th century to cause chemical destruction of nerve roots for analgesic purposes. Few are available for clinical use, and they must be expertly prepared, preferably by a pharmacist, to obtain accurate dilutions.

Phenol

Phenol has been used extensively as a neurolytic agent. It has the following characteristics:

- Poorly water soluble at room temperature, although solubility is improved at higher temperatures
- Very soluble in glycerol, resulting in slow diffusion
- Dissolved in glycerol, is hyperbaric compared with cerebrospinal fluid
- Concentration for typical clinical use varies from 4% to 10%
- Concentrations higher than 5% cause protein denaturation and subsequent necrosis because of perineurial blood vessel injury
- In low concentrations, behaves as a local anesthetic
- In high concentrations, acts as a neurolytic agent
- A common belief is that it has selective effects on small diameter fibers (not myelinated fibers), more specifically motor fibers (muscular tone), A-delta fibers

(fast pain), and C afferent (slow pain). Nevertheless, many authors consider it nonselective.[7]

- Can be used at the intrathecal level, epidural level, peripheral nerve level, and sympathetic level.

Ethanol

Ethanol is the most commonly used and available neurolytic agent. It can be easily obtained in concentrations higher than 95% as 1-mL shots and has the following characteristics:

- It is readily soluble in bodily fluids, diffusing rapidly from the site of application.
- Greater volumes are required to produce neurolysis.
- Application of ethanol is painful because it irritates internal structures.
- At the cellular level it causes lipoprotein and mucoprotein precipitation as it extracts cholesterol, phospholipids, and cerebrosides from nerves.[8]
- At the subarachnoid and epidural level it works on the nonmyelinated areas in the posterior columns, Lissauer tract, and spinal roots.[9,10]
- At higher volumes of injections at the subarachnoid level it may cause spinal cord degeneration.
- Due to its hypobaricity, it reaches a higher concentration immediately after intrathecal administration.
- It can be used for intrathecal and epidural administration, neurolysis of sympathetic ganglions, chemical hypophysectomy, and trigeminal and glossopharyngeal neuralgia.
- It may cause necrosis and cellulitis in adjacent tissues.

Hypertonic Saline Solution

Hypertonic saline solution is not nearly as popular as ethanol or phenol. In 1974 Ventafrida and Spreafico reported using it at the intrathecal level but not achieving long-term pain relief, and all patients returned to the same intensity of pain.[11] The best results were reported by Hitchcock, with pain relief lasting 105 days in one patient.[12]

Glycerol

Glycerol has been used in many concentrations. Histopathologic changes observed included Wallerian degeneration, phagocytosis, and cell degranulation with axonolysis. These were confirmed by electron microscopy.[13]

Ammonium Compounds

In 1942 Bates reported the treatment of neuralgia using a 6% ammonium concentration, causing nerve degeneration with no selective damage, causing diffuse cutaneous abnormalities.[14]

PATIENT SELECTION

To administer a neurolytic agent, patients must be selected carefully, identifying physiopathologic causes of pain, chemical and physical neurolytic properties of the selected agent, and possible side effects. In Mexico, nearly 30% of patients with nontreatable oncologic pain will require a neurolytic procedure for a more effective pain relief. Some consider this a last resort for patients who are not candidates for neurosurgical ablation.[15] Many physicians, however, choose to perform a rhizolysis earlier for a better analgesic effect and no fear of pharmacologic side effects.[16,17]

Usually this technique is reserved for cancer patients with life expectancy of up to 1 year; at that point cancer may have affected some dermatomes in unilateral predominance. The main objective of intrathecal neurolysis is to provoke discrete injuries in posterior cords inside the dural sac. These procedures may present with complications, because neurolytic agents are not selective and motor weakness and incontinence may be present. These effects can be minimized with an adequate neurologic exploration identifying involved dermatomes, an accurate technique in the proper position, and a precise use of hyper- and hypobaric agents (Figures 40–1 and 40–2).[18,19]

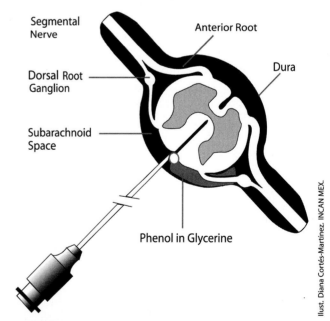

FIGURE 40–1 Lateral supine position used for chemical rhizolysis with intrathecal injection of phenol. Observe the position of the dorsal root. (*Modified from Patt RB, Cousins MJ: Techniques for neurolytic neural blockade. In Cousins MJ, Bridenbaugh PO (eds): Neural Blockade in Clinical Anesthesia and Management of Pain. Philadelphia, Lippincott-Raven, 1998.*)

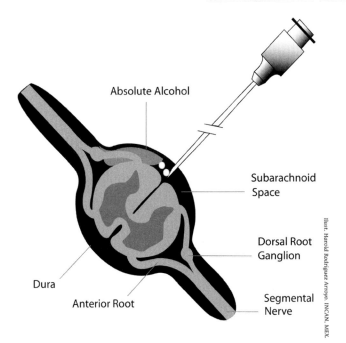

Absolute Alcohol

Subarachnoid Space

Dorsal Root Ganglion

Dura

Anterior Root

Segmental Nerve

Illust. Harold Rodriguez Arroyo, INCAN, MEX.

FIGURE 40–2 Lateral prone position used for chemical rhizolysis with intrathecal injection of alcohol. *(Modified from Patt RB, Cousins MJ: Techniques for neurolytic neural blockade. In Cousins MJ, Bridenbaugh PO (eds): Neural Blockade in Clinical Anesthesia and Management of Pain. Philadelphia, Lippincott-Raven, 1998.)*

TABLE 40–1	Considerations for Subarachnoid Neurolysis
1.	Informed consent from the patient and family
2.	Patient sedation
3.	Selection of neurolytic agent
4.	Neurologic exploration of dermatomes and nerves
5.	Determination of levels of application and number of needles required
6.	Patient positioning
7.	Mapping the sensitivity in the transprocedure area
8.	Follow-up and adjustment of the analgesic selection and dosing, if necessary

ADVERSE EFFECTS

Adverse effects include the following: (1) neuropathic pain, because of high incidence of deafferentation and/or sympathetic participation in which these techniques are not effective; (2) diffuse or nonlocalized pain; and (3) increased risk of sphincter incontinence if the patient had previous dysfunction. The patients and families must be counseled appropriately.

CONTRAINDICATIONS

The procedure is contraindicated when: (1) the patient suffers from incidental pain due to large bone fracture or vertebral collapse (this must be treated in primary form); (2) the patient is unable to maintain the required position; (3) there is secondary pain due to lumbosacral or brachial plexopathy; (4) adequate pain relief posterior to the prognostic block can be achieved with local anesthetics; (5) there is a spinal cord tumor or complete subarachnoid space obstruction in the selected level.[20]

SUBARACHNOID NEUROLYSIS

Subarachnoid neurolysis was first used by Dogliotti in 1931 for treatment of tetanus.[21] Since then, it has been used in other pathologies with controversial results.

It could increase the risk of a malpractice lawsuit if the doctor who performs it has no required expertise. It is often performed in developing countries because it is effective in pain relief and less expensive than pharmacologic treatment. Indications are limited, and a careful and prudent patient selection must be done to achieve good results and minimize complications (Table 40–1). The physician must establish a good rapport with the patient. The patient and family should be fully briefed on all aspects of the procedure, including side effects, the expected results, and the risk of complications such as loss of muscle strength and dysesthesias. In some cases it is prudent to perform a block for diagnosis and prognosis so patients can experience pain relief and recurrent sensations that they would feel permanently after the procedure.

The primary indication is malignant pain with somatic characteristics. It could be preformed in patients with generalized spasticity, in other neurologic pathologies such as multiple sclerosis and superior motor neuron syndrome, and in some specific peripheral neuralgia as well as in neuralgias paresthetica. This block should be ideally implemented only after a block with a local anesthetic to evaluate effectiveness and in the sacral nerve roots to diminish lower sphincter tone due to irritable bladder states.[22,23]

Nevertheless, when performing a rhizolysis, a preganglionic nociception inhibition takes place and interferes with the somatic and sympathetic components. It is recommended that pain in its clinical manifestation must not include more than six dermatomes, in both epidural or subarachnoid techniques; above all we must consider at the moment that we can always reach two dermatomes alongside the ones we want to block due to the diffusion characteristics of the neurolytic agent that may occupy one dermatome from the top and another one from underneath the affected ones. In these cases, for extension that requires blocking many dermatomes, the use of two or three needles and the administration of little volume on each one is recommended until achieving pain relief.[24] We recommend the denervation in more than one section, having an average of two.

It is necessary to inform the patient about immobilization time after the procedure so that a comfortable position is reached, which must be maintained for half an hour to an hour; the neurolytic agent will get better penetration to posterior roots and therefore result in a better pain relief, both with the use of hypo- and hyperbaric agents. There are reports showing that if the patient has mobilization after 15 minutes, small amounts of the neurolytic agent can be found in the cerebrospinal liquid.[25]

The technique used for hyperbaric phenol neurolysis is to lay the patient in lateral position with the painful side down, with an approximate 45-degree dorsal inclination to denervate just a posterior root selection. Considering previous asepsis and antisepsis on the dorsal region, we proceed to use a local anesthetic on skin and then we insert a 20 to 22 French spinal needle directed paramedially or by the midline until the tip of the needle reaches the subarachnoid space to administer phenol. It is suggested to use a 1-mL tuberculine syringe for a slower and more controlled administration. Because phenol tends to crystallize, it is sometimes necessary to submerge the phenol container in hot water to diminish its thickness (Figure 40–3A). With hypobaric agents such as alcohol, the technique involves laying the patient in the same position but with ventral 45-degree inclination

and the same approach to reach the subarachnoid space with the painful area on the upper side (Figure 40–3B). When phenol is being administered the patient can feel an intense pain, perceived on the affected dermatomes, which can be diminished with local anesthetics if it is necessary. The position is contrary to the 45-degree inclination in posterior inclination, the painful area being downside (Figure 40–3C).

It is necessary to perform dermatomal level exploration during the procedure to determine the extension. This can be better performed with the collaboration of a nurse, who determines the muscular strength of the patient, and a dermatome scan for the entire procedure; this must be documented in the postprocedure note. At this point we must evaluate the phenol/alcohol effect and keep in mind the position that the patient must maintain. The needle must be washed in cerebrospinal fluid or local anesthetic at the time of withdrawal of the needle to diminish backache due to a flow of the agent by the tip.

Cervical Subarachnoid Neurolysis

When reaching the cervical subarachnoid level, which technically is more difficult to access than other levels, we can palpate the posterior apophysis and localize intervertebral spaces, with caution at the moment of introducing the needle so as not to damage the spinal cord. Anatomic structures must be identified as the needle penetrates. In certain cases with spinal cord damage there are no apparent complications, only transitory pain on the affected dermatome. In this procedure it is important to ask the patient to perform neck flexion to make the subarachnoid approach easier.

Among the most common complications of lower cervical injections noted are dysfunction and weakness in superior extremities. In upper cervical levels be careful not to touch more than two dermatomes, as complications mentioned previously may occur. The volume is small, considering anatomic characteristics, and having an accurate position of the patient's head depends on the neurolytic agent or adjusting the operating table.[26]

In this level the recommended doses must be no more than 1 mL, and should be 0.05 mL whenever possible. We also suggest a second visualization of the area to reduce the mobility of the procedure because a patient can, with even minimal movements, modify the pressure of the cerebrospinal fluid and therefore the subarachnoid hydrodynamics.

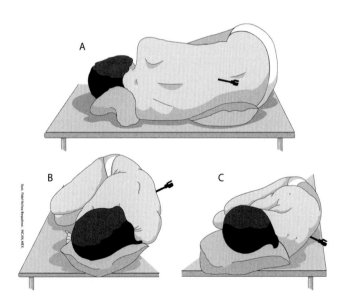

FIGURE 40–3 Position to perform rhizolysis at the thoracolumbar level. *A,* Dorsal view with the needle. *B,* Lateral-prone position used for the subarachnoid administration of alcohol (note 45-degree angle in anterior position). *C,* Lateral-supine position used for the subarachnoid administration of phenol (note 45-degree angle in dorsal position). *(From Patt RB, Cousins MJ: Techniques for neurolytic neural blockade. In Cousins MJ, Bridenbaugh PO (eds): Neural Blockade in Clinical Anesthesia and Management of Pain. Philadelphia, Lippincott-Raven, 1998.)*

Thoracic Subarachnoid Neurolysis

When using thoracic subarachnoid neurolysis we must consider the anatomy of posterior spinous process of the thoracic spine as this is the most difficult site of access due to posterior spinous process enlargement and its acute angle. Here we must use a paramedial approach via intervention with a needle, diminishing the difficulty of subarachnoid space access. In this region neurolysis can be performed quite safely, as at this dermatome level nervous fibers that innervate bladder, intestines, or extremities are not found. Although paralysis of intercostal muscles that rarely cause profound troubles in the respiratory dynamic may occur, at this level we recommend a 1.2- to 2-mL dose at most.[27,28] Compared to the cervical level, this level provides a better result due to a more selective approach. Posterior root injuries may occur due to their anatomic disposition.

Lumbar Subarachnoid Neurolysis

Lumbar subarachnoid neurolysis is used in many countries and may be the easiest treatment to perform to obtain pain relief in the pelvis, perineum, rectum, and genitals, realizing that an adequate neurologic pain exploration must be performed and that it must be used for unilateral pain but also considering vesical or rectum disfunction due to the proximity of sensitive and motor fibers. That is why one must be careful when performing this procedure and it is very important to explain to both the family and the patient the possible complications. Patients who are kept in bed with little mobilization due to neurologic illnesses, old age, cancer, intractable pain, colostomy, or urine deprivation and have the procedure done can experience a high rate of relief and a low rate of complication.[29] However, if symptoms are not taken into account, a physician can cause iatrogenic lesions because the L2 level is where the medullar cone is and the caudal nerves begin, which makes avoiding injuries in posterior roots more difficult.

One of the most commonly used lumbar techniques is the sacral block, which is easy and simple to perform, placing the patient in a sitting position and focusing on the L5-S1 subarachnoid space with a 22 caliber French needle through a paramedian approach. Upon reaching subarachnoid space it is necessary to redirect the bevel of the needle caudally, and then begin injecting the phenol slowly, having the patient lean in a 45-degree inclination to make sure the phenol is deposited only into the posterior roots that are sensorial. In almost every case the patient experiences pain relief after the first dose; the sensitivity trials that should be performed during the procedure at a perineal level are difficult to carry out due to the position. This technique is indicated for painful syndromes with oncologic origins that affect the perineal region, which may or may not include genitals (Figure 40-4).

There are studies on the incidence of vesical dysfunction with neurolytic subarachnoid saddle blocks in concentrations of 7.5%, 10%, and 15%, in which better

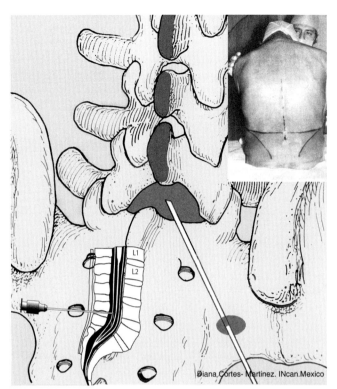

FIGURE 40-4 Patient in sitting position for the subarachnoid administration of phenol in sacral region, with slow administration of hyperbaric agent.

pain relief was observed with higher concentrations. A third of the patients in this report experienced urinary incontinence.[30]

Other complications that need to be considered include the following:

- Infections
- Headache, which is a frequent complication and may persist for weeks
- Spinal cord injury, which is very uncommon
- Posterior spinal artery thrombosis, which is rare but may result in paraplegia
- Weakness or paralysis, which is extremely rare.

EPIDURAL NEUROLYSIS

Although epidural techniques are frequently used by anesthesiologists for surgical procedures, there is very little reported experience of performing neurolysis this way. Reported studies are anecdotal. Previous studies performed in monkeys showed that there was destruction of both the anterior and posterior roots in 6% to 12% of the cases.[31] Two studies performed in cancer patients with 10% phenol as a single dose suggested that one can estimate the required volume of phenol by doing a trial with local anesthetics. For this purpose,

1% lidocaine administered in 2 mL aliquots to a maximum of 8 mL accurately predicted the volume required for epidural neurolysis. Reported results were excellent to good in half of the patients, and only one case of muscular weakness with urinary incontinence was reported. A high percentage of pain relief is reported in many studies, with an average of 3.3 months of pain relief.[32,33]

In 1992 a set of procedures was performed with optimum results in 93% of patients, with minimum volumes and serial repetitions in 2 to 6 daily shots with a maximum volume of 4 mL and a phenol concentration of 5%.[34]

At the National Institute of Cancer in Mexico physicians developed an alternative technique, which consists of verifying that the catheter tip is at the desired position by fluoroscopy with special attention at placing the tip of the epidural catheter at the level of the vertebral spine that corresponds to the middle of the nociceptive area. Epidurography with iohexol is done to determine the extension of the block, and the same volume required to achieve the appropriate spread during the epidurogram is used for the epidural neurolysis. Typically, a 3% phenol concentration is administered in a water-based solution in aliquots of 2 to 4 mL until the total target volume is reached. The patient is asked to remain still for about 15 minutes, then spends 45 minutes with free movement in bed. Later a neurologic and pain evaluation is performed; if pain persists and there is no indication of neurologic injury, then the next dose of 4% phenol is applied; the dose may be repeated with the same concentration or even increased to 5%, but only if pain is still present without neurologic deficit.

If, while using the same criteria for an average of 8 hours a day to make an epidural denervation in selective and sequential segments (which sometimes requires 2 or 3 days of subsequent application until the desired benefit is reached), neurologic alterations present, the procedure must be stopped, epidural space must be washed with an isotonic saline solution, and a steroid must be applied.[35]

This method is used to provide adequate pain control without producing motor deficit. However, if motor deficit develops during the sessions of intermittent injections and pain is still present, one is forced to rule out denervation pain. If this is not the case, one can continue the neurolysis on subsequent days but limit the total volume of each session to the volume that resulted in the motor deficit. In the majority of patients who develop motor deficit, it usually resolves within 72 hours.

In this technique physicians position the patient laterally over the painful side with a 45-degree dorsal angle. Prior to antisepsis and with aseptic technique, the epidural space is reached with the loss of resistance technique using a 22-gauge Tuohy needle. A catheter is then inserted, and the tip is directed, under fluoroscopy guidance, to the appropriate vertebral body corresponding

to the dermatone in the middle of the nociceptive area. When verifying the catheter position it is necessary to use a nonionic contrast medium in small volumes to confirm the diffusion in the epidural space. If you decide to perform the block diagnosis with local anesthetics before administering the neurolytic agent, you must recheck the position of the catheter to avoid migration; this is the reason for using an image amplifier with the contrast media.

Glycerol- or water-diluted phenol should be administrated with a 1-mL tuberculine syringe to minimize resistance. Then position the patient at a posterior angle for the phenol, given its hyperbaric characteristics, to disperse over the posterior roots; this technique, which is different from that used for subarachnoid pain relief, can be observed within 15 minutes of the agent administration. The patient must remain in the same position for at least 40 minutes. When daily administrations are required, the catheter must be rinsed with local anesthetic or saline solution because it could have chemical damage from phenol and glycerol.

Complications

Epidural neurolysis rarely presents complications, but some possible are muscle weakness and urinary incontinence. When applied at the lumbar level, the risk of generating a hematoma is minimal, and laboratory studies such as hematic biometry and coagulation periods could be requested to verify that. The complication rate varies depending on the level of the intervention. They are more common in the cervical and lumbar regions, as shortened spaces between anterior and posterior roots make the technique more difficult. Fortunately there are few reported cases of complications, and they are usually of transitory nature.[36] In cancer patients it is recommended to use magnetic resonance guidance with epidural neurolysis, which helps to confirm the catheter position and identify any infiltration of the spinal cord, because it may cause complications such as epidural hemorrhage, medullar compression, and irreversible neurologic injury.[37]

CONCLUSION

Neurolytic procedures for pain relief are frequently used in underdeveloped countries. They reduce pain intensity, have minimal side effects, and minimize the needed daily amount of opioids and other drugs for pain relief, which is desirable in countries in which poverty is common. Cancer pain is the most frequent indication for neurolysis. It can also be performed in other clinical conditions, such as postherpetic neuralgia, severe muscle spasms, pain secondary to aortic aneurism, and other painful conditions.

The main route of neurolytic agent administration is subarachnoid, due to its fast onset and convenience—the agent affects dorsal roots quickly and the period of immobilization is shorter. As most patients do not tolerate the same position for long periods of time, the epidural approach is preferred when longer periods of immobilization are required.

The most frequently used neurolytic agent in our hospital is ethanol. Ethanol is technically easier to administer intrathecally than hyperbaric neurolytic substances, particularly in patients with oncologic pain. With appropriate patient selection, the rate of pain relief is high and the rate of complications and associated morbidity and mortality is low.

REFERENCES

1. Luton A: Archives generales de medecin, 1863.
2. La Porte G: Les injections d´alcohol dans les neuralgies faciales [Thése]. Paris, 1905.
3. Flesch J: Die Behandlung von Neuralgien mittels Schlössers Alkoholinjektionen. Centralb Grenz Med Chir 12:561–572, 1900.
4. Maher RM: Relief of pain in incurable cancer. Lancet 1:18–20, 1955.
5. Swerdlow M: The history of neurolytic block. In Racz G (ed): Techniques of Neurolysis. Boston, Kluwer Academic Publishers, 1989.
6. Racz GB, Heavner J, Haynsworth R: Repeat epidural phenol injections in chronic pain and spasticity. In Lipton S, Miles J (eds): Persistent Pain. Modern Methods of Treatment, vol. 5. London, Grune & Stratton, 1985, pp 157–179.
7. Smith MC: Histological findings following intrathecal injection of phenol solutions for the relief of pain. Anaesthesia 36:387–406, 1964.
8. May O: Functional and histological effects of intraneural and intraganglionic injection of alcohol. BMJ 2:35, 1912.
9. Labat G: Action of alcohol on the living nerve. Curr Res Anesth Analg 12:190, 1933.
10. Gallagher HS, Yonezawa T, Hay RC, Derrick WS: Subarachnoid alcohol block II: Histological changes in the central nervous system. Am J Pathol 35:679–693, 1961.
11. Ventafrida V, Spreafico R: Subarachnoid saline perfusion, In Bonica JJ (ed): Advances in Neurology, vol. 4. New York, Raven Press, 1974, pp 477–484.
12. Hitchcock E: Osmolytic neurolysis for intractable facial pain. Lancet 1:434–436, 1969.
13. Hakanson S: Trigeminal neuralgia treated by the injection of glycerol into the trigeminal cistern. Neurosurgery 9:638–646, 1967.
14. Bates W, Judovich BD: Intractable pain. Anesthesiology 3:363, 1942.

15. Cousins MJ, Dwyer B, Gibb D: Chronic pain and neurolytic neural blockade. In Cousins MJ, Bridenbaugh PO (eds): Neural Blockade in Clinical Anesthesia and management of Pain, 2nd ed. Philadelphia, JB Lippincott, 1988, pp 1053–1084.
16. Plancarte SR, Velazquez R: Palliative regional anesthesia for hospitalized patients. Curr Opinión Anaesth, 7:444–447, 1994.
17. Plancarte R, Mayer-Rivera F: Regional anaesthesia and medical disease. Curr Opinión Anaesth 13:545–548, 2000.
18. Winnie A, Candido K: Subarachnoid neurolytic blocks. In Waldman S (ed): Interventional Pain Management, 2nd ed. Amsterdam, Saunders, 2001, pp 554–559.
19. Patt R, Cousins M: Techniques for neurolytic neural blockade. In Cousins MJ, Bridenbaugh PO (eds): Neural Blockade in Clinical Anesthesia and Management of Pain, 3rd ed. Philadelphia, Lippincott-Raven Publishers, 1998, pp 1007–1061.
20. Swerdlow M: Neurolytic blocks of the neuraxis. In Patt R (ed): Cancer Pain, 1st ed. Philadelphia, Lippincott, 1993, pp 427–442.
21. Dogliotti AM: A new therapeutic meted for peripheral neuralgias: Injection of alcohol into the subarachnoid space. Pain Clinic 1:197–201, 1987.
22. Khalili AA, Betts HB: Peripheral nerve block with phenol in the management of spasticity. JAMA 200:1155–1165, 1967.
23. Papo I, Visca A: Intrathecal phenol in the treatment of pain and spasticity. Proc Neurol Surg 7:56, 1976.
24. Papo I: Spinal posterior rhizotomia and commisural myelotomy in the treatment of cancer pain. Adv Pain Res Ther 2:439, 1979.

25. Maher RM: Relief of pain in incurable cancer. Lancet I:18–20, 1955.
26. Perese DM: Subarachnoid alcohol block in the management of pain of malignant disease. Arch Surg 76:347–354, 1958.
27. Korevaar WC: Transcatheter thoracic epidural neurolysis using ethyl alcohol. Anesthesiology 69:989–993, 1988.
28. Lloyd JW: Subarachnoid and other clinical uses of phenol. In Racz G (ed): Techniques of Neurolysis, 1st ed. Boston, Kluwer Academic Publishers, 1989, pp 33–44.
29. Ischia S, Luzzani A, Ischia A, et al: Subarachnoid neurolytic block (L5-S1) and unilateral percutaneous cervical cordotomy in the treatment of pain secondary to pelvic malignant disease. Pain 20:139–149, 1984.
30. Ischia S, Luzzani A, Pacini, Meffezzoli GF: Lytic saddle block: clinical comparison of the results, using phenol at 5, 10 and 15 percent. Adv Pain Res Ther 7:339, 1984.
31. Gregg RV, Sehlhorst CS, Liwnickz BH: Histopathology of epidural phenol in the monkey. Abstracts. 7th World Congress on Pain, Paris, 1993, p 93.
32. Ferrer-Brechner T: Epidural and intrathecal phenol Neurolysis for cancer pain. Anesthesiol Rev 8:14–32, 1981.
33. Korevaar WC: Transcatheter thoracic epidural neurolysis using ethyl alcohol. Anesthesiology 69:989–993, 1988.
34. Salmon JB, Finch PM, Lovegrove FTA, Warwick A: Mapping the spread of epidural phenol in cancer pain patients by radionuclide admixture and epidural scintigraphy. Clin J Pain 8:18–22, 1992.
35. Plancarte R: Personal Communication, 1994.
36. Perese DM: Subarachnoid alcohol block in the management of pain in malignant disease. Arch Surg 4:135–144, 1958.
37. Cousins MJ, Dwyer B, Gibb D: Chronic pain and neurolytic neural blockade. In Cousins MJ (ed): Neural Blockade, 2nd ed. Philadelphia, JB Lippincott, 1988, pp 1053–1084.

CHAPTER 41

Management of Cancer Pain in Neonates, Children, and Adolescents

DORALINA ANGHELESCU, MD, LINDA OAKES, RN, MSN, CCNS, AND MARK POPENHAGEN, PSYD

There is no profit in curing the body, if in the process, we destroy the soul.
SAMUEL H. GOLPER, CITY OF HOPE HOSPITAL, DUARTE, CALIFORNIA

The past two decades have brought unprecedented clinical and scientific interest and success not only in the effective treatment of cancer for infants, children, and adolescents, but also an increased emphasis on providing optimal pain management during such treatment. Remarkable improvements in long-term survival of children with cancer have stimulated the need to ensure that these patients endure only minimal suffering during aggressive oncologic treatment, involving chemotherapy, radiation therapy, and surgery, all with an intent to cure. Although successful treatment of a child with cancer is more frequently achieved compared with the outcome in adults, the treatment often means enduring repetitive cycles of chemotherapy associated with painful side effects as well as numerous invasive diagnostic and therapeutic procedures. Even within the current efforts to assess and treat pain, children with cancer continue to report moderate to severe pain. Collins et al. report that both inpatient (86.8%) and outpatient (75%) had moderate to severe pain.[1] The World Health Organization (WHO) reported that 70% of children with cancer suffered severe pain at some point in their treatment and pain was often not recognized or not treated adequately.[2] Findings continue to raise concern that even in leading pediatric hospitals in the United States, 89% of children dying of cancer experience pain, as reported by their parents in after-death interviews.[3] This study further emphasized that parental and clinicians' assessment of children's pain and other distresses may differ, as clinicians did not recognize or treat these children adequately for pain.

PAIN AS A RESULT OF DISEASE AND ITS TREATMENT

Pain causes the most concern and fear for children who are diagnosed with all types of malignancies. Many children think that with a diagnosis of cancer, one is bound to have pain and that little can be done to relieve it. Many survivors of pediatric cancer experience post-traumatic stress as late as 12 years after the completion of successful cancer treatment.[4] The main source of pain for pediatric oncology patients continues to be related to the treatment of cancer[5] including postoperative pain, phantom limb pain, mucositis, infection, chemotherapy-induced pain, and procedure-related pain. Tumor-related pain is generally not the most significant source except at the initial diagnosis, at the time of relapse or during end-of-life care. In summary, most of the pain a child experiences comes from the actual treatment of the cancer, thus mandating the clinicians to simultaneously become skilled in both treatment of the cancer and the related pain. Procedure-related pain is reviewed in Chapter 42.

Nociceptive pain has its source in bones, joints, muscles, skin, or connective tissue and is described as an aching or throbbing sensation. Neuropathic pain results from nerve damage or inflammation and is commonly described as a burning, stabbing, "pins and needles," or shooting sensation, often along the involved nerve tract. The intensity and the duration of pain often greatly exceed the time in which the injury would be expected to resolve. Neuropathic pain symptoms are seen after surgery involving nerves such as amputation or limb-sparing procedures, or related to medications such as vincristine or cyclosporine.

EFFECTS OF UNRELIEVED PAIN IN CHILDREN

Pain is a complex medical problem that can affect the physical and emotional well-being of children. Effective pain management is not only the right thing to do from a moral and ethical perspective; it also minimizes the pain-related physiologic disturbances. Research has shown that the consequences of inadequate pain control are serious undesirable cardiopulmonary, metabolic, hormonal, and emotional systems effects.[6,7] Most of this work has been done studying preterm infants or the corresponding animal model, that of newborn rat pups,[8] while acknowledging that extrapolating the results of animal studies to the clinical world should be done with caution. Evidence has been generated for increased pain sensitivity in neonates. Prolonged or repetitive pain at an early age alters the development of the peripheral, spinal, and supraspinal pain systems. Preterm infants undergoing painful procedures with adequate analgesia had less incidence of adverse neurologic outcomes such as intraventricular hemorrhage compared with those receiving placebo.[9] Unrelieved pain inhibits children's participation in treatment such as deep breathing and physical therapy, leading to further delays in recovery and to increased morbidity and mortality.

Studies have supported the need to avoid the effects of repetitive pain episodes. Taddio et al. evaluated how a painful experience in the early infancy influenced reactions to subsequent pain-generating events.[10] Infants who were circumcised without topical anesthesia showed more behaviors associated with pain during subsequent routine vaccinations at 4 and 6 months of age compared with uncircumcised infants. In infants who had EMLA cream at the site of circumcision, the provision of local anesthetics attenuated the pain response to subsequent vaccinations. Fitzgerald and Beggs[11] looked at how the peripheral nervous system in the newborn is damaged with repetitive pain from heel sticks, and found that the hyperinnervation of the affected tissue for a prolonged period of time after the heel stick seemed to be more profound in infants than in adults.

In view of these research advances, the American Academy of Pediatrics emphasized the responsibilities of clinicians to "expand their knowledge, use appropriate assessment tools and techniques, anticipate painful experiences and intervene accordingly, using a multimodal approach to pain management involving families, and advocating for the use of effective pain management in children."[12]

In summary, the need to overcome obstacles in providing effective pain relief is heightened by new data that suggest that pain experienced during the newborn period may have long-lasting effects on future pain perceptions and behaviors.[8,13-16] Through repeated experiences of pain during childhood, researchers suggest that neurologic changes occur associated with changes in coping responses, eating behaviors, an increased risk of depression, and, in general, a preoccupation with pain.[17] Others have found that undergoing repeated noxious stimulation without a means for escape during early life may lead to children demonstrating learned helplessness behaviors and lack of expression to pain.[8]

Although the extent to which children recall pain and how early pain experiences significantly affect later development of chronic pain remains yet to be determined, the relationship between temperament and pain reactivity is provocative.

Inadequate pain management further complicates the treatment of cancer. Unrelieved pain related to cancer or its treatment will lead to the inability to comply with mouth care (mucositis) and physical therapy (bone or soft tissue pain) or reluctance to taking deep breaths or cough to clear their secretions following abdominal or thoracic surgeries contributing to the risk of atelectasis, lobar collapse, and pulmonary infection.

INFLUENCE OF DEVELOPMENTAL LEVEL

Preschool children are very egocentric in their thinking and believe that all events and sensations originate from their internal world. They have little understanding of cause-and-effect relationships, often misunderstanding the meaning and cause of pain. They may view pain as a punishment for past misdeeds or bad thoughts. Young children need to be repeatedly reassured that procedures and painful experiences are not punishments. Breakdowns in skin integrity from cuts, abrasions, or incisions are extremely threatening to children because of their fears of bodily injury and mutilation. They may believe that all of their body and blood will leak out. Bandages and dressings may hold a special power for children as they "fix the leak" and hold the body in from the environment.

School-age children become more logical and reasonable in their thinking. They are in the process of gaining greater command over their world and tend to be achievement-oriented. Because these children are often organized by rules, they respond well to rituals to cope with painful events. Once these rituals and routines are established, they must be followed consistently to be effective.

Adolescents are capable of abstract thinking and have an understanding of "if-then" relationships. Although capable of adult-level problem-solving, adolescents lack the life experiences that facilitate consistent mature responses. During stressful situations, adolescents may vacillate between adult responses and regression to immature behaviors.

OVERCOMING BARRIERS AND MISCONCEPTIONS OF PAIN IN INFANTS AND CHILDREN

Examination of barriers to effective pain management for children may help to explain suboptimal treatment. Lack of knowledge by children, parents, and health care professionals leads to misconceptions about treatment options, especially regarding the use of opioids potentially leading to addiction. These misunderstandings continue to prevent the timely and appropriate treatment of patients of all ages. Confusion exists regarding two terms associated with the use of opioids: addiction and physical dependency. These terms are often used inappropriately and interchangeably, perpetuating misconceptions. Parents continue to have fears that their children will "get hooked" and will become addicts. It is inappropriate to withhold pain medication from a suffering patient on the theoretical grounds of addiction.[18] As in adults, addiction is a pattern of compulsive drug use characterized by a continuous craving for a drug and the need to use it for effects other than relief of symptoms such as pain. Persons who are addicted use drugs for their mind-altering properties, not for the medical purpose of pain relief. Those fears can be diminished by explaining the difference between using analgesics for mind-altering purposes as opposed to using them for pain.

Another misconception has been the belief that the nervous system is incompletely developed in infancy, and, therefore, infants are incapable of perceiving or remembering pain. Substantial scientific evidence shows that infants perceive and remember pain.[13]

ASSESSMENT OF PAIN IN INFANTS AND CHILDREN

Accurate assessment of pain intensity is a prerequisite for management. A clear standard of care has emerged requiring routine measurement of pain at regular intervals using consistent and valid pain assessment tools. For acutely ill infants, children, and adolescents, this practice includes assessment intervals of at least every 4 hours with reassessment within 1 hour after any pharmacologic and nonpharmacologic intervention. If a new complaint of pain occurs or if existing pain changes in severity or character, a full diagnostic workup is warranted, especially for headache or neuropathic pain.

Children are quite capable of describing many aspects of pain. For children who are able to communicate their discomforts directly, pain assessment is easy to obtain. However, fear, confusion, developmental immaturity, and the severity of illness hinder children's ability to communicate with caregivers. Children should be encouraged to tell caregivers about their pain whenever possible. For older children and adolescents, this can be accomplished much as in adults using a visual or numbered scale. Because children younger than 8 years of age do not have the understanding of the value of numbers to rate the intensity of a symptom, other means of communicating levels of pain are needed.[19, 20]

In the past 20 years several pain assessment scales have been shown to be easily understood by children and clinically useful. Many of these scales use the format of a series of faces ranging from smiling faces that are not showing signs of pain to faces with progressive degrees of distress, aligned along a vertical or horizontal line. Each face is assigned a numerical value reflecting its order within a series of facial expressions (Figure 41–1). Clinicians are cautioned to not confuse rankings of happiness or well-being with that of the intensity of pain when using such tools. Ideally, the best approach is to introduce the tool when children are not in an anxious state. If possible, children should be given the opportunity to define which number is the acceptable pain level for them. In addition to pain intensity, clinicians should evaluate: the quality of pain (throbbing, burning); the location of pain; and aggravating or relieving factors.

For young children and infants who lack the verbal and cognitive abilities necessary to tell their caregivers when they hurt, those methods of assessing pain are inadequate. This is also true with acutely ill children who cannot point to a scale to indicate their pain. For these children, behaviors associated with generalized distress or discomfort have been used to infer pain. Crying is the most common way by which parents and health professionals judge pain in infants and young children, although infants also cry when they are angry, fearful, and hungry. Infants and children demonstrate gross body movements or positioning, ranging from rigidity to thrashing, in association with pain. These observations have been incorporated into pain assessment scales to provide a more objective and systematic approach.

FIGURE 41–1 Faces Pain Scale. *(From Wong DL, Hess CS: Wong and Whaley's Clinical Manual of Pediatric Nursing, 5th ed. St Louis, Mosby, 2000, p 326, with permission.)*

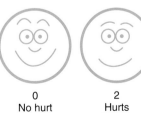

0	2	4	6	8	10
No hurt	Hurts little bit	Hurts little more	Hurts even more	Hurts whole lot	Hurts worst

TABLE 41-1   FLACC Behavioral Scale

Categories	Scoring		
	0	1	2
Face (F)	No particular expression or smile	Occasional grimace or frown, withdrawn, disinterested	Frequent to constant frown, clenched jaw, quivering chin
Legs (L)	Normal position or relaxed	Uneasy, restless, tense	Kicking, or legs drawn up
Activity (A)	Lying quietly, normal position, moves easily	Squirming, shifting back and forth, tense	Arched, rigid, or jerking
Cry (C)	No cry (awake or asleep)	Moans or whimpers, occasional complaint	Crying steadily, screams or sobs, frequent complaints
Consolability (C)	Content, relaxed	Reassured by occasional touching, hugging, or being talked to, distractible	Difficult to console or comfort

Each of the five categories—Face (F); Legs (L); Activity (A); Cry (C); Consolability (C)—is scored from 0 to 2, which results in a total score between 0 and 10.
Copyright 2002, The University of Michigan.

Of these measures, a few have adequate reliability, validity, and clinical usefulness for bedside clinicians. One such tool (Table 41-1) uses the cues to quantify known pain behaviors, specifically the facial expressions, leg position, generalized activity, type of cry, and ease in consoling as means of rating pain behaviors.[21] This tool, known as the FLACC, is an acronym for these components and has been found to have inter-rater reliability and preliminary validity for scoring postoperative pain in children ages 2 months to 7 years. Other researchers have tested the validity of the FLACC by measuring changes in scores in response to analgesics in children younger than 3 years of age including those on a hematology/oncology unit.[22] The reader can refer to a recently published review of available tools for further information on pediatric pain.[23]

PAIN MANAGEMENT TECHNIQUES

Ideally, designated staff such as a pain team should be used to ensure that pain management is a priority within an institution. The multidisciplinary expertise of anesthesiologists, pediatricians, oncologists, pharmacists, psychologists, child life specialists, and physical therapists can be offered directly to those who are suffering cancer pain on a referral basis. Expertise of such clinicians can be used to improve pain management for all infants and children (i.e., the development of standardized protocols useful in promoting consistency in reducing pain, preventing and treating side effects from opioids more promptly, and minimizing dosing errors).

Pharmacologic Therapy

Pharmacologic studies involving children with cancer are still lacking, especially clinical trials of adjuvant analgesics and those exploring oral bioavailability of analgesics.[5] Developmental differences affect the pharmacokinetics and pharmacodynamics of analgesics as well summarized by various authors.[20,24]

Adherence to the World Health Organization analgesic ladder remains the guide for determining the treatment plan.[2] Administering the analgesic by mouth is always preferred, as being the least expensive, invasive, or threatening for the family especially in the outpatient setting. However, for children with cancer who cannot swallow medications, other routes such as intravenous (IV) or transdermal are often used. The intramuscular route is not recommended due to children's fear of needles. Children cannot understand why a shot, which is painful, would help relieve pain. However, for those with poor IV access, subcutaneous infusions of opioids via a small butterfly needle or catheter may be effective with rates of 1 to 3 mL per hour. Rectal administration is discouraged in children, and particularly in those with neutropenia due to the risk of infection.

Acute pain should be treated by regularly scheduled medications sufficient to control pain and by closely monitored titration of the medications in response to the patient's needs. The administration of pro re nata (PRN) medications requires children to be able to communicate their discomfort and might allow them to re-experience pain before the next dose of medication is administered, possibly leading to undertreatment of pain. A PRN schedule is appropriate for children who have intermittent (pain separated by pain-free intervals), unpredictable pain or who have pain related to specific activities such as dressing changes or physical therapy.

Opioid Analgesia

Opioids remain the single most important group of medications for the relief of moderate to severe pain in children with cancer. In patients with known recognized severe pain problems, it is not necessary to slowly advance "up the ladder" to provide relief, allowing to start with IV dosages rather than administer by mouth. Concerns about the safety of administration of opioids to infants and children are not to prevent the clinician from using these when necessary. Opioids are not more dangerous for children than they are for adults when appropriately administered. There are some differences in opioid pharmacodynamics and pharmacokinetics in infants younger than 6 months of age, but adequate analgesia can still be provided safely with appropriate dosages, intervals of drug administration, and rate of administration of parenteral preparations. Even today an excessive and unfounded concern over young children's immature metabolic capacity causing drug accumulation and subsequent adverse effects has been a major deterrent to administering opioids to pediatric patients. Acknowledgment that respiratory depression is a serious and well-known side effect of opioids is appropriate.

Traditionally, the child's weight has been used to determine the starting opioid dose. Numerous variables can influence the appropriate dose for the individual patient. Doses should be individualized on the basis of age, disease status, and previous or current opioid exposure. Higher dosages may be necessary for patients who have been receiving ongoing opioids. The optimal dose should be determined by titration. Patients greater than 50 kg should receive initial dosages using adult tables. As in adults, there is no maximum dose of any

opioid, as the appropriate dose is the one that controls pain with the least amount of side effects. For children who remain alert and are still experiencing pain, it is safe to titrate further doses, using doses equivalent to half the initial dose. Opioid response increases linearly with the log of the dose.[24] Thus a dose increment of less than 30% to 50% is not likely to improve analgesia significantly for those in moderate to severe pain. Very high doses of morphine or its equivalent, as much as 500 mg/kg/hour, may be required in patients with terminal cancer.[5] This wide variability reinforces the need for prompt and individualized attention to unrelieved pain. Table 41-2 provides information about the initial doses of analgesics administered to opioid-naïve patients.[2,20,25-30]

Because ventilatory reflexes to hypoxia and hypercarbia are indeed immature in newborns and develop over the first months of life, use of opioids in this age group requires additional precautions, expertise, and vigilance. Generally, morphine given to infants younger than 6 months of age tends to have a longer elimination half-life and a slower clearance rate. The duration of action of morphine is highly variable among the infant age-group; therefore, opioid titration in young infants must be conservative, with starting doses reduced by approximately 25% to 50% on a per kilogram basis relative to the dosing recommended for older children.[5] The starting dose of oral morphine recommended for older children is 0.2 to 0.3 mg/kg per dose.[5] The infant's response to an opioid dose is to be assessed carefully. Once the infant's response is known, it becomes easier to titrate further doses of opioids effectively and safely.

Morphine is an effective opioid to treat moderate to severe nociceptive pain, both in the immediate-release (short-acting) tablets and parenteral forms, while the sustained release preparations are more convenient for continuous pain. Parents must be taught that these long-acting morphine formulations should not be chewed or broken, which would cause overdosing by

---

TABLE 41-2 Initial Opioid Dosages for Infants and Children

Medication	Route/Method	Initial Dose/Schedule
Oxycodone	Oral only	0.1 mg/kg q4hr
Morphine	Intermittent IV bolus Continuous IV infusion Oral (MSIR)	0.1 mg/kg q3-4hr 0.03-0.06 mg/kg/hr with initial bolus of 0.05 mg/kg 0.15-0.3 mg/kg q4hr
Hydromorphone (Dilaudid)	Intermittent IV bolus	0.015 mg/kg q4-6hr
Fentanyl	Intermittent IV bolus Continuous IV infusion	1-2 µg/kg 1-3 µg/kg/hr
Codeine	Oral	0.5 to 1 mg/kg q4hr

IV, intravenous.

TABLE 41–3   Opioid Equianalgesic Doses

Drug	Equianalgesic dose (in mg/kg)	
	IV/IM	PO
Morphine	10	30
Hydromorphone (Dilaudid)	1.5	7.5
Fentanyl	0.1–0.2	Not available
Oxycodone	Not available	15–30

IM, intramuscularly; *IV,* intravenously; *PO,* per os.

becoming an immediate-release preparation. Kadian is a sustained-release morphine formulation available as capsules that can be opened, and the contained pellets can be swallowed or sprinkled onto soft food.[5] When any sustained-release morphine is given, an immediate-release preparation should be prescribed too, as a means of managing unexpected pain or pain associated with vigorous activity. Immediate-release morphine for such "breakthrough pain" usually should be provided on a PRN basis. Clinicians are to be mindful that chemotherapy-induced renal failure may lead to accumulation of its metabolite (morphine-6-glucuronide), resulting in side effects. Therefore, it may be more appropriate to consider hydromorphone or fentanyl, with no known toxic metabolites, using equianalgesic doses according to the conversion table (Table 41–3).

If unacceptable side effects (pruritus, myoclonus) from morphine occur or if the patient is known to be allergic to morphine, hydromorphone (Dilaudid) may be given using equianalgesic doses according to the conversion

ratios in Table 41–3. Currently hydromorphone has no long-acting oral preparation. However, it can also be used as a continuous subcutaneous infusion due to its high potency and aqueous solubility.

For children who cannot tolerate morphine, oxycodone is an effective alternative. Often compounded with other agents such as acetaminophen (in Percocet), clinicians are to be mindful of the fact that while there is no ceiling dose of oxycodone, there is a maximum daily dose for acetaminophen to avoid the risk of hepatic toxicity (Table 41–4). Therefore, the noncompounded form, oxycodone, may be preferable. Clinicians need to be aware that oxycodone has a shorter elimination half-life in children 2 to 20 years of age compared with adults.[5] For continuous pain, the total daily dose of oxycodone can be converted into the long-acting form OxyContin. As with long-acting morphine preparation, OxyContin is to be taken as a whole tablet. Oxycodone is not available in a parenteral form.

Another opioid that can be an option is fentanyl, with doses described in Tables 41–2 and 41–3. An oral transmucosal preparation is available and has been used in children for preoperative sedation[31] and procedure-related pain.[32] It also has been proven efficacious for control of breakthrough pain in cancer patients[33] and for incident pain.[34] Its very rapid onset of action after intravenous administration makes it attractive for rapid relief of pain. However, its short duration of action means that for other than brief or procedural-related pain, frequent dosages or an infusion would be necessary to provide relief of ongoing pain. The clearance of fentanyl is higher in infants and young children compared to adults.[5] Tolerance and physical dependence may occur within 5 to 10 days of continuous infusions, leading to frequent dose escalation. The clearance is dependent

TABLE 41–4   Orally Administered NSAIDs

Name of Drug	Pediatric Dose (<60 kg)	Maximum Dose/kg/Day	Adult Dose (>60kg)	Maximum Dose/Day
Acetaminophen	10–15 mg/kg q 4–6 hrs PO	75 mg	500–1000 mg q 4–6 hrs PO	4000 mg
Naproxen	5–10 mg/kg q 12 hrs PO	20 mg	250–375 mg q 12 hrs PO	1000 mg
Ibuprofen	5–10 mg/kg q 8–12 hrs PO	40 mg	400–600 mg q 6 hrs PO	3200 mg
Choline magnesium trisalicylate	10–15 mg/kg q 8–12 hrs PO	Information not available	1000–1500 mg q 12 hrs PO	3000 mg
Ketorolac	0.5 mg/kg q 6 hrs IV	Give no more than 5 days	15–30 mg q 8 hrs IV	Give no more than 5 days

NSAIDs, nonsteroidal anti-inflammatory drugs; *PO,* per os.

on hepatic blood flow and may thus be decreased in cardiac failure. A unique problem with fentanyl is that of incidences of chest wall rigidity following rapid IV administration of doses greater than 5 μg/kg. If this occurs, it is best managed by administering a neuromuscular blocking agent, naloxone, or both. No oral formulation is available.

Transdermal fentanyl patches can be useful in treating pain in children when IV access is limited. However, clinicians are to be reminded that the patch with the lowest dose of 12 μg/hour provides the equivalent of morphine IV of 1.2 mg/hour (or 30 mg/day IV or 90 mg/day of morphine orally). Therefore, this method needs to be reserved for those children who have used such an opioid equivalent for an extended time and are likely to need significant doses for at least the next 72 hours. Likewise when the dose needs to be decreased below 12 μg/hour, careful downward titration using fentanyl IV or an oral opioid needs to be provided to prevent withdrawal.

Codeine is an oral opioid used for moderate pain. Nevertheless, since the analgesic effect of codeine is based on its metabolism into morphine and 10% of Caucasians cannot metabolize into morphine, for this group codeine has no analgesic effects.[35]

Methadone is a synthetic opioid with a long and variable half-life following IV or oral administration in children.[5,36] Although useful as a long-acting agent when administered orally in tablet or elixir form, the risk of delayed sedation and overdose compels clinicians to closely assess the child during the first few days until a steady state is achieved.

As in adults, meperidine (Demerol) is best avoided for repeated doses because of the risk of accumulation of its metabolite, normeperidine, which can cause central nervous system stimulation including tremors, muscle twitches, hyperactive reflexes, and seizures. However, low doses can be used for prophylaxis and treatment of rigors with the infusion of amphotericin.

Mixed agonist-antagonist opioids (nalbuphine, butorphanol) have the theoretical advantage of causing less respiratory depression than pure agonists. Their use in severe pain is limited by the ceiling effect and the potential to reverse agonists agents previously given and precipitate withdrawal.[36] Therefore, they are not recommended for use for continuing painful states such as during cancer treatment.

Severe nociceptive pain can often be controlled by intermittent administration of morphine 0.3 mg/kg PO q 3 to 4 hours or 0.1 mg/kg IV q 3 to 4 hours. If the pain is not relieved by this approach, 50% of the above doses can be given every hour until the pain is controlled, and then full doses can be given every 3 to 4 hours to maintain a constant level of pain control. Alternatively, morphine 0.05 mg/kg IV boluses every 5 to 10 minutes can be given with the physician at the bedside until the pain is controlled. Once controlled, a morphine patient-controlled analgesia (PCA) infusion may be started at a rate of 0.02 mg/kg/hour with boluses of 0.02 mg/kg every 10 to15 minutes. Administration can be titrated to the desired effect. Better pain control may be achieved by changing from one opioid to another opioid due to the advantage of opioid rotation and incomplete cross-tolerance. Starting at 100% of the equianalgesic dose is usually not necessary when practicing opioid rotation and may lead to unacceptable side effects or overdose.

When prolonged pain is expected (e.g., early mucositis), it may be more appropriate to start a continuous morphine infusion at 0.01 to 0.04 mg/kg/hour with an initial bolus of 0.05 mg/kg and consider the use of PCA. Continuous infusions of opioids are most preferred to avoid large variations in plasma concentration and to maintain continuous pain relief. Favorable outcomes with PCA have been noted in children as young as 6 years of age, with lower pain scores and less sedation compared with intermittent dosing of opioids.[5,19] A PCA is most effectively used in pediatrics with a basal rate and the ability to add in bolus doses when needed. This method combines the benefits of a continuous infusion with available boluses as needed and gives children some control in their own care. Younger children will need to be reminded and reinstructed regarding the use of the PCA devices including the need to push the bolus button as their pain is starting to increase and not to wait until their pain is at the highest point on the pain scale. Having the basal rate is especially important in providing adequate analgesia while asleep. PCA use has resulted in lower pain scores and better patient acceptance with no increase in opioid use or opioid side effects.[19]

For younger children or those who are developmentally delayed and not cognitively able to understand to self-administer analgesics, some experts advocate for family-controlled analgesia or nurse-activated dosing.[27,37,38] Nurse-controlled analgesia has been shown to be safe for infants and children unable to dose themselves.[19] Because the child's safety is paramount, the clinician is to carefully evaluate parents in terms of their ability to provide parent-controlled analgesia. Parents of children with chronic illnesses such as cancer may wish to retain some control over their child's care during a hospital stay and are often familiar with hospital routines. Clinicians are reminded to evaluate for coexisting medical conditions as well as the use of concurrent sedatives.[39]

Management of Side Effects

Children and adolescents do not necessarily tell their caregivers when they are having side effects. Therefore, clinicians need to ask specifically about these problems.

TABLE 41–5	Prevention and Treatment of Constipation (Oral Doses)
Generic Name	**Dosage/Schedule**
Senna PO	10–20 mg/kg daily or BID
Docusate PO	5 mg/dose (3–12 y old) or 5–15 mg/dose (>12 y old) BID or TID
Bisacodyl PO	5–10 mg/day (3–12 y old) or 5–15 mg/dose (>12 y old) daily
Naloxone PO	3 mg TID titrating up to a maximum of 12 mg TID

BID, twice daily; *TID*, three times daily.

Tolerance to all of these side effects, except constipation, will develop over the first week of starting an opioid. Therefore, symptomatic treatment of the side effect itself should be considered before switching to another opioid as may be useful to minimize these effects.

Constipation is the most frequently reported side effect of opioids, and the risk will not diminish over time. Most children who receive opioid drugs for more than 1 to 2 days should receive regular laxatives (bulk plus a stimulant, such as a senna combination or lactulose) to prevent opioid-induced constipation. Simple stool softeners are not sufficient. See Table 41–5 for dosage recommendations.

Pruritus is a common side effect of opioids. If it occurs, the clinician is to consider an alternative opioid, or add an antihistamine drug such as diphenhydramine (Benadryl), or administer a low-dose IV infusion of naloxone (0.25 µg/kg/hour) carefully titrating to 1 µg/kg/hour to reverse the pruritus without reversal of the analgesic effects of the opioid.[26]

Urinary retention from increased bladder smooth muscle tone and sphincter spasm can develop. Urinary catheterization may be necessary for short-term management.

Dysphoria, drowsiness, confusion, and dizziness can occur initially but usually disappear within a few days. A child who has been in severe pain may be sleep deprived; once the pain is controlled the child may be "catching up" on sleep. This is not a sign of overdosage as long as the patient can be aroused.

If a patient who is receiving opioids experiences nausea and vomiting, it is first necessary to exclude a primary condition as the cause. Nausea and vomiting secondary to opioid use may be treated with one of the following: ondansetron (Zofran) 0.15 mg/kg (PO) or IV with a maximum dosage of 8 mg every 6 to 8 hours, promethazine (Phenergan) 0.25 to 0.5 mg/kg every 4 to 6 hours PO or IV, or diphenhydramine (Benadryl) 0.5 to 1 mg/kg PO or IV every 6 to 8 hours as needed. Ondansetron has no central nervous system depressant effects,

and is the preferred first choice in order to avoid cumulative depressant effects with the opioid.

Respiratory depression is the most feared but least frequently occurring side effect from the use of opioids. Mild respiratory depression can be managed by reducing the opioid dose, whereas with moderate to severe depression, stimulation, airway support, and bag-mask ventilation are to be considered. Naloxone (Narcan), an opioid antagonist, can be used but requires expertise from clinicians in order to prevent excessive reversal of the analgesic effects. Use of a diluted solution is recommended (0.4 mg in 10 mL of normal saline), in 0.5 mL increments IV, and reassess the child's respiratory status. If the IV route is inaccessible, naloxone may be given intramuscularly or subcutaneously. Concurrent airway support and bag-mask ventilation are to be provided as necessary. Further careful observation for improvement of respiratory status without interfering with analgesic effects of the opioid is to be done while titrating subsequent doses. It may be necessary to repeat naloxone after the first response because its duration is shorter than that of most opioids.

Discontinuing the Opioids

Opioid weaning is indicated when the source of pain diminishes and the opioid has been used for more than 2 weeks. A defined plan to appropriately discontinue opioids in infants and children is critical to providing optimal pain management. The clinician is to assure the child and family that this need to carefully decrease the dosages does not mean the child is addicted to the medicines. It means they are temporarily physically dependent on them in the same fashion a child would be dependent on steroids. When a patient is receiving opioid via PCA, the infusion should be stopped or its rate should be reduced while the patient is allowed to continue to self-administer boluses of opioid. The opioid dosage should be reduced by 20% to 30% every 1 to 2 days; however, longer therapy will require slower weaning. A weaning regimen is suggested as follows[40,41]:

- Calculate the total amount of opioid received in 24 hours.
- On the first day, reduce this amount by 20%.
- Wean subsequent doses by 10% per day as tolerated or 20% every 2 days or 30% every 3 days.

Signs and symptoms of withdrawal include sweating, diarrhea, jitteriness, piloerection, agitation, tachycardia, and stuffy nose. Carefully monitoring the signs and symptoms of withdrawal and pain recurrence is necessary, and the opioid dose should be adjusted accordingly. Young infants who have been maintained on opioids for lengthy periods may require a slower wean, such as decreases of 5% to 10% every other day.

Nonopioid Analgesia

Mild nociceptive pain can be controlled by acetaminophen or nonsteroidal anti-inflammatory drugs (NSAIDs). Unfortunately, these medications do have a maximum dose to prevent intolerable side effects, thereby making them inappropriate for treating severe pain (see Table 41–4).[2,20,26-29,42] Acetaminophen (Tylenol) has frequently been used for its analgesic and antipyretic properties; with the advantages of not having NSAID-associated side effects such as gastritis and bleeding. However, this agent is not effective for moderate to severe pain.

NSAIDs are useful for many forms of pain, including, but not limited to, postoperative pain, bone pain (tumor pain or related to administration of granulocyte colony-stimulating factors), and sickle cell crisis pain. All of the drugs used to treat mild nociceptive pain are antipyretic. Prescribing them for neutropenic patients needs to be done collaboratively with the oncologist, since fever can often be the only sign of infection. Because naproxen and ibuprofen inhibit platelet function, these two drugs should be used with extreme caution in patients with thrombocytopenia; choline magnesium trisalicylate (Trilisate) has less antiplatelet effect than naproxen or ibuprofen. Limited data are available regarding the cyclooxygenase 2 (COX-2) inhibitors in children. All NSAIDs should be used with extreme caution in patients with any renal dysfunction, concomitant diuretic use, or hypovolemia, because these agents can precipitate renal failure. The use of NSAIDs should be avoided in patients who are receiving high-dose methotrexate, as the methotrexate clearance can be delayed.[43] Aspirin and choline magnesium trisalicylate should not be used in patients with presumed or confirmed viral infections because of the association between Reye's syndrome and salicylate use.

Neuropathic Pain

Early recognition and aggressive therapy improve the prognosis for the resolution of neuropathic pain. Although some patients report relief using NSAIDs and other nonopioid analgesics, neuropathic pain is less responsive to opioids than nociceptive pain[29,44] or may require dose escalation leading to unacceptable side effects. Anticonvulsants are the mainstay in the treatment of neuropathic pain.[45] Gabapentin (Neurontin) is preferred due to its low side effect profile and no known drug interactions. The initial and maximal dosages are outlined in Table 41–6[2,26-28,44,46] and the clinician can gradually increase the dosage to minimize the side effects. However, it is only available in tablets or capsules. Those can be crushed and prepared in an elixir form too. Other anticonvulsants such as phenytoin (Dilantin) or carbamazepine (Tegretol) are less desirable due to increased side effects and interactions with other medications commonly used in cancer treatment. If the neuropathic pain is not controlled with the maximum dose of gabapentin, addition of a tricyclic antidepressant such as amitriptyline (Elavil) at bedtime can be beneficial. The dose of amitriptyline can be increased every 3 to 5 days until the maximum dosage is reached. An electrocardiogram is recommended periodically during long-term use or if standard dosages are exceeded.[5]

Minimizing the side effects of both these types of medications is achieved best by starting lower initial dosages and doubling the dose every 3 to 5 days until pain relief or the maximum dose is reached. Patients need to be informed that it will take at least 3 days until analgesic effects may be noted. Neuropathic pain syndromes can also respond to sodium-channel blockers such as lidocaine IV or mexiletine PO, or to N-methyl-D-aspartate-receptor antagonists such as dextromethorphan or methadone, but limited data exist in the pediatric population.

Epidural Analgesia

Although initially described and used in adults, epidural analgesia has come into widespread application in the pediatric population especially for postoperative pain control for thoracic, abdominal, or orthopedic surgery of the lower extremities. Comparing this method with intermittent IV doses, epidural analgesia can provide overall comfort with lower pain scores, less muscle spasm, and improved tolerance to physical activity during the

TABLE 41–6 Neuropathic Pain Medications			
Medication	Initial Dose	Maximum Dose	Side Effects
Gabapentin (Neurontin)	5 mg/kg or 100–300 mg TID PO	70 mg/kg/d or 1200 mg TID	Dizziness, ataxia, somnolence, fatigue
Amitriptyline (Elavil)	0.1 mg/kg or 12.5 mg once a day at bedtime PO	1 mg/kg/d	Dizziness, somnolence, dry mouth, cardiac dysrhythmias

PO, per os; *TID*, three times daily.

initial postoperative period. The choice of agents used in the epidural space is similar to those used in adults—either an opioid alone or an opioid/local anesthetic combination (i.e., fentanyl and bupivacaine), which can provide excellent analgesia with less systemic sedation. The maximum recommended bupivacaine infusion rate is 0.4 mg/kg/hour[47] or for infants 0.2 mg/kg/hour.

Chronic Pain Syndromes

Literature relating to long-term pain management problems arising from cancer treatment in children is scant. Chronic pain syndromes include chronic abdominal pain of uncertain origin, complex regional pain syndrome type I, or pain related to steroid-induced avascular necrosis of various joints, neuropathic, and mechanical pain after bone tumor resection, and postherpetic neuralgia. Children may develop scoliosis or various musculoskeletal pain as a result of radiation or surgery to thoracic area. Some patients require chronic opioids or long-term adjuvant therapy for neuropathic pain syndromes such as those having phantom limb pain or neuropathy from chemotherapy associated with nerve damage (i.e., vincristine). Experts feel that chronic pain is best managed by a multidisciplinary team using multimodal interventions of analgesics, physical therapy, and behavioral-cognitive approaches.[5]

The tendency of a chronically ill child to have secondary gain from experiencing pain should not be regarded as an indication that the pain is not real. Nevertheless, it may be necessary to assist the patient and the family in determining limits and responsibilities even within the most functional of families. The responsibility of the individual child, adolescent, and parent as to their roles in the pain management plan is best spelled out in the form of a document signed by the patient and parent (when the patient is a minor). The use of such documents, frequently called "pain contracts," is rare in pediatric practice except for children with sickle cell disease. A therapeutic alliance is made by systematically outlining pain management options actively involving the patient and family. Also the document serves as an agreement on the part of the child or adolescent regarding the need for compliance with all aspects of the treatment plan, including the need to only take medications prescribed by this specialized group and other issues involving safe-keeping of the medications. The process of discussion around such a document can be more therapeutic than the actual signing of the paper as each party accepts their part in the plan to prevent the development of adversarial relationships. An example of such a document is shown in Figure 41–2. This is most important for an outpatient setting. This type of communication needs to include education regarding the medication dosing and schedule plan and the use of a pain diary providing a place to write in dosages for breakthrough pain.

Nonpharmacologic Therapy

Combining nonpharmacologic approaches with pharmacologic interventions optimizes the therapeutic plan. Analgesics attenuate nociceptive activity and are necessary for controlling children's pain, but nonpharmacologic methods are also necessary to mitigate the pain-exacerbating impact of cognitive, behavioral, and emotional factors. Specific nonpharmacologic interventions should be selected for children according to the type of pain, the child's age or cognitive level, and whether the intervention is focused on modifying the child's sensory perception, behaviors, or thoughts and coping abilities.[5]

Health professionals should select the most appropriate pain control interventions for a child from a myriad of physical and psychological interventions (see Table 41–7 for current recommendations).[48,49] The legitimacy for the effectiveness of psychologically based therapies used adjunctively for relieving most types of pain in children and adolescents is well documented. However, these interventions appear to work best in a clinical setting when introduced early in the course of illness as part of a multidisciplinary effort, as a means of giving the patient a sense of control, and "helping the pain medicines work better."

The choice of which nonpharmacologic pain management technique to use varies depending on the age and cognitive abilities of the child as well as previous experiences with such strategies. For example, infants can experience pain relief from sucking on a pacifier dipped in a sweet solution or from tactile stimulation such as rocking or stroking.[48] Preschoolers tend to do better with behavioral techniques that require less cognitive development such as visual distraction, blowing on a pinwheel, counting, or reciting nursery rhymes, while sitting on a trusted caregiver's lap. School-aged children and adolescents alike have fantastic imaginations and are often very able to tune out the environment around them, thereby making them excellent candidates for cognitive-behavioral techniques such as guided imagery, hypnosis, and systematic desensitization, while continuing to benefit from distraction and relaxation exercises.[19] For example, incorporation of sensory components into a combined hypnotherapy and guided imagery exercise during the povidone-iodine (Betadine) wash in preparation for a lumbar puncture, such as "Feel the cool water that the elephant has sprayed against your back" may be a useful way to reduce distress and further deepen the hypnotic state. Ideally nonpharmacologic techniques should be introduced by a skilled health care provider who, prior to the pain experience, empowers the

PAIN MANAGEMENT SERVICE

Your child has been referred to the Pain Management Service to help relieve his or her pain.

What is the Pain Management Service? The Pain Management Service includes doctors, nurses, psychologists, physical therapists, and pharmacists. This group will work with you, your child, and your primary doctor to help relieve your child's pain by having you come to the Pain Clinic when you are outpatient or coming to your room each day when you are inpatient.

The Pain Management Service may use one or several approaches to deal with pain. Pain medications are sometimes called analgesics. More than one analgesic at a time may be prescribed. However, you should not add an analgesic without first checking with a member of the Pain Management Services. The medicines prescribed may include:
- Opioids (narcotics),
- Anti-inflammatory medicines, and
- Medications to treat nerve pain.

Please refer to the Medication Cards for more information about the pain medicine that you are taking. As with all types of medicines, they can cause side effects. If these symptoms occur, notify the Pain Management Service so they can adjust the dosage, change to another medicine, or add another drug to lessen the side effects.

Psychosocial techniques can give you a sense of control over the pain. If recommended, you will be given detailed instructions about how to use these techniques. Some techniques frequently used include the following:
- Relaxation–to alleviate anxiety and reduce muscle tension,
- Distraction–to learn how to focus on something other than the pain,
- Guided imagery–to concentrate on images to relax,
- Play therapy–to provide an outlet for emotions and learn how to cope with pain.

Physical therapy techniques may help reduce the pain of a specific site. These techniques will also help keep you active, independent, and strong, If recommended, you will be given a detailed program of activities which may include the following:
- Exercises–to strengthen weak muscles, loosen stiff muscles, increase blood flow, or help with balance,
- Massage–to decrease swelling, help with relaxation or loosen scar tissue,
- Orthotics (braces)–to support painful or weak joints, immobilize an injury, stretch a tight muscle,
- Transcutaneous electrical nerve stimulation (TENS) unit–for certain types of pain such as neuropathic pain,
- Heat or cold therapy–to decrease swelling or inflammation, loosen tight muscles.

How can I help? To provide consistent and safe pain management, we expect you do the following:
- Follow all parts of the treatment plan developed by the Pain Management Service.
- Store medications safely.
- Take pain medications exactly as prescribed by the Pain Management Service.
- Notify the Pain Management Service immediately about any side effects.(See below for details on how to contact us.)
- Call the Pain Management Service if you feel that a change in the dose or timing of your medication is needed. Do not change your regimen without asking us.
- Keep all appointments with the Pain Management Service and be on time. If your visit will be delayed for a reason you cannot prevent, please call the Pain Management Service physician or clinical nurse specialist (901-495-3300) to see if it is in your best interest to delay your appointment time.
- Expect frequent re-evaluation of the pain problem. It is necessary to monitor the pain and make necessary adjustments in the treatment plan. Appointments will be at least once every two weeks. You may be asked to maintain telephone contact even more frequently.
- Expect to pick up your medications at the hospital. Only in extreme situations will we mail medications to your home. You will receive no more than a two-week supply of any mailed medications.
- Bring all bottles of medication that the Pain Management Service prescribes to each clinic appointment. This will enable us to give you refills.
- You might be asked to keep a written record of when additional medications are taken to help decrease the pain.
- Discuss any over-the-counter or complimentary medicine with the Pain Management Service before using them.
- Remember, as long as the Pain Management Service is prescribing pain medications, no other health care provider should be writing orders for refills or changing your pain medication plan. No changes should be made such as changing the dose of the pain medicines or adding any new pain medicines unless a member of the Pain Management Services is contacted.
- When it is no longer necessary for your child to be followed by the Pain Management, we will tell you and your primary St. Jude doctor will then manage any pain he may have.

Be sure to ask questions related to our recommendations. It is important that you understand the plan. Call the Pain Management Service physician or clinical nurse specialist for any questions or concerns. During normal business hours, call 901-495-4032 and the secretary will contact a member of the Pain Management Service to return your call as soon as possible. During other hours, call 901-495-3300 and ask the operator to page the Pain Management Service physician on-call. Please remain on the telephone line until the physician connects with the call.

Please sign here to indicate you have received the information:

_____   _____   _____
Patient   Parent (if the patient is a minor)   Date

_____
Pain Management Service Member

FIGURE 41–2   Example of a pain management service agreement. *(Copyright St. Jude Children's Research Hospital, October 2002.)*

TABLE 41–7 Nonpharmacologic Approaches to Pain Management

Physical Comfort Measures	Behavioral Techniques
Massage	Relaxation
Heat and cold	Biofeedback
Rocking	Modeling
Pacifier	Desensitization
Acupuncture	Art and play therapy
Transcutaneous nerve stimulators (TENS)	Controlled breathing/ blowing bubbles
Other	**Cognitive Techniques**
Music therapy	Distraction
Meditation and prayer	Guided imagery
	Thought stopping
	Hypnosis

self-talk such as "I'm as strong as Superman; I have had this done before; I know what to do during an IV stick." Positive reinforcement either verbally or with tangible rewards such as stickers are a very important component encouraging future positive behaviors, even if the child experienced difficulties or distress. Uncooperative behaviors should not be punished, and the child should never be threatened or made to feel ashamed of being unable to cooperate due to anxiety or distress. Most importantly, by stressing these techniques as necessary life skills for the child or adolescent to learn, clinicians are providing tools for their patients to use for other medical issues such as nausea, vomitting, and sleep difficulties as well as with everyday distress.

child to employ these skills, while encouraging the parents to act as a coach. Distraction as a means of diverting attention onto something other than the painful stimulus, such as listening to music or a tape of the parents' voices, looking at favorite books or videos, playing video games, or playing with a favorite toy is potentially effective for short procedural pain.

Cognitive-behavioral techniques focus on improving the child's ability to cope with the pain as well as actually decreasing the level of distress that the child experiences in both acute and chronic pain. Another psychological intervention is to encourage the child to pretend to be or to align with a powerful character on television or in a book (i.e., super hero or a positive role model). This diffuses feelings of powerlessness and promotes positive

Implications for Practice

Health care professionals providing care for infants, children, and adolescents with cancer are to systematically assess pain and use both pharmacologic and nonpharmacologic interventions to manage pain. Their role in providing patients and families with factual information about pain and analgesics is an extremely important intervention directed toward breaking down the many barriers to effective pain management. As the outcome of cancer treatment becomes such that cure is more and more possible, clinicians have the fundamental obligation to manage pain and relieve patient suffering as a crucial element of their professional commitment to patient care using the principles outlined in Table 41–8. These are not merely lofty ideals; effective pain management produces a myriad of patient benefits including reduced morbidity and mortality.

TABLE 41–8 Guiding Principles of Pain Management in Children with Cancer

Pain in children is a serious problem and one that is inadequately evaluated and treated.
Children's pain can and should be assessed.
Drug therapy, particularly the use of opioids to alleviate severe pain, is the mainstay of treatment.
Physical, cognitive, behavioral, and supportive therapies should be used to complement drug therapy.
Optimal pain management requires a comprehensive approach to the child to control all the factors that intensify pain and suffering.

REFERENCES

1. Collins JJ, Byrnes ME, Dunkel IJ, et al: The measurement of symptoms in children with cancer. J Pain Symptom Manage 19:363–377, 2000.
2. World Health Organization: Cancer Pain Relief and Palliative Care in Children. Geneva, World Health Organization, 1998.
3. Wolfe J, Grier HE, Klar N: Symptoms and suffering at the end of life in children cancer. New Engl J Med 342:326–333, 2000.

4. Stuber ML: Post-trauma symptoms in childhood leukemia survivors and their parents. Psychosomatics 37:254–261, 1996.
5. Collins JJ, Weisman SJ: Management of pain in childhood cancer. In Schechter NL, Berde CB, Yaster M (eds): Pain in Infants, Children, and Adolescents, 2nd ed. Philadelphia, Lippincott Williams & Wilkins, 2003, pp 517–538.

6. Anand KJS: Relationships between stress responses and clinical outcome in newborns, infants, and children. Crit Care Med 21: S358, 1993.
7. Perreault T, Askin DF, Liston R, et al: Pain in the neonate. Paediatr Child Health 2: 201–208, 1997.
8. Goldschneider KR, Anand KJS: Long-term consequences of pain in neonates. In Schechter NL, Berde CB,

Yaster M (eds): Pain in Infants, Children, and Adolescents, 2nd ed. Philadelphia, Lippincott Williams & Wilkins, 2003, pp 58–70.

9. Anand KJS, Barton BA, McIntosh N, et al: Analgesia and sedation in preterm neonates who require ventilatory support: Results from NOPAIN trial. Arch Pediatr Adolesc Med 153:331–338, 1999.

10. Taddio A, Katz J, Illersich AL, et al: Effect of neonatal circumcision on pain response during subsequent routine vaccination. Lancet 349:599–603, 1997.

11. Fitzgerald M, Beggs S: The neurobiology of pain: Developmental aspects. The Neuroscientist 7:246–257, 2001.

12. American Academy of Pediatrics: The assessment and management of acute pain in infants, children, and adolescents. Pediatrics 108:793–797, 2001.

13. Anand KJS, Gruneau R, Oberlander TF: Developmental character and long-term consequences of pain in infants and children. Child Adoles Psychia Clin North Am 6:703–725, 1997.

14. Johnston CC, Stevens BJ: Experience in a neonatal intensive care unit affects pain response. Pediatrics 98:925–930, 1996.

15. Wong DL, Hockenberry-Eaton M, Winkelstein ML: Whaley and Wong's Nursing Care of Infants and Children, 6th ed. St Louis, Mosby, 1999, p 2040.

16. Zonneveld L, McGrath PJ, Reid G, et al: Accuracy of children's pain memories. Pain 71:297–302, 1997.

17. Ornstein PA, Manning EL, Pelphrey KA: Children's memory of pain. J Dev Behav Pediatr 20:262–277, 1999.

18. Compton P, McCaffery P: Substance abuse. Pain: Clinical Manual, 2nd ed. St. Louis, Mosby, 1999, pp 450–462.

19. Berde C, Masak B: Pain in children. In Wall PD, Melzack R (eds): Textbook of Pain, 4th ed. Edinburgh, Churchill Livingstone, 1999, pp 1463–1477.

20. Berde CB, Sethna NF: Analgesics for the treatment of pain in children. NEJM 347:1094–1103, 2002.

21. Merkel S, Voepel-Lewis T, Shayevitz JR, et al: The FLACC: A behavioral scale for scoring postoperative pain in young children. Pediatr Nurs 23:293–297, 1997.

22. Manworren RC, Hynan LS: Clinical validation of FLACC: Preverbal patient pain scale. Pediatr Nurs 29:140–146, 2003.

23. McGrath PJ, Unruh AM: Measurement and assessment of pediatric pain. In Wall PD, Melzack R (eds): Textbook of Pain, 4th ed. Edinburgh, Churchill Livingstone, 1999, pp 371–383.

24. Yaster, M: Clinical pharmacology. In Schechter NL, Berde CB, Yaster M (eds): Pain in Infants, Children, and Adolescents, 2nd ed. Philadelphia, Lippincott Williams & Wilkins, 2003, pp 71–83.

25. Collins JJ, Grier HE, Kinney HC, et al: Control of severe pain in children with terminal malignancy. J Pediatr 126: 653–657, 1995.

26. Anghelescu D, Oakes L: Working toward better cancer pain management for children. Canc Prac 10(Suppl):S52–S57, 2002.

27. Oakes LO: Caring practices: providing comfort. In Curley MAQ, Molony-Harmon PA (eds): Critical Care Nursing of Infants and Children, 2nd ed. Philadelphia, WB Saunders, 2001, pp 547–576.

28. Oakes LL: Assessment and management of pain in the critically ill pediatric patient. Crit Care Nurs Clin North Am 13:281–295, 2001.

29. Zuckerman LA, Ferrante FM: Nonopioid and opioid analgesics. In Portenoy RK, Kanner RM (eds): Pain Management Theory and Practice. Philadelphia, FA Davis, 1996, pp 111–140.

30. Yaster M, Kost-Byerly S, Maxwell LG: Opioid agonists and antagonists. In Schechter NL, Berde CB, Yaster M (eds): Pain in Infants, Children, and Adolescents, 2nd ed. Philadelphia, Lippincott Williams & Wilkins, 2003, pp 181–224.

31. Feld LH, Champeau MW, van Steenis CA, et al: Preanesthetic medication in children: a comparison of oral transmucosal fentanyl citrate versus placebo. Anesthesiology 71:374–377, 1989.

32. Schechter NL, Weisman SJ, Rosenblum M, et al: The use of oral transmucosal fentanyl citrate for painful procedures in children. Pediatrics 95:335–339, 1995.

33. Portenoy RK, Payne R, Coluzzi P, et al: Oral transmucosal fentanyl citrate (OTFC) for the treatment of breakthrough pain in cancer patients: A controlled dose titration study. Pain 79:303–312, 1999.

34. Gardner NJ: Oral transmucosal fentanyl and sufentanil for incident pain. J Pain Symptom Manage 22:627–630, 2001.

35. Golianu B, Krane EJ, Galloway KS, et al: Pediatric acute pain management. Pediatr Clin North Am 47:559–587, 2000.

36. Chambliss CR, Anand KJS: Pain management in the pediatric intensive care unit. Curr Opin Pediatr 9:246–253, 1997.

37. Lehr VT, BeVier P: Patient-controlled analgesia for the pediatric patient. Orthopaedic Nurs 22:298–305, 2003.

38. Berde CB, Solodiuk J: Multidisciplinary programs for management of acute and chronic pain in children. In Schechter NL, Berde CB, Yaster M (eds): Pain in Infants, Children, and Adolescents, 2nd ed. Philadelphia, Lippincott Williams & Wilkins, 2003, pp 471–486.

39. Monitto CL, Greenberg RS, Kost-Byerly S, et al: The safety and efficacy of parent-/nurse-controlled analgesia in patients less than 6 years of age. Anesth Analg 91:573–579, 2000.

40. Anand KJS, Arnold JH: Opioid tolerance and dependence in infants and children. Crit Care Med 22:334–342, 1994.

41. Anand KJS, Ingraham J: Tolerance, dependence, and strategies for compassionate withdrawal of analgesics and anxiolytics in the pediatric ICU. Crit Care Nurse 16:87–93, 1996.

42. Maunuksela EL, Olkkola KT: Nonsteroidal anti-inflammatory drugs in pediatric pain management. In Schechter NL, Berde CB, Yaster M (eds): Pain in Infants, Children, and Adolescents, 2nd ed. Philadelphia, Lippincott Williams & Wilkins, 2003, pp 171–180.

43. Litalien C, Jacqz-Aigrain E: Risks and benefits of nonsteroidal anti-inflammatory drugs in children. Paediatr Drugs 3: 817–858, 2001.

44. Dellemijn P: Are opioids effective in relieving neuropathic pain? Pain 80: 453–462, 1998.

45. Backonja MM: Use of anticonvulsants for treatment of neuropathic pain. Neurology 59(suppl 2):S14–S17, 2002.

46. Krane EJ, Leong MS, Colianu B, et al: Treatment of pediatric pain with nonconventional analgesics. In Schechter NL, Berde CB, Yaster M (eds): Pain in Infants, Children, and Adolescents, 2nd ed. Philadelphia, Lippincott Williams & Wilkins, 2003, pp 225–240.

47. Macfadyen AJ, Buckmaster MA: Pain management in the pediatric intensive care unit. Crit Care Clin 15:185–200, 1999.

48. Akman I, Ozek E, Bilgen H, Ozdogan T, et al: Sweet solutions and pacifiers for pain relief in newborn infants. J Pain 3:199–202, 2002.

49. Turk DC, Gatchel RJ: Psychological Approaches to Pain Management, 2nd ed. New York, The Guilford Press, 2002.

50. Wong DL, Hess CS: Wong and Whaley's Clinical Manual of Pediatric Nursing, 5th ed. St Louis, Mosby, 2000, p 326.

CHAPTER 42

Management of Procedure-Related Pain in Children

P. De Negri, G. Ivani, F. Tonetti, T. Tirri, P. Modano, and C. Reato

Alleviating pain and anxiety in children is a key component of pediatric care. There is an increasing focus on the recognition, assessment, and management of pain in children of all ages.[1] Barriers to effective pain treatment in children depend on different misconceptions: (1) The myth that children and particularly infants do not feel pain as adults do; we know that children's experience of pain depends on their stage of development, and in the number and types of procedures they perceive as painful and/or frightening[2]; (2) lack of pain assessment and reassessment; it is essential to evaluate children's response to treatment; (3) lack of knowledge of pain management; (4) the concept that pain evaluation in children is time-consuming; and (5) fears of addiction or adverse effects of commonly used drugs.

Children undergo many painful procedures in different clinical environments and are frequently undertreated for their pain.[1] A recent German survey on pain control for pediatric oncology patients showed that according to 17% of physician and 41% of nurses "very often" inadequate pain control still exists. Procedures are the main causes of pain and in 80% of departments a therapy protocol is lacking.[3] Owing to recent emphasis on the benefits of pain management, parents and health care providers expect infants and children to receive safe, effective analgesic treatment for diagnostic and therapeutic procedures.[4] In fact, adequate pain control and sedation ensure the comfort and cooperation of the child, influence the success of the procedure, and affect the child's future attitudes about doctors and medical care.[4,5] Pain experienced by children affected by oncohematologic diseases can be: cancer-related (bone pain, invasion or compression of the central or peripheral nervous system), procedure-related (bone marrow aspiration, lumbar puncture, venous cannulation, sutures and suture removal, etc.), or other therapy-related (mucositis, neuropathy, dermatitis, or skin necrosis due to irradiation or drug extravasation) (Figure 42–1).

Pain during treatment procedures is often identified at the most distressing aspect of the entire cancer experience for a child with cancer, because it characterizes most of the diagnostic and long-term therapeutic procedures.[6] Children's psycho-emotional processing during illness has been recently recognized and characterized by loss of control, anger, and fear, to which pain adds fear of death jeopardizing the sense of survival. Illness and pain provoke a traumatic condition affecting psycho-emotional maturation. The aim of the pharmacologic and nonpharmacologic support is to help children better cope with pain and prevent the healed child from having traumatic effects on his or her future personality structure and behavior (Figure 42–2). To assure the best pain control, support has to be offered right from the first intrusive procedure to avoid anticipatory anxiety,[7] as intense pain has been observed at the beginning of treatment when it is often believed that pain could be better managed. Sometimes pain evaluations had been not often performed and parents considered themselves better judges of their child's pain than professionals.[8]

Currently, managing children undergoing invasive procedures can include the use of sedatives, analgesics, anesthetics, and nonpharmacologic strategies. The goals of therapeutic efficacy and safety must be balanced in all patients.

The use of pharmacologic or psychologic interventions or a combination of the two techniques is strictly determined by the level of anxiety. Pharmacologic and psychologic interventions for procedural distress effectively reduce child and parent distress, and various data support integration of the two approaches. Younger children experienced more distress and warranted additional consideration.[9] Cognitive protocols are effective in relieving procedural distress for a significant number of children, whereas pharmacologic therapies were found to be relatively safe and effective when carefully administered and monitored by medical personnel.[10]

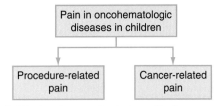

FIGURE 42–1 Causes of pain in pediatric cancer patients.

NONPHARMACOLOGIC INTERVENTIONS

Nonpharmacologic interventions include various physical, cognitive, and behavioral techniques expected to decrease distress and pain through modulation of children's behavior and can be used alone or together with pharmacologic intervention. Cognitive-behavioral therapy has not been applied to very young children (younger than 3 to 7 years) and the severely developmentally delayed. Cognitive-behavioral treatment includes breathing exercises; preparation (to give information about what will be done or what it may feel like, to familiarize with the hospital or medical personnel); relaxation (by biofeedback or progressive relaxation); distraction (the goal is to focus the child's attention away from procedure, e.g., using hypnosis, focusing attention on objects in the room, or joke telling); imagery actively coached by psychologist, parents, or medical staff[11]; and positive reinforcement involving encouragement during the procedure and a tangible reward immediately following the procedure. Some interventions such as providing information before any procedure or positive support after procedure are used more frequently than other techniques such as breathing, distraction, imagery that require more time and training.[12] Clinical hypnosis intervention is able to reduce pain and anxiety in pediatric cancer patients, whereas benefit degraded if patients were switched to self-hypnosis.[13] Nurses play an important role in helping children cope with the stress of the procedure, while anxious parents further contribute to their children's distress.[14] Children experiencing pain prefer the supportive presence of their parents, so nurses might assist and help reduce distress and worry for parents who want to support their children during a painful experience, instead of asking them to "wait outside" until the end of procedure.[15,16] In other studies parents participated in the care of hospitalized children, helping them to cope with emotional support and daily activities, whereas cognitive, behavioral, and physical methods were seldom used.[17] Even young children are able to perceive parents' distress and anxiety, which will increase particularly when the procedure is diagnostic. For this reason it is important to understand the relationship between parents and children and their ability to enhance or interfere with the children's ability to cope. A randomized controlled study involving children with leukemia undergoing lumbar punctures or bone marrow aspiration showed that nonpharmacologic interventions were more effective than pharmacologic interventions in reducing children's distress.[14] Also hypnosis resulted in effectively reducing distress in oncologic children undergoing bone marrow aspiration.[18]

PHARMACOLOGIC INTERVENTIONS

The presence of anxiety and/or pain helps in deciding whether to use a sedative alone, or a regimen also providing analgesia.[19] Any intervention for reduction of pain/anxiety associated with invasive procedures should be based on the age, the developmental level of the child, the type of procedure, the medical status, and the context in which procedure takes place. Maximal accuracy must be taken during the first procedure in order to not allow the development of anticipatory anxiety; in fact

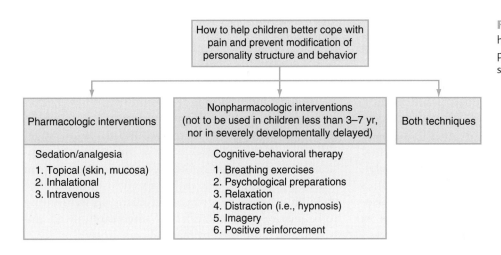

FIGURE 42–2 Options for helping children cope with pain and preventing modification of personality structure and behavior.

inadequate analgesia for initial procedures in young children may diminish the effect of adequate analgesia in subsequent procedures.[20] We still do not know the short- or long-term sequelae of pain experienced by children.

Given the increase in invasive, diagnostic, radiologic, and minor surgical procedures that are performed, the elective and emergency need of analgesia/sedation in the pediatric population has expanded.[21] The safety of the child is, therefore, dependent on the skills of the physician, the venue of sedation, the availability of adequately skilled assistance, the use of appropriate physiologic monitoring, and proper recovery and discharge criteria established for that particular institution or practice.[22]

The first guidelines for sedation were developed in close consultations with the American Academy of Pediatric Dentistry (AAPD) and approved by the American Academy of Pediatrics (AAP). It has used three terms to describe the depth of pharmacologic control: conscious sedation, deep sedation, and general anesthesia.[23] The guidelines also emphasized system issues, including the need for informed consent, appropriate fasting before sedation, frequent measurement and charting of vital signs, the availability of age- and size-appropriate equipment, the use of physiologic support, the need for basic life support skills, and proper recovery and discharge procedures. Unfortunately, the oxymoron "conscious sedation" has resulted in great confusion and allowed practices that were not intended by the original guideline. In 2000, the Joint Commission on Accreditation of Healthcare Organizations (JCAHO) provided definitions for four levels of sedation: minimal sedation analgesia, moderate sedation analgesia, deep sedation analgesia, and general anesthesia. These terms are formally different, but they always refer to the original terms defined by the AAP.[24] The AAP guidelines recognize that the sedation of a patient represents a "continuum": regardless of the intended level of sedation or route of administration, a child may easily move from a light to a deep level of sedation, that may result in loss of the patient's protective reflexes, and are associated with serious risks such as hypoventilation, apnea, airway obstruction, and cardiopulmonary impairment. It means that sedation has to be performed by skilled personnel.

Patients requiring sedation/analgesia for a procedure should undergo a preliminary evaluation, including a review of their clinical history and their physical examination, in order to quantify their procedural risk.[25] Continuous monitoring of respiratory and cardiac function before, during, and after the procedure is critical. Close monitoring insures that any changes in the level of sedation will be detected immediately so that appropriate measures can be undertaken immediately. The on-site equipment to provide continuous monitoring must be age- and size-appropriate for the child being treated.

This equipment should include a pulse oximeter to monitor oxygen saturation, a sphygmomanometer or automated pressure device to monitor circulation, and a stethoscope. Also, electrocardiogram monitoring should be readily available.[25] It is necessary also to include a source of oxygen and a method of administration (nasal cannulae, masks of various sizes), adequate suction (various sized suction catheters), a self-inflating resuscitation bag, a selection of appropriate sized endotracheal (ET) tubes, functioning laryngoscopes and blades, emergency drugs (e.g., atropine, succinylcholine, naloxone, epinephrine, calcium chloride, sodium bicarbonate, cardiac lidocaine), intravenous administration sets and fluids, and a selection of intravenous catheters.

It is crucial to choose the appropriate drugs, doses, and route of administration. Ideally, agents prescribed for pediatric pain management and sedation should produce temporary amnesia, have a rapid onset, short duration of action (for the exact time necessary), multiple options for administration, minimal side effects (e.g., cardiorespiratory), lack of drug–drug interactions, wide therapeutic index, and an available reversal agent.[26]

Selection of a sedative or analgesic must be individualized to meet the patient's particular needs, and no agent or class of agents can be expected to be effective in every patient. The appropriate agent and dose will vary according to the patient and the procedure. Thus, familiarity with different agents and the ability to switch from one to another, in the event of ineffectiveness or adverse effects, is important. When more than one drug or drug class is used, the initial dose of each must be reduced, and the individual patient response may vary. Ineffective or unsafe sedation is clearly tied to inappropriate dosing.

Because the route of administration profoundly affects the ability to control the drug's onset of clinical effect and duration of action, it is an important to consider to avoid undesirable side effects. The following routes of administration are used in pediatric sedation and analgesia:

- Transmucosal (oral, nasal, rectal): Easy to administer but provides less control over the drug's effects; may delay onset and prolong clinical effect in highly lipophilic and aqueous-based agents, for example, certain opioids and benzodiazepines; drugs given via nasal or rectal administration are absorbed more reliably than those given orally.
- Inhalational: Easy to administer but needs specific equipment; provides a satisfactory control on drug's effect that can be also titrated to effect; after the induction, it is easier to obtain an IV access.
- Intravenous: Offers the fastest onset of effect and most reliable delivery of specific degrees of sedation or analgesia (it may be painful to establish IV access in children).[27,28]

- Intramuscular: Offers more complete drug delivery than transmucosal administration, but delivery is painful and less reliable than IV administration.
- Topical application of local anesthetics include EMLA cream (eutectic mixture of lidocaine-prilocaine), Ametop (amethocaine 4% gel), TAC (tetracaine-adrenaline-cocaine), LET (lidocaine-epinephrine-tetracaine), ELA-Max (4% lidocaine cream).

EMLA application substantially reduces pain caused by venous, subcutaneous drug reservoir, and lumbar punctures in children and may therefore be offered to young patients, particularly those repeatedly submitted to such procedures.[29] The topical application of EMLA cream provides highly effective superficial anesthesia,[30] and is extremely useful for pain relief and in reducing children's distress associated with IV insertion.[31] It is highly recommended for every procedure including a needle insertion (e.g., lumbar puncture, bone marrow aspiration); it has to be topically applied at least 60 minutes before performing the procedure and can be applied either by clinicians or even by parents.[32] In fact it has been demonstrated that parent application appears to be as effective as clinician's and also may result in less anticipatory anxiety for younger children.[33] Amethocaine produces similar anesthesia to lidocaine-prilocaine during Port-a-Cath administration in children, with an application time that is half of lidocaine-prilocaine. Nurses perceived that pain was greater for younger children and in males.[34] Lidocaine-prilocaine and tetracaine appear to be comparable for procedural pain relief when used as recommended in children for four different procedures: intravenous cannulation, venipuncture, Port-a-Cath puncture, and laser therapy. Tetracaine resulted more efficacious than lidocaine-prilocaine when both anesthetics were applied for the same amount of time.[35]

Generally, the following classes of agents (alone or in combination) are used in pediatric sedation and analgesia; within each class, agents differ in their duration of action and in their potential for side effects when used alone or in combination with other agents or classes.

Sedatives/hypnotics such as midazolam and propofol resulted extremely useful for patients undergoing non-painful but anxiety-provoking diagnostic or therapeutic procedures, providing varying degrees of amnesia. They are also often used successfully in association with analgesic agents to induce sedation or anesthesia. Intravenous agents such as morphine, fentanyl, remifentanil, and ketamine provide analgesia but not amnesia; when administered with sedatives they are able to offer greater relief from pain and anxiety, but also increase the potential for adverse effects, for example, respiratory arrest or impairment of cardiovascular stability. Midazolam, alone or in combination with morphine or fentanyl, has been first studied for conscious sedation in multiple bone marrow aspirations or biopsies and lumbar punctures.[36] Fentanyl and midazolam have been used as premedication for painful procedures in children with cancer. With proper monitoring they have been used safely in the outpatient clinic setting; midazolam was found to be the drug of preference for the majority of patients.[37]

When bone marrow aspiration or biopsy, lumbar puncture, or combined procedures were performed in a pediatric hematology-oncology clinic a premedication regimen of atropine 0.01 mg/kg, midazolam 0.05 mg/kg, and ketamine 1.5 mg/kg produced superior sedation with a faster onset and recovery and fewer side effects than a meperidine 2 mg/kg and midazolam 0.1 mg/kg combination.[38] The safety and efficacy of an association of midazolam 25 µg/kg and ketamine 0.5 to 2 mg/kg to control pain induced by diagnostic procedures has been evaluated in pediatric oncology patients; midazolam-ketamine association resulted in safely and effectively inducing an efficient brief unconscious sedation with analgesia.[39] The use of midazolam hydrochloride, 0.05 mg/kg, and remifentanil hydrochloride, 1 µg/kg, followed by a remifentanil infusion at 0.1 µg/kg/minute during brief, painful procedures resulted in rapid times to discharge but was complicated by a high incidence of life-threatening respiratory depression.[40] Midazolam, administered as nasal spray, offered relief to children anxious about procedures, such as insertion of a needle in a subcutaneously implanted intravenous port, venous blood sampling, and venous cannulation. Its use, however, may be limited by nasal discomfort in some patients for whom rectal and oral routes might be alternatives.[41] Four propofol-based intravenous regimens (propofol only, propofol plus fentanyl, propofol plus midazolam, or propofol + fentanyl and midazolam) have been administered in order to perform painful procedures in children with cancer. Patients receiving the combination of propofol + fentanyl and midazolam received the least amount of propofol and required the least time to recover. There were no life-threatening complications. Propofol-based anesthesia, when administered by an anesthesiologist had safe and effective results.[42] Children with cancer undergoing bone marrow aspirations and lumbar punctures received a propofol/fentanyl general anesthesia; they experienced significantly less procedure-related pain and distress than did those receiving either EMLA or oral midazolam/EMLA.[43] Propofol anesthesia was effective in optimizing conditions for elective oncology procedures in children, offering adequate comfort and amnesia; it could be safe to use for these procedures in PICU settings as transient hypotension and respiratory depression can sometimes occur.[44] Oral transmucosal fentanyl (OTFC) has been tested for providing analgesia and sedation in children undergoing painful diagnostic procedures; vomiting and itching were frequently observed, but no clinically significant vital sign alterations occurred. OTFC resulted safe and effective in order to relieve pain, but frequency of vomiting may restrict its clinical usefulness.[45] Inhalational agents such as sevoflurane or nitrous oxide are widely used with optimal results. An equimolecular mixture of oxygen and nitrous oxide resulted effective in providing analgesia in a great variety of procedures, such as lumbar puncture and bone marrow aspirations in oncologic patients. Even if the analgesia obtained was satisfactory, this mixture was not effective in all patients, and the best results have been observed in children 3 years old and older. The use of gas mixture seems very safe as no adverse effects have been noted.[46] Nitrous oxide inhalation at concentration of 50% to 70% has been shown its efficacy in alleviating distress during pain-related procedures in children over 6 years old, with minimal side effects and fast recovery time.[47] General anesthesia with sevoflurane, nitrous oxide, and oxygen, when administered for painful procedures in children with neoplastic diseases, was associated with low levels of pain and distress if compared with sedation with midazolam.[48] The outcomes for Conscious Sedation and General Anesthesia for lumbar puncture were similar. Most preferred conscious sedation to general anesthesia also because lumbar puncture in conscious sedation is able to save time and medical resources.[49]

Local anesthetics, when used, are mainly administered through infiltration; they must be given in age-appropriated doses in order to avoid potential cardiac and neurologic toxicity. They can potentiate sedative effects when used with sedatives or narcotics and maximum safe dose should be calculated prior to administration.[2,5]

Psychologic and pharmacologic interventions for pain-related procedure in children are both effective in reducing child and parent distress and there is evidence that support the integration of two approaches.

REFERENCES

1. Liebelt EL: Reducing pain during procedures. Curr Opin Pediatr 8:436–441, 1996.
2. Schechter NL, Berde CB, et al: Pain in Infants, Children and Adolescents. Baltimore, Williams & Wilkins, 1993.
3. Zernikow B, Bauer AB, Andler W: Pain control in German pediatric oncology. An inventory. Schmerz 16:140–149, 2002.
4. Algren JT, Algren Cl: Sedation and analgesia for minor pediatric procedures. Pediatr Emerg Care 12:435–441, 1996.
5. McGrath PA: Pain in Children: Nature, Assessment & Treatment. New York, The Guilford Press, 1990.
6. Macpherson CF, Lundblad LA: Conscious sedation of pediatric oncology patients for painful procedures: Development and implementation of a clinical practice protocol. J Pediatr Oncol Nurs 14:33–42, 1997.
7. Astuto M, Favara-Scacco C, et al: Pain control during dagnostic and/or therapeutic procedures in children. Minerva Anestesiol 68:695–703, 2002.
8. Ljungman G, Gordh T, Sorenesen S, et al: Pain variations during cancer treatment in children: A descriptive survey. Pediatr Hematol Oncol 17:211–221, 2000.
9. McCarthy AM, Cool VA, Petersen M, et al: Cognitive behavioural pain and anxiety interventions in pediatric oncology centers and bone marrow transplant units. Pediatr Oncol Nurs 13:3–12, 1996.
10. Cohen LL, Bernard RS, Greco LA, et al: A child focused intervention for coping with procedural pain: Are parent and nurse coaches necessary? J Pediatr Psychol 27:749–757, 2002.
11. Powers SW: Empirically supported treatments in pediatric psychology: Procedure related pain. J Pediatr Psychol 24:131–145, 1999.
12. McCarthy AM, Cool VA, Petersen M, et al: Cognitive behavioural pain and anxiety interventions in pediatric oncology centers

and bone marrow transplant units. Pediatr Oncol Nurs 13:3–12, 1996.
13. Liossi C, Hatira P: Clinical hypnosis in the alleviation of procedure related pain in pediatric oncology patients. Int J Clin Exp Hypn 51:4–28, 2003.
14. Cohen LL, Bernard RS, Greco LA, et al: A child focused intervention for coping with procedural pain: Are parent and nurse coaches necessary? J Pediatr Psychol 27:749–757, 2002.
15. Broome ME: Helping parents support their child in pain. Pediatr Nurs 26:315–317, 2000.
16. Committee on Psychosocial Aspects of Child and Family Health: The assessment and management of acute pain in infants, children and adolescents. Pediatrics 108:793–797, 2001.
17. Polkki T, Vehvilainen-Julkunen K, Pietila AM: Parents' roles in using non-pharmacological methods in their child's postoperative pain alleviation. J Clin Nurs 11:526–536, 2002.
18. Liossi C, Hatira P: Clinical hypnosis vs cognitive behavioural training for pain management with pediatric cancer patients undergoing bone marrow aspirations. J Clin Exp Hypn 47:104–116, 1999.
19. D'Agostino J, Terndrup TE: Comparative review of the adverse effects of sedatives used in children undergoing outpatient procedures. Drug Saf 14:146–157, 1996.
20. Weisman SJ, Bernstein B, Schechter NL: Consequences of inadequate analgesia during painful procedures in children. Arch Pediatr Adolesc Med 152:147–149, 1998.
21. Algren JT, Algren Cl: Sedation and analgesia for minor pediatric procedures. Pediatr Emerg Care 12:435–441, 1996.
22. Coté CJ: Pediatric sedation outside of the operating room. Problems in Anesthesia 13:468–480, 2002.

23. Guidelines for the elective use of conscious sedation, deep sedation, and general anesthesia in pediatric patients. Committee on Drugs. Section on Anesthesiology. Pediatrics 76:317–321, 1985.
24. Comprehensive Accreditation Manual for Hospitals. Oakbrook Terrace: Joint Commission on Accreditation of Healthcare Organizations, 2000.
25. Sedation Guidelines. In Smith JL (ed): The Hospital for Sick Children 1998 Formulary. Toronto: The Graphic Centre, HSC, 1998, pp 262–266.
26. Coté CJ: Sedation for the pediatric patient. Pediatr Clin North Am 41:31–58, 1994.
27. Ilkhanipour K, Juels CR, et al: Pediatric pain control and conscious sedation: A survey of emergency medicine residencies. Acad Emerg Med 1:368–372, 1994.
28. Tobias JD, Rasmussen GE: Pain management and sedation in the pediatric intensive care unit. Pediatr Clin North Am 41: 1269–1292, 1994.
29. Halperin DL, Koren G, Attias D, et al: Topical skin anesthesia for venous, subcutaneous drug reservoir and lumbar punctures in children. Pediatrics 84: 281–284, 1989.
30. Miser AW, Goh TS, Dose AM, et al: Trial of a topically administered local anesthetic (EMLA cream) for pain relief during central venous port accesses in children with cancer. J Pain Symptom Manage 9:259–264, 1994.
31. Koh JL, Fanurik D, et al: Efficacy of parental application of eutectic mixture of local anesthetics for intravenous insertion. Pediatrics 103:e79, 1999.
32. Bouffet E, Douard MC, et al: Pain in lumbar puncture: Results of a 2-year discussion at the French Society of Pediatric Oncology. Arch Pediatr 3:22–27, 1996.
33. Koh JL, Fanurik D, et al: Efficacy of parental application of eutectic mixture of local

anesthetics for intravenous insertion. Pediatrics 103:e79, 1999.

34. Bishai R, Taddio A, Bar-Oz B, et al: Relative efficacy of amethocaine gel and lidocaine-prilocaine cream for Port-a-Cath puncture in children. Pediatrics 104:e31, 1999.

35. Taddio A, Gurguis MG, Koren G: Lidocaine-prilocaine cream versus tetracaine gel for procedural pain in children. Ann Pharmacother 36:687–692, 2002.

36. Sievers TD, Yee JD, Foley ME, et al: Midazolam for conscious sedation during pediatric oncology procedures: Safety and recovery parameters. Pediatrics 88:1172–1179, 1991.

37. Sandler ES, Weyman C, Conner K, et al: Midazolam versus fentanyl as premedication for painful procedures in children with cancer. Pediatrics 89:631–634, 1992.

38. Marx CM, Stein J, Tyler MK, et al: Ketamine-midazolam versus meperidine-midazolam for painful procedures in pediatric oncology patients. J Clin Oncol 15:94–102, 1997.

39. Pellier I, Monrigal JP, Le Moine P, et al: Use of intravenous ketamine-midazolam association for pain procedures in children with cancer: A prospective study. Paediatr Anaesth 9:61–68, 1999.

40. Litman RS: Conscious sedation with remifentanil and midazolam during brief painful procedures in children. Arch Pediatr Adolesc Med 153:1085–1088.

41. Ljungman G, Kreuger A, Andreasson S: Midazolam nasal spray reduces procedural anxiety in children. Pediatrics 105:73–78, 2000.

42. Jayabose S, Levendoglu-Tugal O, Giamelli J, et al: Intravenous anesthesia with propofol for painful procedures in children with cancer. J Pediatr Hematol Oncol 23:290–293, 2001.

43. Holdsworth MT, Raisch DW, Winter SS, et al: Pain and distress from bone marrow aspirations and lumbar punctures. Ann Pharmacother 37:17–22, 2003.

44. Hertzog JH, Dalton JH, Anderson BD, et al: Prospective evaluation of propofol anesthesia in the pediatric intensive care unit for elective oncology procedures in ambulatory and hospitalized children. Pediatrics 106:742–747, 2000.

45. Schechter NL, Weisman SJ, Rosenblum M, et al: The use of oral transmucosal fentanyl citrate for painful procedures in children. Pediatrics 95:335–339, 1995.

46. Annequin D, Carbajal R, Chauvin P, et al: Fixed 50% nitrous oxide mixture for painful procedures: A French survey. Pediatrics 105:E47, 2000.

47. Kanagasundaram SA, Lane LJ, Cavalletto BP, et al: Efficacy and safety of nitrous oxide in alleviating pain and anxiety during painful procedures. Arch Dis Child 84:492–495, 2001.

48. Crock C, Olsson C, Phillips R, et al: General anesthesia or conscious sedation for painful procedures in childhood cancer: The family's perspective. Arch Dis Child 88:253–257, 2003.

49. Ljungman G, Gordh T, Sorensen S, et al: Lumbar puncture in pediatric oncology: Conscious sedation vs. general anesthesia. Med Pediatr Oncol 36:372–379, 2001.

CHAPTER 43

Forgotten Techniques in Cancer Pain Management

OSVALDO AUAD, MD

".... And I know that the spirit of God is the brother of my own, and that all the men ever born are
also my brothers, and the women my sisters and lovers, and that a kelson of the creation is love..."
"Not a cholera patient lies at the last gap but I also lie at the last gap..."
"Behold, I do not give lectures or a little charity, when I give I give myself."
Walt Whitman, *Leaves of Grass*

Memory and forgetfulness are implicit to all living beings and the societies they constitute. With regard to living beings, memory is being studied by the Laboratory for Neurobiology of Memory of the School of Exact and Natural Sciences of Buenos Aires University, which has presented important works on the subject.[1,2] Psychologist Daniel Schacter[3] described the following as causes of forgetfulness: fugacity, distraction, blockade, fake attribution, suggestibility, oblique memory, and persistence. Thinking of it as a collective phenomenon, it would be irreverent of this author to mention only bibliographic data since memory is also specific to anthropology and social psychology.

BECAUSE WE HAVE FORGOTTEN

This chapter does not intend to be an essay on social phenomena. However, since Argentina was, unfortunately, in the news not only in newspapers but also in major medical and scientific journals such as *The Lancet*,[4,5] I will draw a parallel to what happened there as a way to illustrate it as a consequence of forgetfulness in the society. It is very hard to understand how a country that had the potential to become one of the most developed countries in the world has fallen into such a deep abyss, and it is difficult to predict what the outcome will be.

Argentina has had three Nobel prize laureates in basic sciences: Bernardo Housay (1947), for his discovery of the relationship of the hypophysis with the diabetes and the hydrocarbon metabolism; Luis F. Leloir (1970), for his studies of the enzymes that act in the synthesis of polysaccharides; and Cesar Milstein (1984), for his discovery

of monoclonal antibodies. These Nobel prizes were the corollary of an educational model proposed by President Domingo Faustino Sarmiento (1868–1874), who postulated the need *"to educate the people because ignorance is a crime: citizens have to know what and who they choose."* Sarmiento worked very hard to achieve that objective, but it was only passed into law after his presidency was over in 1884. That law established that primary education should be compulsory, universal, and free. After 1945, the country saw the rise of a populist, authoritarian, demagogic, and messianic model, synthesized in one of its mottos: "canvas shoes yes, books no." The culminating moment that reflected those words was "the night of the long canes" in 1968, during which the police violently expelled professors and world-famous investigators, including foreign scientists, from the classrooms and laboratories of the University of Buenos Aires. The result of this model is that in Argentina—a country that consumes 60 kg of meat per year per person and which is the main producer and exporter of meat, soy, wheat, and dairy—there are children that die of malnutrition.[6] Jeffrey Sachs, one of the world's leading economists and globalization leaders, said in an interview with La Nación, a Buenos Aires daily: "The key is to invest in science and technology."[7] Mary Harney, Irish Minister of Commerce, recently stated: "There is a general consensus that we must create an economy based in knowledge." Ireland devotes 20% of its national budget to education.[8] Recently, the National Academy of Education in Argentina manifested the need to draw teaching out of stagnation (La Nación, September 4, 2003).

Argentine doctors and scientists have made important contributions to the fields of pain and palliative medicine.

In 1953, the Argentinian Federation of Associations of Anesthesia was a founding member of the World Federation of Societies of Anaesthesiologists. In 1974, the Argentinian Association for the Study of Pain was founded as the first Spanish-language branch of the International Association for the Study of Pain (IASP). In 1983, the Prager-Bild Foundation was formed as the first institution in Latin America dedicated to the study and practice of palliative care, following the hospice model developed by Cicely Saunders[9] at St. Christofer's Hospice of London. In 1991, the first hospital-based palliative care services in Latin America were established in two Buenos Aires hospitals: The National Hospital of Pediatrics (Dr. Juan T.Garrahan) and The Hospital of Oncology (Dr. Angel Roffo).

Several scientific contributions are worth highlighting. In 1946, renowned surgeons Drs. Enrique and Ricardo Finochietto published an 18-volume work on surgical techniques,[10] and in the section devoted to anesthesia, they described techniques that were new at the time, such as simultaneous spinal and general anesthesia, continuous spinal anesthesia (modified Lemmon technique), spinal anesthesia in nursing infants and children, thoracic epidural block for the control of postoperative pain, and caudal epidural block for surgery and treatment of pain (Figure 43–1). In 1976, Dr. Jorge R. Schvarcz described stereotactic extralemniscal myolotomy.[11] In 1977, Julio Parada reported on the use of ketamine in subanesthetic doses for the treatment of chronic pain at the XII National Congress of Anesthesia and Reanimation in San Sebastian, Spain.[12] In the early 1980s, this author published reports on treatment of oncologic pain with epidural morphine[13] and the use of epidural clonidine for the treatment of recurring pain. That was the first published work on clonidine use in humans.[14]

There are numerous reasons why a drug, technique, or procedure for relief of cancer pain may have become forgotten over time. They include:

- Very cheap drugs (e.g., intravenous alcohol for postoperative pain).[15]
- Lack of understanding of the working mechanism[16,17] of a clinically proven fact (e.g., ketamine use in subanesthetic doses for chronic pain).[12]
- Some techniques were evaluated and discredited in randomized, double-blind trials (e.g., radio frequency lesion of the dorsal root ganglion).[18]
- In some cases side effects or complications of therapy were worse than the original pathology (e.g., pain in the sensitive area following ethanol neurolysis of the Gasserian ganglion for trigeminal neuralgia[19]; mortality caused by intradural injections of hypertonic saline for cancer pain[20]).
- Interventional therapies were surpassed by the use of oral morphine.[21-23]

- Some techniques have not been published in English (e.g., lumbar epidural block and continuous thoracic block for postoperative pain).[10]
- The medical community decided to leave behind the last resort used by many oncologists and surgeons–the infamous "lythic cocktail"[24,25]—because it was considered a form of covert euthanasia. The lythic cocktail consisted of 50 mg of chlorpromazine, 100 mg of meperidine, and 50 mg of promethazine in a 500 mL solution, which was administered over 6 to 24 hours, until the patient's death. The cocktail was inappropriately and incorrectly used by its creators, with a goal of achieving "hibernation" in neuroplegia.
- Certain substances were declared illegal (e.g., LSD).

FORGOTTEN DRUGS, PROCEDURES, AND TECHNIQUES FOR CANCER PAIN MANAGEMENT

This section summarizes several drugs, techniques, and procedures for cancer pain relief that seem to have been forgotten for various reasons.

Forgotten Drugs

Of the numerous drugs used, we chose to mention the following because they have been—and still are—very useful in our daily practice.

Methotrimeprazine

Methotrimeprazine (or levomepromazine) is an antianemic, tranquilizer, and analgesic.[26] It is a strong tranquilizer that enhances the action of opioid and hypnotic drugs.[27] It is also a strong antihistaminic. It does not provoke euphoria. Patients seem, in a manner of speaking, to part from their pain.[28] This makes it hard to establish whether it is truly an analgesic or an excellent tranquilizer. Because there are problems of tolerance and addiction associated with this drug, it is ideally used in prostrated patients that suffer from pain. Dosing is similar to morphine.[29,30] We currently use this drug in combination with ramifentanil for prevention of opioid-induced nausea and vomiting and to achieve a smooth, sedated awakening.

Meprobamate

Meprobamate is a very useful drug with no known major side effects.[28] It is indicated in patients with reflex muscular spasms as an important part of the pain syndrome. It has very low, almost nonexistent, effect on the cerebral cortex, but inhibits certain thalamic areas. It is especially useful in combination with non-narcotic analgesics and NSAIDs for treatment of musculoskeletal pain. It tends to provoke a slight dependence in high doses and symptoms of withdrawal have been reported when its administration was abruptly interrupted. Nevertheless, it is one of the safest tranquilizers. The standard dose is 200 to 400 mg orally up to 6 times a day. A combination that has given very good results consists of 150 mg of meprobamate and 10 mg of piroxicam (capsules) complemented by 5 to 10 mg of prednisone per day.

Nerve Blocks

Albanese's Technique for Splanchnic and Celiac Plexus Block

Argentinian surgeon Albanese described this technique for splanchnic and celiac plexus block.[31] The splanchnic nerves are located below the diaphragm and in front of the pillars. The lumbar sympathetic chain, semilunar ganglion, and the suprarenal plexus are also located in this space. The advantage of this technique is that all these elements are blocked simultaneously. According to Albanese, the transverse apophysis of the first lumbar would be located at 5 to 6 cm deep, two or three fingers' inclination from the midline, and at three inclinations under the intersection, in the midline, from the prolongation of the axis of the 12th ribs. The bottom of the pleural sac usually reaches from the right the base of the transverse apophysis and from the left it surpasses the inferior edge of the 12th rib by one finger's inclination.

The major splanchnic nerve goes through the diaphragm a little above the plane of the first lumbar transverse apophysis. The minor splanchnic nerve and the lumbar sympathetic chain are located just behind and outside it. In the front and inward lie the semilunar ganglion and the solar plexus. Outward lies the suprarenal gland and its nervous plexus (Figure 43-2). With regard to the cutaneous dorsolumbar surface, the major splanchnic nerve is found approximately 8 to 10 cm deep and 3 to 4 cm from the midline.

The patient is positioned as if for a lumbar puncture. Upon touching the 12th ribs, the axis is extended until it crosses the midline (Figure 43-3). From this intersection, one measures three fingers' inclinations downward, and from there another three outward. At this point, an 8- to 12-cm needle (depending on the size of the patient) is inserted and propelled slightly up and inward until it forms a 10 to 20 degrees angle to the sagittal plane. The transverse apophysis of the first lumbar vertebra is reached at 5 to 6 cm deep. Whether the transverse apophysis is found or not, one continues ahead up to 8 to 10 cm depth of the area of the sympathetic elements. After it is ensured there is no bleeding, the local anesthetic or neurolytic agent is injected. If the tip of the needle touches the lateral face of the vertebral body, it should be moved 1 cm to the side. When the block is indicated, it should be performed bilaterally. We currently only perform the splanchnic block with the guidance of computed tomography.[32]

FIGURE 43–1 Schematic representation of the device for continued sacrococcygeal epidural anesthesia.

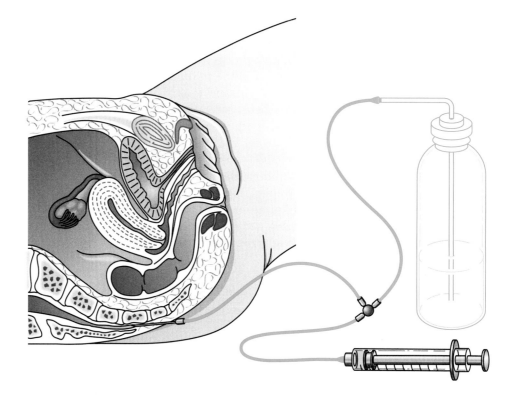

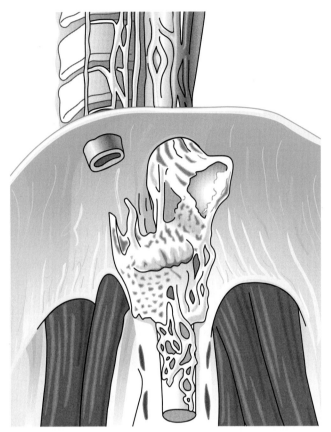

FIGURE 43–2 Descriptive anatomy of the celiac plexus.

Continuous Kulemkaff Block

We described this technique in the prearthroscopic era for the treatment of chronic and neoplastic shoulder pain.[33] This technique achieved pain relief in the shoulder and arm until radiation and chemotherapy took effect or, in the cases of chronic pain, rehabilitation was started. We used Teflon catheter Abbocath #20 and inserted it through a supraclavicular puncture. When we encountered classic paresthesia upon touching a branch of the brachial plexus, we withdrew the needle, leaving the catheter in the plexus. We used small doses of a local anesthetic (lidocaine or bupivacaine) because the goal was to achieve analgesia and not anesthesia. This technique was not prolonged for more than 5 to 7 days.

Continuous Epidural by Infusion

Before we knew of the use of spinal opioids[34] and infusion pumps,[13] we modified Finochietto's technique (Figure 43-4). After tunneling the thoracic, lumbar, and

sacral epidural catheter following our own technique,[14] we connected its end to a microdrip device connected to an intravenous line with 1% lidocaine. The rate of infusion was 10 mL/hour. This technique was used in terminally ill patients for a maximum period of 3 to 4 days.

Neurolytic Blocks

Although we knew of Brompton's syrup, we only began to use morphine regularly after the results of Twycross were published,[35] allowing us to treat our patients in a simple, nontraumatic, effective and, most importantly, economic manner. With time, fentanyl patches appeared, although they were only accessible to the patients of higher socioeconomic status. Our results were similar to those obtained by other authors,[21-23,36] and in our practice, neurolytic blocks were a much used resource.[37] The injection of neurolytic agents is a symptomatic treatment, indicated mainly for neoplastic pain in an advanced disease stage, and whose efficacy is temporary. The ideal neurolytic agent that would induce a permanent and lasting block without destroying nerve fibers is not known at the moment, and every neurolytic agent currently in use has some features that limit their clinical use. The risk of causing permanent neurologic lesions does not justify the use of neurolytic agents for non-neoplastic pain or in patients who are not in an advanced stage of the disease.[37] The effect of the neurolytic block can last for days, weeks, and in some cases, even for several months.

Neurolytic Agents

This section will summarize the neurolytic agents that we have used in our practice or that were reported as used by others. We currently use 50% ethanol for the blockade of the splanchnic nerves and phenol dissolved in water or glycerol.

Ammonium Salts

Several ammonium salts have been used in different concentrations and combinations on the premise that they affect nonmyelinated or small myelinated fibers of somatic nerves, thus eliminating certain types of pain without interfering with other sensory modalities. However, several clinical studies have shown that there is no uniformity in the neurolytic action of these agents.

The possibility of using ammonium salts to induce a sensory but not a motor block was described in 1939 by Steward,[38] but only after the work of Bates and Judovich in 1942 somatic analgesia was described for more than 5000 cases, and ammonium sulfate or chloride (0.75% concentration) started to be used in clinical medicine.[39]

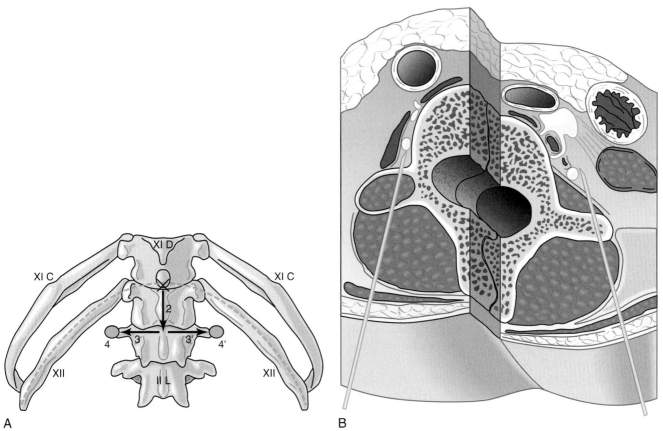

FIGURE 43–3 *A,* Albanese's method for the anesthesia of the splanchnic and related elements. The inward prolongation of the axis of the 12th ribs crosses in the point one of the spinal line. Three inclinations downward, line 2, and three outward, arrows 3 or 3′, and we will be in 4 or 4′, sites for punctioning, in the vicinity of the first transverse lumbar. *B,* Splanchnic anesthesia, "uneven" cut of the dorsolumbar region. To the left, Haertel's method: the injection reaches the sympathetic and the splanchnic nerves between a diaphragmatic pillar and the spine. To the right, Albanese's method, one vertebra below. The injection also affects the semilunar ganglion, efferents of the suprarenal, and part of this same gland.

FIGURE 43–4 *A,* Epidural space descriptive anatomy. *B,* Equipment for the block.

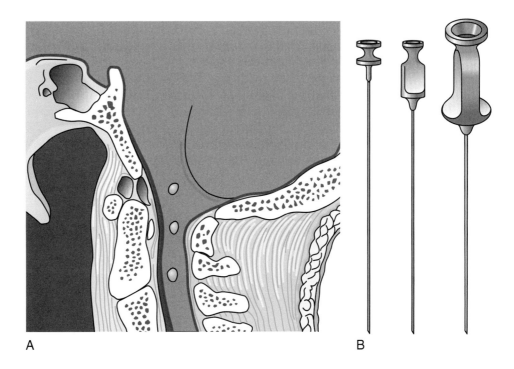

Bonica[40] tried to reproduce those results but they were disappointing at 0.75% concentrations. He increased the concentration to 6% using ammonium sulfate intradurally, with apparently good results. In 1965 Dam[41] published a report of 405 patients in whom he achieved blockade of peripheral nerves with 10% ammonium sulfate.

Wright[42] used 7% to 15% ammonium chloride for treatment of coccygodinia, injecting it in the dorsal tract of sacral nerves IV and V. These results were an encouraging alternative to coccygotomy or dorsal rhizotomy. Miller[43] used 10% ammonium sulfate for treatment of secondary intercostal neuralgia after radical mastectomy or postthoracotomy, achieving analgesia that lasted 20 to 80 days, without observing postblockade neuritis.

Other Neurolytic Agents

In our practice, we have used other neurolytic agents including chlorocresol, silver nitrate, ether, saline solution, cold saline solution, hypertonic saline solution, distilled water, glycerol, and so on. All these neurolytic agents were abandoned because randomized double-blind trials could not prove their benefits as well as because of accidents such as the one caused by the hypertonic saline serum (see below).

Maher[44,45] introduced the use of silver nitrate and chlorocresol. He warned that silver nitrate should not be used routinely but only when the injection of phenol or other neurolytic agent has failed to produce pain relief. It also produced an unwanted side effect by inducing an intense meningeal reaction followed by backache during various days after the blockade. Alexander and Lewis[46] used ether in intradural injections as a hyperbaric neurolytic agent. The doses they administered were of 0.2 mL, which initially produced paresthesia with a feeling of intense burning and later complete analgesia. Ether is very difficult to control, which made the mentioned authors abandon its use.

In 1958 Bridges and Liss[47] reported their results in patients with advanced neoplastic disease. Treatment consisted of the injection of 8 to 10 mL of hot saline solution in the frontal lobe. In 1967, Hitchock[48] published a study of 12 patients treated with intradural injections of physiologic saline serum at 4 degrees. He termed this method saline hypothermia, and it had unexpected results.[49] One year later, he used hypertonic serum at room temperature.[50] As the presence of a hypertonic solution in the cerebrospinal fluid caused intense pain, we had to administer general anesthesia in these patients. This technique caused numerous complications that have been described either as late or permanent. Madrid Arias[51] injected 10% hypertonic saline solution in the Meckel cavity for cases of secondary facial pain or advanced tumors, observing pain relief lasting 2 to 8 days.

In 1959, Jaeger[52] reported the use of hot distilled water injected in the Gasser ganglion for the treatment of trigeminal neuralgia. In 1981, Hakanson[53] introduced glycerol as a neurolytic substance. He used 0.2-0.4 mL, which once injected into the Gasser ganglion produced persistent relief of the pain caused by trigeminal neuralgia without sensory changes. This finding was not repeated by other authors.

Spinal Opioids

Our group was the first to use spinal opioids in Argentina[13] for oncologic or postoperative pain. We experienced several deaths due to late respiratory depression in obstetric patients and in the postoperative period of nononcologic surgery. In a 1981 *Anesthesia & Analgesia* editorial, Bromage warned about the risks of the indiscriminate use of the spinal opioids.[54] These drugs have to be clearly and precisely indicated, and when they are administered patients must remain under medical supervision for at least 6 hours.

Ethanol

It is surprising that ethyl alcohol has not been used more frequently to alleviate pain and achieve sedation. It produces a sensation of well-being as well as moderate analgesia without breathing or circulatory depression, which makes it an almost ideal agent in appropriate circumstances. The vasodilatation and increased diuresis that it causes are also advantageous. Ethanol is completely metabolized at the rate of 10 mL/hour. In appropriately selected patients, ethanol combined with non-narcotic oral analgesics achieves analgesia and the same or greater sense of well-being than that achieved by narcotics. In patients receiving parenteral fluids, a liter of 5% glucose with 50 mL of 95% ethanol achieves pain relief, sedation, and contributes 800 calories. The amount of the infusion can be adjusted as necessary. The recommended amount is 3 L/day, although the usual dose consists only of 1 to 2 L/day.[55]

We now know that the stimulant and sedative effects of ethanol are due to its action on several areas of the central nervous system. The stimulant effect is due to its action on the limbic system, involving numerous neurotransmitters such as dopamine, endorphins, serotonine, gamma-amino butyric acid (GABA), glutamate, cannabinoids and neuropeptide Y. The sedative effect involves glutamate and GABA receptors.[56]

Hallucinogenic Substances

Aldous Huxley already imagined in his books *Brave New World* (1932) and *Island* (1963) the existence of a pill that caused in those who ingested it a state of happiness as well as one of indifference in face of the traumatic situations of life. As years went by, this fantasy became a reality. This heterogeneous group of substances able to cause sensorial alterations was denominated using different terms: hallucinogens, psychomimetics, psychodisleptics, or psychodelics.[57]

The hallucinogens are natural or synthetic substances that traditionally have formed part of religious rituals and magic ceremonies in diverse cultures. It is generally accepted that they do not produce dependence but, their use is associated with the consumption of other substances capable of producing dependence. The hallucinogens can be classified according to their chemical structure or to their similarity with certain neurotransmitters of the CNS.[58] The classification is the following:

1. Group related to lysergic acid. The prototype and best studied hallucinogenic drug is the lysergide, diethylamide of the lysergic acid, LSD 25, or simply LSD.
2. Substances structurally related to the catecholamines, such as mescalin, elemicine, and miristicine. Mescalin is the main alkaloid of the peyote cactus, and it presents some effects comparable to those of the LSD, where the sympathetic-mimetics actions prevail. Elemicine and miristicine are found in nutmeg, and they only possess psychomimetic properties in very high doses. The methoxyamphetamins are amphetaminic variants with hallucinogenic properties.
3. Several natural or synthetic hallucinogens whose chemical structure is closely related to serotonin. One should highlight the indolic or triptaminic derivatives such as psylocibine and psylocine, which are active compounds found in various mushrooms (*Psylocibe*, *Stropharia*, and *Paneolus* genera), bufotenine (5-hydroxi-*N*, *N*-dimethyltriptamine) and similar compounds found in the seeds of some South American legumes.
4. Alkaloids of the harmala (harmine, harmaline, harmalol) are active compounds of South American hallucinogenic drinks called ayahuasca (or caapi or yagé). They are prepared with species of liana banisteria from the jungle. *Peganum harmala*, a plant found in Africa as well as Russian, Syrian, and Indian steppes, is also rich in these alkaloids. Other tryptaminergic derivatives of interest are the ibogaine (alkaloid of the roots and grains of the African plant *Tabernanthe iboga*), and the ibotenic acid and the muscimol, which are active principles with hallucinogenic properties of the *Amanita muscaria* mushroom.
5. Other substances that also produce psychomimetic effects are derivatives of *Cannabis sativa* (marijuana), *Papaver somnifurun* (opium, morphine, heroine), corticoids, sexual steroids, and the anesthetic ketamine.

The discovery of the psychodisleptic properties of the diethylamide of the lysergic acid occurred by chance.

Albert Hofmann, an investigator from the Sandoz Laboratories, synthesized it in 1938 together with other "ergoderivatives" (derivatives from alkaloids of the ergot of the rye). It received the name of LSD 25 (Lysergsáure Diethylamid 25) because it was number 25 of a series. Although initially it did not arouse much interest, Hofmann continued with his study. In 1943, he accidentally absorbed a very small quantity of LSD through the skin that caused slight alterations in perception and he decided to experience the effects of increasing doses in himself.

During the 1950s, the interest in LSD was merely scientific. It was thought it might be of value in studying the physiology of the CNS and the pathogenesis of mental illnesses. It was not yet considered a dangerous drug, or one attractive enough to cause problems of abuse. It was only used among artists and students in restricted circles, with self-exploration objectives or as a means to obtain different perspectives from reality and to develop creativity. In the 1960s, LSD was, together with pacifism and oriental philosophies, one of the most important characteristics of the hippie movement. Many psychiatrists used it to facilitate psychotherapy, especially in patients with lack of self-esteem and rigid defense mechanisms. As with many psychoanalytic techniques, this was not a standard therapy and the form of applying it depended on the therapist.[57] In 1964, Kats and Collins presented a study of 50 patients with intense neoplastic pain. They compared the analgesic effect of LSD with that of the methadone and the meperidine. In the 1970s, its use was declared illegal by the FDA.[59]

Pharmacokinetics

Although LSD is absorbed well by any route, the habitual form is the oral one. It is metabolized by hydroxylation and it is conjugated at hepatic level. Of the total amount ingested, only a small quantity reaches the brain. However, because it is a very potent compound, very low doses are enough to produce psychodisleptic symptoms. Its half-life is 1 to 7 hours. Its effects appear after about 30 to 90 minutes. They reach their maximum approximately 3 to 5 hours after the ingestion and then they begin to decline. The effects can last between 8 and 12 hours and, even for several days. The usual dose is 50 to 200 µg.[57]

Mechanism of Action

Although in peripheral systems the LSD behaves as a serotonergic antagonist, in the CNS it acts as partial agonist of the 5-HT2 receptors, either presynaptic or postsynaptic, mimethizing characteristic effects of the central serotoninergic systems, and inhibiting the activation of serotoninergic neurons of the nuclei of the raphe through the stimulus of the self-receptors.

The subtypes of 5-HT2A and 5-HT2C receptors are those that are involved in this action. The ketanserine blocks some of the specific effects of the LSD. The LSD also activates dopaminergic receptors. Apparently all these actions cause a functional disbalance on different levels (cortical areas, limbic system, etc.) and so they contribute to the distortion of their integrative action.[60]

Clinical Manifestations

In the first moments after ingesting the LSD, a sensation of interior tension that is alleviated by crying or laughing appears. And, depending much on the fellow's expectations, a state of euphoria is experienced. After 2 or 3 hours the characteristic psychodisleptic symptoms appeared, which consists of the psychodelic "trip". Alterations take place in several psychic functions: colors are more vivid, the perception of depth increases and the contours appear clearer, background noises are heard with more clarity and the music perception increases. Colors are perceived as sounds or music in the form of visual images. While sensibility to pain diminishes, the sensibility to temperature and pressure increases. As for the emotional threshold, those who ingest LSD increase their suggestion capacity. In the organization of thoughts, the heedless profusion of ideas that the individual is unable to verbalize orderly and that frequently is referred to as a transcendental perception of the experience is typical. Patients have a pleasant emotional experience with a sensation of euphoria although, in its final phase when hallucinations disappear, they can experience a state of anxiety and even anguish. What draws one's attention is the dysfunction of the personality that takes place after the hallucinations, which corresponds to the despersonalization phenomenon in which the fellow is conscious but has the illusion of not being himself, of being away from his body, and of having lost contact with the environment. Here, one can observe cases of unfolding of personality. We are dealing with a similar state to the one produced by schizophrenia, which justifies the asseveration that these drugs produce an experimental or model psychosis (psychomimetic drugs).[57] Ingestion of LSD produces sympathetic and anticholinergic actions including mydriasis, tachycardia, increased arterial pressure, nausea, vomiting, hyperpnea, pyloerection, hyperreflexia, tremors, muscular discoordination, ataxia, and so on.

Therapeutic Uses

Until the 1980s, LSD had been proposed as an auxiliary in psychotherapy, to help in the treatment of the alcoholism and the addiction to opioids, and as a resource to induce tranquility and to reduce the necessity of opioid analgesics in patients with terminal cancer. In each situation, its use has been abandoned mainly because controlled studies did not show the value of LSD or because all the necessary precautions that had to be taken in order to minimize the bad psychologic reactions dissipated the enthusiasm and made its therapeutic use unattainable.[61]

In 1963, Eric Kast[62,63] started to use LSD in patients with cancer. In presented works, he said that besides being a stronger analgesic than meperidine or methadone (100 μg of LSD produced 92 hours of analgesia, compared with 2 hours produced by 100 mg of meperidine or 3 hours by 2 mg of methadone), LSD possessed psychologic effects that can be summarized in three points: (1) improvement of the depressive state; (2) improvement in sleep; and (3) decrease of anxiety in the face of death.

Several multicenter studies were initiated based on Kast's published results. The most important study was done in 1970 at Maryland Psychiatric Research Center and the Sinai Hospital of Baltimore. As LSD was declared an illegal drug in the United States around the same time, these studies could not be continued or published. Several Argentinian physicians familiar with those early results continued to study the analgesic effects of LSD in cancer patients in Argentina and some of their key findings are summarized below.

The work was centered on the study of patients with cancer. Patient selection was done according to several criteria: (1) life expectancy was at least 3 months; (2) symptoms of marked mental confusion were present; and (3) all patients suffered from intense pain that could be quickly alleviated using analgesic medication. The study was carried out in three stages. The first stage was drug-free and included the patient and family. The second stage was the "psychedelic session," and the third stage was also drug-free and consisted of patient interviews meant to integrate the experiences of the session. The first stage lasted approximately 10 hours and consisted of a series of interviews with the patient and family meant to analyze and resolve any existing communication problems between them. The primordial goal of this phase was to establish a relationship of trust between the patient and the team leader. The second stage began the day before the psychedelic session, with an interview aimed at informing the patient of the states of conscience the LSD could induce. The day of the session, a dose of LSD of between 200 and 500 μg was given to the patient. During the session the patient remained in a comfortable position, listening to preselected music with the eyes covered. During the session that lasted 10 to 15 hours, the patient was accompanied by two therapists and, in the final phase, two family members.

Among the changes that were observed after the sessions, the most frequent one was the improvement in the depressive state and the disappearance of the insomnia. The physical pain sometimes disappeared as well. But the most remarkable effect of therapy was the total transformation that the patients experienced in regard to perceiving the idea of death and a change in their scale of values. Patients experienced new ideas about death, such as the concept of reincarnation, the primacy of spirit over matter, and a loss of interest in earthly possessions. This technique not only caused an overall improvement in the patient's pain and perception thereof, but also better acceptance and coping with impending death, a result also cited by others studying psychotherapeutic effects of hallucinogens.[64,65]

Psychedelic drugs have exposed a strong parallelism that exists among the myths of death and the experiences of death in different cultures. Individuals that know nothing about mythology or anthropology have experienced, under the effect of LSD, complete sequences that are in some cases literal descriptions of the myth of death and resurrection corresponding to a culture other than their own. Persons of European and American descent would without specific preparation narrate sequences of Hinduist or Buddhist mythologies, or passages from the book of the dead. A case described in these studies included a recital of a part of the Apocalypse according to St. John. Also, in several patients who underwent LSD sessions one could appreciate an evolution in their own experiences. At the beginning most of the material that appeared was of a personal character, consistent in dramatic sequences of the part of their early lives following birth. In time, if the sessions continued and the previous problems were resolved, the content of the following experiences was of a transpersonal, religious, and mystic character.[66]

FORGOTTEN NEUROSURGICAL TECHNIQUES

For many years we worked with Schvarcz[11] administering anesthesia to his surgical patients. We were able to appreciate several neurosurgical techniques, such as neurectomy, late rhizotomy by radiofrequency, myelotomy, open or percutaneous cordotomy, comissurotomy, and talotomy.[67] At the World Congress on Cancer in Buenos Aires in 1978, Moricca[68,69] performed practical demonstrations of his technique. All of these techniques were soon forgotten, and not only in the developing world. In a recent IASP syllabus on today's pain therapies,[70] the only interventional therapies mentioned are electrical stimulation with implantable electrodes and reservoir systems for drug supply.

As many of us practice in the developing world, use of interventional and even forgotten techniques is the result of economic limitations of our patients and

countries. These economic limitations make us use all available resources efficiently. We stay updated on the latest developments, and were able to implement the hospice model of care as soon as the works of Saunders,[9] Twycross,[35] Hanks,[71] and others were published and years before those started appearing in the developed countries. Several topics first discussed by us[72,73] were dealt with several years later in the developed world.[74-76] The remainder of this chapter will summarize some of the principles of palliative care that we were able to define based on our own experiences.

SOMETHING TO FORGET: THE PATERNALISTIC MODEL OF THE DOCTOR–PATIENT RELATIONSHIP

In the management of pain in the patient with cancer, we have to face two fundamental realities: the pain itself is only one of the symptoms, and the patients are not the only ones who suffer, but their entire family as well.[35,71] Back in 1985 at the Prager-Bild Foundation,[72] we started the educational and assistance work and treatment aimed at patients with terminal cancer and their families. The objectives—which later became the norm in all palliative care services that were created in Latin America—were guided by the abandonment of the bioethical assistentional paternalistic model,[77] a better comprehension of the processes involved in death, to the improvement and search of techniques for the control of symptoms and to the systematization of psychotherapeutic resources available to patients and their families. Also, we developed therapies of psychosocial reaccommodation of the family after the patient's death.

Our own experiences, as well as the contributions of all those who helped establish palliative medicine, helped define objectives of palliative care that today are the practiced norm in all of Latin America. Some of them go without saying, but it is fundamental to point out that we assist patients of all cultures and races[78,79] that for historical, cultural, religious, and ethnographic reasons, have imposed the so-called bioethical "paternalistic" model of doctor–patient relationship[77] and that to try to modify it has meant the introduction of a radical change in the thoughts and behaviors of doctors and patients. Our conclusions are the following:

Quality of Life[73]: Any patient with a terminal illness should be able to spend this last stage of life free of symptoms, emotionally supported, and feeling sure and content in his or her relationship with doctors and other members of the therapeutic team. The notion of "rehabilitation" is included, that is, when free of symptoms, patients should be encouraged to develop activities to avoid isolation, independent of the natural course of their illness. Doctors should try by every possible means to arrange that the twilight and the final stages of the patient's life occur at their homes, where they can be visited by the members of the therapeutic team and, especially, by all those who want to accompany their loved ones in the end of their lives, without being confined and inhibited at the hospital. The closest family members can be trained to supply oral, sublingual, subcutaneous, rectal, or epidural medication, mobilizing and channeling the desires "to be useful." Besides the quality of life that patients receive by being at home, they also have the benefit of reduced cost compared to a continued hospital stay, which is very often the paramount concern of cancer patients.

Talking about death is not a taboo topic: At the moment, thanks to education and information, sex and sexuality have stopped being regarded as sinful. The same or something similar has happened with death. Socrates wrote "… those who really follow the correct road of philosophy, are directly and for their own will getting ready to die and for death. If this is true and, they have truly been getting ready for death during all their lives it would be, of course, absurd to be upset when the moment so largely contemplated and for which they have been preparing arrives" (Socrates).[80] Also, when conception takes place, the future parents and the siblings—when they exist—are motivated to give the new unborn being "its" place. And the mother is trained not to become distressed, but to speak to the fetus, to make it listen to music and to have her thoughts permanently on that new being still "to be," so that its appearance in the real world is in the least traumatic way possible thanks to its previous existence in the world of ideas. Trying to do a similar work on the family, we motivate, in the other end of life, an almost similar situation: that the passage from life to death is as little traumatic as possible, making a special place for the ones who will no longer be corporally present so that they will remain in the thoughts and memories of their families.

Patients have to be the main characters of their illness and of their death: Patients should be made participants of the state of their illness and of the strategy of palliative care to develop, as well as of the complications or adverse reactions that the latter could cause, requesting their acceptance of the procedures to use or to omit, letting them organize their lives as they please, and not as it seems better to us.

Patients are not forced to accept any treatment, even if refusing it means a shorter life expectancy[81]: We think it is irrelevant to try to discern if this behavior can be classified as passive euthanasia or not. The habitual paternalistic attitude of ordering patients what to do should be set aside and one should respect their decision of how and where to die.

All treatment implies a risk: It is the doctor's obligation to inform and advise patients and their families on the unwanted, secondary effects or complications of radiation and chemotherapy, of oncologic surgery, and of neurolytic blockades. It is the patient's inalienable right to decide, for example, whether to live mutilated by an operation because of tongue or maxillar cancer or to die because of it, but with an intact corporal image.

Patients can die[81]: Medical procedures that are applied in acute, or chronic but recoverable patients, are often inappropriate in palliative medicine. Heart resuscitation, artificial breathing, intravenous infusions, nasogastric tubes, parenteral feedings, antibiotic therapy, and so on, are all routinely applied in patients who have the possibility to return to the state of health. The use of such interventions in terminally sick people, when there are no expectations of improvement of the illness, is generally inappropriate.

Doctors are not forced to preserve life at any cost: Doctors do not have legal or moral obligations to use medications or to apply procedures whose use would prolong suffering toward a certain death. "The obligation of doctors consists more of making an effort in alleviating the pain than in prolonging a kind of life that is not completely human, and that naturally begins to fade."[81,82] Since more than 80% of Latin America's population professes the Roman Catholic faith, it is of utmost importance that the members of the palliative care team be familiar with the ideology and document that sustain this creed so as to make the medical task efficient and, under extreme circumstances, to be endorsed by an institution that in no way can accuse doctors of attempting against human life.[83] Long after we initiated our task in palliative care, the Church promulgated the Encyclical Evangelium Vitae (1995)[84] that says in one of its parts:

"Speaking of her (the euthanasia) it should be distinguished the decision of giving up the so called 'therapeutic savagery', that is to say certain medical interventions no longer appropriate for the sick person's real situation, whether because the results that could be expected are disproportioned or too grievous for the patients and their families. In those situations, when death is considered imminent or unavoidable, one can conscientiously give up some treatments that would only offer a precarious and painful continuation of the existence, however without interrupting the due normal cures for the sick person in similar cases." "Certainly the moral obligation of being treated and cured exists, but this obligation should be valued according to concrete situations; that is to say, it is necessary to examine if the available therapeutic means are provided objectively according to the perspectives of improvement.

The renouncement to extraordinary or disproportionate means is not equal to suicide or euthanasia, rather it expresses the acceptance of the human condition in the face of death." "In modern medicine the denominated 'palliative cares' are booming. They are meant to make suffering in the final phase of the illness more bearable and, at the same time, to assure the patient an appropriate human accompaniment. In this context, the problem of the rightness of the use of the diverse types of analgesics and sedatives available to alleviate the sick person's pain appears, specially when their use involves the risk of shortening life. Indeed, the person who accepts voluntarily to suffer giving up treatments against the pain to preserve full lucidity and to participate—if they are believers—in a conscious way in the passion of the Lord can be worthy of praise but, such 'heroic' behavior should not be considered obligatory for all. Already Pious XII affirmed that it is licit to suppress pain by means of narcotics, in spite of having as consequences limit of conscience and abbreviation of life, if there are no other means and if, under such circumstances, the execution of other religious and moral duties are not interfered. Indeed, in this case death is neither wanted nor looked for, although for reasonable reasons one runs that risk. It is simply sought to mitigate the pain in an effective way, appealing to the analgesics available."

For the sake of those objectives, we have numerous times faced the cruel dilemma of, for example, giving tranquilizers or hypnotics to dyspneic patients with multiple or disseminated lung metastases, or barbiturates as thiopental or midazolam to mitigate the asterixis (or flapping tremor) of the patients with terminal hepatic insufficiency. We have carried out the prescription of such drugs with calmness of conscience, because beyond being endorsed by the papal words, in bioethics this is known as the "principle of double effect"[85]: the one that motivates the act or action is the good effect, and it is carried out because of its benefits; but if, unfortunately and simultaneously, a deleterious action takes place—neither wanted nor looked for—it is ethically correct only if the family of the patient is in complete knowledge and agrees with the procedure. And by no means this behavior can be considered euthanasia because it is substantially different from this, since we are using medications with a clinical purpose, therapeutically indicated, according to adequate pharmacologic doses, and not to provoke death voluntarily and premeditatedly with toxic doses of medications.

"At any cost" also means that, when the course of the illness becomes irreversible, we understand that it is also bad medicine to burden patients and those who are financially responsible for them, with excessive laboratory analysis, imaging diagnostics, and all types of studies and procedures that neither mean nor add absolutely anything to the quality of the patient's life and only satisfy the doctor's desire of handling the case scientifically and professionally.

Predictions of life expectancy should not be made: Making them will imply more an act of chiromancy than one of medicine, since it is common for the life expectancy to be shortened or exceeded due to the influence of many complex and interacting factors.

Truth: The person with a terminal illness, faced with his or her diagnosis, will undergo different stages, each one with specific emotional characteristics: negation, anger, negotiation, depression, acceptance, and so on.[86] Our proposal is the use of the approach of "cumulative truth," that is, truthful information that patients receive gradually. We must always keep in mind "how much they want to know" and "how much they can tolerate." That is to say, doctors should communicate information truthfully, but with affection and sensitivity. Patients will accumulate information and digest it in their own way. Patients will never feel attacked if the information is given in this way.

We understand that to give the information mechanically, with itemized details, even with the prediction of what will come is noxious. The information given in this way becomes an intrusion that increases fear and anguish. The apparently easiest way of communicating information to patients is that of the "hidden lie," using euphemisms: the tumor is a "nodule," and the metastases is "irritation," an so on. To choose this path means falling into a trap, since the bouncing effect of false information will make them lose reliability when patients, feeling deceived, experience the progressive deterioration of their bodies. This situation will generate hostile feelings in the dying patient toward the therapeutic team and will intensify their solitude and isolation.

Communication with patients cannot always be managed with the cumulative truth concept, since there are patients who sometimes restrictively manifest that "they do not want to know anything," that "they will die when God decides it" or "when their time arrives." Primun non nocere, Hippocrates recommended. And in these cases adhering blindly to the concept of telling the truth "under any circumstance" can cause a lot of harm and real damage. It is acceptable to argue that whether or not to tell the truth implies a question of principles. But the ethical and correct posture of respecting the right of the patient to know the truth becomes nonethical if the doctor, when informing the patient of his diagnosis, does not simultaneously offer the necessary help in facing such a difficult, physical, and emotional conflict. When the doctor adopts the position that man is, essentially, a free being, the amount of freedom that such professional exercises inside the permissible limits of society is a question that only the patient can answer. Some patients choose dependence as a form of escape. They are individuals that "choose not to choose", that use their "freedom" only to avoid being free. Odd as such behavior may seem, we respect the freedom that sick people have to not exercise their power of choice.

The members of the palliative care team who make the medical-therapeutic prescriptions with their own ethical values as the only limit for their actions can face a similar ethical conflict of truth-freedom. For example, 500 mL of morphine for oral use for 10 days of treatment cost approximately US$8. Slow-release preparations of morphine at equivalent doses and for the same treatment duration cost US$40 in the same pharmacy, and a catheter is implanted to inject epidural morphine. Besides the cost of hospitalization and the medications used, what is significant is the reimbursement that the physician can receive, since fees that are received for an at-home visit are different from those that can be charged after an interventionist practice, and they are even more expensive if the procedures are not covered by medical insurance. The objective and the result are similar in every situation: the relief of the patient's pain; however, the economic benefit for those who prescribe therapy can vary significantly.

Not to destroy even more than death does: After the patient's death, we are often consulted by the family about their loved one's wish to be cremated. We are fully aware that cremation in the Western society can be viewed as opposite to our anthropologic development. In the 1960s, Ralph Solecki[87] discovered a burial cave in Kurdistan, northern Iraq. Inside he found several Neanderthal remains; they apparently died during an avalanche. One of them, identified as Shanider IV, lay on pollen remains. Arlette Leroi-Gourhan,[88] a French paleobotanist, demonstrated that the pollen came from at least eight types of flowers apparently interweaved with branches of a bush (similar to the pine). No natural development could justify the presence of such vestiges so deep in the cave. This discovery led Solecki to write: "Some human being from the last glacial age must have walked along the hillside with the painful task of gathering flowers for the deceased. Today we find it logical to offer nice things such as flowers to the person who has recently died, but finding flowers in a Neanderthal tomb dated 60,000 years ago is a different thing." The ancient practice of wrapping the corpses in bandages is reminiscent of the fetus being covered by a membrane in the womb; ritual cleaning of the dead body is also reminiscent of cleaning the newborn baby. Even during wars, the opposing sides keep the dead bodies of both their own and enemy forces to give them back to the relatives, and when this is impossible to do, the bodies are put in individual tombs with proper identification.

Every story has to have an ending. But this comes at different times for cancer patients and their family. In psychology this is known as "dual elaboration." Relatives sometimes need to communicate with the dead wherever they may be (such as the Washington cenotaph erected to evoke the missing during the Vietnam War). In the civilizations where cremation is a common practice, it belongs to their culture. Among the Hindus, for example, cremation is a form of purification; the ceremony is performed in the open air, next to a river so that the smoke that symbolizes the soul of the deceased goes to heaven and the ashes to the sea.

Everything we have stated above might be considered rhetoric or comparative anthropology; however, it is, in our opinion, part of the necessary knowledge that does not end at the mg/kg doses administered. If one wants to provide high-quality palliative care, we believe that our task and duty should go beyond prescribing the drugs and finish with signing the death certificate.

REFERENCES

1. Pedreira ME, Maldonado H: Protein synthesis subserves reconsolidation or extinction depending on reminder duration. Neuron 38:863–869, 2003.
2. Mazzuccheli C, Maldonado H, Brambilla R, et al: Knockout of erk1 map kinase enhances synaptic plasticity in the striatum and facilitates striatal mediated lerning and memory. Neuron 4:807–820, 2002.
3. Schacter DL: The Seven Sins of Memory. Boston: Houston Miffin, 2001.
4. Iglesias Rogers G: Policy and people: Major Argentinian health service provider admits accounts corruption. Lancet 356:144, 2000.
5. Iglesias Rogers G: Policy and people: Heart by-pass pioneer's death puts Argentine health care in spotlight. Lancet 356:492, 2000.
6. Iglesias Rogers G: Policy and people: Minister 'ashamed' at malnutrition in Argentina. Lancet 360:2058, 2002.
7. La Nación: 10 de febrero de 2003. Buenos Aires (Argentina).
8. La Nación: 4 de junio de 2003, p 11. Buenos Aires (Argentina).
9. Saunders CM: The challenge of terminal care. Scientific Foundations of Oncology. London, Symingtont & Carter RL. William Heineman Medical Books, 1976.
10. Finochietto E, Finochietto R: Técnica quirúrgica. Tomo III. Buenos Aires: Compañía Argentina de Editores Ediar, 1944, pp 76–100.
11. Schvarcz J: Stereotactic extralemniscal myotology. J Neurol Neurosurgery Psychiat 39:53–55, 1976.
12. Parada J: Actas XII Congreso Nacional de Anestesia y Reanimación, San Sebastián (Spain), 1–5 julio, 1997.
13. Auad AO: Tratamiento del dolor con morfina peridural. Rev Arg Anest 39, 4:321–339, 1981.
14. Auad AO: Clonidina peridural asociada a la morfina en el tratamiento del dolor rebelde. Rev Arg Anest 43:27–34, 1985.

15. Moore DC, Karp M: Intravenous alcohol in the surgical patient. Surg Gyn Obst 80:523–525, 1945.
16. Fisher K, Coderre TJ, Hagen NA: Targeting the N-methyl-D-aspartate receptor for chronic pain management: Preclinical animal studies, recent clinical experience and future research directions. J Pain Symptom Manage 20:358–373, 2000.
17. Eide PK, Stubhaug A, Breivik H, Oye I: Ketamine: Relief from chronic pain through actions at the NMDA receptor. Pain 722:289–291, 1998.
18. Geurts JWM, van Wijh RMA, et al: Radiofrequency lesioning of dorsal root ganglia for chronic lumbosacral radicular pain: A randomised, double-blind, controlled trial. Lancet 361:21–26, 2003.
19. Wikinski J, Bollini C: Complicaciones neurológicas de la anestesia regional periférica y central: Buenos Aires, Editorial Médica Panamericana, 1999, p 30.
20. Lucas JT, Duccker TB, Perot PL: Adverse reactions to intrathecal saline injection for control of pain. J Neurosurg 42:557–561, 1975.
21. Jorgensen L, Mortensen MJ, Jensen NH, et al: Treatment of cancer pain in a multidisciplinary pain clinic. Pain Clin 3:83–89, 1990.
22. Schug SA, Zech D, Dorr U: Cancer pain management according to WHO analgesic guidelines. J Pain Symptom Manage 5:27–32, 1990.
23. Schug SA, Zech D, Grond S, et al: A long term survey of morphine in cancer pain patients. J Pain Symptom Manage 7:259–266, 1992.
24. Laborit H, Huguenard P: L'hibernation artificielle por moyen pharmacody-namiques et physiques. Pres Med 59:1329–1334, 1951.
25. Laborit H, Huguenard P: Practique de l'hibernotherapie en chirurgie et en medicine. Paris: Masson et Cie, 1954.
26. Maxwell DR, et al: A comparison of the analgesic and some other central properties of methotrimeprazine and morphine. Arch Intern Pharmacol 132:60–66, 1961.
27. Beaver W, Wallenstein SL: A comparison of the analgesic effects of methotrimepra-zine and morphine in patients with cancer. Clin Pharmacol Ther 7:436–446, 1966.
28. Sadove M, Albrecht R: The medical clinics of North America (January). Philadephia: W.B. Saunders, 1968, pp 47–53.
29. Sadove M: Chlorpromazine and narcotics in the management of pain of malignant lesions. JAMA 155:626–631, 1945.
30. Hellrich M, Gold MI: Circulatory response to tilting following methotrimeprazine and morphine in man. Anesthesiology 25:662–667, 1964.
31. Finochietto E. y R: opus cit. Técnica quirúrgica.Tomo II, pp 292–293.
32. Rathmell JP, Gallowt JM, Brown DL: Computed tomography and the anatomy of celiac plexus block. Reg Anesth Pain Manage 25:411–416, 2000.
33. Auad AO: Bloqueo de Kulemkaff continuo en el dolor rebelde del miembro superior. Actas III Congreso Argentino Para el Estudio del Dolor. Buenos Aires, 12–14 de octubre, 1978, p 1.
34. Yaksh T, Rudy T: Analgesia mediated by a direct spinal action of narcotics. Science 192:1357–1360, 1976.
35. Twycross RG: Choice of strong analgesics in terminal cancer: Diamorphine or morphine. Pain 3:93–98, 1997.
36. World Health Organization. Cancer Pain Relief and Palliative Care. Geneva: WHO, 1996.
37. Madrid Arias JL: Evolución histórica de los agentes neurolíticos utilizados para tratamiento del dolor crónico.Rev Española Anest Rean 3:197–204, 1984.
38. Stewart W: Effects of ammonium salts on nervous fibres. Am J Physiol 129:475, 1940.
39. Bates W, Judovich BD: Intractable pain. Anesthesiology 3:633, 1942.
40. Bonica JJ: Clinical Applications of Diagnostic and Therapeutic Nerve Block. Springfield, Charles Thomas, 1959, pp 212–213.
41. Dam WH: Therapeutic blockade. Acta Clin Scand 343(suppl):89, 1965.
42. Wright BD: Treatment of intractable coccygodynic by transsacral ammonium chloride injection. Anesth Analg 50:519, 1971.
43. Miller RD, Johnston RR, Hosobuchi Y: Treatment of intercostal neuralgia with 10 per cent ammonium sulfate. J Thorac Cardiovasc Surg 69:476, 1975.
44. Maher RM: Further experiences with intrathecal and subdural phenol: Observations on two forms of pain. Lancet 1:895–899, 1960.
45. Maher RM: Intrathecal chlorocresol in the treatment of pain in cancer. Lancet 1:965–967, 1963.
46. Alexander FAD, Lewis LW: The control of pain. Anesthesiology. Oxford, Hale DH, 1963, p 80.
47. Bridges TJ, Liss HR: Saline lobotomy for relief of pain due to advanced cancer. Cancer 2:322–325, 1958.
48. Hitchock E: Hypotermic subarachnoid irrigation for intractable pain. Lancet 1:133–135, 1967.
49. O'Higgins JW, Padfield A, Clapp H: Possible complications of hypothermic saline subarachnoid injection. Lancet 1:567, 1970.
50. Hitchcock E: Osmolytic neurolysis for intractable facial pain. Lancet 1:434–436, 1969.
51. Madrid Arias JL, Bonica JJ: Cranial nerve blocks. In Bonica JJ, Ventafrida V (eds): Advances in Pain Research and Therapy, vol 2. New York, Raven Press, 1979, pp 347–355.
52. Jaeger R: The results of injecting hot water into the gasserian ganglion for the relief of tic dolouloureux. J Neurosurg 16:659–663, 1959.
53. Hakanson S: Trigeminal neuralgic treated by the injection of glycerol into the trigeminal cistern. Neurosurgery 9:638–646, 1981.
54. Bromage PR: The price of intraspinal narcotic analgesic: Basic constraints (editorial). Anesth Analg 60:461–463, 1981.
55. Gildea J: Relief of pain in postoperative patients. The Medical Clinics of North America (January). Philadelphia, W.B. Saunders, 1968, pp 81–89.
56. Swift RM: Topiramate for the treatment of alcohol dependency: Initiating abstinence. Lancet 361:1666–1667, 2003.
57. Liter M: Farmacología. Buenos Aires, Editorial El Ateneo, 1961, pp 295–298.
58. Schultes RE, Hoffmann A: Plants of the gods: Origins of hallucinogenic use. New York, McGraw-Hill, 1979, pp 172–181.
59. Kast EC, Collins VJ: Lysergic acid diethylan-ide as an analgesic agent. Anesth Analg 43:285–291, 1964.
60. Lorenzo P, Ladero JM, Leza JC, Lizasoain I: Drogadependencias. España, Editorial Médica Panamericana, 1998, pp 215–220.
61. Goodman and Gillman's: The Pharmacological Basis of Therapeutics. MacMillan Publishing, Inc., 1980, pp 560–563.
62. Kast EC: A concept of death. In Aaronson B, Osmonol H (eds): Psychedelics: The Uses and Implications of Hallucinogenic Drugs. New York, Anchor Books, 1970, pp 366–381.
63. Francis G: Pain, death and LSD. A Retrospective of the Work of Dr Eric Kast. Psychedelic Monographs and Essay, vol 5, issue 4. Florida, PM & E Publishing, 1990, pp 114–121.
64. Grof S, Halifax J: The Human Encounter with Death. New York, EP Dutton, 1977.
65. Grot S: LSD Psychotherapy. Alameda, Hunter House, 1980.
66. Fontana AE: In Losada SA (ed): Psicoterapia con Alucinógenos. Buenos Aires,1965.
67. Meyerson BA: The role of neurosurgery in the treatment of cancer pain. Act Anaesth Scand 74(suppl):1109–1133, 1981.
68. Moricca G: Chemical hypophysectomy for cancer pain. In Bonica J, et al: Advances in Neurology, vol 2. New York, Raven, 1974, p 707.
69. Moricca G: Neuroadenolysis (alcoholiza-tion of the pituitary) for intractable cancer pain. In Anesthesiology. Proceedings of the VIth World Congress in Anesthesiology. Excerpta Medica. Amsterdam, 1977, pp 266–269.
70. North RB: Pain 2002. In Fiamberadino MA (ed): An Updated Review Refresher Course Syllabus. Seatle, IASP Press, 2002, pp 221–233.
71. Hanks GW: Opioid analgesics in the management of pain in patient with cancer: A review. Palliat Med 1:1–25, 1987.
72. Bild RE, Germ RM, Auad AO: El cuidado de la persona con enfermedad terminal. Ro 2000 (Roche Laboratoy magazine) 2:5–13, 1988.
73. Auad AO: Aspectos éticos en el trata-miento del dolor y medicina paliativa. Rev Argentina Anest 50:176–182, 1992.
74. Abraham JL: Pain control near the end of life. Pain Clinical Updates, XI 1:1–6, 2003.
75. Feinmann J: Breaking down the barriers to a good death. Lancet 360:1846–1847, 2002.
76. Weiss SC, Emanuel LL, Fairclough DL, Emanuel EJ: Understanding the experience of pain in terminally ill patients. Lancet 357:1311–1316, 2001.
77. Beauchamp TL, Childress JF: Principles of Biomedical Ethics, 4th ed. New York, Oxford University Press Inc., 1994.

78. Riley JL, Wade JB, Myers CD, et al: Racial/ethnic differences in the experience of chronic pain. Pain 100:211–212, 2002.

79. Lasch K: Culture and pain. Pain Clin Update, X 5:1–4, 2002.

80. Platón: Fedón o del alma: Obras completas. Madrid, Ediciones Ibéricas, 1966.

81. Twycross RG: Ethical and clinical objects of pain treatment. Acta Anaesth Scand 74(suppl):83–90, 1982.

82. Pious XII. Exhortaciones y discursos a los médicos. Buenos Aires, Ediciones Guadalupe, 1961.

83. Documentos de la Sagrada Congregación Católica Para la Doctrina de la Fé sobre la Eutanasia. Ciudad del Vaticano y Buenos Aires, 5 de mayo de 1980.

84. Evangelium Vitae. Encìclica de SS Juan Pablo II. Buenos Aires, Ediorial Claretiana, 1995, pp 116–119.

85. Singer P: A Companion to Ethics. Oxford, Basil Blacwell, 1995, pp 297, 303, 413.

86. Kubbler-Ross C: On Death and Dying. London, Tavistock, 1969, pp 34–121.

87. Solecki R: Two Basic Hafts from Northern Iraq Antiquity, vol XXXVII. Columbia University, 1963.

88. Perez FP: El hombre ante la muerte. Madrid, Ediciones Iberoamericanas Quorum, 1986, pp 16–17.

Palliative Care

CHAPTER 44

General Principles of Palliative Care

ROBERT A. MILCH, MD, FACS

Most clinicians are familiar with the World Health Organization's definition of palliative care, a consensus statement first published in 1990: "The active total care of patients whose disease is not responsive to curative therapy. Control of pain, of other symptoms, and of psychological, social, and spiritual problems is paramount. The goal of palliative care is the achievement of the best possible quality of life for patients and their families. Many aspects of palliative care are also applicable earlier in the course of the illness, in conjunction with anticancer treatment."[1] It went on to articulate several core principles of palliative care: it affirms life and regards dying as a normal process; it neither hastens nor postpones death; it provides relief from pain and other distressing symptoms; it offers an interdisciplinary team to help patients live as actively as possible until death; it offers a support system to help the family cope during the patient's illness and in their own bereavement.

This construct well-suited hospice programs, then and now arguably the premier practitioners of coordinated palliative care, but only in a subset of the population: the terminally ill, defined by the Hospice–Medicare Benefit of 1982 as patients with a life expectancy of 6 months or less if the disease follows its usual course. It emphasized care of those with malignant disease, who still comprise the majority of patients in most hospice programs, although each year more people die of heart and lung disease than of cancer. It acknowledged that most patients are referred for this type of service late in the course of their illnesses; even now, the median length of stay in hospice programs nationally is less than 21 days, and 30% of patients die in less than 30 days.[2] Although the Hospice–Medicare Benefit has enabled more dying patients to avail themselves of coordinated, comprehensive palliative care services, other regulations and guidelines of the benefit, misconceptions about them, and strictures regarding compensation have served to limit the numbers cared for and the scope and location of services readily provided.

Recognizing this, spurred by contemporaneous studies such as SUPPORT[3] and from the Institute of Medicine,[4] which documented serious shortcomings in care of the seriously ill, and believing palliative care to be an integral part of—not an alternative to—competent medical care applicable at all points on the trajectory of the patient's experience of illness, leaders in the field re-crafted a working definition of palliative care. "[It] is comprehensive, specialized care provided by an interdisciplinary team to patients and families living with a life-threatening or severe advanced illness expected to progress toward dying and where care is particularly focused on alleviating suffering and promoting quality of life. Major concerns are pain and symptom management, information sharing and advance care planning, psychosocial and spiritual support, and coordination of care."[5]

Hewing to these principles, palliative care has moved "upstream" in health care delivery as it became apparent that, applicable at all stages of the patient's illness, in its broadest context it is independent of curative intent or prognosis. Still, its flagship-hospice remains the focal point of most palliative care in the United States. Providing care for the terminally ill, there are now more than 3400 provider programs in the United States, and in 2002 they served 40% of Americans who died with an antecedent illness.

Importantly, a growing number of patients are benefiting from palliative care services offered by innovative programs in nonhospice settings. More than 30% of academic medical centers and 800 hospitals have palliative care services rendering primary or consultative services in all venues of the hospital, from general medical-surgical to critical care and dialysis units. There are more than 40 approved fellowship programs in palliative care medicine offered by academic centers and community-based hospice programs. More than 1500 physicians have been certified by the American Board of Hospice and Palliative Medicine, and more than 3500 physicians have completed training in the

American Medical Association/Robert Wood Johnson program Education for Physicians in End-of-Life Care (EPEC).[6] Fourteen specialty colleges have endorsed the "Principles Guiding Care at the End of Life," and competency in palliative care is now assessed on the Accreditation Council for Graduate Medical Education certification examination. An increasing number of medical schools now have preclinical and clinical courses on communication skills, advance care planning, self-awareness/professionalism or end-of-life care.

By providing the formal physician training[7,8] and programmatic structures[9] necessary, it is reasonable to believe patients and their families can expect better symptom management and supportive care throughout the course of their illness, bridging the gap between the type of care they want and what they receive.[10]

REFERENCES

1. WHO Expert Committee. Cancer Pain Relief and Palliative Care. Geneva, World Health Organization, 1990.
2. National Hospice and Palliative Care Organization, Annual Report, Washington DC, 2003.
3. The SUPPORT Investigators (Study to Understand Prognoses and Preferences for Outcomes and Risks of Treatment). JAMA 274:1599–1605, 1995.
4. Institute of Medicine. Approaching Death: Improving Care at the End of Life. Washington, DC, National Academy Press, 1997.
5. American Academy of Hospice and Palliative Medicine, Annual Report, Genview, IL, 2003.
6. American Hospital Association, Annual Report, Chicago, IL, 2003.
7. Emanuel LL, von Gunten CF, Ferris FD: The Education for Physicians on End-of-life Care (EPEC) Curriculum. American Medical Association, Chicago, IL, 1999.
8. Larson DG, Tobin DR: End-of-life conversations: Evolving practice and theory. JAMA 284:1573–1578, 2000.
9. Cassel CK et al: Pioneer Programs in Palliative Care: Nine Case Studies. New York, Milbank Memorial Fund, 2000.
10. Singer PA, Martin DK, Kelner M: Quality end-of-life care: Patient's perspectives. JAMA 281:163–168, 1999.

CHAPTER 45

The True Terminal Phase

ROBERT A. MILCH, MD, FACS

No matter how assiduous palliative care has been in the course of progressive illness, the last days and hours of life require renewed, active, often heightened attention to the goals of care: preparation and support of the patient, family, and caregivers through the death and into the early stages of bereavement; and maintenance of the patient's comfort and dignity. Failure to identify—to the extent possible—approaching death risks depriving patients and families of the opportunities for satisfactory life closure and completion of the "taskwork of dying."[1] Loss of control of previously well-managed symptoms, or failure to recognize or prevent the emergence of new ones, can have a devastating effect on all involved, causing distress to the patient and leaving survivors with memories of suffering.

Because the time course of this phase of end-of-life care can be unpredictable and because physicians tend to significantly overestimate survival,[2] the need to recognize its approach is heightened. This allows for review of the plan of care and patient and family choices; anticipation of needs (medications, supplies) that may be required quickly; sensitive discussion of the events that are likely around the time of death, as well as the signs and symptoms of the dying process; and plans for care of the patient after death and provision of support to the caregivers.[3]

GENERAL PRINCIPLES OF DRUG ADMINISTRATION AT END OF LIFE

Review of the medical regimen needs to take place frequently. Medications should be assessed for their appropriateness to the patient's condition, and those not required for symptom management discontinued or their route of administration changed. Almost always antidepressants, anticoagulants, laxatives, cholesterol-lowering agents, antihypertensives, hypoglycemics, vitamins and herbal supplements, antibiotics, and hormonal agents can be stopped (Table 45–1). If the patient has been on corticosteroids for intracranial neoplasm, these may be tapered quickly and stopped; anticonvulsants should be continued if seizures were present previously, or benzodiazepines added, and opiates increased if headache develops. It is important to individualize each plan of care and to involve the family and caregivers in discussion of the rationale for these changes, lest simplification of the plan of care be perceived as abandonment.

As the ability to swallow diminishes, essential drugs should be changed to liquid forms; when swallowing is no longer possible, rectal suppository (PR), subcutaneous (SC), transdermal (TD), or intravenous (IV) administration can be considered. Waller and Caroline[4] write of "The Final Four" of drugs most often used in the true-terminal phase: opiates (usually morphine), benzodiazepines, diuretics, and anticholinergics. These drugs and many others can be administered via the SC route either via indwelling "ports," "butterfly" needles, or syringe drivers, obviating the need for cumbersome intravenous paraphernalia (unless already present) and avoiding the risk of overhydration (Tables 45–2 and 45–3). Moreover, many drugs can be combined in syringes, providing control of a broad spectrum of symptoms with minimal technologic intrusion.

Studies of the symptoms frequently present in the last weeks and days of life note their multiplicity.[5,6] There may be common physiologic changes (increasing fatigue and weakness, decreasing appetite and intake, fluctuating level of consciousness or other neurologic abnormalities, changes in perfusion), as well as more specific symptoms such as dyspnea, "death rattle," dysphagia, and vomiting. Management of each requires assessment, recognizing that they are not diagnoses but symptoms, and then negotiation of a plan of care appropriate to the patient's status and consistent with his or her goals.

TABLE 45–1 Stopping Medications in the Last Hours of Life

Class	Drug	Stop or Continue?	Alternative Routes/Medications
Analgesics	Acetaminophen NSAIDs Weak opioids Strong opioids	Stop Stop oral dosing Stop Continue morphine at $\frac{1}{3}$ oral dose by SC infusion	If needed in patient with bone metastases; to prevent pain on being turned, give indomethacin, naproxen, or diclofenac $\frac{1}{2}$ hour before activity, or use indomethacin gel Low doses of morphine by SC infusion
Antiemetics	Metoclopramide Haloperidol Methotrimeprazine Domperidone Ondansetron	Continue by SC infusion Continue by SC infusion Continue by SC infusion Stop Stop	Metoclopramide by SC infusion Metoclopramide or haloperidol by SC infusion
Laxatives	All categories	Stop	
Sedative-hypnotics	Benzodiazepines (e.g., temazepam)	Stop oral forms	Midazolam IM at bedtime or by SC infusion
Anticonvulsants	Phenytoin	Stop	Midazolam or phenobarbital by SC infusion
Corticosteroids	Dexamethasone	Stop oral dosing	If dosage ≥ 4 mg/day at the time oral dosing is stopped, give by SC infusion, tapering gradually
Diuretics	Spironolactone Furosemide	Stop Stop oral dosing	If given for overhydration (pleural effusion, ascites, severe edema, signs of heart failure) and if patient is catheterized, continue IM or IV dosing every day-BID
Peptic ulcer Rx/prophylaxis	Antacids Sulcralfate H_2 blockers	Stop Stop Stop oral dosing	If symptoms of peptic ulcer, reflux esophagitis, or upper gastrointestinal bleeding are present, continue ranitidine, 50 mg IV QID or by continuous SC infusion
Bronchodilators	Theophylline, etc.	Stop	Albuterol by inhalation with dexamethasone, morphine, and atropine as required by the situation
Urinary sedatives or antispasmodics	Phenazopyridine Oxybutynin	Stop Stop	If dysuria is a problem in the catheterized patient, irrigate the bladder with lidocaine in saline
Antidepressants	Amitriptyline, etc.	Stop	None
Anticoagulants	Warfarin sodium Aspirin	Stop	None
Antihypertensives and other cardiac medications	All categories	Stop	None
Hypoglycemics	All categories	Stop	None
Vitamins	All categories	Stop	None
Antibiotics	All categories	Stop	None
Hormonal agents	Thyroid hormone, tamoxifen, etc.	Stop	None

BID, twice daily; IV, intravenously; IM, intramuscularly; QID, four times a day; SC, subcutaneous.

Modified from Waller A, Caroline NL: Handbook of Palliative Care in Cancer, 2nd ed. Boston, Butterworth-Heinemann, 2000, pp 396–397, with permission.

TABLE 45–2	Drugs That May Be Given by Subcutaneous Infusion
Class	**Preferred SC Drugs**
Opioids	Morphine Hydromorphone Fentanyl
Antiemetics	Haloperidol Metoclopramide Methotrimeprazine Cyclizine
Somatostatin analogs	Octreotide
Sedatives	Midazolam Phenobarbital
Antihistamines	Promethazine Dimenhydrinate Hydroxyzine
Anticholinergics	Atropine Scopolamine
Corticosteroids	Dexamethasone
H_2 blockers	Ranitidine Famotidine
NSAIDs	Ketorolac
Diuretics	Furosemide
Bisphosphonates	Clodronate

Diazepam and chlorpromazine cause subcutaneous inflammation and should not be given by SC infusion.

Subcutaneous drug infusion is contraindicated in cases of severe thrombocytopenia, anasarca, and patient unwillingness.

NSAIDs, nonsteroidal anti-inflammatory drugs; *SC*, subcutaneous

INANITION AND LOSS OF FUNCTIONAL ABILITY

Diminution in functional ability is an accurate prognostic variable for patients with advanced malignant disease. (A good screening question is "Tell me how you spend your day," and when more than 50% of time is spent horizontal in bed or chair, it is a significant prognostic sign). As independence in the activities of daily living (bathing, eating, toileting, ambulation, dressing) is lost, as is unavoidable with weakness and fatigue, the decreased ability to move implies increasing need for care, and strategies need be sensitively negotiated with patients and caregivers for preservation of comfort, dignity, and resources.

This includes frequent repositioning to relieve joint fatigue and skin pressure, passive range of motion movements for limbs, skin care with emollients or lotions, and gentle massage. A hospital bed may allow easier change of position for the patient and hands-on care for the caregiver. Use of a bedside commode expends less energy than trips to the bathroom, and poses less risk for falls. Similarly, disposable diapers can minimize energy expenditure or discomfort in positioning to use a bedside commode or bedpan, and a urinary catheter can prevent skin breakdown from maceration or discomfort from development of urinary retention.

ANOREXIA AND DIMINISHED INTAKE

Loss of interest in food, or failure of the patient to eat or drink, is an emotion-laden subject, frequently a source of great frustration and conflict within the caregiving unit.

TABLE 45–3   Drugs That May Be Combined in a Syringe Driver

Metoclopramide	C	C	C	C			C	C	
Morphine	C	C	C	C	C	C	C	C	C
Methotrimeprazine	C	C	C	C			N	C	
Midazolam	C	C	C	C	N	N	C	C	
Dexamethasone		C		N	C	C	N		C
Ranitidine		C		N	C	C			
Haloperidol	C	C	N	C	N		C	C	
Promethazine	C	C	C	C			C	C	
Octreotide		C			C				C

The letter C indicates that the two drugs are compatible. The letter N indicates that the two drugs are not compatible. If the entry is blank, it means that we have no experience in combining the two drugs and their compatibility is therefore not known to us. If you need to combine more than two drugs in an infusion, use the table to check the compatibilities of each pair of drugs separately. For example, if the patient needs to receive metoclopramide, morphine, and midazolam, check the compatibility of:

Metoclopramide with morphine (= C)

Metoclopramide with midazolam (= C)

Morphine with midazolam (= C)

In the example cited, each pair is compatible, so the combination of all three drugs is compatible.

Modfied from Waller A, Caroline NL: Handbook of Palliative Care in Cancer, 2nd ed. Boston, Butterworth-Heinemann, 2000, pp 528–529, with permission.

Although the causes of anorexia and diminished intake of food and fluids are multifactorial, they are a natural and expected phenomenon of advanced disease. Time needs to be spent helping family understand this is not rejection of their care or "giving up" or "starving to death," and that patients don't die because they stop eating or drinking, but that they stop eating or drinking because they are dying.

Explanation may be helpful that hunger per se is rare, and that a relative fasting state can be beneficial, as a ketotic state induces a semi-euphoria and diminishes pain awareness. Forcing food may induce nausea or vomiting, or pose a risk of aspiration as swallowing becomes more difficult and discoordinated; thus, patients should be offered what they desire and can safely swallow, often in pureed or thickened form, but no more. The question of enteral or parenteral feeding often arises, but there is no evidence that it is beneficial in these circumstances in improving either nutritional status or symptom control or substantively prolonging life.[7]

Similarly, diminished intake of fluids is distressing to families, who may fear the patient will "die of thirst."[8] Again, explanation and reassurance are needed, given that the perception of thirst is not likely related to dehydration but more often to dry mucosal membranes. It can be controlled by allowing sips of such simple liquids (broth, fruit juices, ice pops) as the patient can safely sip and assiduous attention to mouth care, with frequent (every 30 to 60 minutes) applications of commercially available water-based solutions or baking soda mouthwash (1 tsp. salt, 1 tsp. baking soda, 1 qt. warm water).[3] "Artificial saliva" may be painted on the tongue and palate every 4 hours to prevent desiccation and a thin layer of plain petroleum jelly applied to the lips and anterior nares for the same purpose.

The option of parenterally administered fluids, either intravenous or subcutaneous (hypodermoclysis[4]), often arises. They may be considered on a short-term, goal-oriented basis, particularly to reverse delirium or reduce myoclonus. Their injudicious use, however, should be avoided as their burden outweighs their benefit. Particularly in the hypoproteinemic patient, they lead to fluid overload, worsening edema, ascites, and increased lung water leading to more secretions, dyspnea, and cough. They risk needlessly prolonging the dying process while only adding to the symptom burden.[9]

NEUROLOGIC DYSFUNCTION

Some element of neurologic dysfunction always accompanies the last days of life, varying from increasing lethargy and decreasing levels of unconsciousness to agitated delirium or myoclonus. Multiple factors—for the most part irreversible—are usually at play, such as metabolic abnormalities; encephalopathy; hepatic, renal, or respiratory failure; sepsis, paraneoplastic syndromes, or the effects of medications or their metabolites.

Most commonly patients progress from increasing drowsiness through obtundation to a comatose state. Inability to co-respond with the patient can be distressing to families, particularly if there is "unfinished business" or adequate advance planning and preparation have not been done. Because the patient's level of awareness or comprehension may be greater than his ability to respond, families should be advised to speak as though the patient were conscious, even if not participatory. They should be encouraged to say what they feel appropriate, continue to demonstrate affection by gentle touching, and even to give "permission" to die.

Delirium develops in 30% or more of dying patients.[10] It manifests with loss of cognitive function, confusion, restlessness, agitation, and may be associated with "sundowning"(day/night reversal). It may be confused with pain, though the sudden emergence of pain in patients in whom it was previously well controlled is uncommon. Easily reversible causes should be sought, such as urinary retention, fecal impaction, hypoglycemia, or medications such as corticosteroids or short-acting benzodiazepines. If suboptimally treated pain is suspected, a trial of increased dose of opiate should be undertaken; if opioid metabolite accumulation is thought to be the cause (and is more often the case), rotation to another opioid should be made.

It is imperative that terminal delirium be rapidly and effectively managed not only for the patient's sake, but for the caregivers' as well, lest their impressions and memories be of a distressed death. Their support and education about what is happening—and its implications as to the course of the disease—are critical. A calm, familiar environment is helpful to calm the patient, as are verbal and tactile reassurance of presence.

Pharmacologically, benzodiazepines and neuroleptics are the mainstays of treatment. Benzodiazepines, with their anxiolytic, amnestic, muscle relaxant, and antiepileptic properties are useful in the patient who is not hallucinating (visual, auditory, picking at bedclothes). Lorazepam 1 to 2 mg can be given orally or subcutaneously every hour until settled, and then every 4 hours thereafter. A relatively short-acting drug, it may elicit paradoxical worsening of agitation (disinhibition syndrome); this can be managed by using a longer-acting, more sedating benzodiazepine such as diazepam or by a continuous subcutaneous infusion of midazolam (5 mg loading dose, begin infusion at 1.5 mg/hour and titrate by 1 mg/hour to effect).

Patients who are actively hallucinating or who worsen on benzodiazepines should be begun on neuroleptics. Haloperidol can be administered by any route, including subcutaneously, and is most easily titrated. For mild or early-stage delirium or for patients who are "sundowning," 0.5 to 2 mg can be given every 4 to 6 hours and 2 mg at bedtime; for more severe agitated delirium, haloperidol can be upwardly titrated to 10 mg q2h as needed. If more sedation is desired, chlorpromazine 25 to 50 mg can be given every 4 to 6 hours and 50 mg at bedtime and titrated upward, the drug administered PO, PR, or slowly IV. The newer, atypical neuroleptics, such as risperidone, quetiapine, and olanzapine, may be helpful, although they are somewhat more cumbersome to titrate; they are associated with less akithesia and dystonia than haloperidol and thorazine, and there is anecdotal evidence that risperidone may be better suited for agitated delirium or the delirium of dementia (risperidone 0.5 to 1 mg q12h and titrated upward).

Myoclonic jerks usually reflect accumulation of opioid metabolites, often on the background of decreased renal perfusion. If they are mild or infrequent, patients who are semi- or unconscious may not be distressed by them, but family members may be and require explanation as to their significance. They may herald the onset of frank seizures. Myoclonus can be managed by decreasing the dose of opioid (so long as pain remains controlled); rotating to a different opioid, usually at $^1/_2$ to $^2/_3$ the equianalgesic dose; using benzodiazepines such as lorazepam (least sedating), diazepam, or clonazepam (most sedating); or beginning anticonvulsants such as phenytoin (PR, IV) or phenobarbital (PR, IM, IV).

DYSPNEA AND "DEATH RATTLE"

In the final stages of illness, the causes of dyspnea are often multifactorial. It should be assumed that readily remediable conditions, such as effusions or infectious processes, have been assessed and appropriate interventions undertaken. Patients who are actively dying may manifest tachypnea and hyperpnea as a consequence of acidosis, and this difference should be explained to caregivers. The goal of care now is to relieve the tachypnea and anxiety that accompany the sensation of air hunger. A calm environment with support, reassurance, and ongoing presence from caregivers is helpful, as are imaging and relaxation techniques.

The role of supplemental oxygen therapy in these circumstances is controversial. Many dyspneic patients are not hypoxemic, and clinical experience shows many obtain relief from a fan blowing cool air over their face. Those who do have desaturation are likely to benefit somewhat from increased inspired oxygen concentration, special care to control FiO_2 being taken in those with concomitant severe chronic obstructive pulmonary disease and carbon dioxide retention. Nasal prongs are less intrusive and restrictive of communication than masks, but of dubious benefit in patients who are mouth breathing.[11]

In the end, supplemental oxygen is of uncertain help, but its use has become almost a cultural expectation in the United States.

Much of the distress of dyspnea can be alleviated by pharmacologically reducing the rate and work of breathing. Greatest experience has been obtained with morphine, though any agonist opioid can be used, targeting a respiratory rate of 15 to 20 respirations per minute. Those who have been using morphine for pain management will likely need increases of 25% to 50% total daily dose to achieve this effect. Anxiolytics are usually indicated as well, the benzodiazepines being the first-line choices administered on an as-needed basis and often with a standing bedtime dose.

As patients become weaker or stuporous, pharyngeal and upper airway secretions are no longer cleared by their swallowing or coughing. Their accumulation produces a rattling noise with breathing, and although patients are often unaware or not distressed by the noise, it is often disturbing to caregivers. Explanation and reassurance are needed for the family. The patient should be positioned side to side, and the oropharynx gently swabbed. Suctioning is often traumatic and may stimulate more secretions. Anticholinergic drugs begun at the first sign that the process is beginning are helpful (scopolamine 0.4 mg transdermal patch; atropine 0.4 mg SC every 4 to 6 hours), explanation being given as to side effects that might be observed (flushing, dry skin, urinary retention) along with watchfulness for restlessness or excitation.

PAIN

Although tumor-based somatic, visceral, and neuropathic pain per se are present in one half to two thirds of patients dying with cancer,[12] other processes such as agitated delirium, dyspnea, or myoclonus may cause or add to physical discomfort or be interpreted as pain and are equally prevalent. Their presence needs be considered and dealt with as part of ongoing differential diagnosis; thus, urinary retention, which may manifest itself as pain or agitation, is likely better managed with a Foley catheter than with opioid escalation or anxiolytics.

Patients may have incident pain, manifested by moaning or grimacing with hands-on care or movement; this is usually well managed by explaining what is to be done in advance, using gentle and unhurried movements, and anticipating the need for increased analgesia by preemptive dosing of immediate-release pain medication. Patients who have been on nonsteroidal anti-inflammatory drugs (NSAIDs) for bone pain should have them continued in liquid, suppository, or transdermal gel form, decreasing the dose as renal function falters.

Maintenance of satisfactory pain control is of paramount importance at this time. Assessment is often made more difficult as the patient's level of consciousness fluctuates, but indirect indicators such as grimacing or moaning, especially with turning or hands-on care, usually are reliable indicators of suboptimal control. Because even unconscious patients experience pain (as with a general "anesthetic"), patients who have previously required regularly administered analgesics will continue to do so, some in decreased amounts, many in the same or increased amounts.[5] In addition, sudden cessation of analgesic in these patients risks inducing a withdrawal syndrome.

Some conjugates of opiate metabolism accumulate as hepatic and renal function decline, and may be responsible for neurologic toxicity (myoclonus, seizures) or delirium. Thus, consideration should be given to decreasing the total daily dose of opiates by 25% to 50%, so long as pain is still controlled. This is a dose that will prevent withdrawal syndrome while minimizing the occurrence of opioid toxicity.[13]

Patients who have previously used sporadic dosing of analgesics should continue to receive them periodically but liberally, particularly before hands-on care or procedures known to cause distress. Intuitively, patients who are nonverbal or cognitively impaired should not be relegated to PRN dosing regimens.

END OF LIFE

As anticipated death approaches, caregivers often benefit from frequent contact with the physician and other members of the interdisciplinary team. This is the opportunity to revisit the goals of care, reinforce the elements and appropriateness of the plan of care, and clarify any concerns or apprehensions about what is happening. It is also the time to ensure that desired or unique cultural and religious practices are known and understood by all members of the team.

Particularly if death pronouncement is made in the acute care setting, it should be as courteous and unobtrusive as possible.[14,15] Introduction should be made to those in the room and condolences extended to them for their loss. Explanation of the purpose of the examination should be made and visitors given the option of remaining in the room or not. There is no reason to subject the patient to otherwise painful procedures such as sternal rub or corneal stroking to verify death. Assessment should be made of the family's need for further information, direction, or support. A condolence letter from those involved in the patient's care is a gracious gesture greatly appreciated by surviving family members.[16]

Competently and sensitively managed, the last days of patients' lives can be a time of comfort and fulfillment, and the memories engendered a source of solace to the survivors. The physician plays a key role in bringing to the bedside the requisite knowledge, skills, and attitudes to meet the unique needs of this time and, with the other members of the interdisciplinary team, deriving a plan of care that maximizes the opportunity for achieving a defined good outcome.

REFERENCES

1. Byock I: Dying Well: The Prospect for Growth at the End of Life. New York, Putnam/Riverhead, 1997.
2. Christakis N, Lamont N: Extent and determinants of error in doctors' prognoses in terminally ill patients: Prospective cohort study. BMJ 320:469-742, 2000.
3. Module 12: Last Hours of Living. Education for Physicians on End-of-Life-Care (EPEC). American Medical Association, Chicago, IL, 1998.
4. Waller A, Caroline NL: Handbook of Palliative Care in Cancer, 2nd ed. Boston, Butterworth-Heinemann, 2000, pp 393-405.
5. Lichter I, Hunt E: The last 48 hours of life. J Palliat Care 6:7-15, 1990.
6. Ventafridda V, Ripamonti C, DeConno F: Symptom prevalence and control during cancer patients' last days of life. J Palliat Care 6:7-11, 1990.
7. McCann RM, Hall WJ, Groth-Juncker A: Comfort care for terminally ill patients: The appropriate use of nutrition and hydration. JAMA 272:1263, 1994.
8. Parkash R, Burge F: The family's perspective on issues of hydration in terminal care. J Palliat Care 13:23, 1997.
9. Billings JA: Dehydration. In Berger AM, Portenoy RK, Weissman DE (eds): Principles and Practice of Supportive Oncology. Philadelphia, Lippincott-Raven, 1998.
10. Twycross R, Lichter I: The terminal phase. In Doyle D, Hanks GWC, MacDonald N (eds): Oxford Textbook of Palliative Medicine, 2nd ed. New York, Oxford University Press, 1999.
11. Twycross R: Symptom control: The problem areas. Palliat Med 7:1-8, 1993.
12. Lombard DJ, Oliver DJ: The use of opioid analgesics in the last 24 hours of life of patients with advanced cancer. Palliat Med 3:27-29, 1989.
13. Bruera E, Kim HN: Cancer pain. JAMA 290:2476-2479.
14. Weissman D, Heidenreich C: Fast Fact #004: Death Pronouncement. End of Life/Palliative Education Resource Center: (Jan 2005) http://www.eperc.mcw.edu
15. Midland D: Fast Fact #064: Informing Significant Others of a Patient's Death. End of Life/Palliative Education Resource Center: (Jan 2005) http://www.eperc.mcw.edu
16. Menkin E, Wolfson R, Weissman D: Fast Fact #022: Writing a Condolence Letter. End of Life/Palliative Education Resource Center: (Jan 2005) http://www.eperc.mcw.edu

CHAPTER 46

Management of Symptomatic Bone Metastases

GEOFFREY P. DUNN, MD, FACS

The management of symptomatic bone metastases presents one of the greatest tests of interdisciplinary cancer care. In addition to the considerable physical symptom burden of this syndrome and the loss of function, the patient afflicted with bone metastases is also under the psychological burden that stems from the awareness that this disease is almost certainly incurable. The incidence of this problem will undoubtedly increase as newer cancer treatment protocols prolong survival. Because the presence of bone metastases almost always indicates incurable disease, the general principles of palliative care can and should be implemented with alacrity and without ambiguity. For the clinician, the challenge lies in the ability to balance the imperatives of pain control, restoration of function, and promotion of quality of life with a realistic assessment of the patient's tolerance for invasive interventions and the patient's life expectancy. To complete the challenge of palliation, this balancing must be achieved within the framework of the patient's preferences, culture, and personal values.

The availability of effective analgesics, bisphosphonates, percutaneous procedures (vertebroplasty),[1] and radiation therapy have provided alternative avenues for symptom control in patients who are not candidates for operative therapy. Fortunately, much experience has accumulated in the perioperative and operative management of fractures in frail individuals due to the common occurrence of fracture in weight-bearing bones in the geriatric population. Despite the availability of these treatments, the high incidence of cancer pain reported in repeated surveys tragically suggests that they are poorly integrated: The orthopedist may be uncomfortable prescribing opioids for chronic pain; the internist may not be aware of the benefit of bisphosphonate therapy; and the medical oncologist may be too distracted to make a timely referral to an orthopedist.

As an increased number of patients with advanced oncologic illness select hospice and other models of home and nursing home care, it will become increasingly important for all physicians and other health care workers to recognize bone metastasis syndromes and have flexible and practical treatment strategies to offer. Painful bone metastases can present in several clinical contexts. (This chapter will not address management of symptomatic hypercalcemia caused by lytic bone lesions.) The most familiar includes identification of bone metastases at the time of initial diagnosis or later identification in a patient with a known primary. Much less common are presentations of a primary bone cancer or a bone metastasis from a site other than a known primary (e.g., a pattern of skeletal metastasis suggestive of prostate cancer in a person with a previous history of a resection for a favorable colon cancer). This chapter will address patients with an established primary cancer diagnosis who present with painful bony metastases synchronously or metachronously.

INCIDENCE, SITES, AND EVALUATION

Skeletal metastases occur frequently: Approximately 20% of cancer patients can be expected to develop clinical evidence of skeletal metastases during their lifetimes with as many as an additional 50% detected at autopsy.[2] Up to 75% of these patients with metastatic bone disease will have pain.[3] Bone cancer pain is the most common source of pain in patients with malignant disease.[4] Nearly 80% of patients with skeletal metastases who came to a radiation oncology unit reported their pain to be moderate to severe.[5] In one series of patients with skeletal metastases, bone lesions were the initial presentation of cancer in 30% of those reviewed.[6] Cancers of the prostate, breast, lung, kidney, and thyroid account for the majority of cases[7] with breast and prostate cancer accounting for most of these because of their frequency and the relatively prolonged survival of these neoplasms. Bone metastases, however, can occur with any tumor. Lesions of the axial skeleton predominate over lesions of the appendicular skeleton. Appendicular lesions occur more frequently in the proximal aspect of the lower extremities. Prostate cancer will tend to metastasize to the axial skeleton and pelvis through the densely anastomotic venous plexus in these regions.

Pain is the most common symptom of skeletal metastases, typically insidious in onset, progressive, relentless, often awakening a patient at night, and not relieved by changing position. Approximately two thirds of radiographically evident lesions are symptomatic.[8] Increasing pain with function usually portends impending fracture, though fracture without antecedent pain can occur, especially in non–weight-bearing bones.

The presentation of painful bony metastases varies with location. Spinal metastases may remain asymptomatic through the patient's life span, though there are multiple mechanisms including neuropathic processes producing pain with widely varying treatment algorithms (Table 46-1). Pain associated with spinal metastases may be due to bone destruction, raised intramedullary pressure, nerve root compression, muscle spasm, pathologic fracture, spinal instability, or spinal cord or cauda equina compression from bony elements or tumor. Other clues leading to the diagnosis of spinal metastases include kyphotic changes secondary to vertebral collapse and scoliosis secondary to reflex muscle spasm triggered by pain. In addition to sensory neuropathies,

functional impairment (weakness) can be caused by direct tumor invasion of nerve roots, epidural metastases, stretching of the cord or cauda, or compression from collapsed bony elements.

The next most likely sites of bone metastases after the spine are the pelvis and proximal femur. Pain with ambulation will occur with metastases to the weight-bearing portion of the pelvis (acetabulum) and the femur. The high incidence of metastases to the proximal femur is significant not only because of the pain symptom burden but also due to the potential loss of function from pathologic fracture that frequently occurs in that region. Timely recognition of these lesions causing pain, allowing for prophylactic fixation, will prevent the increased technical difficulty and potential complications of treating a pathologic fracture. Upper extremity metastatic disease, usually in the proximal humerus, is much less common than in the lower extremities, although the potential morbidity of fracture is very high due the importance of upper extremity function for daily tasks.

In a hospice or nursing home the presentation of bony metastases may not be appreciated or pursued on the assumption that survival is too limited (the patient "is too far gone") or bone pain symptoms are lost among the others, which are typically numerous and severe.[9] Additional complacency in the pursuit of new symptoms can occur with patients with long-standing bony metastases from breast and prostate cancer who previously had good pain control from hormonal and analgesic therapy. In addition to these potential reasons for delayed recognition, orthopedic implications of bone pain due to metastases may not be known to hospice and nursing home personnel assessing patients.

Following a history and physical, during which a preliminary judgment can be made about overall functional capacity, imaging studies are required to confirm clinical suspicions. The basic study is the plain radiograph, although magnetic resonance imaging (MRI) or computed tomography (CT) will need to be added to fully assess structures such as the spine or pelvis or situations in which neural compromise is present. Pathologic fracture may not always be obvious, though crescendo pain leading up to the time of the break and sudden pain out of proportion to movement or loading are suggestive. A validated scoring system[10] has been devised to assess the likelihood of pathologic fracture based on radiographic features of the metastasis (osteolytic, osteoblastic, or mixed), site of metastasis, type of pain (mild, moderate, pain with activity), and size of lesion on radiograph (Table 46-2).

Technetium-99 positron emission tomography (Tc-99 PET) has been shown to be superior to the more commonly used technetium-99 methylene diphosphonate (Tc-99m MDP) scintigraphy in the detection of osseous metastases[11] because it is a direct reflection of tumor

TABLE 46-1   Pain Syndromes Due to Bone Metastases

Syndrome	Treatments
Bone pain	Chemotherapy, hormonal therapy, nonsteroidal analgesics, opioids, bisphosphonates, steroids, radiation therapy (including radiopharmaceuticals), intercostal and regional block, acupuncture, transcutaneous electrical nerve stimulation
Pain with impending fracture or established pathologic fracture	Weight bearing: Operative reduction/radiation therapy, nonoperative immobilization and analgesics, blocks Non-weight bearing: Radiation therapy, nonoperative immobilization and analgesics, blocks Vertebral: Analgesics, blocks, vertebroplasty
Spinal instability or collapse	Operative fixation
Cord compression	Operative decompression, steroids, radiation therapy, chemotherapy

TABLE 46–2 Mirels Scoring System

Variable	Score		
	1	2	3
Site	Upper limb	Lower limb	Peritrochanter
Pain	Mild	Moderate	Functional
Lesion	Blastic	Mixed	Lytic
Size	$<\frac{1}{3}$	$\frac{1}{3}-\frac{2}{3}$	$>\frac{2}{3}$

Example: A lytic lesion of the humerus involving ¾ of the cross-sectional diameter with pain on motion = Mirels score of 10. (A score of 9 or above suggests a probability of fracture high enough to warrant prophylactic fixation. A score of 8 suggests a 15% probability of impending fracture, and a score of 7 or less suggests a low probability of fracture, allowing for nonoperative management.)

metabolic activity rather than increased mineral turnover, which can result from other, nonmalignant conditions. In situations in which neurologic compromise is secondary to the metastatic process, MRI is the study of choice. Tumor markers should be obtained in situations in which hormonal therapy or chemotherapy is anticipated for treatment. Baseline serum calcium, total protein (for correct interpretation of calcium levels), and phosphorous levels should be obtained if bisphosphonates are to be used to treat bone pain.

In addition to the immediate offer to treat bone metastasis pain, usually nonsteroidal anti-inflammatory medication (i.e., ibuprofen) and/or opioids for pain, there are three immediate concerns the clinician should address: (1) Is there a pathologic fracture? (2) Is there an impending pathologic fracture? and (3) Is there neurologic compromise (cord compression)? If the answer to any of these is yes, orthopedic consultation should be considered. Pathologic fracture may not always be obvious, though crescendo pain leading up to the time of the break, sudden pain out of proportion to movement, or loading are suggestive.

SELECTING TREATMENT

Patients found to have bone metastases, with few exceptions, will have incurable disease. Evaluation for treatment and treatment, itself, may add to the burden of illness in cases of homebound patients with far-advanced disease. Other patients anticipating disease-directed chemotherapy or hormonal therapy may fear that attention to the management of symptoms or orthopedic complications of illness may distract their treating physicians from the primary goals of disease remission and increased survival. In contrast, some patients and physicians may have an unwarranted sense of resignation about the management of skeletal metastases resulting in lost opportunities to better prepare themselves for the remainder of the illness.

The concept of enhancement or preservation of quality of life as a legitimate primary clinical goal is well supported by the majority of medical specialties.[12] Although metastatic bone disease is notorious for its negative impact on the quality of life for cancer patients, Cheng[13] points out that existing instruments for measuring quality of life outcomes for procedures treating metastatic bone disease are inadequate and are hampered by the current reliance on physician reported outcomes.

Balancing disclosure to the patient of progression of ultimately lethal disease and the preservation of sense of hope is the cardinal test of a physician's communication skill when providing palliative care. To do this, the physician must willingly communicate accurate information about the specific problems related to bone metastasis as well as more general knowledge about the nature of the underlying disease and its prognosis while observing and acknowledging the impact of this information on the patient.

Many treatments are effective at achieving immediate goals (e.g., surgical reduction of a fracture). However, it may be less obvious if achievement of the immediate goal will contribute to enhancement of quality of life promoted by durable pain relief, increased function, and freedom from additional burdens (cost, adjuvant therapies, distraction from pressing personal matters). To achieve these longer term goals, the physician should take the opportunity managing pain well allows to encourage the patient to seek guidance in addressing important issues by discussing them with other consulting physicians, social workers, those entrusted with the patient's spiritual care, and family members.

MANAGEMENT OF SELECTED SYNDROMES

Painful Bony Metastases

Palliation of the patient with painful bone metastases begins with the patient's complaint and should not be deferred until radiographic evaluation is completed. Once the necessity for operative intervention is ruled out by clinical examination and radiographic evaluation, pharmacotherapy and radiation therapy are the mainstays of management of pain from skeletal metastases. In presentations consistent with impending or established pathologic fracture, management of pain should not be deferred in anticipation of operative intervention.

Pharmacotherapy

The numerous mechanisms of bone pain and the variety of neoplasia metastasizing to bone provide numerous targets for pharmaco-therapeutic intervention for the relief of pain. Depending on the status of the disease, the tolerances and wishes of the patient, any single agent or a combination of these agents can be used for the management of pain in addition to other goals of therapy such as prolonged survival (chemotherapy), amelioration of hypercalcemia (chemotherapy, bisphosphonates), improved appetite (steroids), or control of fever (nonsteroidals). Cytotoxic chemotherapy, hormonal therapy, nonsteroidal anti-inflammatory drugs (NSAIDs), steroidal agents, opioid analgesics, bisphosphonates, and calcitonin have all been used for the relief of painful bony metastases. All of these modalities have the potential for major side effects, including death, which have to be anticipated in this vulnerable patient population with major comorbidities. The therapeutic nihilism sometimes directed toward the "terminal" patient in the nursing home and hospice settings should not blind the clinician to cytotoxic treatments known to be highly effective against certain cancers, such as small cell carcinoma and lymphomas. By contrast, anti-inflammatory medications such as ibuprofen, available over the counter, can lead to renal compromise, gastrointestinal hemorrhage, and platelet dysfunction.

Hormonal therapy has a potentially important role for control of bone pain in cancers of the breast, prostate, and endometrium and referral to an oncologist should be definitely considered, especially in cases in which it was not previously used. The patient should be cautioned that initiation of these therapies can be followed by a "flare" of bone pain prior to obtaining durable relief.

NSAIDs (Table 46-3), included in the first step of the World Health Organization step-ladder[14] for cancer pain control, are known to be effective in the management of cancer pain.[15] They can be given concurrently with opioids but should not be given to patients receiving corticosteroids or anticoagulants and thrombocytopenic patients. NSAIDs should be avoided in patients with renal impairment, congestive heart failure, and liver disease. Extreme caution is also advised in the treatment of the elderly. The risk of renal impairment from NSAIDs is increased in patients with advanced age, preexisting renal impairment, heart failure, hepatic dysfunction, hypovolemia, concomitant therapy with other nephrotoxic agents (including diuretics), and elevated of angiotensin II or catecholamine levels.[16] Toxicity is the most significant factor limiting long-term use.[17] Major complications are not necessarily preceded by minor ones.

When opioids are included in the treatment regimen, common opioid side effects should be anticipated and discussed. Constipation is an opioid side effect to which

TABLE 46-3 Nonopioid Analgesic Agents

Generic name	Recommended Starting Oral Dose (mg)*	Dosing Schedule	Maximum Oral Dose (mg/day)	Comments
Celecoxib (Celebrex) COX-2 inhibitor	650	Q 4-6 hr	4000 (short term)	No effect on platelet aggregation
Choline magnesium trisalicylate (Trilisate)	500–1000	Q 12 hr	4000	Little effect on platelet aggregation. 500 mg/5 mL liquid
Ibuprofen (Motrin, Advil)	400	Q 6 hr	3200	100 mg/5 mL suspension
Ketoprofen (Orudis)	25	Q 6-8 hr	300	
Ketorolac (Toradol)-IV	15–30	Q 6 hr	120	Use no longer than 5 days due to serious risk of gastrointestinal bleeds. If less than 50 kg, renal dysfunction, or >65 y.o. use 15 mg Q 6 hr. Healthy adults use 30 mg Q 6 hr
Nabumetone (Relafen)	1000	Q 24 hr	2000	Minimal platelet aggregation effects
Naproxen (Naprosyn, Aleve)	250	Q 12 hr	1025–1375	125/5 mL suspension
Salsalate (Disalcid)	500–1000	Q 12 hr	4000	Minimal platelet aggregation effects
Tramadol (Ultram)	25–50	Q 4-6 hr	400	Slow titration, avoid selective serotonin reuptake inhibitors (SSRIs)

Nonsteroidal anti-inflammatory drugs and COX-2s should be avoided in the elderly and congestive heart failure (CHF) due to risk of renal failure and gastrointestinal bleeds.
*Should be reduced by $1/2$ to $2/3$ in the elderly, those on multiple drugs, or those with renal insufficiency. Some patients may require or tolerate less or more.
Courtesy of James B. Ray, PharmD.

tolerance does not develop and should be prophylaxed against with a stimulant laxative. Nausea is a frequent side effect of opioids that can usually be prevented by use of an antiemetic in patients with a history of opioid-induced nausea. Stimulants (methylphenidate [Ritalin]) can be used for opioid-induced sedation. Counseling about and prophylaxis for possible opioid side effects increases compliance. Reassurance that use of opioids for management of cancer pain will not cause addiction is frequently necessary to increase compliance. Because of the potential for dose-limiting side effects and reluctance of many patients to escalate opioid doses, a strategy using the least amount of opioid necessary for relief of pain is employed. Nonopioids and other treatment modalities can be used with opioids for "opioid sparing" to accomplish this. A particularly difficult problem in the use of opioids for bone pain is the management of "breakthrough" pain, usually incident or functional pain (pain that is exacerbated by activity). The doses of systemic opioids necessary to provide pain relief during these episodes, which is usually only partial relief, often result in disabling side effects that undermine overall quality of life. More rapid-acting opioids or delivery systems can partly overcome this problem, but when this phenomenon presents itself, consideration should be given to other modalities of treatment, including surgery and radiation therapy.

Although many patients and orthopedists are familiar with oxycodone as a component of frequently prescribed compound medications for orthopedic conditions and postoperative pain, they may not be aware that the acetaminophen content of these drugs (325 mg) limits their use for bone cancer pain. The maximum 24-hour allowance for acetaminophen in an adult without liver disease or heavy alcohol consumption is 3000 mg. The amount would be even less in the elderly. In a compound such as Roxicet or Percocet, containing 325 mg of acetaminophen and 5 mg of oxycodone, the maximum daily amount of oxycodone that could be given as an agent compounded with acetaminophen without incurring acetaminophen toxicity would be less than 50 mg—far short of what is often required for the effective relief of bone cancer pain. In instances in which oxycodone is to be prescribed, using the uncompounded form is recommended to avoid potential acetaminophen toxicity and to provide greater flexibility in dosing for breakthrough pain and conversion to long-acting forms (OxyContin).

Two other medications encountered commonly in orthopedic and hospital practice, dolophine (Darvocet) and meperidine (Demerol), have no role in cancer pain management because of potential side effects of their metabolites that can occur in the presence of renal compromise, particularly in the elderly.

The pronounced anti-inflammatory properties of steroids (hydrocortisone, dexamethasone) have made them useful for the treatment of pain occurring with widely disseminated bone metastases, or as an adjunct to management of pain complicated by neural compromise, especially if there are other symptoms such as anorexia, nausea, and generalized malaise that may also respond to them. Their use must be considered in light of several possible significant side effects that include immunosuppression, peptic ulceration, hyperglycemia, psychological disturbances, and myopathy. Prophylaxis against peptic ulceration is provided by concurrent use of a proton pump inhibitor.

Bisphosphonates have been approved for the treatment of malignant hypercalcemia and the reduction of orthopedic complications of breast cancer and multiple myeloma. Up to 50% of patients with symptomatic bone metastases treated with bisphosphonates report relief of bone pain.[18] Because of all of these actions, this class of drugs has become a significant addition to the pharmacopoeia of palliative care. The common denominator of these effects is the inhibition of osteoclastic bone resorption, though numerous mechanisms have been proposed about how this activity influences tumor biology. In the bisphosphonate group, pamidronate and clodronate have been studied the most, pamidronate being 10 times more potent than clodronate. Both agents can be given intravenously or orally, though the parenteral route is better tolerated and preferred for single-dose therapy for the management of bone pain. Pamidronate has emerged as the most commonly used agent and is usually dosed 90 to 120 mg as a single infusion when given for bone pain. Unlike pamidronate, which *cannot* be given subcutaneously, clodronate can,[19] allowing it to be given in settings where intravenous access is not possible. Newer, more potent bisphosphonates that can be given orally and transdermally are in development.

Adverse side effects of bisphosphonates include nausea; transient, flu-like cytokine release syndrome with fever, myalgias, and leukopenia; hypocalcemia (increased risk in patients with previous neck radiation or thyroidectomy due to diminished parathyroid hormone production); tissue damage from extravasation from intravenous sites (with pamidronate and other amino bisphosphonates); and renal impairment. Renal dysfunction is a relative contraindication to bisphosphonate therapy requiring a diminished dose or increased infusion time. All patients should be well hydrated prior to bisphosphonate therapy.

Recent studies[20] showing a decrease in urinary excretion of products of bone resorption (pyridinoline and deoxypyridinoline) correlating with improved pain scores following pamidronate infusion suggest that monitoring urine markers of bone resorption will help identify those patients who would continue to benefit from therapy.

Except for chemotherapy and hormonal therapy, the available regimens for relief of bone cancer pain work indirectly through their effects on the peripheral and central nervous systems, the host inflammatory response, or osteoclastic activity. A discrete bone cancer pain mechanism, not simply a combination of generalized inflammatory and neuropathic states, has been proposed recently that recognizes heightened neural sensitivity to nociceptive impulses and as of yet unidentified humoral substances.[21] This pain model could broaden the pharmacologic repertoire for pain control to include antineuropathic agents and future, more selective pharmacologic approaches to bone cancer pain management.

Although the overwhelming majority of metastatic bone pain syndromes uncomplicated by impending or established pathologic fracture respond well to systemic pharmacotherapies, regional or axial analgesic delivery strategies using opioids anesthetics, and N-methyl-D-aspartate antagonists (e.g., clonidine) should be considered in cases of regional excessive disease burden with poorly controlled pain or when unacceptable side effects from systemic therapy occur in patients who are not candidates for surgery or disease modifying treatments such as radiation or chemotherapy.

Radiotherapy

Radiotherapy is highly effective treatment for the management of bone cancer pain and should be considered a possible future option for pain management in any patient with known bone metastases. An extensive analysis by McQuay et al.[22] of 13 trials showed that at least 49% of patients achieved 50% pain relief (range 28 to 81%) and 30% had a complete response at 1 month post radiation therapy. The median duration of complete pain relief was 12 weeks.

When recommending radiation therapy for the relief of pain to a patient, it is important to differentiate this goal from the goal of remission or cure, as the patient may know of someone cured of cancer because of primary radiation therapy. Patients also should understand that pain relief following radiation therapy may not be immediate (sometimes a delay of 3 weeks), especially if given in small fractions over a longer period of time. Analgesics and/or dexamethasone (an effective analgesic therapy for bone pain) should be prescribed as radiation therapy is planned, but may need to be tapered if treatment is effective. Some patients will be reluctant to undergo radiation therapy for palliation of pain because of misconceptions about radiation side effects. A frequently asked question, regardless of the site of planned treatment, is, "Will I lose my hair?"

General considerations for radiation therapy include life expectancy and performance status of the patient; cell type, size, and location of the tumor; prior radiation treatment; ease of access to treatment facility; likelihood of the patient's ability to cooperate with positioning;

potential side effect profile; and the risk/benefit ratio of radiation treatment compared with other therapies.

No particular regimen has been shown to be superior when accounting for effectiveness and minimal toxicity, because of differences in trial methodology and the problems of interpreting the impact of concomitant therapies. In the United Kingdom, palliative radiation for bone metastases is generally given in single fractions, while in the United States, multiple fractions are preferred despite several studies that show[23,24] single fraction therapy is very effective for the palliation of bone pain. The advantage of single fraction therapy is not to be underestimated for patients with far-advanced illness during which the logistics of daily transport, the reimbursement limitations of the Medicare hospice benefit, and time spent in the health care environment collectively become a disincentive for pursuing this treatment.

In a review by Frassica, external beam radiation therapy is completely or partially effective for the relief of pain from bone metastases in approximately 70% of cases.[25] One retrospective[26] analysis showed that pain relief was related to radiation dose, regardless of tumor cell type, with the exceptions of carcinoma of the kidney and nonsmall cell carcinoma of the lung. Other studies have confirmed renal carcinoma's radio-resistance.[27] Myeloma, on the other hand, is quite sensitive to radiation, even at relatively low doses.

For patients with extensive bony metastases, large field radiation, encompassing as much as half of the body, or radioisotopes can be given under the condition that the patient does not have compromised hematopoietic function (>3000 WBC, > 100,000 platelets). For external beam radiation, some effects can be avoided by excluding the area from the field while others can be anticipated and prophylaxed against with antiemetics and antidiarrheals. If both halves of the body are to be treated an interval of 6 weeks for recovery of stem cell function has to be planned between treatment of each half.

Strontium 89 (Sr-89) is an analog of calcium that allows its uptake in the bone matrix resulting in suppression of osteoblastic activity that effectively relieves the pain of bone metastases.[28] It is given as a single-dose intravenous injection. Patients should be advised that they may experience a flare in pain 2 to 4 days following dosing, and should this occur their systemic analgesics can be up-titrated as needed. Myelosuppression is much milder than with other radiopharmaceuticals. Dosing can be repeated at 6-month intervals if myelosuppression has not occurred and if treatment is effective. Onset of pain relief occurs within a month and can last several months. It can be used in outpatients who are continent without extra radiation precautions. Delayed onset of relief and high cost are disadvantages. Both these issues must be considered in cases of very limited life expectancy (less than 6 weeks) When discussing these therapies with patients who are in this range of estimated survival, the health care provider should be prepared to conduct or arrange an honest and empathic discussion about prognosis.

Physiotherapy

Physiotherapy includes several treatment approaches that mitigate cancer-related pain. O'Gorman[29] outlined guidelines for the physiotherapy assessment and treatment of cancer pain in terminally ill patients. These principles emphasize whole patient assessment, regular follow-up, realism, safety, flexibility in the face of progressing illness, and willingness to involve friends and relatives in treatment planning and delivery. Physiotherapies useful in the treatment of cancer pain include exercise, massage, relaxation training, heat and cold therapies, acupuncture, electrotherapies, and splinting. Rehabilitation in this setting refers to maximizing the patient's potential and the restoration of the person, not improving physical strength and endurance.

Both acupuncture and transcutaneous nerve stimulators may improve pain in intractable pain in dying patients[30] though there are no prospective studies demonstrating the efficacy of either of these treatments for the relief of metastatic bone pain. There is retrospective evidence that acupuncture is effective for the relief of pain and reduced opioid requirements in a group of 339 cancer patients treated at a pain clinic, of whom some were presumed to have pain from bone metastases.[31] Increased mobility was also reported in this group. Acupuncture appears to have diminishing effect with increasing burden of neoplastic disease, perhaps because of the maximal stimulation of pain-relieving endogenous opioids (whose release is thought to be stimulated by acupuncture) that has already occurred or loss of endogenous opioids in these patients.

Splinting and use of collars can be used to diminish functional (incident) bone cancer pain, though care has to be taken to properly fit and pad them due to the increased risk of skin break down and nerve compression in this malnourished population.

Pain from Impending or Established Pathologic Fracture

The possibility of pathologic fracture should always be in the back of the clinician's mind when treating patients for bone cancer pain. Pathologic fracture may not always be obvious, though crescendo pain leading up to the time of the break and sudden pain out of proportion to movement or loading are suggestive of fracture. Pain that worsens with weight-bearing and relieved by rest is suggestive of impending fracture. The Mirels scoring

system (see earlier section) can be used to determine likelihood of pathologic fracture (see Table 46-2) as a basis for selecting therapy. Prophylactic treatment has been recommended for lesions more than 2.5 cm in diameter or greater than 50% of the bone cross section. Metastatic lesions of the proximal femur are at greatest risk for fracture of long bone lesions.[32] There is widespread agreement that fixation of an impending fracture is technically easier, less painful, and less likely to be associated with complications than fixation of an established fracture.

The decision to recommend prophylactic surgery for metastatic carcinoma to bone can be very difficult due to the four categories factored into decision making. These factors, as outlined by Rougraff,[33] are: (1) biologic activity of the tumor (some thyroid and prostate carcinomas metastatic to bone are associated with survivals in excess of 2 years), (2) responsiveness of the bone tumor to disease-directed therapy (chemotherapy and radiation therapy), (3) anatomic site of the tumor (weight-bearing versus non–weight-bearing and size of cortical defect), and (4) patient factors that include co-morbid illness and degree of anesthetic risk, expected cancer survival, and patient needs and expectations. Indications for prophylactic surgery based on patient considerations are of necessity harder to pin down than frank fracture, but include reasonable life expectancy (no consensus on this yet exists), prospect for improvement of the patient's lifestyle (often not completely assessed), prospect of facilitating general care (often not discussed due to fear of broaching future physical decline), and sufficient nondiseased regional bone allowing fixation (sometimes the only reason openly discussed for *not* doing surgery). Rougraff gives a clinical rule of thumb that patients with appropriate and unchanged cognitive skills and acceptable liver and kidney function typically benefit from a surgical intervention before their demise. Contraindications surgery include general categories related to anesthetic risk, far advanced disease or imminent demise, severe malnutrition, active infection, and reasons more specific to orthopedic postoperative care and rehabilitation: agitated delirium, peripheral venous thrombosis, and inadequate suitable bone for reconstruction.

The choice of operative fixation includes various forms of internal fixation and resection with or without prosthetic replacement. The use of methyl methacrylate as an artificial matrix has greatly enhanced the possibilities of operative fixation as well as direct relief of pain when used for vertebroplasty (cementoplasty) for bony collapse. Mega-prostheses are increasingly being employed to address the problem of recurrent or progressive disease in patients with increasingly long survival. Loss of fixation from recurrent and progressive cancer requires a different approach to operative fixation than the treatment of traumatic fracture in nondiseased bone. These differences may not be apparent to some orthopedists who may have much trauma experience, but few cancer patient referrals.

Pain from Spinal Metastases

Metastatic disease of the spine has been found in 36% of patients who died from cancer although a significant number of instances of vertebral collapse (22%) in this series had a nonmalignant etiology.[34] Not all pain from metastatic bone disease of the spine is due to localized pain from individual metastases—back pain in patients with spinal metastases can also be caused by spinal instability, nerve root or cord compression, or a combination of these (Table 46–4). Spinal instability accounts for back pain in approximately 10% of patients with disseminated cancer.[35] The Harrington classification[36] stratifies spinal metastases according to degree of bone involvement, neurologic compromise, and vertebral body collapse. Each of the five classes has specific therapeutic implications (Table 46–5). Most metastatic diseases of the spine occur anteriorly in the vertebral body with implications for the approach to operative reconstruction.

Generally, for operative reconstruction, an anterior approach is used. A posterior approach is used to complement an anterior approach in cases of severe destruction encompassing the posterior elements.

Back pain is almost invariably the presentation of spinal cord and cauda equina compression. Paresis follows these symptoms in this palliative care emergency. Anesthesia and urinary retention are late signs of spinal cord compression (SCC), and neurologic compromise at presentation is associated with a diminished chance of full neurologic recovery.[37]

Failure to control spinal pain with opioids or a precipitous rise in opioid requirements should alert the practitioner to the possibility of SCC. One series[38] demonstrated survival was significantly better for patients presenting with good functional status. In this

TABLE 46–4	Mechanisms of Pain Due to Spinal Metastases and Treatment Selection
Disruption of vertebral cortical bone with direct extension to surrounding non-neural soft tissue	Radiation therapy, analgesics, regional block
Nerve root compression or invasion	Radiation therapy/steroids, analgesics, laminectomy
Pathologic compression fracture	Analgesics, vertebroplasty, operative reduction in cases of instability or neural compromise
Spinal instability	Operative fixation
Cord or equina compression	Radiation therapy/steroids, operative decompression, analgesics

TABLE 46–5 Harrington Classification of Spinal Metastases with Treatment Options

Harrington Class	Treatment Options
Class I—No significant neurologic compromise	Analgesics Local radiation Chemotherapy*
Class II—Bone involvement without collapse	Analgesics Local radiation Chemotherapy
Class III—Neurologic compromise in the absence of bony involvement	Analgesics/steroids Local radiation Chemotherapy
Class IV—Vertebral collapse or instability without significant neurologic compromise	Analgesics Operative intervention Vertebroplasty Local radiation
Class V—Vertebral collapse with major neurologic compromise	Analgesics/steroids Operative intervention Local radiation Chemotherapy

*For chemosensitive tumors in patients with good performance status.

series 32% of 166 patients admitted to the hospital with malignant spinal cord compression died before discharge and the median survival was 82 days. Seventy-nine percent of those discharged returned to home. Because of increasing survival times for breast and prostate cancer, it is likely that the incidence of SCC will increase. Heightened attention to performance status at presentation of patients with SCC unbiased by therapeutic nihilism will lead to more realistic expectations about survival, selection of treatment, and discharge disposition.

Considerable community resources are necessary for the care of SCC patients discharged home as the burden of care will increase for the large majority of these patients. Secondary medical problems that can be anticipated in this patient group include pain, constipation, urinary retention and infection, and decubitus ulcers. These secondary problems should be acknowledged as part of developing an individual treatment algorithm at presentation.

CONCLUSION

The act of palliating symptomatic bone metastases represents one of the most challenging and gratifying exercises in interdisciplinary care. This problem is ideal for the interdisciplinary model because of the many dimensions that are touched by it. Treatments make no sense without some understanding by patients and families of the context of advanced oncologic illness, while the future of the illness may seem senseless without the relief that treatment can offer. It is an exciting time to improve our collective skill in the treatment of painful bony metastases. New avenues of personal, social, and spiritual inquiry to better tailor treatments are developing while new understandings of the biology of cancer and the physiology of pain will bring the process of healing in closer alignment to the process of nature itself.

REFERENCES

1. Predey TA, Sewall LE, Smith SJ: Percutaneous vertebroplasty: New treatment for vertebral compression fractures. Am Fam Physician 66:611–615, 2002.
2. Mirra JM: Bone Tumors. Malvern, PA, Lea and Febiger, 1989, p 1498.
3. Vainion A, Auvinen A, et al: Prevalence of symptoms among patients with advanced cancer: An international collaborative study. J Pain Symptom Manage 12:3–10, 1996.
4. Portnoy RK, Payne D, Jacobsen P: Breakthrough pain: Characteristics and impact in patients with cancer pain. Pain 81:129–134, 1999.
5. Janjan NA, Payne R, Gillis T, et al: Presenting symptoms in patients referred to a multidisciplinary clinic for bone metastases. J Pain Symptom Manage 16:171–178, 1998.
6. Katagiri H, et al: Determining the site of primary cancer in patients with skeletal metastasis of unknown origin. Cancer 89:533–537, 1999.
7. Cramer SF, Fried L, Carter KJ: The cellular basis of metastatic bone disease in patients with lung cancer. Cancer 48:2649–2660, 1981.
8. Galasko CSB: Skeletal metastases and mammary cancer. Ann R Coll Surg 50:3–28, 1972.
9. Mercadante S, Casuccio A, Fulfaro F: The course of symptom frequency and intensity in advanced cancer patients followed at home. J Pain Symptom Manage 20:104–112, 2000.
10. Mirels H: Metastatic disease in long bones: A proposed scoring system for diagnosing impending pathological fractures. Clin Orthop 249:256–264, 1989.
11. Peterson JJ, Kransdorf MJ, O'Connor MI: Diagnosis of occult bone metastases: Positron emission tomography. Clin Orthop Relat Res 415S:S120–S128, 2003.
12. Cassel C, Foley K: Principles of Care of Patients at End of Life: An Emerging Consensus among the Specialties of Medicine. Report sponsored by the Milbank Memorial Fund. December, 1999. Available at http://www.milbank.org/. Accessed July 28, 2004.
13. Cheng EY: Prospective quality of life research in bony metastatic disease. Clin Orthop Relate Res 415S:S289–S297, 2003.
14. World Health Organization. Cancer pain relief and palliative care. Report of a WHO expert committee [World health Organization Technical Report Series, 804]. Geneva, Switzerland, World Health Organization, 1990, pp 1–75.
15. Levy M: Pharmacological treatment of cancer pain. N Engl J Med 335:1124–1132. 1996.
16. Jacox A, Carr DB, Payne R, et al: Mangement of Cancer Pain. AHCPR publication No.94-0592: Clinical Practice Guideline No. 9. Rockville, MD, U.S. Department of Health and Human Services, Public Health Service, March 1994.
17. Pace V: Use of non-steroidal anti-inflammatory drugs in cancer. Palliat Med 9:273–286, 1995.
18. Coleman RE: How can we improve the treatment of bone metastases further? Curr Opin Oncol 10(Suppl 1):S7–S13, 1998.
19. Walker P, Watanabe S, Lawlor P, Hanson J, Pereira J, Bruera E: Subcutaneous clodronate: A study evaluating efficacy in hypercalcemia of malignancy. Ann Oncol 8:915–916, 1997.
20. Vinholes J, Guo C-Y, Purohit OP, et al: Metabolic effects of pamidronate in patients with metastatic bone disease. Brit J Cancer 73:1089–1095, 1996.
21. Clohisy DR, Mantyh PW: Bone cancer pain. Clin Orthop Relate Res 415S:S279–S288, 2003.
22. McQuay HJ, Carrol D, Moore RA: Radiotherapy for painful bone metastases: A systemic review. Clin Oncol 9:150–154, 1997.
23. Bone Pain Trial Working Party: 8 Gy single fraction radiotherapy for the treatment of metastatic skeletal pain: Randomized comparison with a multifraction schedule over 12 months of patient follow-up. Radiother Oncol 52:111–121, 1999.
24. Steenland E, Leer JW, van Houweligen H, et al: The effect of a single fraction compared to multiple fractions on painful bone metastases: A global analysis of the Dutch Bone Metastasis Study. Radiotherap Oncol 52:101–109, 1999.
25. Frassica DA: General principles of external beam radiation therapy for skeletal metastases. Clin Orthop Relate Res 415S:S158–S164, 2003.
26. Arcangeli G, Micheli A, Arcangeli G, Giannarelli D, et al: The responsiveness of bone metastases to radiotherapy: The effect of site, histology, and radiation dose on pain relief. Radiother Oncol 14:95–101, 1989.
27. Onufrey V, Mohiuddin M: Radiation therapy in the treatment of metastatic renal cell carcinoma. Int J Radiat Oncol Bio Phys 11:2007–2009, 1985.
28. Robinson RG: Strontium-89—Precursor targeted therapy for pain relief of blastic metastatic disease. Cancer 72:3433–3435, 1993.
29. O'Gorman B, Elfred A: Physiotherapy. In Simpson UM, Budd K (eds): Cancer pain management. Oxford, Oxford University Press, 2000.
30. Pan CX, Morrison S, Ness J, et al: Complementary and alternative medicine in the management of pain, dyspnea, and nausea and vomiting near the end of life: A systematic review. J Pain Sympt Manag 20:374–387, 2000.
31. Filshie J, Redman D: Acupuncture and malignant pain problems. Eur J Surg Oncol 11:389–394, 1985.
32. Harrington KD: Orthopaedic management of extremity and pelvic lesions. Clin Orthop 312:136–147, 1995.

33. Rougraff B: Indications for operative treatment. In Ward WG, Peabody TD (eds): Orthopedic Management of Metastatic Disease. Orthop Clin North Am 31:567–575, 2000.

34. Wong DA, Fornasier VL, MacNab I: Spinal metastasis: the obvious, the occult, and the impostors. Spine 15:1, 1990.

35. Galasko CSB, Sylvester BS: Back pain in patients treated for malignant tumors. Clin Oncol 4:273–283, 1978.

36. Harrington KD: Current concepts review: Metastasic disease of the spine. J Bone Joint Surg Am 68:1110, 1986.

37. Shapiro WR, Posner JB: Medical versus surgical treatment of metastatic spinal cord tumors. In Thompson RA, Green JA (eds): Controversies in Neurology. New York, Raven Press, 1983, pp 57–65.

38. Cowap J, Hardy JR, A'Hern R: Outcome of malignant spinal cord compression at a cancer center: Implications for palliative care services. J Pain Symptom Manage 19:257–264, 2000.

39. Mirels H: The classic: metastatic disease in long bones: A proposed scoring system for diagnosing impending pathological fractures. Clin Orthop Relate Res 415S: S4–S13, 2003.

CHAPTER 47

Management of Dermatologic Problems

LUCIA L. SCARPINO, MS, RN, CWOCN

PRESSURE ULCERS

Definition and Staging

Pressure ulcers represent a type of tissue damage caused by prolonged pressure or other forces, such as friction and shear. Pressure ulcers occur over bony prominences on the sacrum, coccyx, ischium, heels, trochanter, occiput, malleolus, scapula, and elbows. Pressure ulcers are staged according to the depth of tissue injury. According to the Agency for Health Care Policy and Research Clinical Practice Guidelines[1,2]: (1) Stage I: an observable pressure-related alteration of intact skin whose indicators as compared with an adjacent or opposite area on the body may include changes in one or more of the following: skin temperature (warmth or coolness), tissue consistency (firm or baggy feeling), sensation (pain, itching). The ulcer appears as a defined area of persistent redness in lightly pigmented skin, whereas in darker skin tones, the ulcer may appear with persistent red, blue, or purple hues. (2) Stage II: partial thickness skin loss involving epidermis or dermis, or both. The ulcer is superficial and presents clinically as an abrasion, blister, or shallow crater. (3) Stage III: full-thickness skin loss involving damage to or necrosis of subcutaneous tissue that may extend down to, but not through, underlying fascia. The ulcer presents clinically as a deep crater with or without undermining of adjacent tissue. (4) Stage IV: full thickness skin loss with extensive destruction, tissue necrosis or damage to muscle, bone or supporting structures (e.g., tendon, joint capsule). Undermining and sinus tracts may also be associated with Stage IV pressure ulcers. (5) Unstageable ulcer: the depth of tissue damage is not visible due to necrotic or slough tissue.

Risk Factors for Skin Breakdown

Extrinsic Factors

- Pressure: Perpendicular force on tissue causes the capillaries in the dermal layer to collapse, leading to the ischemic process.
- Shear: Parallel force, which causes tissue to slide and twist, therefore disrupting blood vessels in the area.
- Friction: External force exerted when the skin is dragged across a surface.
- Moisture: Prolonged exposure to moisture will result in the softening and wrinkling of the skin.

Intrinsic Factors

- Nutritional status: vitamin C, zinc, and mineral deficiency and hypoproteinemia, hypoalbuminemia, and cachexia.[3]
- Impaired oxygen perfusion related to anemia, hypotension, and circulation.
- Immunosuppression.
- Obesity.
- Chronic medical conditions/drug therapy: corticosteroids.
- Immobility: related to pain, sedation, mental status, and paralysis.
- Aged skin.

Prevention of Pressure Ulcers

- Sleep surface: pressure reducing or relieving (static air mattress, dynamic sleep surface, low air loss, fluid air).
- Maintain turning schedule every 1 to 2 hours.
- Use positioning devices to prevent bony prominences from touching.
- Use pressure-relieving seat/wheelchair cushion. Limit time in chair to 2 hour intervals. Reposition every 15 minutes.
- Position head of bed at or below 30 degrees to reduce sacral pressure.
- Elevate foot of bed to minimize shearing forces.
- Use turning sheets for positioning.
- Use trapeze to assist with repositioning and minimize shear.
- Use elbow/heel protectors.

- Cleanse skin with nonirritating, nondrying soap.
- Hydrate all skin surfaces with moisturizing lotion every 8 hours and as often as necessary.
- Protect skin from urine/fecal incontinence. Use skin protective barrier creams, fecal/urine collectors, and absorbent diapers/pads.
- Monitor nutritional status using nutritionist, protein, and caloric supplements. The Agency for Health Care Policy and Research[2] recommends 30 to 40 k calories/kg of body weight/day for total calories and 1 to 1.5 g protein/kg of body weight/day for total protein.
- Educate patient and family on skin care and pressure ulcer prevention.
- Donut cushions are contraindicated for prevention.

Treatment Options for Pressure Ulcers

The goal in treating pressure ulcers in the terminally ill is different than in the general patient population. The focus should be less on healing the pressure ulcer, and more on promoting comfort, controlling drainage and odor, and enhancing a patient's quality of life.[4]

- Consider the caregiver's time and ability to perform the care.
- When choosing a treatment option, the main goal is to promote moist wound healing, control drainage, and protect periwound tissue.[5]
- Necrotic tissue impedes wound healing and must be removed.
- Cavities and tunnels must be filled or packed to prevent fluid buildup and abscess formation.
- Heel ulcers with dry eschar and no signs of infection should not be debrided.[6]
- See Table 47–1 for treatment options.

Dressing Types

- Film dressings (semipermeable allowing moisture vapors to pass out of the wound and oxygen to pass

TABLE 47–1 Treatment Options

Wound Type	Dressing Objective	Dressing
Clean, red, minimal exudate	Maintain moist wound environment Protect healing wound base Prevent further trauma	Transparent dressings Hydrogel Hydrocolloids
Clean, red, moderate exudate	Control exudate Maintain moist wound environment Protect healing wound base Prevent further trauma	Foams Hydrocolloids Calcium alginate Hydrofibers
Tan/yellow slough, minimal exudate	Autolytic debridement Maintain moist wound environment Protect healing wound base	Transparent Hydrogel Hydrocolloids
Tan/yellow slough, moderate exudate	Autolytic debridement Control exudate Maintain moist wound environment	Hydrocolloids Calcium alginates Hydrofibers Absorption granules or dressings
Tan/yellow slough, high exudate	Autolytic debridement Control exudate Maintain moist wound environment Protect periwound tissue	Calcium alginates Absorption granules or dressings Foams Hydrofibers
Necrotic/dry eshcar	Remove devitalized tissue Autolytic debridement Enzymatic debridement	Foams Hydrogels Hydrocolloids Enzymatic debriding agent
Cavities with necrotic tissue and exudate	Autolytic debridement Fill dead space Control exudates	Wound fillers Calcium alginates Hydrofibers Enzymatic debriding agent

into the wound; impermeable to microorganisms; maintains a moist environment; promotes autolytic debridement; nonabsorptive; can be used as secondary dressing; may remain in place for 5 to 7 days; examples are: OpSite, Tegaderm, Bioclusive.)

- Foam (soft polyurethane foam for wounds that are minimally to moderately exudating; nonadherent; maintains moist environment; promotes autolytic debridement; can be used as secondary dressing; may remain in place for 1 to 4 days; examples are: Allevyn, Flexzan, Lyofoam.)
- Hydrogel (organic polymers gel with a water content of up to 90%; provides moisture to a dry wound; promotes autolytic debridement; minimal absorption; requires secondary dressing; available in impregnated gauze, gel, and gel sheets; examples are: IntraSite, Vigilon, Restore Hydrogel Dressings.)
- Hydrocolloids (use on low-exudating wounds; absorbs wound drainage and forms a gel; waterproof; maintains moist environment; promotes autolytic debridement; no secondary dressing required; available in granules, powder, and paste; may remain in place 5 to 7 days; examples are: Comfeel, Duoderm, Restore.)
- Alginate (calcium or calcium/sodium salts derived from seaweed; hydrophilic gel produced from the sodium/calcium ion exchange; use on heavily exudating wounds; maintains moist environment; not used on dry wounds or eschar; nonadherent; secondary dressing required; available in sheets or ropes; may remain in place 1 to 7 days; examples are: Sorbsan, Restore Calcicare, Algisite.)
- Enzymatic debriding agents (selective enzymatic ointment used to remove necrotic tissue; wound surface must be kept moist; eschar must be crosshatched with a scalpel for ointment to penetrate tissue and be effective[6,7]; debriding agents are used for 14 to 30 days until necrotic tissue is removed and wound base is clean; examples are: Accuzyme, Santyl, Elase.)
- Silver dressings (broad-spectrum antimicrobial agent, including gram-negative and positive bacteria, fungal organisms, and antibiotic-resistant bacteria; wound surface must be kept moist; effective in wound from 3 to 7 days; various types of silver-impregnated dressings available from alginates, charcoal, hydrofibers, and powders; examples are Aquacel Ag, Acticoat, Actisorb Silver.)

STOMAS AND FISTULAE

Definition

Stoma is a surgically created opening into the abdomen to provide an outlet for the elimination of stool or urine. Fistula is an abnormal opening between organs either internal or internal to external. Fistulae can occur as a result of previous pelvic radiation therapy, tumor erosion, or gastrointestinal (GI) cancer.

Sites/Types of Ostomies

There are several types of ostomies created depending on the extent of the disease and the amount of intestine involved with tumor. The anatomic location of the ostomy will determine the type of drainage eliminated.

Sites

Colostomy (large intestine) sites

- Ascending colostomy: ascending portion of large intestine brought to the skin surface. Stool will be liquid and excreted 90 to 120 minutes after ingesting liquids or food.
- Transverse colostomy: transverse colon brought out to the skin surface. Stool will be liquid to semipasty.
- Descending colostomy: descending colon brought out to the skin surface. Stool will be soft formed and will take on normal preoperative bowel habits.
- Sigmoid colostomy: sigmoid colon brought out to the skin surface. Stool will be formed.

Jejunostomy/Ileostomy (small intestine) sites

- Jejunostomy: jejunum brought to the skin surface. Drainage is watery and copious.
- Ileum: ileum brought to the skin surface. Stool is liquid and excreted 90 to 120 minutes after ingesting liquids or food.

Types

- Loop colostomy or ileostomy. A loop of colon or ileum is brought to the skin surface and stabilized postoperatively with a support device such as a plastic rod or red rubber catheter. Each of these devices remains in place an average of 7 to 10 days, or longer depending on abdominal distension or healing time.
- Double-barrel colostomy or ileostomy. The bowel is divided and both ends are brought out to the skin surface. The proximal end from the mouth to the stoma is the functioning colostomy. The distal portion from the stoma to the rectum is the mucous fistula. The main function of the mucous fistula is to provide an outlet for mucous buildup or drainage produced by tumor. Mucous fistulae can be located anywhere on the abdomen and are often at the base of the abdominal incision.
- End colostomy or ileostomy. Performed after an abdominal perineal resection (APR) where the rectum is removed for rectal cancer. May also be performed in conjunction with the Hartmann's pouch in which

the diseased colon is removed and the rectal stump sewn over and left in place.

Urinary Diversions

- Ileal conduit. This is the most common type of urinary diversion created after bladder removal. A portion of the terminal ileum is separated from the small intestine and the ureters are implanted into it. The ileum is brought to the skin surface, and a stoma is created. Urine will drain from the kidneys through the ureters into the piece of ileum and be collected in an external bag.
- Indiana pouch. This is a continent urinary diversion. An internal reservoir for urine is created from the ascending colon, ileal cecal valve, and terminal ileum. Urine is drained from reservoir with a catheter every 4 hours. Because the urine is collected internally, no external pouch is needed.
- Nephrostomy. A tube is inserted through the flank into the renal pelvis of the kidney. The nephrostomy tube is inserted to provide an outlet for urine when the ureters are obstructed. Nephrostomy tubes are replaced every 2 to 3 months.

Care of the Ostomy

Skin Care

- Skin care is an essential component of ostomy care.
- Check for skin reactions with each pouch change.
- Cleanse the skin with warm, soapy water. Avoid premoistened baby wipes and soaps with oil or moisturizers. These can interfere with the adherence of the pouching system.
- Trim body hair around the stoma with an electric razor every week.
- Pouch covers will prevent skin irritation caused by excessive perspiration under the plastic pouch.
- Ileal conduit care is similar to colostomy/ileostomy care.

Stoma Care

- The stoma should be red and moist. Bleeding will normally occur when cleansing the stoma.
- Avoid trauma and hot water to the stoma if the patient is on blood thinners.
- Stoma swelling may occur from trauma or abdominal pressure.

Replacing/Emptying Pouch

- Change pouch every 5 to 7 days early in the morning when bowel activity is minimal. Immediately change the pouch if the seal is broken and leakage occurs.
- Empty stool, gas, or urine when the pouch is one-third full.
- Urinary diversions or ostomies with high watery output should be placed to gravity drainage bags to prevent overfilling.
- Gravity bags used with urinary diversions should be cleansed daily with half strength vinegar and water.

Odor and Gas

- Pouches are odor proof. Avoid placing pinholes in pouches to eliminate gas, as odors will escape as well.
- Odor eliminators are available to place in pouches to decrease odors.
- Spray air fresheners in the room when emptying stool.
- Avoid gas and odor-producing foods such as asparagus, baked beans, broccoli, brussels sprouts, cabbage, cauliflower, eggs, fish, and onions.
- Avoid using straws, smoking, chewing gum, and drinking carbonated beverages.
- Odors may decrease by adding buttermilk, parsley, spearmint, or yogurt to the diet.
- Over-the-counter anti-gas tablets are available.

Constipation

- Stool softeners or laxatives should be prescribed with opioids to prevent constipation.
- If oral intake is not an issue, increasing fluids and adding black coffee, prune juice, and bran to the diet will prevent constipation.
- Colostomy irrigations can be performed daily with 1000 mL tap water as the patient tolerates.

Diarrhea

- Main goal is to increase the bulk of the stool. Add foods such as applesauce, bananas, boiled milk, rice, cheese, tapioca, and tea to the diet.
- Medications such as Metamucil will increase the bulk of the stool.
- Antidiarrheal medication such as Lomotil and tincture of opium can be given to decrease bowel motility.[8] See Table 47–2 for troubleshooting guidelines.

Care of the Continent Urinary Diversion

- No external pouch is required.
- The skin and stoma is cleansed with soap and water and a dry dressing or bandage is applied.
- The internal pouch must be catheterized every 4 hours around the clock with a clean red rubber catheter.[9-11]
- The internal pouch must be irrigated with normal saline to break up any accumulated mucous.

TABLE 47–2   **Troubleshooting Guidelines**

Problem	Description	Cause	Remedy
Skin irritation Rash	Fine raised red rash around stoma or under wafer	Moisture under wafer	Dry skin well before applying wafer. Use hair dryer on cool setting to dry area (skin and wafer) Change appliance 1 day sooner Check pattern size.
	Red rash, irritation, itching, or burning under the entire wafer	Opening of wafer large, skin exposed to drainage Allergy to wafer or tape	If appliance leaks, change immediately Apply skin prep to skin before applying wafer If rash does not clear up in 5 to 7 days a different type of pouching system may be required
	Fine red rash or irritation under plastic pouch	Moisture under pouch	Pouch cover will keep plastic appliance off skin. Place appliance on outside of undergarment. Apply powder or corn starch under the appliance (not wafer)
Irritated hair follicles (Folliculitis)	Raised red areas under wafer that look similar to acne	Removing hair by aggressively pulling wafer off	Shave hair around stoma with an electric razor with each appliance change Use adhesive remover to remove old wafer Apply skin prep to skin before applying wafer Antimicrobial powder may be applied to the affected area[50,51]
Leakage	Wafer loses its seal on skin, drainage leaks under wafer	Incorrect opening in wafer	Check pattern size before cutting wafer
	Pouch wear time less than 5 days	Urine can melt down the skin barrier on the wafer	After removing wafer, examine for melt down Changing to a more durable wafer may be necessary
	Urine leaks from sides of wafer	Skin folds/creases develop around stoma	A protective skin barrier paste applied to the back of the wafer acts as a caulking to fill in skin folds or creases
		Stoma retracts (pulls in) when in sitting position	If the stoma retracts, a convex (curved) wafer may be necessary Apply an ostomy appliance belt to provide added security
Hernia	Abdomen bulges around stoma	Weak abdominal muscles Lifting heavy objects too soon after surgery	Preventing a hernia is the best remedy. Do not lift over 8 lb the first 6 to 8 weeks following surgery Once healing is complete, begin abdominal exercises to build muscle tone Ostomy support belts are recommended when performing strenuous activity **IMPORTANT NOTE** Support belt needs to be snug, but not constricting, and applied while lying down
Cut on stoma	Cuts on stoma appear as a yellow or white line	Wafer opening too small Wafer not centered over stoma	Check pattern size Enlarge wafer opening as needed Sitting or standing facing a wall mirror may allow a better view of the stoma

(continued)

TABLE 47–2   Troubleshooting Guidelines—cont'd

	Bleeding may also occur from cut on stoma	Tight-fitting clothing may cause excessive pressure against the stoma	Alter clothing to accommodate stoma To control bleeding, apply cold washcloth to cut and apply light pressure for 2 to 3 minutes Contact physician if bleeding persists. Silver nitrate may be applied to bleeding site
Difficulty with urinary night drainage system	Over distension of urinary pouch during sleep, which may cause leakage	Vacuum formation prevents gravity drainage of urinary pouch	Use appropriate adapter to connect the pouch to drainage tubing Stabilize drainage tubing with catheter strap or run tubing down pajama leg Promote drainage by connecting tubing to pouch while there is some urine or air in the pouch Coil tubing to prevent kinks Use night drainage with swivel top to maintain patency of tubing Cleanse night drainage system daily with ½ strength vinegar and water

Care of the Nephrostomy Tube

- Dressings around nephrostomy tubes are changed every other day or as needed.
- The site is cleansed with normal saline if there is no drainage and hydrogen peroxide if crusty discharge is present.
- A split dressing is applied to the site and secured with tape.
- The tube is connected to a leg bag when the patient ambulates and gravity bag at night or if bed bound.
- Secure nephrostomy tube with tape or leg strap to prevent dislodgment. If tube becomes dislodged contact the physician.
- If the nephrostomy tubes fail to drain urine, check tubing for kinks, dislodgment, or blockage.
- If the tube is blocked, contact the physician for irrigation orders. Nephrostomy tube can be irrigated with a maximum of 5 mL of solution at one time.

Care of Fistulae

- Fistulae are managed based on the type of drainage and location.
- External fistulae drain to the skin surface and therefore can be managed by pouching or suction drains.
- Internal fistulae drain from the bowel or bladder to the path of least resistance, usually the vagina, bladder, or rectum. Drains and catheters are used to manage this type of fistula. Vaginal fistulae can be managed by diaphragms, pessary, incontinence pouch, diapers, and skin barrier creams.[12,13]
- The goal for managing fistulae is to prevent skin breakdown, monitor output by containing the drainage, minimize odor, and promote patient comfort and quality of life.[14] When pouching fistulae, follow the same guidelines as ostomy care.
- Drainage pouches for high output fistulae should be placed to gravity drainage to prevent overfilling and pouch leakage. If fistulae are not pouched, skin that is exposed to drainage should be protected with barrier creams.

MALIGNANT LYMPHEDEMA

Definition and Incidence

Malignant lymphedema is tumor growth that impairs the flow of lymphatic fluid, resulting in the accumulation of fluid in the soft tissue. The incidence varies in different types of cancer[15]:

- 1% to 2% of occult cancer, lymphedema is the first symptom to occur.
- 40% incidence following axillary node dissection and radiation therapy.
- 70% incidence following radical lymph node dissection in prostate cancer.
- 50% incidence in recurrent gynecologic tumors.
- 10% are the first symptom of tumor recurrence after breast cancer therapy.
- 25% of cases with Hodgkin's disease develop inguinal blockage of lymph flow.

Signs and Symptoms

- Patient complains of limb feeling heavy and or tight.
- Edema is unilateral.
- Acute onset of edema starts centrally with a peripheral progression.
- Increasing tension pain related to rapid accumulation of fluid.
- Rapid increase in pain indicates infection, bone involvement, or progression of tumor.
- Restricted mobility caused by swelling of extremity.
- Paresthesia and paralysis of the extremity.
- Skin is shiny, cyanotic, or has reddish discoloration; skin temperature may be warm.
- Edema is firm, rubbery, and nonpitting.
- Ulcerations, blisters, and cutaneous fistulae can occur.

Management

The onset of malignant lymphedema occurs within weeks as opposed to benign, which develops over months and years. The treatment should be initiated as early as possible to prevent progression and the discomfort associated with the rapid edema. Treatment options are based on the location and extent of the disease and the severity of the swelling. The goals of treating lymphedema are to prevent infection, reduce limb edema, and improve limb function. Treatment should include:

- Perform skin care to prevent ulcerations and prevent infection.
- Cleanse skin with moisturizing soap or soapless skin cleanser.
- Dry skin well with soft cloth especially between toes, fingers, and folds.
- Moisturize skin daily to prevent drying and cracking.
- Monitor for signs and symptoms of infection and cellulitis: fever, erythema, fungal rash, increased swelling, warmth, and pain.

Trauma Prevention[16–18]

- Avoid punctures, blood pressures, blood draws, intravenous infusions, and injections in the affected limb.
- Avoid cutting nails and shaving.
- Use gloves, insect repellent, and sunscreen when gardening.

- Avoid walking barefoot.
- Avoid standing for extended periods of time.
- Avoid heavy lifting and carrying heavy objects.
- Massage therapy and compression bandaging to mobilize fluids.
- Elevate affected limb with pillows or assistive devices. Refer to physical therapy for manual drainage, compression bandaging, and exercise program.
- Manual therapy mobilizes lymph flow around the blockage into adjacent healthy lymph vessels to promote drainage into the circulatory system.[15,19]
- Compression bandages are applied after manual therapy to prevent the reaccumulation of lymph fluid by improving muscle pumping.
- Exercise programs increase muscle pumping and the amount of lymph fluid drained out of the affected limb. Exercise will also help to maintain the range of motion in the affected limb.

MALIGNANT CUTANEOUS LESIONS

Overview

Malignant cutaneous lesions become apparent when cancer cells progress and penetrate the epidermal skin layer. Tumor growth also infiltrates the vascular and lymphatic systems resulting in tissue necrosis, bleeding, infection, and eventually a fungating, friable, malodorous lesion. The common primary skin lesions are lymphoma, squamous cell, basal cell, and malignant melanoma. Secondary cutaneous lesions commonly occur from metastatic breast, kidney, lung, ovary, colon, gastric, bladder, head, and neck tumors. Five to ten percent of all cancer patients with metastatic disease develop cutaneous lesions.[20,21] Nineteen to fifty percent of women with breast cancer and 3% to 8% of men with bronchogenic carcinoma develop metastatic cutaneous lesions.[22] Malignant cutaneous lesions commonly occur on the anterior trunk. Other areas that may become involved are the pelvis, flanks, posterior trunk, and the head and neck region.

Management

Managing malignant cutaneous lesions may involve treating the metastatic disease with chemotherapy or radiation therapy. In palliative care, we must keep in mind that the primary goal is to maintain a patient's quality of life; therefore, treatment should focus on controlling odor and drainage, preventing bleeding and infection, and promoting patient comfort. As disease progression occurs within the wound, re-evaluating the treatment goals must be considered to determine if interventions are appropriate.

Psychologically, these patients have a visible reminder of their disease progression and impending end of life. Social interaction with family and friends diminishes as a result of the odor and wound drainage. Psychological support for both the patient and caregiver must be considered in managing fungating wounds.[23-25] For treatment options, see Table 47–3.

PRURITUS

Definition and Incidence

Pruritus is a sensation that leads to the desire to scratch. Approximately 10% to 30% of patients with Hodgkin's disease present with pruritus, and 20% to 30% will experience episodes during the course of the illness.[30,31] Five percent to twelve percent of cancer patients experience pruritus in the course of the illness.[32] In addition to Hodgkin's disease, pruritus can be a presenting symptom in oat cell carcinoma of the bronchus, non-Hodgkin's lymphoma, cutaneous T-cell lymphoma, leukemia, squamous cell carcinoma, and central nervous system tumors.[30]

Etiology

Pruritus is associated with primary skin disorders and systemic diseases, as well as cancer therapies and drugs. Primary skin disorders include dry, flaky skin that leads to scratching and eventually injury to the skin; contact dermatitis from soaps and creams, neomycin ointments, local analgesic creams, and alcohol; psoriasis; scabies; lice; and fleas. Systemic diseases include chronic renal failure with uremia; biliary and hepatic obstruction from metastatic disease; pancreatic and liver tumors with or without an increase in serum bile acids often results in pruritus; lymphoma[30,32,33]; burning and intense itching occur on the lower extremities of patients with Hodgkin's disease[34]; lymphomas and leukemias usually have generalized pruritus with or without an associated rash or skin eruption[35-37]; cutaneous tumor infiltrates. Cancer therapy includes chemotherapy and radiation, which affects sebaceous glands, causing dryness that leads to pruritus. Pruritus is also a result of wet or dry desquamation caused by radiation injury; and graft versus host disease after bone marrow transplants. Drugs that can cause pruritus include common drugs associated with skin reactions such as penicillin, sulfonamide, allopurinol, vancomycin, morphine, and codeine.

Pathophysiology

Pruritus and pain, although separate sensations, follow the same nerve pathway.[35,38] Pruritus affects not only the skin, but also the conjunctivae, mucous membranes, and upper respiratory tract. The dermis layer of the skin contains nerve endings, blood vessels, and connective nerve fibers.

When cutaneous nerve networks are stimulated, the "itch-scratch-itch cycle" begins.[30] Chemical mediators

TABLE 47–3 Treatment Options

Treatment Issue	Treatment Goal	Treatment Option
Odor control	Wound cleansing	Wound cleansing
Heavy anaerobic bacteria colonization produces foul permeating odors	Cleanse wound to reduce bacterial load and remove loose tissue debris Treat infection Control odor	Normal saline is a safe cleanser to use. Using a 35-mL syringe with a 19-gauge needle will provide enough pressure to remove nonviable tissue and debris Daily showers with a hand-held showerhead can also accomplish this goal 0.25% Dakin's solution has been shown to decrease anaerobic and aerobic organisms and be effective in controlling odors[22] Hydrogels applied to nonviable tissue will help debride and keep the wound clean through autolytic debridement
	Topical applications Antimicrobial/antibiotic products	Topical application Antimicrobial products (silver dressings) Antibiotic products (metronidazole gel or 500 mg tablets crushed and sprinkled on wound bed. Oral tablets can be mixed with saline to produce a solution for irrigation or to moisten dressings[25-28], silver sulfadiazine to control pseudomonas[29]) Systemic antibiotics for infection
	Maintain environmental factors	Ventilate room Room odor eliminating sprays to room and outer dressing Burn scented candles Remove soiled dressings immediately after wound care
Control Exudate	Dressings	Dressings
Dressing intervention to control drainage as nonviable tissue is debrided	Filter odor and absorb drainage Maintain moist wound environment Prevent maceration of periwound skin Promote autolytic debridement	Dressing moistened with Dakin's or Metronidazole applied to the lesion every 12 hours may be an effective wound deodorizer Select dressings capable of filtering odor and absorbing drainage as it increases with autolytic debridement (alginates; cavity foams; hydrofibers) If dressings are inappropriate, consider pouching technique (contains drainage; contains odor; prevents periwound skin maceration and trauma; eliminates pain from frequent dressing changes)
Periwound skin integrity	Maintain or restore periwound skin integrity Prevent maceration of periwound skin by controlling migration of drainage Prevent periwound skin trauma from adhesives Minimize pruritus and discomfort	Apply appropriate barrier to skin surrounding the wound Hydrocolloids Barrier creams or paste Use absorbent dressing to wick drainage away from skin to minimize contact with the skin Avoid adhesives to skin Secure dressings with binders, stretch netting bandages, ACE wrap Maintain skin hydration Moisturizing creams applied to damp skin will promote skin hydration Increase fluid intake Apply cool compresses to affected areas Increase room humidity Control pruritus Topical anti-inflammatories, antipruritics, or analgesics

(continued)

TABLE 47–3   Treatment Options—cont'd

		Antihistamines Skin barrier creams or products containing calamine Oatmeal baths Educate patient on avoiding skin trauma by scratching or rubbing. Use of cotton gloves to massage area and prevent inadvertent scratching
Control bleeding	Minimize trauma to wound bed and friable tissue	
Bleeding associated with dressing changes	Maintain moist wound	If dressing adherent to wound bed, moisten dressing until easily removed Use appropriate nonadherent dressings with longer wear time to reduce frequency of dressing changes Maintain moist wound base with hydrogels, gel sheets, or moisture-retentive dressings Use gentle cleansing agent and gentle force when cleansing wound
Bleeding associated with tumor erosion, infection, absence of platelets	Control bleeding Assess/treat infection	Hemostatic dressings Gel foam, Surgicel Alginates Silver nitrate
Control pain associated with dressing change		Radiation treatment to tumor site
Anticipatory pain Anxiety	Minimize anxiety	Allow patient to participate in wound care Provide diversionary activities (music, relaxation) Medicate prior to dressing change
Pain associated with dressing change	Minimize pain caused by dressing pain	Topical anesthetic creams, gels or sprays EMLA, lidocaine spray Sublingual analgesics Moisten dressings prior to removal. Use nonadherent dressings, gel sheets, hydrogels Minimize dressing change Gentle cleansing Keep wound base moist Avoid adhesive to periwound skin. Use net dressing, ACE wraps, binders

involved with pruritus are histamine, vasoactive peptides, trypsin, enkephalins, prostaglandins, serotonins.[30,39] Opioids receptors affect pruritus: naloxone may increase or decrease pruritus; morphine can increase pruritus.[33,39] Pruritus increases with dehydration and heat and decreases with cold. Anxiety and boredom increase the perception of pruritus.

Assessment

A complete workup is needed to determine the cause of pruritus. Workup should include:

- History and physical establishing the onset, duration, intensity, sensation, and location of pruritus.
- Medication history should include drug-induced rashes and use of opioids. The physical examination should include skin inspection for color, temperature, turgor, appearance of lesions, and skin condition.
- Diagnostic evaluation should include complete blood workup, renal and liver function studies, tumor markers, and chest x-ray.

Management

Most treatment options for pruritus merely diminish the itching sensation rather than completely resolve the problem. Therefore, the goal in managing pruritus should focus on maintaining skin integrity, controlling environmental conditions, treating underlying diseases, administering drug therapy, and promoting comfort and relief.

Maintaining Skin Integrity

- Maintain adequate nutrition and hydration. Increase fluid intake to 2000 to 3000 mL as tolerated.
- Limit bathing to 10 to 20 minutes a day.
- Avoid hot baths and showers to prevent moisture loss and vasoconstriction from heat, which can intensify pruritus.
- Use mild soaps, bath oils, and oatmeal baths.
- Avoid perfumes, powders, and deodorants.
- Use soft cloths to dry skin. Avoid vigorous rubbing to prevent further skin irritation.
- Apply emollient cream to damp skin after bathing.
- Keep nails cut or apply cotton gloves to prevent skin trauma.

Environmental Control

- Increase room humidity as needed.
- Keep room cool and well ventilated.
- Prevent overheating and sweating. Apply cool compresses or ice packs to relieve severe episodes.

- Encourage patient to wear loose cotton clothing at bedtime.
- Avoid irritating clothing such as woolen and tight-fitting clothes.
- Apply cutaneous stimulation, relaxation, or distraction techniques to reduce patient's emotional stress and focus on scratching.

Treat Underlying Disease

- Pruritus associated with cancer may be resolved by removing or treating of the tumor.[30]
- Electron-beam radiotherapy relieves pruritus caused by cutaneous lymphoma.[40]
- Chemotherapy treatment relieves pruritus associated with Hodgkin's disease.
- Pruritus associated with cholestasis responds with biliary stenting to relieve the obstruction.[36]
- Pruritus associated with candidiasis responds with antifungal powders, creams, or medications.

Administer Drug Therapy

Topical[36]

- Topical corticosteroids are available in creams and ointments. Prolonged use of corticosteroids can cause thinning of the skin and therefore increasing the risk of skin breakdown.
- Topical astringents agents are available in lotions and creams. Astringents containing menthol, phenol, and camphor have an anesthetic effect, which produces a cool and soothing sensation. Examples are calamine lotion, Benadryl cream, zinc oxide, and glycerin.
- Moisturizing agents are available in creams, oils, lotions, and are used to prevent and treat dry skin.
- Bandage wraps impregnated with zinc oxide provide relief by producing a cool and soothing sensation to the skin.

Systemic[37]

- Corticosteroids such as prednisone, Decadron
- Sedating histamine antagonists such as Benadryl
- Nonsedating histamine antagonists such as Seldane, Claritin
- Cholestyramine and opiate antagonists for cholestasis

Pruritus is a difficult symptom for practitioners to treat. Lack of understanding of the cause of pruritus adds to the difficulty of prescribing the appropriate and most effective treatment. Therefore, in caring for the terminal patient, promoting comfort and relieving itching should be the primary foci.

RADIATION-INDUCED SKIN DAMAGE

Overview

Radiation therapy is beneficial in palliation treatment for tumors of the spinal cord, bladder, brain, lung, bone, and managing bleeding and pain. Although technology has improved over the years, mild to severe skin reactions still occur in 95% of the patients. The effects of radiation therapy become apparent after 2 weeks of treatment. Skin reactions to radiation include erythema, progressing to dry or wet desquamation, blistering, and fibrosis of the skin.[38,41]

Types of Radiation-Induced Skin Damage

Erythema

Red discoloration caused by capillary dilatation and increased vascular permeability. Occurs 1 to 3 weeks after treatment initiated.[42,43] Inflammation and edema may be also present in this area. Patients may experience mild discomfort, burning, and itching.[43]

Dry Desquamation

Red to brown hyperpigmentation with resulting dry, scaling, peeling, and itching. Occurs 2 weeks after erythema.[42,43] Tissue injury heals within 2 to 4 weeks after treatment is complete.[32]

Wet Desquamation

Occurs when the epidermal skin layer is injured, causing blistering and sloughing of tissue. Injury occurs 4 weeks after treatment initiated. Pain levels with desquamation vary from mild to severe.[42-44] Tissue injury heals within 4 to 8 weeks after treatment is complete.[32]

Management

The goal in managing radiation-induced skin injury is to maintain skin integrity as long as possible, prevent further trauma to the area, promote moist healing, prevent infection, absorb drainage to prevent maceration, and maintain patient comfort. Patient and family education on skin care and preventing trauma is essential.

Prevent Trauma

- Avoid rubbing skin. Use soft washcloths or hands to cleanse skin. Use Peri bottles or a hand-held shower to cleanse difficult areas. Use mild soaps for cleansing skin.[45]
- Keep skin folds clean and dry to prevent damage from moisture.
- Avoid powders, cornstarch, talcum, perfumes, deodorants, and any product containing metals.
- Keep skin moisturized to prevent drying and cracking. Recommended topical agents are aqueous cream and aloe vera gel.[46,47]
- Cotton clothing should be loose fitting to prevent friction.
- Protect the area from extreme hot and cold temperatures, sun, and wind.
- Avoid adhesives to skin. Tubular net dressing is advised to secure dressings.

Promote Moist Healing

- Cleanse drainage and slough with warm normal saline. Gentle showers will help loosen slough.
- Keep dry wounds moist with hydrogels or hydrogel sheets to enhance autolytic debridement.
- Control drainage from wet wounds with nonadherent foam dressings, absorptive dressings, or alginates.

Prevent Infection

- Asses for signs and symptoms of infection. Culture wound as needed.
- Antibiotic therapy as prescribed by practitioner. Topical use of silver sulfadiazine 1% is recommended.[48]
- Reduce moisture retention when fungal infections are present.[49]

Absorb Drainage

- Use absorptive dressings to control drainage.
- Increase frequency of dressing changes according to the amount of drainage. Two to three times a day is recommended.
- Protect periwound skin from moisture with skin barrier creams if not in the radiation field.

Maintain Patient Comfort

- Topical anesthetics for local pain.
- Use nonadherent dressings.
- Keep wound covered to prevent further trauma and to protect exposed nerves.[49]

REFERENCES

1. Agency for Health Care Policy and Research, U.S. Department of Health and Human Services. Pressure Ulcers in Adults: Prediction and Prevention (AHCPR Publication No.92-0047). Rockville, MD, 1992.
2. Agency for Health Care Policy and Research, U.S. Department of Health and Human Services. Treatment of Pressure Ulcers in Adults (AHCPR Publication No.95-0652). Rockville, MD, 1994.
3. Pieper B: Mechanical forces: Pressure, shear, and friction. In Bryant R (ed): Acute and Chronic Wounds: Nursing Management, 2nd ed. St Louis, Mosby, 2000, pp 221–264.
4. Waller A, Caroline NL: Handbook of Palliative Care in Cancer, 2nd ed. Boston, Butterworth-Heinemann, 2000, pp 91–99.
5. Ovington L, Peirce B: Wound dressings: Form, function, feasibility and facts. In Krasner DL, Rodeheaver GT, Sibbald RG (eds): Chronic Wound Care: A Clinical Source Book for Healthcare Professionals, 3rd ed. Malvern, Pennsylvania: HMP Communications, 2001, pp 311–320.
6. WOCN Society: WOCN Clinical Practice Guideline Series 2. Guideline for Prevention and Management of Pressure Ulcers. Glenview, Illinois: WOCN, 2003, pp 1–52.
7. Bates-Jensen BM: Management of necrotic tissue. In Sussman C, Bates-Jensen BM (eds): Wound Care: A Collaborative Practice Manual for Physical Therapists and Nurses. Frederick, Maryland: Aspen, 1998, pp 139–158.
8. Waller A, Caroline NL: Handbook of Palliative Care in Cancer, 2nd ed. Boston, Butterworth-Heinemann, 2000, pp 99–104.
9. Heneghan GM, Clark N, Hensley BJ, et al: The Indiana pouch: A continent urinary diversion. J Enterostomal Ther 17:231–236, 1990.
10. Gardner J: Urinary diversion with an Indiana pouch. Nursing 24:32c–32h, 1994.
11. Rolstad BS, Hoyman K: Continent diversions and reservoirs. In Hamptom BG, Bryant RA (eds): Ostomies and Continent Diversions: Nursing Management. St Louis, Mosby Year Book, 1992, pp 129–162.
12. Faller NA, Beitz JM: When a wound is not a wound: Tubes, drains, fistulae, and draining wounds. In Krasner DL, Rodeheaver GT, Sibbald RG (eds): Chronic Wound Care: A Clinical Source Book for Healthcare Professionals, 3rd ed. Malvern, Pennsylvania: HMP Communications, 2001, pp 721–729.
13. Rolstad BS, Bryant RA: Management of drain sites and fistulas. In Bryant RA (ed): Acute and Chronic Wounds: Nursing Management, 2nd ed. St Louis, Mosby, 2000, pp 317–341.
14. Davis M, Dere K, Hadley G: Options for managing an open wound with draining enterocutaneous fistula. J Wound Ostomy Continence Nurs 27:118–123, 2000.
15. Weissleder H, Schuchhardt CH: Malignant lymphedema. In Weissleder H, Schuchhardt C (eds): Lymphedema: Diagnosis and Therapy, 3rd ed. Baden-Baden, Germany: Wesel, 2001, pp 231–246.
16. Cope D: Lymphedema. In Camp-Sorrell D, Hawkins RA (eds): Clinical Manual for the Oncology Advanced Practice Nurse. Pittsburg, PA: Oncology Nursing Press, 2000, pp 649–652.
17. Couillard-Getreuer DL, Heery ML: Protective mechanisms: Skin. In Gross J, Johnson BH (eds): Handbook of Oncology Nursing, 2nd ed. Boston, Jones and Bartlett, 1994, pp 421–464.
18. Crane-Okadar: Breast Cancer. In Otto SE (ed): Oncology Nursing, 4th ed. St Louis, Mosby, 2000, pp 113–167.
19. Kalinowski BH: Lymphedema. In Yarbro CH, Frogge MH, Goodman M (eds): Cancer Symptom Management, 2nd ed. Boston, Jones and Bartlett, 1999, pp 457–487.
20. Kelly N: Malodorous fungating wounds: A review of current literature. Prof Nurse 17:323–326, 2002.
21. McDonald AE: Skin ulcerations. In Yarbro CH, Frogge MH, Goodman M (eds): Cancer Symptom Management. 2nd ed. Boston, Jones and Bartlett, 1999, pp 382–396.
22. Bauer C, Gerlach MA, Doughty DB: Care of metastatic skin lesions. J Wound Ostomy Continence Nurs 27:247–251, 2000.
23. Piggin C: Malodorous fungating wounds: Uncertain concepts underlying the management of social isolation. Intl J Palliat Nurs 9:216–221, 2003.
24. Wilkes L, White K, Smeal T, Beale B: Malignant wound management: What dressings do nurses use? J Wound Care 10:65–69, 2001.
25. Woodward L, Haisfield-Wolfe ME: Management of a patient with a malignant cutaneous tumor. J Wound Ostomy Continence Nurs 30:231–236, 2003.
26. Collier M: Management of patients with fungating wounds. Nurs Stand 15:46–52, 2000.
27. Finlay IG, Bowszyc J, Ramlau C, Gwiezdzinski Z: The effect topical 0.75% metronidazole gel on malodorous cutaneous ulcers. J Pain Symptom Manage 11:158–162, 1996.
28. McMullen, D: Topical metronidazole part II: Clinical use in malodorous ulcerating skin lesions. Ostomy Wound Manage 38:42–46, 1992.
29. Barton P, Parslow N: Malignant wounds: holistic assessment and management. In Krasner DL, Rodeheaver GT, Sibbald RG (eds): Chronic Wound Care: A Clinical Source Book for Healthcare Professionals, 3rd ed. Malvern, Pennsylvania: HMP Communications, 2001, pp 699–710.
30. Seiz AM, Yarbro CH: Pruritus. In Yarbro CH, Frogge MH, Goodman M (eds): Cancer Symptom Management, 2nd ed. Boston, Jones and Bartlett, 1999, pp 148–159.
31. Cavalli F: Rare syndromes in Hodgkin's disease. Ann Oncol 9:109–113, 1998.
32. Waller A, Caroline NL: Handbook of Palliative Care in Cancer, 2nd ed. Boston, Butterworth-Heinemann, 2000, pp 115–124.
33. Twycross R, Wilcock A: Symptom Management in Advanced Cancer, 3rd ed. Oxon, UK: Radcliffe Medical Press, 2001.
34. Lober C: Should the patient with generalized pruritus be evaluated for malignancy? J Am Acad Derm 19:350–352, 1988.
35. Goolsby MJ: The elusive itch: Assessment, diagnosis and management of pruritus. AdvNurse Prac 6:61–64, 1998.
36. Lonsdale-Eccles A, Carmichael AJ: Treatment of pruritus associated with systemic disorders in the elderly: A review of the role of new therapies. Drugs Aging 20:197–208, 2003.
37. Millikan L: Treating pruritus: What's new in safe relief of symptoms? Postgrad Med 99:173–176, 179–184, 1996.
38. Porock D: Factors influencing the severity of radiation skin and oral mucosal reactions: Development of a conceptual framework. Eur J Cancer Care 11:33–43, 2002.
39. Lidstone V, Thorns A: Pruritus in cancer patients. Cancer Treat Rev 27:305–312, 2001.
40. Krajnik M, Zylicz Z: Pruritus in advanced internal diseases: Pathogenesis and treatment. Neth J Med 58:27–40, 2001.
41. McDonald AE: Skin ulcerations. In Yarbro CH, Frogge MH, Goodman M (eds): Cancer Symptom Management. 2nd ed. Sudbury, Massachussetts, Jones and Bartlett, 1999, pp 382–396.
42. Mendelson FA, Divino CM, Reis ED, Kerstein MD: Wound care after radiation therapy. Adv Skin Wound Care 15:216–224, 2002.
43. Goldberg MT, McGinn-Byer P: Oncology-related skin damage. In Bryant R (ed): Acute and Chronic Wounds: Nursing Management. 2nd ed. St Louis, Mosby, 2000, pp 367–386.
44. Porock D, Nikoletti S, Kristjanson L: Management of radiation skin reactions: Literature review and clinical application. Plast Surg Nurs 19:185–192, 1999.
45. Roy I, Fortin A, Larochelle M: The impact of skin washing with water and soap during breast irradiation: A randomized study. Radiother Oncol 58:333–339, 2001.
46. Heggie S, Bryant GP, Tripcony L, et al: A phase III study on the efficacy of topical aloe vera gel on irradiated breast tissue. Cancer Nurs 25:442–451, 2002.
47. Olsen DL, Raub W Jr., Bradley C, Johnson M, et al. The effect of aloe vera gel/mild soap versus mild soap alone in preventing skin reactions in patients undergoing radiation therapy. Oncol Nurs Forum 28:543–547, 2001.
48. Belcher AE, Selekof J: Skin care for the oncology patient. In Krasner DL, Rodeheaver GT, Sibbald RG: (eds): Chronic Wound Care: A Clinical Source Book for Healthcare Professionals, 3rd ed. Pennsylvania: HMP Communications, 2001, pp 711–720.
49. Barton P, Parslow N: Caring for Oncology Wounds: Management Guidelines. Convatec Division of Bristol-Myers Squibb, Montreal, Quebec, 1998.
50. Erwin-Toth P: Prevention and management of peristomal skin complications. Adv Skin Wound Care 13:175–179, 2000.
51. Hampton BG: Peristomal and stomal complications. In Hamptom BG, Bryant RA (eds): Ostomies and Continent Diversions: Nursing Management. St Louis, Mosby Year Book, 1992, pp 105–123.

Index

Page numbers followed by f indicate figures; t, tables.